D1573701

M. Engelhardt / A. Dorr (Editors)
Sports Orthopedics

Martin Engelhardt / Alex Dorr (Editors)

Sports Orthopedics

Contributors: Silvia Albrecht, Markus Arnold, Martin Bauer, Roland Biedert, Michael Bohnsack, Hans-Peter Boschert, Angelika Braun, Gerd-Peter Brüggemann, Klaus Dann, Jens Dargel, Moritz Dau, Gregor Deitmer, Michael Dienst, Alexander Disch, Dominik Doerr, Roland Eisele, Hans-Georg Eisenlauer, Martin Engelhardt, Andreas Englert, Jens Enneper, Jürgen Freiwald, Arno Frigg, Ludwig Geiger, Wilfried Gfrörer, Ottmar Gorschewsky, Andreas Gösele, Karlheinz Graff, Casper Grim, Rolf Haaker, Berthold Hallmaier, Dietolf Hämel, Cornelius Heck, Heinrich Hess, Thomas Hess, Beat Hintermann, Hubert Hörterer, Hardy Hüttemann, Volker Jägemann, Axel Jäger, Jörg Jerosch, Thomas Jöllenbeck, Bernd Kabelka, Franz Kainberger, Antonius Kass, Gino M.M.J. Kerkhoffs, Matthias Kieb, Markus Knupp, Dieter Kohn, Winfried Koller, Karl-Heinz Kristen, Sabine Krüger, Michael Krüger-Franke, Andreas Kugler, André Leumann, Ludwig Löffler, Olaf Lorbach, Bernhard Lukas, Andreas Marka, Georg Marvridis, Marlene Mauch, Joern W.-P. Michael, Oliver Miltner, Stefan Nehrer, Georg Neumann, Stefan Nolte, Christian Nührenbörger, Geert Pagenstert, Markus Parzeller, Hans-Gerd Pieper, Christoph Raschka, Iris Reuter, Kirstin Richter, Mathias Ritsch, Thomas Rodt, Lisette Rodt, Bernd Rosemeyer, Christoph Schlegel-Wagner, Peter Schmidt, Rüdiger Schmidt-Wiethoff, Holger Schmitt, Christian Schneider, Michaela Schneiderbauer, Dieter Schnell, Volker Schöffl, Claudia Schüller-Weiekamm, René Schwall, Thomas Schwamborn, Christian H. Siebert, Voker Smasal, Gernot Sperner, Gerhard Sybrecht, Carsten Temme, Sebastian Thormann, Axel Urhausen, Victor Valderrabano, C. Niek van Dijk, Kerstin Warnke, Bernd Wolfarth, Markus Zimmer

NEUNPLUS1 EDITION MEDIZIN

Editors:

Martin Engelhardt, M.D., PhD
Klinik für Orthopädie, Unfall- und Handchirurgie, Klinikum Osnabrück,
Am Finkenhügel 1, 49076 Osnabrück, Germany

Alex Dorr, PhD, Langstr. 192, CH-8005 Zürich, Switzerland

Copyright © 2011 Martin Engelhardt

Originally published as Sportverletzungen by Elsevier GmbH, Urban & Fischer, München, Germany

All rights reserved. This book is protected by copyright. No part of this book may be reproduced in any form or by any means, including photocopying, or utilized by any information storage and retrieval system without written permission from the copyright owner.

The publisher is not responsible (as a matter of product liability, negligence, or otherwise) for any injury resulting from any material contained herein. This publication contains information relating to general principles of medical care that should not be construed as specific instructions for individual patients. Manufacturers' product information and package inserts should be reviewed for current information, including contraindications, dosages, and precautions.

The print of this book was supported by an unrestricted educational grant of Bauerfeind Inc. This financial support had no impact on content of the individual chapters or editorial review.

The editors declare no conflict of interest. Alex Dorr is a full-time employee of Actelion Pharmaceuticals Ltd., which develops and markets drugs unrelated to sports medicine (pulmonary arterial hypertension).

Translation: Alexandra Schröpel, verbum optimum, Prömmelte, Germany
Cover design: Sandra Berhold, LVD Gesellschaft für Datenverarbeitung mbH, Berlin, Germany
Cover photo source: wikipedia.org.
Photographer: Cpl. Michelle M. Dickson (United States Marine Corps), U.S.A.
Line drawing: Henriette Rintelen, Velbert, Germany
Layout/Typesetting: SatzReproService GmbH, Jena, Germany
Printing and binding: Neunplus1 GmbH, Berlin, Germany

ISBN 978-3-936033-39-7

Foreword by Thomas Bach,
Vice-President of the International Olympic Committee and President of the German Olympic Sports Confederation

The importance of sports has grown over the past decades worldwide. This is true for high performance sports as well as for mass sports. On the one hand, top athletes are permanently in the spotlight of the media. On the other hand hundreds of millions of people are going for sports in order to simply enjoy the physical activity, to prevent diseases or to rehabilitate from injuries.

In the high-performance sports no one has ever expected the levels top athletes reaching today. Due to the maximum of training, athletes are close to the limit of human potential. An efficient sports medicine is key for those athletes. Furthermore, sports medicine is also of great importance to the health and the prevention of health of the citizens.

This book offers a comprehensive overview on sports medicine and orthopedics. Beyond the introduction of general aspects of sports medicine, the following chapters are addressing diagnostics procedures as well as the presentation of the most important injuries and overuse symptoms per body part. More than 60 sports specific injuries are introduced.

The majority of authors have served several times as team doctor at World Championships and Olympic Games. They are sharing their experience with us. In the same time they are describing the specific risk of different sports and pointing out how to avoid them.

The IOC and the respective national sport organizations are aware of their responsibility with regard to health protection of the athletes. This is in particular true for young athletes.

The book significantly contributes to the idea of a refreshing sport. Therefore I wish that the book will enjoy a great distribution.

Yours

Thomas Bach

Tauberbischofsheim, March 2011

Preface

People exercise sports to enjoy physical activity, boost their ego, prevent diseases or rehabilitate after accidents and operations and these sportive activities continuously include more elderly citizens. Sports medical supervision requires trained and competent doctors, physiotherapists, sports therapists, and trainers who have a growing need for education and learning of sports medicine. The multidisciplinary sports orthopedics is central to this education.

Expectation of sports medical doctors, physiotherapists, trainers, and athletes is high. Often only single bits of information are available to decide on future sports capacity, change of exposure, or complete stop of sports activity. These decisions are taken by a growing number of office or hospital-based physicians increasingly exposed to sports injuries of any kind. Both top and leisure athletes expect from the treating physician quick answers and quick return to training.

Aim of this book is to document the current standards in all areas of sports orthopedics. The authors describe most common injuries, consequences of abnormal exposure, and overuse symptoms at most important body areas, organs, and age-related characteristics. Besides pathology, diagnosis, and therapeutic options, the authors describe concrete steps of post-traumatic treatments and return to sports.

This book is directed to sports orthopedists, sports physicians, general orthopedists, orthopedic surgeons, general practitioners, students in human medicine and sports sciences, physiotherapists, sports therapists, athletes, and trainers.

This compendium captivates with a list of high profile authors. Next to scientifically active, university colleagues, the authors are league doctors working in top sports. They transmit their invaluable, often more than 20 years of practical expertise in sports orthopedics. The structure of the book allows use as reference manual and educational material of younger colleagues.

We are grateful to all authors' contributions, which besides their challenging, daily work contributed competent chapters for this textbook. Special thanks goes to Mrs Petra Enderlein and her team in Jena, Germany who managed the editorial process and the device company Bauerfeind, Germany who supported us with an unrestricted, educational grant to compile this English version.

At the 25th anniversary of the orthopedics-traumatology society in sports medicine (GOTS), which is a German-spoken society uniting Germany, Austria, and Switzerland and counts more than 1,000 members, awarded this book the 'official GOTS manual' title.

We hope that the compiled information helps with follow-up and care of patients and athletes. Beyond this direct value, we believe that the current edition helps to stimulate transatlantic collaboration and partnership, ultimately resulting in potential future co-authorships with Anglo-American colleagues.

The Editors
Martin Engelhardt, MD, PhD
Alex Dorr, PhD

Osnabruck, Germany, and Zurich, Switzerland
March 2011

Contents

I	**General principles of sports medicine**	
1	Response and adjustment to physical strain	3
2	Age- and gender-specific aspects of sports medicine	9
3	Athletics and diseases	23
4	Medication and anti-doping rules in competitive sports	31
5	Disabled sports	39
II	**Diagnostic procedures**	
6	Clinical and functional examination	49
7	Sonography	55
8	Projection radiography, magnetic resonance and computer tomography	71
9	Arthroscopy	97
10	Clinical biomechanics	115
11	Gait and treadmill analysis	125
III	**Body parts affected by athletic injuries**	
12	Central and peripheral nervous system	141
13	Eyes	181
14	Ears, facial cranium and cervical soft-tissue	199
15	Shoulder joint	207
16	Elbow and forearm	227
17	Hand and wrist joint	235
18	Pelvis and hip joint	251
19	Groin	263
20	Knee joint	273
21	Shank, ankle joint and foot	291
22	The skeletal muscle	323
23	Stress reactions of the bones	333
24	Cartilage	341
25	Tendon injuries	351
IV	**Sport-specific injuries**	
	Endurance sports	
26	Biathlon	361
27	Short track speed skating	365
28	Canoeing	369
29	Running	375
30	Orienteering	381
31	Cycling	387
32	Rowing	391
33	Swimming	399
34	Cross-country skiing	403
35	Triathlon	407
	Strengths sports and power sports	
36	Bobsleigh	413
37	Bodybuilding	417
38	Olympic Weightlifting	421
39	Athletics (Jump and Throw)	425
40	Luge	431
41	Skeleton	437
42	Carving	441
43	Ski jumping	447
44	Sport- and Rock Climbing	451
	Martial arts	
45	Aikido	455
46	Boxing	461
47	Fencing	467
48	Judo	471
49	Karate	477
50	Wrestling	481
51	Sumo	487
52	Taekwondo	491
	Contact sports	
53	American football	495
54	Baseball	499
55	Basketball	507
56	Beach soccer	515
57	Ice hockey	519
58	Soccer	525
59	Handball	531
60	Field hockey	537
61	Rugby	543
	Non-contact sports	
62	Badminton	549
63	Beach volleyball	555
64	Squash	561
65	Tennis	565
66	Table tennis	573
67	Volleyball	577

Technical acrobatic sports

68 Ballet 585
69 Figure skating 591
70 Artistic gymnastics 597
71 Rhythmic gymnastics 607
72 Dance 611
73 High diving 615

Trend sports

74 Inline skating 619
75 Kitesurfing 625
76 Mountain biking 631
77 Paragliding 637
78 Snowboarding 643

Other sports

79 Golf 653
80 Motorsports 659
81 Equestrianism 665

82 Shooting sports 671
83 Sailing 675
84 Sport diving 679

V Rehabilitation

85 Rehabilitation after athletic injuries .. 687

VI Deaths in sports

86 Deaths in sports 713

VII Accompanying measures

87 Nutrition 727
88 Sportswear 751
89 Athletic Footwear 759
90 Ortheses 769

Index 781

I General principles of sports medicine

1	**Response and adjustment to physical strain**	3
1.1	Phase of adaptation	3
1.2	Regeneration	3
1.3	Adjustment to training	4
2	**Age- and gender-specific aspects of sports medicine**	9
2.1	Children and adolescents	9
2.2	Women	17
2.3	Elderly persons	18
3	**Athletics and diseases**	23
3.1	Sports and arthrosis	23
3.2	Sports after endoprothetic treatment	24
4	**Medication and anti-doping rules in competitive sports**	31
4.1	Arterial hypertension	31
4.2	Diabetes mellitus	32
4.3	Asthma bronchiale (bronchial asthma)	33
4.4	Intravenous infusions, injections or infiltrations	34
4.5	Orthopedics and trauma	34
4.6	Substances	34
4.7	TUE – the medical exemption	35
4.8	Consequence for clinical practice	36
5	**Disabled sports**	39
5.1	Definition and classification	39
5.2	Sports for disabled persons	40
5.3	Injuries and overload	42
5.4	Competitive sports for people with disabilities	42
5.5	Conclusion	44

Chapter 1

Response and adjustment to physical strain

Georg Neumann

Physical performance leads to organ stress and restrains functions within the organism. Every physical strain is followed by **residual tiredness**. Hence, performance-oriented training will be oriented towards a training-recreational schedule.

Key to optimal performance are the following functions:

- autonomic nervous system
- cardiovascular system
- energy metabolism
- endocrine system
- immune system
- temperature regulation
- water and electrolyte metabolism

When athletes undergo a too high physical strain, their stress tolerance will be exceeded and they will tire too early. The increasing tiredness will cause the release of power resources and thereby an increased biological effort for strain coverage.

> Only continued training can cope with higher demands and less stress after a specific exercising time.

Feeling well during training is not a reliable signal of regeneration. **Strain** and **regeneration** are the basis of performance enhancing training in competitive sports. Adjustment achieved by training is the crucial prerequisite for the increased capacity of an athlete. In the first 4 to 6 weeks of training the organism will pass through various **changes of condition**.

These three phases of conditional changes are:
- adaptation
- regeneration (recovery)
- adjustment

1.1 Phase of adaptation

Adaptation is the organism's reaction to physical strain. Functional adaptations depend upon type, intensity and duration of strain. The catabolic processes within the energy metabolism lead to the development of functional and later **structural changes** within the strained organs.

1.2 Regeneration

Regeneration restores the homeostasis of the body functions, which will run at their respective, individual speed (➤ Tab. 1.1).

The **anabolic processes** of the energy metabolism will start in the regeneration period. Energy stores will be replenished, the acid-base balance will be normalized, the worn-out cell proteins will be exchanged, the immune system will be reconstituted, and the mental relaxation will be started. In regeneration, the organism is supposed to reach a state that allows continuing training without improper stress. Regardless duration and intensity of the training, musculature should be able to withstand stress. If necessary, this can be achieved by compensation loads.

Insufficient regeneration prevents the body to deal with higher stress intensities during training. Continued training after omitted or too short regeneration will slow down the regeneration process.

Tab. 1.1 Chronological cycle of regeneration after sport stress (average values, modified after Neumann, Pfützner, Berbalk 2005).

4–6 minutes	Complete replenishment of the depleted muscular creatine-phosphate storage
20 minutes	Return to starting point of heart rate frequency and blood pressure
20–30 minutes	Normalization of hypoglycemia; intake of carbohydrates after performance will cause an exceed in blood-sugar increase
30 minutes	Reaching of state of balance of the acid-base balance, lactate concentration has decreased to less than 2–3 mmol/l
60 minutes	Fading of the strong blockade of protein synthesis in exposed musculature
90 minutes	Transition of catabolic into the mainly anabolic metabolism state, increased protein process for the initiation of regeneration
2 hours	First regeneration in tired musculature (start of regeneration in disturbed neuro-muscular and sensor-motor functions)
6 hours – 1 day	Regression of hemo-concentration and compensation of liquid balance, normalization of hematocrit. After long-term load, hypervolemia is typical!
1 day	Replenishment of liver glycogen
1–3 days	Regeneration of the diminished immune defense ("open window")
2–7 days	Replenishment of the muscle glycogen in strained or destroyed musculature (e.g. marathon)
3–5 days	Replenishment of the muscular triglyceride storages with balanced diet
3–10 days	Regeneration of the overstrained muscle fibers in strain-damaged contraction proteins and supporting structures
7–14 days	Reorganization of malfunctioning mitochondria, regeneration of important functional enzymes in aerobic energy metabolism, normalization of the diminished endurance and strength-endurance ability, reaching of maximum oxygen uptake (VO$_2$max) before exposure
1–3 weeks	Psychic recovery from full-organic load stress, starting capability for shorter competitions in the field of short, medium, and long-time endurance (LTE) I–II
4–6 weeks	Completion of regeneration after LTE III and IV exposures for several hours (e.g. marathon, long-triathlon, 100-km-running, long distance triathlon), possible starting capability for repeated long-time endurances

1.3 Adjustment to training

Occasional training is **not** sufficient to trigger adaptation of the body. The organism has various possibilities to compensate for short-time physical strains. For example, heart rate may rise up to 200 beats/min during stress – with or without the development of an athlete's heart.

The body gradually adapts its functional system **during stress** to the required physical response. The organism will re-balance functions and structures in an auto-regulated fashion. Hence, the effort of the body will decrease with repeated stress. During a marathon EKR 1/2, and the mitogen-activated protein kinase p38MAP increase significantly (Yu et al. 2001). This endurance exposure induces myocyte-specific gene transcription.

The **athletic heart** is an example of adaptation in competitive sports. The enlarged heart (cardiomegaly) pumps the same blood volume to the tissue at a lower heartbeat. The **heart rate** reacts quickly and dynamically to changed demands. These effects materialize already after 8 days of training (Neumann and Schüler 1989). Endurance-trained people have a 10–20 beats/min-decreased heart rate.

1.3.1 First stage of adjustment: Changes in the movement program

The fast (type IIa and IIb) and slowly (type I) contracting myofibers adapt their activation to the physical strain. The **adjustment in the nervous system** can be measured electromyographically as increase in efferent motor impulse, increase of super-ordinate motor units frequency of, synchronization of inter- and intra-muscular motor units, increased motor units excitability, and decreased alpha-motoneuron presynaptic blockade (Aagaard and Thorstensson 2002). Consequently, 1–2 weeks after training athletes will notice that **sport-specific motions** will become **easier** and more fluently.

The increased activity of the muscular glycogen synthase **increases the glycogen storage**. The reduced glycogen deficit during performance will shorten the regeneration time. The first stage of adjustment takes about **7–10 days**.

1.3.2 Second stage of adjustment: Increase of the energy storage

In the second stage of adjustment, a clear increase of the energy storages of creatine phosphate and glycogen will develop (Kjaer et al, 2003). The **creatine phosphate stores** (CP) will rise after temporary intense, i.e. alactacid, training impulses and the **muscle glycogen content** will be enhanced after longer aerobic-anaerobic training.

Repeated series training with only 6 sec duration (e.g. 30 m sprints) can increase CP stores. However, aerobic exposures of 120 minutes or aerobic-anaerobic exposures of 70 minutes will be necessary to increase the glycogen stores. Exposures shorter than 1 hour will enhance the glycogen stores only slightly. Only aerobic endurance training of several hours will lead to an increase of the **intra-muscular triglyceride**, as well as an increase of the **mitochondrium mass** (Hoppeler et al. 1973).

If the muscle is charged with **force stimuli** (enhanced resistance) muscular hypertrophy may develop. Resistance loads will increase the intracellular protein synthesis and cause a significant enhancement of structural proteins, such as actin, myosin, desmin, titin, collagen, and others (Goto and Radak 2005).

1.3.3 Third stage of adjustment: Improvement of regular systems and structures

The organism will effectively adjust to the demand because of the regulation experience, especially in **metabolism**. This applies to the proportion of glucose and fatty-acid oxidization, in particular. The course of adaptation will occur autonomously within the organism but can be modulated by modes of training.

Thus, training should be reduced **between the 3rd and 4th week** (20th to 30th day) for an easier function optimization in the muscular structures (Neumann and Berbalk 1991).

1.3.4 Fourth stage of adjustment: Coordination of performance-influencing systems

The vegetative and central nervous systems, the cardiopulmonary system, the electrolyte and energy metabolism, the hormone and immune system belong to the **performance-influencing systems**.

The function balance between the central nervous system and the adaptively changing structure of muscles and tendons will be a time-dependent process, starting **between the 30th and 40th day** of training and lasting for about 2 weeks.

The adjustment processes will interfere with each other during training but they will be completed **after 4–6 weeks of performance training**. The described model of adjustment largely applies to endurance-orientated training and is not applicable to all sports (Neumann and Berbalk 1991).

Tab. 1.2 Adaption of the oxygen up-take and selected muscle enzymes after 5 months of aerobic training (Gollnik et al. 1973).

Function systems	Basic value	After training (4 hours of cycling/week)	Increase
oxygen-uptake	3.81	4.40	13%
oxidative enzymes (Succinate dehydrogenase, SQR, µmol/g)	4.65	9.10	95%
glycolytic enzymes (phosphofruktokinase, PFK, mmol/g)	28.5	59.0	117%

The **degradation** of **protein fragments** worn out by stress is of central significance in the adaptation of the strained muscle. In model evaluations, Mader (1990) assumes an exchange of amino acids within the exposed musculature of 2–6% per training day. The compensation of worn-out muscle proteins of about 2% a day would mean that the complete muscle could change adaptively in its structure in 50 days of training. The **most efficient conversion** in the exposed structures occurs during the **relief-times** of training. In training practice, it has been proven repeatedly that there will be no or only small achievement without sufficient times of relief.

> Omitting relief times is a frequent mistake in training practice.

The **development of maximal oxygen up-take** is a reliable criterion for the time of adjustment (➤ Tab. 1.2). Its development from the fitness-sports level to the competitive-sports level will take **5 months** at least.

References

Aagaard P, Thorstensson A (2002). Neuromuscular aspects of exercise-adaptive responses evoked by strength training. In: Kjaer M, Krogsgaard M, Magnusson P, Engebretsen L, Roos H, Takala T, L-Y Woo S (eds.). Textbook of Sports Medicine. Blackwell Scientific Publications, 2002, p. 70–106. Oxford.

Crameri RM, Langber H, Teisner B, Magnusson P, Schröder HD, Oleson JL, Jensen HCh, Koskinen S, Suetta Ch, Kjaer M (2004). Enhanced procollagen processing in skeletal muscle after a single bout of eccentric loading in humans. Matrix Biol 23: 259–264.

Edgerton VR, Zhou MY, Ohira Y, Klitgaard H, Jiang B, Bell G, Harris B, Saltin B, Gollnik PD, Roy RR (1995). Human fiber size and enzymatic properties after 5 and 11 days of spaceflight. J Appl Physiol 78: 1733–1739.

Gollnik PD, Armstrong RB, Saltin B, Saubert CW, Sembrowich WL, Shepherd RE (1973). Effect of training on enzyme activity and fiber composition of human skeletyl muscle. J Appl Physiol 34: 107–111.

Goto S, Radak Z (2005). Proteins and exercise. In: Molecular and Cellular Exercise Physiology (Mooren FC and Völker K, eds.). pp 55–70. Human Kinetics, Champaign IL.

Han XY, Wang W, Komulainen J, Koskinen SOA, Kovanen V, Vihko V, Trackman PC, Takala TES (1999). Increased mRNAs for procollagens and key enzymes in rat muscle following downhill running. Pflügers Arch Eur J Physiol 437: 857–864.

Hoppeler H, Lüthi P, Claassen H, Weibel ER, Howald H (1973). The ultrastructure of the normal human skeletal muscle. Pflügers Arch 344: 217–232.

Kjaer M, Krogsgaard M, Magnusson P, Engebretsen L, Roos H, Takala T, L-Y Woo S (2003). Textbook of Sports Medicine. Blackwell Wissenschafts-Verlag, Berlin.

Mader A (1990). Aktive Belastungsadaption und -regulation der Proteinsynthese auf zellulärer Ebene. Dtsch Z Sportmed 41: 40–58.

Neumann G, Berbalk A (1991). Umstellung und Anpassung des Organismus – grundlegende Voraussetzung der sportlichen Leistungsfähigkeit. In: Bernett P and Jeschke D (eds.). Sport und Medizin. Pro und Kontra. Zuckschwerdt-Verlag, Munich.

References

Neumann G, Schüler KP (1989). Sportmedizinische Funktionsdiagnostik. 1st edition. Barth-Verlag, Leipzig.

Neumann G, Schüler KP (1989). Sportmedizinische Funktionsdiagnostik. 2nd edition. Barth-Verlag, Leipzig.

Neumann G, Lang M (2003). Zur Quantifizierung der Anpassung an Triathlontraining. In: Engelhardt M, Franz B, Neumann G, Pfützner A (eds.). 16. Und 17. Triathlonsymposium 2001 und 2002. Vol. 13. Verlag Czwalina, Hamburg.

Neumann G, Pfützner A, Berbalk A (2005). Optimiertes Ausdauertraining. 4th edition. Verlag Meyer & Meyer, Aachen.

Riley DA, Bain JL, Thompson JL, Fitts RH, Widrick JJ, Trappe DW, Trappe TA, Costill DL (2002). Thin filament diversity and physiological properties of fast and slow fiber types in astronaut leg muscles. J Appl Physiol 92(2): 817–825.

Yu M, Blomstrand E, Chibalin AV, Krook A, Zierath R (2001). Marathon running increases ERK1/2 and p38MAP targets in human skeletal muscle. J Physiol 536: 273–282.

Chapter 2

Age- and gender-specific aspects of sports medicine

Georg Neumann and Stefan Nehrer

2.1 Children and adolescents

2.1.1 Sports and physical development

Georg Neumann

Early learning of motor activity has a persistent effect on successful sport performance. If acquired technically as child or adolescent, performance of swimming, running, cycling or skiing positively impacts on the later pursuing of this sport. If a sport such as swimming is not acquired in childhood, adults will struggle learning the coordinated movement. However, **fitness capacities** such as endurance and power cannot be trained and stored in childhood and adolescence. They require re-development and training.

Training with high load is hardly useful for children at the age of 10–12 years who plan a later sports career. High loads only lead to motor slowness. At childhood age, the **speed and speed-strength training** together with adapting good technique should be in the center of training.

The potentially high endurance capacity of children has been tested in athletics. In New Zealand, 8-year-old boys are asked to do cross runs of 3–5 km [1.9–3 miles] (Lydiard and Gilmour 1999). For the Kenian runner offspring between the 12th and 14th year of age, training loads of 50–70 km [31–43.5 miles]/week are considered normal; although these high volumes are run very slowly (Saltin et al. 1995). 5 to 13-year-olds absolved marathon runs in 2:55 to 4:37 hours. When these kids were reported more than 30 years ago in the U.S., they were expected to be successful runners as adults. However, none of them reached outstanding success in running as adults.

From an orthopedic perspective, children and adolescents can handle high stress volumes astonishingly well. Since endurance cannot be 'stored', it should only be developed for an age-specific performance target.

In addition to early technique learning, the **development of individual speed characteristics** at juvenile age plays a central role. Early development of basic speed that is stabilized by training will also be useful for later achievements. The other way around it will not be possible to train speed after fitness training.

The **strength development** of children and adolescents is very limited prior to puberty. During this period strength training is not recommended because the risk to **disturb bone development** is too prominent. For both sexes, the effectiveness of strength or strength-endurance training clearly increase only with the rise of endogenous testosterone during puberty.

> **Summary**
>
> Fitness performance (endurance and strength-endurance) can be trained with children only if respecting their actual performance capacity and biological age. Since endurance cannot be stored, training of speed, speed strength and coordination should have priority at the age of childhood and adolescence. The optimum motor learning age (10–12 years) is important for acquiring the correct technique of the sport. Technical-acrobatic sports start with the motor learning training already at the pre-school age. Too heavy training slows down the development of speed and coordination.

2.1.2 Sport-orthopedic aspects

Stefan Nehrer

The performance development in top sports increasingly requires starting target-oriented training as child or adolescent. Popular sports and modern trend sports attract young athletes. Respecting the limits of of the growing organism is key for a successful sports career and normal development of the locomotor apparatus.

Childhood sport-orthopedics not only treats but prevents sports damages and injuries. The **evaluation of sport suitability** as a sports-medical primary examination is of great importance.

Age- and growth-associated orthopedic disease patterns that are enormously influence sport aptitude. Articular changes such as hip dyplasia, osteonecrosis or Salter-Harris fractures can crucially change sports capacity of the joints. Spinal changes such as in spondylolisthesis, Scheuermann's disease or scoliosis will influence the sporting capacity. The growth-associated tension effect will be further accentuated during intensive practicing of sports Sports-medical knowledge is necessary for health risks. Too often we found training with too high loads at a biologically too early age, often ending promising sports careers early. A long-time systematic, age-appropriate training set-up with constant sports-medical supervision can enable a harmonic development of achievements and maintain health and fun in sports.

Structures of the sustentacular and locomotor apparatuses: Development, growth and capacity

The ability to resist mechanical stress without impairment of the sustentacular and locomotor apparatuses (such as cartilage, bones, muscles, tendons and ligaments) is called **capacity**. Crossing this limit either causes an acute damage in trauma or microtraumas that impact on efficiency. The long-term effects of these changes often will not manifest until adulthood for both acute damage and chronic overstrain. The capacity of the locomotor apparatus depends on **the biological age of the child**. Occasionally, the biological and chronological ages may differ up to two years with gender-specifics. Capacity evaluations of the locomotor apparatus can only be based on biological development, e. g. with the help of carpus and iliac-crest x-rays (Risser 1958).

The childhood **bones** have a greater plastic formability; however, even a weak force can cause a fracture. The weak points of child bones are the growth plates, which show enhanced responsiveness to shearing forces but are only secured by fibrous structures (Morscher and Desaulles 1964). Generally, the vulnerability of the growing skeleton is proportional to its current growth speed.

The **articular cartilages** of childhood are more elastic and regenerate easier than adult cartilage. They are less susceptible for overuse damages because of their higher water-binding capacity and stronger thickness. Similar to growth zones, an increased susceptibility of these structures is present especially during hormonal fluctuations during puberty.

The muscle strength increases continuously in childhood age. 6-year-olds show about 20%, 10-year-olds about 40% of the maximum muscle strength of a male adult. Beginning with the 10th year of age, there will be a stronger gender-specific development of the maximum strength.

Ligaments are clearly more elastic as compared to adults, and this is the reason for rare torn ligaments at young age. Bony and cartilaginous ligament tears in the area of the apophysic insertion regions of the tendons are much more common because this transitional zone is mechanically less stable than the ligament or the tendon.

The sports capacity at the age of childhood and adolescence always has to be considered in connection with the **full complexity of the psychophysical development** of the child. The growth process of the organism is impulsive and proceeds with different dynamics in the diverse organ systems. The **pubertal growth spurt** is probably a critical phase for the sporting capacity since it triggers muscular dysbalance in combination with coordinative deficiencies and inharmonic build. The understanding of the coach is key at this critical time period.

Special sport-orthopedic clinical pictures at the age of childhood and adolescence

Pediatric-orthopedic diseases need to be considered in the context of age, growth, and development. Therefore, we differentiate between **growth-associated diseases, age-associated diseases and exposure or sport-induced diseases of the locomotor apparatus**. Typical systemic skeletal diseases are Marfan syndrome, osteogenesis imperfecta tarda, and Ehlers-Danlos syndrome. Children with abnormal mobility, frequent fractures and unstable joints with spontaneous habitual dislocations require special attention; these children require careful evaluation of their sporting aptitude. The age-specific disease disposition needs to be considered if evaluating sport-orthopedic problems.

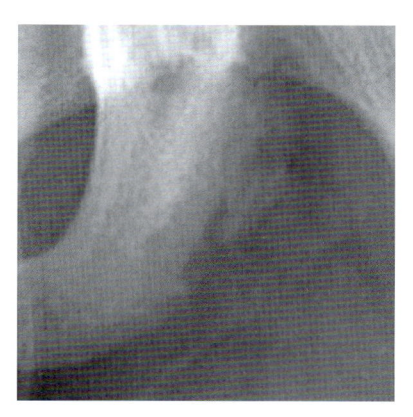

Fig. 2.1 Bowl-like bone retraction at tuber ossis ischii in a 14-year-old artistic gymnast. A slight dislocation and fine-stripped extractions without clear fragmentation of the apophysis can be recognized.

Clinical pictures of the extremities

Hip

Congenital hip dysplasia: This developmental, dysplastic hip disorder clearly limits the capacity of the hip joint. Children in sports with high running load should exclude this dysplasia. Growth retard in the area of the acetabulum with the development of a late dysplasia is typical for the pubertal growth spurt.

Legg-Calvé-Perthes syndrome: The femur necrosis of children peaks around the age of 4 to 6. But the evaluation of the Legg-Calvé-Perthes syndrome is important as it can lead to deformations of the femur. The examination of the free flexibility of the hip joint and radiologic follow-ups until the end of growth are obligatory.

Epiphysiolysis capitis femoris: An atraumatic epiphysiolysis of the femur head with adiposis and development delay in mostly male patients (Froehlich's syndrome). But we have also seen epiphysiolyses increasingly in connection with sports like inline skating or long hikes in rather asthenic children. Chronic, slow dislocation of the epiphysis on the femoral neck and a lasting distortion of the femoral head have been described in connection with soccer. The shape of the femoral head distortion is decisive for the capacity of the hip joint. Other hip-joint diseases are the coxitis types, which can be seen as infection-rheumatoid (coxitis fugax) and also as bacterial arthritis or monarthritis in juvenile rheumatic diseases.

Apopyseal damages of the loin-pelvis-hip region: Apophyses are growth plates in the area of tendon insertions. Growth-associated diseases in the region of loin, pelvis and hip region, primarily the apophyses in the area of the iliac crest involve often the m. rectus femoris, the hamstring, and abductors (Klose and Schuchardt 1980). The apophyseal damages range from little alterations up to complete tears of the tendon insertions, and accordingly the pain projection happens in the region of the groin or the buttocks. The radiologic pathomorphology shows a very variable picture ranging from frail calcific overshadowing in the region of the tendon insertion up to the partial ossification of secondary ossification focuses (➤ Fig. 2.1). Here, differential diagnosis especially in osteolytic processes is key because both infect and tumor-like processes of the skeleton system can cause similar changes (Barnes and Hinds 1972).

Knee joint

Osgood-Schlatter disease: The painful swelling of the tuberosity of the tibia with secondary changes in the region of the apophysis of the insertion of the patellar tendon is often associated with overloads of the knee joint traction apparatus (Kvist and Kujala 1984). The trac-

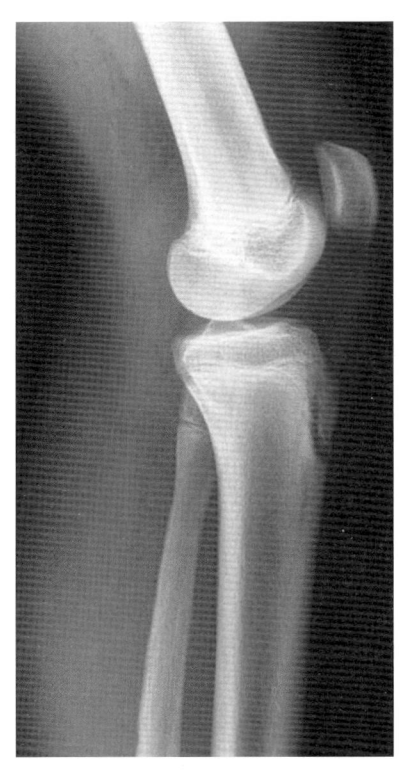

Fig. 2.2 Osgood-Schlatter disease. A fissure and fragmentation of the apophyseal bone core at the Tuberositas tibiae is to be found. This seems altogether definitely clumped with fine-stripped extractions.

tion apparatus is affected by the tibia growth spurt, especially the distal femoral epiphysis, and physical activities, especially in sports like soccer. This can lead lifting and partial tear of the apophysis of the patellar tendon. Ossicles may develop because of secondary ossification disorders (Engel and Winshager 1987) and these may remain painful but can be removed (➢ Fig. 2.2). Treatment is sports pause for knee-wearing sports and recovery of the muscle balance around the knee joint.

Sinding-Larsen-Johansson syndrome: This describes overstressing the insertion point at the distal patella pole and is connected with overusing the traction apparatus of the adolescent knee joint. Calcium-dense, cloddy changes at the distal patella pole, which changes in tenderness, are typical.

Chondropathia patellae: The chondropathia patellae or the anterior knee pain is a complex clinical picture of the adolescent knee joint. Overload of the traction apparatus at growth, changing knee axes, and coordination deficiencies are key for the development of knee pain. Furthermore, changes of the articular capsule such as in plica syndrome, anatomic variations of the patellar shape, or imbalances of the retinaculae patellae soft-tissue can be responsible for anterior knee pain. MRT is indicated for chronic knee pain to exclude patellar or peripatellar pathologies. If MRT is negative, arthroscopy can treat plica infra- or suprapatellaris, or osteochondral focuses in the area of the slide bearing or the patella, respectively. Fixing the traction apparatus into the exposure frame or "envelope" (Scott Dye 1986) is the top-priority. Conservative treatments of condropathias are recovery of the extensor and flexor muscular balance, improvement of intramuscular coordination of the m. quadriceps and the muscular stabilization of the leg.

The long-term prognosis is good at growth and in puberty; surgical interventions are not recommended.

The radiologic analysis of the femoropatellar slide bearing and the patellar shape helps to develop long-term concepts. Release operations and pivot osteotomies of the tuberosity are only sensible after clarifying the individual pathogenetic mechanism.

Discoid meniscus: During development of the knee joint, incomplete formation of the discoid shape especially the lateral meniscus can occur. In such case the complete septating of the lateral compartment stays upright what often causes tears of the central, discoid meniscus. Partial removal of the meniscus shape and, in the case of instability, fixation of instable parts by arthroscopy is recommended. Prognosis for joints requiring complete removal is not very good as it significantly reduces sports capacity.

Osteochondritis dissecans: The etiology of femoral osteonecrosis in adolescents is largely unknown but it is often observed in connection with recurrent traumas or sports-overuse. The integrity of the cartilage cap above the osteonecrosis focus is decisive for the prognosis. Spot boring of the necrosis areas had only limited therapeutic success. The surgical intervention is probably necessary for instable or broken-off fragments with secondary joint disorders. Also the age of the patient is decisive for the therapeutic approach: While osteochondritic focuses before puberty have a good prognosis, especially larger focuses after puberty are connected with marked defects of the joint surface and the formation of a secondary early arthrosis. In these cases, tunnel fixation, osteochondral transplantation (mosaic plastic) or a transplantation of cartilage-cells are recommended.

Habitual and post-traumatic relapsing luxating patella: Recurrent patellar dislocations mostly are connected with a dysplastic change in the area of the femoropatellar slide bearing with valgic knee axes. For therapy it is important whether the patellar luxations caused osteochondral damages at the patella or in the femoropatellar slide bearing. Conservative measures with bandages and muscular stabilization as well as the surgical redirection of the traction apparatus are possible.

Malpositions in the leg axis: Axis formation starts with a distinctive genu-varum condition in the infant and continues as an increasing genu-valgum condition and ends in a normal, slightly valgic condition of the leg axes. Changes of the leg axes in valgus or varus (bow leg or knock-knee) lead to overstrain of the affected joint areas in the knee joint especially with high sports activity. A surgical straightening is strongly recommended in case of axis deviations of more than 7–10°.

Feet

Providing an adequate shoe is the most important prophylaxis during feet development. The shoe should provide adequate support of the hindfoot with a cushioning in tread as well as a leaving foot strike as natural as possible. Shoe corrections and inlays should be tested for their effectiveness in a treadmill analysis. Shoe inlays are made of soft materials such as rubber foam or cork covered with leather. Sever's disease seems to be a typical orthopedic problem with children (Kvist and Kujala 1984). Here, apophysis of the calcaneus is painful and condensation and fragmentation of the epiphysis are visible in x-ray (➤ Fig. 2.3). Soft bedding of the heel and transient sports restrictions offer relief.

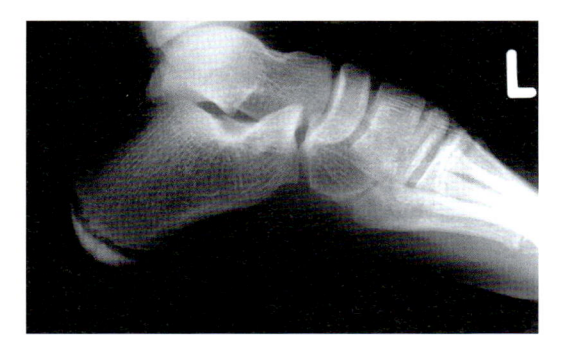

Fig. 2.3 Overuse damage of the calcaneal apophysis with increased sclerosing in the x-ray and broadening of the apophysis in a 12-year-old soccer player.

Clinical pictures of the spine

The spine is the central axis and presents a great challenge regarding diagnosis and therapy of occurring changes, and prevention of sports damages. Up to 64% of top athletes (Wismach 1988) complain about lumbar pain disorders in back-straining sports such as gymnastics; up to 70% of sports exemptions due to changes of their spines. Lumbar pain is often triggered by structural spine or intervertebral disc damages; tumors or infections are rare. Scoliosis, juvenile osteochondrosis (Scheuermann's disease) and spondylolysis/ spondylolysthesis are the most common structural spine disorders. The shape and severity of these clinical pictures are important for the evaluation of sport-aptitude and -suitability. Spinal capabilities and exposure during training requires consultation of athletes and trainers (Junghanns 1980).

Scoliosis: Scolioses or spinal malformations vary between individual sports and ranging from 19% in recreational sports up to higher percentage rates in javelin (Neusel et al. 1987). Incidences of scoliosis range between 0.2 and 4% in orthopedic literature.

Whether one-sided, long-term intensive training leads to spinal malformation has been questioned (Menge 1981). Fixed severe scolioses occur only rarely in sports but are often found in disciplines that are actually prescribed for therapy of scoliosis such as swimming. A continuous clinical and radiological control is important to avoid scoliosis progression. Stereotypical, one-sided exposures with

Cobb angles of more than 10° are not recommended; competitive sports are contraindicated with a Cobb angle higher than 25°.

Juvenile osteochondrosis: Incidence rates range between 0.3 and 8% in normal subjects and reach up to 50% in competitive gymnastics (Pollähne and Steinbrück 1980). Vertebral structural disorders with changes of the intervertebral discs need to be differentiated from juvenile osteochondrosis. The typical changes of the juvenile kyphosis lie in the middle thoracic spine, affect more than three vertebras, and show a kyphosis angle of more than 40° (Puhl et al. 1985). The pathognomonic sign is Schmorl's node in the intervertebral discs. Transient and controlled modifications can be effected on the level of competitive sports for stages 1 and 2. Kyphosing sports and those with high axial load are contraindicated in stages 3 and 4. Stage evaluation, age, scoliosis localization, intensity of exposure, and sport are critical factors (Pollähne 1991).

Spondylolysis and spondylolisthesis: The spondylolisthesis is a ventral dislocation of the vertebral body with its bow roots, cranial articular and transverse processes. The ventral dislocation is possible because of spondylolysis (fissuring) or elongation of the intermediate joint parts (intra-articular portion, isthmus). The dorsal part of the vertebral arch with caudal articular and spinous processes of vertebra stays in anatomic position (Zippel 1980). Vertebral sliding can be triggered by fissure formations of the vertebral arch (spina bifida, retro-isthmic fissure, and malformations of the spine), arthritic changes of the vertebral arch joints in connection with ligament and segmental instability as well as luxation fractures.

Spondylolysis and spondylolisthesis are typically **diagnosed** with sideways x-ray of the lumbar spine or on radiographies that have been turned 45°. Spondylolisthesis is classified according to Mayerding with 4 dislocation stages of cranial to caudal vertebras (Schwerdtner 1980). Shear and pressure stress in the area of the lower lumbar vertebrae and the lumbosacral passage are considered as causes of spondylolysis and spondylolisthesis (Steinbrück 1980). Osseous aberrations and mechanic factors are discussed controversially (Junghanns 1980, Niethard et al. 1997). The occurrence of spondylolyses already at birth is usually negated. In fact, they occur during growth, possibly with the straightening-up for upright walking. Reactive signs with callus formation in adolescents and mostly inactive pseudarthrosis tissue in adults are found in histological examinations. The significantly increased occurrence of spondylolyses and spondylolisthesis in high-performance sports supports the theory of spondylolysis as fatigue fracture (Neusel 1987, Riehl and Bernett 1991, Engelhardt et al. 1997). Micro-traumata and a following stress fracture develop within the intra-articular portion of the vertebral arch a a consequence of mechanic overstrains. A pseudoarthrosis or an elongation of the intra-articular portion can develop, listhesis are often result from reparation attempts (Schiffel et al. 1989). Epidemiologic studies showed spondylolyses and spondylolistheses do occur more often in high-performance gymnastics (Schwerdtner 1980, Wismach 1988), pole-vaulting (Theiss 1980), and javelin (Neusel et al. 1987). In contrast, spondylolyses and spondylolistheses are lower in mixed sports and recreational sports as compared to the general population (Pollähne 1991). Additionally, spondylolysis and spondylolisthesis increase with age.

Children mostly show lumbar myalgic pain symptoms and signs with stress and hyperextension pains. In severe cases, gait disorders and hip-loin traction rigidity might occur. Listhesis is combined with scoliosis in 20–30% and listhesis higher than Mayerding 1–2, malformation is palpable. Children typically develop the picture of a hamstring shortening with a pseudo-Lasègue sign. Cauda syndromes and radicular lesions (mostly S1) are rare. The achieved litheses in childhood age mostly lie in segment L5/S1.

If spondylolysis or spodylolisthesis are existent, conservative **measures** are recommended. Remedial-gymnastics programs can stabilizes musculature and adjust muscular dysbalances . Local physical therapy and temporary stomacher immobilization are possible for pain-dominated cases, although the muscular stabilization should always be preferred. The dorsal spondylodesis or combined procedures are possible for progressive lithesis, therapy-resistant pain syndromes, radicular or caudal symptoms; the indication for surgery must be decided for

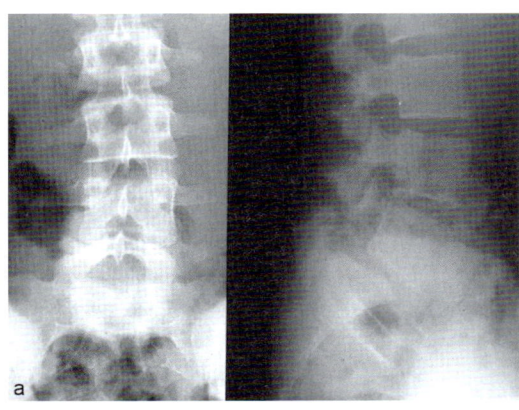

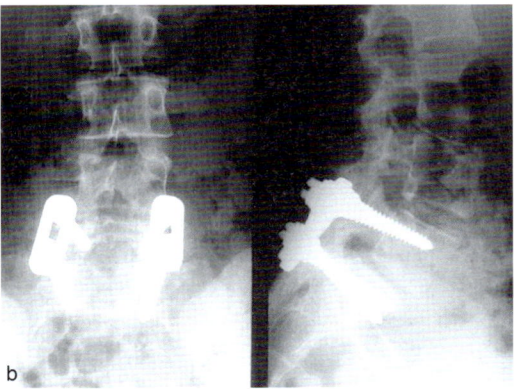

Fig. 2.4 a/b Spondylolisthesis in a young athlete, who had to be stabilized at the age of 15 because of pain and neurologic symptoms and signs. a: pre-operative, b: post-operative.

each case individually. Figure 2.4a/b show a spondylolysthesis before and after stabilization (➢ Fig. 2.4a/b).

Lysis development in childhood age, female gender, dysplastic disorders in the area of the lumbosacral intersection such as a spina bifida, wedge-vertebra development of L5 and a short rounded-down S1 are unfavorable prognostic factors with spondylolysis in terms of spondylolisthesis development. Spine-stressing sports are contraindicated if such changes present. One-sided spondylolyses and minor listheses require a partial sports prohibit for spine-stressing exercises and a clear reduced training amount. Athletes should switch to a less stressing sport. The imposed limited sporting capacity should be monitored with regular x-ray and clinical control. The following sports are particularly unsuitable with spondylolyses: athletics (jumping and throwing disciplines), artistic and competitive gymnastics, trampoline and springboard diving, wrestling and judo, dolphin butterfly stroke, and weight lifting (Steinbrück 1980).

Sports-orthopedic consultation and education in case of spine changes are required trainers, club officials, and athletes. Training intervals and intensity require clarification with the trainer. Learning of new movements – e.g. in gymnastics – can cause misloads of the spine and biomechanical risky movements of the lumbar spine. Supporting measures and coordinative preliminary exercises are recommended.

Incorrect execution of gymnastic exercises in amateur sports carries similar risks for the lumbosacral intersection. Hyperextension movements plus rotation as well as axial compressive stress should be avoided in the case of lyse and listhesis. Conforming expansion and invigoration programs improve the biomechanic situation in the lumbosacral intersection, if a dysbalance and ventral pelvis overturning occurred. A sports prohibit should be expressed partially for certain sports and movements. Patients need to be guided to attractive alternatives. A general sports prohibit is only indicated for severe malformations.

Sport-orthopedic evaluation

Sports-medical evaluation of a child must be geared to the individual development and maturity, and achieved physiologic parameters. Learning of complicated movements seems to be most adequate at elementary school age and should be used for the training of basic techniques. Weights and high compression moments at tendon inserts and apophyses as well as and shear forces at the epiphyses should absolutely be avoided.

A mandatory sports-medical aptitude examination by the sports-orthopedist is indispensable for competitive sports. Rules and training arrangement need to be in line with the child's capacity. Sports physicians and trainers must develop and implement a children-suitable training schedule. In addition to sports, other areas of socials life such as family, friends, and hobbies need to have sufficient space. Training of too many sports at the same time should be avoided because complete exposure triggers overstrain syndromes. Competition in childhood age is important, although it should not be taken too seriously. Long-term development and maintaining of healthy body have clear priority.

Sports ban and competitive-sports ban

In many cases, sports load needs to be lowered transiently or continually, if pathologic child-orthopedic or sport-orthopedic changes are present. A medical certificate for the exemption from school sports or competitive sports should to contain the following information in addition to the diagnosis: permanence, breadth, full or partial exemption, prohibited loads, alternatives, and an examination appointment regarding the sports proscription. The recommendations regarding the sports limitation will be discussed for the individual clinical pictures and often require an individual reconcilement.

Summary
Most sports-orthopedic problems in children are avoidable; too early use of wrong training methods is the most frequent cause. Lyle Micheli summarized the problem of children's sports concisely in a single sentence: "Too much, too soon." (Micheli and Gerbino 1979)

References

Barnes ST, Hinds RB (1972). Pseudotumor of the ischium. J Bone Joint Surg 54A: 645.

Dye SF (1986). Radionuclide imaging of the pastellofemoral joint in young adults with anterior knee pain. Orthop Clin North America 17 (2): 249–262.

Engel H, Windhager R (1987). Der Stellenwert des Ossikels in der Therapie bei Morbus Osgood-Schlatter. Sportverletz Sportschaden 2: 100–108.

Engelhardt M, Reuter I, Freiwald J, Böhme T, Halbsguth A (1997). Spondylolysis and spondylolysisthesis and sports. Orthopäde 26: 755–759.

Junghanns H (ed.) (1980). Die Wirbelsäule in Forschung und Praxis. Vol. 89, Hippokrates, Stuttgart: 41–42.

Klose HH, Schuchardt E (1980). Die beckennahen Apophysenabrisse. Orthopäde 9: 229–236.

Kvist M, Kujala U (1984). Osgood Schlatter's and Sever's disease in young athletes. Duadecim 100: 142–150.

Menge M (1981). Sportartspezifische Belastungsauswirkungen an der Wirbelsäule. In: Rickert (ed.). Sport an der Grenze menschlicher Leistungsfähigkeit. Springer, Heidelberg.

Micheli ML, Gerbino PG (1979). Epidemiology of children's sports injuries. Orthop Trans 3: 88.

Morscher E, Desaulles PA (1964). Die Festigkeit des Wachstumsknorpels in Abhängigkeit von Alter und Geschlecht. Schweizer Med Wochenschr 17: 582.

Neusel E et al. (1987). Röntgenologische Langzeitbeobachtungen bei Speerwerfern der Spitzenklasse. Sportverletz Sportschaden 2: 76.

Niethard FU, Pfeil J, Weber M (1997). Etiology and pathogenesis of spondylolytic spondylolisthesis. Orthopäde 26: 750–754.

Polläkne W (1991). Ergebnisse der Wirbelsäulenschnittauswertung bei Hochleistungsturnern und Hochleistungsschwimmern aus radiologischer Sicht. Dtsch Z Sportmed 42 (7): 292–308.

Polläkne G, Steinbrück K (1980). Wirbelsäulenschäden durch Sport. In Cotta H, Krahl H (eds.). Die Belastungstoleranz des Bewegungsapparates. Thieme, Stuttgart, New York.

Puhl W, Weber M, Wetzel R (1985). Längsschnittuntersuchungen bei Morbus Scheuermann zum Krankheitswert röntgenologischer Veränderungen. In: Junghanns H. Die Wirbelsäule in Forschung und Praxis. Vol. 89, Hippokrates, Stuttgart: 41–42.

Riehl KA, Bernett P (1991). Spondylolyse und Spondylolisthesis im Sport. Dtsch Z Sportmed 1: 12.

Risser JC (1958). The iliac apophysis: an invaluable sign in the management of scoliosis. Clin Orthop 11: 111.

Schiffel et al. (1989). Sportmedizinische Empfehlungen zur Prophylaxe und Belastungsgestaltung bei Sportlern mit Spondylolyse. Med und Sport 29: 244.

Steinbrück K (1980). Die Bedeutung mechanischer Faktoren bei der Entstehung der Spondylolyse. Z Orthop 118: 456.

Schwerdtner HP (1980). Röntgenologische Verlaufskontrollen der Wirbelsäule bei Kunstturnern und -turnerinnen nach langjährigem Training. In: Cotta H, Krahl N. (eds.). Die Belastungstoleranz des Bewegungsapparates. Thieme, Stuttgart, New York.

Theiss F (1980). Typische Verletzungen bei Stabhochspringern unter besonderer Berücksichtigung der Lendenwirbelsäule. Dtsch Z Sportmed: 161–172.

Wismach J (1988). Wirbelsäulenveränderungen bei Kunstturnerinnen. Sportverletz Sportschaden 2: 95–99.

Zippel: Die Spondylolysthesen. Med und Sport 20; 1980: 65–78.

2.2 Women

Georg Neumann

Women had been excluded from long-distance competitions for a long time. The historic break through came with the women marathon world cup in 1983. After the overcoming these historical shortcomings, the best performances of women came close to men.

Objectively, a woman cannot achieve the same top performance as men. Women achieve roughly 10–12 % in comparable endurance sports as compared to men. An outstanding woman can always be ahead of many men.

These performing differences between men and women have several physiological factors:

- build
- endocrine system
- muscular aerobics

  and

- strength potential.

Maximum oxygen uptake (VO_2max) increases with training but will be 10 % lower for women than for men in the same sport. Usually, women are 12 cm (4′ 7″) smaller and weigh 15 kg (33 lbs) less than men in comparable sports. The differences between male and female endurance athletes are only minor regarding adipose (➤ Tab. 2.1).

The testosterone concentration of a female endurance athlete amounts to 1.5–3.2 nmol/l, hence, is 10 to 20 times lower as compared to a male endurance athlete (8.3–34.7 nmol/l). The **lower testosterone level** is the main reason for the **lower strength potential** of women.

Tab. 2.1 Anthropometric data of male and female triathletes, who reached the conveyance status in competitive sports (n = 67*).

Body measurements	Women	Men
size (cm)	171.0 ± 5.5	182.8 ± 5.3
weight (kg)	58.8 ± 5.0	74.2 ± 4.8
adipose (%)	9.6 ± 3.6	9.5 ± 1.6
adipose (kg)	5.7 ± 2.2	7.1 ± 1.3
LBM (Lean body mass) (kg)	53.3 ± 4.4	67.2 ± 4.1
shoulder length (cm)	36.8 ± 2.3	40.9 ± 1.6
breadth of pelvis (cm)	27.7 ± 2.1	28.3 ± 1.5

*Private data of Dr. Gudrun Fröhner, Institute of Applied Exercise Science (IAT), Leipzig.

Female athletes with a higher androgen level, which is produced naturally in the body will be more successful in endurance sports.

Estrogen concentration of the sexually mature female athlete is 5–15 times as high (73–1,652 pmol/l) as compared to a male athlete (20–85 pmol/l). **The fluctuations of the estradiol** concentrations fluctuate in the menstrual cycle and reach 400 pg/ml (1,460 pmol/l) during the ovulation period and 260 pg/ml (949 pmol/l) in the luteal phase. Menstrual cycle may impact on **sports performance**. A higher estradiol concentration allows longer distances for women as compared to men, which is particularly important for any performance depending on fat burning (Bam et al. 1997). If performance training is restarted after pregnancy, women often have higher, long distance performances.

Summary

The performance differences between men and women range between 8–12 % in comparable disciplines. The reasons for these performance differences base on differences in physique, muscular aerobic performance, or hormonal balance. The lower testosterone is the main reason for the lower strength potential of women.

2.3 Elderly persons
Georg Neumann

2.3.1 Preventive use of senior sports

Sports have social, biological, psychological, medical and prophylactic components and adequate sports can be **preventive.** The sports recommendations concentrate on the **reduction of risk factors** or on **protection of the skeleton and musculature.** Sports at rising age will carry higher dangers for bones and muscles and need to be balanced with the benefits of the cardiopulmonary and metabolic systems. Only those therapeutic and preventive measures are considered effective if they prevent an early death (Gillman et al. 1993, Palatini and Julius 1997). Only **endurance sports increasing maximum oxygen uptake** (McMurray et al. 1998) fulfill these prerequisites.

An oxygen uptake of 21–30 ml/kg/min corresponding to 7–10 MET (metabolic equivalent) is considered **medium stress intensity.** In competitive sports training oxygen uptake increases by +30 ml/kg/min (+10 MET) VO_2, i.e. competitive sports training should aim for an average oxygen uptake of 50–60 ml/kg/min.

Running had been for years the dominant leisure sports. Distance runs of 5-160.9 km (100 miles) have turned into running standards of the fitness sector. Leisure and older athletes have given up the ambition of extreme or too-long endurance loads. Running was replaced by more **moderate endurance sports** such as power walking, triathlon, duathlon, cycling, in-line skating, swimming, or cross-country skiing. Currently, versatile and joint-protecting sports, which support weight control and offer prevention. At present, senior citizens adopt **power walking** or **Nordic walking** (Bös 2001, Gerig 2001, Schricker et al. 2003, von Stengel and Bartosch 2003). Competition plays a secondary role for older people; adequate distance is what matters.

2.3.2 Age-dependent change of the organism

The **degeneration** of the motor abilities, strength endurance and speed occurs unequally with increasing age (➢ Fig. 2.5). **Moderate endurance training** is tolerated best in the middle and later age.

Officially, an age class (AC) of senior citizens counts the 40- to 70-year-olds. Senior citizens in training objectively need **longer regeneration periods;** this reduces full training loads and lowers entry into competitive sports.

Body fat analysis over lifetime show that even with sports **body-fat inclusion** in the musculature increases. The body-fat reserves produced naturally increase between 50 and 60 years by an average 2 kg (13–15%). Training only controls little of age-related weight gain.

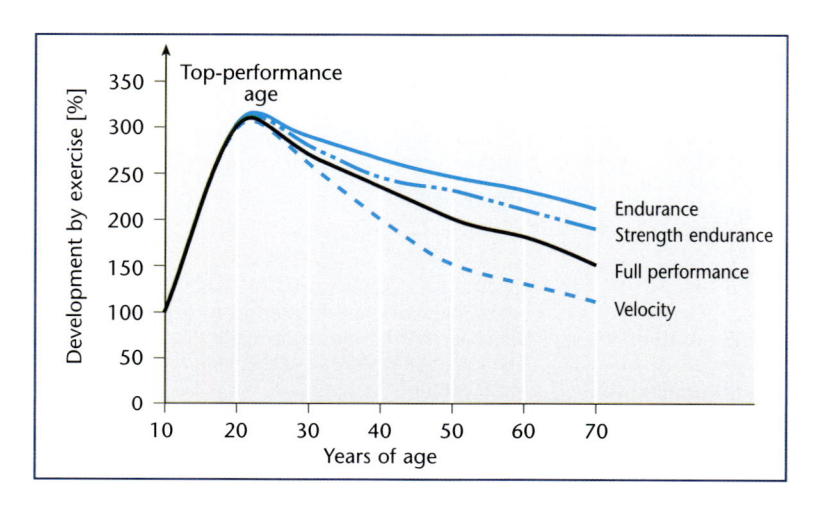

Fig. 2.5 Model presentation of the development and redevelopment of capacities in the aging process. The fitness capacity of endurance can be trained best in age (see Neumann, Pfützner and Berbalk 2007).

2.3 Elderly persons

> The decrease of the active muscle substance is the main reason for the performance decrease starting in the 5th decade of life.

Maximum oxygen uptake (VO$_2$max) decreases with growing age in both sexes. Without training, VO$_2$max decreases between the 25 and 70 years by 8–10% each life decade; with continued training it decreases only 4–5% every year (Heath et al. 1981, Pollock et al. 1987). Endurance running of 2–5 hours/week diminishes 1.1 kg in the long-term average but prevents adiposis (Pollock et al. 1987). Testosterone, which starts decreasing with the age of 25 about 1.2% every year for men (Vermeulen et al. 1996) plays a key role in the age-related fat-deposition.

The decrease of testosterone parallels the **decrease of growth hormone** (somatropin). **Testosterone substitution** with age is approved in certain indications including memory improvement and maintenance of motor activity. The health risks of the testosterone substitution are described minor but prostate-specific antigen **(PSA)** should be monitored. In addition to increased muscle strength, the recreation potency in raises with low testosterone doses in the aging and active man. The usually concealed **erectile dysfunction** is a discrete sign for testosterone undersupply. The testosterone concentration for 35–40% of the more than 65-year-old men amounts to less than 3.5 ng/ml (12.1 nmol/l).

Reduced development of testosterone lets to hypogonadism, reduction of free testosterone, androstenedione and dihydrotestosterone at the age of 40. This is **compensated by an increase of SHBG** (sex hormone binding globulin) and **FSH** (follicle-stimulating hormone of men). In analogy to menopause of women, the reduction of the androgen with age has been called "androgen decline in the aging male", **ADAM**.

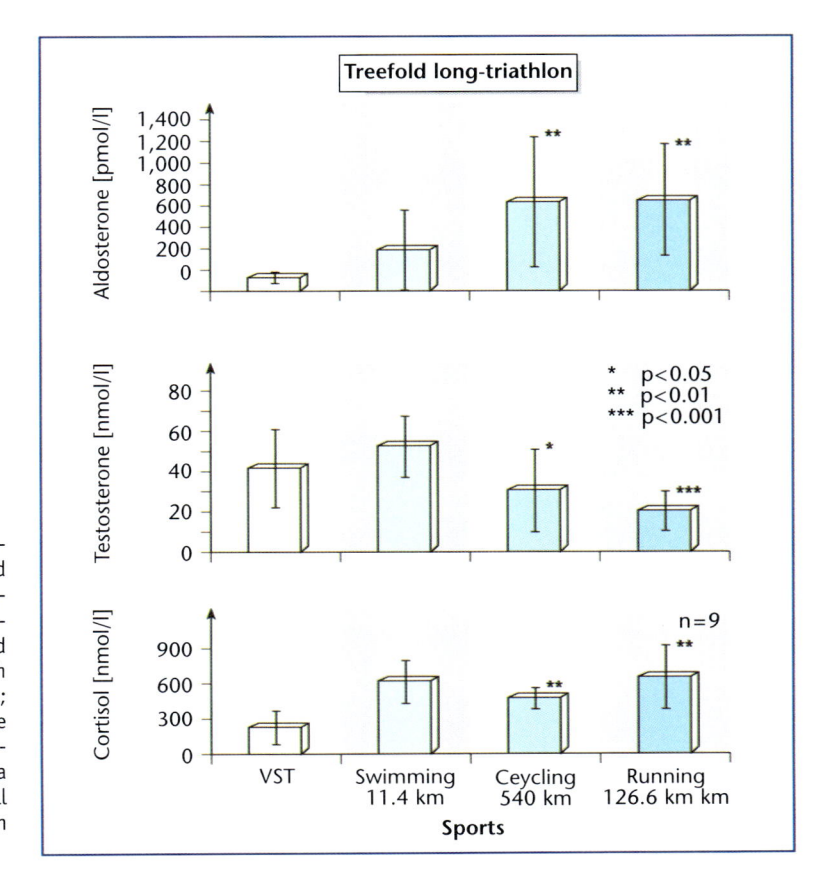

Fig. 2.6 Behavior of aldosterone, testosterone and cortisol at the threefold log-triathlon (11.4 km of swimming, 540 km of cycling, and 126.6 km of running with breaks for sleeping at will; complete time at the average 49 h). After cycling and running stresses, it comes to a significant decrease of the full testosterone (see Neumann and Volk 1999).

Tab. 2.2 Reasonable weekly exposure for senior citizens.

Exposure
■ up to 70 km running training/week or
■ up to 300 km cycling/week or
■ up to 16 km swimming/week

Exogenous testosterone supply is indicated for hypogonadism but stress-caused hormonal undersupply or on individual physiologic marginal cases are debatable. Testosterone concentration decreases after **extreme endurance loads** (Neumann and Volk 1999), thus, real strain duration need to be considered for testosterone monitoring (➤ Fig. 2.6).

Starting at the age of 40 athletes will report more orthopedic problems, if a certain stress level is exceeded (Shephard et al. 1995). **Reasonable loads** in senior sports were examined in running, cycling, and swimming (➤ Tab. 2.2).

Running 80 km per week represents a higher risk for the support and movement apparatus. The orthopedic complaints increase above average with training 8-10 hours/week. Infections occur 15% more often as a result of **immunosuppresion.**

Performance capacity in running competitions differs in each age-class. 80-year-old runners still reach about 50% of the performance of 20- to 30-year-olds (➤ Fig. 2.7).

Specialists often warn about new sports techniques but often proven wrong retrospectively, e.g. skating in cross-country skiing has been used more often by elderly people and has turned out to be more joint-friendly than the classic technique.

Summary

In the 5th decade of life, the gradual reduction of the sporting performance capacity begins, which is mainly conditioned by the reduction of the active muscle mass. The endurance capacity can be trained best with age, while the strength and speed capacities come second. The one-sided running is repressed by moderate endurance and combination sports. At present, versatile loads and especially joint-protecting as well as sporting activities with hardly any injuries are favored, which will help to avoid weight-gaining and promise a preventive effects. Endurance training shows the most preventive effect. Beginning with the 40th year of age androgens decrease. Between 60 and 80 about 22% of men show subnormal complete testosterone and reduced free testosterone. An oxygen uptake of 21 to 30 ml/kg/min (or 7–10 MET) is assumed as a measure for stress intensity in preventive training. This can only be reached by endurance training.

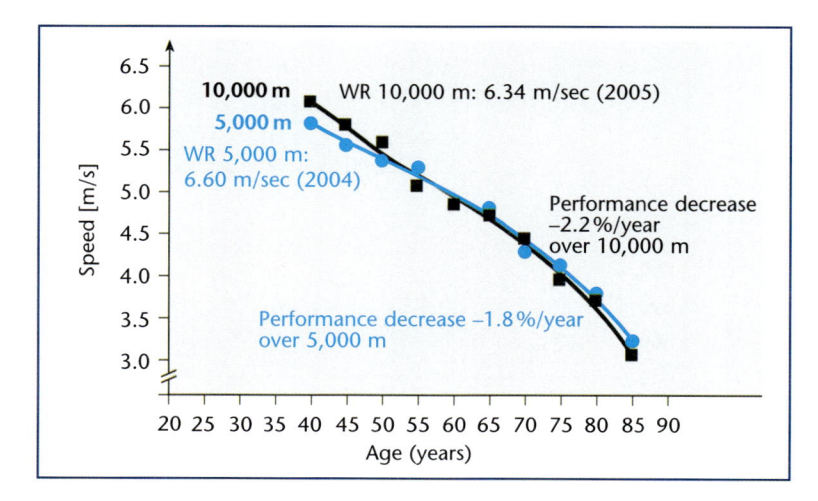

Fig. 2.7 Comparison of running performances in age classes. The absolute performance of 10,000 and 5,000 m decreases in the separate age classes by about 2% each year with growing age, starting with the 40th year of age.

References

Bam J, Noakes TD, Juritz J, Dennis SC (1997). Could women outrun men in ultramarathon races? Med Sci Sports Exerc 29: 244–247.

Bös K (2001). Handbuch für Walking. Verlag Meyer & Meyer, Aachen.

Gerig U (2001). Richtig Walking. BLV-Verlag, Munich.

Gillman MW, Kannel WB, Belanger A, D'Audustino RB (1993). Influence of heart rate on mortality among persons with hypertension: The Framingham Study. Am Heart J 125: 1148–1154.

Heath GW, Hagberg JM, Ehsani A, Holloszy JO (1981). A physiological comparison of young and older endurance athletes. J Appl Physiol 51: 634–640.

Lydiard A, Gilmour G (1999). Mittel- und Langstreckentraining im Jugendbereich. Verlag Meyer & Meyer, Aachen.

McMurray RG, Ainswoth BE, Harrell JS, Griggs TR, Williams OD (1998). Is physical activity or aerobic power more influential on reducing cardiovascular disease risk factors? Med Sci Sports Exerc 30: 1521–1529.

Neumann G, Volk O (1999). Metabole und hormonelle Auswirkungen eines Dreifachlangtriathlons. In: Engelhardt M, Franz B, Neumann G, Pfützner A (eds.). 13. Internationales Triathlon-Symposium Erbach 1998. Vol. 13, pp 21–42. Czwalina-Verlag, Hamburg.

Neumann G, Berbalk A, Pfützner A (2007). Optimiertes Ausdauertraining. 5th ed., Verlag Meyer & Meyer, Aachen.

Palatini P, Julius S (1997). Heart rate and the cardiovascular risk. J Hypertension 15: 3–17.

Pollock ML, Forster C, Knapp D, Rod JL, Schmidt DH (1987). Effect of age and training on aerobic capacity and body composition of master athletes. J Appl Physiol 62: 725–731.

Saltin B, Kim CK, Terrados N, Larsen H, Svedenhag J, Rolf CJ (1995). Morphology, enzyme activities, and buffer capacity in leg muscle of Kenyan and Scandinavian runners. Scand J Med Sci Sports 5: 237–244.

Schricker C, Eichinger W, Lange R (2003). Walking. BLV-Verlag, Munich.

Shephard RJ, Kavanagh T, Mertens DJ (1995). Personals' health benefit of masters athletic competition. Brit J Sports Med 29: 35–40.

v Stengel S, Bartosch H (2003). Nordic Walking. Copress-Verlag, Munich.

Vermeulen A, Kaufmann JM, Giagulli VA (1996). Influence of some biological indices on sex hormone binding globulin and androgen levels in aging and obes males. J Crin Endocrinol Metab 81: 1821–1827.

Chapter 3 Athletics and diseases

Martin Engelhardt and Hubert Hörterer

3.1 Sports and arthrosis

Martin Engelhardt

Degenerative diseases of the support and locomotor apparatuses start to increase with the age of 40. Changed social ideals (sporting and being fit until old age) as well as the increasing life expectancy confront the sports orthopedist with the following questions:
- Does sporting activity result in development of arthrosis?
- May patients with degenerative joint damages carry out sports?
- Which sports are convenient for patients with degenerative joint damages?

3.1.1 Reasons for arthrosis

More than 80% of the people older than 75 years show radiologic arthrosis but only partly with clinical symptoms. Men older than 45 and women older than 55 years carry a higher risk of arthrosis. Besides **age, gender, and genetic disposition** (e.g. hip dyplasia) a number of other risk factors have been identified (Puhl 1996).

The **varus** and **valgus deformities** and **leg-length differences** are significant static-mechanical causes for arthrosis of the lower extremity (hip, knee, and ankle arthroses).

Further possible causes are direct contusions of the articular cartilage, cartilage fractures, and fractures with articular involvement. Joint instabilities after ligament injuries promote the early development of arthrosis.

An increased arthrosis rate has also been detected in patients with metabolic diseases (hyperuricemia, hemochromatosis, ochronoses, etc.).

3.1.2 Sports and arthrosis

The correlation of sports strain and degenerative joint diseases is described controversially in literature.

Some authors reported previously that competitive and top sports do not induce an early arthrosis, however, numerous studies document today an increased arthrosis rate in top sports. Early arthrosis rates have been described for throwing and jumping in athletics, ball sports and martial arts.

> Besides individual disciplines' negative effects on arthrosis, regular physical loads are meaningful for arthrosis patients.

To preserve its mechanic features, every joint requires a **positive-negative pressure**. Regular strain and relief of the cartilage promote the absorption of nutrients from the synovial liquid. On the contrary, immobilization reduces metabolism and increases fat deposition on the sliding surfaces of the articular cartilage.

3.1.3 Preconditions for performing sports with arthrosis

The therapeutic intention requires careful selection of the sports discipline (➤ Tab. 3.1). **Sports with consistent movements** are preferable. Sports with extreme movements, rapid movement sequences, and major impulse loads, all ball sports and martial arts with high risks of injury are not indicated. Specific warming-up and stretching, and strength and endurance exercises lower the risk of injuries.

Tab. 3.1 Therapeutic value of sports disciplines with hip- and knee-joint arthroses (by Zichner and Engelhardt 1997).

Adequate	Conditionally	Inadequate
swimming	golf	tennis
aqua jogging	horse riding	squash
cycling (plain)	jogging	jumping disciplines
bicycle-ergometer training	downhill skiing	ice skating
gymnastics		mountain hiking
hiking (plain)		soccer and other team sports
backcountry skiing		

Start-up and stress pains are a good indication for sports therapy, but movement and rest pains are contra-indications. Arthrosis patients should always focus training on pain-free areas.

Strain has to be significantly reduced if pain and impulse symptoms occur, which are signs of an inadequate stress and capacity. At later stages, systematic rehabilitation training should enhance capacity, while the stabilizing musculature holding the affected joint should be strengthened.

Impulse conditions (activated arthrosis) can be treated with **non-steroidal anti-inflammatory drugs (NSAIDs)** and, if necessary, with **intra-articular injections of steroids**. However, pharmacological treatment cannot rehabilitate an arthritic joint and should focus on pain control.

3.1.4 Sports therapy with arthrosis

Steinau described important aspects of arthrosis sports therapy (Steinau and Suchodoll 1996).

Pain relief together with the positive psychological effects is the most important therapy targets. Group training additionally benefits from pain distraction.

Aqua jogging, **ergometer training** in case of cox arthrosis, and **oscillating movements** with the lower leg in case of gonarthrosis are particularly suitable for movement stimulation. Selective movement exercises stabilize the joint and improve coordination. This reduces joint stress and therefore prevents cartilage abrasion. The spontaneous tonicity change (tonus enhancement of flexor musculature and constraint of extensor musculature) can be improved by movement stimulation.

Systematic training of the cardiovascular system in endurance sports are joint-protecting.

Bradytrophic structures require an extended adaption time and attention to **load dosage**. The loads should preferably not be one-sided and should be about 65% of the maximum strength. Often there is only small window in load dosage. The optimal impulse with bio-positive adjustment and stabilization on a higher level need to be balanced between a too low, performance lowering impulse and a too strong impulse with bio-negative and long-term disturbances.

References

Puhl W (1996). Ätiologie, Pathogenese und Pathochemie der degenerativen Gelenkerkrankungen. In: Zichner L, Engelhardt M, Freiwald J. Sport bei Arthrose und nach endoprothetischem Gelenkersatz. Ciba-Geigy, Wehr.

Steinau M, Suchodoll M (1996). Sporttherapeutische Konzepte bei Arthrose und nach endoprothetischem Gelenkersatz. In: Zichner L, Engelhardt M, Freiwald J. Sport bei Arthrose und nach endoprothetischem Gelenkersatz. Ciba-Geigy, Wehr.

Zichner L, Engelhardt M (1997). Sport und Arthrose. In: Engelhardt M et al. GOTS-Manual Sporttraumatologie. Verlag Hans Huber, Bern: 195–197.

3.2 Sports after endoprothetic treatment

Hubert Hörterer

The endoprothetic treatment of hip, knee, and shoulder joints is a standard procedure in orthopedic surgery today. But increasingly, other joints are treated endoprothetically as well.

Tab. 3.2 Questioning of surgeons about sports and endoprotheses (Hörterer 1985 and 2005).

n = 20	1985	2005
yes	1	17
no	19	3

In the past, analgesia, better flexibility and ability to walk had been the priority, but now often the wish for sporting activity and the continuing of different sports prevails.

Within the last 20 years, the attitude of the surgeons has also considerably changed in favor of the sporting ability (➤ Tab. 3.2).

3.2.1 Influence of sport activity on the prosthesis

Influence of sports intensity and discipline and their impact on the longevity of an endoprothesis are debated vividly in literature. Significant long-term studies haven't been conducted yet (Scholz and v. Salis-Soglio 2002).

Localization of the endoprothesis, different implant types and surgical procedures, and other risk factors complicate interpretation of clinical studies. Different authors see a negative influence of sports load on the implant anchorage and wearing of the tribological pairing (Thompsen et al. 1995, Van den Bogart et al. 1999, Gschwend et al. 2000, Healy et al. 2001).

In recent years, more and more publications report a positive influence of sporting activity on permanent prosthesis-anchorage (Dubs et al. 1983, Widhalm et al. 1990, Hörterer 1991, v. Stempel et al 1992, Jerosch et al. 1995, Engelhardt et al. 1997, Kuster et al. 2000, Scholz and v. Salis-Soglio 2002, Raussen and Zichner 2003, Zentek 2003, Clifford et al. 2005).

Widhalm et al. reported in their hip prosthesis cohort a loosening rate of 57% in non-athletic patients in contrast to 18% in sportingly active patients. Dubs et al. show similar results with 14.3% for non-athletic compared to 1.6% for sportingly active persons; von Stempel shows a loosening of 9.8% and 4.9% respectively. Extremely low loosening rates are reported even for downhill skiing (Hörterer 1991).

Serious stress peaks need to be avoided (Jerosch et al 1995)

> The crucial questions are: Which loads do actually occur in specific sports and what is the effect on the endoprothesis?

There is an **extensive variance** of *in vivo* and *in vitro* studies as well as mathematic models.

Here, assumptions and general experiences are generally used. The *in vivo* results of Bergmann et al. are remarkable (➤ Tab. 3.3; Dubs et al. 1983, Bergmann et al. 2001).

Tab. 3.3 Loads to the hip joint in different activities (Bergmann et al. 1989).

Activity	Strain [SV]
symmetric stand of both legs	0.7
walking	3
jogging 8 km/h	5.5
stumbling	8
lift of the stretched leg	1.6
lowering of the streched leg	2.5

3.2.2 Specific risks

Individual, medical and sport-specific factors need to be balanced (➤ Tab. 3.4).

Tab. 3.4 Factors that have to be considered in sports with endoprotheses.

Individually	Medically	Sport-specifically
■ localization of the prosthesis ■ initial shape of the joint ■ age metabolism ■ pharmaceuticals ■ body weight ■ fitness ■ osteoporosis	■ prosthesis type ■ bones ■ muscles ■ general medical condition	■ fall ■ collision ■ unreasonableness ■ material ■ inappropriate sports ground ■ weather ■ lacking technique

In each sport, dangers are:
- stress peaks and extreme permanence loads
- strong movement amplitudes, abrupt movement changes
- intensive physical contacts, e.g. fall, beat or collision
- excessive intensity of sports activity.

Main risks of sports activity after endoprothetic supply are:
- increased abrasion
- aseptic early loosening
- luxation
- long-term loosening
- prothetic, or rather periprothetic fracture (➢ Fig. 3.1 and ➢ Fig. 3.2).

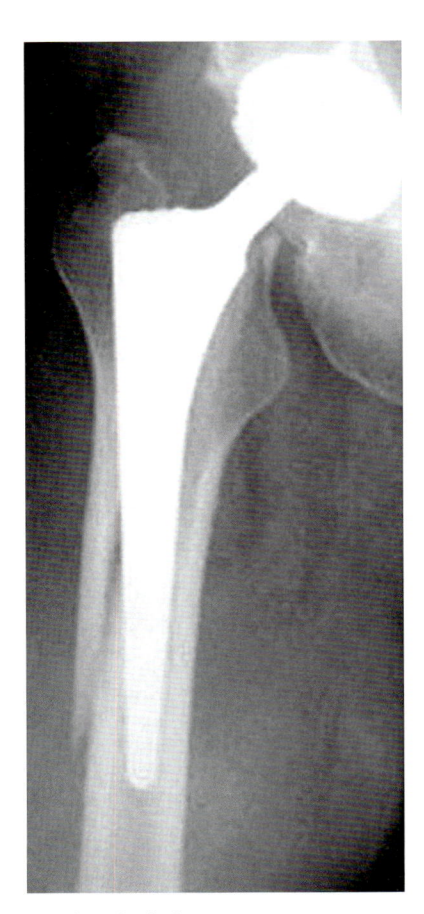

Fig. 3.1 Periprothetic fracture.

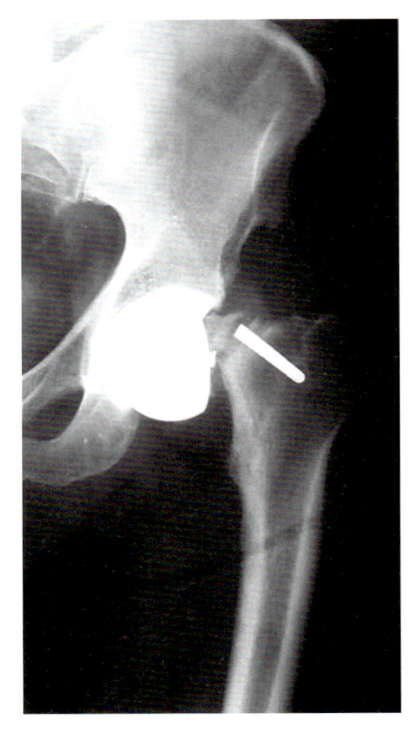

Fig. 3.2 Fracture of a head prosthesis.

3.2.3 Estimation of sports capability

The joint and the endoprothesis itself as well as the individual factors of the patient and sport-specific conditions need to be taken into account if estimating sports capacity. Especially the individual sports and their analogous suitability for the regarding endoprothesis must be considered in addition to contraindications.

Prerequisites

The following prerequisites should be fulfilled:

Joint and endoprothesis
- correct implant anchorage
- osseous integration of the prosthesis
- sufficient joint flexibility
- sufficient ligament stability in knee, shoulder, and ankle
- sufficient muscular stability
- sufficient coordinative abilities.

3.2 Sports after endoprothetic treatment

Individual factors
- normal inflammatory parameters
- no considerable risk factors in general medicine or internal risk factors, such as osteoporosis, metabolic diseases, adiposity, and others
- experiences in the regarding sport.

Sport-specific factors
- no collision stress and uncontrolled movements
- no contact sports
- attention to dangers of falling or collision.

Contra-indications

> Clinically and radiological proven implant loosening, an existing or expected joint infection ban sports.

The following can be considered as contra-indications:
- exchange surgeries
- luxations
- significant leg-length differences
- ligament instabilities
- significant flexibility constraints.

Here, the decision has to be made for each case individually.

3.2.4 Estimation and evaluation of individual sports

The often-used **classification** of sports into adequate, conditionally adequate or inadequate can only present a **rough guideline**. The changeovers are blurred, especially in the conditionally adequate sports. They very much depend on the localization of the prosthesis, of the physician's experiences with the regarding sport, and the rationality of the patient. Geographic aspects also play a role in the estimation of the regarding sport (➤ Tab. 3.5).

3.2.5 Recommendations and advise

> Explaining is better than prohibiting.

Tab. 3.5 Adequacy of different sports for endoprothesis wearers.

Adequate	Conditionally adequate	Inadequate
■ swimming	■ tennis	■ soccer
■ cycling	■ jogging	■ handball
■ rowing	■ golf	■ basketball
■ sailing	■ Cross-country skiing	■ volleyball
■ aqua jogging	■ downhill skiing	■ material arts
■ walking		■ wrestling
■ hiking	■ table tennis	■ high/broad jump
■ gymnastics	■ ninepins/bowling	
	■ equestrianism	

The physician also has to have special sports knowledge in order to advice the patient correctly. It is the physician's task to explain the new situation to the patients and also to slow them in their activities, if necessary. However, one should aim giving back and maintaining fun and joy of the sports activity under the new circumstances. Individual experience and reason used by the patient to perform the sport will probably be determining. The patient must realize that each kind of **serious and competitive sports** is **contraindicated**. The **reintegration** into the according sport is best carried out in a team with a physician, a physiotherapist, trainer or coach, e.g. golf pro, skiing trainers, or others (Hörterer and Kallenbach 1996).

The most intensive individual supervision and security possible is given with a specific technique-tactic-methodology program (➤ Fig. 3.3).

Summary

Sports and endoprothesis can be combined but only in controlled and individually adapted sports activities with consideration of the risk factors.

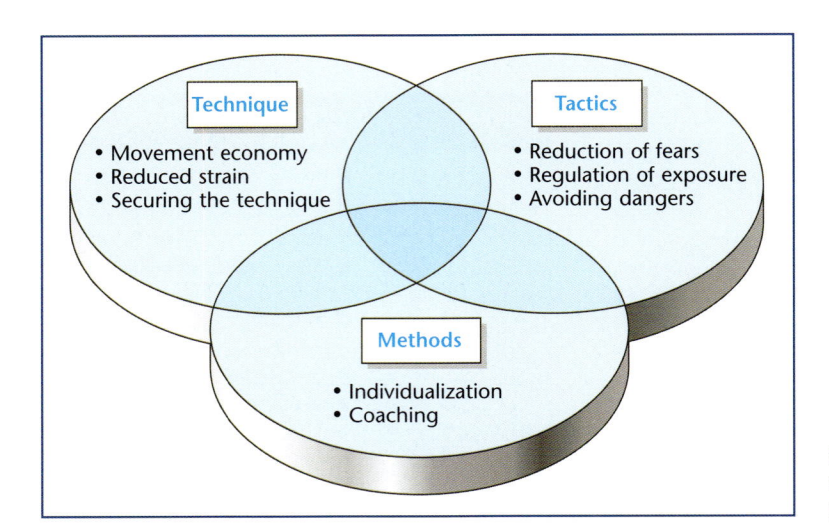

Fig. 3.3 Technique-tactics-methodics program for endoprothesis wearers.

The following picture of a skier with both-sided hip endoprotheses doing heliskiing in Canada shows that exceptions confirm this rule (➤ Fig. 3.4).

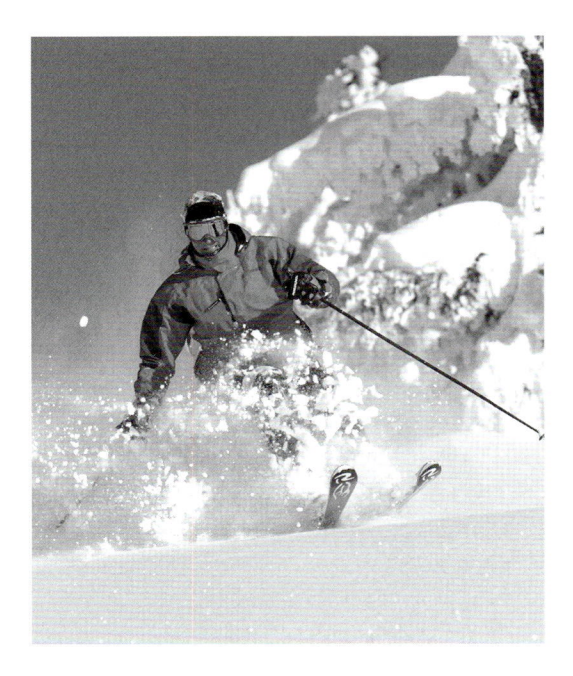

Fig. 3.4 Patient with bilateral hip prothesis (OP right 1996, OP left 1997) at heliskiing in Canada.

References

Bergmann G, Rohlmann A, Graichen F (1989). In-vivo-Messung der Hüftgelenk-Belastung, 1. Teil: Krankengymnastik. Z Orthop 127.

Bergmann G, Deuretzbacher G, Heller M, Graichen F, Rohlmann A, Strauss J, Duda GN (2001). Hip contact forces and gait patterns routine activities. J Biomech 34(7): 859–871.

Van den Bogart AJ, Read L, Nigg BM (1999). An analysis of hip joint loading during walking, running and skiing. Med Sci Sports Exerc 31(1): 13–42.

Clifford PE, William J, Mallon MD (2005). Sports after total joints replacement. Clin Sports Med 2005 (24): 175–186.

Dubs L, Gschwend N, Munzinger U (1983). Sport after total hip arthroplasty. Arch Orthop Trauma Surg 101: 161–169.

Engelhardt M, Hintermann B, Segesser B (1997). Gesellschaft für Orthopädisch-Traumatologische Sportmedizin. GOTS Manual Sporttraumatologie. Verlag Hans Huber, Bern.

Gschwend N, Frei T, Morscher E, Nigg B, Loehr J (2000). Alpine and cross-country horts of 50 patients each, one active, the other inactive in skiing, followed for 5–10 years. Acta Orthop Scand 71(3): 243–249.

Healy WL, Iorio R, Lemos MJ (2001). Athletic activity after joint replacement. Am J Sports Med 29: 377–388.

Hörterer H (1991). Sport und Hüftendoprothetik. Was Ihr Patient wissen muss! TW Sport und Medizin 3: 118–120.

References

Jerosch J, Heisel J, Fuchs S (1995). Sport mit Endoprothese. Was wird empfohlen, was wird erlaubt, was wird verboten? Dtsch Z Sportmed 46: 305–312.

Kuster MS, Spalinger E, Blanksby BA, Gächter A (2000). Endurance sports after total knee replacement: a biochemical investigation. Med Sci Sportd Exerc 32(4): 721–724.

Raussen W, Zichner L (2003). Endoprothese und Sport. Sportorthopädie und Traumatologie 19(3): 207–213.

Scholz R, Freiherr von Salis-Soglio G (2002). Sportfähigkeit nach endoprothetischem Gelenkersatz. Orthopädie 31(4): 423–431.

von Strempel A, Menke W, Wirth CJ (1992). Sportliche Aktivitäten von Patienten mit zementfrei implantiertem Hüftgelenkersatz. Prakt Sport Traum Sportmed 2: 58–64.

Thomsen M, Strachwitz B, Mau H, Cotta H (1995). Werkstoffübersicht in der Hüftendoprothetik. Zeitschrift für Orthopädie 133: 1–6.

Widhalm R, Höfer G, Krugluger J, Bartalsky L (1990). Is there greater danger of sports injury or osteoporosis caused by inactivity in patients with hip prosthesis? Sequelae for long-term stability of prosthesis anchorage. Z Orthop Grenzgeb 128(2): 139–143.

Zentek K (2003). Wer rastet, der rostet! Sport bei Endoprothesenträgern. Orthopaedic Dim, issue 1/2003.

Chapter 4

Medication and anti-doping rules in competitive sports

Sebastian Thormann and Bernd Wolfarth

Chronic illness and competitive sport is in general regarded as a contradiction. However, with proper handling and the improved possibilities for diagnosis and causative treatment of chronic diseases, in many cases an unrestrained physical capacity and therefore the participation in competitive sports is possible. In general, the clinical manifestations of symptoms in chronic diseases such as diabetes mellitus, arterial hypertension and bronchial asthma do not differ between athletes and non-athletic patients. The handling with the disease pattern (clinical picture) and in particular the individual realization of action standards and treatment guidelines poses a specific challenge for the attending physicians, as well as for the concerned athletes.

An extensive capacity checkup, which may be supplemented in particular cases by specific, disease-related aspects, is considered a prerequisite for the permission to participate in competitive sports. The decision-making basis for the sport approval must always involve the exclusion of health disorders caused by the expected, intensive and extensive training. For this purpose, the knowledge of the relationships between performance related training and the respective disease is necessary. In addition, an ideal medical setting has to be carried out, which ensures absolute resolution of symptoms not only at rest but also during exercise. The choice of drugs for the treatment of athletes with reagrds to this must primarily be based on professional principles. After the election of the sufficient drugs needed, it is necessary to reconsider whether agents are registered on the doping list. If this is the case, possible alternatives must be reviewed, and accordingly, if there are no alternative options, a so-called medical certificate of exemption (TUE = Therapeutic Use Exemption) must be applied from the anti-doping-authority, who is responsible for the athlete.

4.1 Arterial hypertension

Hypertension is one of the most common diseases affecting approximately 1 billion people worldwide (1). With progressive age the prevalence of this disease is increasing and is the most common cardiovascular disease in athletes (2).

The diagnosis of arterial hypertension in athletes is the same as for non-athletic persons. Thereby, a unique measurement within the clinical setup should not be taken as diagnostic approach. In this case, repeated outpatient measurements, an exercise test with blood pressure monitoring and eventually a 24-hour-blood-pressure control should be performed (1). At the time of the initial diagnosis an extensive survey of cardiovascular risk factors (family history, lipid metabolism, nicotine abuse, etc.), the exclusion of secondary causes of hypertension (renal artery stenosis, pheochromocytoma, thyroid disease, etc.), and possible endorgan damages must be considered (1; 2).

The treatment should also be conducted under the general principles of antihypertensive therapy. However, frequently in athletes the classical feasibilities of lifestyle modification, such as physical activity enhancement, weight normalization, or optimization of nutrition habits are already exhausted at the time of initial diagnosis.

If the indication for drug treatment is provided, currently ACE inhibitors and accordingly AT1 antagonists or the modern calcium antagonists, are the agents of first choice. If a concomitant use is necessary, these drug classes can be given as a two-combination therapy. If a triple combination is needed a diuretic drug may be added. Because this drug class is recorded on the doping list (http://www.wada-ama.org), a medical exemption would have to be requested. Beta blockers in the antihypertensive therapy of an athlete are classified only as a means of second election.

Especially in the types of sports in which high physical stress plays a significant role, the negative chronotropic effects of beta blockers are counterproductive. In addition, beta blockers as performance-enhancing drugs are listed on the doping list in certain kinds of sports (such as riflery, motorcar sports, etc.) and may only be used on atheletes in these types o sports only after obtaining a medical exemption (3).

Athletes with borderline hypertension or arterial hypertension grade 1 are allowed to participate in competitive sports without limitations (2). However, if a left-ventricular hypertrophy is simultaneously present, a sufficient blood pressure adjustment for intensive exercise (e.g. competition) is a mandatory participation precondition(2). In athletes with higher grades of arterial hypertension (≥ grade 2) exists a contraindication against all static kinds of sports (e.g. weight lifting) at least until a suffient blood pressure control is given. On the condition of an optimal medical setting under regular control physical activity is permitted, in particular, the implementation of traditional life style modifications (e.g. regular endurance training, constant weight) should be noted additionly for static kinds of sports.

4.2 Diabetes mellitus

Globally, diabetes mellitus shows a significant increase in prevalence over the last 10–20 years. This is a result of the increasing physical inactivity and hence the rise in number of overweight individuals, especially in industrialized nations (4; 5). Accordingly, the number of insulin-dependent diabetics is also increasing. In the case of diabetes primarily type I diabetics are seen in competitive sports. The diagnosis of diabetes mellitus in athletes is similar to non-athletic patients. The athletes' pre-participation screening should include an appropriate diabetes screening by fasting glucose measurement and urine stix for detecting glucose and ketones in urine should always be performed, and in case of abnormalities, an oral glucose tolerance test (OGTT) should also be conducted. After the primary diagnosis the main focus is the clarification of any possibly complications in terms of organ damage. For this purpose the cardiovascular risk factors must be reviewed. In addition, a kidney, eye, and neurological examination should be performed.

Given the lack of secondary diseases, there are generally no kinds of sports at which a well-controlled diabetic could not participate. However, in the presence of concomitant diseases the kind of sport should be chosen selectively. In this context, athletes with retinopathy should not exercise e.g. martial arts or weight lifting. Also, patients with diabetic neuropathy should avoid disciplines with the risk of traumatic foot injuries, while those with diabetic nephropathy should not choose activities with a negative impact on blood pressure (6).

Regardless of specific training sessions wihin a sport discipline, the activity recommendation usually consists of at least 2–3 hours endurance training per week, spread into three other sports units (7). Treatment recommendations also target a combination of consistent lifestyle modification and, if necessary, medication. Depending on the type of sport the education and consulting effort for athletic diabetics is high, especially in the initial phase, where there must be a close cooperation between patient, nutrition counsellor and treating physician. In addition to a sufficient basic setting, food supply and medication must be optimized before, during and after exercise. Before initiation of exercise, the blood glucose levels should usually be between 100–200 mg/dl. In case these values are too low, a food supply should be administered followed by a near-time control measurement. In general, the glucose levels decline during exercise so that a regular supply of carbohydrates during exercise is needed. In more complicated cases a regular measurement of load values may be necessary. Especially after long exercise sessions the blood glucose levels should be closely monitored until 24 hours after exposure in order to respond to any fluctuations (6).

If Insulin is used as drug therapy for competitive athletes a medical exemption must be requested. With adequate evidence by diagnostic findings, such exemption is issued for patients with type I diabetes for the duration of their athletic career. Diabetics who are well trained, realize the importance of and consistently maintain lifestyle changes and medication guidelines and who are in an efficient system of self-control and medical supervision by an experienced physician are allowed to participate in sport without restrictions.

4.3 Asthma bronchiale (bronchial asthma)

In competitive sports, asthma bronchiale, exercise-induced asthma and the so-called hyperresponsive bronchial system are among the most common reasons for requesting medical exemptions. The prevalence of exercise-induced asthma in asthmatics is about 90%, for all allergic patients between 30 and 40% and in the general population about 10% (8). In athletes, depending on clinical trial design and type of sport, the prevalence varies widely (8–11). Overall, based on a proportion of about 15–20% of athletes, some deplore continously exercise-induced asthma symptoms (12) while other concerned athletes dependent on external conditions (13). The reported clinical symptoms of athletes vary from typical obstructive respiratory symptoms among submaximal and maximal loads to an irritative cough which can persist after intensive exercise for a longer period of time (14).

Etiologically two main groups attract attention in clinical practice: first, the allergic athletes who are often conspicuous with respiratory problems at an early age and by start of competitive sport activity. Second, there are also experienced older athletes who suddenly develop bronchial hyperreactivity after years of high performance exertion. These athletes often report cumulative broncho-pulmonary infections in their case histories which could play an etiological role for their diagnosis (15; 16).

The diagnosis „asthma bronchiale" can be determined by different examinations. Since the 2002 Olympic Games in Salt Lake City, USA, the International Olympic Committee (IOC) use constantly modified diagnostic targets of an international commission of experts (17; 18). Based on the current version, the decrease of forced exspiratory volume in one second (FEV1) by 10% after specific exercise, or an increase of FEV1 by 12% is sufficient proof of such diangosis. Additionally, the detection of a hyperresponsiveness bronchial system in provocation with methacholine (PD20 < 400 μg) or by EVH test (FEV1 decline > 10%) is accepted as a diagnostic verification. Clinically, in particular allergies, vocal cord dysfunction, side effects of medication, and recurrent infections of the upper and lower respiratory tract should be excluded as differential diagnosis.

Also for athletes, the treatment is according to the guidelines of professional associations and subject to classification of asthma (19). Inhaled corticosteroids such as budesonide are classified as the basic therapy. Depending on clinical symptoms, in mild cases inhaled corticosteroid preparations will be combined with short-acting β2-agonists, which will be taken temporarily 20–30 minutes before exercise. In severe cases, a therapy with a modern combination product of inhaled steroids and long-acting ß2-agonists (e.g. fluticasone/salmeterol) is suitable. Especially in children and adolescent athletes, an anti-inflammatory basic therapy with systemic leukotriene antagonists, such as montelucast, can be administered. In addition to drug therapy, a causal treatment and accordingly the prevention of inducing conditions should be definitely carried out. This includes, for example, desensitization in allergic athletes, avoidance, if possible, of intensive stress during high altitude levels, and the use of a breathing air heater in cold temperatures.

The treatment of asthma in athletes is in due consideration of current anti-doping regulations (20). Although it is considered that the administration of inhaled glucocorticosteroids and β2-agonists show no performance-enhancing effects in lung-healthy athletes (21), some of these drugs are still classified as illegal substances and only certain drugs are approved for the treatment. By the new Prohibited List, effective as of January 1 2011, the inhaled glucocorticosteroids and the two β2-agonists Salbutamol (up to a defined treshold) and Salmeterol are allowed and have only to be indicated on the doping control form in case of a doping control. For other β2-agonists (e.g. Formoterol, Reproterol) the treatment must be requested with a medical exemption. The use of these inhaled ß2-agonists, without exception, is prohibited in and out of competition.

Regardless of the partial complicated requirements for the use of asthma drugs in competitive sports, an optimal therapy and clinical setting should be sought in athletes with clinically verifiable asthma problems(20). With regular clinical monitoring and effective medical treatment no limits for participation in competitive sports exists.

4.4 Intravenous infusions, injections or infiltrations

The Prohibited List of the World Anti-Doping Agency (WADA) is divided into prohibited *methods* and prohibited *substances (http://www.wada-ama.org)*. It is important to understand the various treatments of intravenous infusions and injections in order to adhere to this list and to avoid common mistakes or misunderstanding in treatment in relation to doping controls and regulations.

The Anti-doping regulations make a clear distinction between different intravenous applications and thus it is important to be familiar with the relevant definitions and their formal consequences.

Intravenous infusions are generally prohibited except those legitimately received during hospital admissions or clinical investigations. Only in a few cases, which have to be well documented, infusions are allowed under specific circumstances which include surgery, emergency treatment with resuscitation, blood transfusions in case of substantial blood loss and if medications cannot be given orally due to constant vomiting.

It is important to have a thorough documentation for any medically indicated infusion. The responsible anti-doping authority should be immediately informed about any conducted intravenous infusion as some cases may even require application for a retroactive Therapeutic Use Exemption (TUE). Exercised induced dehydration does not fall under the indications allowing for infusions; however, injections with a single syringe are possible only if the given substance is not forbidden and the total amount applied is below 50 ml.

Infiltrations are permitted so long as the substance being infiltrated is not forbidden

4.5 Orthopedics and trauma

In orthopaedics and traumatology various acute and chronic injuries commonly require treatment which can be given both inside and outside of a clinical setting. The following two treatments should be administered by specialists in specialized clinical surroundings. One modern technique in the treatment of cartilage damage which occurs during sport injuries is the **autologous chondral-/cartilage-cell implantation** (22; 23) which is allowed according to the Prohibited List of the World Anti-Doping Agency and the **PRP = Platelet rich plasma** (24; 25) which is allowed as of January 2011.

4.6 Substances

Analgesics and Glucocorticosteroids (GCS, cortisone)

Treatments given outside of a clinical setting more often refer to substances given orally or by infiltrations. The most often used substances in orthopaedic treatment in sports and sport-related injuries are substances belonging to the group of analgesics (26) and glucocorticosteroids (27).

Regarding Analgesics, non-steroid antirheumatics (NSAR) such as Diclofenac, are allowed when administered topically, orally and also by injection.

Morphine and its derivates are prohibited IN COMPETITION only and require a TUE if their use is deemed necessary. Out of competition they may be administered under careful observation of the respective degradation time.

Local anesthetics are permitted and adrenalin can be administered in addition to local anesthetics but only locally for the treatment of minor injuries.

Apart from analgesics, glucocorticosteroids are the most frequently used substances in the treatment of orthopedic injuries (28). GCS can be added to analgesics and would be permitted when given separately. Generally, the anti-doping rules differentiate between two main methods of administration of GCS: the systemic and the non-systemic application.

Systemic and Non-Systemic Application

A major change in the Prohibited List of WADA, which became effective from January 1, 2011, is the status of **non-systemic** (intra-articular, peri-articular, peri-tendon, epidural, intradermal or inhalativ) **glucocorticosteroids**, which are now permitted and do not require any special declaration of use. Although these non-systemic glucocorticoides are no longer on the Prohibited List, it remains important for athletes who undergo anti-doping testing to mention all treatments while being controlled.

Contrary to the above, all **systemic glucocorticosteroids**, whether administered by oral, intravenous, intramuscular or rectal routes are prohibited In-Competition. If an athlete has been given such treatments they must wait a minimum of seventy-two hours before they may take part at the next competition. However, if an athlete has been given these treatments due to a valid medical reason, the athlete is required to apply for a TUE.

Topical treatments with **glucocorticosteroids** for medical reasons due to problems of the ear, the skin (including iontophoresis/phonophoresis), the gingival, the nose, the eyes and around the anus are permitted. Nevertheless it is essential that athletes who have required such medical treatment clearly state this on the doping control formular.

Glucocorticosteroids, GCS, Cortisone

Systemic applications by oral, rectal, intravenous or intramuscular routes **are prohibited in competition**. If a medical condition necessitates the continuous treatment with systemically administered GCS a Therapeutic Use Exemption is required. This commonly applies to chronic conditions such as Crohn's Disease, Colitis or rheumatic disorders. In case of an emergency treatment with GCS by systemic routes, for example, in case of an allergic shock or for a short extended period out of competition this treatment should be well documented by the attending physician for the prompt notification of the respective anti-doping authority.

Non-systemic applications of GCS (infiltrations intra-articular, peri-articular, peri-tendon, epidural, intradermal or inhalativ) can be administered but should be declared and registered on the doping control form at a sample collection session. This also applies to **topical applications** of GCS such as dermal, nasal, buccal, ophthalmic, otologic or gingival.

It is generally important to name any treatment with GCS at a doping control.

Skeletal muscle relaxants like substances belonging to the group of benzodiazepines are permitted when administered orally.

Growth hormones or growth factors are prohibited at all times, that is in and out of competition.

4.7 TUE – the medical exemption

On examination of the statistics of the National Anti Doping Agency of Germany (NADA) for the year 2010, a total of 4,168 therapeutic use expemptions were issued in Germany alone, of which 272 applications in the context of chronic diseases (e.g. diabetes mellitus, arterial hypertension) were submitted as so-called TUE`s (therapeutic use exemptions). 3,574 so called Declaration of Use (DoUs), formerly ATUEs (abbreviated therapeutic use exemptions), have been submitted for approval or registration on the inhalative use of beta-2-

agonists or inhaled glucocorticosteroids as well as for non-systemic applications of cortisone. Collateral to conventional medical exemptions, 322 certificates of emergency treatments, the administration of infusions and other documents were counted (http://www.nada-bonn.de).

Most of these therapeutic use exemptions were found for diabetics (insulin), patients with arterial hypertension (diuretics/beta blocker), systemic rheumatic/immunologic diseases (systemic steroid dose) or adolescents with ADHD (attention deficit hyperactivity disorder-methyphenidat). For this purpose a comprehensive submission of medical documentations is necessary. The documents are reviewed in accordance with the International Standard for TUE 2010 (WADA) by a multi-member medical panel of anti doping authorities. At least three expert opinions are needed to make a conclusive decision regarding the approval or rejection of the request (http://www.wada-ama.org). With a positive appraisal by the expert advisory board an exemption is most often granted for a period of twelve months, with the possibility of an extension. After this period a re-application is necessary.

4.8 Consequences for clinical practice

The increased demands of anti-doping regulations pose a growing challenge for athletes and in particular for physicians in high performance sports. Although it is the responsibility of the athlete to inform the anti-doping committee of all substances used by the athlete, this burden is usually transmitted to the supervising physician. Therefore, it is essential to become familiar with current anti doping regulations and to ensure that these regulartions are being implemented. Information regarding these regulations, including the latest updates and appropriate procedures can be found on the website of the anti doping authorities (e.g. www.wada-ama.org).

According to the International Standard for Testing, § 7.4.5 (n) medications and supplements taken shall be declared at sample collection sessions by the athlete.

Irrespective of these requirements, just as the wellbeing and health of the athlete remains the underlying factor for success within competitive sports, these same factors including the medical treatment of the athlete represents the underlying responsibility of the physician in clinical practice. Therefore, the priority should always be to treat the athlete/patient with the most appropriate medical solution available. If this is in contradiction with the current anti-doping rules and a medical exemption is not granted at the given time, the optimal/guideline treatment should be given and the athlete may need to be temporarily or permanently withdrawn from competitive sports.

References

(1) Chobanian AV, Bakris GL, Black HR, Cushman WC, Green LA, Izzo JL, Jr., Jones DW, Materson BJ, Oparil S, Wright JT, Jr., Roccella EJ. The Seventh Report of the Joint National Committee on Prevention, Detection, Evaluation, and Treatment of High Blood Pressure: the JNC 7 report. JAMA 2003 May 21; 289(19): 2560–2572.

(2) Maron BJ, Zipes DP. Introduction: eligibility recommendations for competitive athletes with cardiovascular abnormalities-general considerations. J Am Coll Cardiol 2005 April 19; 45(8): 1318–1321.

(3) Vanhees L, Defoor JG, Schepers D, Lijnen P, Peeters BY, Lacante PH, Fagard RH. Effect of bisoprolol and atenolol on endurance exercise capacity in healthy men. J Hypertens 2000 January; 18(1): 35–43.

(4) Koenigsberg MR, Bartlett D, Cramer JS. Facilitating treatment adherence with lifestyle changes in diabetes. Am Fam Physician 2004 January 15; 69(2): 309–316.

(5) Mokdad AH, Bowman BA, Ford ES, Vinicor F, Marks JS, Koplan JP. The continuing epidemics of obesity and diabetes in the United States. JAMA 2001 September 12; 286(10): 1195–1200.

(6) Ting JH, Wallis DH. Medical management of the athlete: evaluation and treatment of important issues in sports medicine. Clin Podiatr Med Surg 2007 April; 24(2): 127–158.

(7) Standards of medical care in diabetes – 2006. Diabetes Care 2006 January; 29 Suppl 1: S4–S42.

(8) Parsons JP, Mastronarde JG. Exercise-induced bronchoconstriction in athletes. Chest 2005 December; 128(6): 3966–3974.

References

(9) Ahad A, Sandila MP, Siddiqui NA. Prevalence of exercise-induced bronchospasm in national hockey players of Pakistan. J Pak Med Assoc 2004 February; 54(2): 96–99.

(10) Farooque SP, Lee TH. Exercise-induced asthma: a review. Practitioner 2003 April; 247(1645): 279–285, 288.

(11) Turcotte H, Langdeau JB, Bowie DM, Boulet LP. Are questionnaires on respiratory symptoms reliable predictors of airway hyperresponsiveness in athletes and sedentary subjects? J Asthma 2003 February; 40(1): 71–80.

(12) Langdeau JB, Boulet LP. Is asthma over- or under-diagnosed in athletes? Respir Med 2003 February; 97(2): 109–114.

(13) Hermansen CL. Exercise-induced bronchospasm vs. exercise-induced asthma. Am Fam Physician 2004 February 15; 69(4): 808.

(14) Sinha T, David AK. Recognition and management of exercise-induced bronchospasm. Am Fam Physician 2003 February 15; 67(4): 769–774, 675.

(15) Sue-Chu M, Karjalainen EM, Altraja A, Laitinen A, Laitinen LA, Naess AB, Larsson L, Bjermer L. Lymphoid aggregates in endobronchial biopsies from young elite cross-country skiers. Am J Respir Crit Care Med 1998 August; 158(2): 597–601.

(16) Karjalainen EM, Laitinen A, Sue-Chu M, Altraja A, Bjermer L, Laitinen LA. Evidence of airway inflammation and remodeling in ski athletes with and without bronchial hyperresponsiveness to methacholine. Am J Respir Crit Care Med 2000 June; 161(6): 2086–2091.

(17) Anderson SD, Argyros GJ, Magnussen H, Holzer K. Provocation by eucapnic voluntary hyperpnoea to identify exercise induced bronchoconstriction. Br J Sports Med 2001 October; 35(5): 344–37.

(18) Anderson SD, Fitch K, Perry CP, Sue-Chu M, Crapo R, McKenzie D, Magnussen H. Responses to bronchial challenge submitted for approval to use inhaled beta2-agonists before an event at the 2002 Winter Olympics. J Allergy Clin Immunol 2003 January; 111(1): 45–50.

(19) National Asthma Education and Prevention Program. Expert Panel Report: Guidelines for the Diagnosis and Management of Asthma Update on Selected Topics – 2002. J Allergy Clin Immunol 2002 November; 110(5 Suppl): S141–S219.

(20) Weiler JM, Malloy C. Asthma and athletes: therapy to compete. Clin Rev Allergy Immunol 2005 October; 29(2): 139–149.

(21) Wolfarth B, Wuestenfeld JC, Kindermann W. Ergogenic effects of inhaled beta2-agonists in non-asthmatic athletes. Endocrinol Metab Clin North Am 2010 March; 39(1): 75–87, ix.

(22) Harris JD, Brophy RH, Siston RA, Flanigan DC. Treatment of chondral defects in the athlete's knee. Arthroscopy 2010 June; 26(6): 841–852.

(23) Komarek J, Valis P, Repko M, Chaloupka R, Krbec M. [Treatment of deep cartilage defects of the knee with autologous chondrocyte transplantation: long-term results]. Acta Chir Orthop Traumatol Cech 2010 August; 77(4): 291–295.

(24) Paoloni J, De Vos RJ, Hamilton B, Murrell GA, Orchard J. Platelet-rich plasma treatment for ligament and tendon injuries. Clin J Sport Med 2011 January; 21(1): 37–45.

(25) Mei-Dan O, Lippi G, Sanchez M, Andia I, Maffulli N. Autologous platelet-rich plasma: a revolution in soft tissue sports injury management? Phys Sportsmed 2010 December; 38(4): 127–135.

(26) Feucht CL, Patel DR. Analgesics and anti-inflammatory medications in sports: use and abuse. Pediatr Clin North Am 2010 June; 57(3): 751–774.

Chapter 5 Disabled sports
Markus Zimmer

Loss of function, disability-friendly sport, and adequate medical care are central to sports for the disabled.

In 1944, Sir Ludwig Guttmann set paraplegic patients into wheelchairs and motivated them to perform sports, such as archery, wheelchair polo, or even wheelchair basketball.

At the same time, veterans performed sports again and motivated their comrades to so-called "sport for the disabled". Parallel to wheelchair sports, today's disabled sports was born.

The question of "Who can perform which sport to which extent?" is the central topic of sports medicine in disabled sports, and it requires not only knowledge of the sport but also knowledge of the disability and care. The athlete will quickly find out whether the physician has access to the area in which the disabled is his own expert.

5.1 Definition and classification

> Every functional disorder restricts sports to the limitations set by the disability, which may apply to physiology, intellect and psychology.

Today, the negative connotation of "damage" has been replaced by **loss of function or residual function**, respectively, which clearly refers to the sport-specific function. ➤ Table 5.1 exemplarily classifies diagnoses of essential functions; this demonstrates that most diagnoses lead to simultaneous loss of several functions.

At a first glance, limitations of motor function seem to be relevant for the orthopedists only. But the complete spectrum of sport-specific orthopedic problems will also impact on people with non-orthopedic functional limitations in sports-medical care.

Functional disorders of the locomotor organs, caused by a motor disability, are:

- loss or dysplasia of limbs
- contractures or joint instabilities
- coordination disorder or paralysis
- muscular atrophy.

Athletes will be assigned to so-called starting groups, which will ensure a comparable functional performance, in order to achieve a fair competition. This classification is an important criterion of disabled sports, which is typically sport-specific.

Irrespective of diagnoses, functional loss is important for the understanding of disabled sports. While the height of a paraplegic fracture does indicate loss of function, the neurological height will be a better descriptor of the functional loss. But the spectrum of functional loss at the same neurological level is very broad even in today's incomplete paralysis. Also disabilities that appear obvious at first, such as amputations of the thigh, vary in residual function. Not only the length of the stump, but also the muscular covering of the stump, biomechanics, scaring and sensibility will influence function significantly.

> Disability is unique to every person and is the basis for any sport potential, risk assessment and therapy. The individual advice must not be limited to orthopedic evaluation only. The whole personality needs consideration with all positive effects of sports including psychologically.

Tab. 5.1 Grouping of disabilities based on functional disorders.

Limitation of function	Mental, psychic	Sensoric	Motor (incl. strength, flexihibility, coordination)	Metabolic, cardiopulmonary
Diagnosis (selection)	Down syndrome mental retardation cerebral palsy condition after breast cancer asthma	Visual impairment blindness deafness cerebral palsy cross-section	Amputations dysmelia cross-section cerebral palsy poliomyelitis	Chron. polyarthritis coronary heart disease asthma diabetes osteoporosis

5.2 Sports for disabled persons

It is key to establish the danger of overload or other damages if structures with lower functionality are taking over full sports function. Based on these considerations, the definition of "disability-friendly sports" has been established (Zimmer 1998). The following updated definition is the basis of today's sports medicine for disabled persons.

> A sport is disability-friendly, if
> - the specific movement sequences will be adapted to the residual function and psychology
> - the residual functions will be strengthened and compensating movements will be trained
> - the risk of injuries will be sport-specifically normal, and it will not be immensely increased by the disability, and an enhancement of the disability will be improbable.

In orthopedics, the **interplay of performance capacity and load** is central and can easily be extended to internal medicine and psychology.
Wolff's law and its extension from the bone to locomotor structures is the foundation of these considerations. The first point represents the danger overload, and the second point represents the problem of too little load, which is often underestimated in the case of disabled persons. If a load is physiological for the structures of the locomotor organs (➢ Tab. 5.2) will only depend on the training condition of the structure.

Tab. 5.2 Physiologic load of the structures of the locomotor organs.

Structure	Load
Bones	Pressure suitable for the axes
Tendons and ligaments	Traction, suitable for the axes in the insertion
Muscles	Innervations adjusted to the load counter draw, adjusted to maximum strength
Cartilages, joints	Rhythmic stress and relief with use of the excursion
Movement segment, movement chain	Appropriate stress

> The physiological conditions require intense survey by the attending orthopedist for each individual disabled person. Then the optimization of ortheses, sports equipment and movement sequences will be carried out in close agreement with coaches and orthopedists.

For example, an female track-and-field athlete with of tendopathy insertion of the Achilles tendon in Athens 2004 complained about increasing pain increased in the insertion area of the Achilles tendon after training with a new orthesis. The examination indicated overextension of the foot by a few degrees in orthograde "knee position". The two matches demonstrate the angle posture that required change in the orthesis (➢ Fig. 5.1 and ➢ 5.2). After adjusting the angle, pain-free, full sports performance was possible again after a short time.

5.2 Sports for disabled persons

Fig. 5.1 Track-and-field sport-orthesis of the right leg at the condition after rotation plasty.

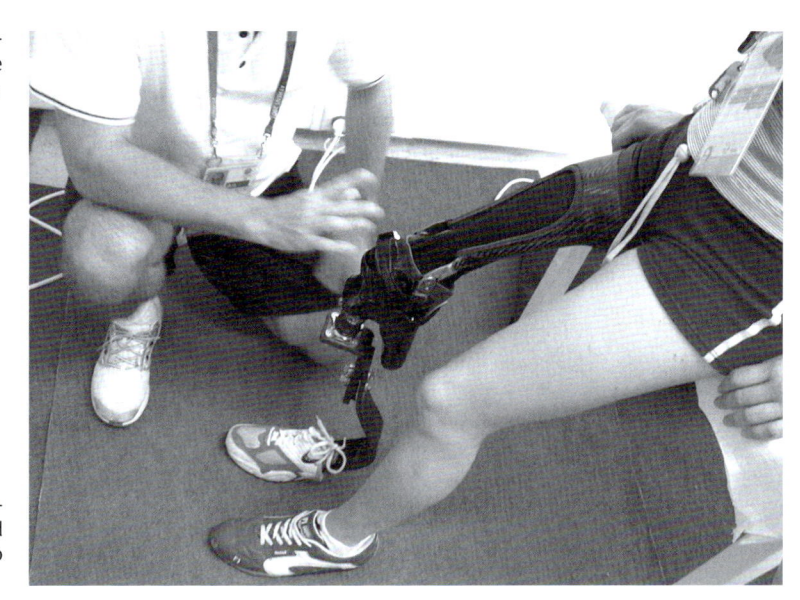

Fig. 5.2 Reduction of the extension of the track-and-field sport-orthesis; shown by two wedged-in matches.

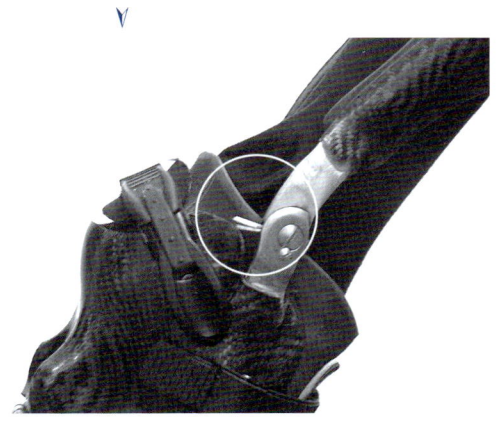

The relationship between load, load capacity, and time course are depicted in ➤ Figure 5.3. This applies to individual structures and the complete movement. At start, reduction of the motor capacity is unavoidable, if motor load is suddenly reduced due to disability or injury, performance of other disabled sports will be affected. The performance will only enhance again with continuous physiologic load increase (recreational period). Only if frequency and degree of load peaks exceeding the capacity will reach a certain level, overuse damages or even injuries occur.

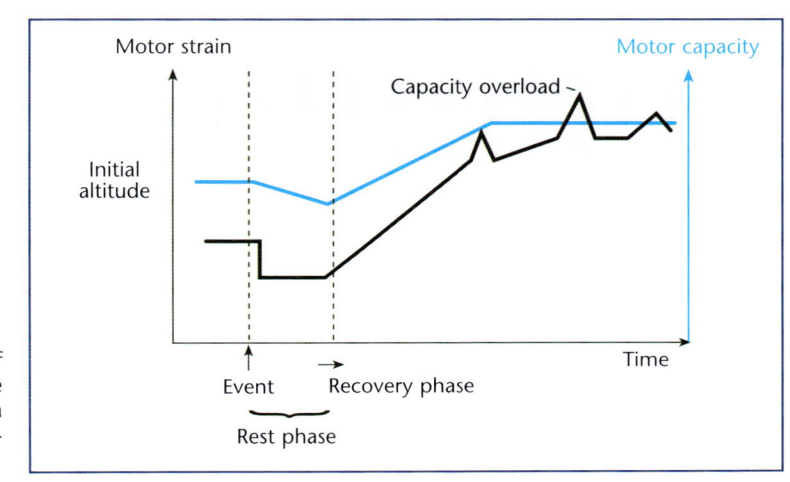

Fig. 5.3 Theoretic scheme of connections between exposure (black) and ability (blue) in a structure or chain of movements.

> Sport is always evaluated as "disability-friendly" or "disability-unfriendly" with regards to functional loss.

Therefore, football tennis, for example, a sport being played analogously to tennis rules but by using the feet, is obviously a sport for persons with disorder of the arm function or arm loss. The load for the lower extremity is as normal and physiologic as soccer. The residual functions, as e.g. balance and coordination, will be trained perfectly. In contrast, a person with amputated lower leg playing football tennis will also train his residual function, but will partially stress the prosthesis unphysiologically.

The large spectrum of available sports and assistive equipment offers the chance for everybody to find the sporting activity appropriate to the residual function (Weber et al. 2001).

Eventually, no generally valid assertion can be made about the evaluation of a sport with regard to a certain kind of disability. The assertion will always be individual and will refer to the individual person, and it should not only involve the motor conditions but also the psychosocial environment and the corresponding geographical range of available sports.

5.3 Injuries and overload

The patterns of injuries and overuse are comparable to non-disabled sports and disability-specific problems can be added.

Typical injury patterns can be transferred to disabled sports (Ferrara and Peterson 2000). Therefore, injuries of the upper ankle joint dominate with 47% in addition to finger injuries with 14% in basketball (Klein 1998). On the other hand, an injury of the lower extremity is not sport-specific in wheelchair basketball due to the disability, but disability-specific injuries will be fractures of the osteoporotic tubular bones at a fall out of the wheelchair. This rather rare incident is easily overlooked, if it is pain-free in line with the paraplegia.

Some typical disability-specific problems are listed in ➤ Table 5.3 as examples that will be important for the treating sport physician.

Tab. 5.3 Disability-specific complications and problems of some disability kinds (selection).

Disability	Typical problems
Amputation	Muscular dysbalance
Dysmelia	Posture asymmetries
Peripheral paresis	Atrophy and local inactivity osteoporosis Gait and other coordination disorders
Paraplegia	Deficient seat control (depending on the lesion zones) Pressure ulcera Contractures Inactivity osteoporosis Infection of the genitourinary tract Vegetative disorders
Cerebral palsy	Insertion tendopathies Contractures
Visual impairment, blindness	increased danger of falls and contusions
Mental retardation	Disturbed orientation
Poliomyelitis	Contractures

5.4 Competitive sports for people with disabilities

Since 1992 in Barcelona, all treated cases during winter and summer Paralympics have been documented consequently.

In ➤ Table 5.4, the increased size of this exceptional international event will be visible. The pressure to perform, the professionalism of the disabled sports, and therefore also the stress for the individual athletes have increased competitors.

> Up today, the stress of persons with disabilities in high-performance sports is pushing the "residual function" to a limit.

Treated cases in Athens 2004 by the medical German medical team added up to 249 primary consultations and 783 drug prescriptions/handouts. 13 guests and 44 attendants were affected in addition to 192 athletes (of 210) of the 249 treated cases (primary consul-

5.4 Competitive sports for people with disabilities

tation with a new disease). The only fracture occurred in a female athlete. One athlete was hospitalized with an infectious disease. 50% were general and internal medicine cases, which indicates a less sport-specific but more climate and environment related problem (➢ Fig. 5.4). Orthopedics was underrepresented with only one third of the cases. The locomotor organs still prevailed in Barcelona and Atlanta (➢ Fig. 5.5). Two eye contusions occurred for the first time in ball sports in Athens. The rest of the cases can be assigned to disability-specific problems, such as decubiti with paraplegia patients or prosthesis wearers.

The essential assertion is demonstrated by ➢ Figure 5.6. It had been defined for all primary contacts whether or not the affected person was handicapped in training and competition capacities. The sporting capacity had been completely withdrawn temporarily only in the fever case. Similar examinations in US American athletes resulted in a normal measure of sports injuries with disabled athletes (Ferrara et al. 2000).

The predominant number of athletes only made use of the medical help for problems not resulting from the exertion of sports, but would possibly limit the maximum performance. The level of sports injuries was normal.

In the overview of the spreading to the individual Paralympics sports, basketball, track and field athletics and cycling stand out with high numbers (➢ Fig. 5.7). Many different factors,

Tab. 5.4 Static data of the summer Paralympics.

	Atlanta 1996	Sydney 2000	Athens 2004
Athletes	3,310	3,838	3,969
Countries	103	125	136
Sports	16	18	19
Attendants	97	113	116
Key: attendants per athlete	0.41	0.45	0.58

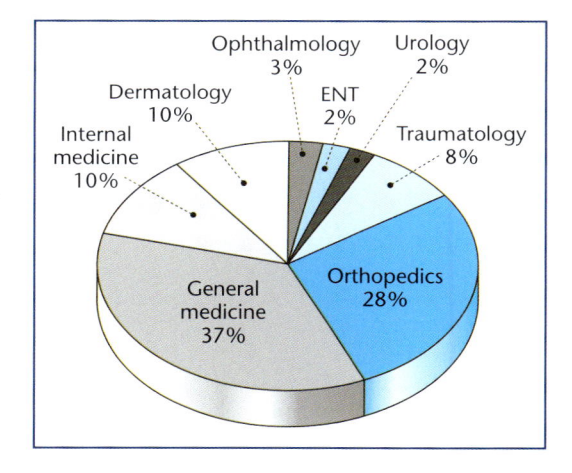

Fig. 5.4 Percental splitting of the 249 first contacts according to medical special subject (Paralympics in Athens, 2004).

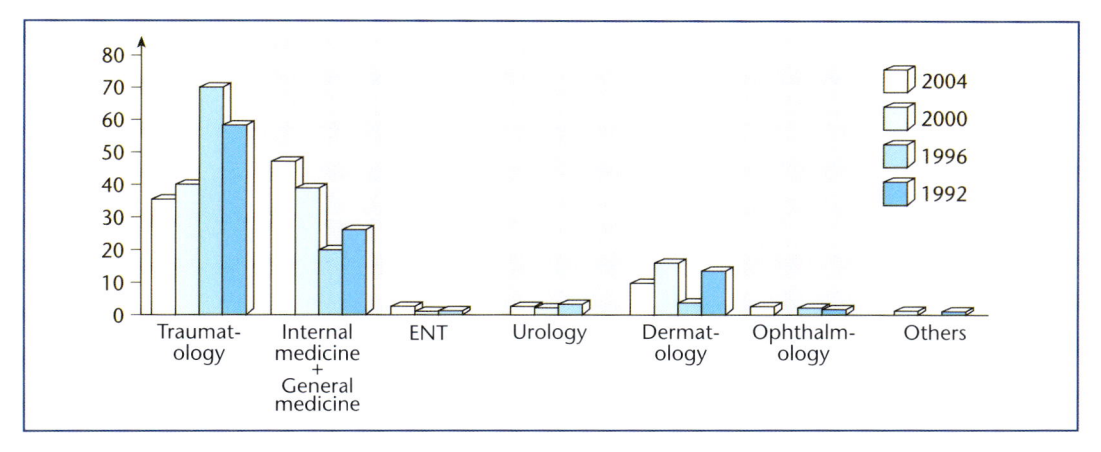

Fig. 5.5 Order of treated cases according to medical special subject, itemized for the German team at the Paralympics in Barcelona in 1992, Atlanta 1996, Sidney 2000, and Athens 2004.

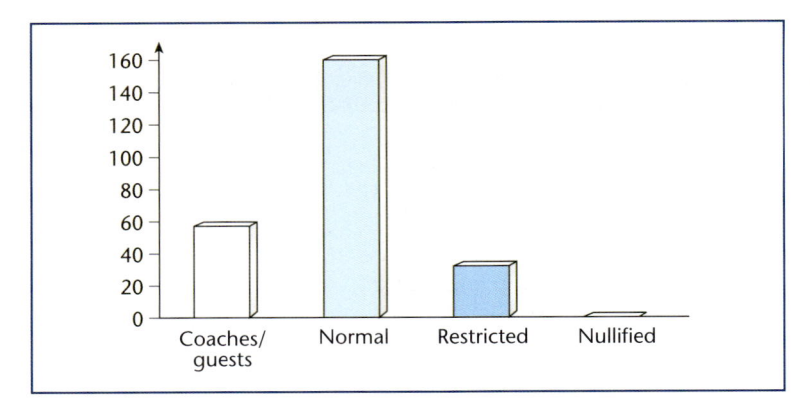

Fig. 5.6 Classification of treated cases (n = 249) in terms of normal, limited and nullified sport capacity of the athlete (Athens 2004).

which have also been clearly different for the four Paralympics Games, are effective, in addition to the number of members of each team. No significant trend could be found. The accumulation of diseases with gastrointestinal infection in a team had clearly been advanced by the spatial closeness of the accommodation of the team, 192 treated cases in 210 athletes and 82% of them without limitation of sporting capacity have clearly demonstrated that sport for persons with disabilities does not often lead to medical problems even at maximum load. In Athens, 23 accidents were documented including one midfoot fracture. Ten of those had occurred during training, nine had occurred during competition.

> High-performance disability sport is not combined with an increased number of medical problems.

5.5 Conclusion

In summary, no significant traumatic or orthopedic diseases occurred in high-performance disability sports.

Currently, the risk comparison with non-disabled sports is not possible given the lack of cohort studies. Moreover, evaluation of disabled sports needs to consider the psychosocial envi-

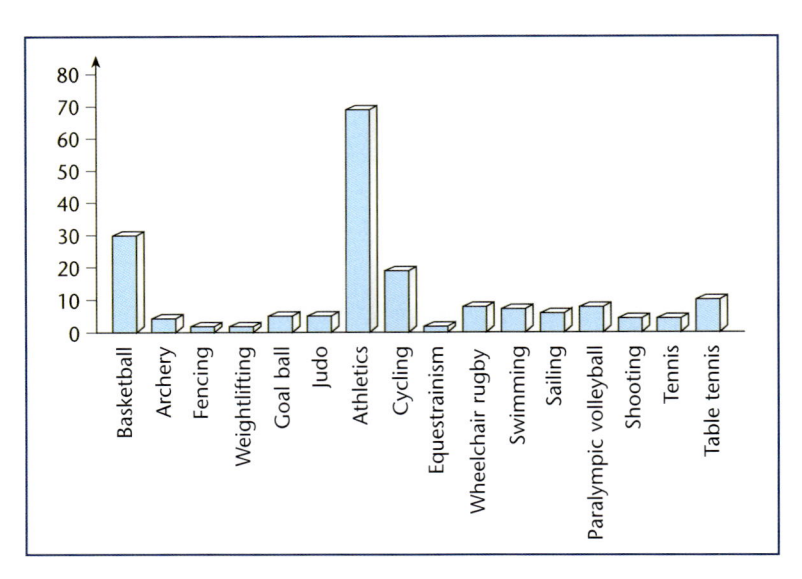

Fig. 5.7 Absolute number of medical first-contacts in each sport.

ronment, for which also no scientific results have been available yet. Only case reports are available. The strengthening of self-confidence and the overcoming of social isolation are key in leisure as in competitive sports.

Every doctor should encourage and motivate sports of persons with any kind of disability. Medical consultation should focus on individual loss of function, sport-specific stress and disability- and sport-specific risks.

> Disabled sports offer the possibility to every person – independent of their loss of function – use of their residual functions and to hold ground in a psychosocial environment. Risks are manageable with medical support. Persons with disabilities need to estimate the risks and evaluate them personally.

References

Ferrara MS, Palutsis GR, Snouse S, Davis RW (2000). A longitudinal study of injuries to athletes with disabilities. Sports Med 2000 21: 221–224.

Ferrara MS, Peterson CL (2000). Injuries to athletes with disabilities. Sports Med 30(2): 137–143.

Webster CB, Levy CE, Bryant PB, Prusakowski PE (2001). Sports and recreation for persons with limb deficiency. Arch Phys Med Rehabil 82: 38–44.

Klein J (1998). Basketball. In: Klümper A (ed.). Sporttraumatologie. Handbuch der Sportarten und ihrer typischen Verletzungen. Ecomed-Verlag, II-3, 1–12.

Zimmer M (1998). Behindertensport. In: Klümper A (ed.). Sporttraumatologie. Handbuch der Sportarten und ihrer typischen Verletzungen. Ecomed-Verlag, II-6, 1–24.

II Diagnostic procedures

6	**Clinical and functional examination**	49
6.1	Anamnesis	49
6.2	Examination	49
7	**Sonography**	55
7.1	Shoulder	56
7.2	Elbow	60
7.3	Hand	61
7.4	Hip joint	63
7.5	Thigh and lower leg musculature	64
7.6	Knee joint	65
7.7	Foot	67
8	**Projection radiography, magnetic resonance and computer tomography**	71
8.1	Sports medical demands	71
8.2	Tendons and muscles	76
8.3	Neurons	78
8.4	Bones	80
8.5	Spine	80
8.6	Shoulder	83
8.7	Elbow	85
8.8	Hand	87
8.9	Hip and groin	89
8.10	Knee	91
8.11	Foot	92
9	**Arthroscopy**	97
9.1	Equipment	97
9.2	Indications and contraindications	100
9.3	Pre-operative preparations	101
9.4	Technique	102
10	**Clinical biomechanics**	115
10.1	Use of clinical biomechanics	115
10.2	Measuring methods and application of selected biomechanical procedures	115

11	**Gait and treadmill analysis**	125
11.1	Introduction	125
11.2	Definitions	125
11.3	Walking on the treadmill vs. gait on a walkway	126
11.4	Observing gait and treadmill analysis	126
11.5	Instrumental gait and treadmill analysis	127
11.6	Kinematic gait and treadmill analysis	127
11.7	Kinetic gait and treadmill analysis	130
11.8	Electromyography	134
11.9	Standardization vs. individualization	135
11.10	Means and limits of gait and treadmill analysis – summary	136

Chapter 6 Clinical and functional examination

Andreas Kugler

6.1 Anamnesis

The following aspects should be part of the anamnesis:
- Exact **circumstances** and **time** of the first occurrence of the complaints, or of the accident, respectively: e.g. warm-up/warm-down, throw/defense, acceleration/landing, fall on outstretched/flexed arm
- **Localization** of complaints
- Characteristics of the complaint or pain, respectively
  - Subjective description, e.g. "The elbow suddenly blocks", "My knee goes away", "The complaints within the knee occur only when running on uneven grounds"
  - Spreading of the complaints (where?)
  - Possibility of triggering or provoking complaints (by what?), e.g. cold/warmth, high rotation in throwing
- **Avoidance strategies** such as evasion movements, tape
- Is this a **primary** or **repeated injury**
- Whether **surgeries** have already been applied (including time, surgeon and intervention)
- Which **diagnoses** have been carried out, so far.

> The better the anamnesis, the better the first preliminary diagnosis.

6.2 Examination

> A standardized clinical examination helps not to miss any pathology.

The following should be considered if examining affected body areas:
- Redness, hyperthermias, swellings, inflammation
- Bruises, hematomas, abrasions, open injuries
- Atrophies, obvious muscle defects
- Malpositions, relieving postures
- (Surgical) scars.

Inspection, **palpation**, and final examination conclude with **functional and diagnostic tests**. Neighboring structures or joints often need to be included in the examination, e.g. the hip for knee complaints, or the cervical spine for shoulder complaints.

6.2.1 Foot, upper ankle and lower leg

Position of the hind foot (valgus/varus) and constitution of the arches (weak foot, hollow foot, spread foot) are part of foot examination. Swellings will point to acute injuries or thrombosis, ruptured Baker cyst of the calf or lower leg. Relevant points of forefoot, mid foot and hind foot, upper ankle joint and lower leg are palpated (➤ Tab. 6.1) with regard to anamnesis and initial examination findings. Points of pain require special attention.

Functional assessment depends on the initial diagnosis and should only be carried out after imaging (e.g. supposed Weber A fracture – no test of ligament stability before radiography).

Tab. 6.1 Palpation points at foot, upper ankle and lower leg with possible tentative diagnoses for pain symptoms and signs.

metatarsal head I metatarsophalangeal joint I	hallux valgus, hallux rigidus, sesamoid-bone fracture/inflammation
metatarsal head II–V	metatarsalgia osteonecrosis
metatarsal diaphysis II, III, IV	stress fracture, fracture
metatarsal V-base	avulsion fracture of the base (peroneus brevis muscle)
os navicular appendage of tibialis posterior muscle	activated os navicular bipartitum tendinitis (e.g. by toeing in)
Bifurcatum ligament	ligament rupture osseous tear
lateral ligament apparatus/distal fibula (LFTA, LFC, LFTP)	ligament rupture Weber A fracture
medial ligament apparatus	ligament rupture, fracture if the inner ankle
ventral joint cavity of the upper ankle joint	impingement OD effusion
distal fibula epiphysis	Injuries of the epiphysis in children
peroneal tendon groove	peroneal tendon luxation
Achilles tendon	rupture bursitis Haglund's exostosis
insertion of calcaneal plantar fascia	plantar fasciitis
syndesmosis	rupture of the syndesmosis
proximal fibula	fibula fracture, maisonneuve fracture blockage of the fibula head
tibial leading edge	tibialis anterior syndrome stress fracture

LFTA = lig. fibulotibiale anterius, LFTP = lig. fibulotibiale posterius, LFC = lig. fibulocalcaneare, OD = osteochondrosis dissecans

The **active and passive movement of individual joints** is compared left to right and to regular values. Depending on initial diagnosis, squeeze or Thompson test talar shift, lateral lift-off or luxation of the peroneal tendon is carried out (➢ Tab. 6.2).

Tab. 6.2 Selection of functional and diagnostic tests of foot, upper ankle and lower leg with according tentative diagnoses.

sqeeze test	injuries of the syndesmosis
talus prolapse	ligament instability (LFTA)
lateral lift-off	ligament instability (LCF)
possibility of luxation of the peroneal tendon	luxation of the peroneal tendon
Thompson's test	rupture of the Achilles tendon

LTFA = lig. talofibulare anterius, LCF = lig. calcaneofibulare

In the squeeze test, the hanging shank is squeezed one hand below the knee joint. Pain in the anterior syndesmosis or the distal membrane interossea indicates syndesmosis injury.

In the **Thompson test**, a plantar flexion triggered by the ventral compression of the calf musculature will indicate (impaired) functionality of the Achilles tendon.

The lateral **ligament stability** will be right-left compared in a lying patient. Shifting the shank dorsally to the talus tests the stability of the ligament talofibulare anterius. Stability of ligament calcaneofibulare is tested overturning the talus with fixed calcaneus.

The gait pattern and foot rolling need to be equally considered.

6.2.2 Knee

Analysis of the standing leg axis, Q angle, muscle atrophies, swellings, spontaneous posterior 90° drawer movement complete the general **examination** of the knee.

Intraarticular effusions (dancing patella) and swelling are differentiated by **palpation**. Soft-tissue swellings indicate bursitides (b. praepatellaris, b. infrapatellaris), Osgood-Schlatter disease, patellar tendinitis or more extensive meniscus ganglia. Diffuse soft-tissue swellings are distinctive of traumas such as tibia head fractures, patellar fractures, complex capsule-ligament injuries.

Relevant palpation points of the knee joint are indicated in ➢ Tab. 6.3. Some of these points yield a quick diagnosis. Pressure pain at the

6.2 Examination

Tab. 6.3 Palpation points of the knee joint.

medial joint cavity
lateral joint cavity
medial parapatellar area
tuberositas tibiae
insertion of internal ligament proximal
insertion of internal ligament distal
external ligament in progression
fibula head
tuberculum Gerdy
lateral retinaculum
lateral patellar facet
pes anserinus
biceps tendon
patellar top
tractus iliotibialis

Tab. 6.4 Selection of functional and diagnostic tests with suspected meniscal lesions.

hyperextension pain
pressure pain at medial and/or lateral joint cavity
Steinmann I and Steinmann II
McMurray sign
Apley sign
Payr's sign
Boehler's meniscus sign

proximal insertion of the patellar ligament indicates a patellar top syndrome and pressure pain at tractus iliotibialis above the lateral femoral condyle an iliotibial band syndrome.

After **testing the active and passive mobility in left-right comparison**, the thigh **muscle tonus** – especially of the m. vastus medialis – is determined.

Thereafter, special meniscus examinations and ligament diagnostics complete analysis of the femoropatellar joint.

Several are of value in **meniscus diagnoses** (➤ Tab. 6.4). In each case, the basis of these tests is to expose the meniscus to pressure and traction forces.

For **ligament injuries**, varus and valgus stresses in flexions of 0° and 30° examine internal and external ligaments, the **Lachman test** in 25° and higher flexion degrees the anterior cruciate ligament, the posterior drawer test the posterior cruciate ligament (➤ Tab. 6.5). Rupture or wrong insertion is diagnosed by testing ligament tension and insertion. The anterior instability can be tested with the **pivot-shift test**, a subluxation of the lateral tibia head during valgus stress and tibial internal rotation, which resets abruptly at increasing flexion and indicates instability. Posterolateral complexes will be assessed in **external-rotation-asymmetry test according to Cooper**. In ventral position, an asymmetry in passive external rotation of the shank in a flexion of 30° will indicate posterolateral damage, in a flexion of 90° an additional damage of the posterior cruciate ligament.

With a preliminary diagnosis, the **femoropatellar joint** is examined again. Beside the lateral patellar facet, the plica mediopatellaris is examined for **pressure soreness**, the patella is tested for **pain on motion**. The patella within the sliding support is analyzed in passive movement, e.g. in order to verify a maltracking. Furthermore, the patella in extension will be pressed with the medial edge into the trochlea femoris, so that the lateral patellar edge rises. In case it does not rise, this indicates a too tight lateral retinaculum. If the patient reacts to this with a muscular avoidance, this indicates a patellar subluxation (**apprehension test**). If the flexion is painful for the patient, the patella in flexion may be pressed medially with the **reposition test according to McConnell**. This removes the pressure from the lateral patellar facet in a subluxation, and patients report a pain reduction.

6.2.3 Shoulder

Examination of the **shoulder** starts with the spine assessing pelvic position, spine shape, and the shoulder girdle with regard to the shoulder and scapula position, muscle atrophies, contour changes, malpositions – especially in the area of the clavicular diaphysis and the lateral clavicula –, swellings or abrasives. Muscle atrophies (e.g. n.-suprascularis entrapment), contour changes (e.g. rupture of the long biceps tendon) or malpositions (e.g. injuries of the acromioclavicular joint, clavicular fractures, shoulder luxations) are often a nearly blind diagnosis.

Shoulder points will be **palpated for pressure pain** (➤ Tab. 6.6) and **functional and diagnostic tests** are carried out (➤ Tab. 6.7).

The **adduction, retroversion and internal rotation of the arms** give a functional orientation; **passive and active mobility** is documented and painful arc is evaluated.

Tab. 6.7 Selection of functional and diagnostic tests with ligament injuries at the knee joint with according tentative diagnoses.

Muscle function	
Test	Impaired muscle
neutral abduction test	supraspinatus muscle
supraspinatus test according to Jobe (empty can test)	suprasoinatus muscle
neutral external rotation test	infraspinatus muscle
external rotation abduction test	infraspinatus muscle
neutral internal rotation test	subscapularis muscle
lift-off test	subscapularis muscle
belly press test	subscapularis muscle
palm-up test/speed test	biceps tendon
Yergason's test	biceps tendon
O'Brian's test	biceps tendon (anchor)
Impingement	
impingement test according to Neer	impingement
impingement test according to Hawkins-Kennedy	impingement
Instability	
anterior apprehension test	anterior instability
posterior apprehension test	posterior instability
relocation test	anterior instability

Tab. 6.8 Palpation points of elbow and hand.

radial epicondyle
ulnar epicondyle
olecranon – ulnar nerve
head of radius
ulnar styloid process
radial styloid process
carpus – especially radial fossa and lunatum
saddle joint of the thumb
collateral ulnar ligament
annular ligament
first extensor tendon compartment
tendon courses

The pathologies of the subacromial area, the acromioclavicular joint, the rotator cuff, the biceps tendon and the biceps-tendon anchor and stability of the glenohumeral joint is tested. A **number of testing alternatives** exist that require individual selection.

The individual **shoulder muscles** tests are:

- Neutral abduction test for the supraspinatus muscle
- Neutral external-rotation test for the infraspinatus muscle
- Neutral internal-rotation test and the lift-off tests for subscapular muscle
- Palm-up test/speed test for the long biceps tendon
- O'Brian test for the biceps tendon anchor

In the lift-off test, the athlete rises the internally rotated arm lying on the back against the resistance of the examiner. In the palm-up test, the arm is almost stretched in the elbow and supinated and rises isometrically against the resistance of the examiner.

Impingement tests according to Neer as well as Hawkins-Kennedy are of value for **impingement** verification.

Glenohumeral joint instability is examined with the drawer test to ventral, dorsal and caudal. The "sulcus sign" indicates caudal instability. The anterior and posterior apprehension tests and the relocation test are the next steps. In the anterior apprehension test, the humerus head is ventralized by 90° abduction of the thumb onto the humerus head from dorsal and an external 90° rotation. The athlete tries to avoid the (sub-)luxation by muscular tension and/or indicates pain with the presence of an instability. The relocation test is only performed after a positive apprehension test. The apprehension maneuver is carried out in dorsal position, while the examiner passively dorsalizes the humerus head and avoids a ventral (sub-)luxation. Earlier pain in the apprehension test or a muscular tension does not appear with instability and indicate shoulder instability.

Instability of the acromioclavicular joint is diagnosed with the piano key phenomenon, a **degenerative affection of the acromioclavicular joint** with the horizontal abduction test with pain indication in the acromioclavicular joint.

6.2.4 Elbow and hand

As with other body areas, hands and elbow are examined for redness, hyperthermia, inflammation signs, swellings, atrophies, bruises, hematomas, abrasions, open injuries, malpositions, poor or relieving postures and surgery scars. Callosity of the hand requires special attention to identify problems related to gripping a racket.

Palpation points (➢ Tab. 6.8) are examined thoroughly, mobility in all directions right-left compared, and ligaments are tested for stability. Functional and diagnostic tests are carried out (➢ Tab. 6.9), if needed.

Tab. 6.9 Selection of functional and diagnostic tests of elbow and hand with according tentative diagnoses.

ligament stability PIP/DIP joints in stretching	instability/ligament rupture
ligament stability MCP joint in flexion	instability/ligament rupture
ligament stability lig. collaterale ulnae	instability/ligament rupture
Watson's test	scapholunate instability
shear test	lunotriquetral instability
extension DIP under fixation in medial phalanx	injuries of the extensor terndon
extension PIP under fixation of basic phalanx	injuries of the extensor terndon
flexion of fingers with fixation of medial joints	injuries of the extensor terndon (deep)
flexion of fingers with fixation of neighboring fingers	injuries of the extensor terndon (superficial)
extension test of the forearm	ulnar epicondylitis
Mill's test	radial epicondylitis
Cozen's test	radial epicondylitis
stress test of varus/valgus	ligament instability elbow

DIP = distal interphalangeal joint, PIP = proximal interphalangeal joint, MCP = metacarpophalangeal joint

6.2.5 Pelvis, hip and spine

Traumas of the spine require screening for prevertebral hematomas and swellings. The spine is completely palpated in dorsal position and neural status is tested.

Great trochanter, spina iliaca anterior superior, the tendon starting points, such as the rectus femoris muscle, the adductor longus and magnus muscle, the iliopsoas muscle and the rectus abdominis muscle, and the inguinal ligament are palpated. Iliosacral joint testing excludes an inguinal hernia.

The **clinical functional tests** that are important for sports orthopedics/traumatology are limited to determining mobility of the hip in bilateral comparison, testing the compression pain, the forward flexion phenomenon of the sacroiliac joint (SIJ), the triggering of the snapping in a coxa saltans or an articular clicking in a labrum lesion and with according questions regarding the determining of the antetorsions of the femoral neck in abdominal position. Tendinopathies in this region are verified by movement tests against resistance.

Summary

A structured anamnesis followed by standardized, careful clinical examination often enables a clear diagnosis. This avoids unnecessary examination steps, wrong diagnostics and saves time.

References

Backup K (2000). Klinische Tests an Knochen, Gelenken und Muskeln. Thieme, Stuttgart.

Hedtmann A, Heers G (2002). Klinische Diagnostik. In: Gohlke F, Hedtmann A (eds.). Schulter. Reihe: Wirth CJ, Zichner L (eds.). Orthopädie und orthopädische Chirurgie. Stuttgart, Thieme, 76–97.

Neumann C, Weigel B (2005). Wirbelsäule. In: Weigel B, Nehrlich M (eds.). Praxisbuch Unfallchirurgie. Springer, Berlin.

Niezold D, Ferdini RM (2002). Klinische Untersuchung. In: Wirth CJ (ed.). Fuß. Reihe: Wirth CJ, Zichner L (eds.). Orthopädie und orthopädische Chirurgie. Thieme, Stuttgart, 11–19.

Welk E, Martini AK (2003). Klinische Untersuchung. In: Martini A-K (ed.). Ellbogen, Unterarm, Hand. Reihe: Wirth CJ, Zichner L (eds.). Orthopädie und orthopädische Chirurgie. Thieme, Stuttgart, 28.

Wirth CJ (2005). Klinische Diagnostik. In: Kohn D (ed.). Knie. Reihe: Wirth CJ, Zichner L (eds.). Orthopädie und orthopädische Chirurgie. Thieme, Stuttgart, p 61.

Chapter 7 Sonography

Ludwig Löffler

The development of imaging revolutionized medical progress. X-rays initially focused on fractures and bone malpositions leading to the development of orthopedics as separate discipline. A comparable revolution arose with the development of imaging procedures in the soft-tissue, namely sonography and magnetic resonance tomography (MRT). In the past 20 years, orthopedic surgery has focused on reconstruction of capsule-ligament injuries, tendon and muscle lesions. Earlier diagnosis of soft-tissue damages is possible by sonography or MRT.

Sonography of the locomotor apparatus and MRT has developed almost simultaneously. While MRT is reserved for radiologists, ultrasound diagnostics have proved of value for soft-tissue injuries in the hands of practicing sports physicians. Sonography comes with lower costs, rapid availability, dynamic examination and lateral comparison, as well as the option to carry out repeated examinations during treatment.

This has turned sonography into the "stethoscope of the sports medic". Therefore, diagnostics of shoulder injuries without sonography are unthinkable in particular with regards to high sensitivity in differentiating tendon and capsule-ligament injuries (Löffler 2001, 2005a, 2005b). Therapy has become more and more specific and successful because of differential diagnoses. The same applies to muscle injuries, overuse problems of knee and Achilles tendon, clarification of inguinal pain or undetermined hand and elbow pains. In individual cases, sonography may substitute radiography or may spare radiography in children.

A good instrumentation with a high-resolution transducer (7.5 MHz at least), an excellent training and knowledge of the anatomy are the preconditions for a safe sonographic diagnosis recognizing reference structures correctly. The examining physician must be aware of possible sonographic examinations errors; the dynamic examination should be fully explored, and lateral comparison starting with the healthy side is obligatory (Löffler 1988, Dumbs and Kunz 1990, Jerosch and Marquart 1993, Graf and Schuler 1995).

Principles for the ultrasound examination of athletes:
- Precondition: high-frequency transducer (7.5–2 MHz)
- Implementation:
  - Attention to landmarks
  - Findings in two levels
  - Dynamic examination
  - Lateral comparison

Sonography of the locomotor apparatus focuses on simple and compound joints, capsule and ligament injuries, tendon and muscle injuries/disorders and soft-tissue injuries, swellings or diseases such as lipomas, lymph node diseases, neurinomas and subcutaneous hematomas.

Sources of errors in sonography of the locomotor apparatus:
- Transducer tipping
- Lacking connection (advance!)
- Incorrect description of the reference structures
- Over- or under-radiation of the transducer
- Bad resolution of the transducer (too low frequency)
- Pressure on the transducer too high (e.g. in muscle imaging)
- No dynamic examination

7.1 Shoulder

7.1.1 Indication

Shoulder diseases are differentiated into injury, overuse, and functional complaints. Injury will affect bones (fractures of humeral head, socket, scapula, clavicula and acromion), the tendons (ruptures of rotator cuff and long biceps tendon), or soft-tissue as in the ventral or dorsal labrum lesion. Typical overuse lesions typically appear at bursa subacromialis, rotator cuff insertion tendinoses, long biceps tendon, and the dorsal or cranial labrum region. Functional pain will hardly show any structural changes in ultrasound or MRT. Dynamic examination should be applied with the option of instability diagnostics. ➤ Tab. 7.1 summarizes sonography areas of the shoulder joint.

7.1.2 Standard level and regular finding

Sonographic examination of the shoulder starts with imaging the long biceps tendon by placing the transducer ventral and longitudinal above the sulcus bicipitalis (➤ Fig. 7.1 a, b). The sulcus with the biceps tendon lies inside tuberculum minus and majus, which is hardly distinguishable from the retinaculum. The biceps tendon is round and 2–3 mm thick (Dondelinger 1996, Fornage 1988, Löffler 2005a).

To visualize subscapularis muscle with insertion at the tuberculum minus, the arm is rotated outwards keeping the same transducer position. This dynamic examination is important to detect tears only visible in motion. The subscapularis tendon is a little more echogenic than the musculature and moves together with the tuberculum minus.

Next, the arm is rotated inwards and retroflected. This yields the picture of the supra or infraspinatus tendon. The so-called beak pattern presents itself at the vertical position of the transducer as an echogenic tendon running along the tuberculum majus. The same tendon shows itself as ring pattern in the horizontal position of the transducer as an echogenic, evenly bordered and homogeneous structure. The tendon runs parallel to the contour of the humeral head.

Tab. 7.1 Structures and joints of the shoulder accessible to sonography.

long biceps tendon
rotator cuff/bursa
labrum
capsule
head contour
shoulder joint/coracoclavicular ligaments

The subdeltoid bursa presents a thin limiting lamella between supraspinatus tendon and deltoid. A dynamic examination offers an additional diagnostic support of small tendon defects.

Next, the transducer is moved to dorsal (➤ Fig. 7.2 a, b). The dorsal glenoid edge with the labrum is represented primarily in addition to the contour of the humeral head with the echopenic suffusion (hyaline cartilage). The labrum is an echogenic triangle lying directly on the sound shadow of the dorsal edge of the glenoid cavity, tightly nestling to the humeral head and not participating in the movement. The infraspinatus tendon lies above the labrum. The muscle has a lower echogenicity than the tendon and shows a ripple.

The ventral labrum display is carried out in the incision of the pectoralis edge. With the patient lying on the back, the arm is slightly abducted and rotated outwards and the transducer is set ventrally above the humeral head or the edge of the glenoid cavity. The ventral labrum shows as an echogenic triangle, which will sit directly on the osseous edge of the glenoid cavity. The subscapularis muscle or the coracobrachialis musculature and the deltoid, respectively, move above.

The transducer is set parallel to the clavicula and above the palpable joint cavity for the image of the shoulder joint. Acromion and clavicula are represented with the joint cavity and the enveloping capsule.

7.1.3 Pathology

Biceps tendon

An echopenic halo is detectable in every form of effusion or biceps tendinitis (➤ Fig. 7.1 d). The tendon is roughened, deformed and broadened in advanced degenerative cases. An

7.1 Shoulder

Fig. 7.1 Sonography of the biceps tendon. a: transducer position. b: normal findings. c: rupture if the long biceps tendon. d: tendinitis. e: luxation of the biceps tendon.

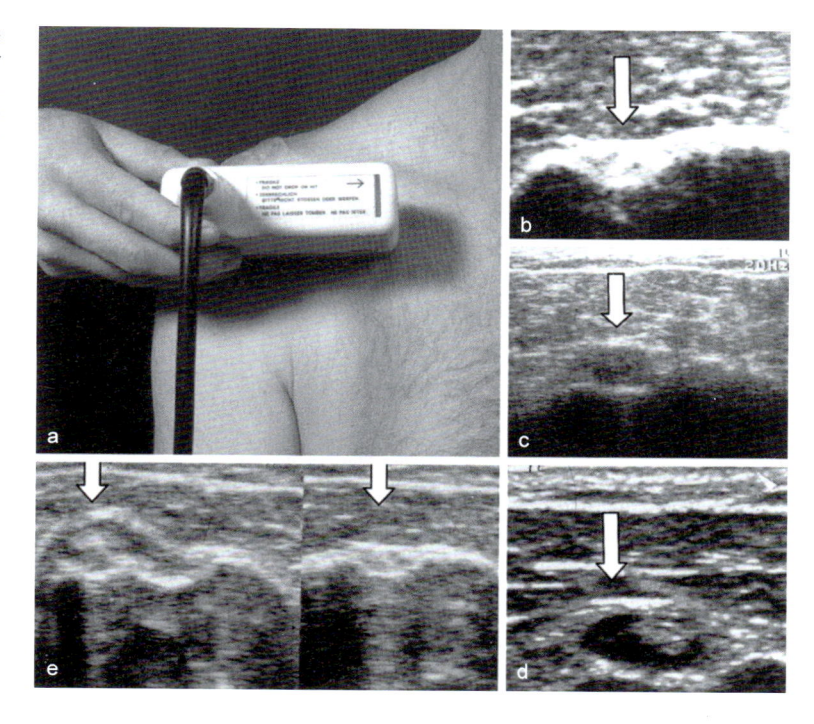

Fig. 7.2 Sonography of the dorsal labrum. a: transducer position. b: normal findings. c: labrum rupture.

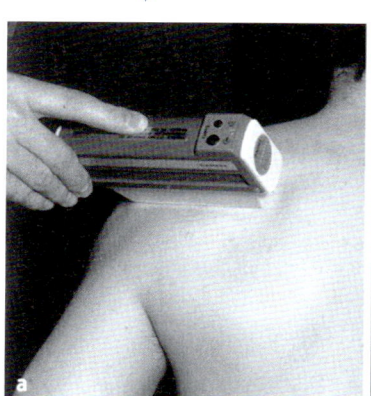

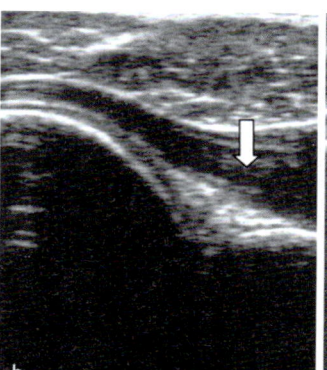

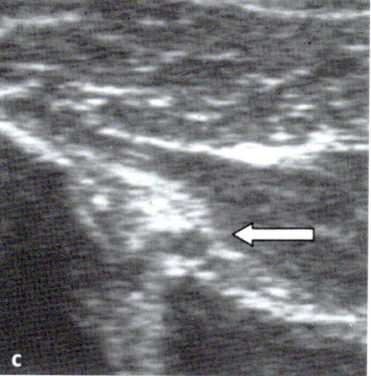

empty sulcus forms at luxations of the biceps tendon; the tendon rides over the tuberculum minus (➤ Fig. 7.1 e). If the sulcus is empty, we refer to a biceps-tendon rupture, at which additionally an effusion will show in the fresh injury (➤ Fig. 7.1 c); in older injuries, the retinaculum is caved in. The dorsal transducer position is advisable for more extensive effusions. Here a capsule detachment is found beneath the infraspinatus musculature.

Bursitis

Bursitis refers to broadened bursa filled with an echo signal deprived fluid line of several millimeters between rotator cuff and deltoid muscle. The bursa may have a breadth of several centimeters at a defective rotator cuff.

Rotator cuff defect

Clear and unclear criteria exist suggesting a rotator cuff defect. Clear criteria are the loss of tendon tone with bursal line reversal (concave), defect with an echogenic tendon stump, bone roughening, fatty degeneration of the muscles with atrophy, and increased echogenity (dorsal transducer position). The movement of the tendon stump reveals in the dynamic examination with inward and outward rotations.

Tendinitis
In tendinitis, the tendon is swollen (thicker than 5 mm), broadened and has rather low echogenicity. If echogenic inclusions are detected (sound shadows), we refer to a tendinitis calcarea. Only if calcium carbonate causes a sound shadow, it is visible in x-ray.

Fracture
If a step is detected at the tendon insertion with a concomitant edema, this indicates a tuberculum majus fracture. In this particular case, sonography is often superior to x-ray imaging in early diagnosis. Small steps are equally found in degenerative changes and older rotator-cuff defects.

Labrum defect
The labrum is defined as an echogenic triangle at the osseous glenoid cavity. Defects present with a deformed, off-lifted or dislocated (dynamic examination) echogenic triangle or if the osseous glenoid cavity is roughened or broadened.

Dorsal labrum defects are frequent. Degenerative changes are characterized as stump, roughened and increased echogenic or deformed structure (➢ Fig. 7.2 a–c).

Dorsal Luxation
Dorsal luxation with latching often presents at a dorsal transducer position with a bulged humeral head (lateral comparison) and loss of rotation. If steps at the contour of the humerus head are detected, this is referred to the so-called Hill-Sachs lesion, which is indicative of a previous luxation (➢ Fig. 7.3 a, b).

Shoulder joint destruction
In shoulder joint destruction, the clavicula is elevated more than the shaft breadth. Additionally, effusion and broadening of the joint cavity is detected (➢ Fig. 7.4 a–d).

Arthrosis/necrosis
Stress-induced arthroses or necroses at the lateral end of the clavicula are characterized by effusion without malposition (➢ Fig. 7.5 a–c).

Muscle atrophy
A rotator-cuff defect should always be excluded if diagnosing a supraspinous or infraspinous muscular atrophy (lateral comparison). Occasionally, a weakness of this muscle group occurs in younger patients. The activity of musculature can be tested in M-mode. If an inactive musculature is found further neurological or MRT clarification is required to exclude spinalglenoid ganglion as cause of suprascapular nerve lesion.

If for inexplicit functional shoulder pain no structural changes are detectable by sonography or imaging, a selective instability diagnosis should be carried. The ventral and dorsal subluxation tendency or the sulcus sign, respectively, should be documented by sonography as signs of a hyperlaxity/hypermobility of the shoulder, especially in younger athletes. Sometimes also a deformation of the ventral or dorsal labrum, a slight reactive effusion in sulcus bicipitalis or a swelling of the insertion of the supraspinatus tendon and a discrete broadening of the bursa can be found. Mostly, this is characteristic for overuse in throwing and overhead sports, and swimming. Partial tears superficial supraspinatus tendon are common side symptoms. X-rays or MRT should exclude subacromial shortage.

Sonography can only be used as a screening method with swellings or suspected tumors; only rarely a differentiation is possible, as with lipomas (fusiform echogenic structure subcutaneously). Ganglia are found mostly above the AC joint (➢ Fig. 7.4 d). Spinoglenoid ganglia are better accessible by MRT. Distinctive effusions and bursitides can be clearly recognized as such and can also be distinguished from the villonodular synovitis.

Shoulder stiffness
Idiopathic shoulder stiffness is visible only as a slight effusion in sulcus bicipitalis. Posttrau-

7.1 Shoulder

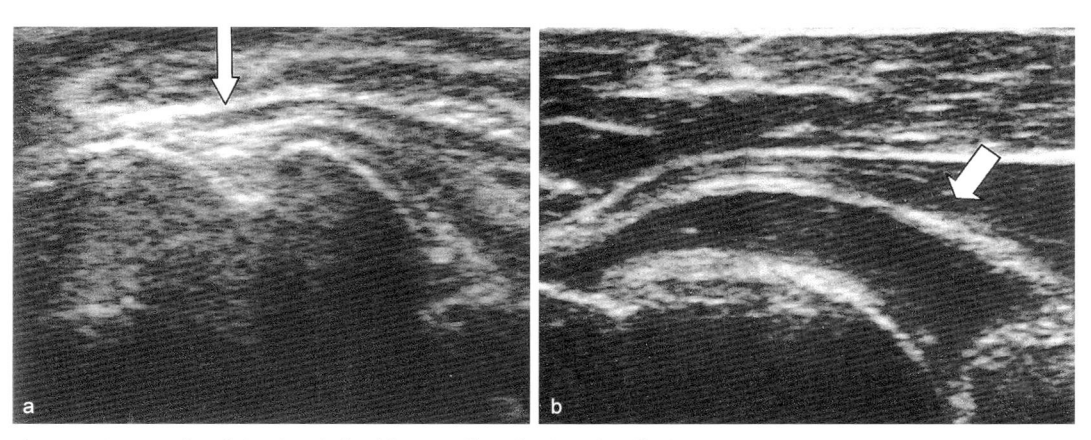

Fig. 7.3 Sonography of the dorsal shoulder. a: Hill-Sachs dent. b: effusion.

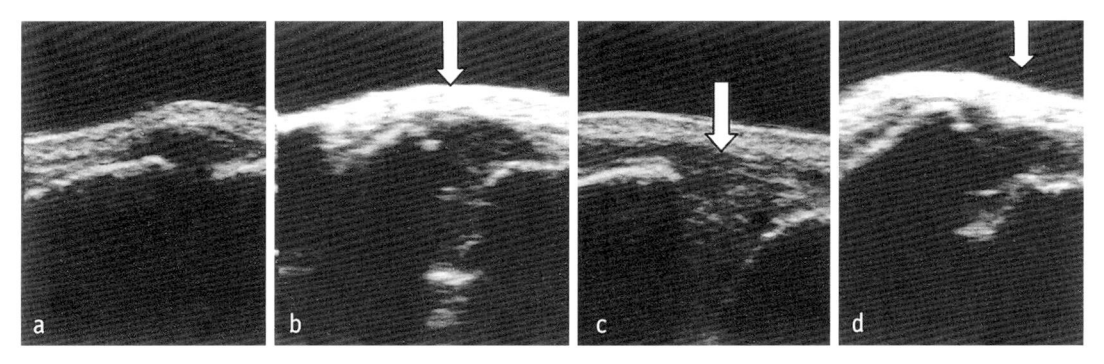

Fig. 7.4 Sonography in a shoulder joint injury. a: normal findings. b: Tossy I: effusion and widening of the joint cavity. c: Tossy II: slight raise of the clavicula. d: Tossy III: clear raised standing of the clavicula.

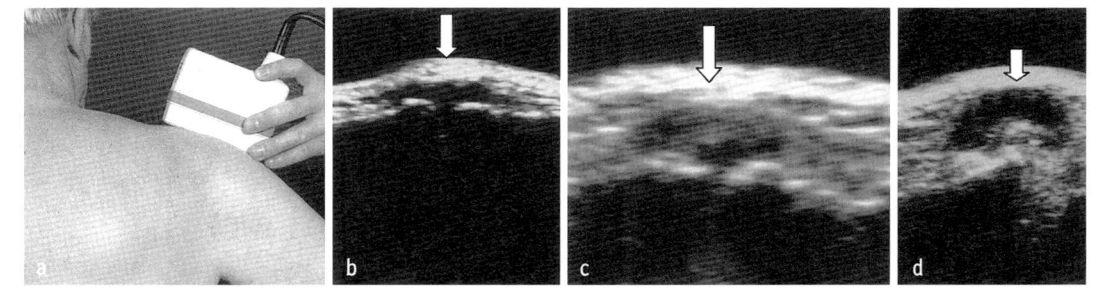

Fig. 7.5 Sonography of the shoulder joint. a: transducer position. b: normal findings. c: effusion. d: ganglion.

matic or reactive capsulitis are characterized by changes at the rotator cuff or contour of the humeral head (roughening in case of arthrosis). A hooked dorsal subluxation or luxation can be presented by sonography in the dorsal standard layer in lateral comparison.

7.2 Elbow

7.2.1 Indication

Pain, swellings and movement limitations occur after injury of the elbow. One needs to differentiate a subcutane soft-tissue swelling, intraarticular effusion, or a bursitis olecrani. Sonography only serves as a screening method in fracture diagnosis and needs validation by X-ray or MRT. Post-traumatic intraarticular effusions require further evaluation, if an osseous injury (fracture, osteochondral chipping, osseous tendon tearing, previously or currently existent luxation) is excluded (Löffler 1988).

Tab. 7.2 Structures and joints of the elbow accessible to sonography.

capsule
humerus/radius/ulna
fossa olectani
fossa coronoidea
coronoideus process

Elbow overuse symptoms are often accompanied by movement limitations and unspecific pressure pain. Intraarticular findings (effusion), possibly in connection with loose bodies, will require further sonography follow-up. Similarly, an epicondylitis at the radial or ulnar epicondyle, calcifications of the tendon insertions in the area of the forearm-extensor or forearm-flexor musculature or triceps, and edema of the supinator muscle require sonography clarification. ➢ Tab. 7.2 summarizes the affected and structures of the elbow accessible to sonography.

7.2.2 Standard level and regular finding

The elbow will preferably be examined in full extension. The transducer will be set lengthwise and crosswise in a flexor-sided position with a picture of the capitulum humeri, radius head, the fossa coronoidea and the ulna. Radially, the capsule will lie tightly against the radius head and the capitulum humeri. The coronoid process, the fossa coronoidea or olecrani and the brachialis muscle that is running above show in the ulnar image (➢ Fig. 7.6 a

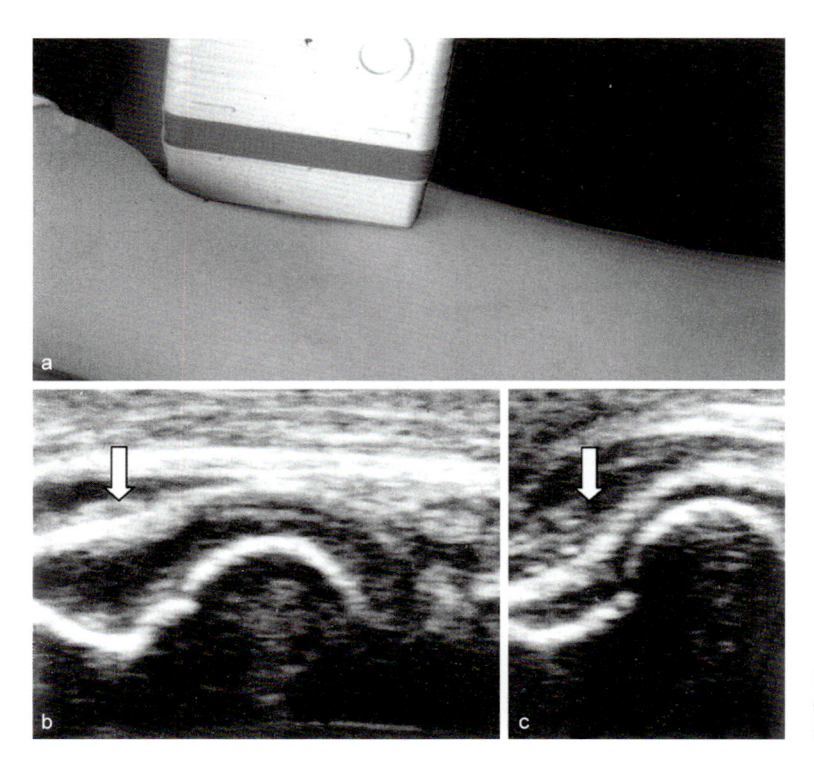

Fig. 7.6 Sonography of the elbow. a: transducer position. b: effusion. c: normal findings.

7.3 Hand

cause a sound shadow. Overlapping in the area of osseous structure indicates a **fracture**, often accompanied by hematoma or effusion.

Tendinitis of flexor or extensor insertions present as an echo-deprived signal, broadened tendon insertion low of fibers. Pressure pain at the radial or ulnar epicondylitis occurs often concomitantly (➢ Fig. 7.7 a–c).

The ulnar nerve comes as an echo-deprived signal and can be displayed in **subluxations** (crosswise transducer position).

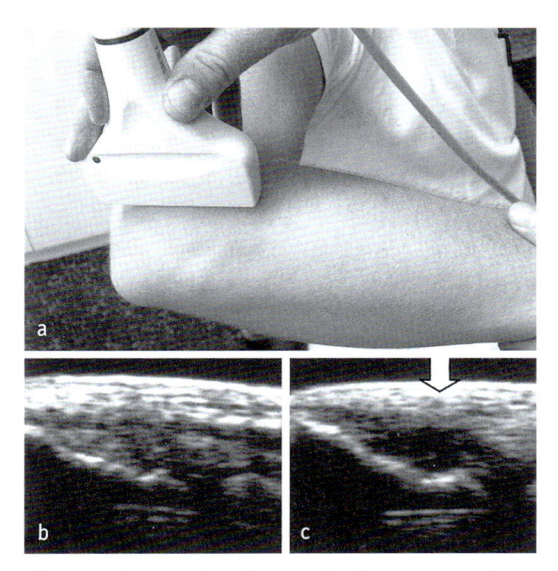

Fig. 7.7 Sonography of a tennis elbow. a: transducer position. b: normal findings. c: tennis elbow.

and c). The crosswise image is recommended for the inhibition of the extensors. Here, the capitulum humeri and the trochlea humeri are found as a curved line with the tightly adjacent capsule.

The fossa olecrani of the flexed elbow is displayed dorsally in two layers for the examination of effusion and loose bodies. In regular findings, the capsule is tightly boud, the content of the fossa is echogenic, and the fossa bottom constitutes an echogenic ligament. The transducer is set parallel to the forearm at the epicondylus for the picture of the epicondylus radialis. The extensor tendons of the forearm are echogenic and insert at the epicondylus radialis or ulnaris (forearm flexor). Starting from these insertions, the musculature of the forearm flexor and the forearm extensor can be traced with appropriate positioning of the transducer.

7.2.3 Pathology

If the capsule is off-lifted in the lengthwise and crosswise picture and an echo-deprived signal, liquid line exists between capsule and bone, we refer to an effusion (➢ Fig. 7.6 b).

Flexor-sided **loose bodies** are found mostly in the fossa coronoidea; they are echogenic and

7.3 Hand

7.3.1 Indication

The classic injury mechanism for hand injuries is the fall onto the hyper-extended wrist joint, which presents clinically with a swelling, painful movement limitation and malposition. Songraphic detection of effusion with the detachment of the joint capsule from the osseous structures is the most sensitive findings. Step formation at the wrist bone or radius base indicates a fracture, which requires further radiographic clarification. Typical soft tissue swellings are tendon and ligament ruptures, such as thumb ulnar collateral-ligament ruptures, ring-ligament injury of the flexor-tendons, and effusion with tendon swelling (see Dondelinger 1996).

Overuse symptoms of the hand mostly affect the tendons. A tendinitis stenosans in the first extensor tendon groove of the extensor tendon (de Quervain) can be differentiated by sonography from changes of the bone structure. In a trigger finger, we find a halo around the tendon next to a swelling of the tendon. The trigger finger may be differentiated from the hygroma of the tendon sheath. Tendinitis of the extensor-tendons is rare, but also present with a liquid line. Luxations of the extensor-tendons can be pictured dynamically. Insertion tendinoses with typical edemas occurs especially in the area of the flexor carpi ulnaris tendon at the pisiform bone. The carpal tunnel syndrome often presents with inflammations of the flexor tendons next to the narrowing median nerve.

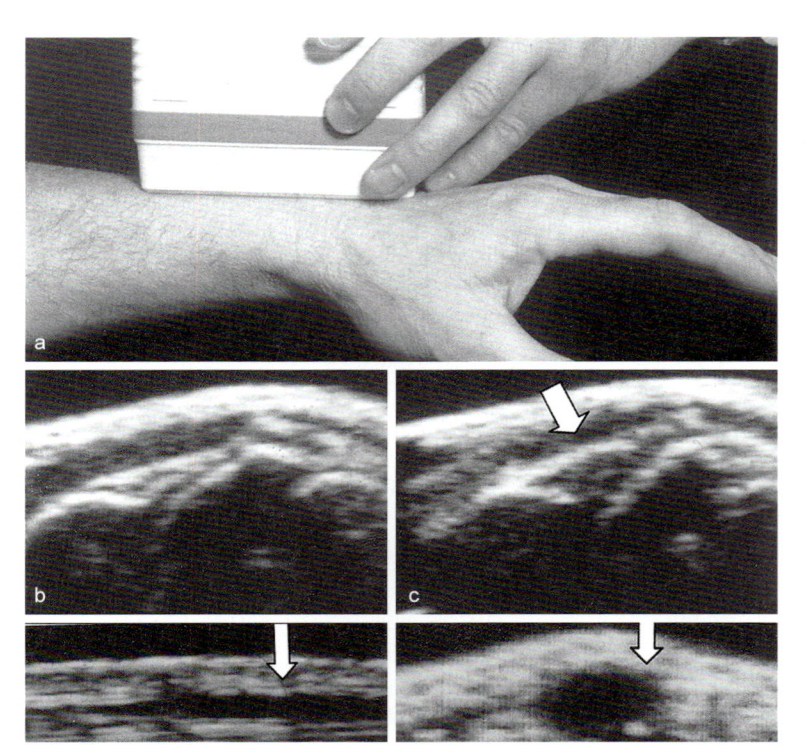

Fig. 7.8 Sonography of a wrist. a: transducer position. b: normal findings. c: effusion. d: tendinitis of the extensor tendons. e: ganglion.

7.3.2 Standard level and normal findings

The hand is extended and lies on a table or the examination couch. The transducer is set dorsally length- and crosswise. The extensor tendons displays adjacent to the subcutaneous tissue and joint capsule. The wrist joints are echogenic and trigger a sound shadow. On the flexed side, the median nerve presents as a 1–2 mm echo-deprived signal and thick stripe between the echogenic retinaculum and flexor tendons (under movement of the fingers) (➢ Fig. 7.8 a and b). The flexor tendons are pictured lengthwise and crosswise in the palmar fold in connection with the joint capsule of the metacarpophalangeal joints of the fingers. In motion, the tendons can be distinguished from the joint capsule. The collateral ligaments present echogenic bridges above the joint cavity.

7.3.3 Pathology

We refer to an **effusion** at the detachment of the joint capsule from the bone and echo-deprived signal structures between capsule and bone (➢ Fig. 7.8 c).

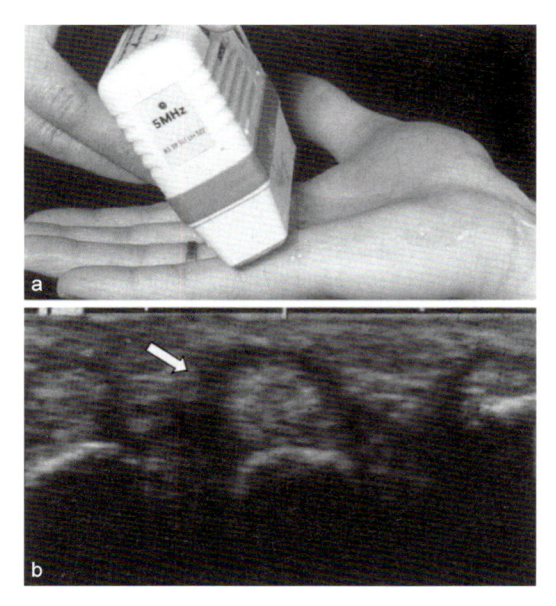

Fig. 7.9 Sonography of the flexor tendons of the finger. a: transducer position. b: tendovaginitis.

Step-formation at the bone with concomitant hematoma or periost detachment indicates a **fracture** and requires further radiographic clarification.

Tendinitis is associated with a swelling of the tendon, increased echogenicity and a liquid line (halo) (➢ Fig. 7.8 d and ➢ Fig. 7.9 a, b). **Ligament lesions** show a defect with echogenic rim, broadening of the ligament structure, loss of tone and concomitant hematoma. The instability examination under dynamics is helpful. A sandglass shaped narrowing of the median nerve between the retinaculum and the flexor tendons is typical for **carpal tunnel syndrome**.

Ganglia are evenly bordered, with an echo-deprived signal, are connected to joints and trigger a sound increase. They are compressible, hence, distinguishable from exostoses (➢ Fig. 7.8 e).

7.4 Hip joint

7.4.1 Indication

Inguinal pain is differentiated from pain triggered by accidents or overuse. In most cases, injury clearly limits movement of the hip joint.

Firstly, femoral neck and pelvis fractures need to be excluded by radiography. Tearing injuries of the abductors, the rectus femoris (often tearing of the apophysis) or other muscle and tendon injuries can be distinguished by sonography. Effusion and malposition accompany injuries at the symphysis (Gerber et al. 2000).

Stress-triggered pain emanating from the hip joint presents with effusion into the joint. Irritation of the tendon insertions, e.g. at the abductors, presents with edema and broadening of the insertion. Calcifications in the region of the muscle or tendon insertions indicate for a myositis ossificans as a sign of a previous injury. Buristis is less often detected by sonography as clinically expected (bursits trochanterica).

Fatigue fractures of pelvis or femoral neck presenting as ejection of the cortical bone or of periost in connection with an effusion are unlikely to be detected by sonography. They require radiological diagnosis. This applies equally to transient osteoporosis, which shows an effusion in the hip joint.

Tab. 7.3 Structures and joints of the hip accessible to sonography.

| femoral head |
| femoral neck |
| capsule |
| iliopsoas muscle |
| rectus femoris muscle |
| sartorius muscle |

➢ Tab. 7.3 will summarize the structures that are accessible to sonography.

7.4.2 Standard level and regular findings

For the examination of the hip joint, the patient lies with his back on the examination couch with the hip joint extended as far as possible in a medium rotation. The transducer is set ventrally at the height of the hip, corresponding to the angle of the femoral neck. Three muscle groups show as reference structures: sartorius muscle, rectus femoris muscle, and iliopsoas muscle lying directly above the hip joint. The joint capsule covers the femoral head and neck as an echogenic ligament. The femoral neck shows a concave osseous structure with sound shadow, the head of femur is convex and supplied with cartilage coating (echo-deprived signal).

7.4.3 Pathology

Effusions are referred to as a convex lift-off the joint capsule above the femoral neck (capsule distention); the content of the joint capsule has an echo-deprived signal depending on the effusion cause (➢ Fig. 7.10 a and b).

The loose bodies present themselves as echogenic structure with sound shadow; this is also true for **calcifications of the tendon insertions or the musculature**, especially at the insertion of rectus femoris muscle. **Muscle ruptures** show a defect with hematoma, a wavy contouring of the muscle structure as a sign of the tone loss as well as an echogenic muscle stump.

A **deformation of the femoral head epiphysis**, especially in adolescents of the ages between 5 and 10 years, indicates Legg-Calvé-Perthes syndrome. The epiphysis is decreased in height and the ball is deformed, depending on the stage also chunkily disintegrated. An effusion

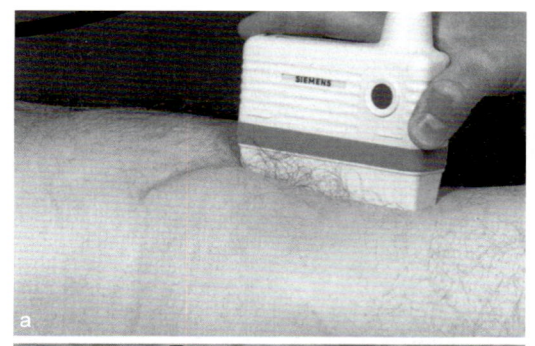

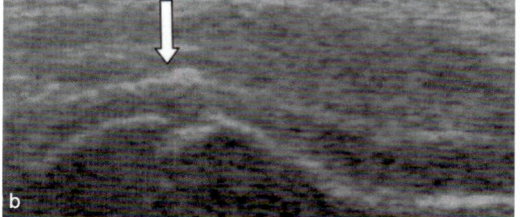

Fig. 7.10 Sonography of the hip joint. a: transducer position. b: effusion/epiphyseal Salter-Harris fracture.

as well as a small overlapping in the area of the epiphyseal cartilage is found in the **epiphyseolysis**, primarily in the beginning stage.

ual therapy, ranging from short restraint with analgesia up to surgery. Mainly, the duration of the stoppage and the general prognosis of the injury are important for the athlete (Reimers and Gaulrapp 1988).

In addition to injury-caused muscle disorders, muscle disorders caused by overuse are differentiated. The chronic compartment syndrome at the shank shows an echogenic milk-glass effect and a fascia-like swelling indicating edema forming. Muscle atrophies are pure inactivity atrophies. Causes such as neurological disorders require follow-up with an appropriate specialist. Tendon ruptures causing muscle atrophy can be displayed by sonography, which is indicative for overall activity. The M mode is in addition to the B mode particularly useful. A complete loss of the muscle function may have a neurogenic as well as a structural cause (tendon tear).

Muscle diseases are distinguished into dystrophy, atrophy and spinal muscle atrophy. Only structural changes of the musculature are displayed in sonography without further differentiation.

Musculature swellings that are not muscle-conditioned are typically at the calf (Baker's cyst), a leg-vein thrombosis or a tumor.

7.5 Thigh and lower leg musculature

7.5.1 Indication

Primarily injury-caused and, less often, overuse changes can be differentiated. With muscle injuries, longitudinal injuries are differentiated from transversal injuries. The direct muscle injuries, such as contusions, contusion traumas and bruises, are referred to as transversal injuries. In longitudinal injuries, extreme tears trigger rupture of the musculature and are classified into four grades. Strain trauma presents (clinically) with painful muscular rigidification. Rupture of the muscle fiber presents with broadened and swollen musculature, whereas muscle bundle rupture has additionally a hemorrhage and extensive functional loss. A complete functional loss of the respective muscle group occurs at the tearing, e.g. of the adductor longus muscle. These muscle injuries need sonographic differentiation and individ-

7.5.2 Standard level and regular findings

Muscle diagnostics should examine every muscle in the area of thigh and shank in two layers (lengthwise and crosswise), dynamically, and in lateral comparison. The osseous reference structure (femur or tibia) is placed in both layers (narrow echogenic band). Three layers can be detected: first, the subcutaneous fatty tissue shows, second, the echogenic ligament of the fascia, and third, the typical ripples of the musculature (fish bone pattern). The muscle septa are echogenic, comparable to the cortical substance of the bone. A differentiation between muscle venter and muscle bundle is possible, muscle fibers can only be displayed microscopically (➢ Fig. 7.11 a).

7.5.3 Pathology

Muscle rupture presents with hematoma and echogenic muscle stump, which is flexible un-

Fig. 7.11 Sonography of a muscle injury of the abductors. a: normal findings. b: muscle-fiber rupture. c: muscle-bundle rupture. d: muscle detachment of the Sartorius muscle. e: muscle detachment of the adductor longus muscle.

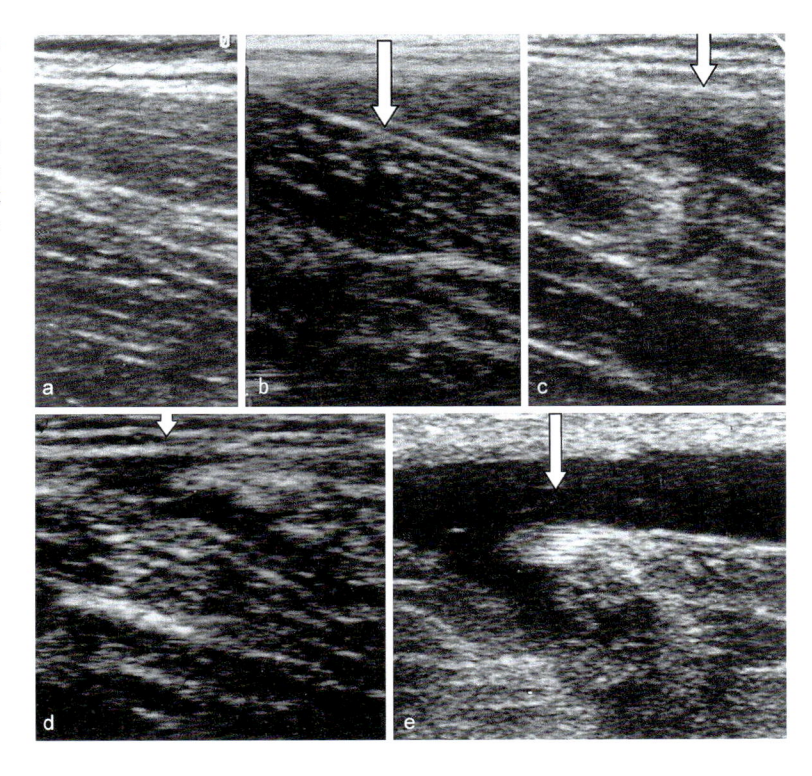

der dynamic examination. The muscle bundle shows a tone loss. The different shapes of fiber, bundle and complete muscle rupture exhibits a broadened and swollen the musculature with more extensive hemorrhage at functional loss (➤ Fig. 7.11 b–e).

In contrast, **muscle contusions** loose echographic signal, the bundle is broadened, and the structure is washy (milk glass effect). The typical ripple cannot be displayed any longer. If an echogenic structure is detected in the sound shadow, this is referred to **myositis ossificans** (often not defined borders). Lager **hematomas** after muscle injuries are echosignal deprived, sharply defined, compressible, and show interior echoes only if organized.

We refer to a **myopathy**, if a diffuse echogenic washy muscle structure with strong sound absorption is present and conditioned by fat inclusion. Scar formations as well as inferior perfusion need consideration in differential diagnosis.

7.6 Knee joint

7.6.1 Indication

At the knee joint, we differentiate between accident- and overuse-triggered symptoms. However, knee sonography has not the same power as compared to the shoulder, but still is valuable in particular cases (Graf and Schuler 1995).

A swollen knee is the first sign of knee injury. Intraarticular effusions and subcutane soft-tissue swelling (bursitis) can be differentiated by sonography. An effusion in the upper recessus always indicates an intraarticular injury, mostly cruciate-ligament-meniscus injuries or osteochondral injuries. These require appropriate, further diagnostics.

In the event of effusions, capsule-ligament and tendon injuries require exclusion. The quadriceps tendon presents at the upper pattelar pole and the patellar tendon at the lower patellar pole. In case of a suspected patellar luxation,

Tab. 7.4 Structures and joints of the knee accessible to sonography.

patellar tendon
quadriceps tendon
femoral role
internal and external ligaments
patellar top/tuberositas tibiae
vessels and nerves
gastrocnemius muscle

the medial retinaculum is treated separately. Meniscus injuries show the typical changes in addition to the effusion, especially in the area of the posterior horn.

Knee joint disorders caused by overuse are indications for sonography. These include the tendopathy of the quadriceps tendon, the patellar top syndrome or tendinitis of the patellar tendon. In children, Osgood-Schlatter disease requires differentiation from patellar tendinitis.

Degenerative meniscopathies caused by overuse show changes at the posterior horn with distortion and increased echogenicity. Accessory symptoms are effusion in the upper recessus, Baker's cyst in the hollow of the knee, as well as the exterior meniscus ganglion. Prepalletar bursitides can be distinguished according to localization. With ostechondral lesions, only capsule edema is detected prior occurrence of narrowed joint cavity or osteophytic protrusions.

Baker's cysts and tumors often trigger a swelling sensation in the knee hollow.

➤ Tab. 7.4 summarizes the structures of affected knee joint areas, which are require assessment.

7.6.2 Standard level and regular findings

The patient is examined in dorsal or ventral position, depending on the structure to be examined, with a widely extended or slightly flexed knee.

On the extended side, the transducer is set length- and crosswise above the quadriceps tendon and the patellar tendon. The according tendons are displayed above the osseous reference structures such as femur and patella, patella and tibia head, respectively. The patellar slide bearing is examined at a maximum-flexed knee joint with the transducer set crosswise. The tendons are echogenic, homogeneous, and few millimeters thick; the slide bearings shows an angle of 135°, an echo-deprived signal, and medial-lateral steady cartilage coating. The collateral ligaments at the medial and lateral joint cavity are echogenic and lie directly subcutaneously on the according joint cavity. Menisci are examined from dorsal at a slightly flexed knee joint in dorsal or ventral position, and appear as an echogenic homogeneous triangle in the joint cavity. The hyaline cartilage has an echo-deprived signal and coats the femur. The cartilage of the tibia head cannot be visualized.

The knee hollow is presented length- and crosswise, medial and lateral. The vessels are lateral reference structures. The popliteal notch sits medial between gastrocnemicus muscle and semimembranosus muscle, where Baker's cyst is to be searched for.

7.6.3 Pathology

If the joint capsule or the quadriceps tendon in the upper recessus is detached and a broad echo-deprived or echo-free signal exists between tendon and femur, this is referred to an **effusion**. If an echogenic structure with sound shadow is found, this indicates a **loose body**. Villus formations in the area of the synovialis indicate chronic or older effusion or even a rheumatic disease.

A **tendinosis of the quadriceps tendon** presents as a swelling, in decreased echogenicity and in diminished fibers. A tendon lesion presents as local defect with echo-signal deprived hematoma; the tendon stump is echogenic, wave-contoured as a sign of tone loss and mostly broadened. The **dynamic examination** is helpful. At a ligament lesion, the ligament is broadened and shows an echo-deprived defect zone with echogenic ligament (➤ Fig 7.12 a and b).

If the **meniscus** is degenerated, it shows similar to arthroscopy or MRT changes of form and structure. The meniscus is inhomogeneous, increasingly echogenic and diminished, deformed, blunt, torn at the basis or shortened.

7.7 Foot

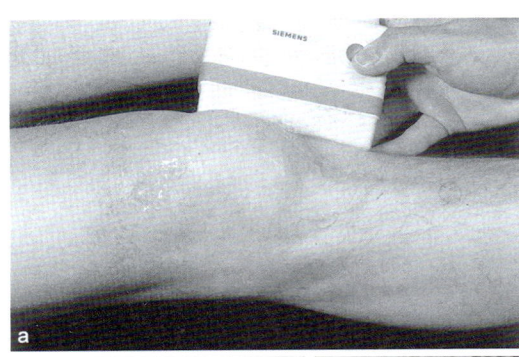

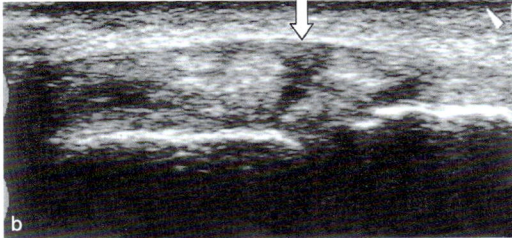

Fig. 7.12 Sonography of the knee joint. a: transducer position. b: rupture of the intraarticular ligament.

Tab. 7.5 Structures and joints of the foot accessible to sonography.

tibia/talus
extension tendons
flexion tendons
Achilles tendon
peroneal tendons
TFA/CF ligaments
syndesmosis
plantar fascia

We will speak of a **ganglion** or a **cyst**, if an echo-signal deprived, evenly bordered structure with sound amplification exists.

An articulation can be sonographically displayed. If the angle in the patellar storage is smaller than 135°, we refer to a **dysplasia of slide bearing**; if the cartilage coating is narrowed or used up, this indicates a femoropatellar joint arthrosis. In the gonarthrosis we find osteophytal protrusions and lifted-off of the capsule or a capsule edema at the medial and lateral joint cavity in addition to the joint-cavity narrowing.

7.7 Foot

7.7.1 Indication

Every foot injury inevitably needs a radiographic examination but sonography of swollen lower and upper ankle joint differentiates between intraarticular effusions with capsule lift-off and capsule-ligament injuries. This applies particularly to the area of the anterior talofibular ligament (TFA), the calcaneofibular ligament (CF), the syndesmosis and the medial ligament of talocrural joint. Often, tendon injuries, Achilles tendon and extensor tendons, are often diagnosed incorrectly. A sonographic picture shows a complete or incomplete tendon rupture or tendon sliding tissue changes. This applies equally to the peroneal tendons and the plantar aponeurosis (Löffler 2001).

Detection of soft-tissue changes at the foot caused are the strength of sonography.

Tendinitis of the tibialis anterior tendon, the tibialis posterior tendon, the peroneal tendons and Achilles tendon are central examinations. In the area of the Achilles tendon, different inflammations can be distinguished such as general tendinitis, peritendinitis achillea, insertion tendinoses, and bursitides. Effusions and stress fractures can be displayed by sonography but require further radiographic clarification.

➢ Tab. 7.5 summarizes the affected structures of the foot that are accessible to sonography.

7.7.2 Standard level and regular finding

The examination of the upper ankle joint begins with the joint cavity between tibia and talus. The transducer is set lengthwise at the ankle (➢ Fig. 7.13 a). Tibia and talus present as narrow echogenic ligament with capsule, extensor tendons, and the tibial anterior tendon laying above. The extensor and flexor tendons are displayed length- and crosswise depending on the anatomy. Typically, they are homogeneously echogenic with a small echo-signal deprived line. The classification works primarily by movement of the corresponding structure (upper and lower ankle joint, toe flexor and extensor).

The presentation of the capsule-ligament apparatus is important for differentiation. The anterior talofibular ligament presents as double-contoured echogenic ligament between fibula and talus and runs parallel to the foot sole. The examination usually works only with flow line. The transducer is set parallel to the foot sole; fibula and talus with tuberculum innominatum serve as reference structures. The calcaneofibular ligament is displayed laterally dorsal under the peroneal tendons; it inserts at the calcaneus, is echogenic and 2–3 mm thick (➤ Fig. 7.15 a and b). The deltoid ligament is also echogenic and double-contoured; it consists of three structures and runs from the medial malleolus to the navicular, to the calcaneus and dorsally to the talus. In general, injuries occur in the ventral or medial part, rarely in the dorsal part. The syndesmosis shows a 2 mm thick ligament between tibia and fibula, echo-signal deprived, double-contoured, and slightly rising from lateral to medial. The transducer is set with advance distance diagonally distal between tibia and fibula (➤ Fig. 7.14 a and b).

The Achilles tendon is examined length- and crosswise (➤ Fig. 7.16 a and b). Normally, it is 5–7 mm broad, has a homogeneous echo-deprived signal, lies directly subcutaneous and is evenly bordered. At the calcaneus insertion, it runs a little bend and therefore has an echo-deprived signal at this point.

7.7.3 Pathology

We refer to **upper ankle joint effusion**, if an echo-signal deprived capsule detachment occurs ventrally with a sound increase at the talus (➤ Fig. 7.13 b).

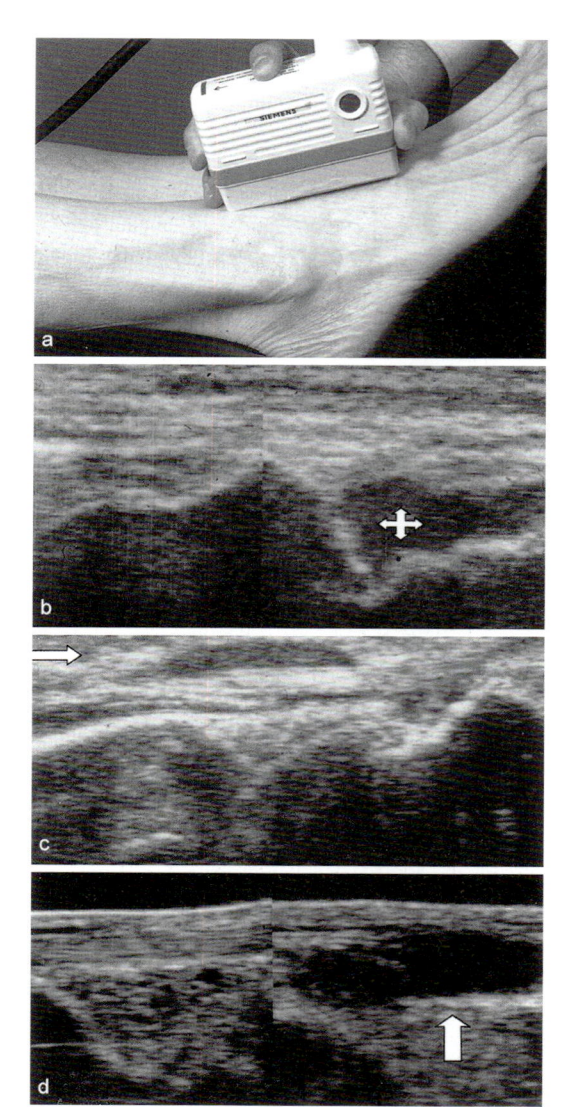

Fig. 7.13 Sonography of the foot: tibialis-anterior tendon. a: scanner-head position. b: effusion upper ankle joint. c: tendinitis. d: rupture.

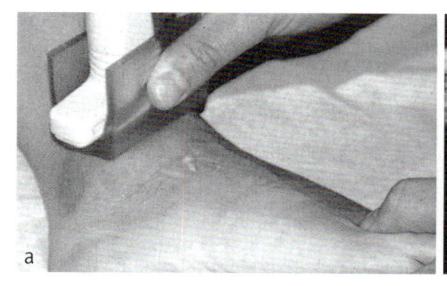

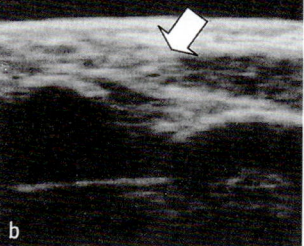

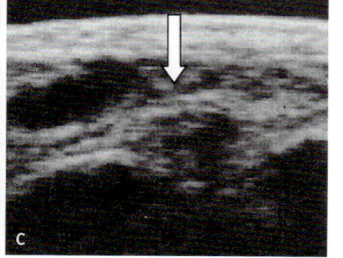

Fig. 7.14 Sonography of the foot: syndesmosis. a: transducer position. b: normal findings. c: fresh rupture.

7.7 Foot

Fig. 7.15 Sonography of the foot: calcaneofibular ligament.
a: transducer position. b: normal findings. c: ligament lesion.

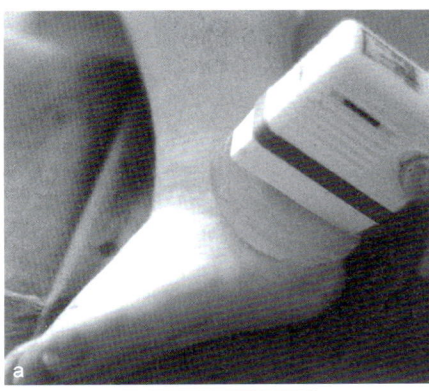

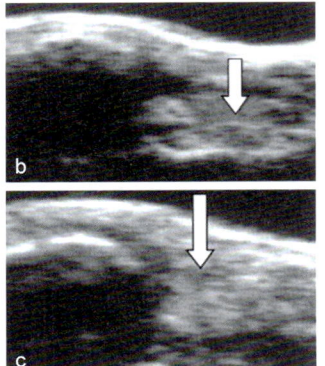

The typical finding of a **ligament lesion** is the defective ligament course with echogenic edge, hematoma, tone loss of the ligament structure, edema, and swelling of the surrounding tissue. **Tendon ruptures** exhibit an echo-deprived signal and hematoma. In addition to the tendon defect, a wavy contoured echogenic strong tendon stump presents with the tendon stump in the rupture being clearly broader than the regular tendon (➤ Fig. 7.13 d, ➤ Fig. 7.14 c, ➤ Fig. 7.15 c).

In a **tendinitis**, the tendon is swollen and shows a halo that is an echo-signal deprived line in the slide bearing (➤ Fig. 7.13 c). The tendon becomes increasingly echogenic and often shows a fusiform swelling, e.g. in tendinitis of the Achilles tendon (➤ Fig. 7.16 c and d). A broadened fascia is found especially at the calcaneus insertion, similar to the patellar top syndrome, in fasciitis plantaris as cause for the plantar pain of the sole of the foot.

In a **bursitis**, we find an echo-deprived signal, evenly bordered structure between tendon and bone, e.g. at the insertion of the Achilles tendon.

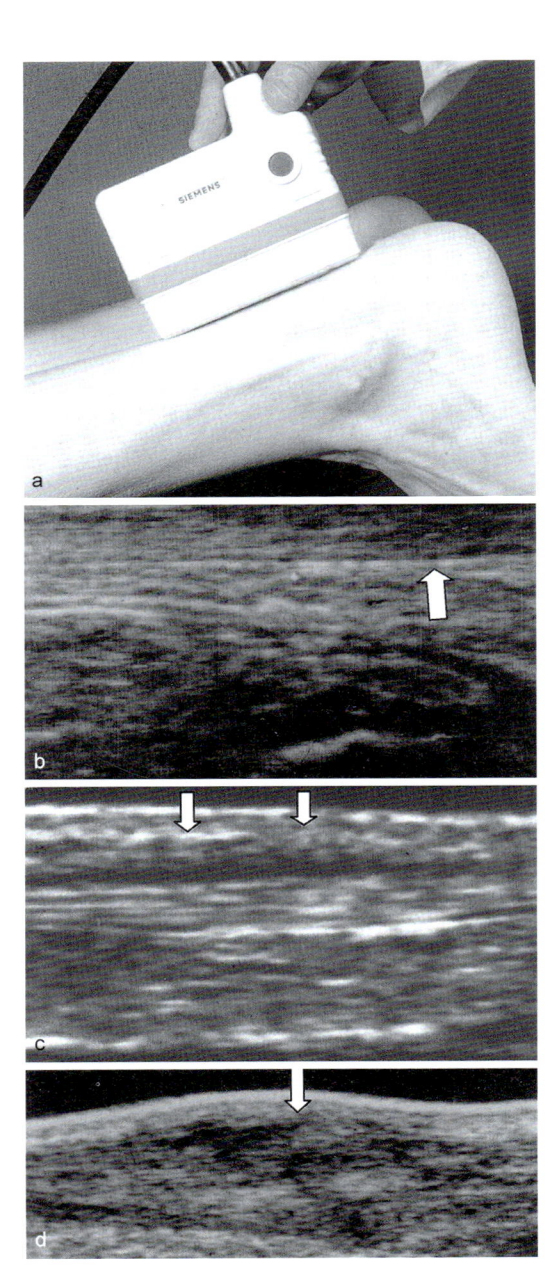

Fig. 7.16 Sonography of the foot: Achilles tendon.
a: transducer position. b: normal findings. c: peritendinitis. d: Achilles tendinitis/partial rupture.

Summary

Sonography allows focused access to soft-tissue structures of the locomotor apparatus; it links anamnesis and clinical examination with radiodiagnostics. Ultrasound examination has advanced new diagnosis but earlier, preliminary diagnosis often requires confirmation by imaging. This allows a focused therapy as early as possible. Follow-ups as well as healing results become more objective. Sonography of the locomotor apparatus is superior to MRT if using dynamic examination, lateral comparison, anamnesis, and clinical findings. Sonography convinces by its low costs and quick availability, and is of value for tendon and soft tissue diseases. MRT remains unrivaled intra-articular imaging, tumor diagnostics, and mass defects of the rotator cuffs. However, sonography is superior to MRT in muscle and tendon injuries.

The development of sonography at the locomotor apparatus still continues. The future lies in a further improvement of transducer resolution, a further differentiation of the soft-tissue findings considering vessels (Doppler sonography). This will further increase sensitivity and specificity of sonographic diagnostics.

References

Dumbs B, Kunz B (1990). Sonographie des Bewegungsapparates. Hans Huber Verlag, Bern.

Dondelinger RF (1996). Peripheral musculoskeletal ultrasound atlas. Thieme, Stuttgart.

Fornage BB (1988). Ultrasonography of muscles and tendons. Springer, Heidelberg.

Gerber AT et al. (2000). Sonographie des Bewegungsapparates. Thieme, Stuttgart.

Graf R, Schuler P (1995). Sonographie am Stütz- und Bewegungsapparat bei Erwachsenen und Kindern. 2nd ed. Chapman and Hall, London.

Gruber G, Konemann W (1997). Sonographie des Stütz- und Bewegungsapparates. Chapman and Hall.

Jerosch J, Marquart M (1993). Sonographie des Bewegungsapparates. Biermann Verlag, Zülpich.

Löffler L (1988). Ultraschalldiagnostik am Bewegungsapparat. Thieme, Stuttgart.

Löffler L (2001). Die sonographische Diagnostik der Kapselbandverletzung. Sportorthopädie, Sporttraumatologie 17: 148–152.

Löffler L (2005a). Die sonographische Diagnostik der Schulter. Sportorthopädie, Sporttraumatologie 21: 15–22.

Löffler L (2005b). Sonographie. In: Grifka J (ed.). Praxiswissen Halte- und Bewegungsorgane. Sportverletzungen – Sportschäden. Thieme, Stuttgart, p. 7–14.

Löffler L, Kayl W (1988). Überlastungsschäden der unteren Extremität durch Sport. Sportverletzungen – Sportschäden 2: 147–152.

Marcelies S, Daenen W, Ferrara MA (1996). In: Dondelinger RF (ed.). Peripheral musculoskeletal ultrasound atlas. Thieme, Stuttgart.

Reimers CD, Gaulrapp H (1988). Muskel- und Sehnensonographie. Deutscher Ärzte Verlag, Cologne.

Chapter 8

Projection radiography, magnetic resonance and computer tomography

Franz Kainberger and Claudia Schüller-Weidekamm

8.1 Sports medical demands

Motivated by the radiographic supervision at the Olympic Games (starting in Atlanta in 1996), imaging has been integrated into an interdisciplinary sports-medical supervision concept.

8.1.1 Indication

Radiographic examinations are key to traumatology and orthopedic supervision of top- athletes. The sport-specific imaging documentation of morphologic and functional abnormalities observed in training and physiotherapy is key.

Evidence-based referral criteria have been specified as standard by the EU (Referral Criteria) and the American College of Radiology (ACR-Appropriateness Criteria) (Frühwald et al. 2006, Loose et al. 2006). Furthermore, sport-specific referral diagnoses (➢ Tab. 8.1) can be framed. The way to better standards in patient supervision and a reduction of costs was demonstrated with the help of Canadian recommendations for primary care (Ottawa ankle and knee rules, etc.).

The primary examination mostly consists of conventional radiographs. Sonography (So) and magnetic resonance tomography (MRT) are used in increasingly – for example, in achillodynia – as primary procedures to directly represent tendon and muscle changes as well as internal joint changes.

For some radiographic indications (as at the spine), clinical "red flags" have been defined, which especially concern neurological signs or neoplasia-suspected palpable swellings.

Measures of therapy in the shape of imaging-controlled infiltration techniques are primarily carried out controlled by ultrasound in the case of complex anatomic relations or low-grade morphologic changes (Hall and Buchbinder 2004).

8.1.2 Examination Techniques

Almost all morphological findings are detectable on static radiographic, CT or MRT images. Functional tests on a regular basis, e.g. rotation in the humero-glenoid joint are possible with sonography. This applies similarly to other special problems such as at the wrist. MRT function studies are more extensive and therefore rarely used in practice. They are carried out either by stringing together static images of a movement that have been digitally post-processed (so-called pseudomovies) or by way of kinematic MR techniques ("MR radioscopy") with exceptional fast sequences.

In **projection radiography** (conventional radiographic images), digital procedures based on the principle of phosphor-storage-disc technology or by means of direct radiography are qualitatively superior to the traditional film/screen procedure because of the higher contrast and image post-processing. Also length and angle measurements are digitally more accurate than analog technology. Special projection technologies such as the Frik tunnel image at the knee joint, the "held" images of different joints under weight or different special images of the occipitocervical junction have been replaced successively by more significant tomographic technologies. Images made of a patient in standing position or in certain flexion positions (e.g. parade images of the patella) as well

Tab. 8.1 Sport-specific assignment criteria for projection radiography (X-ray), sonography (So), computer tomography (CT), magnetic resonance tomography (MRT) and nuclear medicine (NM). The order is defined as primary (P), continuative (C) or "after observation" (aO).

Question	Modality	Degree of recommendation	Commentary
tendon overstrain syndrome including tendon rupture	X-ray MRT	indicated (P) indicated (W) indicated (W)	sonography for tendovaginitis and tendopathies in achillodynia and other superficial tendons Additionally, X-rays for predisposed factors or malpositions of the axes, respectively
muscle rupture	So X-ray MRT	indicated (P) indicated (P) indicated (W)	Smaller hematomas can evade the sonography detection. Radiographies are sensitive for calcifications and avulsion MRT is best procedure for classification timely recognition of soft-tissue sarcomas by documentation of solid tissue parts, additional picture controlled preoperative biopsy, if necessary
ligament injury, impingement, joint trauma	X-ray So MRT	indicated (P) indicated (W) indicated (W)	radiographs for the diagnostic of malpositions including a bony impingement; in special cases, stress (tolerance) radiographs are expedient superficial ligaments will be directly presentable with high-resolution So MRT and possibly MR arthography are the most sensitive procedure for ligament injuries, osseous or soft-tissue impingement, meniscus or discus lesions, and cartilage damages
stress or insufficiency fracture	X-ray MRT CT NM So	indicated (P) indicated (W) indicated (W) indicated (W) indicated (W)	earliest detection with MRT by means of bone marrow edema and periosteal reaction bone scintigraphy primarily applicative for multiple fractures (also torture) sonography for the picture of cortical interruptions in special situations (e.g. rip fracture)
conventional fractures	X-ray CT MRT So	indicated (P) indicated (W) indicated (W) indicated (W)	survey radiograms in two layers, possibly supplemented by special radiographs such as the scaphoid series for suspected scaphoid fracture or oblique radiographs of the tibia head, constitute the basic examination CT is a tomographic examination with multiplanar picture MRT serves the demonstration of traumatic bone-marrow edemas by contusion ("bone bruises"), primarily sonography for projection-radiographically problematic findings, if complex tomogram-procedures are not available
occult fractures	X-ray MRT CT NM	indicated (P) indicated (W) indicated (W) indicated (W)	Fractures with clinically uncertain signs and projection- radiographically negative findings because of discrete radiographic signs that are not presentable as free of overlapping (such as at the rips) in a narrower sense, the un-shifted scaphoid fracture and other carpus fractures as well as the gomphosis of the fracture of the femoral neck
nerve-compression syndromes	So MRT X-ray	indicated (P) indicated (P) indicated (W)	for the picture of causative bony or expansive structures
vessel injuries	So CT MR angiography	indicated (P) indicated (P) indicated (W)	efficient first diagnosis with CT including CT angiography, in non-acute cases also with Doppler So MR angiography for intima damages with thrombosis that are often caused by overuse

as functional images of the spine in inclination and reclination still remain standard procedures. The radiation exposure of digital procedures constantly diminishes due to technological improvements. Compared to the film-based technologies, radiation is lower at the extremities and generally higher at the trunk. Criteria of the optimal imaging quality are an adequately sized examination area (including the neighboring joints or at the spine of the neighboring junction area, respectively), a good luminosity and – in order to save dose – a reduced signal-to-noise ratio at check-ups.

MRT has been established for practically all sport-specific syndromes as a procedure with highest diagnostic informative value given its excellent soft-tissue contrast. MRT is perfectly applicable for the imaging of osseous changes, especially of bone-marrow edemas. Picture documentation in all three spatial planes is carried out by default in all peripheral joints, with the exception of the hip. Contrast agents may be applied i.v. for inflammatory, expanding processes, and intra-articularly imaging in line with MR arthrography (Zanetti et al. 1999). The informative value of the MRT at acutely post-traumatic tissue swellings is limited give the diffuse edema formation (➢ Fig. 8.1). In general, devices with field strengths of 1.0–3 tesla (and high gradient field strengths, concomitantly) are used due to technological enhancements. Devices with lower field strength will achieve better results for numerous problems than projection radiography, sonography or CT. Physical limits are reached in terms of spatial resolution (acuity of signs), duration of the examination (and with that the rate of movement artifacts) as well as the size of the presentable field (field of view). The same applies to models with which an examination in standing position will be possible. 3-T devices have the advantage of a better spatial resolution, which mainly is of high advantage for cartilage presentation; on the other hand, they have the disadvantage of the higher extent of costs and examination. Several special sequences are available for the imaging of the hyaline cartilage, which have been developed towards an exact regional quantification (mapping) and a biochemical image analysis (especially with the dGEMRIC method). The invasive catheter angiography for diagnostic use has nearly completely been substituted by MR angiography together with Doppler sonography. A range of further MR technologies such as analysis of the oxygenation of muscle tissue is rarely used in practice. Contraindications for the MR examination are pace makers and other bio-stimulators, ferromagnetic contaminants as well as implants. With implants examination is only possible, if they are approved for the according field strength (more information under www.MRIsafety.com).

Computer tomography is carried out with multidetector technology. Because of the spatial, sub-millimeter resolution in all three space lay-

Fig. 8.1 Rupture of the tendon of the extensor digitorum longus muscle with fiber dehiscence and hematoma after a minor trauma (jogging) based on a hyperflexion trauma in playing volleyball, years ago. a: extensive posttraumatic soft-tissue edema on a T2-weighted fat-suppressed MRT picture with additional contusion edema of the ventral tibia edge (arrow). b: The dehiscence due to retracted curled fibers (arrow) are shown better in the corresponding sonographic picture. T = tibia.

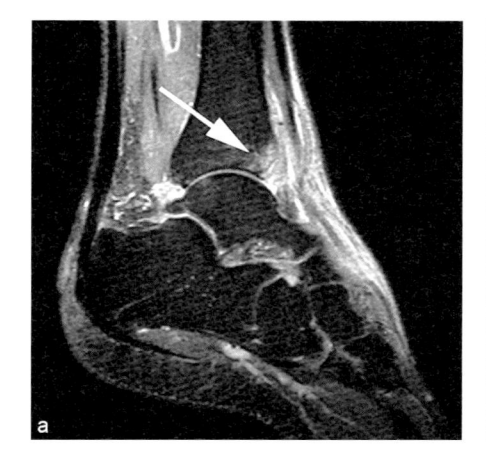

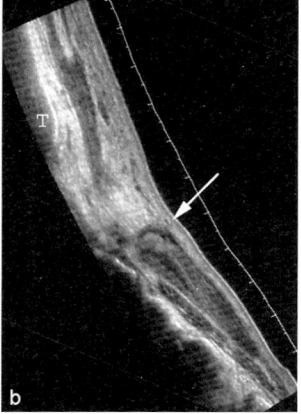

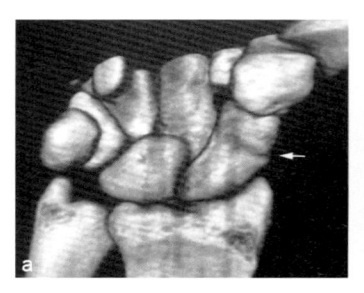

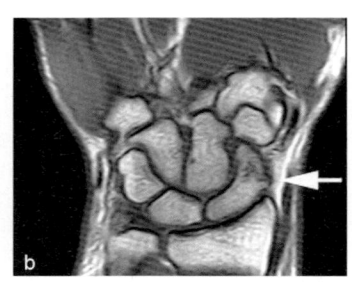

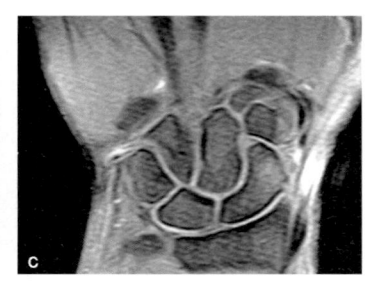

Fig. 8.2 Conventionally radiological occult scaphoid fracture. a: Discrete notched deformation (arrow) on a volume-reconstructed set of CT picture data. b: T1-weightedly, a spongy bone fracture (arrow) is to be found via MRT. c: T2-weighted MRT picture of a traumatic edema of the distal third.

ers, multi-planar layer slices and volume reconstructions can be generated (➤ Fig. 8.2). The spine and other skeleton segments can be examined from thoraco-abdominal and cranial CT examination in poly-traumatized patients. This avoids overview radiograms. The evaluation of such multidimensional image data sets requires experience. Metal artifacts are clearly lower, which allows post-operative implant check-ups. radiopaque material is administered intraarticular in CT arthrographies, which gives highly detailed resolution, if MR arthrographies (e.g. with carriers of pacemakers or implants) are contraindicated. CT-rotation error analysis is carried out by standardized cuts at the three large joint areas of the lower or, to less extent, at the upper extremity in lateral comparison. More sensitive detector systems have drastically reduced the exposure to radiation of a single slice image. However, the collective dose in Europe or North America continues to increase given the extended anatomic examinations and advanced indications.

The **measuring of bone density (osseous densitometry)** is indicated for persons with osteoporosis (underweight and endocrine disorders), but not for stress fractures that develop mainly due to training errors. Lowered density values have been reported for female gymnasts and ballet dancers, mostly with secondary amenorrhea. Conversely, the anabolic effect of weight training or fencing has been documented by densitometry. The dual energy x-ray absorptiometry (DXA) should be preferred over other densitometric procedures because of its higher degree of standardization, validation, and lower radiation exposition. Increasingly, DXA is applied in sports medicine to determine the body fat percentage ("body composition"), for instance for cross-country skiers (Larsson and Hendriksson-Larsen 2008). Alternatively (not in sports medicine, but for diagnostics of morbid adiposity), MRT is used for body fat diagnosis.

The vessel image with color Doppler sonography, MR or CT angiography is rarely used in sports medicine. Indications are cervical spine traumas (vertebral dissection), overuse damages such as ulnar artery hypothenar hammer syndrome of martial artists, or deep vein thrombosis of weight lifters or skiers, and anatomic variants (such as kink formation of the iliac arteries of cyclists).

8.1.3 Diagnostic consequences

The mostly three- to five-stepped quantification systems can be deviated from characteristic patterns of use as a result of direct or indirect macro or micro traumas.

Picture analysis of "movement chains"

Next to traumatic injuries, indirectly reacting strength vectors exist in so-called critical zones. They are part of one of the two large chains of movement ("kinetic chains") of the muscle skeleton system, the musculo-tendino-osseous or ligamentary-interosseous chain. The analysis of such changes, with or without neurovascular concomitant changes, provides the basis of a "radiographic status" of indirect sports damages or sports traumas. In the process, **cardinal symptoms ("footprints")** are not subject to an isolated interpretation, but mostly have to be interpreted in context with other concomitant changes. The risk of ruptures or fractures can be estimated based on extrinsic (extra corporal) and intrinsic parameters, whereupon radiographic examination results present important – because they are often directly ascertainably and also quantifiably – intrinsic factors. In further succession, image information of this kind can be used for sports-medical decisions to rehabilitation (avoiding the inadequate rehabilitation syndrome), in single cases also for the resuming of training ("return to play").

Tab. 8.2 Frequent and rare causes of pseudo-tumors of sportsmen.

- fat tissue necrosis after banal trauma
- foreign body reaction
- chronic hematomas
- inflammatory pseudo-tumor (pseudo-tumor in the narrower sense)
- Morel-Lavallée lesion of the proximal thigh (chronic hematomas after injury of fascia lata)
- myositis ossificans in the sub-acute phase (before the late phase with calcification)
- pseudo-aneurysms
- tumerous calcinosis

- **Malalignment:** axial aberrances are circumscribed or apply to several elements of one movement chain. The causes are congenital or gained (mostly traumatically) and affect mainly bones and ligaments. Avulsions involve bone marrow edemas or a traumatic usur with directly inserting ligaments (with fibrocartilaginous transition zone), with ligaments that irradiate indirectly into the periost with a continuing tear along the bone surface (sleeve lesion). In chronic status images, concomitant muscular atrophies can often be observed, which sometimes may escape the clinical examination.
- Any accumulation of liquids, especially **edemas and swellings**, **at tendons and muscles** indicates overuse reactions (above all, tendon overuse syndromes) or ruptures, respectively. They require MRT confirmation or projection-radiography, especially in the form of shadows of the fat lines or fat bodies. Solid processes of expansive character will mostly be **pseudo tumors**, but can also relate to rarely occurring malign tumors and require pre-operative biopsy. Pseudo tumors are mostly MRT incidental findings after a (not memorized) trauma and rarely have characteristic appearance (➤ Tab. 8.2). **Nerve entrapment syndromes** are diagnosed at predisposed places, mostly osteofibrose channels, by means of delicate edemas or fibrozation as well as an atrophy of the supplied musculature.
- At the joints, formations of effusions and synovial swellings are mostly degenerative and result of overuse. They can be recognized by MRT and sonography, with high sensitivity. The knee and upper ankle joint can also be visualized by projection radiography. Post-traumatic synovitis develops due to direct tears of mucosa with hemorrhage or incarcerations of the synovial plicae and is regarded as a chronic inflammatory secondary sign of a joint trauma. A post-traumatic synovitis can be diagnosed hardly by radiography (as opposed to arthroscopy). A joint effusion can also indicate a ligament rupture, provided that not only an extracapsular located ligament is affected.
- **At cartilaginous structures:** Overuse damages of fibrous-cartilaginous tissue of menisci or disci go along with damages of the dermatan or keratan sulfate side-chain collagenic fibers. These processes are observed by MRT given the higher content of chemically free hydrogen protons. At the hyaline cartilage, surface defects or inhomogeneities of the deeper layers or of the border lamella are not always detectable by arthroscopy. They can be quantified on the basis of the narrowing of the joint cavity or the cartilage ligament and the contrast changes, respectively.
- **At the bone, a bone marrow edema** is an important sign of overuse or of the injury. Bone marrow edema are also observed in oteonecroses, inflammations, neoplasias or neuropathies, and can be differentiated by localization, form and structure together with the clinical context. Traumatically caused bone contusions ("bone bruises") or avulsions are degenerated, subchondral edemas or early stage of osteonecrosis (bone-marrow edema syndrome) (➤ Fig. 8.2). At trauma, impaction edemas and avulsion edemas are differentiated based on

location and form. The latter are observed at tendon insertion points; their signal intensity depends on the severity of the acting force.

Differential diagnosis

Differential diagnoses of a sport damage or sport trauma are:

- Neoplasias of the bones (most often osteoid osteomas and Ewing's sarcoma) or soft tissue, mass lesions or osteodestructions
- Inflammatory rheumatic diseases, mainly seronegative spondylarthropathies (as Reiter's syndrome and other reactive arthritides), less often also infectious diseases
- Battered child syndrome suspected at every morphological unusual form of a trauma, especially if different anatomic regions or temporally asynchronous (recognizable by the callus formation) are affectedMetabolically conditioned changes, insufficiency fractures as consequence of osteoporosis or other demineralizing osteopathies, periarthropathically localized calcificating tendinitis (hydroxylapatite disease) of the rotator cuff or the trochanter region of the hip.

8.2 Tendons and muscles

8.2.1 Indication and examination

Sonography is the primary examination for painful functional limitations or sudden injuries; MRT is more in-depth information (➤ Fig. 8.1, ➤ Fig. 8.3 and ➤ Fig. 8.4). Additional information especially regarding calcifications, post-traumatic residues and a malalignment, can be gained by conventional radiograms. Special projection-radiographic procedures for the presentation of osteofibrose channels in the tangential path of rays, as the sulcus image of the proximal humerus or the carpal tunnel image, are imprecise and, as to the expressiveness of the different tomographic procedures, they have become unusual. Exercise tests after forced load are a special MR technique in order to document edemas, especially as an indication of a compartment syndrome. The thermography has sporadically been carried out in order to measure an over-

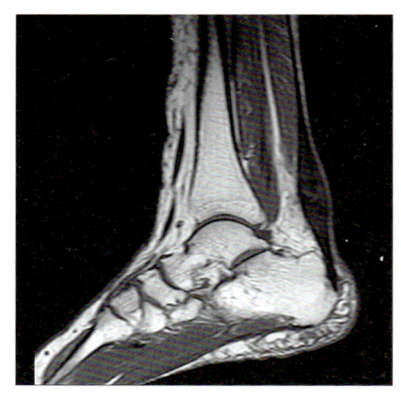

Fig. 8.3 High-grade tendinosis of the Achilles tendon with spindle-shaped swelling in the middle third (MRT).

use-conditioned development of heat of individual muscle groups and underlying training fields. No standardized indications have been described for the CT.

8.2.2 Radiographic diagnosis

Changes of the musculo-tendino-osseous movement chain run uniformly in all anatomic regions. In addition to changes due to direct force effect, points of special, mostly eccentric load after an extension movement (critical zones) are known as a result of indirect effects at many tendons and muscles, which require specific radiographic follow-up. A typical time interval with increased rupture risk can be defined (vulnerable phase), at least theoretically. With regard to age, the critical one at childhood age is located at the epiphyseal plate, at the age of adolescence it will be located at the apophysis, in active athletes of young grown-up age at the muscle, and at the degeneratively predamaged tendons starting with the third decade of life. Stage-like radiological image patterns may be deduced this way.

Tendon changes can be summarized under the term of **tendon overuse syndromes** (Kainberger et al. 2001).

- Earlier stages will be associated clinically with pains depending on movement; the radiographic examination is negative.
- Inflammations of the tendon gliding tissue will have to be observed with regard to the anatomic factors in the form of a ten-

8.2 Tendons and muscles

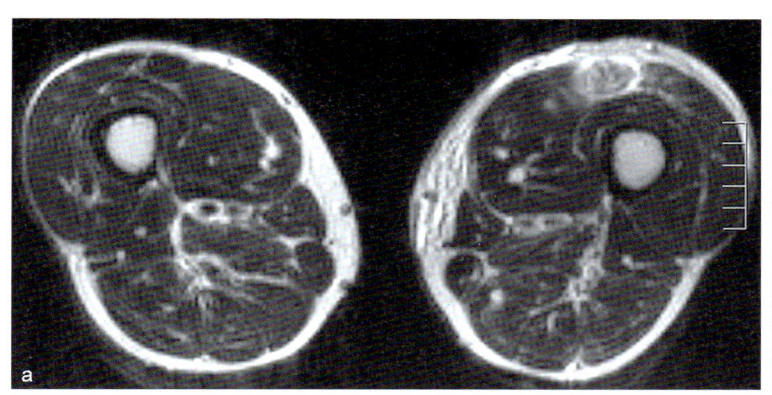

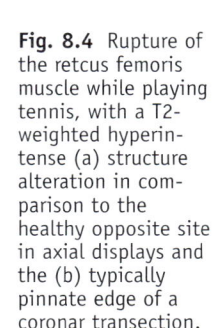

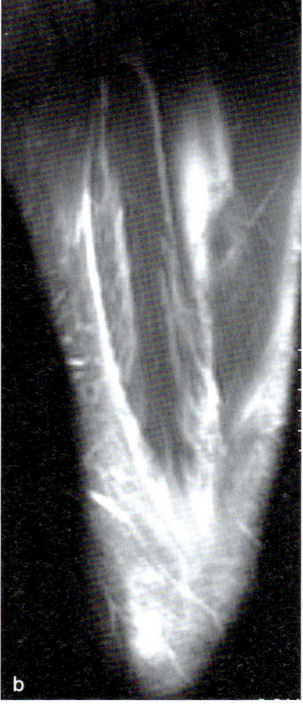

Fig. 8.4 Rupture of the retcus femoris muscle while playing tennis, with a T2-weighted hyperintense (a) structure alteration in comparison to the healthy opposite site in axial displays and the (b) typically pinnate edge of a coronar transection.

dovaginitis, peritendinitis or bursitis with edemas or effusions. In chronic stages, more or less distinct fibrous-marked reactions are found at the foot as tendovaginitis stenosans.

- Degenerative damages of the tendon tissue occur: 1) as tendinosis (> Fig. 8.3), i.e. micro-traumatically conditioned collagen fiber damages with a swelling, 2) in line of a compression syndrome (impingement) with structure inhomogeneities due to edema or necrosis zones (e.g. Haglund's deformity or impingement of the rotator cuff), or 3) as enthesiopathy (fibro ostosis) because of abnormal traction with edema and later traction osteophytes. Special forms of enthesiopathy at the age of adolescence will be the diverse apophysis lesions and the periostal desmoids (Nehrer et al. 2002). Osgood-Schlatter disease, apophysitis calcanei and the little leaguer's elbow with a liquid-filled bursitis and later irregular ossicles will count into the first category. The periostal desmoid, an irregularity that sometimes bears a striking resemblance to malign tumors with all imaging procedures or a subcortical lysis are mostly localized at the distal posterior femur metaphysic. The tendolipomatosis clinically asymptomatic special form of degeneration occurring at the quadriceps tendon and at the wrist.
- Ruptures with signs of dehiscence or of the hematoma can develop from tendinoses, in some regions also as a consequence of an impingement (Kannus and Josza 1991). Sonography and MRT contribute to the risk assessment of a rupture (Nehrer et al. 1997).

Signs of the hematoma are a radiological cardinal symptom in **muscle lesions** because of direct force effect (contusions). Strains or tears will develop because of indirect force effect; their "critical zones" of increased rupture risk are at the biarticular muscles of the lower extremities with strong bellies (rectus femoris muscle, semitendinosis muscle, etc). The "vulnerable phase" is mostly during the third decade of life because of excessive sports performance. Strains or tears may be graduated MRT, partly also by sonography:

- Mild forms ("first degree strains") are microfiber ruptures (less than 5%) associated with signs of the edema or "feathered" limited hematoma. Similar edemas have been described in addition to the microfiber ruptures with muscle soreness.
- Changes are distinct with forms of moderate degree ("second degree strains"), the partial ruptures (> Fig. 8.4).
- Serious third-degree forms or complete ruptures go along with a retraction of the torn fibers.

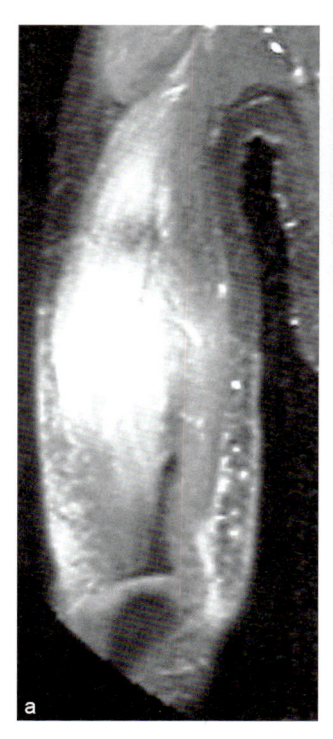

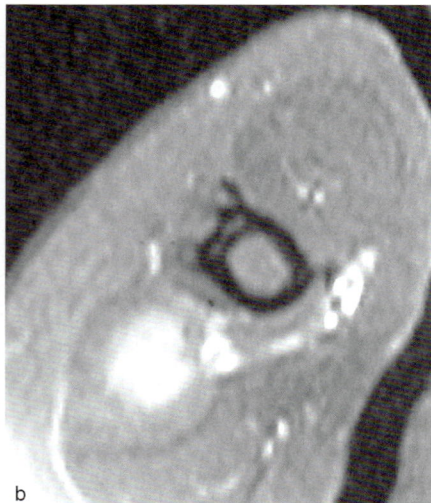

Fig. 8.5 Non-traumatic myositis ossificans at the humerus in stage 1, MRT picture. a: T2-weighted fat-suppression sequence. b: After administration of contrast medium.

- Congenital varieties, either as incidental findings, or accessory muscles, hypo- or aplasias going with clinical symptomatic: special examples are the soleus muscle accessories or a volume increase of the elbow musculature.

Special forms of muscle lesions:
- Hernias with a swell can be detected by sonography.
- Acute or chronic compartment syndromes with edema or volume increase.
- Neuronal loss due to neuropathy with fatty transformation of muscle tissue.
- The traumatic myositis ossificans proceeds in three stages: the acute (➢ Fig. 8.5) or pseudo-inflammatory, the subacute or pseudo-tumor, and the chronic phase.
- Chronic modular inflammatory reactions occurring after a rupture mostly at the rectus femoris muscle can be observed with the inflammatory pseudo-tumor (➢ Tab. 8.2). They can hardly be distinguished from malign neoplasias; they are distinguished by moderate enrichment of contrast medium (Boutin et al. 2002).
- A T2-weighted severely signal-intense liquefaction can be detected by MRT with rarely calcifying myonecrosis that may be conditioned traumatically, toxically or neurologically.

8.3 Neurons

Morphologic changes, such as chronic-relapsing inflammations are detectable around neurons, which today can be represented with high resolution, in sports-associated neuron entrapment syndromes. They are localized in osteo-fibrous channels or musculo-tendinous structures shaped in loops. The causal lesion, such as a post-traumatic malalignment, a neighboring nerve-compressing synovialitis of a joint or a tendon sheath, or a variety of close muscles or muscle tendon insertions is documented less often (➢ Tab. 8.3 a and b). Sonography (also called neuro-sonography here) and MRT are indicated as primary procedures.

The non-inflammatory form of the Parsonage-Turner syndrome is a compression syndrome at the shoulder typically found in volleyball players and other throwing athletes with constriction of the incisura scapulae. Mostly, painless infra-spinatus atrophy appears. Another phenomenon associated with throwing sports is the compression of the axillaris neuron by means of the quadrilateral space syndrome.

8.3 Neurons

Tab. 8.3 Radiographic characteristics of separate typical sports-associated neuron entrapment syndromes

a) Upper extremity

Nerve	Localization	Local changes	Muscular changes	Coordination of movements
supra-scapular nerve	spino-glenoid notch	post-traumatic osseous deformations	atrophy of the infra-spinatus muscle, muscle edema	repetitive forced movements, anterior shoulder luxations
	incisura suprascapularis	suprascapular ganglion (after tear of the labrum), swollen transversum scapulae ligament, hypertrophy of the subscapularis muscle	atrophy of the infra-spinatus and supraspinatus muscles	volleyball, rarely basketball
axilliary nerve	spatium axillare laterale (quadri-lateral space)	post-traumatic scars, ganglia, venous vessel plexus	atrophy of M. teres minor or M. deltoideus	throwing sports
ulnar nerve	sulcus of the ulnar nerve	edematous scars, swollen nerve, sulcus osteophytes	epitrochlearis muscle as norm variant	repetitive valgus flexion movements
	Guyon's canal	signs of inflammation in the shape of edemas or effusions	anomalies of the ulnar flexor musculature in the insertion area	hamulus fracture, overuse conditioned synovitis of the pisotriquetral joint
median nerve	distal humerus	Struthers' ligament	–	–
	pronator teres muscle	anomalies of the tendon insertions of superficial flexor digitorum muscle or the lacertus fibrosus	hypertrophy of the pronator teres muscle (global or one of the heads)	forearm pronation
	carpal tunnel	tendosynovitis of the flexor tendons, deformation of the nerve, vaulting of the retinaculum	proximal origin of the lumbricales muscles	flexion and grasping movements, repetitive forearm rotation running

b) Lower extremity

Nerve	Localization	Local changes	Muscular changes	Coordination of movements
sural nerve	fibula-sided distal calf	peritendinitis of the Achilles tendon, swollen fibula tendon vaginas, post-traumatic scars		running
posterior tibialis nerve	tarsal tunnel	post-traumatic deformations or scars, tendosynovitis	accessory muscles: flexor digitorum accessorius longus muscle, peronaeo-calcaneus internus muscle	running
plantar medial nerve	knot of Henry	signs of the hyperpronation or the hindfoot valgus, post-traumatic malpositions		jogger's foot

8.4 Bones

8.4.1 Indication and examination

Fractures are primarily clarified projection-radiography and MRT. Occasionally, a periostal hyper-vascularized callus formation is detected by sonography. The bone scintigraphy, which has primarily been considered sensible for the detection of stress fractures is rarely indicated (➤ Tab. 8.1). Also the DXA is generally not indicated. For the exact fracture classification, CT is still helpful, the same as it is for the detection of the osseous knitting.

8.4.2 Radiographic diagnosis

The **classic (high-energy) fractures** can generally classified according to their degree:

- Bone contusions ("bone bruise") accompanied by bone marrow edema – the edema by impaction and edema by avulsion
- Cancellous bone fractures (at compression)
- Fissures and fractures in the actual sense with cortical interruption
- Post-traumatic osteolysis are old osseous stress reaction, e.g. in weight lifters at the acromial end of the clavicula.

Stress fractures typically result from increased traction or flexion (compression). Direct osseous stress is rare (e.g. hamulus or other hand bones in golfing). Compression-conditioned stress (e.g. at the tibia plateau) and muscular-traction-conditioned forms (due to fatigue of the agonist muscle, e.g. at the os pubis) are more common (Chevrot et al. (1998). According to the Wolff's law, every change in form and function of a bone changes the interior architecture and exterior configuration. MRT should be carried out with thin slices. Bone marrow edema are early and cardinal symptoms showing the strongest intensity at the fracture line and decrease proximal or distal (➤ Fig. 8.6). Painless, stress conditioned bone marrow edemas are frequent and temporary adaption (e.g. in joggers or after the removal of a plaster cast). It recovery without interrupting sporting activities is possible, as long as no changes are detected on T1-weighted images (Arendt and Griffith 1997). However, entheseal stress edemas are bad prognostic sign (with a high probability terminating a sports career). Bone scintigraphy or positron emission tomography (PET) measure activity of the osteoblasts and, hence, bone reaction to a micro-trauma are positive signs with slight timely retardation (Steingruber et al. 2002). A fracture line or callus formation can be detected with conventional x-ray and CT or MRT. Therefore, stress fractures can be classified by MRT (➤ Tab 8.4; Anderson and Greenspan 1996, Fredericson et al. 2006). To understand whether an unspecific bone marrow edema is an early stress reaction without fracture or a not yet malign tumor, correlation with clinical, sport-specific risk factors is indispensable.

8.5 Spine

8.5.1 Indication and radiographic examination

Predominantly, it comes to traumatic lesions at the cervical spine (CS), in acute situations a CT should be carried out without time delay. First, the indication for MRT will arise from neurologic symptomatology, secondly from indications to discoligamentary hyper extension injuries, and thirdly from a suspected vertebralis dissection. Overuse damages will be found alongside at the thoracic and mainly the lumbar spine (LS). The distinction of the very frequent myalgias or of the unspecific gluteal pain will not always be easy for the radiographic clarification; "red flags" of clinical diagnostics (e.g. neurological deficits) have been described as helpful.

Fractures often develop in the frame of a hyperflexion-hyperextension trauma and present the most frequent indication at the cervical spine promoted by trend sports with jump movements or high speeds (motor sports, kite surfing, and others). They are examined in the acute phase via CT under non-emergency-based conditions with conventional x-rays as primary procedure. At the CS, special attention is paid to the complete examination area; amendatory pictures with elevated arm or with oblique path of rays are made in case of overlap by shoulder soft-tissue.

8.5 Spine

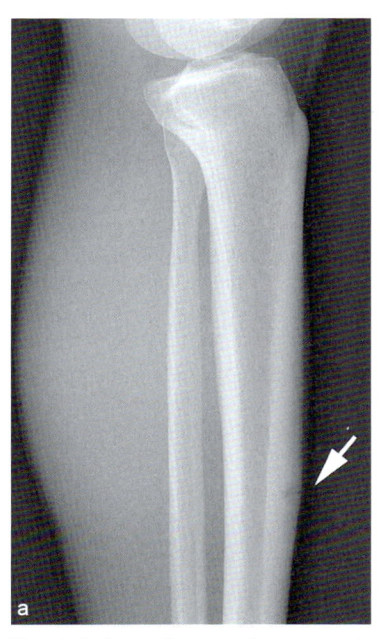

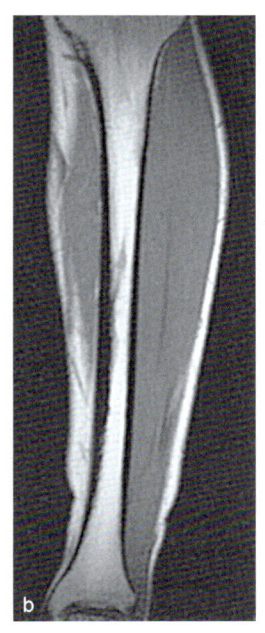

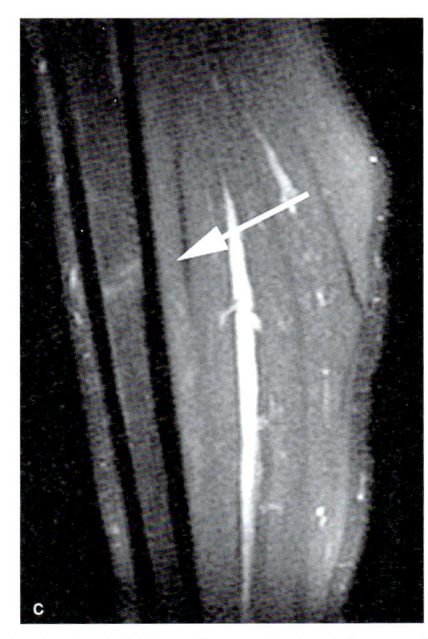

Fig. 8.6 Stress fracture of a soccer player. a: Conventional radiological, clearly visible swollen cortical substance of the tibia. b: A rather vertically oriented edema is shown by MRT. c: Horizontal fracture line (arrow) that will be visible in MRT after some weeks.

Tab. 8.4 Classification of stress fractures (according to Arendt and Griffiths 1997).

Degree	Conventional x-raying	MRT
normal	w.d.	w.d.
1	w.d.	STIR +
2	w.d.	STIR + T2w +
3	benign periosteal reaction	T1w and T2w + STIR without cortical interruption
4	benign periosteal reaction or interruption	T1w and T2w with fracture line

w.d. = without distinctiveness

Trauma complications in form of **neurological damages**, hematoma of the cervical bone marrow, lesions of the plexus brachialis, rarely also injuries of the vertebralis vessels, all require MRT clarification and/or angiography.

Osseous stress reactions in form of spondylolysis at the caudal spinal cord is most frequently detected in athletics, dancing and other activities with lumbar hyperextension. Conventional survey and function radiograms are the primary examination; an additional spotfilm of the lumbosacral junction or oblique images can be requested in case of unclear findings (➤ Fig. 8.7). MRT distinguishes an acute stress reaction of chronic congenital shape that requires quick treatment for adolescents with lower back pain, for adults facing a planned fusion surgery, and for the detection of possible additional herniated discs. The diagnosis can be made with CT; healing processes can additionally be documented with the help of the osseous bridging. Stress fractures of the os sacrum are rare and can be found in excessively practiced running, basketball or volleyball, and also in aerobics (excessive load transmission from axial skeleton to the lower extremity). MRT is the imaging method of choice; survey radiograms are often negative (Sommer et al. 2003).

Invertebral disks, ligament and joint injuries, interspinal ligament lesions and ruptures of facet joints are often connected with abrupt rotation movements or a hyperflexion in adolescent athletes. The MRT is the method of choice.

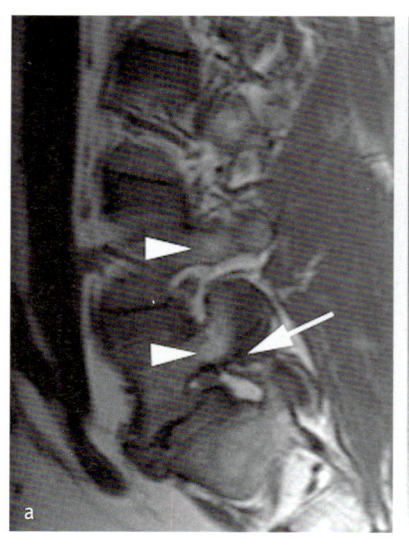

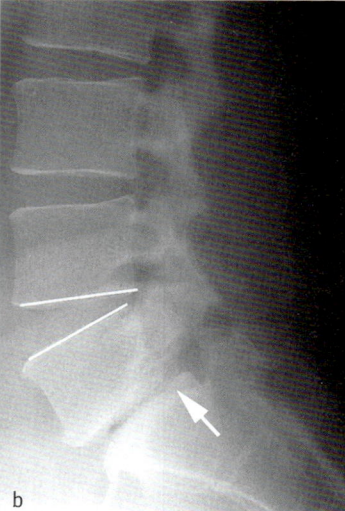

Fig. 8.7 Spondylolysis. a: MRT detected lysis fissure (arrow) and degenerative yellow-bone-marrow conversion (arrow heads) in the pedicles of L5 and, to a lesser extent, also L4. b: Beside the anterolisthesis degree I, an increased detachment of the discus area L4/L5 (line marking) is seen at the opposite of the degeneratively narrowed lumbosacral motion segment (inclination picture).

Overuse of the sacroiliac joints resulting from asymmetric exercise can be detected by radiography. Edemas, hypertrophies of the piriformis muscle (piriformis syndrome), or leg length discrepancy are detected and quantified by MRT. Subchondral edemas of a sacroiliac joint are common and should not be confused with a rheumatic sacroiliitis.

Conventional overview and function radiographs are indicated as primary examination for **degenerative secondary damages**; follow-up by MRT is recommended.

8.5.2 Radiographic diagnosis

The effect of high kinetic energies and high muscle strengths on spinal movement is central to gymnastics, monotone-repetitive patterns in rowing, or asymmetric force effects in golf and cricket. **Spinal Injuries** should be classified by the following three **criteria** (Mintz 2004):

- Instability (fracture classification according to Magerl, ligament ruptures of the posterior elements)
- Impingement (neutral or vascular structures)
- Impairment (functional loss, mostly pain-conditioned with potential chronic-degenerative damages)

The assessment of the "spinal capacity", i.e. opening width of the spinal canal is essential for the estimation of **impingement** since congenital or idiosyncratic narrowness increase damages of the bone marrow or spinal verves (➤ Fig. 8.8). Bone marrow contusions are associated to stenoses. Disco-ligamentous hyperextension injuries are visible in MRT as T2-weighted, hyperintense edema. The three stages (partial rupture of the annulus fibrosus, ruptures of the longitudinal ligaments and posterior ligament and joint capsule ruptures) can be differentiated by high-resolution technology.

Congenital malformations and junction disorders require radiographic differentiation from syndromes. Cervical fused vertebras in Klippel-Feil syndrome, occipito-cervical assimilated vertebra and variants of os odontoideum are contra-indications for contact and other sports. Lumbosacral assimilated vertebra or diverse mild "junction disorders" may lead to later degenerations. An incomplete closing of the topmost sacral segment is often associated with spondylolysis.

Spondylolysis, apophysis, and scoliosis are characteristics of **overuse damages**; accelerated growth ("growth spurt") contributes to their development.

Spondylolysis develops at the beginning school age and is mostly localized at the fifth lumbar vertebra, rarely in higher and other vertebras.

Fig. 8.8 Incomplete quadriplegia after fall in a tennis match with a hit of the back of the head against the boards. a: CT, no bone trauma but constitutionally narrow spinal channel with additional narrowing by dorsal spondylophytes. b: MRT hyperintense bone marrow contusion and contusion edema of the vertebral bodies at the same height.

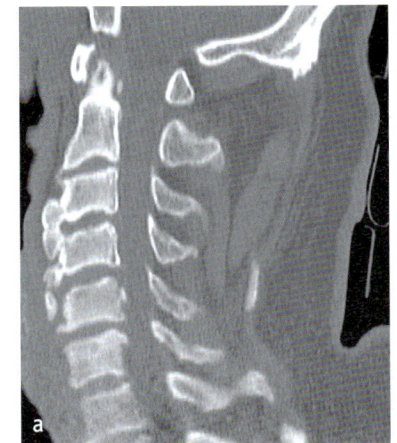

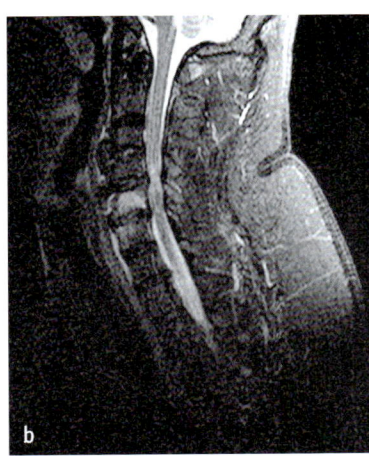

Multisegmental forms are detected as well. A congenital dystrophy of the lumbosacral junction is one of the causes (Vialle et al. 2005) and detected by radiography. The confirmation of an interruption vertebral arch in a LaChapel's dog figure (also called "Scotty dog") requires CT confirmation. Regarding therapy and prognosis, an early phase with good prognosis is distinguished from a late phase in which the opening of the spondylolysis fissure is more than 3 mm. Signs of hypermobility can be detected by functional x-rays (Engelhardt et al. 1997). In further succession, an isthmic spondylolysthesis (vertebral gliding) can develop; and is graduated into four stages (by the sagittal diameter of the vertebral body below) according to Meyerding.

Apophyseal damages are observed as microfractures of the deck plates of the vertebral body or as atypical Scheuermann's disease especially in power athletes, skiers and track-and-field athletes (Ogon et al. 2001).

Intervertebral disk damages are found in young sportsmen, while a height reduction of the disk space and a hypointense dehydration of the nucleus pulposus is recognized on T2-weighted MRT images as early signs. Conventional X-rays in ante or retro flexion position documents segmental movement disorders in hyper- or hypo-mobility or instability.

8.6 Shoulder

8.6.1 Indication and examination

Sonography or MRT continuously monitor **tendopathy of the rotator cuff**, which is often triggered by an impingement.

At the **instability**, MRT and MR-arthrography are required for pre-operative clarification, while present effusion after recent trauma can serve as "natural contrast medium". At the MR-arthrography, image sequences are taken in three layers in dorsal position of the patient – axial, parallel, and vertically on the scapular layer. Additional images are required with the arm set in ABER (abduction and external rotation) position.

CT is a useful tool for classification of **fractures**. CT is also indicated in specific cases for therapy planning of calcifying tendinitis. Often a standardized trauma-series (true a.p. projection tangential-glenoidal, true lateral projection transscapular, axial-axillary projection and a.p. picture of the humerus in inward and outward rotation) is made by projection-radiography.

For the **acromioclavicular joint**, conventional survey images are useful together. In addition, anterior-posterior pictures under traction of the arms are important for the recognition of any instability at the post-traumatic state.

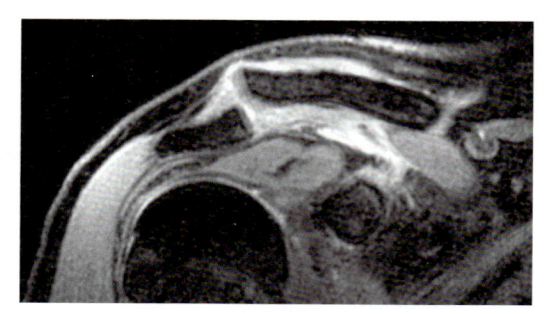

Fig. 8.9 Traumatic rupture of the AC joint with rupture of coracoclavicular ligament (MRT).

8.6.2 Radiographic diagnosis

At the rotator cuff, tendinosis and later ruptures develop after increased or asymmetric traction forces, an impingement, or both.

Acute irration of the tendon synovium is often a consequence of forced training and presents with small liquid accumulations in the bursa subdeltoidea and in the humeroglenoidal joint.

At **impingement**, interpretation of tendon radiological findings needs consideration of the environmental structures:

- The subacromial impingement can be estimated by conventional radiograms exactly adjusted in the anteroposterior path of rays (with the central ray bent craniocaudally by 20° at the tangentially hit glenoid) and on the basis of the subacromial opening (normal value >1 cm). The morphology of the acromion is categorized in three forms (even, bent, and hook-shaped) according to Bigliani. However, reproducibility of radiographs and MRT is moderate. Moreover, the bent of the acromion to lateral (acromial downslope with type A < 10° and type B > 10° according to MacGillivray) and the osteophytes are assessed subacromial or at the acromioclavicular (AC) joint. A raised stand of the humerus head indicates rupture of the rotator cuff. Changes of the rotator cuff can be classified by MRT according to Neer.
- Rare forms of the subchondral impingement, structural disorders of the subscapular tendon or post-traumatic, disposition-conditioned deformation of the coracoids process are found.
- The postero-superior glenoidal impingement, also called internal impingement, occurs in throwing sports and is accompanied by tendon, the joint capsule and the humerus head edema in the junction zone of the supraspinatus to the infraspinatus tendon and are detectable by MRT.
- In contrast to these "absolute" compression forms, "relative" impingement in bodybuilders can be found with a gain of rotator cuffs volume, often intensified by anabolics.

Degenerative tendon changes are detected by sonography or MRT most often as tendinoses in the shape of heterogeneous structural inhomogeneities in the central segment of the supraspinatus tendon. This tendon is 15 mm wide in the ventrodorsal diameter (Teefy et al. 2000). Insertion degenerations with osteophytes at the tuberculum majus are associated with a rupture of the rotator cuff in 75% (Wohlwend et al. 1998).

Ruptures of the rotators are classified or quantified as follows:

- At partial ruptures, a circumscribed central, profound or superficial defect is present. Concomitant degenerative osteophytes are detected in the vicinity. A thinning can be observed by MR-arthrography, though only with joint-sided profound forms.
- At complete rupture, the degree of severity is specified by the extent of the gap. Small (<1 cm), moderate (1–3 cm), large (3 to 5 cm), and massive (>5 cm) gaps are differentiated (Stoller et al. 2004). They will develop mostly chronically, rarely acutely, typically at excessive outward rotation of the arm.
- PASTA (partial supraspinal tendon avulsion) lesions are a special form of overuse at the supraspinal tendon, which is exposed to strong mechanical forces.
- Osteochondral lesions of the humerus head at the junction between caput and tuberculum majus may develop by friction stress and will be marked by a circumscribed subchondral edema with mostly profound partial rupture.
- At the subscapular tendon, ruptures and degenerations are often accompanied by edematous swelling. Luxation of the long biceps tendon caused by the roof-forming subscapular tendon of the sulcus intertubercularis requires special attention.

Long endurance tendon ruptures are often associated with atrophy of the affected muscle belly. The supraspinatus muscle is particularly vulnerable to atrophy, which can be quantified by MRT or sonography. The degree of severity is based on the shape changes (convex = normal, flattened = moderate atrophy, concave-subsided = severe atrophy). An alternative classification developed by Goutallier applies to the fat content of the atrophied muscle (0 = no intramuscular fat, 1 = some fatty streaks, 2 = less fat than muscle tissue, 3 = gat equal to muscle tissue, 4 = more fat than muscle tissue; Goutallier et al. 1994).

Changes in the rotator interval and in the sulcus intertubercularis are characteristic for the **long biceps tendon**:

- Interval lesions trigger ruptures of the neighboring supraspinal and subscapular tendon with post-traumatic, hemorrhage-induced synovitis. Subcoracoid bursitis is a typical concomitant finding.

- Microinstability summarizes irritant conditions in rotator vicinity and mostly result from a capsule insufficiency of the superior or medial glenohumeral ligaments and come with edema and small tears of the tendons or labrum (Stoller et al. 2004).

- Hidden lesions are insufficiencies of the musculoligamentary "roof" of the sulcus intertubercularis accompanied by a medial subluxation of the biceps tendon, which are recognizable by circumscript edemas (Bennett 2001). A dislocation of the biceps tendon can develop and comes with extensive synovitis or effusion.

- Tendinoses, partial, and complete ruptures of the long biceps tendon are often difficult to diagnose without clinical correlation. Typically, they come with degenerative changes within the osteofibrose canal (biceps tendon pulley).

The long-term consequences of a luxation are detected best by MR arthrography. The articular labrum, the glenohumeral ligaments and the shape of joint bodies can be detected; the assessment of the hyaline cartilage remains difficult. SLAP lesion and labral cysts are special labrum ruptures (➤ Tab. 8.5) in addition to the most frequently found cartilaginous or osseous Bankart lesions. The HAGL lesion (humeral avulsion of the inferior glenohumeral ligament) is the best-known capsule rupture and is detected as J-formed ligament defect at coronal MR images.

Degenerative changes with erosions and subchondral cysts or sclerosings are found at the **AC joint**; this can be the case for weight lifters in massive-destructive form with osteolyses. traumatic capsule ruptures and can be documented by high-resolution MRT; this often identifies coracoclavicular ligament ruptures.

Tab. 8.5 Forms of SLAP lesions (superior labrum anteroposterior), whose development will also be influenced by form variants of labrum articulare (Stoller et al. 2004).

I	degenerative plucking apart
II	ablation of the biceps anchor
III	basket handle tear of the labrum without defect of the biceps tendon anchor
IV	basket handle tear of the labrum reaching into the biceps tendon anchor
V	Bankart lesion that dissects the labrum up to the biceps tendon anchor
VI	unstable radiate ruptures or flap tear with complete ablation of the biceps trendon
VII	SLAP lesion that reaches into the middle glenohumeral ligament
VIII	type-II-SLAP lesion reaching into the posterior labrum
IX	complete circumference of the rupture comprising the labrum

8.7 Elbow

8.7.1 Indication and examination

Conventional radiographs are the primary examination of this complex joint (trochoginglymus). Different inflammatory and degenerative sports damages can be recorded directly via sonography and MRT (Steinbach et al. 1997, Miller 1999).

- **Lateral epicondylitis** associated with overhead movements (tennis elbow, also with golfers, rowers and at diverse leisure-time activities such as gardening or needle-work)

are the main reason. The radial collateral ligament is intensely stretched during the whole flexion movement.
- the **medial epicondylitis** (golfer's elbow, thrower's elbow) and the laterally localized osteochondritis dissecans (with gymnasts and throwers)
- **damages around the olecranon** (posterior tennis elbow, hyperextension syndrome or student's elbow)
- **ventral overuse reactions** (with bodybuilders and weight lifters) often occur at the distal biceps tendon. Clinical assessment can be impeded at partial rupture and a local edema or if the lacertus fibrosus is still intact.

Generally, patients are examined in dorsal position with medium- and high-field MRT.

The CT is used in case of complex fractures and dislocations, as this is the case with fractures of the coronoid process or with lateral instabilities.

8.7.2 Radiographic diagnosis

The **lateral epicondylitis** at the carpi radialis brevis muscle (ECRB) is an edema, inflammatory reaction even long time after clinical improvement. Edema can be differentiated from granulation tissue (associated with worse clinical outcome) by administration of contrast medium (Steinborn et al. 1999; ➤ Tab. 8.6). A traction osteophyte is detected at late stage disease on conventional radiographs . An inflammatory-frazzled radiocapitular meniscoid is detected by MRT. Degenerative changes of the annular ligament and a consecutive lateral instability are only indirectly (e.g. laterodorsal effusion) detectable by radiography. A traumatic

Tab. 8.6 Stadia of the epicondylitis lateralis humeri (ECRB = M. extensor carpi radialis brevis; Stoller et al. 2004).

I	reversible inflammation
II	irreversible damage at the origin of the ECRB muscle
III	rupture at the insertion tendon of the ECRB muscle
IV	secondary changes with fibrosis or calcifications, respectively

Tab. 8.7 Stadia of the osteochindrosis dissecans (Stoller et al. 2004).

I	hyaline cartilage faultless
II	stable lesion: prominent separation best with radiopaque material enhancement
III	unstable lesion: liquid in the separation belt (best detectable arthrographically)
IV	ablated fragment (corpus librum)

rupture at the proximal part of the lateral ulnar collateral ligament (LUCL) with dorsal subluxation of the radius and a clinically measurable pivot shift phenomenon is observed at the posterolateral rotator instability according to O'Driscoll. The LUCL, which inserts dorsally at the crista supinatoria of the proximal ulna shaft and is compared to the anterior knee joint ligament, is part of the radial collateral ligament complex together with the radial collateral ligament, which will reach to the annular humeral ligament, and the accessory collateral ligament.

An **osteochondritis dissecans**, called Panner's disease with occurrence in childhood age, is observed at the capitulum humeri, an area scarcely supplied with blood, as a consequence of increased lateral pressure stress (➤ Tab. 8.7). A subchondral stress edema with osteochondral tissue damage is a leading symptom; corpora libra can be observed rarely.

The **medial epicondylitis** (➤ Fig. 8.10) is part of a degenerative valgus stress overload (VSO)

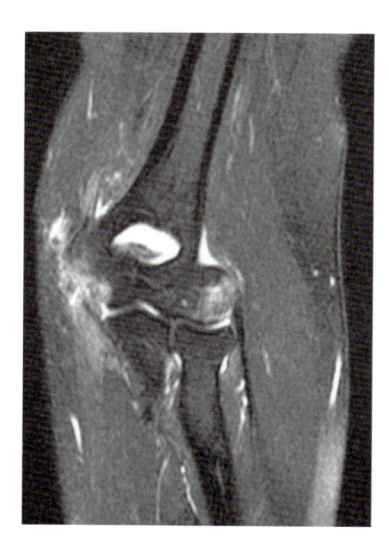

Fig. 8.10 Rupture of the medial collateral ligament with collateral contusion edema of the capitulum humeri (MRT).

syndrome with medial traction and lateral pressure stress, and it will primarily apply to the middle of the anterior bundle of the three-bundled medial collateral ligament, which inserts medially from the coronoid process at the sublimis tubercle. Formations of edemas and later degenerative-inflammatory changes or defects dominate the radiographic image, in severe cases accompanied by stress-conditioned regional synovialitis within a small recessus under this ligament. An edema, a partial rupture or a hypertrophy with compartment syndrome is observed at the pronator teres muscle as a consequence of excessive rotation movements such as in golfing. Overuse reactions with subchondral edema and later possibly with cysts are observed laterally as a consequence of the valgus stress. The little leaguer's elbow, a traction apophysitis of the epicondylus medialis with a ligament-formed bone marrow edema develop due to valgus stress. Overuse reactions along the ulnar nerve, which can be subjected to large traction as well as a compression and subluxation within the cubital tunnel, is detected by edema formations (MRT) or by dynamic sonography. Sometimes a thick-bellied anconeus epitrochlearis muscle causes the ulnar compression on MRT images. Rare triceps tendon ruptures are recognized best by complete dehiscence in flexed position.

A **bursitis olecrani**, e.g. as consequence of a direct trauma, or a fibroostosis at the insertion point of the triceps muscle with or without traction osteophytes (olecranal spur) mostly is associated with repetitive hyperextension movements. Corpora libra will be found with higher probability in the fossa olecrani, as a consequence of an osteochondrosis dissecans, a synovial chondromatosis or a released arthrotic capsule osteoma. They may easily be overlooked on radiographs because of their position in deepness of the fossa. They must be distinguished from a rare os supratrochleare in the insertion zone of the triceps tendon.

Ventrally localized changes will mainly apply to the **distal biceps tendon** positioned superficially to the brachialis muscle, which inserts complexely at the tuberositas radii and at the muscle aponeurosis (lacertus fibrosus). **Hematomas after a tendon rupture** can be mistaken as a pseudotumor. An increased filling pressure of a swollen bicipito-radial bursa can cause a compression of the posterior interosseous nerve. In rare cases, certain muscle hypertrophies can cause ventral neuron compression syndromes: the directly medially positioned pronator teres muscle at the median nerve, and the dorsally positioned supinator muscle, which circularly surrounds the radius with its insertion tendon, the Frohse's arcade, at the radial nerve. The changes are discrete (with stagnant soft-tissue edemas and an atrophic volume reduction of the affected muscles) on MRT pictures.

8.8 Hand

8.8.1 Indication and examination

Radiographs belong to the primary examinations of the hand (except tendon changes).

- Soft-tissue, overuse damages of larger tendons or tendon sheaths are readily detected by MRT. Vessel stenoses, vasospasm or thromboses of hypothenar hammer syndrome are detectable by MR angiography.
- Exactly adjusted, conventional radiographs readily detect carpal instabilities. Midcarpal instability can be diagnosed by transillumination and are helpful to prove a click phenomenon. Ligament lesions are detected by MRT and MR arthrography.
- Conventional radiographs are taken of osseous injuries and sports damages in the shape of degenerations or osteonecroses require exact adjustment for the detection of instabilities. A four-parted radiograph series (scaphoid quartet) is produced for the os scaphoideum positioned obliquely in every spatial level.

8.8.2 Radiographic diagnosis

Radial-sided stress phenomena mostly triggered by excessive grasping movements in throwing sports, rowing (oarman's wrist) or diverse leisure-time activities (gardening, etc.), are:

- Morbus de Quervain affects tendons of the abductor policis longus muscle or the extensor policis brevis muscle at the first (radial) tendon. Tendon swellings are observed in addition to a characteristic effusion of

the tendon sheath. The thicker tendon of the abductor pollicis longus muscle can contain several fascicles surrounded by hyperintense connective tissue and should not be confused with a tendinosis.
- The intersection syndrome is characterized by soft-tissue edema of the distal forearm, which is triggered by excessive flexion-extension movements. The trigger point is proximally (some inches) of the Lister's tubercle, where the muscles of the second tendon drawer (extensors radialis longus and brevis muscles) cross with the first ones.

Ulnocarpal stress phenomena or posttraumatic status in this so-called ulnocarpal area are:
- The ulnocarpal impaction goes along with acute or chronic mechanical stress signs as edema or sclerosis, especially at the ulnar-sided os lunatum. Concomitantly, ulnar heading or ulna-minus variant can be present. Changed signal intensity of the hyaline cartilage coat or of the central discus articularis signal degenerative sequels.
- Lesions of the discus triangularis and its suspension apparatus are diagnosed by MRT; thin coronary layer conduction can be helpful. Since 1989, they have been classified into a traumatic (class 1 with ulnar or radial avulsion or a central laceration, respectively) and a degenerative form, developing in the frame of an ulnocarpal impaction (class 2 with a neighboring chondromalacia) (➤ Fig. 8.11). Contrary to the asymptomatic radial-sided communicating defects, ulnar-sided discus lesions are clinically relevant in 50% of the cases. They should not be confused with ligamentum subcruentum within the interior of the discus, which will be broader here (Pfirrmann and Zanetti 2005). MR-arthrography will be the most certain measure for diagnosis.
- The tendovaginitis of the extensor carpi ulnaris muscle develops as a consequence of repetitive ulnar abduction movements or due to subluxation brought forward by an ulna-minus variant. All stages of tendon overuse – in rare cases up to a rupture – are observed via sonography or MRT. A central rotund hyperintensity, which is formed by an intratendinous septum continuing from both muscle bellies, must not be misinterpreted as degeneration (Pfirrmann and Zanetti 2005).

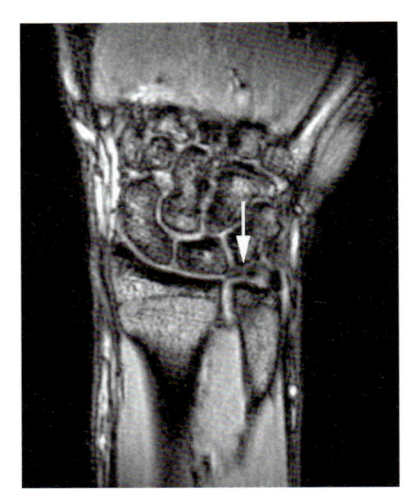

Fig. 8.11 Traumatic rupture of the triangular discus in its central segment (arrow), to be classified as 1A according to Palmer (MRT).

- Overloading of the distal movement chain of the flexor carpi ulnaris muscle, which will cover the insert tendon at the os pisiforme, the pisohamate ligament and the hamulus to the basis of the ulnar metacarpalia, with regional inflammation signs in close neighborhood of the ulnar neuron and its distribution. Instability of the os pisiforme is typical.
- The traumatic distal radioulnar joint instability is hard to diagnose by conventional-radiology, easiest on strictly laterally adjusted images. A deformation of the sigma-formed radial joint surface has been described as characteristic on axial CT images. Additionally, ruptures of the ligaments are recognized by MRT.

Among the traumatic carpal instabilities, the scapholunary (SL) dissociation is the most frequent form, triggered by an intercarpal-ulnar or -supinaotry movement. As with other instabilities, a malalignment, especially in the shape of a joint cavity expanded to more than 3 mm between os scaphoideum and os lunatum (Terry-Thomas sign) is observed on conventional radiographs. A direct detection of a ligament rupture is possible by MRT in special thin layers or by MR arthrography. The typical three-layer framework with the according broader dorsal and the volar part that is most important for stability as well as a small central part, which has the SL the same as the lunotriquetral ligament and requires exclusion of false positive findings. The SL dissociation is the mildest form of the perilunar instabilities, whose other phenotypes can be diagnosed directly via MR as a continuing effusion or irregular and thinned ligament structures. Due to chronic stress of the SL ligament, a subchondral cyst can develop in the ligament insertion area of os lunatum (Stäbler et al. 2000).

For **fractures**, MRT signs of hematomas and the detection of a fracture line are typical (➤ Fig. 8.2). Hamulus avulsions at the os hamatum may easily be overlooked, and are best detected by CT.

Osteonecroses of the os scaphoideum or the os lunatum (Kienbock's disease) require MRT clarification, while in many cases the administration of contrast agents is sensible to evaluate vitality of the bone tissue. The middle stages of necrosis are characterized by CT changes of the cancellous bone structure. The stage-oriented application of all three procedures is necessary for classification (at the lunatomalacia).

Changes at thumb and fingers are:

- The skier's thumb (also gamekeeper's or breakdancer's thumb, also occuring in Nordic walking) is a strain or rupture of the ulnar collateral ligament in the first carpometacarpal joint. The changes are detected by high sensitivity sonography. Ruptures are differentiated as partial or complete ruptures (most often in form of UCL tear; Hergan et al. 1995).
- At the fingers, a frequent injury of the palmar plate of the capsule insert of the proximal interphalangeal joints by hyperextension in ball-athletes is observed and can e documented by sonography. In climbing or baseball, degenerations and tears of the flexor tendons or the belonging pulleys (A1–A5) with a resulting chronic scar formation in the form of a trigger finger are common (Klausner et al. 2002). Pulley tears are quantified by sonography regarding phalanx-tendon-distance. The osseous avulsion of the flexor tendons is called rugby finger, which in many cases is detectable by conventional radiology.

8.9 Hip and groin

8.9.1 Indication and examination

Groin pain (osteitis pubis) or ventral hip pain is one of the main sport-specific diagnoses. These complaints correspond up to one fifth of the assigned cases in soccer players triggered by repetitive operating shear forces. Furthermore, apophysis avulsions at the hip joint are typical, especially in adolescent soccer players. A **pelvis overview radiograph** (preferably standing) is the primary indication. This can be amended by a **faux profile image** (display of the anatomic relation between acetabulum and femur head), and an **image according to Dunn** (Biedert and Netzer 2005).

Procedures with hip-joint pain or pubalgia, summarized under the syndrome of "sportsman's groin" are:

- MRT for detection of effusions or edemas in muscles or bones and differential-diagnostic regarding pain transmitted from lumbar or sacral. MR arthrography of the hip joint can be considered for labral lesion, corpus librum, or osteochondral lesion after hip luxation.
- CT for the classification of an osseous trauma
- Sonography for the detection of larger effusions, dynamic documentation of a snapping phenomenon, or tissue weakness along the inguinal canal. However, penetration depth of the ultrasound can be limited. The diagnostics of labrum acetare – though visible by sonography – has not been established.

8.9.2 Radiographic diagnosis

Radiography focuses on the early detection of coxarthrosis and predisposing factors and traction effects of the musculature. These traction forces are very strong at the hip/groin and act in complex movement patterns, to the bone as well as the canalis inguinalis and its vicinity.

At the **hip joint**, small subchondral edemas are an important sign of **internal lesions**. At the dysplasia arthrosis, the femur head is anterolateral luxated with eccentric narrowing of the joint cavity and osteophytosis. Consequences of the femoroacetabular impingement in form of

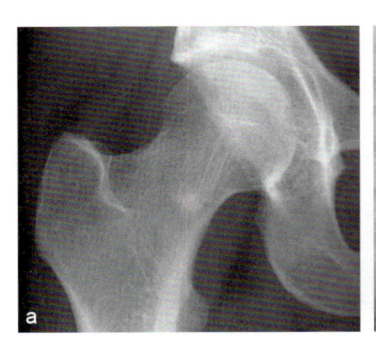

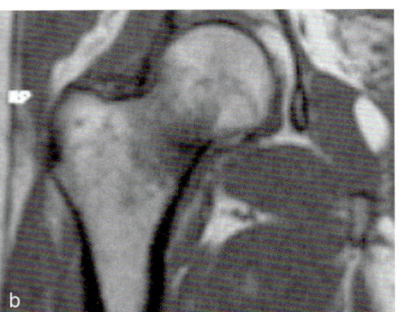

Fig. 8.12 Female inline skater with with hip pain for several months because of a stress fracture. a: conventional radiographic detection of the sclerosed fracture. b: MR tomographic display of the stress fracture surrounded by an edema.

labrum lesions, paralabral or subchondral cysts, corpora libra and others are found at the non-dysplastic coxarthrosis. The labrum lesions are rarely acute, mostly chronic and often combined with a narrowing and irregularity of the lateral hyaline cartilage. The anterolaterally directed shear forces of the femur head or an impingement are the main cause for these pathologies.

Muscle lesions are observed with differently pronounced diffuse or feathered **edemas**:

- A strain, sometimes also an avulsion of the two-headed rectus femoris muscle, the most often affected part of the quadriceps muscle, are associated with edema and later a characteristic subfascial fibrosing due to fibers of the caput reflexum (indirect head of sulcus supraacetabularis at the upper edge of the acetabulum).
- At the zone of origin of the dorsal thigh musculature (hamstrings), edemas of the tendon, of the subtendinous bone and the bursa can be detected. Such changes will also be observed at avulsion fractures, also at chronic avulsion lesions. At the latter, the existence of an edema will be helpful in order to differentiate irregularities or ossicles from norm variants.
- At the gluteus medius muscle, the according changes can be observed in its distal third above the trochanter major. A liquid-filled bursa retrotrochanterica is typical.
- Stress-conditioned edemas are found in the abductors, especially at the proximally positioned adductor minimus muscle and the neighboring ventral hip muscles. Edemas in the environment of the os pubis can also occur at stress fractures or, in rare cases, as osteomyelitis.
- At the snapping hip, edemas are MRT-leading symptoms: inflammation of the tractus iliotibialis and the bursa trochanterica and edema underneath the iliopsoas tendon.

No radiological findings exist for muscularly conditioned **instabilities of the pelvic ring** or a psoas-conditioned secondary pelvic tilt (though the muscle structure and thickness are detectable with sectional image procedures).

Neoplastic changes – especially hemangiomas, fibromatoses and neurinomas in the age group of young athletes – require consideration in differential diagnosis.

Stress reactions or fractures after trauma, such as avulsions of trochanter major are found at the adolescent bone.

Typical localizations of stress reactions are:

- at the femoral neck (> Fig. 8.12) primarily at the inner side at Shenton's arch
- at the os pubis at the upper and lower branches of the pubic bone and under the symphysis. As is other stress fractures, the edemas are osseously and can reach adjacent muscle bellies of the abductors or hip muscles. Residues after Malgaigne's fracture, which include the rami ossis pubis, may hardly be distinguished from a stress fracture by conventional radiography. A "plucking apart" of the symphysis region on conventional radiographs can be observed as a consequence of a gracilis-adductor syndrome.

Important differential diagnoses are cancerous changes such as the osteoid osteoma, bone cysts and the fibrose dysplasia.

A "sportsman's hernia" or "groin disruption" can be documented by dynamic sonography. CT herniography are not recommended given the high radiation exposure.

8.10 Knee

8.10.1 Indication and examination

Besides conventional radiographs, the MRT is increasingly considered as the primary examination. The CT is indicated for osseous trauma classification, sonography for superficial soft-tissue changes. For the diagnosis of the femoropatellar pain syndrome, complete leg images in standing position and tangential images of the patellar slide bearing in flex positions (parade images) are recommended. Axial CT images can be produced under exertion of the quadriceps muscle to detect muscular imbalance.

8.10.2 Radiographic diagnosis

Typical findings at the extensor apparatus of the knee joint are:

- Upper patellar spur at the insertion of the rectus tendon
- Swelling of the patellar ligament (jumper's knee), which can be graduated by sonography according to Fritschy (Fritschy and de Gautard 1988)
- Soft-tissue edema between the lateral epicondylus of the femur and the tractus iliotibialis (runner's knee)
- Signs of edema or fibrosis at Hoffa's fat pad
- Damage of the patellar joint cartilage: Deep tissue degeneration of this thick cartilage may escape arthroscopic detection. The cartilage ulcera developed by a downshear movement of the patella (lunge lesions), positioned in the opposite joint surface of the femur are clear signs of degeneration (➢ Fig. 8.13). Classification of cartilage defects for clinical purposes is generally according to Outerbridge (➢ Tab. 8.8; Sanders and Miller 2005).
- A swelling of the peripatellar plicae, e.g. as consequence of a subluxation with impaction, post-traumatic synovialitis, or congenital plica mediopatellaris is not rudimentary. However, it triggers a friction synovitis or infrapatellar fat pad in running sports.

Lesions of the ligaments, the menisci (➢ Fig. 8.14), the joint capsule and the subchondral bones, are so-called **internal injuries of the knee joint.** The dorsolateral or dorsomedial capsule structures are called posterolateral or posteromedial corner. Certain injury patterns are classified for the amendment of clinical functional tests based on the MRT findings. This is especially important for the spread of the bone marrow edema where the causative power impact is mostly complex. These classifications (e.g. according to Hayes) are a useful continuation of the "unhappy triad" concept according to O'Donoghue (Hayes et al. 2000). If MRT image cannot be assigned to a pattern, an arthrosis is likely. The five most frequent injury patterns are:

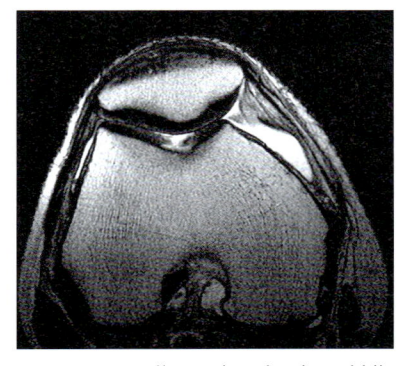

Fig. 8.13 Deep cartilage ulcer in the middle of the patellar joint surface of the femur (lunge lesion; MRT).

Tab. 8.8 Classification of cartilage damages (chondromalacia) of the knee joint (modified according to Sanders and Miller 2005).

		Cartilage thickness	Cartilage structure	Diameter
I	irregular surface	swelling or thinning <50%	inhomogeneous structure, cartilage edema	
II	superficial fissures	thinning >50%	no involvement of the subchondrium	<1.5 cm
III	deep fissures	permanent cartilage loss	no involvement of the subchondrium	>1.5 cm
IV		permanent cartilage loss	with signal alteration of the subchondrium	

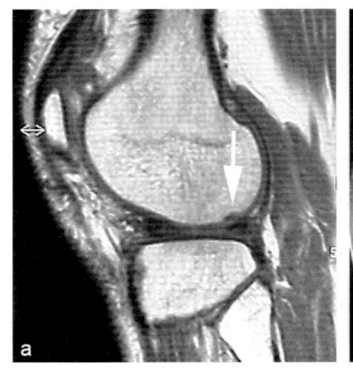

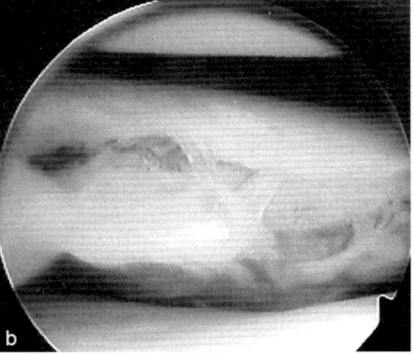

Fig. 8.14 Degenerative rupture of the lateral meniscus. a: MRT: meniscus hyperintensely changed in all its segments, to be hardly differentiated from the surroundings. Neighboring, a chronic cartilage defect (arrow) at the femur. b: arthroscopic correlate of the layered structure.

- The pivot shift injury (anteromedial rotator instability), resulting from flexion, valgus position and outwards-rotation of the tibia. At least half of all patterns can be assigned to it. The anterior cruciate ligament, the medial collateral ligament and the menisci are affected. The contusion foci lie in the lateral femoral condylus and in the lateroposterior tibial condylus; also the posteromedial tibia may be affected by a contrecoup injury.
- A varus hyperextension trauma is much rarer (less than 10%) and leads to anterior cruciate ligament rupture with instable posterolateral corner. The popliteofibular ligament that is the most important stabilizer of the posterolateral capsule is directly detected by high-resolution MRT.
- A flexion trauma with posterior tibial translationis associated with an isolated rupture of the posterior cruciate ligament. Because it is twice as thick and twice as resistant as the anterior cruciate ligament, partial ruptures are observed more frequently than complete ruptures.
- An isolated valgus stress is rare and affects the cruciate ligaments as well as the medial collateral ligament. The contusion foci lie in the lateral femur and tibia condylus.
- In a lateral patellar (sub)luxation with spontaneous reposition, the bone contusion appear at the lateral femoral condylus and at the medial patella. A retinaculum rupture is recognized as an edematous swelling, sometimes also by a feathered limited rupture of the distal vastus medialis obliquus muscle. Concomitantly, a rupture of the medial collateral ligament and perhaps the anterior cruciate ligament may be present.

In many cases, clinical **asymptomatic changes** are found in athletes. Retropalletar chondropathies of young basketball players and meniscus ruptures (13% with the ones younger than 45 years and 36% with the older ones) belong to those. They should not be considered as norm variant, but as degenerative process. The finding of a meniscocapsular separation, which is identified correctly in only about 10% by means of MR tomography, will be difficult diagnostically, given its complex anatomy.

8.11 Foot

8.11.1 Indication and examination

Conventional radiographs are sensible primary examination, especially for documentation of traumatic or post-traumatic changes. Stress images for the detection of a fibular ligament rupture have been widely substituted by MRT. Special, oblique adjusted images are useful for the anteromedial osseous impingement (van Dijk et al. 2002). The MRT should also be indicated at chronic post-traumatic instability of the ankle joint in order to distinguish rare mechanical forms from more frequent functional forms. The CT clarifies osseous traumas. Complex injury patterns are typical with soccer payers (soccer's ankle), whereas in practice the primary task is to distinguish the acute trauma from the multiple pre-existing defects.

Sonography is the primary procedure of choice for tendon changes; increasingly, MRT is used in order to apprehend the complexity of certain tendon changes and associated concomitant changes.

8.11.2 Radiographic diagnosis

Different sports damages at the hindfoot are often part of **hyperpronation syndrome according to Clement** (Clement et al. 1984). Pronation posture of the calcaneus affects an asymmetric tension – which primarily is recognized at sagittal MRT images – of the Achilles and internal malleolus tendons, soft-tissue edema of the sinus tarsi and effusion in the upper ankle joint (Ulreich et al. 2002). Later, overload damages of the spring ligament may appear. A degenerative pseudotumor of the anterior distal tibiofibular syndesmosis or a medial tibial stress syndrome is ascribed to hyperpronation.

Ruptures of lateral ligament stabilizers, especially of the anterior talofibular ligament, can be diagnosed with MRT after subluxation of the talus. The same applies to lesions of post-traumatic, mostly edematously swollen or interrupted distal **tibiofibular syndesmoses** and the **osteochondritis dissecans tali** that can be categorized into four degrees of severity (> Tab. 8.7). Different classifications at the talus are in use (Stoller et al. 2004). A ventrolateral regional synovitis, possibly with a pseudomeniscoid leading to a soft-tissue impingement and "kissing" osteophytes is diagnosed, especially after the application of contrast agents (lateral gutter syndrome). **Ruptures of the talocalcaneal ligaments**, especially of the cervical tali ligament occur with severe forms of subluxation and can be recognized by edema with undelineated ligament structures.

Ruptures of the deltoid ligament are typical for eversion injuries. MRT is used for detection of injury complexity with concomitant fibula fractures, or ruptures of the spring ligament, bifurcatum ligament, tibialis posterior tendon or retinaculum flexorum.

The **anteromedial osseous impingement of the upper ankle** (with soccer players, orienteering runners, and others) is characterized by traction osteophytes at the capsule insert points, e.g. in the shape of a so-called talus nose, irregularly contoured articular sockets and a local synovialitis.

Mainly, a tendovaginitis of the flexor hallucis longus muscle is observed, caused by forced flexion movements (soccer, ballet) at the **posterior impingement**; at acute overuse, an edema of the os trigononum (> Fig. 8.15) and swelling of the posterior talofibulare ligament is observed.

Repetitive flexion movements lead to **overuse syndrome of the large flexor tendon**. The tibialis anterior tendon may also be affected at eccentric stress load. Injuries of this tendon can occur with sudden hyperflexion traumas (> Fig. 8.1). Injuries of Lisfranc's joint are suspected because of edema or effusion medially to the os metatarsale II base; Lisfranc's ligament rupture requires exact, thin layers.

The different **plantar overload damages**, the proximal and distal plantar fasciitis, hypertrophy of heel fat pads and concomitant edemas

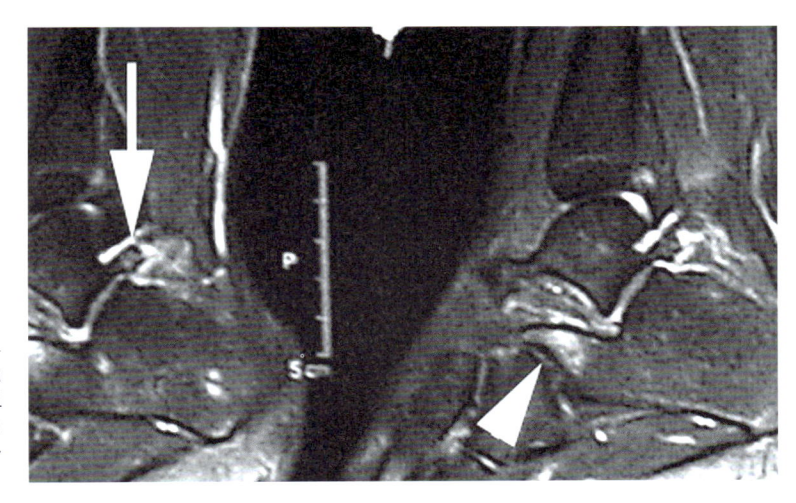

Fig. 8.15 Blotched stress edema of os trigonum (arrow) at a ballet dancer with additional traumatic edema (arrow head) in the anterior calcaneal process (MRT).

and swellings, with traction osteophytes at the tuberculum mediale of the calcaneus (anterior calcaneal spur) are detected by MRT. Tubercular edematous swelling marks rupture of the plantar fascia, which is difficult to detect by sonography.

The **fifth tarsometatarsal joint** is disposed to overuse. A liquid line in sonography or MRT characterizes tendovaginitis or bursitis along the fibullaris brevis tendon. Osseous stress reactions of the four segments of the os metatarsale V (avulsion of the fibularis brevis tendon, metaphyseal Jones fracture, proximal-diaphyseal stress fracture and distal-diaphyseal dancer's fracture) are detected by MRT.

Edemas, joint effusion, and osteophytes are found with **changes of the metacarpophalangeal joint of the hallux**, such as the hallux rigidus, the turf toe syndrome conditioned by forced dorsal flexion, and stress reactions of the sesamoid bones. Radiographic discrete changes are observed at diagnostically relevant structures, so that the correlation with the clinical findings is decisive.

References

Anderson MW, Greenspan A (1996). Stress fractures. Radiology 199: 1–12.

Arendt EA, Griffith HJ (1997). The use of MR imaging in the assessment and clinical management of stress reactions of bone in high-performance athletes. Clin Sports Med 16: 291–306.

Bennett WF (2001). Subscapularis, medial, and lateral head coracohumeral ligament insertion anatomy. Arthroscopic appearance and incidence of "hidden" rotator interval lesions. Arthroscopy 17: 173–180.

Biedert R, Netzer P (2005). Femoroazetabuläres Impingement beim Sportler. Sportorthopädie – Sporttraumatologie 21: 195–200.

Boutin RD, Fritz RC, Steinbach LS (2002). Imaging of sports-related muscle injuries. Radiol Clin North Am 40: 333–362.

Breitenseher MJ, Metz VM, Gilula LA, Gaebler C, Kukla C, Fleischmann D, Imhof H, Trattnig S (1997). Radiographically occult scaphoid fractures: value of MR imaging in detection. Radiology 203: 245–250.

Chevrot A, Drape JL, Godefroy D, Dupont AM, Gires F, Chemla N, Pessis E, Sarazin L, Minoui A (1998). Stress fractures. In: Masciocchi C, ed. Radiological Injuries of Sports Injuries. Springer, Berlin Heidelberg New York, pp 235–249.

Clement DR, Taunton JE, Smart GW (1984). Achilles tendinitis and peritendinitis: etiology and treatment. Am J Sports Med 12: 179–184.

Engelhardt M, Reuter I, Freiwald J, Böhme T, Halbsguth A (1997). Spondylolyse und Spondylolisthesis und Sport. Orthopädie 26: 755–759.

Fredericson M, Jennings F, Beaulieu C, Matheson GO (2006). Stress fractures in athletes. Top Magn Reson Imaging 17: 309–325.

Fritschy D, Gautard R (1988). Jumper's knee and ultrasonography. Am J Sports Med 16: 637–640.

Frühwald F, Imhof H, Kletter K (2006). Orientierungshilfe Radiologie. Anleitung zum optimalen Einsatz der klinischen Radiologie. Verlag der österreichischen Ärztekammer, Wien.

Goutallier D Postel J, Barnageau J, Lavau L, Voisin M (1984). Fatty muscle degeneration in cuff ruptures: pre- and postoperative evaluation by CT scan. Clin Orthop Relat Res 304:78–83.

Hall S, Buchbinder R (2004). Do imaging methods that guide needle placement improve outcome? Ann Rheum Diss 63: 1007–1008.

Hayes CW, Brigido MK, Jamadar DA, Propeck T (2000). Mechanism-based pattern approach to classification of complex injuries of the knee depicted at MR imaging. Radiographics 20 Spec No: S121-134.

Hergan K, Mittler C, Oser W (1995). Ulnar collateral ligament differentiation of displaced and nondisplaced tears with sonography and MR imaging. Radiology 194: 65–71.

Kannus P, Jozsa L (1991). Histopathological changes preceding spontaneous rupture of a tendon. A controlled study of 891 patients. J Bone Joint Surg Am 73: 1507–1525.

Kainberger F, Ulreich N, Huber W, Bernhard C, Müllner T, Nehrer S, Imhof H (2001). Das Sehnenüberlastungssyndrom: Bildgebende Diagnostik. Wien Med Wochenschr 151: 509–512.

Klauser A, Frauscher F, Hochholzer T, Helweg G, Kramer J, Zur Nedden D (2002). Diagnose von Überlastungsschäden bei Kletterern. Radiologie 42: 788–798.

Larsson P, Henriksson-Larsen K (2008). Body composition and performance in cross-country skiing. Int J Sports Med (epub ahead).

Loose R, Stöver B, Müller W-U (2006). Orientierungshilfe für radiologische und nuklearmedizinische Untersuchungen. Empfehlung der Strahlenschutzkommission. H. Hoffmann GmbH – Fachverlag, Berlin.

Miller TT (1999). Imaging of elbow disorders. Orthop Clin North Am 30: 21–36.

Mintz DN (2004). Magnetic resonance imaging of sports injuries to the cervical spine. Semin Musculoskelet Radiol 8: 99–110.

Nehrer S, Breitenseher M, Brodner W, Kainberger F, Fellinger EJ, Engel A, Imhof F 81997). Clinical and sonographic evaluation of the risk of rupture in the Achilles tendon. Arch Orthop Trauma Surg 116: 14–18.

Nehrer S, Huber W, Dirisamer A, Kainberger F (2002). Apophysenschaden bei jugendlichen Sportlern. Radiologe 42: 818–822.

Ogon M, Riedel-Huter C, Sterzinger W, Krismer M, Spratt KF, Wimmer C (2001). Radiologic abnormalities and low back pain in elite skiers. Clin Orthop Relat Res 390: 151–162.

Pfirrmann CW, Zanetti M (2005). Variants, pitfalls and asymptomatic findings in wrist and hand imaging. Eur J Radiol 56: 286–295.

Sanders T, Miller M (2005). A systematic approach to magnetic resonance imaging interpretation of sports medicine injuries of the knee. Am J Sports Med 33: 131–148.

Sommer B, Pauleit D, Altmann D (2003). Stressfraktur des Os sacrum bei einem Basketballleistungssportler. Rofo 175: 569–570.

Stäbler A, Spieker A, Bonel H, Schrank C, Glaser C, Petsch R, Putz R, Reiser M (2000). Magnetresonanztomographie des Handgelenks – Vergleich hochauflösender Sequenzen und unterschiedlicher Fettunterdrückungstechniken an Leichenpräparaten. Rofo 172: 168–174.

Steinbach LS, Fritz RC, Tirman PF, Uffman M (1997). Magnetic resonance imaging of the elbow. Eur J Radiol 25: 223–241.

Steinborn M, Heuck A, Jessel C, Bonel H, Reiser M (1999). Magnetic resonance imaging of lateral epicondylitis of the elbow with a 0.2-T dedicated system. Eur Radiol 9: 1376–1380.

Steingruber IE, Wolf C, Gruber H, Gabriel M, Czermak BV, Mallouhi A, Jaschke W (2002). Stressfrakturen bei Athleten. Radiologe 42: 771–777.

Stoller D, Tirman P, MA. B, Beltran S, Branstetter R, Blease S (2004). Diagnostic Imaging Orthopaedics. Amirsys, Salt Lake City.

Teefey S, Hasan S, Middleton W (2000). Ultrasonography of the rotator cuff. A comparison of ultrasonographic and arthroscopic findings in one hundred consecutive patients. J Bone Joint Surg Am 82: 498–504.

Ulreich N, Kainberger F, Huber W, Nehrer S (2002). Die Achillessehne im Sport. Radiologe 42: 811–817.

van Dijk CN, Wessel RN, Tol JL, Maas M (2002). Oblique radiograph for the detection of bone spurs in anterior ankle impingement. Skeletal Radiol 31: 214–221.

Vialle R, Schmit P, Dauzac C, Wicart P, Glorion C, Guigui P (2005). Radiological assesment of lumbosacral dystrophic changes in high-grade spondylolisthesis. Skeletal Radiol 34: 528–535.

Wohlwend J, van Holsbeeck M, Craig J (1998). The association between irregular greater tuberosities and rotator cuff tears: a sonographic study. Am J Roentgenol 171: 229–233.

Zanetti M, Jost B, Lustenberger AS, Hodler J (1999). Clinical impact of MR arthrography of the shoulder. Acta Radiol 40: 296–302.

Chapter 9

Arthroscopy

Dieter Kohn and Michael Dienst

9.1 Equipment

Arthroscopy is worldwide the second most common surgical treatment at the musculoskeletal system after osteosynthesis. Storz pioneered joint surgery with the development of the first high-quality and robust arthroscopes.

In the 1970s, Storz combined a Hopkins rod lens system with a light transmission via fiberglass. A decade later inside view into the joint was replaced by video viewing on screen. This important simplification initiated the development of complex intraarticular surgery. Until today arthroscopic surgeons requires a fundamental, technological knowledge. This know-how guarantees optimal surgery and right reaction to intraoperative technical problems.

9.1.1 Imaging system

Arthroscopes with optical fiber cable, light source, video camera with control unit, and monitor enlarge the image of the articular area.

Arthroscope

The image creating lens system and the light transmitting glass fibers are combined in a metal pipe. The arthroscope will project a circular area, the so-called visual field.

The aperture determines the size of the visual field, which depends on the refraction index of the surrounding medium and the arthroscope. Hence, gas-filled joints offer a larger visual field than liquid-filled joints.

Wide-angle arthroscopes reach an aperture of about 120°. Similar to photographic cameras, a large opening angle induces image distortion. The central ray is the angle bisector of the opening angle. If the central ray runs parallel to the instrument axis, the viewing angle decreases to 0°.

Knee joint arthroscopy typically uses viewing angles of 30° or 70°. In rotating such angle optics around the optical axis, the larger the chosen viewing angle of the instrument. Therefore, a rotation of the arthroscope around its axis will correlate with "looking around" within the joint without the risk of cartilage injury.

70°-arthroscope has a large visible area by rotation. However, the 70°-arthroscope is difficult to maneuver in the joint (Kohn 1997) because visual field does not allow a forward view anymore. These physical preconditions make the **30°- optics** the preferred instrument in clinical practice. Navigating 30°-angle optics requires thorough training (Kohn 1991) and the **70°- optics** is mostly used for posterior recessus of the knee joint and for inspection of the glenohumeral ligaments in the shoulder joint.

Instruments with an **external diameter of 4 mm** are most appropriate for the knee joints of adults. The **2.7 mm arthroscope** is the preferred choice for knee joints of children up to 10 years. Additionally, the 2.7 mm arthroscope allows full inspection of very narrow joints of adults.

The 4 mm arthroscope is preferred for shoulder and hip joint. 2.7 mm or 1.9 mm arthroscopes are recommended for the wrist. Today, Hopkins rod-lens systems still remain superior in terms of image quality to flexible fiberoptical systems.

Arthroscopes are always used with a protective **trocar sheath**, which penetrates the the periarticular tissue. This metal sheath surrounds the arthroscope shaft and is bolted against the arthroscope with a quick release. The internal sheath diameter is larger than the external diameter of the arthroscope. The space between the arthroscope and the sheath is used for irrigation. A blunt and a sharp trocar will be delivered with the trocar sheath, and they will fit exactly into the sheath, can also be bolted against it and whose end will jut out of the sheath.

In clinical jargon, which is used in the following, "arthroscope" refers to the combination of trocar sheath/arthroscope whereas the expression "optics" refers to the optical instrument.

Lighting

A halogen or xenon lamp is the **light source**. The trend goes to weaker light sources to match the higher sensitivity of modern video cameras. However, a light reserve is still useful for the production of printer images or if using older light cables with transmission loss. Therefore, high performance (ca. 300 W) lamps with a daylight-adequate color temperature of about 6,000 K are recommended.

Light transmission to the arthroscope occurs via a **light guide cable**. Fiberglass optic cables transmit enough light and can be autoclaved and are less expensive than liquid-filled fiber optics. Light source and video unit should come from the same manufacturer as the light intensity of modern systems is controlled by the camera. Long light guide cables of at least 2 m will give the arthroscopist enough freedom of operation.

Video chain

Photo diodes will convert light signals into voltage fluctuations in the chip camera. We recommend a camera with highest resolution and zoom lens. The **zoom function** is necessary when operating 2.7 mm or 1.9 mm arthroscopes to create monitor format-filling images. The zoom option is useful at high precision surgery.

The camera must have an **automatic aperture control** to deliver an optimally illuminated picture and to protect the chip from overexposure.

High-resolution color monitor with anti-glare screens visualize the analogue or digital images.

9.1.2 Lavage

Only after filling the joint space with liquid, joints can be subject to arthroscopy. Generally, electrolyte-containing **Ringer's lactate** is used to support the cartilage metabolism (Reagan et al. 1983). Today, compressed air has widely been abandoned after the lethal embolisms. Also, use of glycine solution is contraindicated because of temporary blindness (Burkhart et al. 1990).

An intraarticular pressure of ca. 50 mm Hg is sufficient for capsule distension. This pressure can be achieved with high hanging rinsing-fluid bags but **pumps** are best practice. Modern pumps are generally equipped with a pressure sensor and automatically cut off the inflow into the joint after reaching the selected maximum pressure. Pressure control has proven reliable with different customary pumps, maximal flow volume rates, however, still remain unreliable (Muellner et al. 2001).

High flow volumes will improve the visibility. The flow into the joint should be directed via the arthroscopic sheath. This rinses of particles and clears vision. The **intraarticular pressure** in the joint can be increased shortly up to to 200 mmHg at vision interference by bleeding arterial vessels. The extremity's bulging and hardening of an arthroscoped joint is a warning signal requiring immediate pressure reduction. Otherwise a **compartment syndrome** can develop.

9.1.3 Documentation

A postoperative protocol immediately prepared after the intervention, ideally with **visual documentation** is good clinical practice. The exact position and extent of cartilage defects should be described for clinical and scientific questions. However, their value must be considered with care given variability (Oakley et al.

2003). Even though exact mapping protocols are available (Hunt et al. 2001), their time consuming effort makes routine implementation questionable.

Intraarticular findings require objective documentation and **PC technology** facilitates image documentation (photographs and videos). Digital image quality is generally sufficient for patient records, publications and presentations and renders classical photography obsolete. Digital storage media and programs are of great advantage for archiving, order and search of images (Johnson 2002).

Digital image processing may help to increase quality but may introduce bias, if not falsify the original image. Hence, its use is problematic if guidelines for scientific imaging are not followed. Movies are helpful for medical education purposes and visualization of extraordinary findings.

9.1.4 Additional instruments

A sterilizable camera-arthroscope, a probing hook and a rinsing liquid draining system are necessary for every arthroscopy (Kohn 1991 and 1997). Furthermore, repositioning of the arthroscope requires changing counterbraces and canulas.

Probing hooks require adaptation to the field of ooperation. Overlong hooks are necessary for shoulder and hip, miniaturized probing hooks are required for wrist and ankle joint. A marking on probing hooks allows comparing length.

A **cannula of size 1** should be used for pre-probing and is superior to a Kirschner wire since reflux from the canula indicates their intraarticular location.

Shoulder and elbow joints can be arthroscoped from opposing sides. This requires a **Wissinger rod,** which is an overlong, blunt trocar embedded into the arthroscope sheath. This allows perforation of the opposite articulated wall. A sheath is retrogradely attached to the rod and the rod is then pulled backwards. This positions the sheath opposing to the fist access and may serve e.g. as inflow channel for rinsing liquid or as working channel of motorized instruments.

So-called **switching rods** fit precisely on the arthroscope and inflow sheath and allow exchange of the arthroscope and inflow sheath. This turns the previous liquid inflow into the arthroscope and vice versa. Standard size switching rods can be used in all joints except the wrist.

The use of a cannulated trocar sheath system is of advantage especially for shoulder and hip joint. While such systems will be used mostly for the arrangement of additional portals in the shoulder joint, they will also be used for the arrangement of standard portals in the hip joint. With implementation under arthoscopic control, they will offer the advantages of exact portal placement and minimization of iatrogenic extra- and intraarticular lesions.

Special instruments are needed for arthroscopic surgeries such as meniscus resection and reconstruction, synovectomie, cruciate ligament reconstruction, and resecting and reconstructing of the joint cartilage.

Manually operated instruments

Arthroscopic instruments are **atraumatic for the joint cartilage** given their adapted shape and design (Glinz 1989). Loss of instrument pieces or breakage within the joint is inacceptable. Manually operated instruments such as suction tube, biopsy forceps, grasping forceps, knives, scissors, punches, suture instruments, knot pushers, awls and curettes are a key for arthroscopy.

The most frequently used resection instrument is the **cutting forceps**, which allows contouring resection and provides the surgeon with a feel for tissue texture. Suction punches combine the suction tube and cutting forceps, which allows convenient aspiration of tissue fragments. However, this will be difficult in narrow joints. Small arthroscopy knives allow working even in narrowest joint segments but carry the risks of cartilage injuries or instrument damage.

Recently, a number of **new manually operated special instruments** in particular for meniscus suture, reconstruction of rotator cuffs and shoulder stabilization have been developed. Besides classic instruments for inside-out and outside-in suture instruments, complete internal suture and one-hand instruments are available for knee arthroscopy.

Difficult to access posterior horns of the menisci may require expensive implants, or combination with a classical meniscus seam. New systems for thread passage, thread management and anchor placement are equally efficacious as classical arthroscopic shoulder and rotator cuff seam techniques. Initially, they often were too voluminous and ineffective but new needle-conducted systems significantly advanced this surgery.

Motorized instruments

The **basic principle** of motorized instruments is the combination of a suction tube with a rotating blade. Tissue is aspired and stabilized at the suction tube; the rotating blade will cut it off. The suction force, the engine speed, the shape of the cutting window and blade as well as the contact pressure will decide about the efficiency of the motorized instruments. Oscillating instruments and an easily adjustable vacuum are indispensible. Some manufacturers have integrated a **coagulation function** into the instrument tip of motor-driven fraises, which saves repositioning of the fraise in case of bleedings and thereby accelerates the surgical surgery. For example, we recommend use of an angled cutter blade in a narrow knee joint for the equalization of the posterior horn of the medial meniscus. In the hip joint, the arthroscoper will reach fossa acetabuli only with an overlong and angled shaver for resection of a ruptured capitis femoris ligament.

High frequency instruments

High frequency instruments which operate in an electrolyte-containing medium experience a renaissance. Contrary to the routine use of electronic instruments in the subacromial area, today's use for other joints has been optional. **Bipolar** instruments have been introduced recently and advantages and disadvantages of both monopolar and bipolar systems still remains a matter of debate (Edwards et al. 2002).

Application ranges from electro-coagulation, tissue ablation during synovectomy, meniscectomy and soft-tissue debridement to focused heat shrinking of tissue and cartilage equalization (Barber et al. 2002). Temperature in the tissue, penetration depth and duration of the application will determine outcome. **Collagen shrinking** is at 65–75°C. Higher temperatures cause collagen disaggregation and no effect is detectable at lower temperatures.

Monopolar instruments require a neutral electrode attached to the patients skin. Bipolar instruments do not require an additional electrode. Cell death in the capsule and the ligaments or in the synovial tissue up to 3–5 mm in depth are triggered by the **heat development** at the top of the instrument. However, this is tissue dependent and reaches merely 0.5 to 3 mm in hyaline cartilage. High frequency instruments for the resection of tissue are alternatives to the mechanical instruments but their use for chondroplasty, capsular shrinking or shrinking of elongated ligaments is controversial (Owens et al. 2002, Shellock 2001). Recently, movable high frequency instruments have been introduced for hip and shoulder joints. Laser instruments require balancing high cost and higher risks as compared to high frequency instruments.

9.2 Indications and contraindications

9.2.1 Indications

Purely diagnostic arthroscopy is rare today and is only used if clinical and imaging examination or contradictory findings of imaging procedures cannot resolve a clinical problem. However, any diagnostic arthroscopy is always ready for surgery. Arthroscopic analysis of the hyaline joint cartilage consistency and meniscus maybe required for high tibial osteotomy. If MRI does not provide definite diagnosis hemarthros at a ligament-stable knee joint can require arthroscopic clarification. Similarly, relapsing joint dysfunction of unknown origin may be an indication for arthroscopy.

If **arthroscopic surgery** offers similar results it will be superior to open surgery based on lower morbidity or even better efficacy.

Nowadays, most **arthroscopic knee operations** are equal or even better than open surgeries. Typical arthroscopy interventions are meniscus resections, seams and replacement, splitting of the lateral retinaculum patellae, reconstruction or reefing of the medial retinaculum patellae, and partial or complete synovectomy. The arthroscope has turned into an indispensable tool for the reconstruction of the **cruciate ligaments**. While the replacement of the anterior ligament by autologous or allogenic tendon or tendon-bone transplants is carried out in most cases as arthroscopic procedure, combined arthroscopic/open surgeries compete for the posterior ligament interventions. Surgical repair of complex knee instability requires a knee surgeon experienced in both arthroscopic and open surgery.

Surgery can treat traumatic **cartilage defects** with autologous cartilage-bone transplantation, opening of the medullary cavity and autologous chondrocyte transplantation. The autologous cartilage-bone transplantation – also called "mosaic plasty" or "OATS" (osteochondral autograft transfer system; Hangody 1994, Bobic 1996) – the Pridie drilling, micro-fracturing and abrasion arthroplasty are carried out under arthroscopic view. The transplantation of autologous cartilage cells requires covering with a periosteal flap via arthrotomy. Arthroscopic transplantation of chondrocytes is possible if using so-called "matrixes" (Erggelet 2003).

Knee and **shoulder joint** have seen a similar devolopment. Arthroscopic subacromial decompression, removal of free bodies from the glenohumeral joint, synovectomy and bursectomy are now arthroscopic standard of care and have replaced open surgery. The thermal shrinking of the lax shoulder-joint capsules does not offer long-term efficacy. Recurrent instabilities and capsular necroses have been reported. Arthroscopic surgery still competes with open surgery for treatment of post-traumatic shoulder instability. Reconstruction of the rotator cuff and transposition of the long biceps tendon are possible under arthroscopic view.

Arthroscopy of the **hip joint** has clearly improved over time (Dienst 2005) and has improved diagnosis of hip diseases. Labrum damag, ligament capitis femoris injuries and pathology in femoroacetabular impingement are now established indications for arthroscopic interventions.

9.2.2 Contraindications

Every **infection**, abrasion, furuncles or incompletely healed incisions are contraindications of arthroscopy.

Neoplasms adjacent to joints carry the risk of tumor cell dissemination into the joint. Hence, neoplastic diseases are excluded from arthroscopy and two-plane radiographs are required for each arthroscopy. Every invasive action including arthroscopy is ineligible with an **algodystrophy**.

9.3 Pre-operative preparations

9.3.1 Informing

Similar to other surgeries, arthroscopy is associated with risks:

- infection
- thrombosis or embolism
- injury of nerves and vessels
- surgery-specific complications.

Arthroscopic complications are but not limited to breaking of instruments postoperative hemorrhage after incision of lateral retinaculum and synovectomy. Potential open invasive interventions after arthroscopy are **extremely important** and patients need to consent to instant invasive alternatives in case of technical problems.

Meniscus lesions can be reconstructed, which implies a 6-week postoperative splinting of the treated leg.

Microfracturing, pridie drilling or abrasion plasty may require postoperative decompression of hematomes. Arthroscopic surgeries of the anterior cruciate ligament or anterior shoulder reconstruction may end in technically irresolvable complications, which require open surgery.

The same applies to subacromial decompression and reconstruction of the rotator cuff. During preoperative discussion switching from the arthroscopical to open technique should be explained to the patient not as a catastrophe but as a modification of the operation technique with identical final result. Hence, informing the patient by the surgeon himself is of great advantage in arthroscopy but not always feasible.

9.3.2 Diagnostics

MRT is only necessary if clinical and radiographic examination remain inconclusive. Surgery for osteochondrosis dissecans is best performed with pre-operative MRT. Generally, the MRT readout increases with the expertise of the requisitioning physician. The radiologist requires a precise question to choose the best image mode and correct interpretation of the images (Sherman et al. 2002).

The pre-arthroscopic **radiographic examination** is necessary in case of osseous injury implications, joint adjacent bone tumors, and algodystrophy. A Frik tunnel view is needed if free loose bodies of the knee are suspected. We recommend side-to-side comparison of tangential patellar views in case of patellofemoral problems.

9.3.3 Analgesia and anesthesia

General anesthesia offers the best conditions to arthroscopy as unwanted movements of the arthroscoped joint are avoided. Peripheral innervations and perfusion can directly be tested postoperatively.

Regional anesthesia allows hip, knee, and ankle interventions. Spinal anesthesia, however, limits post-operative mobilization – one of the great advantages of arthroscopy – due to postdural puncture.

After arthroscopic meniscus suture, peripheral motor function and sensibility should be examined immediately as irritation of the saphenous or peroneal nerve, respectively, have been described. Early examination carries the greatest potential success for restitution. Peridural anesthesia is of advantage in the postoperative phase after synovectomy or separation of adhesions in the knee joint. The necessary passive mobilization of the joint can be carried out pain-free and effectively.

Knee and ankle joint interventions not only require analgesia of the according joint. In addition, the thigh is anesthetized so that the patient tolerates the pneumatic tourniquet. The proximal nerve blockages, such as the "three-in-one block" at the thigh, do not translate into a full knee joint analgesia. Therefore, they should not be used routinely and reserved for the expert.

Local anesthesia for arthroscopy means anesthesia of portals of entry and the joint space. Analgesia of about 30–60 minutes may be expected after the binding of the drug to receptors produced naturally in the body. Joint distension with hydrous fluid is possible. The maximum dose of the local anesthetic must not be exceeded. Generalized seizures and even a case of death are known **complications**.

The **interscalenar blockade** represents an alternative to general anesthesia.

9.4 Technique

9.4.1 Knee joint

Arthroscopic surgeries at the knee joint will usually be carried out with a 90° flexed knee with a fixed thigh. Intervention at the lying, freely movable leg will offer some advantages for complex surgeries as the reconstruction of the posterior cruciate ligament or combined surgeries as for collateral ligament reconstruction.

The **pneumatic tourniquet** should be attached within the thigh holder. A routine inflating of the tourniquet is not necessary. The tourniquet will complicate the finding of bleeding sources and the evaluation of synovial changes. It could possibly lead to paresthesias in the post-operative phase. The fear of nerve or muscle damage caused in the longer term by the effect of pneumatic tourniquet could not be confirmed (Nicholas et al. 2001). On the other hand, surgeries such as arthrolysis or synovectomy with the use of motorized instruments with strong suction effect are only feasible with supply tourniquet. Therefore, the tourniquet is inflated in case of deterioration vision and occasional if exceptionally strong fixation of the thigh is needed.

Portals

The portals should be large enough to allow penetration with an arthroscope or an addi-

9.4 Technique

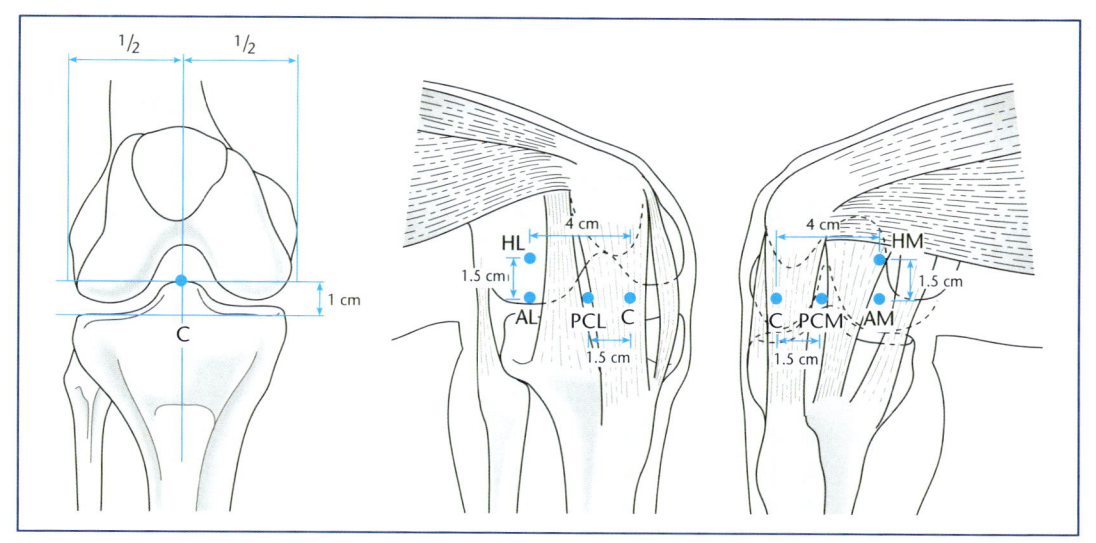

Fig. 9.1 Central portal and further important portals to the knee (C = central, PCM = paracentral medial, AM = anteromedial, PCL = paracentral lateral, AL = anterolateral, HL = high lateral, HM = high medial).

tional instrument but no loss of intraarticular pressure should occur and fluid extravasation should be avoided. Hence, the **skin incisions** are about 8 mm for the arthroscope portal and 5 mm for instrument portals.

All skin incisions should follow **cleavage (Longo's) lines** to minimize scaring. The cleavage lines run horizontally near the joint space. Preprobing of planned instrument portals with a needle allows exact positioning of the portals. Arthroscopic incisions may be closed at the knee with a skin closure strip and sterile wound dressing. **Drainage** of irrigation liquid within the first postoperative hours is desired.

The **central portal** is routinely used for knee arthroscopy (➤ Fig. 9.1). It allows almost complete examination of the joint space without repositioning of the arthroscope. The position is defined by osseous landmarks. A defined position for the most important instrument portals will be possible after the central portal has been established first. Proceeding can be symmetrically for operations at the medial and lateral meniscus, which shortens the learning curve of these procedures. The fibers of the patellar tendon are gently pushed apart at the central portal which avoids postoperative complaints. The different areas of the meniscus can be assigned directly to the separate portals (➤ Fig. 9.2).

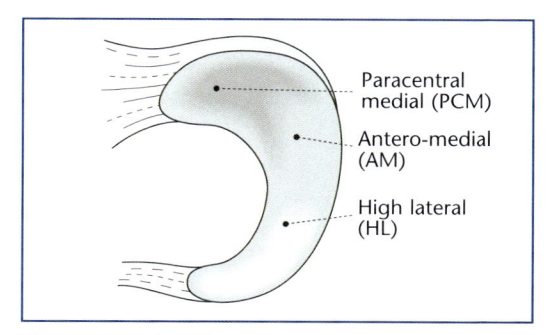

Fig. 9.2 Portals to the diverse parts of the inner meniscus. The procedure for the external meniscus will be symmetric.

The reconstruction of the posterior horns of the meniscus and the posterior cruciate ligament reconstruction will require a good survey of the posterior joint recessors. A **posterior "trans-septal" portal** has been described, which includes perforation of the posterior median knee septum with arthroscope and instruments (Ahn et al. 2003) and the resection of the septum for improved visibility (Louisia et al 2003).

Diagnostic arthroscopy

After establishing the central portal and applying the 30°-arthroscope, the joint will be filled with distension fluid up to an **operating pressure** of 50 mmHg. An out flow cannula is placed in the superiomedial recessus and connected with a drain hose and role clamp. Arthroscopy will be carried out under continuous **liquid flow**. The diagnostic 'roundtrip' must follow an **exact pattern** in order to not "forget" parts of the joint space (Kohn and Adam 2005). To achieve optimal coordination the valgus and varus opening of the joint spaces will be carried out by the surgeon himself and not by an assisstent (Kohn 1995).

Palpation of the anterior cruciate ligament and the hyaline-cartilaginous joint surfaces are part of every diagnostic knee joint arthroscopy. Estimation of ligament tension of the anterior cruciate ligament with a probe requires some experience.

Often **diagnosis of a fresh cruciate ligament injury** is not an easy task. The ligament will tear within the intact synovial tube and this may simulate an intact cruciate ligament. Only palpation hints to the underlying problem. Another problem remains estimation of the extent of a partial rupture. This can often better be assessed at preoperative examination under anaesthesia by side-to-side comparison than by arthroscopy.

Assessment of the meniscus surfaces and classification of meniscus ruptures, however, is well characterized. We advise using the classification system according to Warren (Warren 1990) for the exact **localization of meniscus lesions**.

In case of damage of the hyaline joint cartilage, the so-called **chondromalacia,** the simple grading system of Noyes (Noyes 1989) is of value if used in combination with a diagram depicting injury position and size. Grade I chondromalacia, the softening of the cartilage, is determined with a probing hook. Broken and frayed cartilage surface indicates a grade IIA but will not be deeper than half of the cartilage thickness. The damage is more profound in grade IIB but is not including the complete cartilage layer. In grade III, subchondral bone lies bare.

Complete knee joint arthroscopy gives **insight into both dorsal knee recesses**. This is possible in almost every joint if using the central portal. If the lesion is suspected in the posterior recess, e.g. longitudinal rupture of the posterior meniscus horn or loose bodies, we recommend a 70°-optics. The 30° wide angle optics is sufficient for all other cases.

Operative arthroscopy

Meniscus operations

Arthroscopic meniscectomy is the meniscus resection surgery of choice. The resection of damaged meniscus parts under preservation of a stable peripheral ridge is the fundamental principle. Complete punching of the meniscal ring equals functionally a total meniscectomy.

Total **meniscectomy** results in **osteoarthritis** of the affected joint after 10–15 years. The risk of early osteoarthritis is also present after partial meniscus resection. Hence, **refixation** of the detached meniscus part should be considered. Only meniscocapsular reinsertion produces excellent results for periods of 10 years or longer. Good, medium-term results are obtained with suture of a longitudinal rupture in the vascularized peripheral third of the meniscus.

Introduction of new implants has shortened time and helped to avoid additional dorsal incisions in meniscus reconstruction. However implant-related complications have been reported (La Prade and Wills 2004). In most cases, the primary stability of sutures is not achieved with these implants.

Treatment in case of MRT detectable lesions but preserved meniscus surfaces still remains a matter of debate. If the patient expresses pain at the joint space some authors suggest partial resection by arthroscopy; others recommend preservation of the complete meniscus. In rare circumstances, a meniscus ganglion can be peeled off during an open surgery if arthroscopy detects intact meniscus surfaces. Generally, partial resection of the meniscus with opening the ganglion from intraarticular is necessary. If during operation ganglion content drains into the joint, the ganglion may be debrided arthroscopically from the joint side. A torn lateral discoid meniscus is resected in part and a stable marginal ridge is preserved.

Postoperative MRT has detected bone marrow edemas in asymptomatic patients within the first year after meniscectomy (Kobayashi et al. 2002). The clinical relevance of the changes is unclear. Osteonecroses of the femur condyles have been described after arthroscopic meniscus surgeries; but no causal coherence could be established. (Faletti et al. 2002, Pape et al. 2004). Hence, we will pay attention to such reports as this may affect indication and post-operative therapy of arthroscopic meniscectomy.

Knee extension apparatus

The patellofemoral joint can be inspected from full extension to 120° of flexion. Arthroscopy gives more information as non-invasive imaging in concurrent damage of the hyaline joint cartilage and malposition of the patella in relation to the trochlea femoris. Therefore, arthroscopy is indicated if exact pre-operative analysis of the extensor apparatus is required or imaging produces contradictory or unclear results (Pidoriano and Fulkerson 1997). The **patello-trochlear joint** is examined from the central portal first and then again after the transfer of the arthroscope to the superomedial portal. Only the additional proximal view allows complete assessment of the joint surfaces and the patello-trochlear joint contact.

Synovectomy

If arthroscopy detects a compact, thick pannus without villous formation, open synovectomy is the preferred choice. Arthroscopic synovectomy is more time consuming but as effective as open surgery and allows access to both posterior joint recesses.

The **minimal periarticular soft tissue trauma** at arthroscopic portals, which are small in comparison to arthrotomy, simplifies postoperative rehabilitation, provides a superior cosmetic result and facilitates the repetition of the procedure in case relapse. In general, full range of motion and the ability to walk should be restored two weeks after arthroscopic synovectomy of the knee joint.

Cruciate ligament reconstruction

Both cruciate ligaments are accessible by arthroscopy whereas the collateral ligaments aren't. Therefore, **only isolated lesions** of the cruciate ligaments are recommended for arthroscopic treatment.

Medium-term results after cruciate ligament suture were disappointing, thus, **primary ligament replacement** is the procedure of choice. Similarly, prosthetic substitutes of the cruciate ligaments provided unfavorable medium-term results. Autologous bone-ligament-bone or tendon transplants are standard of care today. Allogenic transplants are reserved for special indications and revision procedures (Kueche et al. 2002).

A fundamental question remains the intraoperative use of an image intensifier or the use of a navigation system (Julliard et al. 1998). Fluoroscopic control and navigation will improve the precision of **insertion of the ligament grafts** (Kohn et al. 1998), which is important for post-operative mobility and stability. The ligament replacement material must not collide with the wall or the entrance of the fossa intercondylaris even in full extension. The course of the graft should be impingement free (Howell and Clark 1992).

Only parts of the **posterior** cruciate ligament are visible as synovial tissue covers the femoral insertion. The cruciate ligament fibers are additionally covered ventrally by **Humphry's ligament**, the anterior meniscofemoral ligament. If the arthroscope is inserted into the posteromedial recess and if the instrument points in a lateral direction, the medial ridge of the posterior cruciate ligament appears and can be followed to caudal. At a suspected posterior cruciate ligament injury, the ligament is palpated with the probing hook and examined for freshly ruptured fiber bundles. The differentiation of complete versus incomplete rupture is generally not possible by arthroscopy alone. The reconstruction of the posterior cruciate ligament is carried out using tendon material from the knee extensor apparatus or pes anserinus tendons.

Joint cartilage

The condition of the hyaline joint cartilage is indicative for prognosis. Smooth undamaged cartilage surfaces indicate a good **prognosis** of a knee joint injury or disease whereas damaged surfaces are predictors of poor outcome.

Although arthroscopy is still associated with a **risk** for the joint cartilage, the portals have little impact on the soft tissue. Less experienced surgeons might damage the hyaline joint cartilage with the arthroscope or instruments. Even a skilled surgeon resecting the posterior horn of the internal meniscus in a small joint with tight ligaments is in danger to damage the cartilage. The **cartilage lesions** must be considered as "silent" danger of arthroscopic surgery, which will not be recognizable immediately as a complication but has long-term negative effects.

Joint cartilage requires visual inspection and palpation during arthroscopy, which is still the most reliable method for the diagnosis of cartilage damage but offers only limited therapeutic options. Surgical treatment options are best for traumatic localized, circumscribed lesions at the femoral condyles (Spaglione et al. 2002). Arthroscopically controlled surgery in osteoarthritis, however, still remains a matter of discussion (Moseley et al. 2002).

Cartilage fragments may lead to locking. Decaying cartilage parts will cause synovitis with effusion and pain. Osteochondral fragments floating freely in the joint will be nourished by joint liquid and can even grow. The removal of such loose bodies will be an easy but very successful arthroscopic operation. Any fragile or loose cartilage fragments prone to imminent detachment should be removed.

Shaving of irregular cartilage surfaces at a chondromalacia grade II has been abandoned as at best it would only cause a short-term improvement but may trigger further thinning of the hyaline-cartilaginous layer.

Breaking of the subchondral sclerosis zone may create **scar cartilage (fibrocartilage)**. Drill, awl and burr will be used for this intervention and are known as **Pridie drilling** (Muller and Kohn 1999), **micro-fracturing** (Steadman et al. 2003) or **abrasion arthroplasty** (Johnson 2001). Retrospective uncontrolled surveys indicate a long-term improvement of the clinical complaints.

Cartilage-bone transplantation using small osteocartilaginous cylinders from less important, nonweightbearing zones is a relatively new technique. Short-term results of animal experiments after this procedure have been promising (Lane et al. 2001). Furthermore, transplantation of extracorporally cultivated cartilage cells (ACI) should induce new formation of hyaline cartilage. These cells are first removed from intact cartilage zones

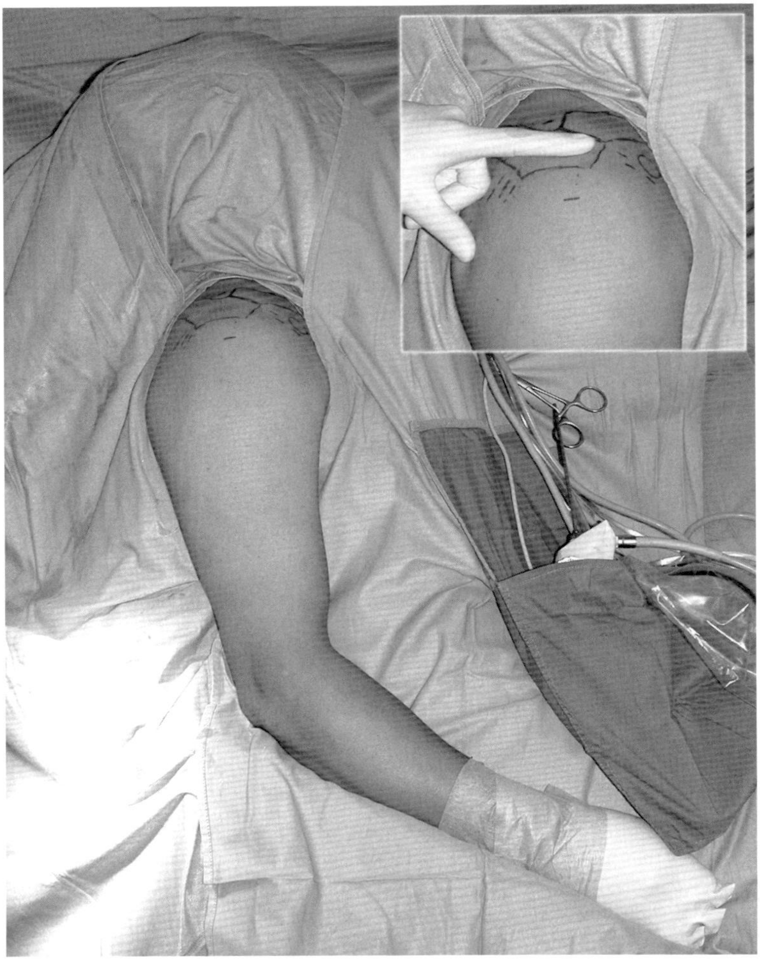

Fig. 9.3 Sitting position for shoulder arthroscopy. Aim is the nearly horizontal positioning of the acromion.

9.4 Technique

kept in culture for some weeks and multiplied and then transplanted back into the periostal lamella.

9.4.2 Shoulder

Shoulder arthroscopy after knee arthroscopy arthroscopy belongs to the most frequent arthroscopic procedures in orthopedics and traumatology. It is an important diagnostic tool for the assessment of the glenohumeral joint structures and the subacromial space.

The intervention can be performed in a lateral position or in the so-called beach chair position. This allows better traction without help of the assistant and a good overview of the posterior accesses. The beach chair position is advantageous becaus it is in accustomed anatomic orientation and allows for an easy transition from arthroscopic to open procedures. In the lateral position, attention should be paid to a thorough **axillary protection** of the opposite side and a permanent control of the traction force at the arm. The expression beach chair position actually is misleading as the patient has a more sitting position with the torso erected to 70–80° (➢ Fig. 9.3). The more horizontal direction of the acromion avoids working "uphill" all the time and allows better access from dorsal. Especially dorsal covering and covering at the neck must allow access to medial portals that lie further dorsomedially, the Neviaser portal for the rotator cuff, and the superior labrum portal. In a sitting posture the lateral shoulder region has to be kept free, which requires secure fixation of the torso and the head. An arm holder allows special joint postures.

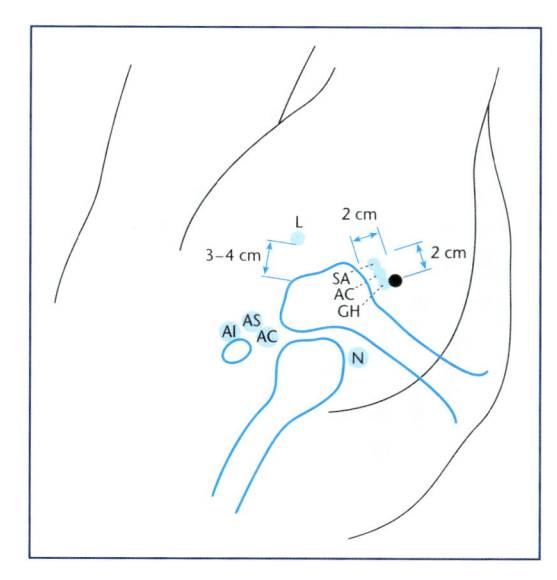

Fig. 9.4 Portals to the shoulder joint: "Classic" dorsal portal (black spot), dorsal portals for of operative arthroscopy in the glenohumeral joint (GH), AC joint (AC) and subacromial area (SA), lateral portal (L) and anterior portals to AC resection (AC), anterosuperior (AS) and anteroinferior portal (AI).

Portals and diagnostic arthroscopy

The arthroscopy of the shoulder starts with **marking** of the osseous landmarks and the possible portals since orientation can be impeded later by increasing soft-tissue edema (➢ Fig. 9.4). The first diagnostic roundtrip will happen through a **dorsal portal**, 2 cm caudal and 2 cm medial of the dorsolateral acromion corner (Kohn 1997). A further superolateral portal 1 cm caudally and 1 cm medially of the acromion corner fits working at the rotator cuff and in the subacromial space. Additional medial and lateral portals are useful to inspect the lateral end of the clavicula.

The anterior-superior and anterior-inferior portals are used as **ventral standard portals** for the glenohumeral joint. These portals are created under arthroscopic supervision from the outside to the inside or alternatively with the Wissinger rod from the inside outwards.

A probe is introduced via one of the anterior portals for the diagnostic circuit through the glenohumeral joint. All joint areas are consequently inspected and palpated; the transposing of the optics to ventral and the probing is obligatory with unclear findings or suspected change in the dorsal joint area.

Lateral portals are used for the arthroscopy of the subacromial space. The "classic" lateral portal lies about 3–5 cm laterally of the acromion ridge and 1–3 cm dorsally from the ventrolateral acromion corner. Additional lateral portals can be set up further ventral or dorsal for works in the area of the rotator cuff as well as for the management of suture material (Gartsman 2003). An additional anteromedial portal directly ventral of the acromioclavicular joint is useful for the resection of the lateral clavicula.

The **Neviaser portal** in the cavity between acromioclavicular joint and spina scapulae is used for the insertion of the suture material into the rotator cuff and the upper labrum as well as for instruments for working in the area of the fossa supraspinata.

Improved imaging – especially since the introduction of the **MR arthrography** – has made diagnostic shoulder arthroscopy a rare procedure. Chronic shoulder pain, snapping phenomena and instabilities, which will remain unclear even after extensive, non-invasive diagnostic measures still require arthroscopic clarification. The pathologic changes of the upper labrum and biceps tendon insertion still remain difficult to diagnose with imaging (Imhoff et al. 1992).

An accurate classification of SLAP lesions is hardly possible even with MR tomography. Partial rupture of the biceps tendon and its suspension as well as injuries of the joint capsule and its ligaments can often only be adequately assessed by arthroscopy. In contrast to the static radiologic examination, arthroscopy gives insight to dynamic functional examinations. The diagnostic superiority of arthroscopy often makes it an initial part of an open surgery, which is adapted to the arthroscopic findings, if needed.

Operative arthroscopy

The list of indications for arthroscopic surgery in the glenohumeral joint, the subacromial space and acromioclavicular joint continues to expand with further development of arthroscopic technologies and instruments.

A classic indication for shoulder arthroscopy is the presence of one or several **loose bodies**.

Arthroscopy offers the possibilities of puncture, inspection, biopsy and therapy by synovectomy or chondroma removal in case of **synovial diseases** such as chondromatosis or rheumatic synovitis.

Arthroscopic capsulotomy has already replaced mobilization under anaesthesia for adhesive capsulitis in stages II and III with lasting movement limitations (Warner et al. 1996). However, the narrow joints will be harder to treat by arthroscopy.

The increasing arthroscopy experience in the shoulder joint and correlation with clinical findings has contributed to the understanding of the different **forms of impingement**. Though the indications for subacromial decompression (Ellman 1987) at a classic outlet impingement have distinctively decreased, intrinsic forms of impingement such as the subcoracoidal impingement in golfers, the posterosuperior impingement in throwing athletes (Jobe 1995) and the anterosuperior impingement with lesions in the area of the rotator interval require special attention. Only the arthroscopic inspection and functional examination confirms diagnosis. Arthroscopic removal of calcium depots is indicated in **tendinosis calcarea**; only in few cases, an acromionplasty will be additionally necessary.

As decribed above, arthroscopy will provide the "golden standard" of diagnostics also for the origin and the intraarticular course of the **long biceps tendon**. Though the MR arthrography has improved preoperative diagnostics, only arthroscopy with palpation of the tendon and its anchor will deliver the decisive information about a lesion of the upper labruma degeneration, partial rupture or synovial infiltration of the tendon and about lesions in the area of the biceps tendon at the entry into the sulcus bicipitalis (Snyder et al. 1990, Weishaupt et al. 1999). Though the arthroscopic treatment of the upper labrum lesions is clearly superior to open surgery, best procedures of biceps tenodesis in the area of the sulcus bicipitalis require further discussion.

In shoulder instability arthroscopy provides information about collateral damage as e.g. the size and position of a Hill-Sachs lesions or allows to make a decision for an arthroscopic or open procedure by identification of ventroinferior osseous lesions of the glenoid rim (Burkhart and De Beer 2000). Depending on the kind of shoulder instability, the arthroscopic stabilization will be a fast and successful procedure.

Recent development of suture instruments and suture anchors has led to advance in arthroscopic rotator cuff reconstruction. Though the arthroscopic procedure is technically demanding, expensive, and time-consuming for the beginner, it protects the deltoid muscle.

Endoscopic lateral clavicula resection is established since the early 1990s. It can be carried out from the subacromial space (Gartsman 1993) or purely intraarticularly (Flatow 1995). The decision for lateral clavicula resection is made preoperatively based on radiological and clinical symptomatics and, if required, with infiltration tests.

9.4.3 Hip

After the wrist joint, arthroscopy of the hip belongs to the most challenging arthroscopic surgery procedures (Dienst et al. 2002). The arthroscopic access is more difficult and the manoevrability of the arthroscope and instruments is limited in comparison to other joints.

Diverse **anatomic characteristics of the hip joint** are responsible for this restriction:

- a thick soft-tissue coating
- proximity of two neurovascular bundles
- a strong joint capsule
- a small synovial space
- the permanent contact of femur head and acetabulum, and
- the additional sealing of the "deep" joint part by the acetabular labrum

Without traction at the leg, the joint surfaces of acetabulum and femur are only separated by a thin liquid film.

Especially the anatomy of the **acetabular labrum** has an impact on set up of the arthroscopy portals. Traction forces raising often to more than 400–500 N are required for the separation of femur head and joint socket. Only this allows pulling away the labrum far enough from the femur head to insert arthroscope and instruments (Byrd and Chern 1997).

Traction leads to an increased tension of joint capsule and intrinsic ligaments, the iliofemoral ligament, the ischiofemoral ligament and the pubofemoral ligament. This decreases the joint space distal to the acetabular labrum. Because of that arthroscopy of the **peripheral joint area without traction** with a freely movable hip joint will provide great advantages (Dienst et al. 2001).

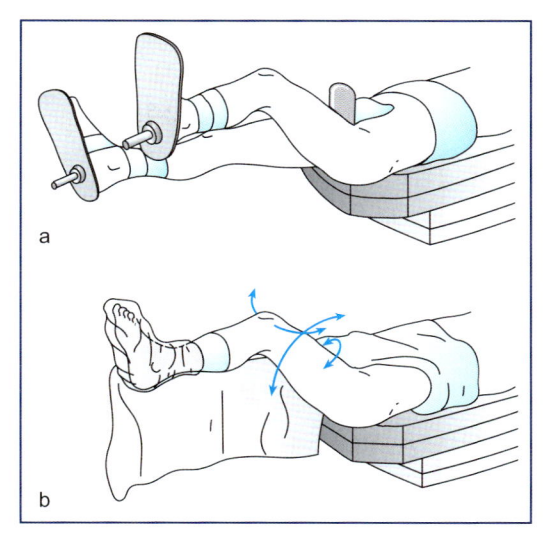

Fig. 9.5 Supine position for arthroscopy of the central compartment (a) and peripheral compartment (b) of the hip joint (according to Dienst et al. 2002).

The described anatomic conditions led to the classification of the hip joint into two arthroscopic compartments (Dormann and Boyer 1999). The **central compartment** includes the acetabulary joint surface, the fossa acetabuli with pulvinar and capitis femoris ligament and the primarily loaded joint surface of the femur head. The **peripheral compartment** includes the acetabular labrum, the intraarticularly located femoral neck with its synovial folds, a large part of the synovial lining and the joint capsule with its intrinsic ligaments and the zona orbicularis.

The patient may be positioned on his back or side for hip arthroscopy (➤ Fig. 9.5a and b). A radiolucent extension table is used for the **dorsal position** (Byrd 1994) and special extension devices for the **lateral position** (Glick et al. 1987). The pelvis is placed in a way that the countertraction rod is lateralized and pressed against the proximal thigh of the hip. The foot will be cushioned with one to two cotton-wool bandages and tightly fixed in the traction shoe. A slight external rotation of 10–20° without abduction of the leg is the recommended **posi-**

tion of the hip joint during arthroscopy of the central joint area.

The joint should be rotated neutrally for the setup of the portals in order to preserve the anatomic relations and keep neurovascular bundles away from the portals (Dienst 2005).

Portals and diagnostic arthroscopy

After the marking of the osseous landmarks, an **image intensifier** is useful to establish the first portal. With adequate experience it is possible to set up all further portals under arthroscopic observation. In general, hip arthroscopy requires three portals for each compartment to inspect and treat hip joint pathologies (Dienst 2005).

The **central compartment** can be examined via a ventral, ventrolateral and dorsolateral portal (➢ Fig. 9.6 a). Damag of the ventrolateral labrum-cartilage junction can be found and treated with shaver and instruments only in combination with the ventral and ventrolateral portal. Pathologic changes such as loose bodies, synovitis and ruptures of the capitis femoris ligament are often found in the fossa acetabuli are only accessible via ventral and dorsolateral portals. The set-up of two portals may be sufficient in dysplastic and very lax joints.

A ventral, proximal, and distal ventrolateral portal (➢ Fig. 9.6 b) is required for the **peripheral compartment**. Three portals are particularly advantageous for the treatment of femoroacetabular impingement. This allows correct resection of the head-neck junction under protection of the blood vessels.

As in all other joints, the inspection of the different joint areas should be standardized in the hip joint. First, the central compartment will be examined under traction. This allows an optimal positioning of pelvis and lower extremities achieving a good joint distraction. The traction will be reduced and the hip joint will be flexed or extended to different angles, rotated or abducted for the arthroscopy of the peripheral compartment.

The **bi-compartmental** approach ensures a more complete evaluation of pathological changes. The arthroscope is inserted via every portal in both joint compartments. A change between the 30° and the 70° optics is necessary. The 70° optics is the main optics especially in the central compartment for inspection of the labrum and the junction between labrum and facies lunata. The 30° optics is mainly used for the fossa acetabuli and the peripheral compartment.

Operative arthroscopy

The **list of indications** for hip arthroscopy has constantly grown since introduction of high-resolution MRT and MRT-arthrography.

Labrum lesions, **cartilage damage** at the junction between labrum and facies lunata and **loose bodies** are recognized preoperatively. Traumatic **labrum ruptures** are rare and their significance requires further clarification such as the femoroacetabular impingement.

The radiologic diagnosis of a **rupture of the capitis femoris ligament**, often seen in athletes after an acute abduction, adduction and rota-

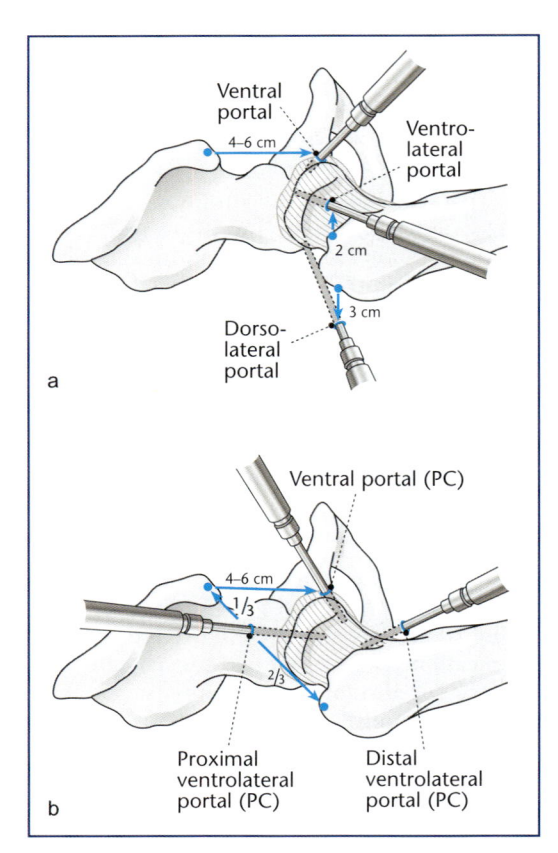

Fig. 9.6 Portals to the central (a) and peripheral (b) compartments of the hip joint.

tion trauma as well as after repeated microtraumas, remains problematic despite MR arthrography. Arhroscopy will be the procedure of choice for direct assessment and therapy; the results of smoothing and resection have been convincing.

Arthroscopy will diagnose correctly a suspected **synovial disease** such as chondromatosis, pigmented villonodular synovitis and aseptic or septic (early stage) synovitis with inspection and biopsy. In addition, the results of the arthroscopic synovectomy and chondroma removal will be good or very good.

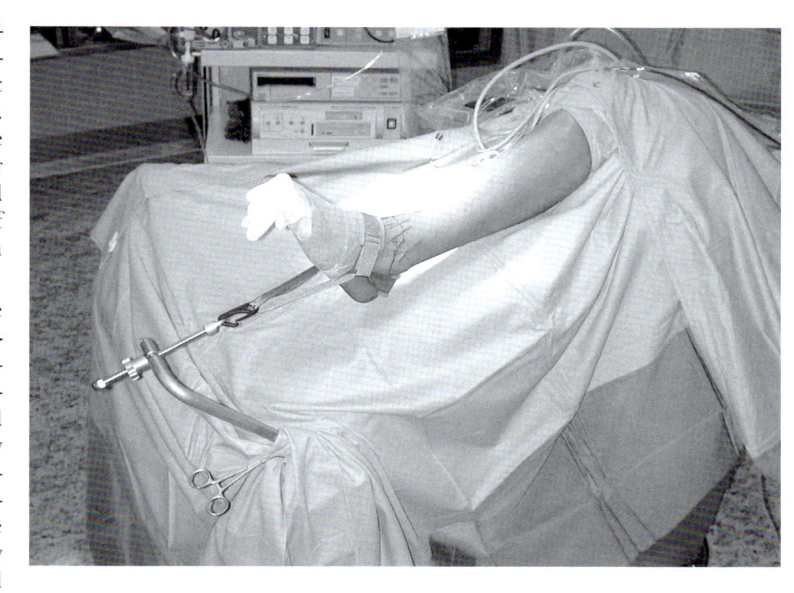

Fig. 9.7 Non-invasive distraction for arthroscopy of the ankle.

9.4.4 Ankle

Arthroscopy of the ankle joint can be carried out in **dorsal position** with a supported or with a hanging lower leg (➤ Fig. 9.7). Different **distraction procedures** are available such as non-invasive distraction devices and simple manual distraction by an assistant (Kohn 1997). Invasive distraction procedures such as osseous distraction should only be reserved for special cases such as arthroscopic arthrodesis.

Portals and diagnostic arthroscopy

Special care must be taken if setting up ankle portals given the vicinity to neurovascular structures (➤ Fig. 9.8). Similar to the elbow, a **safe portal zone** does **not** exist. Identification and marking of the osseous, tendinous and neurovascular structures are carried out prior to the intervention.

The joint will be punctured and filled with fluid from **anterolateral** lateral to the tendon of the peroneus tertius muscle at the height of the joint cavity. For the creation of the portal, a skinfold will be formed, the incision will be carried out strictly superficially and the subcutaneous tissue will be spread by a blunt clamp. The capsule penetration will occur with an blunt trocar. After initial diagnostic analysis using the 30° optics, the **anteromedial portal** is set up medially to the tendon of the anterior tibial muscle. Neurovascular structures as the

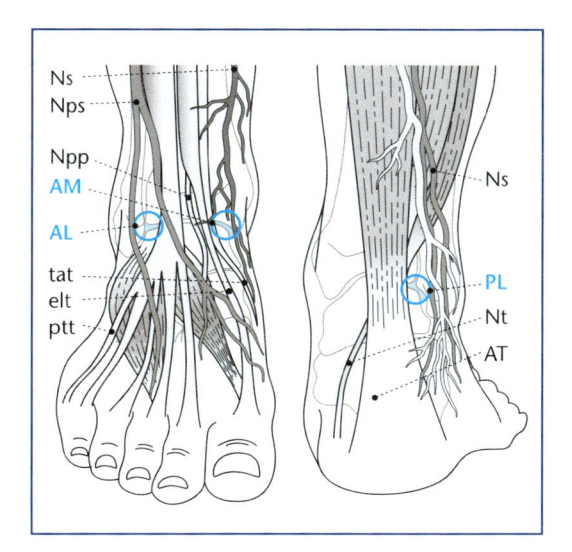

Fig. 9.8 Standard portals to the ankle: anteromedial (AM), anterolateral (AL) and posterolateral (PL) portals. N. peroneus superficialis (Nps), n. saphenus (Ns), n. peroneus profundus (Npp), tendon of the tibialis anterior (tat), tendon of the m. extensor hallucis longus (elt), tendon of the m. peroneus tertius (ptt), n. tibialis (Nt), Achilles tendon (AT) (with regard to Kohn 1997).

suralis nerve lying in the area of the portals must be identified by diaphanoscopy.

The inspection of the medial talomalleolar joint, the medial talus trochlea and the tibial leading edge will be carried out via the anterolateral portal. After the changing the arthroscope to anteromedial portal, the optics are pushed through the notch of Harty into the posterior joint chamber after distraction. A further working portal can be created from **posterolateral** directly lateral to the Achilles tendon at the height of the posterior jointline.

Operative arthroscopy

A frequent indication for arthroscopy of the ankle is the **anterolateral impingement** as a consequence of a distortion trauma. Scar tissue in the area of the anterolateral capsule (**meniscoid**) can often be detected. Typical changes, such as swelling and inflammatory changes of the joint capsule at MRT are indications for this.

Traumatic and non-traumatic causes will lead to **osteochondral lesions** of the talar dome. Arthroscopy allows an exact inspection of the integrity and stability of the osteochondral lesion. This will be important for further decision-making regarding operative technique. The formation of **osteophytes of the tibial leading edge** especially in sports with repeated ankle stress such as soccer will lead to a painfully limited dorsal extension. These osteophytes can be removed arthroscopically. Recently, tendoscopies of the peroneal tendons in patients with persisting posterolateral pain have been reported (Van Dijk and Kort 1998).

References

Ahn JH, Chung YS, Oh I (2003). Arthroscopic posterior cruciate ligament reconstruction using the posterior transseptal portal. Arthroscopy 19: 101–102.

Barber FA, Uribe JW, Weber SC (2002). Current applications for arthroscopic thermal surgery. Arthroscopy 18: 40–50.

Bobic V (1996). Arthroscopic osteochondral autograft transplantation in anterior cruciate ligament reconstruction: a preliminary clinical study. Knee Surg Sports Traumatol Arthrosc 3: 262–264.

Burkhart SS, Barnett CR, Snyder SJ (1990). Transient postoperative blindness as a possible effect of glycine toxicity. Arthroscopy 6: 112.

Burkhart SS, De Beer JF (2000). Traumatic glenohumeral bone defects and their relationship to failure of arthroscopic Bankart repairs: significance of the inverted-pear glenoid and the humeral engaging Hill-Sachs lesion. Arthroscopy 16: 677–694.

Byrd JWT, Chem KY (1997). Traction versus distension for distraction of the joint during hip arthroscopy. Arthroscopy 13: 346–349.

Byrd JWT (1994). Hip arthroscopy utilizing the supine position. Arthroscopy 10: 275–280.

Dienst M, Gödde S, Seil R, Hammer D, Kohn D (2001). Hip arthroscopy without traction: In vivo anatomy of the peripheral hip joint cavity. Arthroscopy 17: 924–931.

Dienst M, Gödde S, Seil R, Kohn D (2002). Diagnostische Arthroskopie des Hüftgelenks. Operat Orthop Traumatol 14: 1–15.

Dienst M (2005). Hip arthroscopy – technique and anatomy. Oper Tech Sports Med 13: 13–23.

Dienst M, Seil R, Kohn D. Safe arthroscopic access to the central compartment of the hip. Arthroscopy (in print).

Dormann H, Boyer T (1999). Arthroscopy of the hip – 12 years of experience. Arthroscopy 15: 67–72.

Edwards RB, Lu Y, Rodriguez E, Markel M (2002). Thermometric determination of cartilage matrix temperatures during thermal chondroplasty: comparison of bipolar and monopolar radiofrequency devices. Arthroscopy 18: 339–346.

Ellman H (1987). Arthroscopic subacromial decompression: Analysis of 1–3 years results. Arthroscopy 3: 173–181.

Erggelet C, Sittinger M, Lahm A (2003). The arthroscopic implantation of autologous chondrocytes for the treatment of thickness cartilage defects of the knee joint. Arthroscopy 19: 108–110.

Faletti C, Robba D, de Petro P (2002). Postmeniscectomy osteonecrosis. Arthroscopy 18: 91–94.

Flatow EL, Duralde XA, Nicholson GP, Pollock RG, Bigliani LU (1995). Arthroscopic resection of the distal clavicle with a superior approach. J Shoulder Elbow Surg 4: 41–50.

Gartsman GM (1993). Arthroscopic resection of the acromioclavicular joint. Am J Sports Med 21: 71–77.

Gartsman GM (2003). Shoulder Arthroscopy. Saunders, Philadelphia.

Glick JM, Sampson TG, Behr JT, Schmidt E (1987). Hip arthroscopy by the lateral approach. Arthroscopy 3: 4–12.

Glinz W (1989). Neben den bekannten gibt es auch heimliche Gefahren bei der Arthroskopie. Arthroskopie 2: 37–40.

Hangody L (1994). New possibilities in the management of severe circumscribed cartilage damage in the knee. Magy Traumatol Orthop Kezseb Plasztikai Seb 37: 237–243.

Howell SM, Clark JA (1992). Tibial tunnel placement in anterior cruciate ligament reconstructions and graft impingement. Clin Orthop 283: 187–195.

Hunt N, Sanchez-Ballester J, Pandit Ravi et al. (2001). Chondral lesions of the knee: A new localisation method and correlation with associated pathology. Arthroscopy 17: 481–490.

Imhoff AB, Perrenoud A, Neidl K (1992). MRI bei Schulterinstabilität – Korrelation zum Arthro-CT und zur Arthroskopie der Schulter. Arthroskopie 5: 122–129.

Jobe CM (1995). Posterior superior glenoid impingement: Expanded spectrum. Arthroscopy 11: 530–536.

Johnson DH (2002). Basic science in digital imaging: Storage and retrieval. Arthroscopy 18: 648–653.

Johnson LL (2001). Arthroscopic abrasion arthroplasty: A review. Clin Orthop 391: 306–317.

Julliard R, Lavallee S, Dessenne V (1998). Computer assisted reconstruction of the anterior ligament. Clin Orthop 354: 57–64.

Kobayashi Y, Kimura M, Higuchi H et al. (2002). Juxta-articular bone marrow signal changes on magnetic resonance imaging following arthroscopiy meniscectomy. Arthroscopy 18: 238–245.

Kohn D (1991). Arthroskopie des Kniegelenkes. Urban und Schwarzenberg, Munich.

Kohn D (1995). Arthroskopie. In: Bauer R, Kerschbaumer F, Poisel S (eds.). Orthopädische Operationslehre Band II/2. Thieme, Stuttgart.

Kohn D, Busche T, Carls J (1998). Drill hole position in endoscopic anterior cruciate ligament reconstruction. Knee Surg Sports Traumatol Arthrosc 6: 13–15.

Kohn D (1997). Diagnostische und operative Arthroskopie großer Gelenke. Thieme, Stuttgart.

Kohn D, Adam F (2005). Arthroskopie. In: Wirth CJ, Zichner L (eds.). Orthopädie und Orthopädische Chirurgie, Knie. Thieme, Stuttgart.

Kuechle DK, Pearson SE, Beach WR et al. (2002). Allograft anterior cruciate ligament reconstruction in patients over 40 years of age. Arthroscopy 18: 845–853.

La Prade RF, Willis NJ (2004). Kissing cartilage lesions of the knee caused by a bioabsorbable meniscle repair device. A case report. Am J Sports Med 32: 1751–1754.

Lane JG, Trontz WL, Ball ST et al. (2001). A morphologic biochemical and biomechanical assessment of short-term effects of osteochondral autograft plug transfer in an animal model. Arthroscopy 19: 856–863.

Louisia S, Charrois O, Beaufis P (2003). Posterior "back and forth" approach in arthroscopic surgery on the posterior knee compartments. Arthroscopy 19: 321–325.

Moseley JB, O'Malley K, Peterson NJ et al. (2002). A controlled trial of arthroscopic surgery for osteoarthritis of the knee. N Engl J Med 347: 81–88.

Muellner T, Menth-Chiari WA, Reihsner R et al. (2001). Accuracy of pressure and flow capacities of four arthroscopic fluid management systems. Arthroscopy 17: 760–764.

Muller B, Kohn D (1999). Indication for and performance of articulate cartilage drilling using the Pridie method. Orthopäde 28: 4–10.

Nicholas SJ, Tyler, TF, McHugh MP (2001). The effect on leg strength of tourniquet use during anterior cruciate ligament reconstruction. A prospective randomised study. Arthroscopy 17: 603–617.

Noyes FR, Stabler CL (1989). A system for grading articular cartilage lesions at arthroscopy. Am J Sports Med 17: 505–513.

Oakley SP, Portek S, Szomor Z et al. (2003). Accuracy and reliability of arthroscopic estimates of cartilage lesion size in a plastic knee simulation model. Arthroscopy 19: 282–289.

Owens BD, Stickles BJ, Balikian P et al. (2002). Prospective analysis of radiofrequency versus mechanical debridement of isolated patellar chondral lesions. Arthroscopy 18: 151–155.

Pape D, Seil R, Kohn D, Schneider G (2004). Imaging of early stages of osteonecrosis of the knee. Orthop Clin North Am 35: 294–303.

Pidoriano AJ, Fulkerson JP (1997). Arthroscopy of the patellofemoral joint. Clin Sports Med 16: 17–28.

Reagan BF, McInerny VK, Treadwell BV, Zarins B, Mankin HJ (1983). Irrigation fluids for arthroscopy. J Bone Joint Surg (Am) 65: 629–631.

Spaglione NA, Miniaci A, Gillogly SD et al. (2002). Update on advanced surgical techniques in the treatment of traumatic focal articular cartilage lesions in the knee. Arthroscopy 18: 9–32.

Shellock FG (2001). Radiofrequency energy-induced heating of bovine capsular tissue. Temperature changes produced by bipolar versus monopolar electrodes. Arthroscopy 17: 124–131.

Sherman PM, Penrod BJ, Lane MJ et al. (2002). Comparison of knee magnetic resonance imaging findings in patients referred by orthopaedic surgeons versus nonorthopaedic practitioners. Arthroscopy 18: 201–205.

Snyder SDJ, Karzel RP, Del Pizzo W, Ferkel RD, Friedman MJ (1990). SLAP lesions of the shoulder. Arthroscopy 6: 274–279.

Steadman JR, Briggs KK, Rodrigo JJ et al. (2003). Outcomes of microfracture for traumatic chondral defects of the knee: Average 11-year followup. Arthroscopy 19: 477–484.

Van Dijk CN, Kort N (1998). Tensoscopy of the peroneal tendons. Arthroscopy 14: 471–478.

Warner JJP, Allan A, Marks PJH, Wong P (1996). Arthroscopic release for chonic refractory adhesive capsulitis of the shoulder. J Bone Joint Surg 78-A: 1808–1816.

Warren RF (1990). Meniscectomy and repair in the anterior cruciate ligament-deficient patient. Clin Orthop 252: 55–63.

Weishaupt D, Zanetti M, Tanner A, Gerber C, Hodler J (1999). Lesions of the reflection pulley of the long biceps tendon. MR arthrographic findings. Invest Radiol 34: 463–469.

Chapter 10

Clinical biomechanics

Andreas Gösele-Koppenburg and Marlene Mauch

Recording of human motion is an important instrument of orthopedics and sports medicine. The importance of locomotor functional analysis – especially injuries, overuse, and their prevention – is increasing in sports medicine. This trend is further fostered by the availability of new diagnostic tools resulting from a combination of different medical specialties, in particular, orthopedics, biomechanics, and sports sciences.

The clinical motion analysis uses an extensive repertoire of proven and validated examination techniques. Developing hard- and software help handling clinical routine. Still biomechanical examinations are time consuming and come with significant material and financial cost, which restrict their use to specialized centers.

Here, cost efficacy determines which method can address clinically relevant questions.

Quantifiable methods such as isokinetics are superior to standard clinical analysis (inspection, palpation, muscle function tests) in detecting movements or forces more precisely. Results of such quantifiable methods allow more focused therapy.

Hence, knowledge of the diagnostic tools and interpretation of their results is of great importance for the practicing sports physicians and therapists.

10.1 Use of clinical biomechanics

Use of clinical biomechanics can be very manifold and reaches well beyond the limits of clinical daily diagnostic especially if investigating cause of injuries and diseases. Combination of modern and traditional diagnostics is particularly important in the age of demystified medicine and increasing technical possibilities. This applies equally to causal research of overuse complaints, complaints after injuries, and the diagnosis of movement disorders, supervision and evaluation of therapeutic interventions, as well as to therapy planning.

The functional examination may serve **different intentions**:

- quality control after conservative therapy or after surgical procedures
- definition of the degree of severity of a functional disorder
- the objective comparison of competing therapeutic methods
- the examination of rehabilitation success
- quantitative examination of the effect of ortheses, arch supports and foot wear.

Simple gait-analytic examinations with a standardized set of parameters will provide answers to questions left open by conventional clinical diagnostic procedures. This additional information helps the clinician in informed therapeutic decision-making. Clinical motion analysis is not competing with clinical standard diagnoses; it is enhances the repertoire of available techniques.

10.2 Measuring methods and application of selected biomechanical procedures

Three-dimensional movement analysis with high-speed or infrared cameras, gathering of pressure or force dynamic-kinetic parameters, or recording of muscle activity by electromyography (EMG) has revolutionized biomechanical diagnostics. This allows better quantification of movements and diagnosis of pathological movement. Strong diagnostics result in optimal and personalized therapy and therefore improve therapeutic outcomes. This protects the athlete of injuries and shortens rehabilitation.

10.2.1 Kinematic motion analysis

Three-dimensional gait analysis provides an important insight to pathobiomechanics or pathophysiology of complex gait and movement disorders, which is the basis of any adequate therapeutic decision. High-duty processors and digital imaging of gait-analytic systems are frequently found in today's medical facilities.

Kinematic movement analysis illustrates distance-time progressing of body parts and quality of the movement execution. The kinematic movement analysis is more accessible for less scientific-oriented users as compared to dynamic-mechanical evaluation of the foot strike (cf. pressure measuring).

Nowadays 2D and 3D systems are readily available. Most high-resolution, digital high-speed video cameras use **2D systems**, which record movements in the frontal and sagittal layer. Optoelectronic stereophotogrammetric systems analyze **3D motions** with stroboscopic light sources and reflecting markers. In general, 2D systems are less precise (radiography rate, monitoring level) but are far more widespread in clinical routine.

Use of the according systems and costs has been discussed controversially in literature (Sheldon 2004); both are afflicted with measuring faults. In the end, users must decide themselves which question is answered by what analysis.

Important aspects of data collection and evaluation have been described (Capozzo et al. 2005). In addition, gait and running analysis is discussed by Walther (➤ Chapter 11).

10.2.2 Plantar pressure measurement

The foot as lowest articular point of the human motion chain is the ultimate interface between human being and environment. Kinetic movement analysis and electronic pressure measurement under the foot are important for an assessment of the movement process and stress. Measuring ground forces will unravel involved forces. The pressure measurement may **localize effecting forces** at discretely anatomic position underneath the foot. This helps to uncover overuse or injury patterns the lower extremity, development of shoe inlays or arch supports. Hence, pressure measurements will provide valuable information for therapeutic decisions and follow-ups of etiopathologies.

Forces and pressures are important variables in **kinetic gait analysis**. Forces describe the interaction between two bodies, while pressure and pressure distribution are forces affecting a surface. The unit of force is Newton (N), defined as the force that is necessary to accelerate a body of 1 kg by 1 m/s^2. The pressure is calculated from the quotient of force and area in Pascal (Pa) or Nm^2. One Pascal equates to a force of 1 N/m.

Functionality and systems

The functionality will be similar in all pressure measuring systems: the external force, which will be carried out by the foot on the ground or on the measurement plate or measurement sole, will lead to a deformation of a body. This deformation will be translated into electric signals and will be measured.

Different measuring systems will be available on the market, and they will be distinguished regarding their technical specifications (different sensor technologies) and their preferred applications (different devices). Mainly, **three different technologies** will be available: Today resistive or capacitive sensors, in rare cases also piezoelectric sensors, are consulted for the measuring of the pressure dispersion.

The **resistively working sensors** will consist of two conductive layers that will have a defined contact surface available. The affecting force will increase the contact surface and decrease the electronic resistance. The functional principle of the systems with resistive sensors will be the same everywhere; still the sensor will be differently built in parts and differently arranged within the measurement platform or measurement sole.

The **capacitive sensors** (condensator) will consist of two electrically conductive plates that will be separated by a non-conductive element (dielectric). The capacity will be determined by the distance of the plates and the conditions of the dieletricum between the plates. If a force affects the condensator, the distance of the plates to each other will change, and so will also the electric resistance. These changes will be measured by the system.

Piezoelectric quartzes that will have the condition of being statically charged afterwards will be used in **piezoelectric technology**. The molecular lattice structure will be disarranged by external pressure, so that electric charges at the surface of the body will develop. These will be proportional to the operating force and electronically measurable (Orlin and McPoil 2000).

The diverse sensors will be used **in measurement platforms or flexible insoles**. Measurement platforms will be embedded in a running track or a treadmill ergometer and will be used for barefoot measurements. This way, they will be basically limited to the application in the laboratory. The way of construction will often secure an increased robustness as well as a higher spatial resolution and metering time period than flexible insoles. Still, the application of pressure measurement platforms may lead to distortions of the movement exposure, because the athlete will be required to hit the plate in a certain area, and this will possibly have to go along with an adaption of the gait rhythm. This problem can be faced by covering the platform or a pressure measurement plate integrated into a treadmill. Covering the platform will be accompanied by the difficulty that distortion of the measured signal will occur because of dampening effects of the covering material; the running on an ergometer will often be criticized because it is not considered to correspond to the "natural" manner of movement of the runer. Flexible insoles, on the other hand, may be used under field conditions and conduce to the examination of the plantar pressure within a shoe and therefore to making conclusions about the effects of different shoe constructions or insole provisions.

The achieved **spatial resolution** of the pressure measuring systems will usually range between 0.5 and 4 sensors/cm², the **metering time period** of few individual measurements by the second amount to 500 Hz. A scrolling process in normal walking speed will take about 0.7 sec. The time in which the foot will have ground contact will be considerably shorter in running or sprinting. 25 to 50 Hz will be considered sufficient for normal walking movements. It should be made a point, though, of a clearly higher measuring frequency of up to 250 Hz in the treatment of athletes, in order to be able to exactly analyze the tread, support and roll phases sufficiently (Rosenbaum and Becker 1997, Best 2003).

Measures

Different measures that characterize the foot strike taken from the data acquired during pressure measuring ground contact while standing, walking or running can provide additional information.

The data of the complete **foot surface** is classified into **anatomically justifiable subareas (templates)**. Identical measurements are assessed in these templates. Diverse methods ranging from a purely visual identification of separate pressure tops to the use of software-based algorithms for the recognition of different foot areas based on the geometry of the foot print can be used. According to the examination aim and question, the anatomic structures of the foot will be differentiated and classified in four to ten templates. This results in a medial and lateral heel template, one or several metatarsal templates, two or five forefoot templates, and two or more toe templates. ➢ Figure 10.1 shows a classification of nine anatomically functional templates according to Maiwald (2008).

Calculated **parameters** can be divided in **global measures** that calculate all exposed sensors and **local measures** that provide force and pressure in individual templates. Generally, the calculation of the pressure measures is carried out by dividing the measured force values of a sensor by its sensor surface. Pressure values varies according to spatial resolution of the measurement system because the size of the sensor is a decisive criterion for the development of the resulting pressure values at constant end force on a structure (Rosenbaum and Becker 1997).

Maximum force (F_{max}, N): The force values of all sensors within a template add up and the maximum determines the complete foot strike process. Mostly, F_{max} will be standardized to the body weight (FW) of the racer and expressed as a multiple of FW (kg). The measurement parameter will show the peak load in the complete foot strike.

Maximum/medium pressure (P_{max}, kPa): This value represents the peak pressure values of a sensor, a template or the complete ground contact.

Force-time integral (FTI, %): The sum force values of all sensors within a template is divided by the value of force-time integral of the complete pressure matrix. FTI is expressed as percentage and will represent the template's relative part, i.e. anatomic structure of the foot strike. The relative load analysis allows interindividual comparison between homogeneous groups due to normalization to the body weight or the size of the foot surface.

The **loaded surface of the foot** is measured barefoot to evaluate arch foot development and detection of other foot problems/deformities. In this case loaded sensors is summed up allowing calculation of the loaded surface.

The **relative contact time (rel CT, %)** expresses the foot strike. The number of individual images is divided by the number of complete foot strike process images.

Center of Pressure (CoP): The CoP describes the pressure balance point of the currently loaded sensor matrix. For pressure measurement plates, the CoP complies with the contact point of ground reaction force. A sequence of individual images is recorded continually during the foot strike process. The local and timely course of CoP can be visualized by help of a connecting line after finishing the foot strike process. CoP is often used as a characteristic measurement of hindfoot movement and foot function (Cornwall and McPoil 2003).

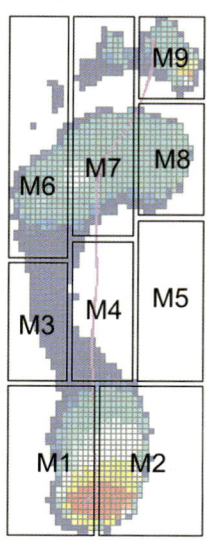

Fig. 10.1 The pressure dispersion image will be divided into anatomically functional templates (according to Maiwald 2008) and allows evaluation of local measurements.

Clinical implementations

Pressure measurement can provide useful insights into **load distribution between injured and uninjured, pre- or posttraumatic/operative movement patterns**. In sports, **convenience of running shoes** is critical and can be assessed by pressure measurements. (Henning and Milani 2000). Additionally, pressure measures can determine the efficiency of orthopedic shoes (Baur 2004). Based on the pressure measurements injury patterns recurring especially in running sports can be quantified and qualified and therapies tailored (Grau 2001). Pressure measurement is used to characterize causes and therapeutic options of diabetic feet (Leung 2007).

Critical consideration of pressure measurement

Reliability of pressure measurement data is user dependent. The walking speed, the walking distance, the shoe, the underground or the number of steps that will be measured and evaluated will influence the result. Measuring conditions must keep constant in order to compare data. Additionally, good measuring results will depend on the quality of the sensors. Therefore, calibration of the sensors is key.

> **Summary**
>
> Load distribution during step movement can be measure with pressure dispersion. Combined with clinical examination pressure measurements provide a powerful diagnostic tool. In order to interpret biomechanics of the foot correctly, anatomy of the lower extremity is critical.

10.2.3 Strength diagnostics

In addition to the kinematic and kinetic movement analysis, strength diagnostics is an important component of clinical biomechanics. Power diagnostics assesses the **effects of a training or rehabilitation process on power parameters** (improvement/change) and **strength** level of the patient or athlete in comparison to different groups or general norm data. For comparative measurements strength level should be measure without prior information of fitness condition. Strength diagnostics has a central role in documenting rehabilitation success.

Indirect measurement methods such as circumference measurements of extremities or muscle function tests quantifies muscle strength in the clinic, in sports science and training Indirect measurement methods have a lower reproducibility than apparative measurement methods (Sole et al. 2007, Chevilotte et al. 2008). Therefore, different biomechanical measurement systems have established in strength diagnostics for a longer time that can detect the strength level of individual muscles or muscle groups. Use of measurement systems requires a case-by-case decision depending the underlying problem and application.

Isokinetics

Isokinetic strength measurement is an established diagnostic tool in therapy and rehabilitation. Isokinetic strength measurement allows **dynamic and static strength determination of individual muscle groups** as well as **diagnostics of muscle dysbalances**. Thus, this technique is critical in both high-performance sports and rehabilitation medicine (➤ Fig. 10.2).

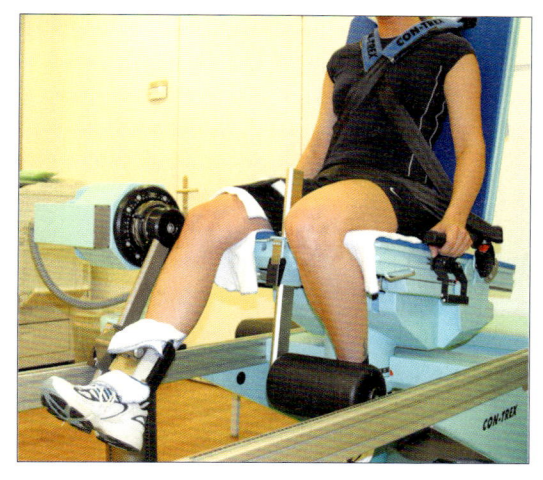

Fig. 10.2 Isokinetic strength measuring instrument (photo: crossklinik Basel).

Mechanism of Isokinetics

Isokinetic (i.e. same strength) measuring is carried out based on an constant movement speed and corresponds to the contraction speed of the muscle. Strength (moment of force) will be executed over the complete movement area against a variable, individually adjusted resistance. This allows joint-angle specific strength detection as well as the strength evolvement under different load conditions.

Different technical systems are available: **Microprocessor-controlled electrical and electromagnetical drives**. Mechanically, hydraulically or pneumatically controlled isokinetic systems are uncommon.

Measured values

The rotation effect of the affecting force on the lever arm – the moment of force – quantifies the static and dynamic forces of an isokinetic device. The external moment of force is the most frequently used parameter in isokinetic tests. Further parameters can be calculated such as power, flexor-extensor relation, right-left differences or relative forces.

Maximum moment of force in relation to the angle position: Maximum moment of force will present a decisive power-determining biomechanical parameter for flexion and extension movements, internal and external rotations as well as abductions and adductions. Gravity influences maximum moment of force and supports downwards and exacerbates upwards movements. Most new isokinetic devices correct for gravity.

Movement speed: The contraction speed determines the angle position/muscle length and moment of force. Muscle strength depends on the speed of length change: the higher the contraction speed the lower is the resulting maximum moment of force.

Mechanical power: The mechanical power is the product of maximum moment of force and angle speed. Physical power will be estimated by the moment-of-force value at a preset angle speed. The power will decrease with the increase of the angle speed; power maximum can only be reached with very high speed, thereafter power is decreasing.

Evaluation of different parameters

Correlation between different isokinetic parameters (e.g. max. moment of force) and the sporting performance have been tested (Impellizzeri et al. 2007). The data relative to body weight allow interindividual comparisons. Functional relations allow assessment of strength variables, e.g. agonistic and antagonic strength values, or of right-left differences. Functional asymmetry and muscular dysbalance (divergence from the standard value) need to be differentiated. To interpretation such findings the profile of the athlete or the clinical history of the patient toned to be considered. Right-left differences of non-athletes of more than 10% are clear sign of a dysbalance. However the same difference is interpreted as a functional dysbalance in long-jumper or soccer players. Similarly, a 66% relation of knee extensor and flexor is "normal" for a non-athlete, the strength relation for these muscle groups are clearly different in a sprinter.

Limitations of isokinetics

Isokinetic data reproducibility is often criticized. While reproducibility of knee and hip is judged as reliable data from joints a higher degree of freedom, e.g. shoulder or ankle joint require cautious interpretation (Meeteren et al. 2002).

Isokinetic measurements of various device manufacturers are often subject to interdevice variability. Ratios or lateral differences are reliable. Furthermore, increased braking and accelerating forces at high angle speeds or the moments of inertia at long levers may distort results and produce measurement artifacts. In addition to device- errors the subjectivity of the examiner, incorrect positioning and fixation of the test person and training effects contribute to biased isokinetic data.

Jump Tests

Elasticity is a power-determining factor in many sports is routinely detected with force measurement plates. At the measurement of springiness, different jump forms are carried out. These are counter movement jump (CMJ), the squat jump (SJ) (➢ Fig 10.3), the drop jump (DJ), one-legged jumps or jump series. Here, the estimation of the reactive movement behavior (springiness) is acquired by **jump height** and **time of ground contact**. These two parameters determine the strength-time. The jump height can either be calculated from the jump impulse or the flight time. The time of ground contact is easily determined from the strength-time curve. Additionally, the maximum achieved power, a parameter that had not been detectable with previous measurement systems (Grossenbacher et al. 1998).

Procedure of springiness measurement

The formula $h = {}^1/_2\, g\,(t/2)^2$ deuced from kinetics will serve the **calculation of the jump height via the flight time**. This procedure is still relatively **inexact**; the measurement errors lies at up to 25% and can be significantly influenced by the adopted posture. An artificially lengthened flight time might be caused by possible differences of foot, knee and hip joints in jumping and landing.

The **calculation of the jump height by means of the jump impulse behavior** (integration of the strength-time course) **and the maximum body speed** is wide spread. The jump height can be calculated more exactly via the jump-impulse method. In addition, the parameters of maximum speed of the body balance point and the maximum as well as relative jump power can be investigated by means of the strength-time

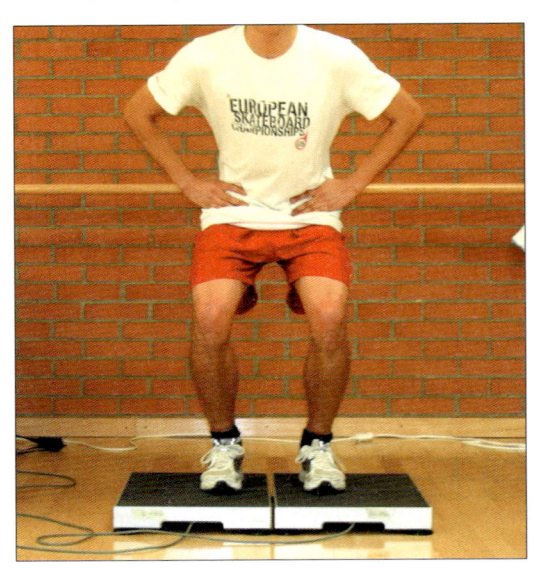

Fig. 10.3 Measuring of springiness with a force platform (photo: crossklinik Basel).

curve. The maximum and relative jump power is important parameters for the **assessment of the elasticity**. It is reached at the point where the steepest point in the power-time curve will be reached (most strength per time unit). This parameter provide more exact values than the maximum jump height in the assessment of elasticity and do not depend as strongly on the acceleration distance, the anthropometric sizes and coordinative abilities of test persons.

There are differences between coordinative deficits and missing elasticity by an intra- and inter-individual comparison of jump height and jump power, which would not be possible by the sole examination of the jump height.

Interpretation of the power values

The interpretation of the power values depends on the profile of the according sport. Therefore it is more sensible to interpret the absolute values in sports that have to raise strength against resistance (throwers, opponents). On the other hand, the relative values are interesting in sports in which the own body has to be accelerated (artistic gymnastics).

The positive acceleration distance (s_pos), the maximum jump height (s_max), as well as the (relative) maximum power (Pmax) is decisive parameters in the analysis of springiness.

These parameters give information about functional relations in the elasticity abilities. This is calculated by the relation between maximum jump power of jumps using both legs and the sum of the maximum jump powers of one-legged jumps left and right ($[P_{max}$ both sides/ (P_{max} left + P_{max} right) $-1] \times 100$). By means of this index, the powers of a person can be compared with a comparison group (sport-specific standard values). If the bilateral deficit is higher than the one of the comparison group, the tested person is stronger one-legged than in using both legs. If, on the other hand, the values of the index are lower than the ones of the comparison group, the test person is stronger both-legged than one-legged. Based on these results, it is possible to give recommendations for training.

A careful interpretation of the bilateral deficits has to be carried out with side differences of the one-legged jumps of more than 10%, because falsely deep sums may be the result of the one-legged jumps.

Another parameter for the evaluation of springiness power is presented by the **effect of pre-stretch**. Passive energy is stored in the elastic structures by stretching during the strike-out movement for the jump movement, which in general lead to a higher jump height at the counter-movement jump (CMJ) when taking off. This parameter is calculated by the differences of jump heights (cm) of the counter – movement jump (CMJ) and the squat jump (SJ) (CMJ – SJ). The differences between 4 and 8% are considered as normal. At a difference of more than 8%, a very effectively coordinated movement execution at CMJ or insufficient maximum power ability will be assumed. At differences of less than 4%, ineffective movement coordination at CMJ or a missing implementation of the maximum strength into movement can be assumed. The interpretation of the results of this measurement parameter has not been scientifically proven yet.

Possibilities and limits

Springiness diagnostics will offer the possibility to quantify the fitness ability of "elasticity". Furthermore, it will allow the uncovering of coordinative deficits, and therefore offer a basis for intra- and inter-individual comparisons (standard data), as a basis for training recommendations, for the detection of training effects and, finally, for the possible prevention of injuries, for example by the uncovering of side differences.

For comprehensive and focused functional diagnostics, comparing the results with isokinetic strength devices or EMG maybe needed.

> Both the isokinetically collected forces as well as the forces recorded via the strength measurement plate are important parameters for the performance assessment of a patient or athlete. Ideally, the results should be taken into consideration together with findings of other biomechanical test methods, such as the kinematic or kinetic gait analysis or the muscle activity (EMG).

10.2.4 Electromyography (EMG)

Electromyography (EMG) measure the electric muscle activity (excitation and contraction conditions of the musculature). In clinical biomechanics, the connections between the frequencies or the amplitudes of the registered electric signals and the strength of a muscle is examined to diagnose the movements of the athlete and – if required – to optimize them.

We distinguish clinical and kinesiology EMG. In **clinical EMG**, the nerve conduction velocity and the discharge rates of the motor units as well as the characteristics of individual action potentials, regarding duration, amplitude and shape, will be examined via wire and needle electrodes. In **kinesiology EMG**, the connection between muscle actions, movements and strengths is examined. In contrast to clinical EMG, superficial electrodes are applied to the skin above the muscle, which deduce the activity of large and superficially located muscles. The implementation of fine wire electrodes is necessary for small and deeply located muscles. Kinesiology EMG is applied almost exclusively to clinical biomechanics.

Functionality

The activation of a motor nerve via acetylcholine release at the neuromuscular junction leads to an action potential at the muscle fiber. The activated discharges depend on the contraction intensity and are transmitted along the muscle fiber membrane. Via the electromechanical coupling, they lead low discharge rates and tetanic contractions of the myofilaments at a sufficiently high frequency. The activated potential changes, which have been created at the muscle fiber membrane at can be detected by the help of the applied electrodes. The EMG signal represents an extracellularly deducted signal of all action potentials of the active motor units (➤ Fig 10.4).

The technical specifications, the positioning of the electrodes and the detailed EMG analysis are described elsewhere (e.g. Konrad 2005, De Luca 1997).

Use

The EMG provides **insights into the inter and intra-muscular coordination**, i.e. for the timely relation of the activation of individual muscles, for the coactivation of muscles, i.e. how many muscles are involved at the same time, and with regard to different innervation patterns in movements. This allows **measuring** and comparison **of agonistic and antagonistic muscles**.

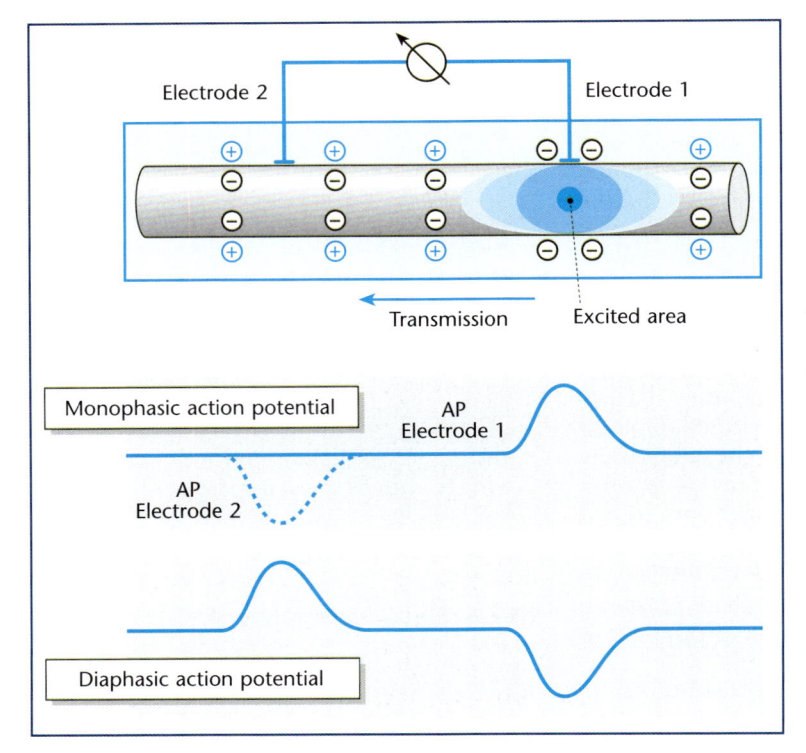

Fig. 10.4 Derivation of a nerve fiber with two extracellular electrodes. An action potential runs from right to left over the nerve fiber (top), the excited area has just reached electrode 1. At electrode 1, the green drawn out potential development will be measured (middle line). When the action potential finally reaches electrode 2, the green dashed potential course will be measured. The separate potential courses of the middle line are monophasic action potentials each. The diphasic action potential (bottom) is measured between electrodes 1 and 2 as complete potential course.

In addition to the clinical diagnosis of muscle diseases (myopathies) as well as the qualitative assessment of damages and regeneration, orientating **evaluations of muscle activities during certain movement courses** can be carried out via EMG in line with functional anatomy. The complex movement analysis, in which EMG are seen in connection with kinematic and dynamic-kinetic measurement methods, finally provides information about the movement quality and can be used to optimize movement (Karamanidis et al. 2004).

Restraints and limits

Besides the multiple possibilities and areas of application, EMG has its limitations. The problem of EMG regarding a high measurement artifact risk has been discussed intensely. The EMG signal depends on the muscle length and the position of the electrodes. Different measurement artifacts can appear because of large movement amplitudes and high accelerations or because of sweat production. A different number of electrodes are applied depending on number and positioning of the derived muscle activity. Each of the electrodes is connected to a measurement device (analog-to-digital converter, amplifier) by a cable. The cabling and application of the electrodes can cause a limitation of the natural movement execution. In recent developments, this problem has been encountered by the implementation of radio-controlled signal transmission. After all, the high acquisition costs have to be calculated and balanced, accompanied by the costs for sets of consumables for the implementation in the clinical field.

> EMG data have their own limitations and should be integrated into comprehensive functional diagnostics.

References

Baur H (2004). Effektivität und Wirksamkeit einer funktionell-dynamischen Schuheinlagenversorgung im Sport. Dissertation, Wirtschafts- und Verhaltenswissenschaftliche Fakultät der Universität Freiburg.

Best W (2003). Druckverteilungsmessung im Überblick. Orthopädieschuhtechnik 7/8: 33–41.

Cappozzo A, Croce DU, Leardini A, Chiari L (2005). Human movement analysis using stereophotogrammetry. Part 1: theoretical background. Gait Posture 21: 186–196.

Chevillotte CJ, Ali MH, Trousdale RT, Pagneno MW (2009). Variability in hip range of motion on clinical examination. J Arthroplasty 24(5): 693–697.

Cornwall MW, McPoil TG (2003). Reliability and validity of center-of-pressure quantification. J Am Podiatr Med Assoc 93: 142–149.

De Luca CJ (1997). The use of surface electromyography in biomechanics. J Appl Biom 2: 135–163.

Grau S (2001). Objektivierung des Zusammenhangs von Verletzungen und biomechanischen Bewegungsmerkmalen in der Sportschuhforschung am Beispiel chronischer Achillessehnenbeschwerden bei Läufern. Dissertation, Fakultät für Sozial- und Verhaltenswissenschaften der Universität Tübingen.

Grossenbacher A, Bourban P, Held T, Marti B (1998). Schnellkraftdiagnostik mit einer Kraftmessplatte: Ergebnisse bei Spitzensportlern. Schw Zschr Sportmed Sporttraumat 46: 150–154.

Henning EM, Milani TL (2000). Pressure distribution measurements for evaluation of running shoe properties. Sportverletz Sportschaden 14: 90–97.

Impellizzeri FM, Rampinini E, Maffiuletti N, Marcora SM (2007). A vertical jump force test for assessing bilateral strength asymmetry in athletes. Med Sci Sports Exerc 39: 2044–2050.

Karamanidis K, Arampatzis A, Brüggemann GP (2004). Reproducibility of electromyography and ground reaction force during various running techniques. Gait Post 19: 115–123.

Konrad P (2005). The ABC of EMG. Noraxon Inc. U.S.A.

Leung PC (2007). Diabetic foot ulcers – a comprehensive review. Surgeon 5: 219–231.

Maiwald C (2008). Der Zusammenhang zwischen plantaren Druckverteilungsdaten und dreidimensionaler Kinematik der unteren Extremität beim Barfußlauf. Dissertation, Technische Universität Chemnitz.

Meeteren J, Roebroeck ME, Stam HJ (2002). Test-retest reliability in isokinetic muscle strength measurements of the shoulder. J Rehabil Med 34: 91–95.

Orlin MN, McPoil TG (2000). Plantar pressure assessment. Phys Ther 80: 399–409.

Rosenbaum D, Becker HP (1997). Plantar pressure distribution measurements. Technical background and clinical applications. Foot Ankl Surg 3: 1–14.

Schmidt RF, Thews G (1997). Optimax-Physiologie. Bild-CD. Berlin, Springer-Verlag.

Sheldon RS (2004). Quantification of human motion: gait analysis – benefits and limitations to its application to clinical problems. Journal Biomech 37: 1869–1880.

Sole G, Hamrén J, Milosavljevic S, Nicholson H, Sullivan SJ (2007). Test-retest reliability of isokinetic knee extension and flexion. Arch Phys Med Rehabil 88: 626–631.

Chapter 11

Gait and treadmill analysis

Thomas Jöllenbeck

11.1 Introduction

Walking and running are the most natural ways of human locomotion. The powers necessary for the propulsion are mainly produced in the lower extremities and forces necessary for the maintenance of balance are produced in the upper extremities resulting in a complex interaction of the entire locomotor apparatus. The force transmission is carried out via the foot as the final link of the kinematic chain and it is done passively in the foot plant as well as actively in the footprint. The basic facilities of walking and running as well as the derivative or modified forms of movement compose the foundation of motion and performance for a high number of sports. Modern gait analysis, the related procedures, standard values, and gait pathologies are mainly based on the studies of Perry (2003), Whittle (2002) and Winter (1991). A consistent analysis standard has not been achieved yet, although gait analysis is considered a well-developed subject area with its own specific societies (GCMAS: Gait and Clinical Movement Association, ISPGR: International Society for Posture and Gait Research; Rosenbaum 1999).

The motion analysis elements of gait analysis and recently also treadmill analysis are a comprehensive diagnostic instrument for the presentation of the dynamics and complexity of human walking and running. Motion analyses had been reserved for university institutions and for competitive athletes in specifically equipped high-performance centers in earlier times. However, it found its way into medical diagnostics in recent years. A complete motion analysis of walking and running as an objective instrumental procedure includes a range of biomechanical measurement methods with a number of measurable motion parameters. Its objective precision contrasts with the subjective motion description, which is widely spread in the therapeutic field.

11.2 Definitions

Gait analysis is the systematic recognition of human gait and its parameters. The run analysis as a special form of gait analysis synonymously deals with human running. Gait and run analyses cover a wide spectrum of application. Their aims are:

- Description and definition of the "normal" and pathological walking and running
- Optimization of motion processes
- Detection of improper strain and overstrain for the prevention of medical conditions and for the treatment of impairments or after injuries, accidents or surgeries
- Efficiency review of processes of rehabilitation
- Development and inspection of therapeutic appliances (Rosenbaum 1999).

The observing (subjective) gait analysis is being distinguished from the instrumental (objective) gait analysis (Perry 2003).

The observing gait analysis is based on a systematic screening with the steps of information structuring, schematic observation and interpretation for the detection of deviations from the standard and their causes (Götz-Neumann 2003, Perry 2003).

The instrumental gait analysis basically involves three different complementary analytical approaches (Winter 1991). Kinematics describes

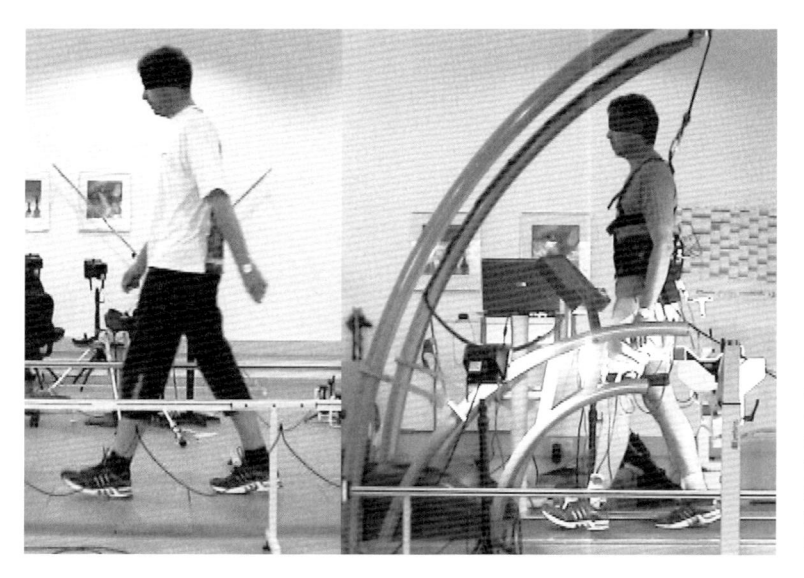

Fig. 11.1 Left: gait analysis on a gangway by 2 force plates (Kistler). Right: treadmill analysis by integrated force plate (Zebris FDM-T), 3D-ultrasound motion analysis (Zebris) and insole foot pressure measurement (Novel).

the temporary process of a motion in a space with the associated quantities such as distance, time, angle or velocity. Kinetics is concerned with the reasons for motions and thus with the effect of forces and momenta on amount and direction. Electromyography (EMG) describes time, duration and intensity of a muscular activity. An efficiency review of the gait by the detection of energy consumption is also partially mentioned as a fourth approach (Perry 2003).

The treadmill analysis as a special form of gait analysis enlarges the spectrum of analyses by the virtually stationary walking and running on a treadmill at variable velocities and tilting of the gait surface (➣ Fig. 11.1).

11.3 Walking on the treadmill vs. gait on a walkway

The treadmill enforces a constant speed of walking or running, while walking on a walkway conforms to the normal gait with arbitrary speed that is variable in every single step. Therefore, irregularities in the gait pattern of the test persons must be compensated in every step on the treadmill. Surveys mainly show that the results of gait analyses on walkways and treadmill analyses are not directly comparable (Vogt and Banzer 2005). There is an increased uncertainty with existent impairments or at a higher age (Schache et al. 2001). Additional differences in kinematics parameters such as cadence, time of standing or hip angle (Alton et al. 1998) as well as in kinetic parameters such as the force values at medial support or in footprint phase exist and complicate interpretation and comparability (White et al. 1998).

Standardization is one of the treadmill advantages in addition to the number of analyzable step cycles with a stationary measurement subject. A run-in phase is necessary for adaptation; nonetheless, patients with stronger impairments of the locomotor apparatus are sometimes unable to walk on the treadmill. In any case, the patient must be protected against falls.

11.4 Observing gait and treadmill analysis

The observing gait and treadmill analysis is the simplest form and is established in therapeutic diagnosis. The assessment of the motion process by observation does not require any further instruments. Systematic observation charts and analysis schemes are available (Perry 2003). However, such an analysis remains totally subjective and is of limited value. The limited spatio-temporal cognitive ability enables the observer to apprehend motion details only insufficiently and in limited detail. Several repetitions with accordingly directed attention and also from different perspectives are necessary to cover all criteria. Additional synchronic video recordings from several perspectives orthogonally to the running direction allow a slowed and repeated observation of individual motion sequences. The use of a treadmill can guarantee constant conditions for the entire observation process. The subjective assessment of the results often leads to minor compliance of different observers (Vogt and Banzer 2005).

11.5 Instrumental gait and treadmill analysis

The instrumental gait and treadmill analysis is more complex (Winter 1991). It requires time and the competent handling. In return, the instrumental motion analysis is an objective procedure, and provides reliable and valid information that goes far beyond the possibilities of the observing analysis.

Independently from the chosen method, implementation of synchronized video cameras in dorsal and/or lateral is always recommended to correlate the 2- or 3-dimensional line drawings to motion picture.

Special attention should be paid to partial motions and part of the body where the abnormality begins. The kinematic chain allows ascending as well as descending directions of effect in its construction and coupling as well as due to the number of degrees of freedom.

11.6 Kinematic gait and treadmill analysis

The standard method of kinematic analysis is the image-guided recording of motion by video camera and computerized evaluation (Rosenbaum 1999).

The treadmill allows evaluation of numerous step cycles in high resolution and image definition. Compromises have to be made between the size of the image section, resolution, image definition and the number of the analyzable steps or rather the number of the required repetitions. The variance of the individual repetitions and steps and acquired parameters is generally higher than on the treadmill. The aim or question determines the number and alignment of the video cameras. The frame rate of common video cameras is limited to 50 fields or 25 progressive scans/s, but modern digital high-speed cameras allow frequencies of up to 1,000 progressive scans/s. Their use is recommended for fast movements as in running, although specific programs are necessary for recording and analysis (e.g. Contemplas™, Simi™, Qualisys™, Dartfish™).

First, markers have to be applied to the test persons to calculate the kinematic parameters. The evaluation is carried out half- or full-automatically but comes with significant post-processing efforts. Step length, step frequency and cadence, gait speed, duration of support and swing phase as well as the extent of motion of the joints and the motion processes of the body parts are standard parameters (Rosenbaum 1999).

11.6.1 Video and 2D motion analysis

Only one or two cameras are required for the simple form of observing or 2D motion analysis, and these cameras are adjusted in and/or

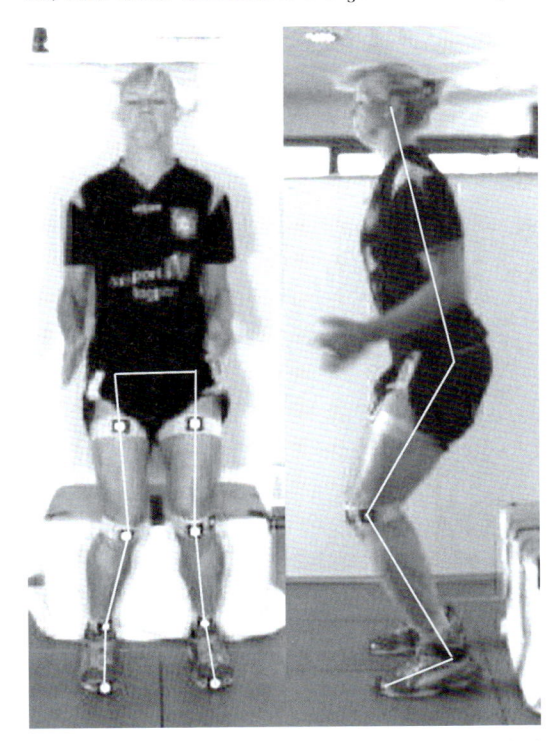

Fig 11.2 2D high-speed video analysis as simplified kinematic illustration of foot, leg, hip, knee, ankle, and torso position.

orthogonally to the running direction. The motion behavior is evaluated in slow-motion or single-frame shooting. Kinematic parameters such as angles, lengths, and distances can easily and quickly be measured; velocities is recorded with time. The synchronous presentation of comparison exposures is also possible. A simple calibration in the camera level, e.g. by help of a simple scale or a one-dimensional calibration grid, is primarily necessary for the determination of metric data. The use of marker points improves precision of the analysis (➤ Fig. 11.2).

The following recommendations can be given for the positioning of video cameras in standing, walking or running: observation from dorsal is recommended, if the pronation or supination behavior of the feet with or without shoes, the leg posture, the pelvic tilt or the posture of the upper body is analyzed and only one camera is available. A lateral camera position is recommended for roll-off behavior, runner type, foot, knee or hip flexion and extension, tilt of the upper body or the arm movement. An enlargement of the section or a focusing on the required body region, e.g. the foot is meaningful in both cases.

A dorsal and a lateral position are generally recommended, if a second video camera is available. The lateral observation should preferably be carried out on the problematic side, even though the side of observation is mainly irrelevant. The contra-lateral side is only observed at a very slow gait with a step length smaller than foot length. If necessary, the contra-lateral camera position should be added first, and then the frontal camera.

11.6.2 3D motion analysis

2 cameras, better 4 or more cameras are required in an angle of 60–120° to each other and 30–45° angle to the running direction for a complex 3D analysis. Precise calibration of the motion space by a three-dimensional cali-

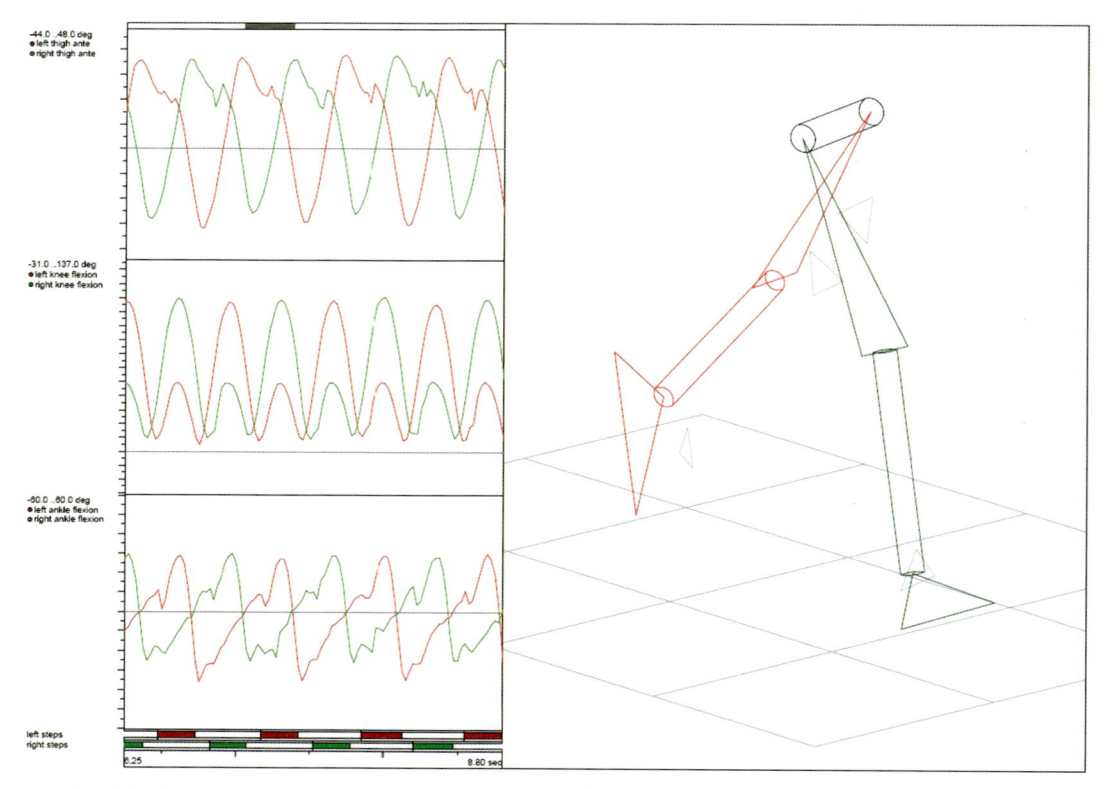

Fig 11.3 3D ultrasound motion analysis on treadmill at 12 kph [7.5 mph]. Left: Angle-time-gradient from thigh (top), knee (middle) and ankle joint flexion (bottom). Left and right are plotted in red and green, respectively in sagittal view. Right: 3D motion picture.

bration grid is a mandatory set-up condition. This grid consists of as many single spots as possible. Markers are stringently required for an at least semi-automatic evaluation. Reflecting markers and lately also LED markers are recommended and optimize the tracking of individual marker points in addition to colored sports. A too low spatial resolution of the cameras or a too low camera frequency is a limiting factor for 3D video analysis. Automatic tracking is still problematic since other body parts cover marker spots, which often significantly increases post-processing efforts.

The 3D-ultrasound motion analysis (e.g. Zebris™, Lukotronic™) is available as immediate information system (➢ Fig. 11.3) and is an alternative to the image-guided video analysis. The single or 3-fold markers consist of ultrasound sensors and present the referenced body points as space coordinates in an online line drawing with high precision; the frequency is limited to 100 Hz. Infrared camera systems (Vicon™) have become popular in recent years, which show any number of body spots as space coordinates with high precision. They measure frequency by 4 or more cameras. Although these systems are very expensive, they seem to establish as state-of-the-art. Markers with spacers are often used for better identification of body spots. These underlie diverse effects of inertia, especially with high velocities of movement or motions with impact momenta. Therefore, data must be smoothed by filtering to compensate movement artifacts. Infrared- and ultrasound-based systems also provide a calibration that allows an assignment of markers to 3D space coordinates. The uses of as many cameras as possible at infrared systems or of so-called multiple reference markers at ultrasound systems address the problem of covered markers and allow better immediate feedback. Data are available as 3D line drawings and can be turned into every required perspective. They can be watched as frame or animation for all mentioned procedures. Furthermore, only 3D systems provide the option to visualize rotating motions of individual body parts or to record rotating motions, e.g. in shot put or golf.

Systems based on radio-controlled inertial sensors (Biosyn™) or motion recorders completely free of markers (Biostage™) are new on the market. These procedures will certainly enhance the spectrum of kinematic motion analysis in near future, although data are still lacking.

11.6.3 Important analysis parameters

Important information of the motion behavior, e.g. track width, foot position at foot plant and footprint, or also the gait or running stability can already be assessed in the simple video. The complex 3D motion analysis provides a large number of objective, kinematic parameters that ensure correct motion diagnosis and comparison across various recordings. This is important for movement optimization in competitive sports and rehabilitation; it cannot be achieved with sufficient precision by 2D motion analysis.

The observation in the major motion levels, i.e. in the frontal, sagittal and transversal level, independently from the used systems is recommended for the motion analysis. Differences in lateral comparison that indicate unilateral deficiencies or improper strain deserve special attention – regardless of the perspective.

Frontal level

Specifically the behavior in the dorsal foot plant and footprint is of interest in the frontal level. A narrow track width possibly indicates an increased pronation risk, while a wide track width indicates an increased supination risk. Close observations of the initial ground contact and the subsequent lowering motion of the foot show whether an unusual pronation or supination movement is present (➢ Fig. 11.4). The direct comparison with the barefooted roll-off motion is of specific importance and shows if the outside structure of the shoe or the foot posture is initially responsible for improper movements. This also allows tracking the efficiency of shoe treatments. Inward or outward rotation of the foot in the footprint requires special attention as this may indicate problems at the ball of the foot and hallux.

The leg positioning and the pelvic tilt in their processes as well as in the lateral comparison are further important characteristics. A distinct change of the leg posture – especially in the main phases of exposure in foot plant and footprint – indicates possible instabilities and additional strain on the knee joint. These instabilities might have different causes, such as

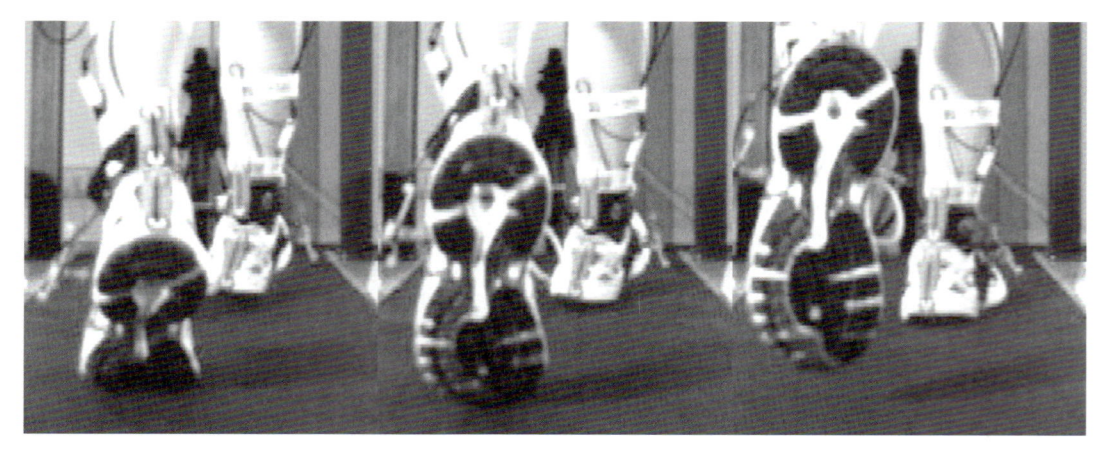

Fig. 11.4 Treadmill analysis of foot movement with high-speed camera. Foot rolling (right) at 10 kph (6.2 mph), instantly after (middle) and after foot rolling (right). Time lapse: 50 ms.

muscular deficiencies in at the knee or hip joint. An enhanced pelvic tilt or lowering during ground contact on the contra-lateral side suggests muscular deficiencies of the muscles stabilizing the hip on the side of the standing leg. Short and medium term problems can be the result of overstrains in the muscle-tendon apparatus or due to a changed range of spinal motion especially in the region of the lumbar spine. Leg length differences in standing and in motion can also be visible due to the pelvic tilt.

Sagittal level

Primarily, the motion process and the extent of motion of the propulsion-effective kinematic chain of ankle, knee and hip joint are of specific importance in the sagittal level. Movement modifications or impairments of a joint partner influence the others and more or less have to be compensated by them. Further parts of the locomotor apparatus such as the contra-lateral side, pelvis and spine are also affected, if this is not achieved completely or to the same extent on all sides. If the knee angle at ground contact does not show a sufficient flexion-extension motion, the reduced impact absorption increases strain on the hip. A distinction by line drawing is useful. The anatomical pivot point of the knee joint lies behind the connecting line of hip joint and ankle joint. This leads to a straightly extended knee joint being overextended in the line drawing. The pelvic tilt, the tilt of the upper body and the arm-swinging movement are further important parameters.

Additionally, a typing in hindfoot, midfoot and forefoot runners can be deduced from the roll-off behavior in running. The velocity of plantar flexion after the foot plant can provide first indications for muscular or neuronal deficiencies, e.g. a weakness of the dorsal flexor. The extent of the plantar flexion of the hallux in foot printing can indicate the involvement and ratio of the hallux in the push-off motion, on the other hand.

Transversal level

The posture of the foot as well as the pelvic posture and pelvic rotating deserve special consideration in the transversal level. Malpositions can be identified easily. Especially rotating motions that are unrecognizable in the sagittal or frontal level become visible in the transversal level and provide important indications for the causes of motion abnormalities. Thus, a leg posture turned inward or outward in motion dynamics can be conditioned anatomically and by an increased inward and outward rotating of upper and lower leg. This difference only becomes visible in 3D motion analyses.

11.7 Kinetic gait and treadmill analysis

11.7.1 Dynamometry

The recording of force-time procedures of motion by multi-component force plates (e.g.

11.7 Kinetic gait and treadmill analysis

AMTI™, Bertec™, Kistler™) is a standard method of kinetic gait and run analysis (Rosenbaum 1999). In general, they are embedded in a walkway and are stationary. Ground reaction forces in all three dimensions as well as the line of force application and duration of the support phase are the standard parameters. Asymmetries can be shown easily and causes can be limited in the lateral comparison with at least two force plates arranged in a row, and also kinematic parameters such as step length, duration of support and swing phase or gait velocity can be detected. In addition to the required number of repetitions for reliable results, the requirement of the plates being uninfluenced by the test persons and only met by one foot each on the entire surface is the disadvantage of the stationary arrangement.

The lines of force application show the position of the body's center of gravity as perpendicular to the force plate. Their course can show the foot posture and can also indicate deficiencies in the roll-off motion with different roll-off lengths; an assignment to the foot structure is not possible, though.

The time-power curves (> Fig. 11.5) in walking show the altitude of the strain response in the foot plant, the push-off force and the dynamic of the motion in the vertical line due to the differences between the typical two maxima and the minimum. The retarding force impact during strain response and the acceleration force impact during the footprint phase in the running direction have to be distinguished from each other in altitude and course. The forces directed transversely to the running direction show the distance of the perpendicular of the point of gravity to the contact point at the ground during a step in measure and course. The according impulse can be calculated easily from the force-time curves as important measure of force transmission and thus of motion dynamics.

Analysis of force-time curves

A unilaterally reduced dynamic of the vertical force due to lower maxima and a higher minimum analytically indicates a deficiency of this side of the body (> Fig. 11.5). Unilaterally higher impulses transverse to the running direction during the unilateral standing phase show a deficiency on this side of the body and imply a shift of the point of gravity as an evasive motion to the contra-lateral side of the body. Comparably lower retarding or acceleration force impacts in

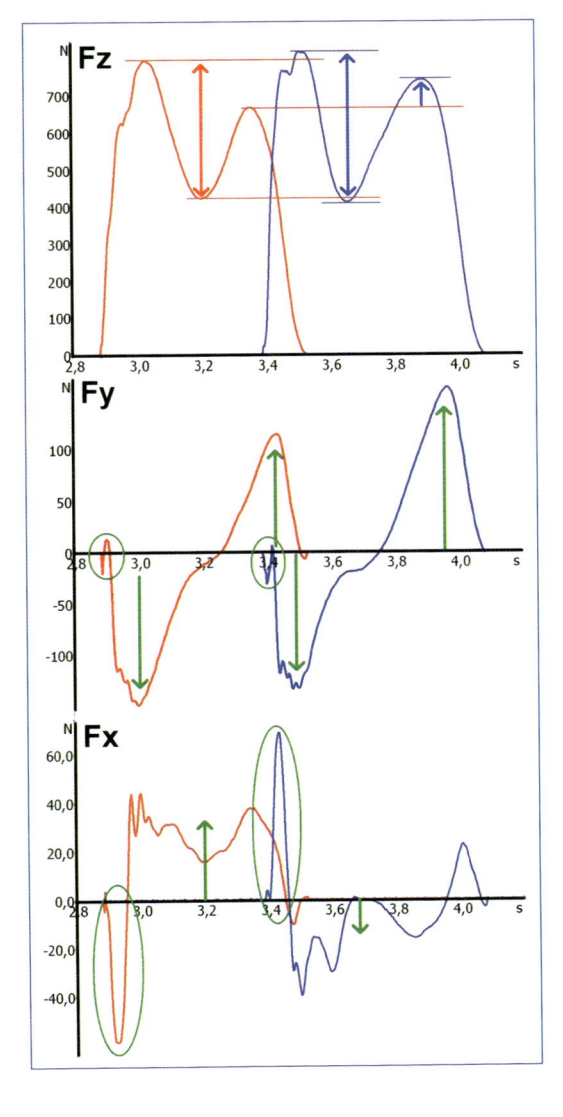

Fig. 11.5 Gait analysis: time-power-curves, floor reaction force (Fz) vertical (top), Fy in running direction (middle), and Fx transverse to running direction (bottom), left (red), and right (blue). Analysis a) Fz (top): left dynamic and impulse from reduced, i.e. sick side left, b) Fy (middle): left acceleration and following break movement right reduced, i.e. problem in foot print left, c) Fx (bottom): impulse during supporting phase left bigger than right, i.e. problem left in weight transfer to right. Additional, inward turn (green oval) of both feet at floor contact (bottom) with stabilizing movement (middle).

running direction indicate deficiencies in foot plant or footprint. The often present short initial force peaks in and/or transversely to the running direction contrary to the normal force direction indicate that the foot at the end of the motion of demonstration at the foot plant in running direction "falls" backwards and transversely to the running direction inwards on the ground. The cause needs detection with those peaks being specifically high at the resulting momenta for the ankle joint. A comparison to the barefooted gait is necessary in order to assess the influence of shoes.

Altogether, force-time curves are an important indicator for possible impairments. The results can identify the affected side of the body and the deficient motion phase. The causatively affected part of the body cannot be determined, though.

Treadmills with integrated one-dimensional (H/P/Cosmos™, Kistler™) and three-dimensional (Bertec™) force plates have been available for a few years now, which provide forces and mean values for many step cycles. Nevertheless, the analytical options are limited for the one-dimensional variants because of missing forces in and transversely to the running direction. Reactive treadmills that compensate the disadvantages of the constant treadmill velocity are currently in development.

The calculation of joint momenta by inverse dynamic is generally possible, if kinetic and kinematic data are available (Winter 2005). A complete multi-dimensional dataset and according software are the precondition. Nonetheless, the effort for this is still intense and position of the joint spots is still relatively imprecise (➤ Fig. 11.6).

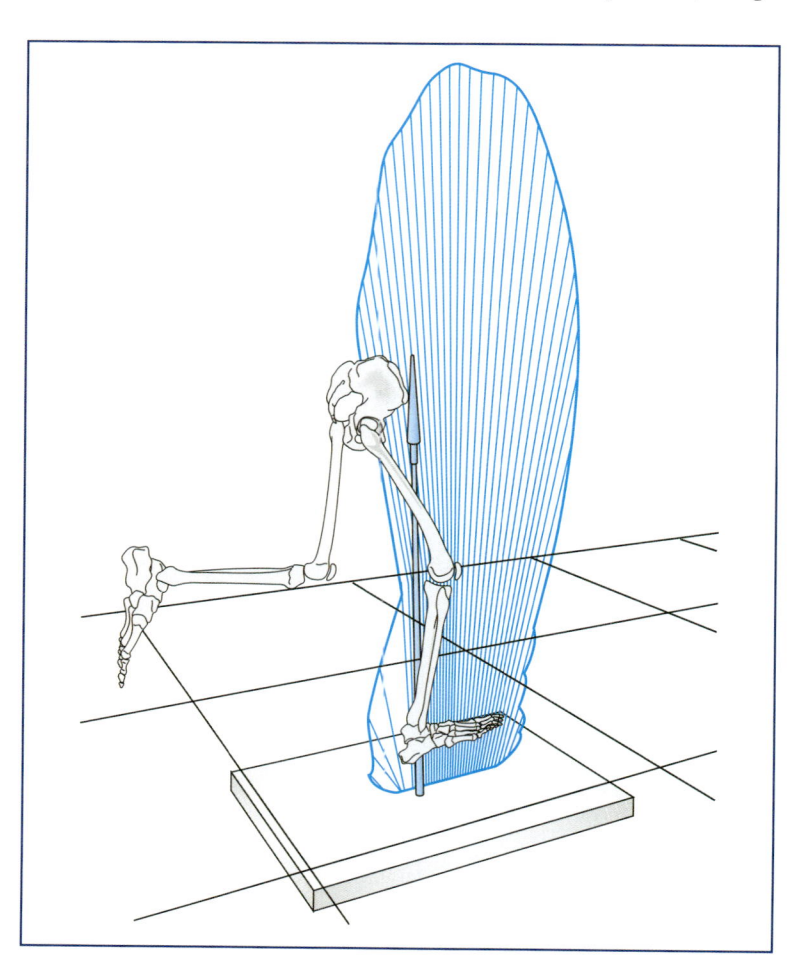

Fig. 11.6 Vector graphic illustrating floor forces during running (Walther M., 2009).

11.7.2 Pedography

Pedography as imaging procedure of kinetic analysis for feet problems is an established procedures especially in shoe orthopedics. Force plates (Novel™, Zebris™ and others) or insoles (Novel™, FastScan™, Medilogic™, TecScan™, Zebris™ and others) record the pressure-time processes under the foot sole. Force plates are usually stationary and embedded in a walkway; they primarily serve the recording of the strain characteristics under the soles of the feet (Rosenbaum 1999). Similar to force plates, this platform has to be calibrated exactly and uninfluenced. Treadmills with integrated force plates (Zebris™) have been available for some time, which allow a stationary analysis of many step cycles and thus a reliable image of walking and running behavior. Foot pressure measurement insoles are mobile and are used as shoe inserts. They examine the interaction between foot, shoe and underground. Measurements can be static in standing or dynamic in walking or running. The foot can be analyzed as a whole or divided in stress-bearing areas. In addition to the medial and maximum pressure, the duration of exposure, force and impulse process, point of pressure gravity and the roll-off behavior are available measurement parameters. There is the option to vary speed and tilt of the running surface with the treadmill, and additional important kinematic parameters such as step length and track width, foot position and length of the gait line as well as resulting information about gait symmetry and gait stability are available.

So far, there have not been any generally applicable guidelines for the evaluation of pedographic measurements. The lateral comparison in standing can uncover shifts of the point of gravity. Barefoot measurements are helpful as a base for the assessment and limitation of problem areas and pathologies as for the shoe and insole treatment. The efficiency of such treatment can be checked by foot pressure insoles (➤ Fig. 11.7).

In addition to the medial and maximum pressure images, the roll-off behavior is primarily significant. The extent of concordance with gait-typical movement patterns primarily shows in walking in addition to the possibility to identify the foot shapes and deformations.

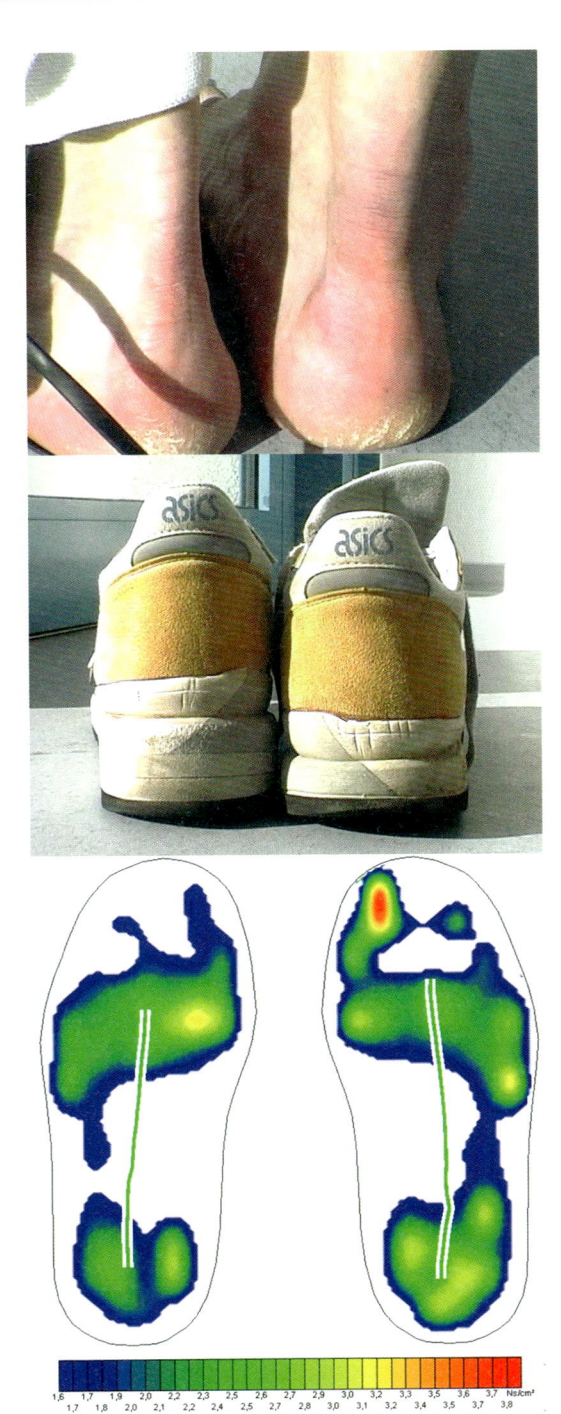

Fig. 11.7 Treadmill analysis at 14 kph [9.3 mph], Achilles tendon inflammation (top right), shoe elevation 1.5 cm [2 in] (middle), pedography maximum pressure picture (bottom). The elevating shoe inlay left is too high.

The cyclogram (> Fig. 11.8) provides important information on gait stability and gait symmetry. The force-time curves determined by the pressure process show the vertical reaction forces between ground or shoe and foot and allow the calculation of the vertical impulse, but they are less precise than the ones of force plates. The type-intrinsic features such as pronation movement in hindfoot runners, exposure of the external side in midfoot runners or of the ball in forefoot runners can be well assessed in running in addition to the identification of the running type, and countermeasures can be implemented in the case of improper strain. The comparison between walking or running barefooted and wearing shoes at the use of a treadmill provides important information on the influence of shoes.

Most results of the kinetic analysis require interpretation in the context with the entire movement, while prominent pressure peaks can be assigned definitely to a foot problem. Although the force transmission in walking and running is carried out via the foot, it only represents the last link of a complex kinematic chain with the aim of moving the body's point of gravity. Therefore, cause of abnormalities should be searched in the foot or in the respective leg.

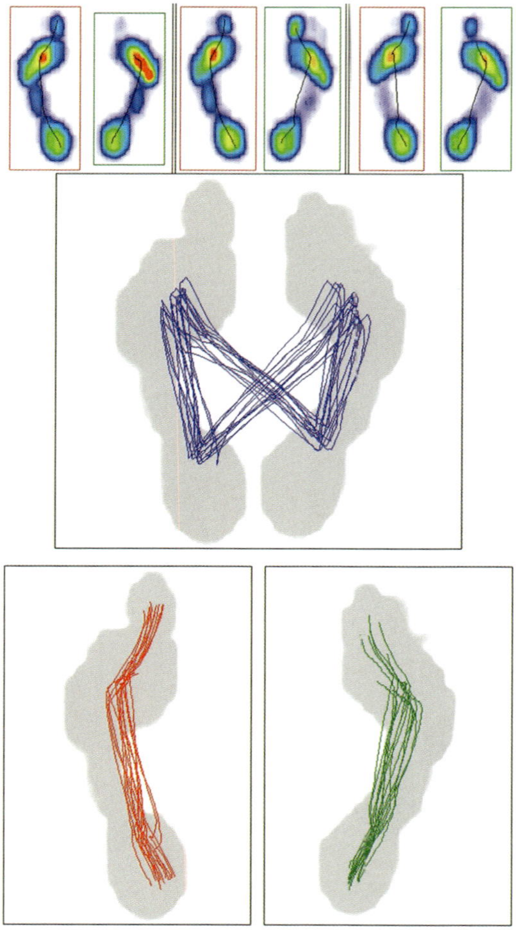

11.8 Electromyography

A muscle function analysis can be excluded by surface electromyography (e.g. Noraxon™, Biovision™) as extension of the kinetic or kinematic gait or run analysis. This complex method can help to diagnose which muscle is active at what time and for how long with which activity and in which intra- or inter-muscular interaction. Such information can help to display muscular, neuronal or sensomotor abnormalities and provide possible explanations for kinetic or kinematic abnormalities. Electrodes are placed on the muscle, intensified (by 1,000 to 5,000 times) and transmitted by a cable or by radio. Recording frequency is high (>1 kHz). However, only muscles close to the surface of the skin are captured by this method. The use of needle electrodes is not applicable in gait and run analysis and would also only be able to record a small pool of muscle fibers. Electromyography is very susceptible for physical, biological, electrochemical and electromechanical interferences because of the low signals. Movement artifacts arise especially in the dynamic examination. Thorough application and evaluation are necessary for the prevention or reduction of interference (Hermens and Freriks 1999, Feiwald et al. 2007).

The anterior tibialis muscle, the peroneus longus and brevis muscle, the medial and lateral gastrocnemius muscle and the soleus muscle can be deduced for the muscle function analysis of the flexors and extensors of the foot. The determination of the maximum EMG is recommended before the data collection in or-

Fig. 11.8 Treadmill analysis (Zebris FDM-T) with pressure picture at touch-down (insert, top), cyclogram (butterfly) with length of gait lines and transition left and right (middle) and middle release diagram with separate gait line (bottom).

11.9 Standardization vs. individualization

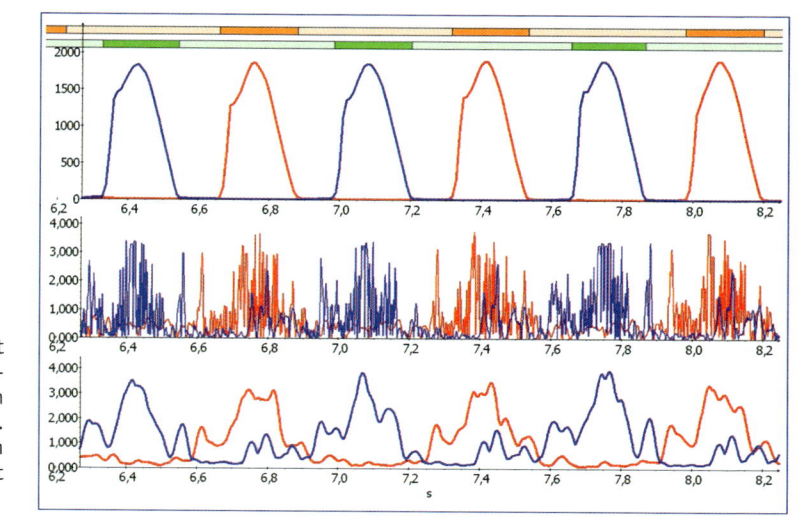

Fig 11.9 Treadmill analysis at 16 kph (9.9 mph) with power-time-curve (top) and EMG of m gastrocnemius med. (middle). Envelope of power spectrum (bottom), left (red) and right (blue).

der to allow a comparability of the data also in lateral comparison. Time and duration as well as the amplitude of the signal are the available measurement parameters.

The unilateral evaluation mainly shows to what extent a muscle is activated according to time and amplitude of its function. Reduced or lacking activity of the peroneus muscle allows detection of a weak dorsal foot flexor. The lateral comparison also allows assessment of the activation symmetry (➤ Fig. 11.9). Differences in the activation pattern, in the temporary process as well as in the amplitude indicate functional deficiencies with causes that have to be clarified (Freiwald et al. 2007). The function analysis of other muscles and muscle groups can be structured analogously.

In addition, electromyography allows to a certain extent also the identification of parameters for the muscular fatigue or strain, for the inter- and intra-muscular coordination or for the triage, recruitment and frequenting of fiber types during muscular innervations. These topics that are highly complex also in analysis and that are still in scientific discussion are not to be treated further at this point.

11.9 Standardization vs. individualization

Standard curves and values are key to automatization of data processing (see Freiwald and Engelhardt 2002). They are a great help in the presentation and understanding of complex coherencies such as gait and treadmill analysis and allow assignment of current results (Fiot 2010). In this respect, every deviation from the standard primarily deserves special attention.

However, approx. 32 % of all test persons previously selected as "normal" are subsequently stigmatized as "non-standard" because their movements deviate from the standard curve by more than one standard deviation. Human individuality is mainly expressed in the deviation from a standard and not in the conformity with it. A distinct type of deviation from the standard is the individual maximum performance of top athletes.

The high complexity of a movement such as human walking or running contains numerous degrees of freedom and therefore allows accordingly many solutions. Human movement underlies the principle of economy and efficiency; it is also marked by high variability and ability of compensation. This is expressed in motion deficiencies, effects of fatigue or strain, as well as in a natural motion variety and a utilizing of the degrees of freedom. No steps being identical in all details can be found by measurements. Pathologies are only one of many causes.

Therefore, the assessment of a movement according to its individual regularity seems to be more important than the standard comparison. Thus, there is generally no reason to change a symmetric but non-standard movement, unless pathological malpositions or impairments are present. In the case of asymmetries in walking or running, however, the method should not primarily be determined by bringing both sides to a cover due to a standard process, but rather by approximating the obviously deficient side to the contra-lateral one. The solution is an individual standardization.

11.10 Means and limits of gait and treadmill analysis – summary

Gait and treadmill analysis is a reliable instrument for the extension and confirmation of medical diagnosis. Modern instruments drastically reduced the effort of gait and treadmill analysis and results are available instantly.

Abnormalities in the dynamics of walking or running motions are uncovered by kinematic or kinetic analyses. Early intervention prevents or delays impairments of the locomotor apparatus. In terms of rehabilitation, changes and remaining deficiencies become measurable and allow support of therapeutic measures.

Force-time curves show problematic motion phases. Pedography helps in the assessment of the roll-off behavior and the identification of improper strain or overstrain in the area of the foot. Kinematic procedures ranging from video analysis to 3D motion analysis and electromyography support the search for causes of abnormalities and help to address questions of treatment approaches.

Respective limitations of the used measurement methods need to be balanced with their possibilities. Although kinematics can describe the movement of the body in spaced and time with extreme precision, no information is provided about the effecting forces or the activity of the muscles that are involved in the movement. Kinetics, however, provides exact data regarding the force-time process and the impulse of a full body movement, but it does not detect body movements and involved muscles. Therefore, individual methods such as pedography for the diagnosis of the roll-off behavior or a 2D video analysis for the identification of the knee angles in foot plant and footprint give concise answers to specific questions. A gait and run analysis for the creation of a complex cause-and-effect correlation can only be facilitated by the simultaneous use of several measurement methods.

References

Alton F, Baldey L, Caplan S, Morissey MC (1998). A kinematic comparison of overground and treadmill walking. Clin Biomech 13: 434–440.

Fiot, Forschungsinstitut für Orthopädietechnik. Angewandte Ganganalyse. http://www.fiot.at/start.php?Page=Projekte/Ganganalyse/Publikationen/AGW/ (22.12.2010).

Freiwald J, Baumgart C, Konrad P (2007). Einführung in die Elektromyographie, Sport – Prävention – Rehabilitation. Balingen, Spitta.

Freiwald J, Engelhardt M (2002). Stand des motorischen Lernens und der Koordination in der Orthopädisch-traumatologischen Rehabilitation. Sport Orthop Traumatol 18: 5–10.

Götz-Neumann K (2003). Gehen verstehen – Ganganalyse in der Physiotherapie. Thieme, Stuttgart-New York.

Hermens HJ, Freriks B (1999). Seniam CD – European recommendations for surface electromyography. Roessingh Research and Development, Enschede.

Perry J (2003) Ganganalyse – Norm und Pathologie des Gehens. Urban & Fischer, München-Jena.

Rosenbaum D (1999) Klinische Ganganalyse in der Orthopädie und Traumatologie. In: Jerosch J, Nicol K, Peikenkamp K, Rechnergestützte Verfahren in Orthopädie und Unfallchirurgie. Steinkopff, Darmstadt, pp. 145–158.

Schache AG, Blanch PD, Rath DA, Wrightley TV, Starr R, Benell KL (2001). A comparison of overground and treadmill running for measuring the three-dimensional kinematics of the lumbo-pelvic-hip complex. Clin Biomech 16: 667–680.

Vogt L, Banzer W (2005). Instrumentelle Ganganalyse. Deutsch Z Sportmed 56(4): 108–109.

Walther M (2009). Gang- und Laufbandanalyse. Aus: Engelhardt M. Sportverletzungen. Elsevier, München.

White SC, Yack HJ, Tucker, CA & Lin HY (1998). Comparison of vertical ground reaction forces during overground and treadmill walking. Med Sci Sports Exerc 30: 1537–1542.

Whittle MW (2002). Gait analysis – an introduction. 3rd Ed, Butterworth-Heinemann, Oxford.

Winter DA (1991). The biomechanics and motor control of human gait. 2nd Ed, Waterloo Biomechanics, Waterloo.

Winter DA (2005). Biomechanics and motor control of human movement. 3rd Ed, Wiley, Waterloo.

III Body parts affected by athletic injuries

12	**Central and peripheral nervous system**	141
12.1	Injuries of the central nervous system	142
12.2	Injuries of the spine and the spinal cord	154
12.3	The peripheral nervous system	161
13	**Eyes**	181
13.1	Sports for children and adolescents	181
13.2	Non-competitive, popular and health sports	183
13.3	Competitive and high-performance sports	186
13.4	Sport-specific eye injuries	187
13.5	Conclusion	195
14	**Ears, facial cranium and cervical soft-tissue**	199
14.1	Injuries in the area of the ear	199
14.2	Facial cranium	201
14.3	Cervical soft-tissue	204
15	**Shoulder joint**	207
15.1	Arthroscopic minimally invasive procedures	207
15.2	Open surgery procedures	217
16	**Elbow and forearm**	227
16.1	Sports injuries	227
16.2	Overuse syndromes	229
17	**Hand and wrist joint**	235
17.1	Anatomy and kinematics	235
17.2	Epidemiology and etiology	236
17.3	Fractures	236
17.4	Ligament injuries in the wrist	240
17.5	Injuries of the TFCC	242
17.6	Injuries of the finger joints	243
17.7	Tendon injuries	245
17.8	Nerve impairments	247
17.9	Tendinitides	247
17.10	Overstrain syndromes at the wrist joint	248

18	**Pelvis and hip joint**	**251**
18.1	Anatomy and biomechanics	251
18.2	Pelvic injuries	251
18.3	Hip injuries	255
19	**Groin**	**263**
19.1	Biomechanics	264
19.2	Hernias	264
19.3	Psoas syndrome	267
19.4	Iliopectinea bursa	268
19.5	Entrapment syndrome	268
19.6	Adductor syndrome	270
20	**Knee joint**	**273**
20.1	Anatomy	273
20.2	Biomechanics	274
20.3	Injuries	275
20.4	Overuse impairments of the knee joint	286
21	**Shank, ankle joint and foot**	**291**
21.1	Fractures of foot and ankle	291
21.2	Stress fractures of shank and foot	297
21.3	Tendon injuries of the foot	301
21.4	Ligament injuries of foot and ankle	310
22	**The skeletal muscle**	**323**
22.1	Structure and control of muscle system	323
22.2	Classification of muscle injuries	324
22.3	Mechanisms and causes of injury	324
22.4	Pathobiology of muscle healing	324
22.5	Diagnostics of muscle injuries	327
22.6	Treatment of acute muscle injuries	327
22.7	Relapsing/chronic muscle injuries	330
22.8	Compartment syndrome	331
22.9	Prevention of muscle injuries	331
22.10	Muscular dysbalances	331
23	**Stress reactions of the bones**	**333**
23.1	Etiology	333
23.2	Diagnostics	334
23.3	Differential diagnosis	336
23.4	Therapy	337
23.5	Prevention	338

24	**Cartilage**	341
24.1	Basics	341
24.2	Cartilage treatment	343
24.3	Strategies of cartilage treatment	348
25	**Tendon injuries**	351
25.1	Anatomic-physiological basics	351
25.2	Tendon diseases	354

Chapter 12
Central and peripheral nervous system

Iris Reuter

There is sufficient evidence for the beneficial effects of exercise but with the increasing popularity of sports activities the number of acute and overuse sports injuries rise. About one and a half million of sports injuries are registered in Germany each year (Schneider et. al 2006). Injuries of the musculoskeletal system are well known, but sports injuries can also affect the central and peripheral nervous system. Due to improved education injuries of the head and the cervical spine after falls are well known. In contrast overuse injuries of the peripheral nervous system are rarely considered.

The percentage of sports-related injuries among all reported injuries of the central and peripheral nervous system is estimated at 2.9% to 42.7% (Lang and Stefan, 1999). The great variance suggests that the incidence of sports related injuries of the nervous system needs to be reassessed.

The risk of suffering from a head injury varies between the different types of sports. Falls and direct contact with the opponents in martial arts can lead to traumatic injuries of the brain and the spinal cord. Sports activities such as handball, American football, soccer, rugby, hockey and ice hockey imply a high risk of traumatic sports injuries (Cantu & Müller, 2000). However, also in Asian martial arts head injuries may occur due to falls outside the mats or technically incompetent throws.

Falls are frequent in biking (Road and mountain bike), horse riding, skiing, snowboarding (Cantu & Müller, 2000), motor sports, inline skating, artistic gymnastics, trampolining and diving. The incidence for head injuries in in-line-skating is reported to range between 5% and 17% (Jerosch & Heck 2005) but only 2.6% of the inline skater wear a helmet.

People engaged in leisure time sports have often poorer and less suitable equipment than professional athletes and are at a higher risk for injuries. Injuries of the head and spine account for 28% of the injuries in skiing and snowboarding (Tarazi et al. 1999). Snowboarders suffer more often from head injuries than skier. This might be explained by the fact that the snowboarder, in particular beginners, fall more often backward and hit the ground with the back of the head (Siu et a. 2004; Levy & Smith 2000). The incidence of head injuries in skiing is around 10% (Hörterer 2005).

The risk for injuries in horse riding is especially high when both, horse and rider fall due to potential contact of the rider with the horseshoes or the body of the horse. Cross country riding is associated with the highest risk of falls and injuries. About 1% of the athletes who take part in endurance competitions sustain an injury. 31% of the injuries are related to the face and the brain and 20% to the shoulder girdle. C. 80% of riders who require hospital treatment have injuries of the skull or/and the brain. In contrast to the high risk of head injuries, only 50% of the riders wear a riding hood.

Paragliding and kite surfing are considered as new and trendy and are most popular among young people but they are not without risk. The risk of head injuries decreased significantly (4%) after implementation of the obligation wearing a helmet. In contrast the risk of sustaining a spine injury is still alarming (Bohnsack & Schröter 2005). Head injuries occur most often during landing or are due to technical difficulties in mastering the paraglider. Pilots, unable to change the direction of the paraglider, hit obstacles i.e. trees, rocks in their way.

The injury rate in kite surfing adds up to 7.0/1000 hours with an increased risk for injuries during jumping. The incidence of head injuries amounts to 13.7%. Head injuries are attributed to the inability to detach the kite from the harness. The fixed board often hits the head of the surfer (Petersen et al. 2005). A helmet is worn by 7% of the athletes.

In mountainbiking we observe a gender specific effect regarding injuries. While men suffer from 6.8 injuries/1000 hours on the bike, females have 12 injuries during that time (Kronisch & Pfeifer 2002). Female athletes fall more often than males and they leave the bike more often over the top of the handlebar.

The impact of the ground after falling forward over the handlebar in bicycling is associated with the highest risk of skull and facial bone fractures. The injury profile of mountain bikers especially during downhill riding is more severe with 2.6% combined skull and brain injuries (Arnold 2005) and c. 55% facial bone fractures. Mountain bikers and cyclists without helmet sustain the most severe injuries. Leisure time bikers have the highest risk for severe injuries since they wear helmets in 56% only. For medical reasons helmets with faceguards and compulsory helmet use for all cyclists, and particularly mountainbikers is required.

Artistic gymnasts are prone to spine injuries. Trampolining has become popular during recent years, and the number of injuries has increased with the popularity. Most common are fractures to the lower extremities but injuries of the spine, especially the cervical spine are also frequent. The majority of injuries occur on the body of the trampoline, but falls on to the frame or the springs are often reported. Athletes performing a somersault are at risk of falling off and landing on or outside of the mat. Athletes who are falling of the trampoline have an increased risk for head injuries. In accordance gymnasts who fall during vaulting or fall off the balance beam during flic-flacs or somersaults have an increased risk for head injuries. Finally, dismounting from the uneven bars or the balance beam can lead to severe injuries.

In diving uncontrolled contact with the board can result in severe head injuries. This happens most often when athletes jump off the hand stand position. 300000 head traumas are recorded per year (Frommelt 1995), 8% can be allocated to sports related injuries.

The popularity of a certain sport and the body of rules and regulations of sports activities affect the frequency of injuries. Significant more athletes play American football in the USA compared to Europe and its popularity is reflected in the total number of injuries related to American football. In the past the incidence of head and cervical spine injuries was very high but a modification of the rules which has forbidden the tackling with the head has significantly reduced these injuries.

Diagnosis and treatment of sports-related head injuries does not differ from head injuries which are not sport-related.

12.1 Injuries of the central nervous system

The injuries of the skull are divided in penetrating and non-penetrating head injuries and spine injuries. There are two major mechanisms underlying brain injuries the direct blow and the contrecoup. The direct blow applies a force to the head and produces an injury at the side of the force. The contrecoup injury is due to an acceleration of the brain while the cranium decelerates. A blow to the front of the head might cause a contrecoup injury to the occipital lobe. Rotational acceleration injuries result often in a torsion of the blood vessels and might cause more severe injuries. Helmets might protect against direct blow injuries but it is difficult to protect the brain against the acceleration/deceleration injuries which are associated with shear forces. Rotational movements can also lead to a twisting of the cerebral hemisphere on the brainstem.

12.1.1 Penetrating head injuries

Penetrating head injuries are characterised by a direct connection between brain and scalp, thus there is no barrier between the intracranial and extracranial compartment. Skull impression fractures with dislocation of the bone towards the brain, fractures of the skull of the brain and the penetration of sharp foreign bodies might lead to the rupture of the dura. Most often a focal impact (i.e. a puck) causes focal damage of the brain with consecutive bruises of the brain tissue. Typical late complications are secondary bleedings and infections, such as meningitis, phlegmona and brain abscess.

> Note that minor external wounds may be misleading and initial clinical symptoms might be mild or missing.

Each penetrating head injury requires surgical treatment. The injury has to be cleaned in an operation theatre and proper antibiotic coverage is needed. Tetanus vaccination coverage has to be checked. Exploration of a penetrating skull fracture at the place of the accident is absolutely prohibited.

Penetrating skull fractures occur frequently in horse riding with aggravation of the injuries by a kick of the horse shoes or in bicycle races when bikers fall without wearing a helmet. Fabio Castelli died at the Tour de France in 1995, when he came off his bike while racing downhill. He dashed against a stone which resulted in a penetrating skull fracture. Despite of this devastating incident the professional bikers were against an obligation to wear a helmet. 2003 Andrei Kivilev died of his brain damage after a fall with low speed. Motor sports proved to imply a high risk for head injuries as well. Pole vaulters also have a potential risk for head injuries when they fall backward. Athletes with high risk for head injuries include hang gliders, paragliders, gymnasts, trampoline athletes and figure skaters. However, the risk of spine injuries outweighs the risk of brain injuries. Some spectacular falls occurred in pair figure skating with the female skater falling during pair lifts especially upside down lifts, rotational lifts or headbanger lifts. Professional boxers still do not wear a head protection thus they are at risk for severe acute and chronic head injuries. Punches to the orbit or the root of the nose lead often to fractures of the facial bones and the base of the skull.

12.1.2 Non-penetrating head injuries

Non-penetrating head injuries are characterised by an impact of the skull without tears of the dura mater. Two mechanisms are observed: the compression trauma and the acceleration/deceleration trauma. In compression trauma a direct force impacts on the fixed skull which results in a focal brain damage i.e. hematoma or contusion.

Acceleration

If the head is not fixed, acceleration and deceleration forces might be imparted on the head. Violent accelerations might be not absorbed by the cerebrospinal fluid which surrounds the brain. While the movement of the skull is stopped the brain moves further and hits the bone (coup), more severe damage develops on the other side of the skull (contrecoup). The negative pressure on this side leads to tears of blood vessels and soft tissue. Forces might cause linear, rotational or angular movement of the brain or a combination of all types of movements. Linear accelerations result in lower relative movements between brain and skull, while rotational and angular movements result in more severe brain trauma. The midbrain and the diencephalon are the brain structures most affected by rotational forces. Rotational and angular accelerations, i.e. caused by a punch against the chin during a boxing match, lead to huge relative movements of brain and skull and generate tearing of blood vessels and extensive structural brain damage. The direction of the imparted force contributes as well to the damage which is to expect. Brain damage in the basal ganglia, corpus callosum and white matter is caused by sagittal impact on the head. Combined rotational and translational forces produce sever combined head and spine injuries. 20% of the American and 17% of the Canadian ice hockey players sustain at least one head injury during their careers.

12.1.3 Skull and facial fractures

A skull fracture is a break of one or more bones of the skull. Five types of skull fractures are recognized: linear fractures, skull fractures with impression, depressed skull fractures, diastatic skull fractures and basilar skull fractures.

Linear fractures are most common and frequently in the frontal or temporo-parietal area; surgery is rarely required.

Skull fractures with impression result from a focal blunt trauma, often associated with a tear of the dura (penetrating head trauma).

Depressed skull fractures usually resulting from a blunt trauma, account for 11% of severe head injuries. Broken bones are displaced inward and might damage the brain. Compound depressed skull fractures occur when there is a laceration over the fracture resulting in the cranial cavity being in direct contact with the outside environment. The dura mater is torn. The risk of brain damage is high. Surgery is most often required to lift the bones.

Diastatic fractures occur when the fracture transverses the sutures and result in widening of the sutures

Basilar skull fractures are breaks of the base of the skull (4% of severe head in juries). They are often associated with severe damage of blood vessels and soft tissue. Blood is often found in the sinuses and the ethmoidal cells. Cerebrospinal fluid leaks in 80% of basilar skull fractures from the nose or ears. Although the leaking stops in 70% within a week, there is a high risk of developing a meningitis.

> The prognosis of skull fractures depends on the injuries of blood vessels and brain structures.

12.1.4 Facial fractures

Facial fractures are often found in falls with a bike, a motor bike or in contact sports and often associated with traumatic brain injuries. In descending sequence fractures of the mandibula, combined fractures of the os zygomaticum and maxilla, os ethmoidalis and isolated maxilla fractures are found. The classification of the facial fractures is based on the mapping of these fractures by Le Fort. Accordingly they bear his name and are known as Le Fort Fractures grade 1–3.

Tab. 12.1 Classification of the facial fractures according to Le Fort.

Fracture	Structures involved
Le Fort 1	Horizontal maxillary fracture, separating the maxilla from the palate
Le Fort 2	Pyramidal fracture, crosses the nasal bone and the orbicular rim
Le Fort 3	Craniofacial disjunction

Facial fractures may disturb jaw function and can lead to disfigurement. Additionally painful neuralgias may occur. The cranial nerves might be affected as well. Frontobasal injuries might compromise the olfactory nerve, fractures of the orbita the optical nerve, facial fractures the trigeminal nerve, clivus fractures the abducens nerve and petrosal bone fractures the facial and vestibulocochlear nerve.

Compression of the optical nerve by a piece of bone might require surgical decompression in case of visual deterioration. Comparably, surgery is recommended in facial palsy without signs of improvement. However, the damage to the facial nerve happens most often at the time of the injury. Subsequently, the effect of surgery is minor. Patients with lesions of the optical nerve and the facial nerve should receive corticoids. Peripheral injuries of the oculomotor nerve might result in mydriasis but an intracranial rise of brain pressure has to be excluded. Neuralgias of the cranial nerves have to be treated equally to neuralgias of peripheral nerves. Symptomatic treatment includes the use of antiepileptic drugs such as gabapentin, pregabalin, carbamacepine, sometimes in combination with amitriptyline.

12.1.5 Intracranial/extracerebral bleedings

Extracerebral bleedings are closely associated with scull fractures.

Epidural hematoma

In 90% the epidural hematoma is associated with a skull fracture, especially temporal skull fractures might tear the middle meningeal artery with release of blood between the skull and the dura mater. Thus, the location of the hematoma is intracranial but extracerebral and most often unilateral temporal, rarely infratentorial (➤ Fig. 12.1). The epidural hematoma often appears lentiform and might cause a huge compression of brain structures. Dependent on the age of the patient and the localisation of the bleeding the mortality might reach up to 50%, epidural hematomas which are infratentorially located have a mortality of 70%.

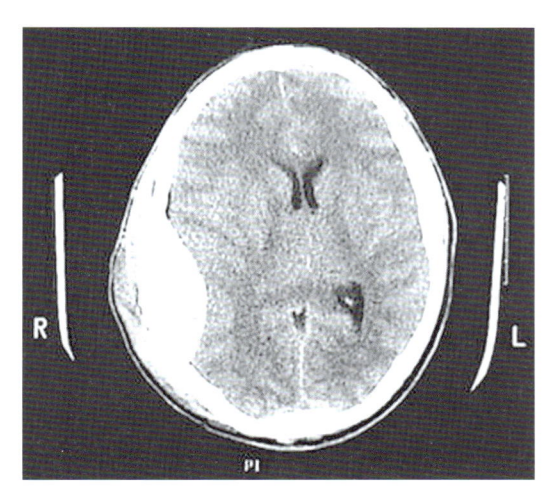

Fig. 12.1 Epidural hematoma.

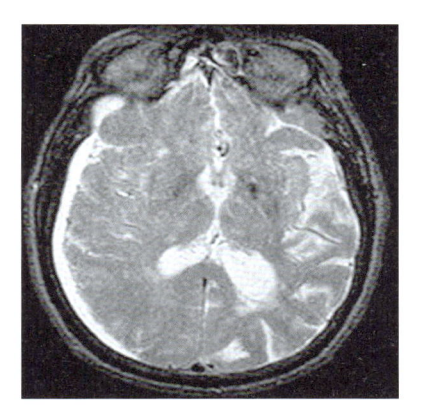

Fig. 12.2 Supdural hematoma.

The "so-called typical clinical course of symptoms" which is cited in the literature include an initial loss of consciousness, followed by a lucid interval which is followed by a rapid clinical deterioration. However, this sequence of events applies to 20% of patients only.

Subdural hematoma

Ruptures of the bridging veins from the surface of the brain towards the dural sinuses may release blood beneath the dura. Subdural hematoma might the only injury (70%) but occurs in combination with epidural hematoma in about 10%.

Subdural hematomas frequently result from rotational (angular) acceleration injuries. Rotational forces are often associated with a torsion of blood vessels. Besides a direct punch to the head a collision with a puck or a ball travelling with high speed might cause these injuries.

Subacute or chronic subdural hematomas did not play an important role in sports medicine so far. With an increasing number of elderly subjects participating in sports activities, the percentage of persons with significant concomitant diseases increases (➢ Fig. 12.2). Physicians are confronted with a growing number of patients with an increased bleeding risk due to medication or a medical condition. Therefore the development of a chronic SDH has to be considered. ➢ Table 12.2 shows the key symptoms of an acute and a chronic SDH.

Tab. 12.2 Symptoms of acute and chronic subdural hematoma (SDH).

Acute SDH		Chronic SDH	
symptoms	%	symptoms	%
Loss of consciousness	80	headaches	80
Pupils unequal	51	Loss of consciousness	53
Optic disc edema	16	hemiparesis	45
hemiparesis	49	Pupils unequal	24
abducens nerve palsy	5	Oculomotor nerve palsy	11
		hemianopia	7

Intracerebral hematoma

Intracerebral hemorrhage (ICH) is a subtype of an intracranial hemorrhage that occurs within the brain tissue itself. Intracerebral bleedings due to trauma occur in 10–45% of head injuries (➢ Fig. 12.3 a and b). Although penetrating head traumas or depressed skull fractures are frequently the origin of intracerebral bleedings, acceleration/deceleration imparted to the head might also result in intraparenchymal bleedings. Even apparently minor traumas might be devastating and irrevocable. Intraparenchymal and intraventricular hemorrhages are to distinguish. Shearing forces strong enough to tear intracerebral

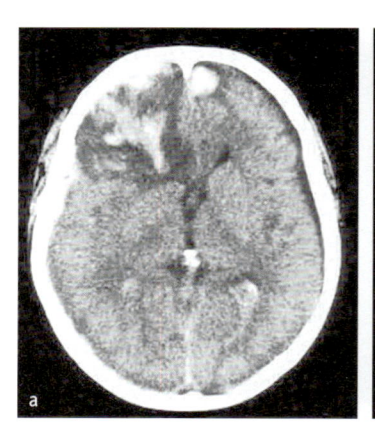

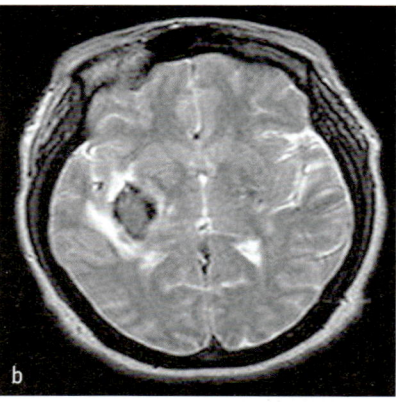

Fig. 12.3 a and b: Contusion bleeding.

blood vessels within the brain substance result in intracerebral hematoma. Central bleedings of the white matter, basal ganglia and the cerebellum also occur without concussion related bleedings and are frequently related to punches. Diffuse intraparenchymal damage of the brain caused by destruction of the fine capillary network around the neurons and the network of neurons results in an interruption of oxygen and glucose supply and interconnecting axons. Intraparenchymal bleedings due to vascular disruption are often multiple and related to falls. Prone to this type of injuries are elderly people with a history of vascular disease. Small bleedings around the third and fourth ventricle so-called Duret-Burner-bleedings occur after blunt head traumas and may occur between some hours to some days after the incident.

Bleedings are present in 95% of fatal head injuries. Bleedings due to contusions are caused by depressed skull fractures, contre-coup injuries and herniations.

Traumatic damage to the central area of the brain (basal ganglia, brain stem, corpus callosum) can be found without marked violation of the coverings of the brain and are the result of the shear forces acting on the brain and tearing of the branches of the medial cerebral artery. The predestined locations of contusions are the temporal and frontal lobe. Biomechanical studies have shown that the shape of the skull tends to focus the shear forces in the frontal and temporal lobe and also to produce damage on the side of the head opposite to where the blow is struck. Although the brain is encased within a bony shell and floats in the cerebrospinal fluid, the complexity of the neuronal network makes it vulnerable. Focal minor impacts are followed by a brief disturbance of neuronal function, more serious shearing forces lead to tearing of axons and death of neurons. Besides the initial injury a secondary damage may result from hypoxia by respiratory failure, ischemia by the surrounding brain edema and raised intracerebral pressure. Patients with intraparenchymal bleedings have symptoms that correspond to the functions controlled by the area of the brain that is damaged by the bleedings. Other symptoms include those that indicate a rise in **intracranial pressure**.

The risk of death from an intraparenchymal bleed in traumatic brain injury is especially high when the injury occurs in the brain stem or medulla oblongata. These areas harbor vital functions such as the control of breathing and blood circulation. Surviving patients often develop a coma vigile. Hemorrhages in the cerebellum have a high risk of a rise in intracranial pressure.

12.1.6 Traumatic subarachnoid hemorrhage

Subarachnoid hemorrhage (SAH) occurs in 30% of patients with traumatic brain injury and carries a poor prognosis if it is associated with deterioration in the level of consciousness (➤ Fig. 12.4). The blood is most often located over the parietal lobe but can be found in all fissures and cysterna. In contrast to spontaneous subarachnoid hemorrhage the sympto-

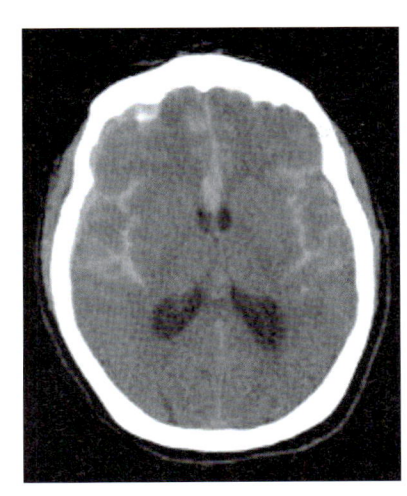

Fig. 12.4 Subarachnoid bleeding.

matic bleedings are more often located over the convexity of the brain. Subarachnoidal hemorrhage at the tentorium cerebelli with associated brain stem damage implies a poor prognosis. Since the fissures are wider SAH is easier to detect on CT scans in elderly. Vasospasms are a complication of SAH and occur often with blood in the basal cisterns. With increasing severity of the hemorrhage the risk of vasospasms rises. Further complications are the inadequate ADH release, electrolyte disturbances, pathological ECG, seizures and obstruction of cerebrospinal fluid resulting in a hydrocephalus.

12.1.7 Traumatic damage to the blood vessels

Dissection of a blood vessel is a separation of the layers of the artery wall. Blood can enter into the space between the inner and outer layers of the blood vessel. Subsequently, the diameter of the blood vessels narrows and might result in a stenosis or occlusion of the blood vessel. Carotid artery and vertebral artery dissections are caused by rapid deceleration with resultant hyperextension and rotation of the neck. Vertebral artery dissection is less common than carotid artery dissection (Bassetti et al 1996, Pelkonen et al. 2003). Intradural dissection are rare and most often a progression of extradural dissections (Pelkonen et al. 2004). It is thought that the internal carotid artery is stretched over the upper cervical vertebrae. Strangulation is an additional risk factor for vertebral artery dissection. Sometimes minor traumas result in a dissection of a blood vessel, i.e. a collision with waves. The distinction between traumatic and spontaneous artery dissections is sometimes difficult. The incidence of spontaneous dissections is estimated at 2–3/100,000. A coincidence of the trauma with a spontaneous dissection might be more likely when the trauma was very mild. A genetic disposition for artery dissection can be found in patients with Marfan syndrome, Ehlers-Danlos syndrome, autosomal dominant polycystic kidney disease, pseudoxanthoma elasticum, fibromuscular dysplasia, and osteogenesis imperfecta type I.

Complications of artery dissection are thromboses, embolism, pseudoaneurysms (aneurysma spurium).

The injury of the artery wall is a predestined site for blood clots. Emboli emerge from blood clots, which break off and travel through the arteries towards the brain and might block blood supply of the brain. Emboli, originating from the dissection are thought to be the cause of infarction in the majority of cases of stroke in the presence of carotid artery dissection. The dissection rarely leads to an immediate occlusion of the artery. Thus, early stroke after the dissection is less frequent.

The dissection might lead to a pseudoaneurysm, which is a balloon like bulge of an artery. The force of the blood pushing against the injured wall can cause an aneurysm.

If the dissection of the artery extends into the intradural space subarachnoid hemorrhage might occur. The risk is higher in vertebral artery dissection than in carotid artery dissection (1–3%).

Symptoms: About 66% of the patients complain about local symptoms only. Pain of the neck radiating to the head is one of the most common signs and sometimes the only symptom of the dissection. Headaches are also frequently reported. Patients with carotid dissection complain more often of frontal headaches while patients with vertebral dissections report more often occipital headaches. The character of the headache is most often throbbing.

Focal signs of a carotid dissection may be an ipsilateral Horner syndrome (decreased pupil size and drooping of the eyelid) or paresis of the hypoglossus nerve (sometimes an involvement of the facial nerve, the lingual nerve, accessory nerve or the chorda tympani are observed. The deficits of the caudal cranial nerve are possibly due to pseudoaneurysms or to the disturbance of capillaries providing the blood supply of the nerves.

The range of neck movements is often reduced and might mislead the physician to diagnose a distorsion of the neck.

Ischemic symptoms are either due to a complete occlusion of the blood vessels or to emboli. However, even a complete occlusion of an artery remains asymptomatic because bilateral circulation keeps the brain well perfused. Thus, hemodynamic stroke is less frequent in arterial dissection.

About 60% of patients with acute artery dissection do not show any ischemic symptoms initially, but 80% develop permanent or transient ischemic symptoms (transient ischemic attack) within one week after the event.

If an ischemic stroke occurs, the neurological deficits refer to the brain areas involved: Carotid artery: i.e. contralateral, hemparesis, aphasia.

Vertebral arteria: visual loss, unsteadiness, ataxia, difficulties in swallowing and speaking (dysarthria), autonomic symptoms.

Diagnosis:

Finally, the diagnosis can be made by duplex sonography in 90% of patients, however the initial duplex sonography might be normal in up to 31% of the patients (Arnold 2008). Especially, the examination of the internal carotid artery is difficult and a dissection might be missed (➢ Fig. 12.5).

The best results are obtained by magnetic resonance tomography with a 1.5 or better 3.0 Tesla machine applying a high field technique. If the angiogram without contrast (Time of flight) cannot clarify the condition of the blood vessel, a contrast enhanced MRI angiography should be included (Phan et al. 2001). The best results are achieved in the T1 setting using a protocol known as "fat suppression". The intramural hematoma is confirmed by a hyperintense sickle like structure.

Conventional angiography might be necessary in some cases of vertebral artery dissection. Collateral blood flow or diagnosis of a general disease of the blood vessels can be made by a conventional angiogram.

Treatment:

The goal of treatment is to prevent the development or continuation of neurologic deficits. Patients have to admitted to a stroke Unit and require monitoring.

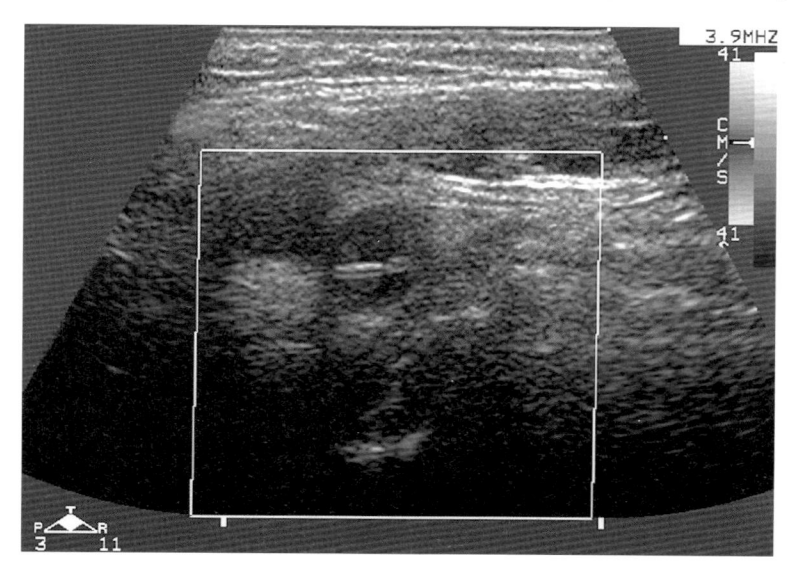

Fig. 12.5 Dissection.

Treatments include observation, anticoagulation, stent implantation and carotid artery ligation. Thrombolysis treatment with rtPA to dissolve blood clots is possible within a time frame of 3–6 hours. Local intravasal thrombolysis might be considered in selected cases. Stenting involves the catheterization of the affected artery and the insertion of a mesh-like tube. Stenting might be considered in special cases when the lumen of the blood vessel is extremely narrow or an aneurysm has to be sealed. Stenting and insertion of coils might be also performed if there is an intradural extension of the dissection or an aneurysm. It is not clear whether the procedures translate into an improvement of the clinical outcome.

There is also no evidence that anticoagulation is superior to platelets inhibitors or vice versa. The most common treatment schedule in Germany for secondary prevention of stroke in artery dissection is the anticoagulation for 3–6 months, followed by life long treatment with 100 mg ASA.

For prevention of blood clots anticoagulation is the treatment of choice, however presence of intradural dissection is a contraindication for anticoagulation. Treatment is usually with either antiplatelet drugs such as aspirin or with anticoagulants such as heparin or warfarin. The general outcome is quite good, over 75% of patients recover completely.

The development of a Carotis-sinus cavernousus fistel is the most dangerous sequelae of an intradural extension of a carotid artery dissection. Symptoms are a unilateral chemosis with retroorbital swelling and venous congestion. Patients complain of reduction of visual arcuity. Additionally the oculomotor, trochlear, abducens nerves might be compromised which results in a limitation of ipsilateral eye movements. mydriasis or ptosis. Impairment of venous blood flow might lead to intracerebral bleedings. Treatment: endovascular occlusion with coils.

12.1.8 Traumatic brain injury

Concussion

A concussion is a traumatic brain injury induced by an impulsive force transmitted to the head resulting from a direct or indirect impact to the head, face, neck, or elsewhere. It is the most common traumatic brain injury. In the most recent literature the term traumatic brain injury replaces the term concussion. Concussion is often interchangeably used with the term mild traumatic brain injury. Clinical symptoms indicating that a concussion has taken place are physical signs such as loss of consciousness, amnesia, behavioural changes (i.e. irritability), cognitive impairment (i.e. slowed reaction times), sleep disturbances (i.e. drowsiness), somatic symptoms (i.e. headaches), nausea and dizziness.

There are different grading systems in grade 1–3 in use, which classify the severity (mild, moderate, severe) of the head trauma according to the time of unconsciousness. Some authors have the grading system disputed. Although, the idea of grading the seriousness of a concussion at the time of injury for better prediction of the outcome is attractive, it has been abandoned by many clinicians because the scales were not research based. Furthermore, the grading system was sometimes misleading. In the past it has been generally accepted that loss of consciousness denoted more severe injury. However, patients might have sustained severe brain injury without being unconscious. However, loss of consciousness has still some meaning in the clinical routine.

Brief loss of consciousness (LOC) does not correlate with severity of the head injury but the presence of prolonged LOC (>1 min). Retrograde amnesia is also not relevant for the severity of the disturbed brain function. However, anterograde amnesia, especially lasting more than 6 hours, the duration of confusion, the presence of fatigue, cognitive deficits or balance problems have a predictive value for the severity of the brain injury. Probably, the outcome of a concussion is best determined by the nature, burden and duration of symptoms.

The diagnosis of a mild traumatic head injury is always challenging for the physician.

On one hand symptoms might have a rapid remission leading to an underreporting of mild brain injury. On the other hand symptoms might occur later and more severe brain injuries are misdiagnosed as mild brain injury. 11% of subdural hematomas might be treated as TBI because of a lack of symptoms within the first 24 hours after the trauma.

Pathophysiological mechanisms:

There is no structural damage of the brain in concussion but an interruption of brain function maybe due to a disruption of synapses and axonal disturbances.

Pathophysiology:

Mild TBI does not lead to immediate axonal loss or proteolysis but brain function is disturbed. Axonal swelling might occur and 2 to 3 hours after the accident protein S and NSE indicating neuronal damage rise. Increases of the S-100B are also found in contusions of the thorax and bone fractures (Biberthaler et al. 2001). The time of the axonal swelling and loss of microtubuli is very long in humans. Subsequently, even after a mild brain injury the cells show a higher vulnerability for some time. A second trauma during this sensitive stage might cause severe brain damage (Biasca et al. 2007).

Cerebral contusion

A contusion is a type of traumatic brain injury (TBI) that causes bruising of the brain tissue. Cerebral bruises are often associated with microhemorrhages, which are leaks of small blood vessels into the brain. Contusions are present in 20–30% of severe head injuries. Patients show loss of consciousness or drowsiness and have neurological deficits, hemiparesis or speech disorders. Intracranial pressure might rise and may result in herniation. Stretching of the extremities indicates a life threatening condition.

Clinical symptoms last longer than 24 hours. Patients show often a delirium when they wake up and are disorientated. Sometimes they develop psychosis. Epileptic seizures might occur as well.

Diagnosis:

The full extent of the injury may not be completely recognized immediately. The diagnosis of a head injury is made by conducting a physical examination, which includes neurological testing and diagnostic tests. During the examination, the physician obtains a complete medical history of the patient and of witnesses and asks how the injury occurred.

Imaging:

Although for a diagnosis of concussion the scan has to be without any structural damage, concussion might be present in setting of other structural injuries such as fracture.

Patients with neurological signs, loss of consciousness and very long lasting amnesia should undergo a CT or MRI scan. There is a debate about the indication of a CT or MRI scan. According to the Zurich guidelines (➢ Table 12.3) no scan is required in patients with concussion.

Tab. 12.3 Zurich guidelines.

1.)	athletes with symptoms should be removed from play
2.)	no athlete with symptoms, at rest or with exertion, should continue to play
3.)	young athletes need to be treated more conservatively
4.)	there is no role for CT or MRI in concussion
5.)	a multidisciplinary approach to management is useful

Tab. 12.4a Glasgow-Coma Scale.

Response	Observed response	Score
Eye opening	Spontaneously	4
	In response to voice	3
	In response to painful stimuli	2
	Does not open the eyes	1
Verbal	Orientated, converses normally	5
	Disorientated, confused	4
	Utters inappropriate words	3
	Incomprehensible sounds	2
	Makes no sounds	1
Motor	Obeys commands	6
	Locates painful stimuli	5
	Flexion and withdrawal to painful stimuli	4
	Abnormal flexion to painful stimuli (decorticate response)	3
	Abnormal stretching to painful stimuli (decerebrate response)	2
	Makes no movements	1

Tab. 12.4b Severity of head injury.

GCS-points	Severity
13–15	mild
9–12	moderate
3–8	severe

In patients with drowsiness or neurological symptoms the scan has to be repeated after 3-6 hours, even when the initial scan was clear.

Patients with cerebral contusion often show bleedings on the MRI and multiple lesions due to contusions of the cortex (Coup-Contrecoup injuries). Brain edema might be present in severe brain injury.

Glasgow Coma Scale is used to rate the extent of injury and chances of recovery. The scale (3–15) involves testing for three patient responses: eye opening, best verbal response, and best motor response. A high score indicates a good prognosis and a low score indicates a poor prognosis.

Acute management of the athlete with head injury

Even mild traumatic brain injury might have serious sequelae und a hematoma might develop even days after the injury. Athletes who lost consciousness should not take up the competition the same day again. The prerequisites for immediate return to the contest or practice are that the athlete did not loose consciousness and do not show any retrograde or antegrade amnesia. The athletes have to be assessed for balance, reaction, orientation and neurocognitive symptoms. Concussion symptoms are often more notable when the patient is trying to perform at high level. Therefore, a short exercise test should be performed prior to returning to the competition. Each athlete who perceives headaches or any symptoms after returning to the competition has to be taken out of the competition.

When an athlete suffered from a loss of consciousness or the athlete is disorientated, reports blurred vision or dizziness and cannot remember the events prior or after the accident concussion should be suspected. A careful medical examination has to take place. The athlete has to be removed from the competition or the practice. Vital signs have to be assessed, airways, breathing and circulation have to be checked (ABC).

The transport should be conducted to the next hospital suitable for the care of patients with head and spine injury. Transportation should be fast and with consideration. Transport by airway is not always the best solution. In case of a severe traumatic brain injury intensive care medicine is requested. The patient might need arteficial ventilation, an intravenous catheter, administration of catecholamines and brain edema treatment. X-rays of the cervical spine and thorax and a cCT-scan have to be performed.

Note the high coincidence of head injury and chest trauma and pelvic trauma. All athletes with moderate and severe traumatic brain injury should have x-rays of the lung, cervical spine, pelvic and an ultrasound scanning of the abdomen.

The treatment of extracerebral injuries is often urgent due to high blood loss. Therefore, operative treatment of these injuries has to happen first. Sometimes, the treatments of the intracerebral and extracerebral injuries have to be carried out simultaneously. If no surgical procedures are necessary the patients has to be monitored for 24 hours, analgesics and antiemetics are given on demand. When patients suffer from severe nausea intravenous fluids are given.

Prognosis

The outcome of TBI depends on the cause of the injury and on the location, severity, and extent of neurological damage. Outcomes range from good recovery to death.

Return to sports activity

Even mild TBI can lead to headache, confusion, difficulty concentrating or with multitasking, mood alteration, sleep disturbance, vertigo, short-term memory loss and anxiety. Most often the symptoms resolve completely within days. Some patients have persistent symptoms that last 6 months or more. When symptoms persist greater than a few days postconcussive syndrome should be considered.

Patients without any pathological morphological sign in the MRI scan have also to be checked by a physician for subtle neurological symptoms.

Second impact syndrome (SIS)

Although the second-impact syndrome is a rare condition but it might have devastating effects on the brain. There is still some disagreement about the pathophysiology. It seems that it occurs prior to complete recovery of a previous concussion and leads to cerebral edema by cerebrovascular dysregulation. The worst case is the subsequent herniation. Young athletes below the age of 18 and children are at higher risk to experience a SIS. Zemper et al (2003) reported that athletes having suffered from a TBI have a 6times increased risk of suffering a second brain injury. 39% of athletes who experienced a SIS with poor outcome had not been recovered from the first trauma at the time of the second trauma (Boden et al. 2007).

Returning to physical activity and participation

Taking care for an athlete might be challenging. Athletes have a very high motivation to return to participation, they rather hide symptoms or minimize health problems. Although there might be third party interests influencing the athlete and making it difficult to ascertain a correct medical history. Further, athletes taking part in contact sports experience many impacts during a game or practice and might not remember any special hit or kick. The physician should also consider that many athletes want to perform at an extremely high level of physical activity. Thus some symptoms might be still interfering with the athletes' performance at this level and might delay full recovery. Therefore, athletes have to be supervised after returning to training.

An athlete who suffered a brain injury and lost consciousness or showed symptoms indicating a disturbance of the brain function has to be removed from contest and practice. Athletes should not return to physical activity on the same day. After the first mild concussion athletes might return to sports activity after being well for one week, after a moderate concussion athletes should abstain from sports for at least 2 weeks after being well. In severe brain injury athletes should be off for 6 weeks and return after being well for 1 week. After the second concussion athletes have to be well for two weeks after a mild TBI prior to return to competition sports. Athletes have to be 6 weeks off after a second moderate head trauma and being well for 1 week prior to participation in practice. In case of a second severe concussion athletes have to be completely off for the season and return the next year. If a third concussion happens, patients with mild TBI have to be off for 6 weeks and return after 1 week being well, with moderate TBI have to be off the rest of he season and with severe TBI patients have to desist from contact sports.

If the athlete is felt to be symptom free without the use of medication and the physical examination is completely normal, a neurological assessment including balance tests, reaction time measurements and neurocognitive testing should be conducted.

Athletes without loss of consciousness might also have experienced a concussion. A short physical and neurological examination has to be conducted (Kelly et al. 1997). The athlete needs to be fully orientated regarding person, time and situation and should be able to recall the events of the contest. To control memory the athlete has to recall 3–5 words immediately and after a delay of 5 min. Another test for working memory is the digit span backward. These tests do not require any specific tools and are easily conducted and interpreted by lay persons. A short exercise test including some jumps and a short sprint complete the examination. If the athlete manages all tasks without headache, vertigo or other symptoms they are allowed to participate again. A further check of the athlete 10 to 20 min later is to recommend hence some symptoms occur later.

Note, every athlete with a traumatic brain injury who seems to be less concentrated, slowed down and does not perform as usually, has to be taken off the contest. The athlete is at high risk to suffer a second traumatic brain injury.

The decision to return to the match has to be made in some sports activities under pressure of time. While in some team sports the athletes can be replaced for some minutes and then return again, i.e. in soccer players cannot return. Some football and ice hockey clubs in USA and Canada use Laptop supported tests for assess-

12.1 Injuries of the central nervous system

ing memory, attention, reaction time and information processing speed. A baseline test is performed in all players prior to the season. After a concussion athletes have to be serially tested, sometimes sideline the pitch (Lovell et al. 2006). The test results have shown that symptom-free athletes need up to 7 days to regain the cognitive level prior to the brain injury. Children and adolescents might need more time (Adirim 2007).

Besides head injuries acrobatic flights, paragliding and parachuting can have major impact on the brain. Some components of the programme like spirals lead to gravitation forces up to 5 G and provoke dizziness, nausea, decreased ability to respond which might result in a crash.

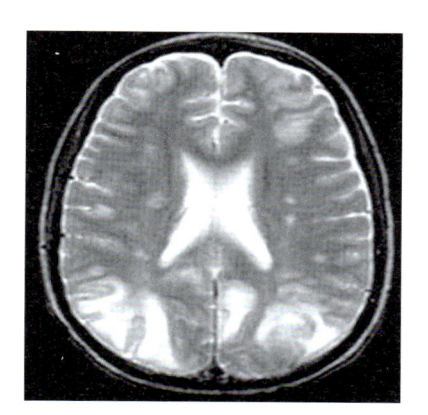

Fig. 12.6 Encephalopathy of a boxer.

12.1.9 Chronic cumulative effects

Besides acute symptoms after brain injury there is increasing concern about cumulative effects of concussions. On the extreme side, boxers are well known to be at risk of developing permanent neurological deficits. Jordan et al (2000) found among a group of former boxers in 20% signs for a chronic brain damage with cognitive and motor deficits and behavioural disturbances. The most pronounced form is the encephalopathia pugilistica. Clinical manifestation reminds to Parkinson's disease, the pathological characteristics resemble Alzheimer's disease. The risk of developing an encephalopathia pugilistica correlates with the duration of a boxer's career, the number of punches to the head and a poor performance. Otto et al. (2000) showed an increase of the concentration of protein S-100 in plasma after hitting the head of boxers. The plasma concentration correlated directly with the number and the impact of the punches and inversely with the cognitive performances. Possibly the protein S might serve as a marker for an estimate of chronic brain damage. Chronic traumatic encephalopathy was also described in retired professional football players who had a history of 5 and more concussions. McKee et al confirmed a neuropathological distinct tauopathy.

While the encephalopathia pugilistica (➤ Fig. 12.6) can be referred to repetitive concussions there is a separate concern about athletes sustaining routine injuries while playing American football, ice-hockey or soccer. In Germany soccer is a very popular sport comparable with American football in the USA. There is some disagreement whether heading the ball might result in chronic brain damage. While some authors describe emotional and cognitive deficits (Baroff 1998; Witol and Webbe 2003) and cognitive deficits (Baroff 1998) in soccer players, Putukian (2000) could not confirm cognitive deficits in players during a season. In contrast the studies of Baroff and Witol & Webbe have shown a correlation between cognitive deficits and the number of headings. Players who performed many headings had a higher risk of a concussion. A ball kicked with moderate impact from a distance of 10m has a power of 100 kPa. Therefore, heading technique has to be practised for prevention of chronic head trauma.

In summary excellent technical skills are prerequisites for the prevention of head injuries. The equipment has to be optimized and should be worn not only by professional but also by non-professional athletes. Protectors and helmets have to be worn. The efficacy in preventing TBI by helmets has been generally accepted (Wesson et al. 2000). There is still the need for further information and improvement of acceptance. 30% of inline skaters do not wear helmets because of visual appearance. The equipment is often very expensive and adolescents and their parents cannot afford it. Besides technical skill and equipment external factors i.e. weather and the condition of the streets or the pitch in out door sport have to be considered. Further the rules of some sports activities influence the rate of concussions and some specific sports equipment. Experienced surfers do not use a board leash in kite surfing and prefer a rolleash. The rolleash keeps contact with the board by a 3–5 m linen or fabric tape. Athletes using a boardleash have an increased risk of being hit by the board. Therefore athletes should wear a helmet and a protective vest.

> TBI are most often caused by a fall or a blunt direct trauma to the head. Besides fractures extra- or intracerebral bleedings may occur. Shearing forces might result in dissections of blood vessels and lead to an ischemic stroke. The extent of the brain damage is often to assess more clearly some hours after the event. Following sports activities are associated with increased incidence and prevalence of TBI, contact sports activities, horse-riding, paragliding, skiing, snowboarding, biking, motor sports. Athletes who had suffered from loss of consciousness or had shown neurological symptoms have to abstain from sports activities. Only athletes who are symptom-free can participate in practice and competition. Frequency and severity of concussion can be reduced by improvement of technical skills and equipment, especially wearing helmets.
>
> Besides external factors a genetic disposition seems to make some people more vulnerable. Recently a mutation in the CACNA1A calcium channel subunit gene was detected and linked to malignant brain edema and the apolipoprotein –E-ε4-Allel plays probably a role in the development of long-term effects.

12.2 Injuries of the spine and the spinal cord

The **incidence rate** of spinal cord injuries is 1.5–5/100,000 (Ngouchi 1994) and about 60% of spine injuries are associated with **spinal cord injuries**. **Penetrating spinal cord injuries** results from stitch, tears, high-speed trauma, or bone fragments that penetrate the dura mater. Indirect, external force triggers **non-penetrating spinal cord injury**. The **severity** of the spinal cord damage depends on biomechanics, duration of impact on the spine, and pre-existing pathologies (spondylolysis, spinal stenosis). Cervical spine injuries are most frequent, followed by thoracic and lumbar spine injuries. Individual sports have their own, characteristic injury pattern, e.g. cervical spine injuries are more frequent in snowboarding as compared to skiing. In contrast, cauda equine and conus medullaris syndromes are rare in snowboarding. This injury pattern is a result of the snowboarding technique. Both legs are fixed on the board, which lowers the risk of thoracic and lumbar spine injuries but increases the risk of cervical spine injuries. Other contributing risk factors are the sport skills (amateur versus professional sports), climate, and environment, e.g. street condition in a bike race. The details of an accident, direction and impact on the spine help predicting the sequelae of an injury. Again, **individual preconditions** such as a scoliosis may aggravate the damage.

12.2.1 Biomechanical mechanisms

In humans, the cervical vertebrae are small and accommodate a large range of movements. Contrary to humans, animals may have very strong necks carrying a heavy head. Some sports increase the weight bearing of the neck such bridging movements in wrestling. The neck absorbs force impacts or sustains huge torque loads. The neck musculature arises from the lower cervical spine and the upper thoracic vertebral arches to control and support the head. The mobility of the atlanto-occipital and atlanto-axial joints accounts for 50% of the cervical spine mobility.

Atlanto-occipital movement
    Flexion: 15°
    Extension: 15°
    Side flexion: 5–10°
    Rotation: no

Atlanto-axial movement
    Rotation: 45°
    Flexion: 10–15°
    Extension: 10–15°
    Lateral gliding
    Vertical approximation

C2–C7 motion
    Combined movements
    C5–C6 mainly flexion
    C6–C7 mainly extension

Range of motion extension/flexion: 55°
 Rotation
 Lateral flexion

12.2.2 Mechanisms

Forced excessive motions, including abnormal anteflexion, retroflexion, rotation and acceleration of the spine or direct compression result in spinal cord injury. Combination of forced excessive motions and compression are equally possible.

Compression fractures: The force is transmitted vertically on the head by a blow or a fall, which results in compression, impression, and skull fractures associated with spinal cord compression. Falls on the head often result in cervical spine injuries at a level of C1/C2.

Hitting the ground while jumping into shallow water, a punch on the chin or front of the head, fall, or whiplash lead to a **retroflexion** of the head. Such retroflexion injuries: ruptures of the longitudinal ligament, ruptures of the discs, ventral luxation, compound fractures of the dens or luxations of the dens. Fractures of the facet joints are frequently found. MRI reveals necrosis and bleeding in the central area of the spine. Vertebral artery injuries may occur as well.

Impact on the occipital part of the head leads to **anteflexion** trauma. Typically, the cervical spine is flexed and impact is axial. Spinal cord injuries are less frequent and occur mainly with the head in an extreme anteflexion. Extreme anteflexion may cause subluxation or dislocation of the vertebrae, ventral compression of the spinal cord, or damage of the posterior funiculi. Representative examples are falling backward from a horse or falling backward while snowboarding. This typically happens to beginners.

Rotational forces trigger vertebral dislocation fractures of the lower thoracic, and lumbar spine. Lesion of the cauda equine and conus are characteristic concomitant injuries after spinal cord compressions.

Combined flexion and rotation trauma, subluxations, luxation with unilateral disc protrusions, or slipped discs follow most often a severe whiplash injury. This often results in compression of the spinal cord with subsequent central spinal cord damage.

Whiplash injury is a posterior and subsequent anterior acceleration and often results in fractures of the processus transversus. Spinal cord injuries are rare.

In contrast, combined dorsal flexion and rotation of the spine is often associated with central cervical spine necrosis. Ligament tears in the area of the thoracic spine are common. Here, cerebral contusions are frequently observed.

12.2.3 Sport-specific injuries

Falls or physical contact with opponents in contact sports is the main cause for spinal cord injuries.

Diving

Diving injuries account for a high incidence rate of catastrophic injuries. Diving into shallow water and hitting the ground of the pool is the most frequent cause. In competitive diving, athletes perform spectacular and difficult dives including somersaults and twists. In order to obtain high scores, divers try to increase the difficulties of their dives. They may loose orientation and hit the board with the head. Diving accidents are typically more frequent in sun shine states where many private pools exist and people enjoy water sports on lakes, rivers, and the ocean. Alcohol is a confounding factor and contributes to poor judgment of the water depth. Typical spinal injury in diving is the cervical fracture between C4 and C6 with a complete loss of motor and sensory function and a poor prognosis for recovery.

Skiing

Specific injuries in **skiing** are related to the thoracic and lumbar spine. With the number of skiers increasing, the frequency of ski accidents rises equally. Attempting jumps, poor landings, loosing control while speeding or hitting trees or rocks are the most common causes. Other contributing factors are poorly prepared, overcrowded slopes with fast skiers colliding into slow skiers, cross runs, and obstacles located just over the edge of the slope. Poor skiing skills, lack of physical fitness, and unsuitable equipment as well as alcohol and overestimation of their own capabilities are tightly linked to skiing accidents. Associated injuries in other parts of the body are present in more than a half of the subjects with spine fractures. Therefore, an examination of extremities, thorax, pelvic girdle, abdomen and the head is required for a safe transport and management of the injured person.

Snowboarding

Snowboarding involves a variety of styles. Free ride is easily accessible and might qualify the athlete to perform more difficult forms of snowboarding such as free style, alpine or half pipe. Free-riding might already include acrobatics and aerial tricks.

Big air competitions are contests where riders present their jumps and tricks in the air. They try to attain jumps with sizable height and distance and clean landing. The aerial tricks hold a high risk of falling. After a failed heel side turn the rider might land on his back, which can result in serious head and cervical spine injuries. Injuries of the wrist are more often associated with cervical spine fractures in snowboarding than injuries of the knee, which is common in skiing.

Ski-jumping

Ski-jumping is a highly specialized sport and performed by few people. It is a competitive sport and rarely performed by amateurs. Severe injuries are seldom due to the high skill level of the jumpers and the fact that it is not a mainstream sport. Usually the preparation of the in-run and the landing area is good. The equipment has been improved. Therefore, spine fractures are rare. Young athletes at the age of 15–17 years with poor judgment who attempt longer jumps than those for which they are physically qualified have the highest risk of spinal injuries. At the end of the season when athletes try to surpass personal best distances they take a higher risk and test their limits. Consequently, the frequency of injuries rises towards the end of the season.

Equestrian injuries

25% of **equestrian injuries** are associated with cervical spine and cauda equine damage. One third involve the cervical spine and two-thirds the thoraco-lumbar junction. Head and facial injuries are very common in horse riding; head and spine injuries often occur concomitantly.

American football

Prior to the change of the game rules in **American football**, spinal fractures occurred often. In recent years, quadriplegia has decreased remarkably. The mechanism of spinal fractures is axial loading with the cervical spine slightly flexed. Axial loading occurs when the head is abruptly stopped and the rest of the body continues moving in its initial trajectory. The neck is stuck in between the head and body. The improvement of the equipment has reduced the rate of injuries. Historically, the helmet and the fulcrum of the single-bar-face mask contributed to hyperextension resulting in cervical spine fractures. Furthermore, the ban of spearing, head butting and face tackling has decreased neurological injuries. Neck rolls do not prevent cervical fractures but may protect against spinal root traction.

Rugby

Rugby is associated with a high risk of spine fractures. The most vulnerable age for injuries is between 15 and 21 years and are often related to dangerous play. The front row players bear the highest risk of injury. Therefore, the rules were changed for the young players. Young players have to keep the head and shoulders above hip level. The rules should be also applied in recreational sport. Furthermore, neck strengthening is an important measure to reduce injuries and devastating results.

Ice hockey

In contrast to other contact sports, **ice hockey** carries an increasing risk of spinal cord injuries with quadriplegia. The helmet does not alter the dynamics of the neck during a collision. Fractures of C5 and C6 are typical for ice hockey (➤ Fig. 12.7). Cervical spine and trans-

Fig. 12.7 a and b: Compression fracture of a ice hockey player.

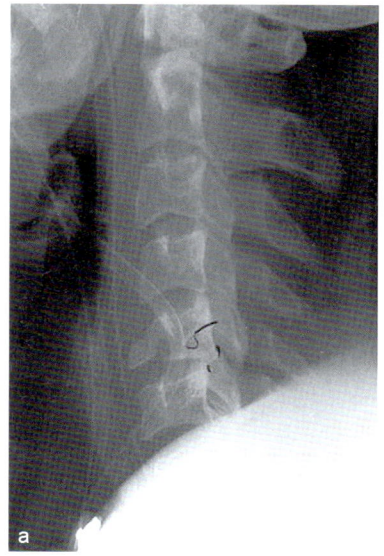

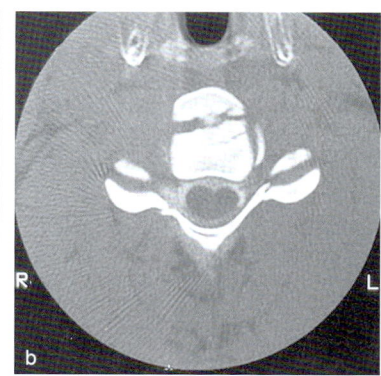

verse processus fractures are the sequelae of backward body checks. **Most severe injuries** result from contact between players and boards (Mölsa et al., 1999). The mechanism is an axial load during flexion while the player hits the boards. Therefore, checking from behind into the boards is forbidden now but does still happen. Cross-checking and high sticks are also linked to serious head and neck traumas.

Paragliding

Spine injuries are predominant in **paragliding** accidents. Zeller et al. (1992) evaluated a series of 489 paragliding accidents. They reported 125 fractures of the thoraco-lumbar junction. Schulze et al. (2000) reported spinal fractures in 62% of injuries. Pilot errors are the main contributing factors responsible for 93% of the accidents. Launching and landing imply high injury risks. Inadequate technical skills during launching – especially reverse launch in higher winds – might deflate the wing and result in crash. Modern recreational wings will inflate without pilot's input. Good piloting techniques reduce the frequency and severity of deflations. Deflations in low altitude can result in serious injuries due to the ground impact. A stall during landing can lead to a landing outside of the landing area. Collision with trees or rocks is a further risk for paragliders. The pilot tries to absorb the shock of the landing with the feet. If the pilot fails to land correctly, compression and shearing forces impart on the thoracolumbar junction and might cause a fracture and a cauda/conus syndrome. Although spine injuries decreased after introduction of back protectors they account still for 31% of the injuries in paragliding.

Trampolining

Trampolining has been considered as a high risk sport regarding cervical spine injuries which led to ban of trampolining in schools. In recent years trampolining has become more popular again. The risk profiles of using trampolines in competitive sports and in leisure activities differ. Athletes taking part in competitive sports are highly trained but they try to perform complex acrobatics, which can lead to falls and accidents. Thus, they might be unable to complete a combination of rotations around the longitudinal and lateral axis producing somersaults and twists and land on the head or the neck. Contact with the bed with a hyperflexed neck while attempting a backward somersault might result in a severe cervical spine injury. Uncontrolled landings on the back or buttock also might impart compression on the spine. Less trained subjects have even more difficulties to control the bouncing movements.

Furthermore subjects might fall off the bed and land on the mat or the end deck of the trampoline. The trampolines in competitive sport have padded end decks and spring covered with pads. The terms and regulations of international competitions require 200mm thick mats on the floor for 2 m around the trampoline. However, the rules vary between the countries and the requirements are less strict in some national competitions. Safety aspects are less thought in leisure activities and falls might cause more severe injuries. The double mini-trampoline has also a higher risk of injuries. It has a flat bed and a slope end. Specific skills are needed to jump on to trampoline and to dismount on to the mat. Very small trampolines are popular in families with children. If those are not properly secured they may tumble over when children bounce up and down.

Artistic Gymnastics

Although safety issues have improved in **artistic gymnastics** and age limits should prevent children from performing at a level they are not physically qualified for, spectacular accidents still happen. Landings including somersaults and incomplete twists might result in falls on the neck or head. The impact on ground transmits a huge force on the head and the cervical spine; the force depends on the power, the speed of the rotations, and altitude of the equipment (e.g. high bar). Falls on the equipment may also cause severe injuries i.e. hitting the lower bar of the uneven bar with the neck or the balance beam during a flic-flac with the head. Failed vaults might result in falls on the equipment and imply a high injury risk for the upper cervical spine. In artistic gymnastics and trampolining, injuries of the upper cervical spine account for the majority of severe injuries.

Biking

Spine injuries result most often from falls with high speed and collisions with stationary obstacles or other **bikers**. Bad weather, poor road conditions, and team racing increase the risk of fall. Falling over backwards or head over the handlebar generates a direct impact on the spine. Dirt bike and down hill racing are special risk factors.

Falls also account for the majority of severe spine injuries in **motor sports**, especially in motocross. Jumping in motocross freestyle increases the risk of loosing 3D, kinaesthetic control in the air. Thus, risk of fall and spinal injury is high.

12.2.4 Classification of spinal cord injuries

Spinal edema, **spinal contusion**, and **intramedullary hemorrhage** are three classic spinal cord injuries. Spinal cord edema excludes a structural damage of the spinal cord and is associated with a favorable neurological outcome. Neurological deficits are reversible and transient. Spinal cord contusions represent a structural damage of the spinal cord. Axonal edema, synaptic disruption, endothelial damage, neuronal necrosis and demyelination might occur. Neuronal damage and edema extend centrifugally and may stretch across several segments. Cord contusion shows a less favorable outcome. Spinal cord hemorrhage may be patchily or spiky and is associated with more severe neurological deficit, usually resulting in residual symptoms. Complete spinal cord injury is associated with poor neurological outcome.

Posttraumatic syringomyelia is one of the possible posttraumatic complications. Tubular central intramedullary hemorrhage is rare. Compression of the spinal cord occurs if a piece of bone, cartilage, spinal disc or soft tissue is dislocated and narrows the spinal canal. The criteria for a compression of the spinal cord are fulfilled if the dislocation of the vertebrae obstructs more than 50% of the spinal canal or more than 30% of the width of the vertebrae at the injured level. Bone splinters, disc material and hematoma may lead to an additional compression of the spinal cord. The final neurological outcome depends on the duration and the severity of the compression of the nervous structures. Mechanical fragments require instant removal.

The initial phase of a spinal cord injury is often characterized by a **spinal shock**. Clinical signs are absent muscle jerks, flaccid muscle tone, loss of motor function and sensation, and loss of bladder control. The spinal shock is often followed by a **quadriplegia** or paraplegia depending on the segment involved. The level of sensory loss indicates roughly the level of the injury. Besides loss of sensori-motor function, autonomic symptoms may occur such as pathological sweating, bladder and bowl dysfunction, and abnormal cardiovascular reflexes. Autonomic dysreflexia is a potentially life-threatening clinical syndrome consisting of acute episodes of excessive, uncontrolled sympathetic output. These uncontrolled bouts of sympathetic output can cause transient and pronounced elevations of blood pressure. In rare cases, this can lead to serious sequelae such as hypertensive intracerebral hemorrhage. Autonomous dysreflexia are often triggered by noxious stimulus such as distended urinary bladder or fecal impaction. Despite hypertension, sudden onset of orthostatic hypotension is a typical complication in spinal cord injury above T5. Patients with quadriplegia resulting from cervical spine lesions are at risk of respiratory failure.

> Transient quadriplegia is a syndrome physicians are now more aware of than previously.

Transient quadriplegia, also called cervical neurapraxia (Torg 1990) presents with a transient posttraumatic paralysis of the motor and/or sensory tracts of the spinal cord. Some patients complain only about burning hands and arms, and occasionally, the legs. Symptoms persist on average for 10–15 minutes although neurological deficits up to 48 hours are reported. Flexion of the neck enhances symptoms. Young men have a higher risk than females to sustain a transient quadriplegia. Congenital stenosis of the spinal canal, cervical disc problems, a ligamentous or bone abnormality, or ligamentous instability are revealed in 50% of the patients. Torg et al. stated that the young individual suffering from cervical neuropraxia with or without quadriplegia is not predisposed to permanent neurological deficits (Torg, 1990). Today, the syndrome is a variant of the central spinal cord syndrome. A thorough follow-up is needed in athletes with transient quadriplegia such as plain cervical spinal films with flexion and extension views, CT-and/or MRI. Somato-sensory potentials complete the assessment and may reveal dysfunction of the spinal cord. If no evidence of a spinal cord injury is detected, athletes may return to competition. However, up to 50% of athletes returning to their sport experience a further episode. A direct blow to the head resulting in a sudden flexion or hyperextension of the head often precedes the symptoms.

Athletes with bony or ligamentous abnormalities of the cervical spine should not participate in contact sports due to their risk of developing a transient quadriplegia. Clinical examination, plain X-ray, MRI and electrophysiological testing should be performed. The diagnosis of the initial SCI is critical in order to predict an accurate functional prognosis. Thus, special sequences of the MRI such as diffusion weighted scan or magnetic transfer imaging might help to recognize even mild spinal cord trauma.

12.2.5 Assessment of athletes with spinal trauma

Athletes should be assessed immediately after the accident; the main complaint needs to be recognized quickly. The **location and description of pain** often indicates its origin and helps with diagnosis. Athletes who recover quickly and are pain-free within minutes are allowed to return to the competition as long as they do not show any neurological symptoms and can move their neck freely.

Athletes showing the following symptoms require discontinuation of competition:

- Lhermitte-sign
- Paraesthesias
- Sensory-motor deficits
- Pain provoked by sneezing, coughing or head movements
- Pain between the scapulas.

> The neck should not be moved in unconscious athletes.

Patients who are awake can be examined further. Patients are asked to move their head forward, backward, to the right, and left side. For a better location of the damage, the examiner moves the head into side flexion combined with rotation into flexion or extension with the opposing shoulder is depressed. This maneuver approximates the neuroforamina. Increase of pain during this maneuver may indicate irritation of a nerve root, foraminal encroachment, adhesions around the dural sleeve and / or changes in the facet joint and capsule. Overpressure applied to the head causes foraminal compression and provokes pain in patients with an encroachment of the nerve root. Careful traction might ease the pain in case of compression of nervous structures.

According to the NASCIS-III trial the administration of 30 mg/kg bodyweight methylprednisolone with subsequent administration of 5.4 mg/kg bodyweight per day as permanent drip is recommended in patients with spine trauma without major concomitant diseases. Long-term treatment with methylprednisolone enhances the risk of severe infections.

A neurological screening test is mandatory. Muscle strength, reflexes and sensation have to be checked. If the examination of the neck is clear, the brachial plexus will be examined. Rapid diagnosis using plain x-ray and CT/MRI scans is necessary for improvement of the neurological outcome. Transportation of the patient with pain and neurological symptoms requires a spinal board or a stretcher. Head and neck need to be stabilized. Breathing has to be secured in patients with quadriplegia. Operative treatment is needed in patients with unstable fractures, spinal cord compression, ligamentous instability, and luxations. Physiotherapy and occupational therapy are implemented early. Rehabilitation depends on the severity of the injury and the structures involved. Strengthening of the anterior and posterior neck muscles prior to returning to practice and competition is strongly recommended.

12.2.6 Overuse injuries of the spine

Slipped discs, facet joint damage, ligamentous instability, and spondylolisthesis are found more often in athletes who are active in sports with abrupt rotation or hyperflexion. There is rarely any damage to the nervous system. The most frequent overuse injury is the spondylolysis (Soler & Calderon 2000). Spondylolysis is a defect of the neural arch, usually in the pars interarticularis. Although spondylolysis is a congenital defect, it is not found in newborns and frequently diagnosed at the age of six years and most often localized at the level of L5. Decreased stress tolerance of the pars interarticularis of the vertebral arch increases the risk of developing spondylolysis. Thus, spondylolysis can be considered a stress fracture. Among the European population spondylolysis is estimated at 5–7%, in 4% an isthmic spondylolisthesis develops (Gangu 2002). Spondylolisthesis is defined as a slipping of one vertebra forward another. Between 10 and 14 years and during the growth spurt, the grade of spondylolisthesis progresses.

Clinical symptoms of spondylolysis and spondylolisthesis are dull backache, deep dull buttocks pain sometimes with radiation towards the sciatic nerve, aggravation of pain by activity, sciatica, spasms of the hamstrings and the erector spinae muscles and increased lumbar lordosis. It is important to distinguish pseudoradicular and radicular pain. Since pain increases always with physical activity, symptoms might mimic a claudicatio spinalis. Symptoms of a claudicatio spinalis are most often reported by patients with spondylolisthesis or by patients who have additional slipped disc or a spinal stenosis.

Patients with spondylolisthesis often show a pronounced lordosis of the lumbar spine. Persistent loss of sensation or motor function is rare, and should raise some doubts regarding the diagnosis. Vigorous physical activity might play a role in the pathophysiology. The following sports put a high strain on the neural arch and make the development of a spondylolysis more likely.

- Sport with repetitive hyperlordosis of the lumbar spine such as: wrestling, artistic gymnastics, throwing a javelin, basketball, volleyball, rhythmic sports gymnastic, swimming butterfly, and diving
- Sports with repetitive rotation such as canoeing, playing golf or throwing
- Sport with impact of high muscular power on the neural arch, i.e. bodybuilding, wrestling and hockey
- Sports requiring a huge range of movement between the local spinal segments, such as

American football, dancing, figure skating, and some disciplines such as high jumping or throwing a javelin.

Typical imaging diagnostics are lumbar-sacral section with plain x-ray, ap and tangential views (LaChapel's 'scotty dog' figure), CT scan, and MRI. The MRI has advantages regarding the information on the width of the spinal canal or the condition of the discs.

Treatment

Treatment aims at strengthening the muscles of back and abdomen, improving technical skills and stretching of the hamstrings. Anti-inflammatory drugs should be administered for a short-term. Training should be restricted for a period of time. If pain continues despite decreased activity and treatment, a brace and a break in sports activities have to be considered. Surgical treatment has to be considered when the fissure is 3 mm or more, otherwise a fusion is very unlikely. Spondylolisthesis grade 3 also requires surgical treatment. The same applies for patients with neurological deficits. Unfavorable factors are abnormalities of the spine. Sport, which involves axial loading, extreme hyperextension and rotation of the lumbar spine, is not suitable for athletes with spondylolisthesis. Running, swimming backstroke, biking (excluding mountain bike and dirt bike), and Nordic Skiing are recommended. Assuming there are no other spine abnormalities, sports capacity is restored after surgery.

Stress fractures of the os sacrum are rare but have been reported in long distance running, aerobics, basket- and volleyball. A pseudoradicular pain characterizes them. Pain of the iliosacral joints with and without hypertrophy of the piriformis muscle might also mimic a radicular pain.

> **Summary**
> Injuries of the spine are frequently associated with spinal cord injuries and head injuries. Depending on the mechanism of the accident specific spinal cord injury patterns may develop. The clinical symptoms in the initial phase of a spinal cord injury correspond to a spinal shock. The initially predominating flaccid paresis is often followed by a spastic paraparesis or tetraparesis. Injuries of the spine are most often caused by falls, with either high speed or collision with stationary obstacles. Depending on the location (head, neck, buttocks) and the intensity of the impact, injuries might occur rather in the upper, middle or lower part of the cervical spine. Congenital abnormalities of the spine are often associated with a transient quadriplegia. Overuse injuries of the spine result from repetitive lumbar hyperextension and increases the risk of a spondylolisthesis.

12.3 The peripheral nervous system

Acute injuries of the peripheral nervous system can be caused by hematoma, compression, tears, ischemia and strains (Lang & Stefan). Overuse injuries of the peripheral nervous system are less frequent (Menger 1992), their incidence correlates with the training load of the athletes. Medical history, localization and characteristics of the pain and the assessment of neurological deficits lead to the diagnosis. The neurological examination includes testing of muscular strength, muscle jerks, sensation and trophic condition.

Plain X-rays, CT-scan, MRI-scans support the medical examination. While the CT scan is superior to the MRI in the assessment of the bone, the MRI shows the details of nerves structures and soft tissue much better than the CT scan. The 1.5 Tesla machines are still limited regarding the resolution of the images. While the 1.5 Tesla scanner remains to be optimal for imaging the brachial plexus (motion artifacts), the 3 Tesla scanner provides an adequate resolution to evaluate nerve injuries. Most of the peripheral nerves are small and show only subtle imaging findings. The generation of 3 Tesla machines has improved the assessment tremendously. Furthermore, 7 Tesla scanners pave the way into clinical assessment although they are predominantly used in research. Lesions of the nervous system are typically shown in T1 weighted images without fat suppression and in T2 weighted images with contrast and fat suppression. Details of the adjacent tissue are shown in T2 weighted imaging with suppression of fat and flow artifacts.

The MRI will identify most pathological states of the spinal nerves or the brachial plexus especially tumors or other space occupying lesions (i.e. hemorrhages). The majority of tumors take up gadolinium. However, some inflammatory neuropathies show the same pattern. Compression of the nerval structures, i.e. the ischiadicus nerve is characterized by a hyperintense signal. A thoracic outlet syndrome can be identified by displacement and constriction of nerve bundles. Transectomies of nerves with greater diameter can be visualized by MRI, while those of small nerves are easily missed. Nerves without structural damage but with altered function are not distinguished from healthy nerves on routine MRI. High-resolution ultrasound is a new approach to nerve lesions. Recently, the resolution of the new ultrasound machines has been much improved by using new linear probes with high emission frequencies. The new software applications supported these developments. The combination of ultrasound imaging (B-scan) with color-coded power-duplex-sonography provides further information.

The sonography is already an alternative to the MRI in the diagnosis of carpal tunnel- syndrome and cubital tunnel syndrome. The sonography shows most often the etiology of the compression such as ganglia, accessory muscles, and aberrant blood vessels. The sonography identifies as well whether an injury of a nerve requires surgical intervention. During surgery the sonography might support the identification of nerve endings, after surgery the sonography helps to control the healing and might show the early development of neuromas.

Damage of a nerve can result in demyelination or in loss of axonal fibres or both. Thus, nerve conduction studies might show a slowing of the nerve conduction velocity or a reduction of the muscle sum potentials or a combination of both. EMG studies will not be of value in acute damage of the nervous system until at least 10 days have passed after the onset of symptoms. However, they yield complementary information and differentiate neurogenic from myopathic processes. Furthermore EMG studies are of value in the diagnosis of chronic conditions and might be helpful regarding the decision of surgery. They also give information about the severity of the process and the temporal profile and might indicate recovery processes.

Injury of the brachial plexus

Motor bike accidents or illegal tackling in American football lead often to injuries of the brachial plexus. The injuries are frequently related to punches or the continued use of now illegal blocking and tackling techniques involving the head as first contact. The typical underlying mechanism of the resulting injury is a stretch-pinch syndrome of the brachial plexus. Players complain of pain located in the supraclavicular region or report a radiating pain between the shoulder bladders. Depending on the severity of the injury the pain might radiate towards the hand and numbness and paraesthesias of the hand might occur. If motor deficits are present they might last for minutes only but with increasing severity of the injury the deficits need weeks or months to recover. In some cases the damage is irreversible (➤ Table 12.5). The tearing of the upper

Tab. 12.5 Classification of nerve injuries according to Sneddon.

Severity	Definition
Grade 1 Neurapraxia	Physiologic interruption of function, transient dysaesthesia or weakness, full recovery within 2 months
Grade 2 Axonotmesis	Degeneration, interruption of some axonal fibres within an intact neurolemmal sheath, full recovery within 3 months
Grade 3 Axonotmesis with damage of the neurolemmal sheath	Interruption of axonal fibres and interruption of the neurolemmal sheath, persisting motor and sensory loss, electrophysiological abnormalities, recovery potential c. 60%
Grade 4 Neurotmesis	Disruption of the neurolemmal sheath, but some parts of the nerves might be intact, poor recovery between 30–60%
Grade 5 Neurotmesis	Complete separation of the nerves, regarding the brachial plexus with torn nerve roots, recovery potential max. 30%

brachial plexus and the C5 and C6 nerve roots without motor deficits are called stingers or burners (Kuhlmann et al. 1999). However, motor deficits can be easily missed, when the strength of the muscles is not tested separately. Players who have suffered from such injuries repeatedly have often mild to moderate deltoid muscle paresis. Wrestlers are at risk of suffering a brachial plexus injury when the opponent uses the Nelson grip and the head is forced into a lateral position.

The upper paresis of the brachial paresis leads to a deficit of the abduction and external rotation of the shoulder, a paresis of the elbow flexors including the brachioradial muscle, the supinator muscle, partially of the triceps muscle and the hand extensor muscles. The muscle tone is flaccid and the arm inward rotated. If the C7 nerve fibres are affected as well the function of the triceps muscle, the pronator teres muscle and the flexor carpi radialis are affected.

Lesions of the lower plexus involve the C8 and Th1 nerve roots. They result in a paresis of the intrinsic hand muscles and of the long finger flexors. The clinical characteristics are a claw-hand with hyperextension of the fingers in the metacarpal-phalangeal joint and flexion of the phalangeal joint and dorsal extension of the hand joint. The sensation of the ulnar division of the hand and the ulnar-innervated forearm are disturbed.

The distinction between supraclavicular and infraclavicular lesion of the brachial plexus is also important. Injuries involving the roots or trunks occur in the supraclavicular portion of the plexus and lesions involving the cords or terminal nerves in the infraclavicular plexus. Supraclavicular lesions are more common than infraclavicular plexopathies and are less likely to show complete recovery. In cases of severe trauma simultaneous injury to the root such as root avulsion may occur. Sometimes distinguishing root avulsion from a pure plexopathy may be difficult. Clinical symptoms pointing to the diagnosis of root avulsion are severe weakness, loss of sensation, Horner syndrome, evidence of spinal cord injury.

The sparing of the sensory nerve conduction responses on electrodiagnostic testing in the context of severe sensory loss might indicate a preganglionic lesion.

Lumbar puncture might further clarify whether root avulsion occurred.

Non-operative treatment includes immobilization with the arm abducted at 60 degree and electrotherapy.

Operative treatment is required in patients with neurotmesis. Depending on the damage reconstruction of the nervous structures, transplant techniques or nerve transfer techniques might be used.

Sometimes muscle transfer techniques are required.

Prevention of brachial plexus injuries: strengthening of neck and shoulder girdle muscles, improvement of technical skills, modification of rules, improvements of equipment.

A differential diagnosis to brachial plexus injuries is the neuralgic neuropathy. It is the most common form of plexopathy although it might be misdiagnosed. Neuralgic amyotrophy is an immune-mediated plexopathy characterized by an acute onset of pain, followed by motor deficits.

An intense physical work out is often reported by patients prior to onset of the symptoms i.e. long swimming in cold water. Other risk factors are: immunization and wet weather. The incidence is 1.64/100,000. Amyotrophic neuralgia may occur, although definite precipitating events are not always identified.

65% of patients complain either of pain radiating from the shoulder to the arm or a deep dull ache. The location of the pain correlates with the neurological deficits and is aggravated by movements. Pain usually persists for several hours or even weeks. Muscle atrophy and weakness are delayed in onset and begin often c. 2 weeks after onset of symptoms. Sensory loss is present in 66% of the patients (Tsairis et a. 1972). Bilateral brachial plexus involvement (2%), isolated involvement of the radial, long thoracic, suprascapular, axillary, anterior interosseus nerve has been reported (Rubin 2001). EMG studies do not reveal a typical pattern, investigation of the CSF reveals an elevation of protein at times but is otherwise normal. Antibodies against myelin could be identified in the blood of patients. Thus, neuralgic amyotrophy is not an overuse injury but an inflammatory condition. At risk are rather young adults male more often than female. Therapy is typically conservative (reduction of physical activity, passive movements, warmth). With decreasing pain, active physiotherapy replaces the passive movement therapy. Corticosteroids help to reduce pain but there are no controlled studies proving that they might alter the course of the disease. The prognosis is generally good 36% recover completely within one year, at the end of the second year 75% and after three years 89% of patients show a restitutio ad integrum.

Suprascapular neuropathy

The suprascapular nerve is a motor nerve arising from the upper trunk from the brachial plexus (C4–C6) passing through the suprascapular notch on the upper border of the scapula to supply the supra- and infraspinatus muscles. The suprascapular nerve travels proximally underneath the transverse superior ligamente and distally under the inferior transverse ligamente. The nerve leaves the fossa supraspinatus laterally of the spina scapulae and enters the fossa infraspinatus. There are two entrapment syndromes known, one proximal lesion in the region of incisura scapulae and one inferior lesion at the level of the spinoglenoidal protuberantia.

Etiology: Blunt trauma with direct impact on the scapula, punch in martial arts or injury with the stick (hockey player), anterior luxation of the shoulder i.e. in American football, falls during biking. The nerve is most often injured by trauma with excessive forward movement of the shoulder.

Etiology of chronic overuse injury: entrapment syndrome proximal as well as distal lesion. Tennis player, javelin, artistic gymnastics, handball, volleyball, archery (Hashimoto et al. 1983), weight training (Goodman 1983), cable pull training, and dancing.

The distal lesion is most often found in volleyball players (Ferretti et al. 1998; Colonna et al. 1999) and baseball players (Cummins et al. 1999). An inflamed bursa can be found in the region of the entrapment resulting from chronic pressure.

Clinical symptoms: Acute injury, pain at rest with increase of pain at night time.

Chronic entrapment syndrome: pain in the posterior shoulder, deep, ill-defined location, increase of pain on shoulder movements, painless palsy of the infraspinatus muscle, weakness and atrophy of the supra- and infraspinatus muscles, which is easily missed. Proximal lesions lead to both a palsy of the supraspinatus and infraspinatus muscle. The supraspinatus muscle initiates arm abduction and the infraspinatus muscle external rotation.

Symptoms might be provoked by repeated sequence of movements including external rotation of the arm combined with arm abduction followed by internal rotation of the arm towards the contralateral side or by fast and excessive forward movement of the stretched arm (i.e. serving in tennis, goal-throw, javelin throw, shatterball in volleyball). Even in dancing a painless infraspinatus palsy has been reported when powerful abduction and external rotation of the arms were required.

Diagnosis: medical history, weak abduction and external rotation.

Tests: M. supraspinatus: abduction of the loose-hanging arm.

M. infraspinatus: external rotation of the arm with flexed elbow, optimal testing in prone position.

Cross-body-test: A positive test result indicates a lesion in the region of the incisura scapulae (scapular notch). The patient put the hand on the contralateral shoulder and lifts the elbow of the injured side to the horizontal level. The examiner pulls the elbow towards the healthy side provoking an intense pain.

Treatment: If symptoms occur for the first time: conservative for a limited period of time

When symptoms persist, especially in cases of suspected bursa surgery is indicated. The ligaments will be cut in patients with very severe nerve damage, nerve transplantation might be considered.

Prognosis: good.

Long thoracic nerve

The long thoracic nerve is a purely motor nerve arising from the ventral rami of the C5, C6, C7 spinal nerves. The nerve is at risk for pressure lesions because of its long course along the chest. The nerve runs beneath the clavicle and travels down the chest wall anterolaterally and innervates the serratus anterior muscle.

Etiology: Trauma or vigorous physical activity.

Carrying of heavy backsacks, climbing harness or weight vests.

Excessive shoulder movements, repetitive abduction above 90 degree of the arm with retraction of the shoulder: basketball, back stroke, golf, archery, tennis, skittles, baseball, tennis, squash, wrestling.

Symptoms: dull pain.

Winging of the scapula.

Diagnosis: Winging of the scapula is demonstrated by having the patient extend the arm forward and push the hands against a wall. The scapula elevates from the chest wall.

EMG studies: fibrillations in the anterior serratus muscle.

Treatment: Conservative, very good.

Surgery: neurolysis of the nerve when lesions persist.

Nerve transplantation: end-to-end coaptation of the long thoracic nerve to the dorsal scapular nerve.

If all treatment approaches mentioned so far fail muscle replacement operations will be performed i.e. fixation of the shoulder by using the latissimus dorsi muscle or transfer of the pectoral muscle or fixation with the contralateral scapula by using a fascia graft.

Axillary neuropathy

The axillary nerve arises from C5 and C6 fibers. The posterior cord of the brachial plexus divides into the radial and axillary nerves. The axillary nerve travels below the shoulder joint and innervates the teres minor muscle an external rotator of the arm. The axillary nerve courses behind and lateral to the humerus and divides into the branches innervating the deltoid muscle. A small cutaneous nerve supplies the skin above the shoulder. Etiology of lesions: Humerus dislocation or fractures, entrapment syndrome, quadrilateral space. The quadrilateral space is formed by the humerus, teres major, teres minor, long head of triceps. The axillary nerve and the posterior humeral circumflex artery pass posteriorly through the quadrangular space (Francel et al. 1991).

Symptoms: paraesthesia and pain of the shoulder and down the arm, aggravated by abduction, extension and external rotation, especially with overhead activity.

Sensitivity to pressure in the area of the quadrilateral space.

Sensory motor deficits have been reported rarely. Paladini et al.(1996) and Oberele et al. (1999) identified a quadrilateral space syndrome as reason for treatment resistant shoulder pain in basketball and volley ball players. Athletes with overhead activities such as weight lifter, javelin, baseball players, and softball players have also an increased risk for a quadrilateral space syndrome (pitcher).

Diagnosis: medical history, neurological examination, electrophysiological studies, angiography, transient blockage of the posterior humeral circumflex artery esp. with abducted and externally rotation of the arm.

Treatment: When non-operative treatment regimes fail surgical treatment is indicated, surgical decompression most often fibrous bands entrap the axillary nerve. Prognosis good, >90% full recovery (Timothy et al. 2008).

Musculocutaneous nerve

The musculocutaneous nerve arises from the C5, C6 and C7 fibres and leaves the lateral cord of the brachial plexus as sensory-motor nerve. The musculocutaneous nerve supplies the coracobrachialis, biceps and brachialis muscle. It continues in the forearm as purely sensory nerve.

Etiology of lesions:

Trauma: martial arts, American football, rugby, hockey. Punch or blow to the upper arm that might lead to secondary swelling of the soft tissue and compression of the nerve. Sudden onset of pain.

Retroflexion of the half abducted arm might lead to a tearing of the nerve (Judo, wrestling).

Acute onset of symptoms was also observed in throwers who complain of a sudden pain and sensory deficit of the forearm.

Overuse injuries: Repetitive flexion of the arm with heavy weight load (weight lifter), backstroke in tennis.

Clinical symptoms:

Acute traumatic lesion: Weakness of the coracobrachial, brachial and biceps muscle. Weakness of elbow flexion with the forearm supinated, weakness of supination with flexed elbow.

Chronic condition: no weakness of the coracobrachial muscle, but weakness of the biceps and brachialis muscle.

Additionally pain, paraesthesia and sensory deficits of the forearm.

Entrapment at the level of the biceps aponeurosis, sensory deficits and dysaesthesia of the lateral forearm. Tennis players have an increased risk to suffer from this type of entrapment syndrome.

Diagnosis: Electrophysiological studies, fibrillations in EMG studies, EDS differentiate the lesion of the musculocutaneous nerve from C5 radiculopathy. The SNAP is normal in C5 radiculopathy but abnormal in musculocutaneous neuropathy.

Sonography, clinical tests.

Treatment: Since non-operative treatment is only in 30% of patients with musculocutaneous nerve lesions due to trauma successful, surgical treatment is recommended. In contrast patients with overuse injury of the nerve should receive non-operative treatment. Immobilization in mildly flexed arm position and antiphlogistic drugs. If non-operative treatment is not successful surgical decompression or i.e. resection of a part of the biceps aponeurosis might be suitable.

Radial nerve

The radial nerve arises from the C5 to the Th1 nerve roots and supplies the extensor muscles of the arm. Compression of the radial nerve may occur at different levels, i.e. humerus, elbow, forearm and wrist. Fibrous bands, the radial artery and vena, the tendon of the extensor carpi muscle and the arcade of Frohse might compress the nerve. Alterations of the bone or a bursitis bicipitoradialis have to be excluded.

Proximal lesion:

Etiology: Compression of the nerve at the lateral triceps head, at risk are swimmers, golfers, weight lifters, tennis players, and powerful throwing of a ball. The nerve might be damaged by vigorous arm exercise involving contraction of the triceps muscle.

Symptoms: Pain along the extensor muscles and the forearm accompanied by paraesthesia and weakness of the extensor muscles.

Diagnosis: Neurological examination, electrophysiological studies, sonography.

Treatment: Surgical decompression.

Distal lesions: Supinator syndrome (Posterior interosseous nerve).

Compression of the ramus profundus (posterior interosseous nerve) a purely motor termination of the radial nerve in the forearm. The PIN supplies the supinator muscle and the wrist and finger extensors. The nerve might be entrapped at the Arcade of Frohse, the most superior part of the superficial layer of the supinator muscle, which is a fibrous arch over the posterior interosseous nerve. The arcade of Frohse is the most frequent site of posterior interosseous nerve entrapment, and is believed to play a role in causing progressive paralysis of the posterior interosseous nerve, both with and without injury.

Unusual vigorous repetitive movements, exercises against resistance, alternating pronating and supinating movements. Sport activities such as tennis playing, throwing or backstroke might lead to a muscular compression of the nerve. Fencing put high demands on the forearm muscles, especially beginners complain often about pain of the forearm, motor deficits are rare.

Backhand, thrown with high impact with the arm involving stretching of the arm from a flexed and internally rotated position.

Mechanical damage by lateral friction are cause of a radialis nerve lesion but important regarding the medical care of athletes.

Symptoms: pure motor deficits involving the supinator muscle, the extensor carpi ulnaris, finger extensors and thumb extensor, excluding brachioradial, triceps and carpi radialis muscle.

Intense elbow pain when the recurrent sensory nerve supplying the elbow joint mimicking a lateral epicondylitis.

Diagnosis: neurological examination, sonography, EMG examination shows fibrillation potentials in the aforementioned muscles, reduced amplitude of the radial CMAP and normal SNAP.

Treatment: Non-operative treatment: non steroidal antiphlogistic drugs, reduction of physical activity of the arm, cold packs, potential administration of corticoids

Purely sensory lesion

The superficial sensory branch of the radial nerve supplies sensation to the dorsolateral hand and the dorsal aspects of the first three digits. Compression might occur between the tendon of the brachioradial muscle and the extensor carpi radialis muscle. Compression at the wrist level by local trauma or compression.

Diagnosis: medical history, Nerve conduction studies (NCV) shows reduced or absent superficial radial sensory nerve action potential (SNAP).

Symptoms: burning pain, paraesthesia, numbness of the dorsolateral hand.

Ulnar nerve

The ulnar nerve arises from C8 and Th1 nerve roots. The fibres which form the ulnar nerve travel with the medial cord. The ulnar nerve follows first the axillary artery, courses to the extensor side and enters the ulnar sulcus at the level of the elbow. The compression of the nerve in the cubital tunnel is the most common cause of ulnar nerve entrapment. Luxation or fractures of the elbow are risk factors for a cubital tunnel syndrome. Further entrapment syndromes are found at the level of the wrist. After leaving the cubital tunnel the ulnar nerve follows its leading muscle to the wrist, where the nerve travels through the fibro-osseous tunnel connecting the pisiform and hamate wrist bones. As the nerve emerges from Guyon's canal, it divides into a deep terminal branch, which is purely motor and a superficial terminal branch. The deep terminal motor branch supplies all ulnar-innervated hand- muscles. The superficial branch supplies sensation to the medial distal half of the palm and the palmar surfaces of the 4th and 5th finger.

Cubital tunnel syndrome

Etiology: Lesions of the ulnar nerve caused by repeated flexions of the elbow in individuals with hypertrophy of the triceps muscle, fibrous bands between olecranon and epicondylus and hypertrophy of the extensor carpi muscle (passage of ulnar nerve).

Athletes who have to stretch the arm from a flexed position are prone to a cubital tunnel syndrome. Predisposed are baseball pitcher, thrower, handball keeper, and volleyball player. Due to an insufficient use of the sticks in cross country skiing, beginners complain often about pain and symptoms which can be referred to a cubital tunnel syndrome. Remote elbow trauma with and without fracture predisposes to later development of entrapment neuropathy in the elbow.

Symptoms: Sensory complaints including paraesthesias, decreased sensation and pain in the ulnar division of the hand. Pain may be also located in the forearm and elbow. Muscle weakness might involve the interossei, abductor dig. minimi, adductor pollicis and flexor pollicis brevi muscles. When weakness is chronic, atrophy might occur and a clawhand might develop.

Diagnosis: Nerve conduction studies, decreased ulnar CMAP and NAP, Conduction block of motor fibers localized to the elbow region.

Sonography, plain X-ray

Treatment: Non-operative treatment has been recommended a first line treatment including immobilization, splinting, casting, non-steroidal antiphlogistic medication, improvement and modification of stroke and throwing techniques, and use of the sticks. In the past surgeons were afraid to disturb the sequence of movements and worsens the performance of an athlete by transfer of the nerve to a ventral position. However, Andrews (1995) could show that 50% of the athletes returned to competition sports 12 weeks after neurolysis and ventralization of the ulnar nerve.

Independent of the type of treatment it is necessary to identify any predisposing pathology such as epicondylitis, alterated collateral bands, ganglions, lipomas, fibrous bands or an epitrochlear muscle.

Entrapment syndromes at the level of the wrist

Etiology: Pressure on the wrist or hyperextension of the wrist as seen in cycling. However, artistic gymnastics and climbers have their hands often in an extended hand position. Cross country skiers with powerful push off, complain often about pain.

Baseball pitcher show often lesions of the distal ulnar nerve due to repeated impact on the hand.

Symptoms: Entrapment of the ulnar nerve in the Loge Guyon involves often both the deep and the superficial branch leading to motor and sensory deficits.

Pure Motor deficits: Lesions of the deep branch of the ulnar nerve can occur prior and after the nerve supplying the hypothenar leaves.

Proximal lesion: clawhand, all muscles of the hypothenar and in addition the adductor pollicis muscle and the flexor dig. brevis, development of a typical clawhand without disturbance of sensation.

Distal lesion: hypothenar not involved, but clawposition of the long finger extensors and weakness of the thumb muscles.

Diagnosis: Medical history, EMG, radiogram or CT-scan of the wrist in order to check the wrist bones especially the hamate bone for fractures. It is the most commonly fractured bone when golfers hit the ground hard. Usually, it is a hairline fracture at the base of the hook like process, often missed on plain X-rays. Pain is aggravated by gripping. There is a tenderness over the hamate and sometimes numbness of the fifth finger as well partial involvement of the ring finger. Weakness of the fifth finger may occur.

Results of EMG studies depend on the terminal branches involved.

Treatment: Non-operative.

Hoyt reported a series of 117 cyclists who underwent a non-operative treatment schedule with use of splints, padding, modifications of the handlebar, special padded gloves, improvements of the biking technique with change of gripping and position. Improvement of the bikes also contributed to a reduction of injuries i.e. there is a huge collection of mountain bikes available with full suspension (Patterson et al., 2003)

The equipment has to be checked and individually tailored to the needs of the athlete. Sometimes immobilization and administration of corticoid medication is necessary.

Surgical decompression when non-operative treatment fails.

Median nerve

The median nerve arises from C5 to Th1 and contains fibers from all parts of the brachial plexus. It travels along the ventral part of the arm and supplies all hand- and finger flexors. There are several entrapment syndromes known: carpal tunnel syndrome, pronator teres syndrome and Kiloh-Nevin syndrome (Anterior interosseus syndrome).

Etiology: The pronator teres syndrome is a proximal entrapment syndrome. It is presumed that the median nerve is compressed where it passes between the two heads of the pronator teres muscle. Potential causes for the compression of the median nerve are a local trauma, a fibrous band running from the pronator teres to the flexor digitorum superficialis muscle and repetitive pronation of the forearm which leads to hypertrophy of the pronator teres muscle.

Sports activities which require a powerful closing of the hand and repetitive pronation bear the risk for athletes to develop a pronator teres syndrome.

Symptoms: pain and paraesthesia of the forearm. At an early stage of the disease pain after exercise, in advanced stages pain at rest. Rarely motor or sensory deficits.

Diagosis: medical history, neurological examination, EMG studies, sonography.

Treatment: Non-operative reduction of activity kryotherapy, non-steroidal antiphlogistic drugs.

Surgical treatment: neurolysis.

Anterior interosseus syndrome (Kiloh Nevin Syndrome)

Etiology: Frequently direct injury of the nerve by fractures of the forearm or secondary soft tissue swelling, less often compression of the nerve by overstraining of the forearm muscles

i.e. playing skittles or training with an expander for the hand.

Symptoms: patients are not able to flex the distal finger joint of the thumb, indexfinger and middle finger.

Diagnosis: sonography, EMG.

Treatment: Recovery most often without specific treatment.

Surgical treatment required in patients after trauma or without recovery. Surgical exploration often reveals a fibrous band crossing the nerve, less often an interossea artery.

Carpal tunnel syndrome (CTS)

Distal entrapment syndrome

Injury caused by fractures with tearing, partial or complete transection of the nerve

Compression of the nerve provoked by repetitive hand stretching- and flexing

Tennisplayers or squashplayers with poor technique, badminton, cycling, and forceful gripping (baseball pitcher, expander, racket). 30% of wheelchair users suffer from CTS, up to 70% show a pathological distal motor latency.

Symptoms: intense nocturnal pain, burning, paraesthesia along the radial fingers, in advanced stage pain during the day.

Motor deficits regarding abduction and opposition of the thumb followed by muscle atrophy

Diagnosis: medical history (characteristic), neurological examination, EMG/NCS.

Treatment: Immobilization, non-steroidal antiphlogistic drugs. Local corticoid injections, modification of hand position during biking, biking uphill with less weight load on the hands.

Surgical treatment: motor deficits and failure of non-operative treatment schedules.

Further lesions of the median nerve

Neuroma of the ulnary digiti proprius nerve of the thumb caused by compression of the nerve at the thumb in bowlers (bowler's thumb) or baseball pitchers. Touch results in painful paraesthesia reminding to an electrical stimulus. Neuroma is easily to find by palpation and confirmed by test with local anesthesia. Treatment: Padding of the thumb, surgical treatment. However, competitive sports activities have to be given up most often.

Compression of the palmaris proprius nerve in tennis players and squash players results in pain at the radial part of the index finger. Compression of the digital nerves requires a modification of the finger position and padding of the racket.

Lesions of the truncal nerves

Intense training of the rectus abdominis muscle might lead to a compression of the intercostal nerves. Athletes complain of pain along the rectus abdominis muscle, which is provoked or aggravated by contraction of the muscle. An injury of the aponeurosis has to be considered as differential diagnosis.

Sciatic nerve

The sciatic nerve arises from the nerve roots L4 to S3.

Etiology of sciatic lesions: direct trauma, fractures of the hip, femur with and without dislocation of bone fragments (i.e. bike accidents). Typical traumatic injuries of the sciatic nerve are transections of the nerve or strain on the nerve with bleedings within the nerve.

Symptoms: proximal lesions of the nerve lead to paresthesia of the feet, most often lateral. The peroneal part of the sciatic nerve is more vulnerable than the tibial part. Violent cramps of the dorsal thigh may occur.

Treatment: Non-operative treatment is indicated in case of a neurotmesis, if the structure of the nerve is damaged and the neurolemmal sheath is interrupted, operative treatment is required.

Compression of the sciatic nerve caused by prolonged sitting during biking, rowing or kayaking might cause damage. Chronic damage of the sciatic nerve results from repeated compression of the nerve i.e. during meditation sitting in the lotus-posture or practicing weight lifting. Long distance riding does infrequently provoke damage of the sciatic nerve. The area of the piriformis muscle is predisposed for such lesions. The nerve is also at risk of compression between the trochanter minor and the femur. Slim subjects are more prone for entrapment syndromes.

Symptoms: Pain in the area of the sciatic foramen, increasing with flexion and internal rotation of the thigh. Paresthesia of the feet accompanied by intense pain in the gluteal region are characteristic. The peroneal division is more vulnerable than the tibial division of the nerve. If sensory symptoms are ignored motor deficits especially a foot drop might develop. Additional risk factors are wet and cold conditions. Differential diagnosis is an irritation of the ischiogluteal bursa or the sciatic bursa. Subjects suffering from an inflamed ischiogluteal bursa complain of local pain inside of the thigh radiating to the dorsal side of the thigh. The pain caused by an inflamed sciatic bursa can be mistaken for sciatica.

Treatment: Non-operative treatment with modification of the seating position. Padding of the saddle, strengthening of the muscles.

Ruptures of the hamstring muscles especially of the semitendinosus muscle might compress the sciatic nerve and lead to sciatic paresis. Operative approach is indicated with suturing of the muscle tear and evacuation of the hematoma.

Lesions of posterior cutaneous femoral nerve

The nerve arises from S1 to S3 and travels together with the lumbosacral plexus, leaving sometimes together with the inferior gluteal nerve. It provides sensation to the bottom, the perineum and the skin inside of the thigh.

Long distance biking may provoke paresthesia on the back of the thigh.

Pudendal nerve

The pudendal nerve arises from the nerve roots of S2 to S4. It passes through the sciatic notch and descends towards the perineum and divides into the inferior anal nerves (sphincter ani) and the perineal nerves which provide sensation to the perineum and in men to the penis. The deep location of the nerve protects it from injury, but severe trauma (falls with a motor bike, bicycle) i.e. pelvic fractures might lead to stretch injuries, compression and sometimes even to transection of the nerve. Prolonged compression by long biking on a hard and small saddle increases the pressure of the pelvic floor and indirectly in the alcock canal leading to immobility of the nerve and causing dysfunction.

A forward inclined saddle might press the dorsal penis/clitoridis nervi to the symphysis causing numbness of in the innervated region. Due to the position of the saddle mountain bikers have a higher risk for the injury than road racer. There are two underlying pathophysiological mechanisms, either the perineal nerves are directly damaged or the pudendal artery or pudendal vene (Goodson 1981) are occluded. While deficits and pain related to vascular compression recover quickly after decompression, those related to primary demyelination might take weeks or months to recover (Vogt et al. 2005). A similar dysfunction was reported in females and is due to a damage of the clitoridis nerve. Bikers who ignore the numbness of the perineum or the genital area risk persistent loss of sensation in this area (Leibovitch and Mor 2005). Although there is a correlation between the severity of the damage and the bodyweight the duration of the compression is of paramount importance. However, some bikers already experience numbness in this area after 60 min biking (Schwarzer et al. 1999). Up to 61% of bikers completing more than 400 km/week report numbness of the penile shaft or the scrotum during and after biking, 21% complain of an erectile dysfunction. Andersen and Bovim (1997) found these problems in 22% of bikers participating in a long distance race. 13% of the participants suffered from erectile dysfunction up to 1 month after the race. Braun et al (2000) reported a close correlation between numbness of the perineal and genital area, erectile dysfunction and quantity of the training. Athletes spending more than 20000 km on a bike were three times more likely to become impotent than gender and age matched non-biking subjects. Diabetic subjects have a higher risk that symptoms become permanent. Perineal numbness is also known in female bikers and according to Lasalle (1999) 34% of female bikers suffers from such symptoms.

The most important treatment is to stop the compression of the neurovascular structures.

Prevention of pudendal nerve compression: Horizontal saddle position or decline by 1 to 3 degree. The legs should not be completely stretched, when the pedal is at the deepest point in order to support the bodyweight,

Frequent change of position, broader and padded saddle (Vogt et al. 2005, Sommer et al. 2001). Cutting out parts of the saddle has not proved to be useful (Dettori et al. 2004).

Obturator nerve

The obturator nerve arises from the L2 to L 4 nerve roots. The nerve passes behind the psoas muscle, descends into the pelvic and exits through the obturator foramen. The anterior ramus travels between the adductor brevis and the adductor longus muscle distally, the posterior ramus runs underneath the adductor longus to the adductor magnus muscle. The obturator nerve innervates all adductor muscles and supplies sensation to the upper medial thigh.

Etiology of lesions: The nerve can be compressed by fat tissue bulging into the obturator canal, this applies to weight lifters.

Further possible reasons for compressions of the obturator nerve are obturator hernia or a hernia of the adductor muscle.

Injuries of the adductor muscles can cause pain in the innervation area of the obturator nerve. Sports involving stretching and powerful abduction-adduction movements, such as speed skating or cross country skiing. Entrapment of the nerve in a gap of adductor brevis muscle fascia in rugby players has been described.

Symptoms: Damage of the obturator nerve results in a weakness of the adductor muscles and sensory loss of the upper medial thigh. Ambulation is difficult and gait is disturbed by preponderance of the abductor muscles. Pain of the groin and the medal thigh is characteristic.

Diagnosis: Medical history, careful clinical examination excluding motor and sensory involvement other than what can be attributed to the obturator nerve, loss of the adductor jerk, MRI, sonography.

Therapy: according to the underlying mechanism, in case of mechanic compression: neurolysis

Prevention: Gymnastics, Stretching and strengthening training of the abdominal muscles.

Femoral nerve

The femoral nerve arises from L1 to L4 and innervates the iliopsoas muscle and the knee extensors. The nerve supplies sensation to the medial lower leg.

Etiology of lesions: Sudden extension and flexion of the hip joint, i.e. artistic gymnastics, parachuting, judo, karate, dancing and somersaults. Especially dancing requires at times maximal stretching of the hip with flexion of the knee which might damage the nerve by abrupt stretching within the inguinal canal. Sometimes intraneural bleedings occur. An abrupt stretching of the femoral nerve might also occur in cross country skiing when the athletes slips while skiing uphill.

Ischemic lesion of the femoral nerve in elder athletes, male with severe osteochondrosis of the spine are more prone to that damage. Biking has been proven to be disadvantageous.

Biking has to be stopped and the position changed as soon as numbness or weakness or both are noticed.

Rare conditions: Compression of the femoral nerve by strong quadriceps muscle

Biking uphill against great resistance, especially elderly athletes are affected which makes an additional vascular factor more likely. The presence of diabetes mellitus increases the sensitivity of the femoral nerve.

Isometric contraction of the quadriceps muscle, especially the lateral vastus muscle is affected. Iliopsoas muscle and hip flexion are intact.

Coagulopathies: hematomas in the area of the iliopsoas muscle (Medical history, drugs such as ASA, warfarin).

Symptoms: Weakness of knee extensors.

Mild weakness of hip flexion.

Disturbed sensation of the ventral thigh and the medial lower leg.

Decreased or lost patellar jerk.

If the clinical examination suggests an involvement of the iliopsoas muscle a plexuspathy has to be considered, weakness of the adductor muscles requires an additional damage to the obturator nerve.

Treatment:

Operative treatment: Space occupying lesions, hematomas, lack of recovery, or suggested intraneural bleedings

Non-operative treatment: restriction of sports activities, immobilization, physiotherapy

Prognosis: good- if the damage is due to repeated controlled stretching.

Poor- if the damage was caused by abrupt stretching without muscular control, due to frequent intraneural bleedings and tearing of fascicles.

Saphenous neuropathy

The femoral nerve divides after emerging under the inguinal band into motor and sensory branches. The major sensory division descends within Hunter's canal and leaves the canal at the level of the knee. It supplies sensation to the medial lower leg.

Compression in the Hunter's canal results in sensory loss or paresthesia of the lower leg. Young male subjects surfing for hours are at risk.

Patellar neuropathy

Damage of the infrapatellar branch of the saphenous nerve at the level of the femoral condylus:

Etiology of lesion: knee surgery, risk of damaging this branch is especially high during operations involving the medial part of the knee (capsule and ligaments).

Symptoms: Sensory loss of the medial part of the knee and below

Pain triggered by touch of the scar, patellar neuropathy is in 60% of patients temporary, in 40% persistent. Increase of pain by exercise which prevents reuptake of sports activities in some athletes.

Treatment:

Non-operative: local injection with cortison, medical treatment with antiphlogistic medication or pregabaline.

Operative treatment: Transectomy of the branch, cave. Neuroma of the scar.

Lateral femoral cutaneous neuropathy

Pure sensory nerve arising from the dorsal divisions of the ventral primary rami of the L2–L3 spinal nerves.

The nerve passes under the inguinal ligament and pierces the fascia lata, divides into anterior and posterior branches and supplies sensation to the anterolateral thigh. Anatomic variations regarding the course are frequent.

Etiology of lesions: Entrapment near the inguinal ligament, additional risk factors: Adipositas, wearing of tight corsets or belts. Weightlifters and divers are at risk of developing lateral femoral cutaneous neuropathy.

Exercising on the uneven bars especially tired athletes or athletes with poor technical skills.

Symptoms: Meralgia paresthetica, pain, burning sensation with variable loss of sensation in the anterolateral thigh, exacerbation by flexion of the hip, getting out of a chair and walking.

Sometimes hypersensitivity.

Diagnosis: clinical examination, typical area of decreased sensation, tenderness in the area of the inguinal ligament, which might serve as a trigger point and might precipitate symptoms, patients often rub the area for relief.

Injection of the trigger point with local anesthetics, which reliefs pain immediately.

Therapy: sometimes spontaneous recovery by avoiding tight belts and trousers or by losing weight.

Non-operative treatment: injection of local anaesthetics (see diagnosis), administration of pregabalin, Gabapentine, improvement of technical skills (artistic gymnasts performing on uneven bars).

Operative treatment: Resection of a neuroma, or neurolysis of the nerve in case of suggested entrapment syndrome.

Peronaeal nerve

The common peronaeal nerve, arising from L4 to S2, follows the biceps femoris muscle and branches from the sciatic nerve at the level of the knee and moves toward the lower lateral portion of the popliteal fossa, where two cutaneous sensory nerves emerge. The peronaeal nerve travels in juxtaposition to the fibula and passes through a tendinous arch formed by the peronaeus longus muscle and divides then into the deep and the superficial peroneal nerve. The deep peroneal nerve innervates all extensors of the foot and digits and supplies sensation to the skin of the first and second toe. The superficial peroneal nerve innervates the peronaeus longus and brevis and provides sensation to the lateral and dorsal surface of the foot.

Etiology of entrapment symptoms: Compression at the level of the head of the fibula or hypermobility, compression of the nerve on its course between the peronaeus longus muscle and the fibula, compression by adjacent structures of the knee or a baker cyst, compression of the peronaeal nerve by the fascia at the level of the fibula, especially well known in runners. Rapid increase of training load and too strong pronation of the foot (esp beginners), long surfing with compression of one leg and abduction of the other leg.

Ankle sprain, mild trauma results often in deficits of the superficial peronaeal nerve, severe trauma is more likely to affect the deep peroneal nerve.

Tight shoes, especially skiing boots, hiking boots, skaters.

Compression of the terminal sensory branch of the superficial sensory nerve passing beneath the lower retinaculum with consecutive numbness of the skin in the first interdigtal space.

Compression of the nerve by fixing a key to the shoe (runners)

Damage of the distal branches of the deep peroneal branch by playing soccer.

Symptoms:

Common peroneal nerve

Pain accompanied by cramps

Loss of sensation in the first interosseum space and at the lateral division of the foot

Foot drop with supination due to motor deficits.

Superficial peroneal nerve

Pain and cramps along the lower leg towards the foot

Loss of sensation dorsal foot, increasing with exercise

Sometimes swelling

Weakness or loss of pronation

Deep peroneal nerve

Foot drop

Since the division of the sciatic nerve into a tibial and femoral part is often proximal to the knee and prior to the division into two separate branches the peronaeal part of the sciatic nerve might be injured at the level of the thigh and mimic a distal peroneal lesion.

Compression of the dorsal cutaneous intermedius nerve results in pain along the mediolateral foot. Tight or hard skiing boots, climbing boots or skaters.

Another possible compression syndrome occurs around the hallux. The combination of osteophytes and too tight and hard shoes lead to loss of sensation of the medial hallux and pain around the toe. Therapy: padded shoes, improvement of running skills, insoles for better distribution of pressure.

Anterior tarsal tunnel syndrome

Compression of the sensory-motor branch of the deep peroneal nerve beneath the cruciate ligament.

Symptoms: Pain, loss of sensation in the first interosseum space and mild weakness of the extensor digitores brevis muscle . Although most often no convincing reason for the clinical symptoms can be identified, athletes with tight and hard shoes suffer more often from these symptoms. Female dancers with high heels and runners with very high training load belong to risk groups as well (Schon and Baxter 1990)

Therapy: suitable shoes and padding of the shoes.

Diagnosis: clinical examination, EMG studies.

Sural nerve

The sural nerve arises from the medial cutaneous nerve (sometimes peroneal nerve) and sometimes from the lateral cutaneous sural nerve. A ganglion or compression caused by the rim of the skiing or climbing boots or lacing of dancing shoes. Symptoms: Pain and paresthesias of the lateral foot. Frequent change of shoes and special padding.

An entrapment of the sural nerve has been observed at the aponeurosis of the lower leg and cause pain radiating along the achillic pain.

Tibial nerve

The tibial nerve arises from the L4 to S3 nerve roots. At times the division of the sciatic nerve happens at the level of the infrapiriform foramen. The tibial nerve innervates all flexors of the foot and all intrinsic muscles of the toes apart from the extensor muscles of the toes. The terminal branches are the rami calcanei, the medial and lateral plantar nerve .Sensory loss of the sole of the foot.

Tarsal tunnel syndrome

Compression of the nerve behind the internal malleolus. An upper (compression of the tibial nerve) and a lower tarsal tunnel syndrome (compression of the medial or lateral plantar nerve) have been described.

Etiology: Trauma of the ankle, inflammation of the tendons and synovialitis i.e. rheumatic arthritis.

Repeated dorsal flexion and -extension combined with pronation might provoke pain and paresthesia. valgus deformity of the foot and a insufficient arche contribute to the symptoms. The differential diagnosis which has to be ruled out is a fasciitis plantaris.

Compression of the medial plantar nerve (Jogger's foot). Symptoms: pain, paraesthesia, claw toes, often no objective deficits.

Diagnosis: examination, sonography, MRI, electrophysiological assessment, CT scan for assessment of the bones.

Treatment: Non-operative. antiphlogistic medication, cortison, loose-fitting shoes.

Lesions of the lateral plantar nerve: pain and paraesthesia in the area of the medial calcaneus bone, lesions of the medial plantar nerve: navicular bone, medial arche, lesions of the anterior calcaneal branch paraethesia and pain of the hallux, lesions of the lower calcaneal branch causes pain of the heel.

Morton metatarsalgia

Isolated damage of the interdigital sensory terminal branches with development of a neuroma. Women are predominantly affected and patients with flat foot.

Symptoms: Burning plantar pain, maximal at the level of 3rd or 4th toe. In early stage pain occurs during exercise, in advanced stages at rest. The condition does not seem to be more common in athletes but they seek earlier and more frequent for help. Diagnosis: clinical examination: extreme pain can be provoked by rubbing of the metatarsal heads. Injection with local anesthesia abolishes the pain immediately.

Treatment:

Non-operative: insoles with retrocapital support, local application of anesthetic drugs and cortisone and administration of medication for neuralgia (pregabalin, gabapentin).

In 80% of patients conservative treatment is successful. If non-operative treatment fails operative excision of the neuroma is indicated (Greensfield et al 1984).

Secondary damage of the peroneal and tibial nerve occurs in compartment syndrome. Pressure and ischemia are the reasons for sensory-motor deficits. Trigger for compartments syndromes are high trainings load or sudden increase of training to which the athletes was not adapted. Modification of training conditions such as running uphill or downhill might provoke the symptoms.

Tab. 12.6 Compartment syndromes.

Compartment-Syndromes	Affected nerves	Functional Deficits
Tibialis anterior syndrome Anterior compartment syndrome	Deep peroneal nerve	Foot and toe extensors, numbness of the first interosseum space
Lateral compartment syndrome	Superficial peroneal nerve	Pronation, peronei muscles
Deep posterior compartment syndrome	Tibial nerve	Claw toes and talipes cavus
Anterior compartment syndrome of the thigh	Saphenous nerve	Paraesthesia and loss of sensation of the lower leg
Posterior compartment thigh	Sciatic nerve	Rarely motor deficits

Non-operative treatment: Early stages: Reduction of training load or immobilization, modification of training

Advanced stages: operative treatment to protect neurovascular structures and muscles

Exercise-induced muscle damage

Rhabdomyolysis occurs after intense strenuous exercise. Milder muscle damage after exercise results from overtraining (Toumi et al. 2003). The exercise-induced myopathy is less known. The histological findings resemble those of the cortison-induced myopathy. The oxidative-glycolytic muscle fibres are mainly affected. The athletes complain of fatigue, pain and feeling of heaviness provoked by mild exercise involving the proximal muscles. Symptoms occur as a part of the overtraining complex but may also occur in subjects with a history of muscle diseases (Chaussain et al. 1992).

In subjects with exercise-induced muscle pain inflammation (myositis, polymyositis) and metabolic disorders have to be ruled out (mitochondrial myopathy, McArdle-syndrome)

Athletes with exercise-induced myopathy have to reduce their training load. Quantity of the training has to be reduced as well as the quality of training requires modification. Thus, the components of the training need to be altered. Strength-training, training of explosive power and training at high running speed have to be avoided.

Athletes might support recovery by eating more protein, sleeping sufficiently and reducing stress levels.

Injuries of the peripheral nervous system result from stretching, compression, tearing or ischemia. Repetitive movements often lead to overuse injuries. Nerves in exposed location or nerves piercing through muscles are at high risk for overuse injuries. Diagnosis includes medical history, neurological examination, electrophysiological testing and imaging studies. Treatment and prevention of peripheral nerve injuries include improvement of technical skills and optimization of the equipment. Athletes with damage to the peripheral nervous system do rarely return to high competition sports.

Dystonia in athletes

In the past there has been a lot of discussion whether dystonia in athletes is of psychogenic origin or somatic. Recent studies have supported the hypothesis of an somatic origin of exercise-related dystonia, although, psychological aspects play an important role and may worsen the condition. Dystonia is a movement disorder which is characterised by involuntary turning and twisting movements with abnormal posture. Exercise-related dystonia can be classified as task specific dystonia. The abnormal movements occur only during sports and are most often constrained to a specific movement, i.e. sprinters experience a stiff leg when they push off the starting block. The pathophysiological mechanism behind seems to be an abnormal activation of the neurons of the basal ganglia. The primary motor cortex shows insufficient activation while the secondary motor cortex shows too much activation. The dystonic movements may spread to other muscles not involved in the early stages of the disease. The

Tab. 12.7 Sports specific injuries.

sports	lesion of the peripheral nerve
dancing	suprascapular nerve femoral nerve superficial peroneal nerve sural nerve Morton neuroma
baseball	suprascapular nerve radial nerve musculocutaneous nerve median nerve (pronator-teres-Syndrom) ulnar nerve plexopathy
pitcher	Proper palmar digital nerve (neuroma)
arching	digital nerves median nerve long thoracic nerve
american football	stinger C5/C6 radiculopathy brachial plexus Thoracic outlet-Syndrome median nerve ulnar nerve radial nerve sciatic nerve peroneal nerve (dislocation of the knee)
frisbee	radial nerve
soccer	obturator nerve peroneal nerve tibial nerve
weightlifting	Stinger (C5/C6 radiculopathy) brachial plexus ulnar nerve radial nerve median nerve Carpaltunnel Syndrome musculocutaneous nerve thoracodorsal nerve long thoracic nerve femoral nerve entrapment of intercostal nerves (rectus abdominal muscle)
golf	median nerve digital nerves ulnar nerve
handball	ulnar nerve (elbow)

Tab. 12.7 (Continued).

sports	lesion of the peripheral nerve
hockey	Stinger (C5/C6 radiculopathy) brachial plexus axillary nerve peroneal nerve tibial nerve tarsaltunnel-syndrome
inline skating	superficial peroneal nerve
martial arts (judo, Karate, kick-boxing, taekwondo)	direct punch or kick ulnar nerve median nerve accessorial nerve long thoracic nerve peroneal nerve Morton neuroma
skittles, bowling	ulnar proprius digital nerve (thumb)
climbing	brachial plexus (backsack) axillary nerve long thoracic nerve suprascapular nerve obturator nerve tarsaltunnel Syndrome
running	peroneal nerve tibial nerve tarsaltunnel-Syndrome terminal branches of the tibial and peroneal nerves (foot) Morton neuroma lateral cutaneous femoral nerve Saphenous neuropathy Compartment Syndrome rhabdomyolysis
biking	Loge Guyon (ulnar nerve) Carpaltunnel-syndrome (median nerve) Cubital tunnel syndrome (ulnar nerve) Pudendus nerve Posterior cutaneous femoral nerve
Rhythmic artistic gymnastics	Supinator syndrome (radial nerve) Femoral nerve Lateral cutaneous femoral nerve
wrestling	Stinger (C5/C6 radiculopathy) Brachial plexus Axillary nerve Long thoracic nerve Suprascapular nerve Ulnar nerve, Carpaltunnel-syndrome

Tab. 12.7 (Continued).

sports	lesion of the peripheral nerve
Rugby	Axillary nerve Obturator nerve
shooting	Long thoracic nerve
swimming	Long thoracic nerve
Cross country skiing, nordic skiing	Femoral nerve Obturator nerve Ulnar nerve
skiing	Radicular symptoms thoracic and lumbar spine
snowboarding	Radiculopathies cervical spine Brachial plexus
surfing	Saphenous neuropathy Peroneal nerve
diving	Lateral cutaneous femoral nerve
tennis	Radial nerve (supinator syndrome) Suprascapular nerve Thoracic outlet syndrome Lateral cutaneous antebrachii nerve Digital nerves
volleyball	Suprascapular nerve Axillary nerve
Yoga	Sciatic nerve

exercise-related dystonia may also lose the specificity and occur during other movements or even at rest. Exercise-related dystonia is triggered rather by repetitive movements than by exhausting and straining exercise. Hence, golf players, tennis players, cricket players, and baseball pitcher. However, exercise-related dystonia has also been observed in runners and sprinters. The athletes suffering from dystonia complain of disturbance of the movement sequences, but also about pain. The complaints are often misconstrued and a muscle injury is considered.

In contrast to other types of exercise-related dystonia the involuntary movements in golfers are well known and are called "Yips". The involuntary movements occur during putting. During the crucial hit of the ball sudden jerks, a tremor or freezing of the movement may occur preventing the athlete from putting the ball. EMG studies have shown a muscular hyperactivity with a co-contraction of agonists and antagonists. The abnormal movements are more likely to appear during putting downhill, breaks from the left side or in a competitive situation (Smith et al. 2003). Golf players suffering from exercise related dystonia have a firmer grip and a higher heart rate while playing. Their performance regarding putting is worse. Anxiety has a negative effect on the dystonia and the performances of the golfers. The problem is of general interest since 32 to 47% of serious golfers suffer fro some type of dystonia. Athletes with high training load and many years of practice are prone to develop exercise-related dystonia (Sachdev 1992; Bawden and Maynard 2001). Since there is still no satisfying therapy many players retire from competition sports. Therefore, it seems to be important to avoid the development of dystonia by a diversified training.

Cricket player show an abrupt dorsal extension of the hand, followed by a flexion disturbing the accuracy of the movement.

Tennis player experience an inhibition of the movement with a co-contraction of the forearm muscles. The dystonia occurs most often during serving and playing backhand. Players complain of pain in the forearm. Sometimes it is difficult to distinguish between a supinator syndrome (posterior interosseus neuropathy) and an exercise-related dystonia.

Long distance runners experience dystonic movements while running with high speed. The lower leg rotates internally and the foot is supinated. The running rhythm is definitely disturbed and prevents the runner from keeping up the speed. Sometimes the athletes cannot continue with running and have to break off the training or to give up the competition. Predisposed are runners with very high training load and many years of practice. Similar to golfers a diversified training might help to prevent the development of dystonic movements. Although dystonia in runners is not a rare phenomenon the problem is often mistaken for a muscle cramp.

Treatment of exercise-related dystonia is difficult. All approaches to tackle the symptoms of dystonia may interfere with the performance of the athletes. The treatment regime is multimodal. Drugs such as benztropine or trihexyphenidyl can be used. A focal selective chemical denervation with botulinumtoxin A might be considered. However, it is very difficult to choose the right dosage since the dystonic movements are not always present, but when they break through they might be violent. Therefore, a dosage of botulinum toxin that stops the movements would probably weaken the muscle too much and interfere with the performance of the athlete. Since a monotonous training with high training load seems to be a risk factor for the development of a dystonia a modification of the training is necessary. The training has to be more diversified, physiotherapists and sports therapists try to change movement patterns. In addition psychological aspects might play a role. Athletes often develop anxiety and expect failure. Therefore, psychologists will work with the athletes to support their self esteem and reduce anxiety.

References

Adirim TA (2007) Concussions in Sports and Recreation. Clin Ped Emerg Med. 8: 2–6

Andersen KV, Bovim G (1997) Impotence and nerve entrapment in long distance amateur cyclists. Acta Neurol Scand. 95 (4): 233–240.

Arnold MP (2005) Mountainbiken. Orthopäde 34: 405–410.

Arnold M, Baumgartner RW, Stapf C, Nedeltchev K, Buffon F, Benninger D, Georgiadis D, Sturzenegger M, Mattle HP, Bousser MG (2008) Ultrasound diagnosis of spontaneous carotid dissection with isolated Horner syndrome. Stroke 39(1): 82–86.

Bailes JE, Cantu RC (2001) Head injuries in athletes. Neurosurgery. 48: 26–45.

Bailes JE (2005) Experience with cervical stenosis and temporary paralysis in athletes. J Neurosurg Spine. 2: 11–16.

Baroff GS (1998) Is heading a soccer ball injurious to brain function? J Head. 13: 45–52.

Bassetti C, Carruzzo A, Sturzenegger M, Tuncdogan E (1996) Recurrence of cervical artery dissection. A prospective study of 81 patients. Stroke 27(10): 1804–1807.

Bawden M, Maynard I (2001) Towards an understanding of the personal experience of the "yips" in cricketers. J Sports Sci. 19: 937–953.

Beghi E, Kurland LT, Mulder DW (1985) Brachial plexus neuropathy in the population of Rochester, Minnesota, 1970–1981. Ann Neurol. 18: 320–323.

Biasca N, Maxwell WL (2007) Minor traumatic brain injury in sports: a review in order to prevent neurological sequelae. In: Weber & Maas (eds.) Prog Brain Res. 161: 263–291.

Biberthaler P, Mussack T, Wiedemann E et al. (2001) Evaluation of S-100ß as a specific marker for neuronal damage due to minor brain trauma. World J Surg. 25: 93–97.

Boden BP, Tacchetti RL, Cantu RC, Knowles SB, Mueller FO (2007) Catastrophic head injuries in high school and college football players. Am J Sports Med. 35: 1075–1081.

Bohnsack M, Schröter E (2005) Verletzungsmuster und sportartbedingte Belastungen beim Gleitschirmfliegen. Orthopäde. 34: 411–418.

Bookvar JA, Durham SR, Sun PP (2001) Cervical spinal stenosis and sports-related cervical cord neurapraxia in children. Spine. 26: 2709–2712.

Braun M, Wassmer G, Klotz T, Reifenrath B, Mathers M, Engelmann U (2000) Epidemiology of erectile dysfunction: results of the "Cologne Male Survey". Int J Impot Res. 12: 1–7.

Cantu RC, Mueller FO (2000) Catastrophic football injuries: 1977–1998. Neurosurgery. 47: 673–677.

Chaussain M, Camus F, Defoligny C et al. (1992) Exercise intolerance in patients with McArdle's disease or mitochondrial myopathies. Eur J Med. 1(8): 457–463.

Colonna S, Montagna P, Orlandi V et al. (1999) Suprascapular nerve neuropathy in volleyball players. An epidemiological study in a young group of volleyball players and the results of a case treated with neuroylysis. Med. Sport. 52/1: 35–40.

Cooper MT, McGee KM, Anderson DG (2003) Epidemiology of athletic head and neck injuries. Clin Sports Med. 22: 427–443.

Cummins CA, Bowen A, Andersen K et al. (1999) Suprascapular nerve entrapment at the spinglenoid notch in a professional baseball pitcher. Am J Sports Med. 27/6: 810–812.

Dettori JR, Koepsell TD, Cummings P, Corman JM (2004) Erectile dysfunction after a long-distance cycling event: association with bicycle characteristics. J Urol. 172: 637–641.

Ekman R, Welander G, Svanstrom L, Schelp L, Santesson P (2001) Bicycle-related injuries among the elderly a new epidemic? Public Health. 115: 38–43.

Ferretti A, De Carli A, Fontana M (1998) Injury of the su-prascapular nerve at the spinoglenoid notch: The natural history of infraspinatus atrophy in volleyball players. Am J Sports Med. 26/6: 759–763.

Francel TJ, Dellon AL, Campbell JN (1991) Quadrilateral Space Syndrome: Diagnosis and Operative Decompression Technique. Plast Reconstr Surg 87: 911–916.

Frommelt P (1995) Neurologische Erkrankungen. In: Sozialmedizinische Begutachtung in der gesetzlichen Rentenversicherung. Verband Deutscher Rentenversicherungsträger, Fischer, Stuttgart. 409–415.

Gangu A (2002) Isthmic spondyloslisthesis. Neurosurg Focus. 13 (1) E1.

Goodman GE (1983) Unusual nerve injuries in recreational sports. Am J Sports Med. 2: 224–227.

Goodson JD (1981) Pudendal neuritis from biking. N Engl J Med. 304: 365.

Greenfield J, Rea J, Ilfeld F (1984) Morton's interdigital neuroma. Indications for treatment by local injection versus surgery. Clin Orthop. 185: 142–144.

Hashimoto K, Oda K, Kuroda Y, Shibasaki H (1983) Case of suprascapular nerve palsy manifested as selected atrophy of the infraspinatus muscle. Clin Neurol. 23: 970–973.

Hörterer H (2005) Carving-Skifahren. Orthopäde 34: 426–432.

Hoyt CS (1976) Ulnar neuropathy in bicycle riders. Arch Neurol. 33: 372.

Jerosch J, Heck VC (2005) Verletzungsmuster und -prophylaxe beim Inline-Skating. Orthopäde 34: 441–447.

Jordan BD (2000) Chronic traumatic brain injury associated with boxing. Semin Neurol. 20: 179–185.

Kelly JP, Rosenberg JH (1997) The diagnosis and management of concussion in sports. Neurology 48: 575–579.

Kelly JP (2000) Concussions in sports and recreation. Semin Neurol. 20: 165–171.

Kuhlman GS, McKeag DB (1999) The "burner": A common nerve injury in contact sports. Am Fam Phys. 60/7: 2035–2042.

Kronisch RL, Pfeiffer RP (2002) Mountain bike injuries: an update. Sports Med. 32(8): 523–537.

Kronisch RL, Pfeiffer RP, Chow TK (1996) Acute injuries in cross-country and downhill off-road bicycle racing. Med Sci Sports Exerc. 28(11): 1351–1355.

Lang C, Stefan H (1999) Sportverletzungen des Nervensystems. Fortschr Neurol Psychiat. 67: 373–386.

LaSalle M, Salimpour P, Adelstein M, Mourtzinos A, Wen C, Renzulli J et al. (1999) Sexual and urinary tract dysfunction in female bicyclists. J Urol 161: 269.

Leibovitch I, Mor Y (2005) The vicious cycling: Bicycling related urogenital disorders. Euro Urol. 47: 277–287.

Levy AS, Smith RH (2000) Neurologic injuries in skiers and snowboarders. Sem Neurol. 20: 233–245.

Lovell MR, Iverson GL, Collins MW, Podell K, Johnston KM, Pardini D et al. (2006) Measurement of symptoms following sports-related concussion: Reliability and normative data for the post-concussion scale. Applied Neuropsychology. 13 (3): 166–174.

McAdams TR, Dillingham MF (2008). Surgical Decompression of the Quadrilateral Space in Overhead Athletes. Am J Sports Med 36(3): 528–532.

McCrea M, Guskiewicz KM, Marshall SW, Barr W, Randolph C, Cantu RC et al. (2003) Acute effects and recovery time following concussion in collegiate football players: The NCAA concussion study. JAMA. 290 (19): 2556–2563.

McCrory P, Bell S (1999) Nerve entrapment syndromes as a cause of pain in the hip, groin and buttock. Sports Med. 27 (4): 261–274.

McCue FC III (1982) The elbow, wrist and hand. In: Curland (ed.) The Injured Athlete. Philadelphia, JB Lippincott.

Menger H (1992) Affektionen peripherer Nerven im Sport. Dtsch Zeitschr Sportmed. 43: 44–58.

Mölsa JJ, Tegner Y, Alaranta H et al. (1999) Spinal cord injuries in ice-hockey in Finland and Sweden from 1980 to 1996. Int J Sports Med. 20: 64–70.

Mumenthaler M, Stöhr M, Müller-Vahl H (2003) Läsionen peripherer Nerven und radikulärer Syndrome. Thieme, Stuttgart.

Noguchi T (1994) A survey of spinal cord injuries resulting from sport. Paraplegia. 32: 170–173.

Oberle J, Kuchelmeister K, Schachenmayr W (1999) Axillarisparese nach Squash-Spielen. Nervenarzt. 70: 750–753.

Otto M, Holthusen S, Bahn E et al. (2000) Boxing and running lead to rise in serum levels of S-100 protein. Int J Sports Med. 21: 551–555.

Paladini D, Dellantonio R, Cinti A (1996) Axillary neuropathy in volleyball players: report of two cases and literature review. J Neurol Neurosurg Psychiatry 60: 345–347.

Patterson JM, Jaggars MM, Boyer MI (2003) Ulnar and median nerve palsy in long-distance cyclists. A prospective study. Am J Sports Med. 31: 585–589.

Petersen W, Nickel C, Zantop T, Zernial O (2005) Verletzungen beim Kitesurfen. Eine junge Trendsportart. Orthopäde. 419–425.

Putukian M, Echemendia RJ, Mackin S (2000) The acute neuropsychological effects of heading

in soccer: a pilot study. Clin J Sport Med. 10: 104–110.
Sachdev P (1992) Golfers' cramp: clinical characteristics and evidence against it being an anxiety disorder. Mov Disord. 7: 326–332.
Saunders RL, Harbourgh RE (1984) The second impact syndrome in catastrophic contact-sports trauma. JAMA. 252: 538–539.
Schneider S, Schmitt H, Tönges S, Seither B (2006) Sports injuries: population-based representative data on incidence, diagnosis, sequelae and high-risk groups. Br J Sport Med. 40: 334–339.
Schon LC, Baxter DE (1990) Neuropathies of the foot and ankle in athletes. Clin Sports Med. 9: 489–509.
Schulze W, Hesse B, Blatter G, Schmidtler B, Muhr G (2000) Verletzungsmuster und -prophylaxe beim Gleitschirmfliegen. Sportverl Sportschad. 14: 41–49.
Schulze W, Richter J, Schulze B, Esenwein SA, Büttner-Janz K (2002) Injury prophylaxis in paragliding. Br J Sports Med. 36: 365–369.
Schwarzer U, Wiegand A et al. (1999) Genital numbness and impotence in long-distance cyclists. J Urol. 161: 178.
Siu TL, Chandran KN et al (2004) Snow sports-related head and spinal injuries: an eight-year survey from the neurotrauma centre for the Snowy Mountains. Austral J Clin Neurosci. 11(3): 236–242.
Smith AM, Adler CH et al. (2003) The "yips" in golf: a continuum between a focal dystonia and choking. Sports Med. 33: 13–31.
Soler T, Calderon C (2000) The prevalence of spondylolysis in the Spanisch elite athlete. Am J Sports Med. 28: 57–62.
Sommer F, Schwarzer U, Klotz T, Caspers HP, Haupt G, Engelmann U (2001) Erectile dysfunction in cyclists. Is there any difference in penile blood flow during cycling in an upright versus a reclining position? Eur Urol. 39 (6): 720–723.
Tarazi F, Dvorak MF, Wing PC (1999) Spinal cord injuries in skiers and snowboarders. Am J Sports Med. 27: 177–180.
Torg JS (1990) Cervical spinal stenosis with cord neurapraxia and transient quadriplegia. Clin Sports Med 1990(2): 279–296.
Toth C (2008) Peripheral nerve injuries attributable to sport and recreation. Neurol Clin. 113: 89–109.
Toumi H, Fitzsimons DP, Best TM (2003). Exercise-induced myopathies. Basic Appl Myol. 13(4): 163–170.
Vogt S, Schumacher YO, Bültermann D, Heinrich L, Blum A, Schmid A (2005) Urologische Probleme im Radsport. Sportorthopädie-Sporttraumatologie. 21: 95–97.
Wesson D, Spence L, Hu X, Parkin P (2000) Trends in bicycle-related head injuries in children after implementation of a community-based bike helmet campaign. J Pediat Surg. 35: 688–689.
Witol AD, Webbe FM (2003) Soccer heading frequency predicts neuropsychological deficits. Arch Clin Neuropsychol. 18(4): 397–417.
Zeller T, Billing A, Lob G (1992) Injuries in paragliding. Int Orthop. 16: 255–259.

13 Eyes

Dieter Schnell

Eyesight is key to sports and any injury of the eye is devastating for the athlete. Man absorbs 85 to 95% of all environmental stimuli via the eye (Schnell 1996). In sports, visual feedback controls and corrects body movement. Contrary to lay assumptions that visual control is critical in the phase of learning, visual feedback is a key component when fine-tuning movements especially in the **automation phase** (Schnell 1996 and 1997). A **decrease or even failure of visual functions** of one or both eyes drastically impacts on **the capacity to execute sport** and considerably increases **risk of injury**.

> Protection of the eyes is the sports physician key duty in medical care of athletes at all performance levels.

Principally, we can distinguish three areas of sports:

- sports for children and adolescents, including school sports
- mass, recreational and health sports, as well as
- competitive and high-performance sports.

These three sports areas present different demands to the organ of sight and also bring along different dangers.

13.1 Sports for children and adolescents

The first physical activities of infants and toddlers may already be called sports. Current research shows that **physical activity in the shape of coordination exercises** presents the highest stimulus to interconnect synaptically nerve cells that are present at birth.

The visual system is pivotal to normal development of movements because **blind children** have a far **lower compulsion to move** than those with optimal sight (Mc Graw 1935, Scherer 2005, Schnell et al. 2009).

Sports at **preschool age** and eventually **school sports** optimize the physical activities of children. Hence, enjoying movements and sports should not be diminished by fears or even accidents.

In general, school sports constitute the first **systematic athletic training of the body**, which lays the foundation for life-long exercise activity. This contributes to vitality and health maintenance in a long-term fashion.

Numbers of accidents in school sports in Germany are alarming. In 2003 about 640,000 sport accidents have been registered in school sports (Scherer 2005). The head had been involved in about 86,000 (13%) of those accidents. Approximately 12,600 students (2%) suffered eye injuries (➢ Tab. 13.1).

The **increase of eye injuries** by 42% within the last 10 years is worrisome. The fact that especially **contusions, concussions and ruptures** have increased is a matter of concern (➢ Tab. 13.2; Scherer 2005). The accident frequency of male students exceeds with 70% by far the 30% of female students.

Most accidents were triggered by other students (28%) or a ball (25%); self-injury only accounted 8% of the cases. Further causes for accidents had been the sports terrain (6.5%) or the racquet (3%) (➢ Tab. 13.3).

Tab. 13.1 General head and eye injuries in school sports 2003 (Scherer 2005).

	Total number	Percentage of accidents related to number of accidents	Percentage of accidents in relation to all students
total number of students	17,443,636		
total of accidents	642,078	100%	3.6%
head injuries	86,487	13.5%	0.49%
eye injuries	12,599	1.96%	0.07%
in-patient eye injuries	186	0.029%	0.001%
increase of eye injuries 1993 to 2003	from 8,900 to 12,599 (by 3,699)	by 41.56%	increase by 0.02%
eye injuries boys	8,571	68%	0.049%
eye injuries girls	4,028	32%	0.023%

Tab. 13.2 Kinds of eye injuries in school sports (Scherer 2005).

Kind of injury	Frequency 1993	Frequency 2003	Decrease and increase 1993 to 2003
contusions, traumas	3,000 (33.71%)	5,350 (42.46%)	+2,350 (78.33%)
ruptures	2,900 (32.58%)	4,650 (36.9%)	+1,750 (60.34%)
bruises, soft-tissue shears	1,900 (21.35%)	1,650 (13.1%)	−250 (−13.16%)
others	1,100 (12.36%)	950 (7.54%)	−150 (−13.64%)
total accidents	8,900 (100%)	12,600 (100%)	3,700 (41.57%)

Tab. 13.3 Causes for eye injuries in school sports (Scherer 2005).

Cause of accident	Total number	Percentage
other person	3,545	28.1%
ball	3,126	24.8%
injured persons themselves	967	7.7%
ground	838	6.6%
racket	387	3.1%
others*	3,738	29.7%
total	12,599	100%

*other play and sports equipment, plants, objects, e.g. missiles as stones, snowballs, etc.

Optimized eye protection in school sports should follow below measures:

- Spectacle wearers should use sports goggles for contact sports, which should not be removed at any time during school sports.
- Protective glasses should be worn during exercise of particularly eye-injuring sports such as boxing, soccer, handball, basketball and hockey.
- Sports teachers should be aware of any handicaps of their students including virtual or actual monocular vision, forced postures of the head (with paralytic strabismus and nystag-

mus) or limitations of physical capability because of therapies interfering with vision (wearing of e.g. bi- or tri-focal glasses, shut-taping of one eye, or administration of pupil-dilating drops). Individual solutions are key to limit accidents and keep school sports risk free as possible and maintain fun and optimal performance.

Tab. 13.4 The five most frequent sports in which eye injuries have occurred in school sports (Scherer 2005).

Exercised sport	Number of eye injuries	Number in percent
soccer	1,579	12.52
basketball	612	4.90
hockey	516	4.10
handball	451	3.57
volleyball	415	3.28
others	9,026	71.63
total	12,599	100.00

Soccer ranked first on the list of injury-frequent sports with 13% of eye injuries, followed by basketball with 5%, hockey, handball with 4% each and volleyball with approximately 3% (➤ Tab. 13.4).

13.2 Non-competitive, popular and health sports

2 to 4% of all eye injuries occur in adult sports (MacEwen 1989, Rompe et al. 1981, Zagelbaum 1993, Zagelbaum et al. 1994) with approximately 1% of all sports injuries affecting eyes (Kahle et al. 1993, Toppel 1972, Pashby 1997).

The incidence of **eye injuries in sport activities** reaches **6 to 26 per 100,000 people.** 100,000 hours of sports account for 10 to 20 eye injuries (Genovese et al. 1990, Schnell 1987). One third of the eye injuries in sports are moderate to severe, two thirds are mild. About 25% of the eye injuries require **in-patient clinic treatment** (Erie 1991, Genovese et al. 1990, Jones and Tullo 1986, Jones, 1987, MacEwen 1987 and 1989, Schnell 1987). The number of cases of **loss of sight in sports** fluctuates **between 7 and 12%** (Fong 1994, Pashby 1985, 1989 and 1992, Rapoport 1990, Schnell 1987).

A 17 year study in Cologne found that **most frequent injuries** in sports are eye contusions (more than 50% of the cases) followed by injuries triggered by foreign objects, infections and irritations, chemical and physical impacts as well as cut and spear wounds (➤ Tab. 13.5; Erie 1991, Fong 1994, Genovese et al. 1990, Labelle et al. 1988, MacEwen 1987 and 1989, Rapoport 1990, Schnell 1987, Zagelbaum 1993).

Tab. 13.5 Eye injuries and other impairments of the eye region in sports exercise (own statistics of 17 years, n = 632 athletes; Schnell 1997).

Eye injuries	Number
eye contusions	51.1%
injuries by foreign bodies	12.5%
radial, chemical and physical effects	11.9%
cut and spear injuries	5.8%

Tab. 13.6 The absolute and relative eye injuries of individual countries most frequent in men (Erie 1992, Easterbrook 1992, Zagelbaum 1993, Fong 1994, Schnell 1996, Jendrusch 2004).

Country	Absolutely most frequent eye injuries in sports	Relatively most frequent eye injuries in sports
Australia	squash, badminton, Australian football	squash, Australian football
Canada	baseball, squash, racquetball, badminton	squash, racquetball
Germany	soccer, tennis, volleyball, squash, ice hockey	water polo, squash
France	baseball, soccer, tennis, squash	baseball, squash
United Kingdom	squash, soccer, badminton, tennis	squash, tennis
Ireland	football, rugby, squash, badminton	rugby, squash
U.S.A.	baseball, racquetball, pool sports	ice hockey, racquetball

Country-specific variations are detected (➤ Tab. 13.6). In countries exercising **squash and ice hockey without eye or face protection** eye injuries are most common.

> Disciplines involving racquets, balls or pucks are most dangerous as they cause 55% of the eye injuries. Small balls are more prone to injuries than large balls. Small balls reach higher speeds and impact on the eye from a shorter distance.

Soccer has the highest number of eye injuries in Germany, which is a reflection of its popularity. In terms of frequency, **water polo, squash and ice hockey** carry the highest danger of eye injuries. Hence, **safety goggles** or face mask are strongly recommended for all three sports in training as well as in competition.

The dangers of eye injuries caused by balls are much higher depending on the sport at up to 94% and occur more often **with small balls**. The reason is not the fact that small balls fit easier into the eye socket, but the higher speed and the smaller distance to the eyes.

> Small inelastic full balls mostly lead to injuries in the area of the anterior eye segment; hollow balls cause more damage in the area of the vitreum, retina and optic nerve.

The eye is hung up elastically and eludes backwards up to a certain degree in a collision but it is more or less strongly compressed, decompressed and hyperextended depending on the impact force.

Hollow balls have a **suction effect** given the direct impact all around the orbita in the repulsive phase. This suction primarily leads to injuries of the **posterior segments** of the eye (➤ Tab. 13.7).

The injury risk by the individual sports varies drastically. Water polo, squash and tennis as well as badminton carry far higher eye injury risks (➤ Tab. 13.8).

Most severe injuries are:
- retina hemorrhages (➤ Fig. 13.2) and detachments
- choroid ruptures
- optic nerve sheath hematomas
- blow-out fractures and
- bursts of the eyeball.

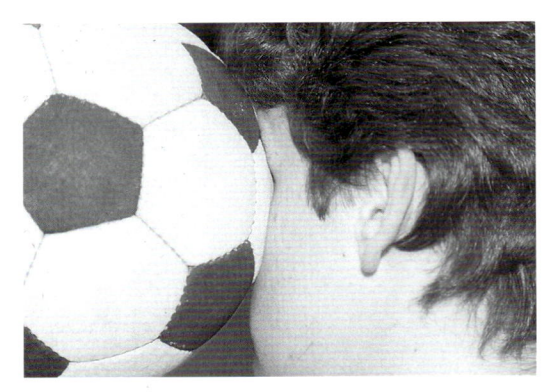

Fig. 13.1 A soccer ball also "fits" into the eye (by deformation).

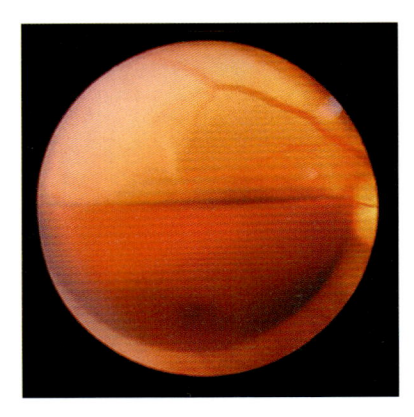

Fig. 13.2 Preretinal hemorrhage after soccer injury.

Modifications of sports equipment lead to a **reduction of severe eye injuries** in some sports. Therefore, the handles, the peaks and the plates of **skiing sticks** have been modified to avoid injuries (➤ Fig. 13.3 a and b): in the depicted case no important organ was observed and after the removal of the stick with the peak the child quickly recovered.

Routine follow-up by the ophthalmologist is of great importance after eye injuries. Many impacts lead to unnoticed damages that only become visible at a later stage.

> No eye injury – whatever its degree – should be underestimated! A late blindness after a contusio bulbi of moderate degree is unforgivable and, above all, avoidable.

Tab. 13.7 Causes, locations, stages and consequences of injuries in sports (Kroll et al. 1083, de Lucia 1985, Kirchhoff and Kroll 1991).

Cause of injury	Location of injury	Stages of injury	Consequences to the eye
small full balls (badminton ball, baseball, golf ball, snowball, puck)	anterior and middle segment of the eye	1) compression phase: sagittal shortening to 50%, incipient equatorial broadening	damages at cornea, conjunctiva, lens, ciliary body, iris, iridocorneal angle and anterior part of the vitreous body
		2) decompression phase: effect of repulsion, equatorial broadening to 128% (pear-shaped)	tears in the iris, peripheral retina, iridocorneal angle, vessels, rupture of zonule fibers
		3) hyperextension phase: sagittal enlargement to 112% (ellipsoidal)	hemorrhages, lens luxations, tears of the iridocorneal angle, vitreous body detachments, rarely vitreous body-retina problems
		4) oscillation phase: the eye oscillates	tears, dislocations of the lens, hemorrhages, damages of the iridocorneal angle, iris and lens
large hollow balls (soccer ball, handball, basketball)	(anterior) middle and posterior segment of the eye	1) compression phase: broadening under decrease of length of the eyeball	injuries of eyelids, conjunctiva, cornea, iris, ciliary body
		2) first repulsion-suction phase: suction between iris and vitreous body, length increase of the eye by low pressure	injuries of iris, lens (subluxations), ciliary body, tears of the peripheral retina, vessel tears, hemorrhages
		3) second repulsion-suction phase: between vitreous body and retina	Berlin's edema, preretinal, subretinal and intraretinal hemorrhages, formation of retinal holes, detachments, choroidal tears
racket	anterior segment, orbita and facial bones	1) compression phase: sagittal shortening, equatorial broadening	contusion of the anterior eye segment and the osseous eye socket (orbital, blow-out fracture), choroid and bulb ruptures
		2) decompression phase: lengthening of the eyeball	hematomas, lid swellings, lens luxations, optic nerve sheath hematomas
finger, arm, foot	anterior segment of the eye and its appendage	acute injury	contusions, lid injuries, ruptures of the lacrimal canal, cornea, conjunctiva, aclera-ocular-muscle injuries

Tab. 13.8 Accidental injury risk for the eyes in sports Jendrusch et al. 2004).

Sport	Injury risk
water polo	11 times
squash/racquetball	8.0 times
tennis	5.9 times
badminton	5.5 times
ice hockey	2.8 times
swimming	2.2 times
hockey	2.1 times
judo	2.0 times
table tennis	1.1 times
handball	1.05 times
karate	1.0 times
basketball	1.0 times
volleyball	0.9 times

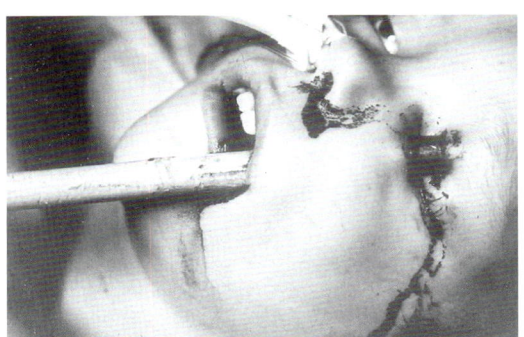

13.3 Competitive and high-performance sports

Principally, the same injuries are found in high-performance sports as in mass, recreational and health sports. But eye injuries are **more frequent and more severe** in certain sports.

Revision of guidelines reduces eye injuries in professional sports. For example, eye injuries in **ice hockey** dropped after banning high sticks. The frequency of eye injuries in many countries dropped after introduction of mandatory eye or face protection. No loss of sight has been reported anymore since eye protection became mandatory in Canada in 2000 (Pashby 1987, 1988 and 1992).

Habit and fashion often oppose the accident prevention and guideline revisions. German squash players still reject safety goggles although several severe injuries as well as loss of sight continue to occur every year. In contrast, eye injury frequency drastically dropped in the US after protective eyewear became mandatory (Vinger 1990).

As opposed to mass, recreational and health athletes, the competitive and high-performance athletes earn their living by sports. So it should be especially important for them to protect themselves of eye injuries in sports. Interestingly, German ice hockey professionals still neglect **eye protection** in training. Eye protection is only mandatory **in competition**.

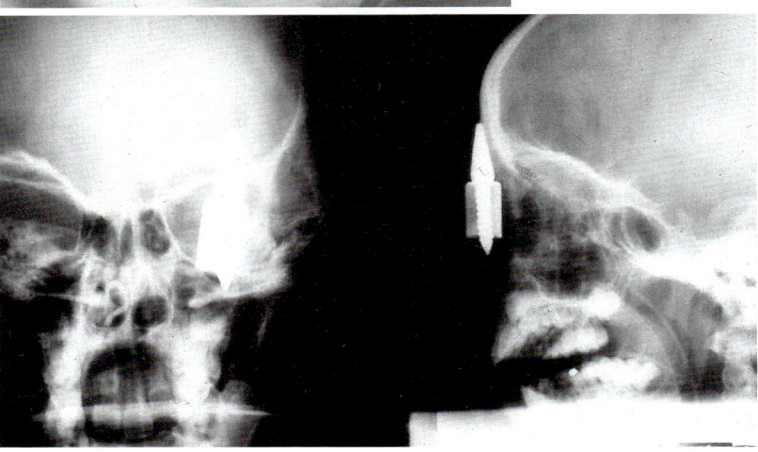

Fig. 13.3 a and b: Skiing stick injury of a girl in 1967 without lasting damages.

Another difference to non-professional athletes is the responsibility of the physician to **maintain the condition** of the competitive or high-performance athlete, no matter how severe the eye injury is.

Athletes with eye injuries can maintain fitness on a stationary bicycle. **Jogging** is not recommended after eye injuries. The concussions of the eye can accelerate **the vitreum** up to 4–5 G (Draeger and Dupuis 1975), which can cause **retinal hemorrhages** and vitreum-retina problems.

Ruptures of the lacrimal tunnels of volleyball and basketball players (➢ chapter 13.4.26), **retrobulbar emphysemas or infections** of waterpolo players and swimmers especially with herpes viruses, ubiquitous germs and fungi, as well as racquet injuries in tennis and badminton doubles are observed more frequently than in amateurs sports.

Even today, **contact lens damages by anoxia** are surprisingly frequent in sports although excellent soft as well as hard lenses are available by now. Still many athletes wear only slightly gas-permeable contacts and do substantial mistakes during maintenance of the lenses.

> Overnight use of contact lenses is not recommended due to the increased cornea infection and risk of damage.

Overnight-wearing of highly gas-permeable **contact lenses is not recommended** because the **cornea is more stressed in intensive sports exercise** and requires recreation during night (Fong 1994, Holden 1985, Holland 1994, Reim 1977, Schnell 2003). Occasional wearing over night hardly does any damage, though. In **orthokeratology** a hard, relatively thick lens is worn over night, which like a brace constricts and changes the cornea. This is not recommended for similar reasons (Schnell 2003).

Corrective laser treatment is also **problematic** in professional athletes. Indications are very strict and surgery technique has to be adapted to individual sports requirements. Only an experienced sports ophthalmologist should advise a professional athlete; the coach should always be included in the consultation. Our work group maintains an own section of "Refractive Surgery in Sports", which is available upon request.

13.4 Sport-specific eye injuries

In addition to protective eyewear the optimal **optical correction is the most important preventive measure** of eye injuries in sports (Jendrusch et al. 1999, Jendrusch and Heck 1999 and 2000, Jendrusch et al. 2004).

13.4.1 American football

Although football has superseded baseball in popularity long ago, it still is at the bottom of the scale of most frequent eye injuries. The mandatory **helmet protects** the eyes in an excellent way. Only helmet loss or another player grabbing through the lattice, which strictly speaking is forbidden can cause injuries in the face and at the eyes. There is no direct danger for the eyes by the spheroid "ball"; shots against the head can indirectly lead to concussions of the eyes.

13.4.2 Badminton

Shuttlecocks reach speeds of more than 200 km/h. In general, the rapid retardation only leads to severe eye injuries at close distance. The **racquet of the teammate** in a double might cause serious injuries especially if no optimal sports goggles are worn (Easterbrook 1992, Jones 1993, Kahle et al. 1993, MacEwen 1989, McWhae and LaRoche 1990, Schnell 1987, Jendrusch and Heck 1999, Jendrusch et al. 2004, Schnell 1978). **Contusions and defects of the corneal surface layer** present the most frequent injuries of the eye.

13.4.3 Baseball

With **more than 43,000 eye injuries per year** baseball leads the list of most frequent eye trauma in the U.S.A. (Zagelbaum et al. 1994). The injuries are almost exclusively caused by the inelastic baseball and in general affect the **anterior eye segment**. The clubbed bat does not play a crucial role here (Erie 1991, Zagelbaum 1993, Zagelbaum et al. 1994). Significantly less eye injuries in baseball have been registered in Canada (Easterbrook 1992, Labelle et al. 1988).

13.4.4 Basketball

Basketball is the most frequent played sport on earth. Elbows, hands and fingers of opponents and teammates are the most frequent causes of mostly **superficial eye injuries**. The relatively large hollow ball only exceptionally causes contusions or erosions. Injuries of the eyelids also occur in addition to damaged conjunctival and corneal surface layers; **ruptures of the lacrimal canal** are common (Kahle et al. 1993, Zagelbaum 1993).

13.4.5 Boxing

Boxing ranks on the fourth place of eye injury frequency in Germany. **Ruptures of the lid skin (cut)** are the most frequent in addition to **eye contusions**. Enzenauer and colleagues uncovered that only 5% had to be admitted to in-patients care; one of them **lost his eyesight because of a bulbus rupture** (Enzenauer and Mauldin 1989).

> Recurring eye contusions of boxers accumulate in more severe damages.

Lens dislocations and cataracts (➢ Fig. 13.4) are found frequently in professional boxers of higher weight classes. Giovannazzo et al. (1987) had found eye injuries in 66% of the cases in New York and Wedrich et al. (1993) in **76% of asymptomatic boxers** in Vienna. 58% of them showed decline in visual acuity as well as damages at the iridocorneal angle, at the lens, the macula and the retina. Some authors found unusual **retinal changes** in a high percentage, which often needed laser treatment (Carter and Parke 1987, Maguire and Benson 1986).

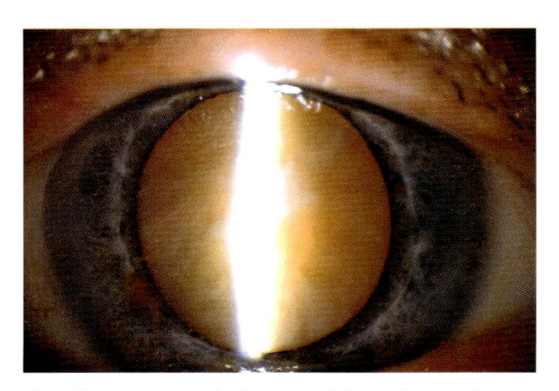

Fig. 13.4 Cataract of a heavy-weight professional boxer (before surgery).

13.4.6 Bungee jumping

In general, bungee jumpers jump a height of 50 to 90 m to feel a euphoria effect although **no endorphins** are released; only **cortisone level rises** (Loew et al. 1993).

> The higher the fall the higher the danger of eye complications such as lens, ciliary, vitreous and retinal damages.

Cerebral blood congestion is a major issue in bungee jumping. The pressure of thorax is transferred to eye and brain via the nonvalvular jugular veins during headfirst free fall. The braking, which is relatively abrupt despite the elastic cord and the successive rebound increases the pressure on eye and brain. This causes **intra- and preretinal hemorrhages** (➢ Fig. 13.7) and **vascula occlusions** with axonal congestion, so-called **cotton wool spots.** This can cause permanent deterioration of visual acuity and in individual cases even virtual loss of sight, if occurring centrally.

13.4.7 Cricket

Cricket being almost exclusively restricted to former British Empire can cause severe injuries such as **retinal detachments** or even **bursts of the eyeball** (Coroneo 1985). In New Zealand, this sport yields 30% of all eye accidents in sports, which requires a **stay in hospital** (Aburn 1990).

13.4.8 Ice hockey

Stick and incompressible hard-rubber disk (puck) extremely threaten all segments of the eye, if no eye or face protection is worn (Labelle et al. 1988, Myles et al. 1993, Pashby 1985, 1987 and 1988).

In Germany, most eye injuries up to **loss of eyesight** and **eye bursts** occur as adults wear no face protection during training. Protective gear in training is not mandatory and perceived as weak by teammates. Without eye protection, injuries such as the simple erosion, retina-choroid degenerations and ruptures (➢ Fig. 13.5), up to **blow-out fractures** (by the stick), lens dislocations and severe bulbus ruptures occur commonly.

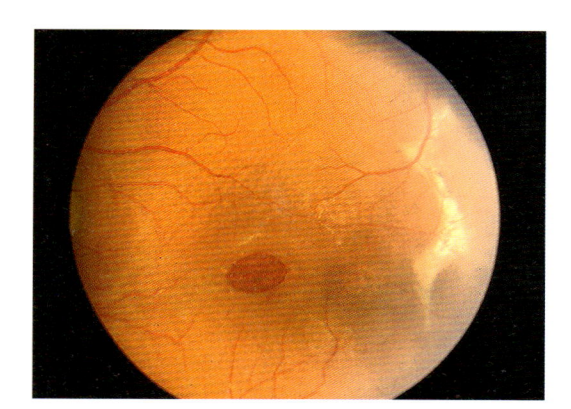

Fig. 13.5 Central retinal hole after severe contusion injury of an ice hockey professional without eye protection by a puck (remaining visual acuity 5%). Typical consequences of contusion injuries of a special form of choroid rupture (retinopathia sclopetaria) at the right edge of the image.

The most frequent eye injuries in soccer are skin injuries, conjunctival and corneal injuries.

Shot from close by the hollow ball has the described **suction effect** with influences to the posterior eye segment. Nevertheless, severe eye injuries are relatively rare.

In absolute terms, eye injuries in soccer sport are in first place in our statistic. In relation to the frequency of the exercise of the sport, we find this sport only in the ninth place for adults, far behind basketball, volleyball and handball (➤ Tab. 13.9). Unfortunately, only few of the athletes with defective vision wear the according correction, which leads to lack of movement precision and higher injury risks.

The number of eye injuries has decreased immensely since mandatory eye protection is prescribed **for adolescents** in training as well as in competition and for adults in competition. In Canada, serious and most serious eye injuries dropped from 300 to 19 per year after consequent **facemask enforcement**. The losses of eyesight have decreased from about 20 (not including a high estimated number of unknown cases) to 0 (Pashby 1987, 1988, 1992).

Table 13.9 Absolute and relative frequency of eye injuries in the individual disciplines in the area of Cologne and in Bergisches Land (own statistics n = 632 sports injured).

Order of sports	Frequency of eye injuries in percent in relation to the frequency of exercising the sport	Approximate frequency of exercising the sport (projection)
1) squash	0.153%	7,200
2) ice hockey	0.130%	11,100
3) tennis	0.085%	71,400
4) field hockey	0.084%	21,300
5) boxing	0.082%	14,700
6) basketball	0.050%	47,500
7) volleyball	0.033%	111,500
8) handball	0.010%	160,000
9) soccer	0.006%	1,216,600
10) equestrianism	0.005%	320,000
11) water polo	0.005%	180,000
12) gymnastics	0.003%	436,600
13) others	0.035%	430,000
total	0.010%	3,027,900

13.4.9 Fencing

One of the sports with relatively frequent occurrence of eye injuries despite intensive protection is fencing. Strict interpretation of rules by the referee has an impact on the likelihood of eye injury. Every **veering away of the head**, every **loss of the mask** involves a risk of eye injuries. Goggles worn underneath the mask offer additional protection.

13.4.10 Soccer

Soccer is the most popular ball game in European countries. Similar to basketball most injuries are caused by elbows, hands, fingers and heads. Surprisingly, hardly any eye injuries are caused by leg and foot of the opponent or teammate (Erie 1991, Gregory 1986, Harada et al. 1985, Schnell 1987, Sherwood 1989, Zagelbaum 1993).

13.4.11 Golf

Eyes injuries are rare. In failed hits the ball may be flung into the own eye or may hit an opposing player or spectator. Shot from close by the nearly incompressible small ball can cause **severe injuries of the anterior and middle eye segment**, ranging from hematomas, erosions of the lids or conjunctiva and cornea, to damages of iris and iridocorneal angle and lens dislocations.

Therefore, **golf goggles** should protect the eyes like sports goggles. With **presbyopia**, distance glasses should be used for the tee; **corrections** for distances of 2 m to 40 cm are needed for putting and for writing down the results. The corrections for medium and close distances can either be applied in front of the distance glasses in the form of half-glasses, or the distance glasses are exchanged with multifocal glasses.

Recently golf goggles became available with unbreakable glasses, which **can be folded forwards**. Also **frontally attachable filters** are available for the improvement of contrast in bad weather conditions or as sun and UV protection (➤ Fig. 13.6 a and b).

Acid-filled golf balls are also used in some countries. These might burst in a collision and can cause chemical burns (Farley 1985, Nelson 1970). Sports goggles also protect extensively of this danger.

13.4.12 Paint ball

If the recommended face protection or eye protection is not being used eyes are at increased risk of injury in this war game (Anders 1994). **Corneal erosions and contusions** occasionally also injuries of the eyelids can occur.

13.4.13 Team handball

The frequency of eye injuries in handball is underestimated. The highest risk exists for the **goalkeeper**, whose eyes are much endangered at throws of field players as well as at 7-meter throws (the distance to the thrower often is only 2–3 m). Surprisingly, no rules of protective eyewear have been established yet for goalkeepers.

> Reaction time is often too short to protect the eyes or the head given the short distance to the goal and the high speed of the ball. Thus, sports goggles are urgently recommended.

Field players, though more rarely than goalkeepers, also suffer from severe to serious eye injuries caused by fingers, hands, arms, elbows and balls.

Contusion and suction occur often given the important acceleration of the ball, which is usually by far superior to soccer balls. **Iridocorneal angle, lens, vitreum, retina** (➤ Fig. 13.7) and **optic nerve** often suffer most severe damages here.

Though handball only ranges at the eighth or ninth position of all eye injuries in our sports

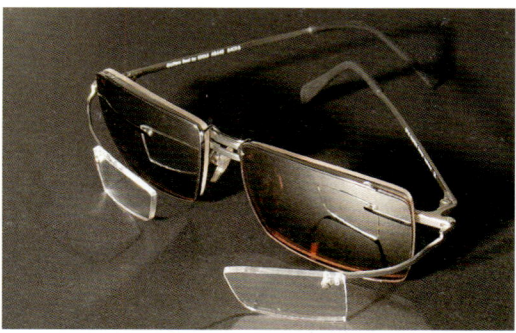

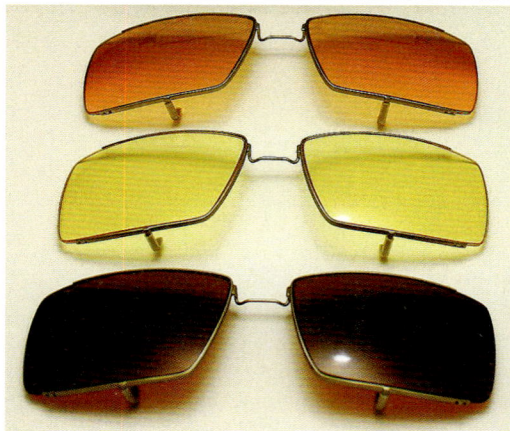

Fig. 13.6 a: Special golf goggles with multifocal or near-vision parts (right glass for the distance, left glass slightly folded back). b: Diverse contrast and sun filters.

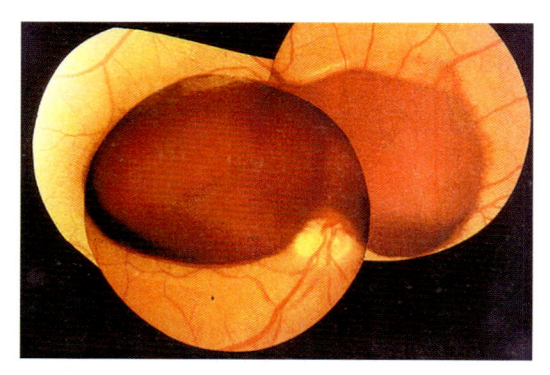

Fig. 13.7 Sub-, intra- and preretinal hemorrhage with choroid rupture of a goalkeeper by a ball in seven-meter throw.

accidents' statistic (Jendrusch 2004), the injuries caused by a (hand)ball are mostly very severe. Also, handball sport is the most frequent cause of eye injuries for **women** (Gregory 1986, Schnell 1987, Jendrusch 2004).

13.4.14 Hockey

The inelastic, hard-hit hockey ball often causes injuries at the anterior eye segment. **Injuries of the lens and iridocorneal angle, orbita fractures** and **bulbus ruptures** occur based on the inelastic nature of the hockey ball and the transgressive movement of the stick at the height of the eyes. Amateurs are particularly prone to these injuries in contrast to professional athletes (Reim 1977, Schnell 1987, Pashby 1987 and 1988, Erie 1991, Kahle 1993, Zagelbaum 1993).

13.4.15 Sport at altitude

The past years have seen an increased boom of sport at altitude. This led athletes reaching significant altitude faster and faster – mostly using helicopter transfers.

Given the drastically shortened acclimation, **mountain altitude sickness** often occurs with subsequent rare cases of **brain edemas, brain and eye hemorrhages**. Also **changes of rods, cones and macula** have been found recorded in patients with mountain altitude sickness.

From an altitude of 4,000–5,000 meters threaten visual loss due to drought intolerance of contact lenses of the eyes and circulatory problems.

Many athletes risk their lives because of the mountain altitude sickness or at least the option of ascending more and more new peaks.

Currently, **intraocular pressure** could serve as an indicator for mountain altitude sickness. The eye tension obviously runs parallel to the pO_2 level of the blood. Should both descend, the athlete is at the risk of mountain altitude sickness (Pavlidis et al. 2004).

Another risk for the eye consists in the **intensive solar radiation** at high altitudes. UV radiation is further intensified by snow and ice reflection. **Glacier goggles** with absorption of 94-97% as well as 100% **UV protection** are indispensable. Whoever suffered the extreme **snow blindness** caused by intensive UV radiation never forgets again light or UV protection in the mountains.

13.4.16 Running

Running primarily on hard ground (marathon, etc.) can cause oscillation frequencies of more than 25 Hz. These oscillations can **accelerate the vitreous body** up to 4 G. Ultimately, **vitreum-retina problems** or even detachment is the consequence (Draeger and Dupuis 1975). Therefore, running on soft ground (forest ground, etc.) at least in training is strongly recommended especially for high-risk **groups such as myopics**. Retinal examination is recommended for prevention. Nordic walking does not present a risk.

13.4.17 Martial arts

Wrestling, Judo, Karate, Taekwondo, as well as other European and Asian martial arts lead to eye injuries with frequencies and severities. Severity of eye injuries is mainly determined whether sparring is performed with or without contact. The most frequent injuries are **macerations of the eyelids, conjunctival hemorrhages and corneal erosions**. So far, it has not been common to wear sports goggles in martial arts. Often referees can play a critical role in reducing risk of eye injury by early intervention in the sparring. A strict interpretation of the rules is active eye protection.

13.4.18 Kite surfing

This relatively new surfing sport uses the wind to pull a rider through the water on a small surfboard or a kiteboard. Kite surfing involves some risks for the eyes. The most frequent are impact with handle of the kite. The board or kite rarely causes injuries. Injuries caused by other kite surfers become more frequent on small lakes with little free, individual space.

Light contusions up to **most serious injuries of all eye segments** including bulbus ruptures can occur during kite surfing.

Sports goggles and helmets absorb impact of severe collisions and are strongly recommended. In addition, protective eyewear absorbs **light and UV** on bright days reflected by the water surface. Goggles should fit tightly around the eyes to reduce scattered radiation from the water.

Other athletes can be endangered by kite surfers as well. The board can reach important speed and can cause very serious eye and head injuries in unnoticed swimmers, divers, water skiers or surfers. Large swimmer's goggles (➤ Fig. 13.8) provide a certain protection.

13.4.19 Equestrianism

Branches at rides through the forest induce the most frequent injuries in horse riding. Here, **sports goggles** provide very efficient eye protection. Injuries by the mane of the horse, the hand holding the reins or course obstacles are rare. The hooves of kicking horses cause severe and most serious injuries.

13.4.20 Swimming

Indoor as well as outdoor pools are often disinfected with chlorine, which js why light **chemical burns** occur frequently. These chemical burns are characterized by **corneal stippling**, which mostly disappear within half a day. The swimmers experience blurred eyesight and feel a slight scratching of the eyes. Hence, **swimmer's goggles** protecting the eyes are routinely recommended. Goggles even offer the possibility of wearing contact lenses (Schnell 2002 and 2003).

The swimmer's goggles of high-performance athletes are smaller than the eye socket, keep the water resistance low and fit very tightly. The swimmer tosses them off directly upon finishing the competition. Given this tight fit we recommend **large goggles** (➤ Fig. 13.8) for mass, recreational and health sports in chlorine as well as in open waters. Goggles are strongly recommended for open waters where surfers, kite surfers, sailors and motorboat drivers can provoke great risks to swimmer. **Contact lenses** should be removed after swimming, cleaned and reapplied only after a recreational period.

13.4.21 Squash

The same small squash playing field makes this sport particularly exposed to eye injury from both racquet and the ball. Squash balls can be accelerated to an astonishing 300 km/h. They differ in hardness and require a dynamic way of playing. The balls are often hit in the height of breast or head. Contrary to other sports head involvement is more than 50% of the squash accidents with 60–90% ball-triggered injuries (Labelle et al. 1988, Kahle et al. 1993). The eyes are affected in about 25% of the cases (Gregory 1986, Schnell 1987). The elastic nature and the quick slow down of the ball result rarely in serious eye injuries. Typically, **erosions, corneal and conjunctival hemorrhages** occur. However, **racquet-triggered injuries** representing 5–10% of all cases can be **serious** – including reported cases of eyeball rupture.

Protection goggles in squash have not yet been internationally introduced; thus, eye damages or loss of eyesight continue to be reported every year. All eye injuries in squash could be prevented with optimal sports goggles (Kroll et al. 1983, MacEwen 1989, Genovese et al. 1990, Kirchhoff and Kroll 1991, Vinger 1990 and 1993, Kahle et al. 1993, Zagelbaum 1993, Schnell 1987, 1996 and 1997, Jendrusch 2002 and 2004). Hence, it is particularly disappointing that the German squash association is still resisting to mandatory protective eyewear. Every eyesight loss in squash is potentially avoidable with simple eye protection.

13.4.22 Surfing

Surf board, boom, mast and sail can lead to serious or severe injuries of the surfers themselves or of unnoticed swimmers. Below the water surface the blade can hit with high speed and injure extremities of swimmers. **Large swimmer's goggles** (➤ Fig. 13.8) can provide certain protection to swimmers and surfers but are rarely worn. The major risk factor remains

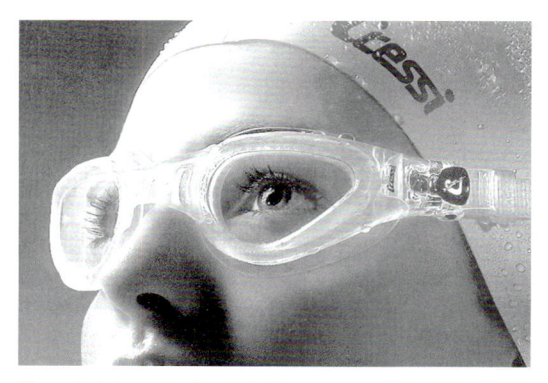

Fig. 13.8 Large swimmer's (protection) goggles.

the board and its blade, which can reach high speeds (Colin et al. 1984, Lawless et al. 1986).

The **most frequent injuries** are mild and develop if the surfer **falls** onto mast, boom or sail.

> Swimmers' accidents triggered by surfers are often serious and include lens dislocations, blowout fractures, retinal hemorrhages, choroid, retina and optic nerve ruptures.

13.4.23 Sport diving

Diving masks offer an excellent protection of eye. Not surprisingly eye injuries are extremely seldom in sport diving.

Missed **pressure compensation** at the descent can cause facial and eye **barotrauma** which include skin and conjunctiva hemorrhages. Generally, these hemorrhages are not very painful and heal relatively quickly.

> Neglect of decompressing times is dangerous.

Divers diving during the zerohour – the time that enables them to surface directly without stopping at designated depths and without having to observe decompressing times – only take low risks of suffering a decompression disease. **Pyknic persons**, however, might already suffer such a trauma even with the adherence of decompressing times because nitrogen stores earlier and more intensively into the abundant adipose tissue than in normal subjects. In part, they already have to observe decompressing times within the zerohour but have to extend decompressing times when diving exceeds the zerohour.

In **decompression sickness**, also known as caisson disease, the disintegrating nitrogen leads to **nervous, retinal choroidal and vascular damages** in the area of the eyes and the rest of the body. While no crucial damages have been found in divers who always remained within the zerohour (Harada et al. 1985, Scholz et al. 1991), **vascular changes** in the shape of vascular obstructions (enlarged arterioles and microaneurysms) as well as **damages of the macula pigment** have been described in divers with a history of decompression symptoms. The more often such symptoms had been experienced, the earlier they occurred with up to 50% of divers being affected (Polkinghorne et al. 1988, Day 1994).

> Every diver who has suffered a decompression trauma should also consult an ophthalmologist.

Examinations of the retina, fluorescence angiography, visual reaction time and examinations of blue-visibility reveal the kind and degree of damage (Curley and Butler 1987, Scholz et al. 1991, Day 1994, Schnell 2002 and 2003).

In general, **soft contact lenses** are recommended for the correction of defective vision of divers above and under water. Long-time wearers of hard contacts may also dive with their contact lenses after previous practice in their home pool (Holland 1994, Schnell 2002 and 2003). However, **hard contact lenses** can signal disintegrating nitrogen under the lenses at a beginning decompression trauma (Guldner and Vola 1987, Socks 1988, Holland 1994). The 3–6 min half-life period of corneal gas satiety under hard lenses is almost identical to blood, so that nitrogen bubbles can emerge in blood vessels and nervous tissue parallel to the emerging gas bubbles under the lens (Holland 1994). An immediate reaction by observance of sufficient decompressing periods is often life-saving. Soft contact lenses do not show a similar effect.

Artificial eyes have to be taken off before since the high pressure in the diving mask can trigger implosion.

> Narrow iridocorneal angle and glaucomas are absolute contraindications for diving. Similarly, patients with advanced diabetic retinopathies, maculopathies and angiopathies should not practice diving.

The ophthalmologist should decide about the necessary duration of a sport restriction after eye surgeries, especially of cataracts and glaucomas.

13.4.24 Tennis

Tennis ranks third to fifth in eye injury frequency. **Adolescents** especially in the begin-

Table 13.10 Equipment of sports goggles for contact sports.

Frame
■ It has to be stable in all parts, unbreakable and cushioned all around (= coated), including – if there are any – the hinges and sidepieces.
■ It must not have any sharp edges, has to sit firmly at the head (e.g. by webbed sidepieces, rubber bands or other constructions) and must not be far protruding, but without reducing the field of vision.
■ The nose pad should have a supporting surface of 300–400 mm^2 at least.
■ The frame has to be large enough and sit high enough to brace at the osseous eye socket at a frontal impact, so that the eyes are not contused (➢ Fig. 13.10).
■ The internal notch of the border of the glasses has to be higher than the external notch, so that the disks cannot fall out to the inside but only to the outside.

Glasses
■ They have to be made of unbreakable special glass, plastics or polycarbonate, so that they cannot break.
■ They should preferably be vaulted outwards to not hit the eyes in a collision.
■ The rims of the disks must not be cut sharply in order to avoid cut injuries.
■ While exercising sports in the sun, the disks must provide protection of glare (absorption of 75 to 97%) and UV light (100%).

ning of their tennis career should always wear **sports goggles**.

Injuries by tennis balls are far more frequent than by racquets. Ball injuries are often light to moderate **changes in the anterior eye segment**; racquets often cause **orbital fractures** and serious or **most serious eye contusions**.

Eye injuries are rare in singles matches but their frequency increases in doubles. Balls bouncing off the own racquet or the one of the teammate or the racquets themselves can impact the eye, before the player is able to protect it. Therefore **sports goggles for contact sports** (➢ Tab. 13.10, ➢ Fig. 13.10 a and b) are recommended at doubles and in sunlight fitted with the necessary light and UV protection.

13.4.25 Gymnastics

Gymnasts seldom suffer eye injuries. Nevertheless, concussions of jumps or dismounting can lead to damages particularly in cases of **myopia** (Draeger and Dupuis 1975). **Eye injuries** can occur **at support or safety positions** in training by PE teachers, coaches or comrades.

Long exercises, in which the body is positioned above the head, such as handstands and (yoga) headstands, shoulder stands etc. should be avoided. **Damages of the visual field** similar to glaucomas occur in athletes who had performed yoga headstand over a longer time period (Rice and Allen 1986). The transfer of the **pressure from the chest** to the jugular brain and eyes veins can damage the eye.

13.4.26 Volleyball

Eye injuries in volleyball occur often especially by impacting fingers, hands, arms and elbows of teammates. **Ruptures of the lacrimal canals** (➢ Fig. 13.9) as well as skin and conjunctival injuries can occur.

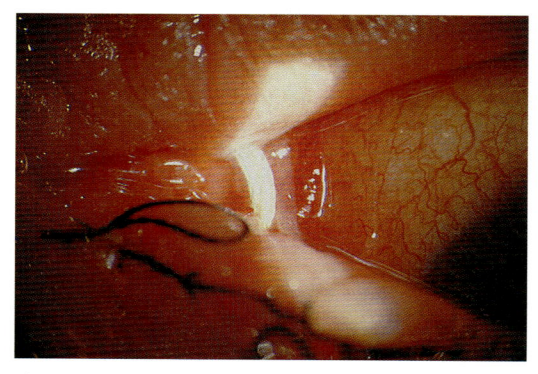

Fig. 13.9 Rupture of the lacrimal canal treated with a plastic ring probe and sutured skin wounds (injury cause by the finger of a team mate in volleyball).

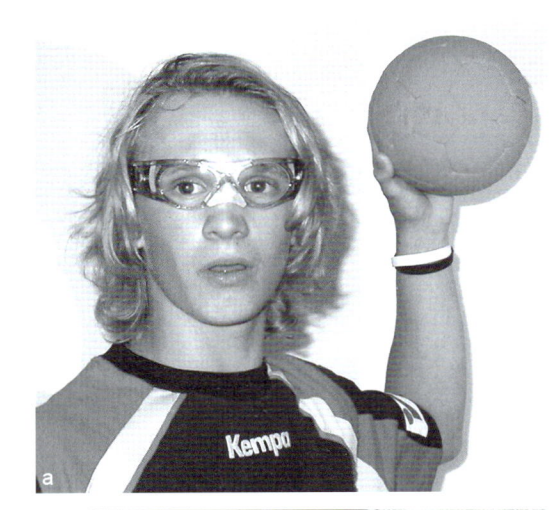

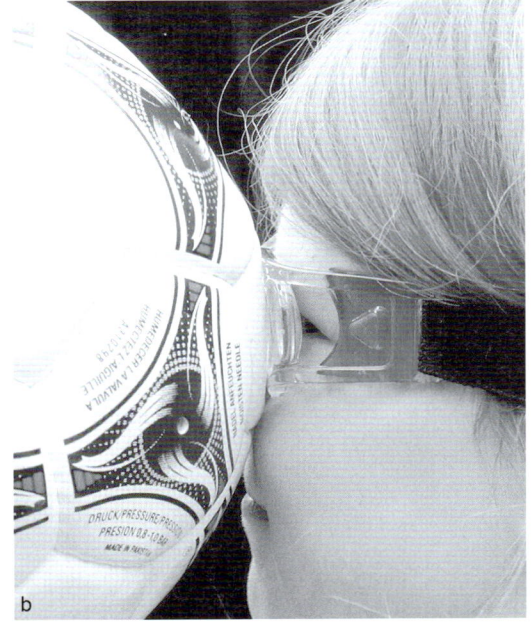

Fig. 13.10 a: A handball player with sports goggles for contact sports. b: The sports goggles optimally brace at the osseous rims of the orbita in a frontal collision, the outwards vaulted glasses do not touch the eye.

13.4.27 Water polo

Water polo has the **most frequent eye injury risk**. Water polo has an 11-times elevated risk (Jendrusch 2004) and clearly ranks above squash (8 times higher). Hands, arms, elbows and balls can injure the eyes mild or moderately. **Large sports goggles** (➤ Fig. 13.8) bracing the orbital bones without pressure on soft parts of the eye – this might in case of collisions increase of the risk of injuries – are strongly recommended.

Similar to swimming **corneal stippling by chlorine** and bacterial or viral **eye infections** are common. **Contact lenses** should be removed after water polo, cleaned and reapplied only after a recreational period.

13.4.28 Winter sports

Skiing goggles or masks offer reasonable eye protection. However, only few **snowboarders** or **figure skaters** wear protection goggles. Lights to moderate contusions are often reported. Optimal visual acuity is pivotal for high-performance skiing (Jendrusch et al. 1999, Senner et al 1999, Jendrusch and Heck 2000).

The **optimal lighting** is important for accident prevention and overall performance. Contrast-improving or light-decreasing goggles or mask offer adequate help (Senner et al. 1999, Lingelbach and Jendrusch 2003).

Contusions of the head and eyes can lead to hemorrhages and even retinal detachment. Draeger and Dupuis found that indirect traumas at vitreous body-retina border can trigger retinal damages or detachments (Draeger and Dupuis 1975). Altered knobs, plates and peaks of skiing sticks can greatly reduce the risk of eye injury.

13.5 Conclusion

Eye injuries in sports are relatively rare (1% of total reported injuries) but have a great impact on physical performance given the importance of vision. **Protective eyewear** can reduce eye injuries more than 90% (Vinger 1990 and 1993, Schnell 1996 and 1997). Hence, athletes that do not require corrective glasses and do practice dangerous sports should wear protection goggles, masks or helmets (Nelson 1970, Schnell 1987, Labelle et al. 1988, Genovese et al. 1990, Erie 1991, Easterbrook 1992, Pashby 1989 and 1992, Vinger 1993, Kahle et al. 1993, Zagelbaum 1993).

Coaches, doctors and officials should make sure those athletes suffering from eye diseases, eye injuries or are recovering from eye surgeries practice sport only with a consulting ophthalmologist.

Athletes at risk such as myopics, athletes suffering from eye diseases as well as athletes with family history of retina-vitreous body diseases should regularly undergo eye examinations. This is equally important for wearers of contact lenses as damages can develop unnoticed.

References

Aburn N (1990). Eye injuries in indoor cricket at Wellington Hospital: a survey January 1987 to June 1989. New Zealand Med J 103 (898): 454–456.
Anders N (1994). Augenverletzungen durch Gotcha. Klein Monatsbl Augenheilkd 204: 54–543.
Applegate RA (1992). Set shot shooting performance and visual acuity in basketball. Optom Vis Sci 69 (10): 765–768.
Carter JB, Parke DW (1987): Unusual retinal tears in an amateur boxer. Arch Opthalmol 105 (8): 1138.
Colin J, Fily J, Bonissent JF (1984). Accidents oculairesde la planche à voile. Presse médicale 13 (4): 224.
Coroneo MT (). An eye for cricket. Ocular injuries in indoor cricketers. Med J Austr 142 (8): 469–471.
Curley MD, Butler FK Jr (1987). Visual reaction time performance preceding CNS oxygen toxicity. Undersea Biomed Research 14 (4): 301–310.
Day RT (1994). Pupil cycle time in the long-term neurologic assessment of divers. Undersea Hyperbaric Med 21 (1): 31–41.
de Lucia PR, Cochran EL (1985). Perceptual information for batting can be extracted throughout a ball's trajectory. Perceptual and Motor Skills 61 (1): 143–150.
Draeger J, Dupius H (1975). Mechanische Faktoren bei der Auslösung der Amotio retinae. Klein Mbl Agenheilk 166: 431-435.
Easterbrook M (1992). Getting patients to protect their eyes during sports. Physic Sportsmed 20 (7): 164–170.
Enzenauer RW, Mauldin WM (1989). Boxing-related ocular injuries in the United States Army, 1980 to 1985. South Med J 82 (5): 547–549.
Erie JC (1991). Eye injuries. Physic Sportsmed 19 (11): 108–122.
Farley KG (1985). Ocular trauma resulting from the explosive rupture of a liquid center golf ball. J Am Optom Assoc 56 (4): 310–314.
Fong LP (1994). Sports-related eye injuries. Med J Austr 160 (12): 743–747.
Genovese MT, Lenzo NP, Lim RK, Morkel DR, Jamrozik KD (1990). Eye injuries among pennant squash players and their attitudes towards protective eyewear. Med J Austr 153 (11, 12): 655–665.
Giovinazzo VJ, Yannuzzi LA, Sorenson JA, Delrowe DJ, Campbell EA (1987). The ocular complications of boxing. Ophthalmol 94 (6): 587–596.
Gregory PT (1986). Sussex Eye Hospital sports injuries.Brit J Ophthalmol 70 (10): 748–750.
Guldner D, Vola JL (1987). Tests ophthalmologiques en plongée profonde à saturation. Bull de Sociétés d Ophthalmol de France 87 (4): 463–465.
Harada T, Hirano K, Ishii M, Ichikawa H (1985). Bilan sur 164 cas des traumatismes oculaires dus à certains sports. J Franc Ophthalmol 8 (6/7): 455–458.
Holden BA, Sweeney DF (1985). Effect of long-term extended contact lens wear on the human cornea. Invest Ohthalmol Vis Sci 26: 1489–1501.
Holland R (1994). Kontaktlinsen beim Tauchsport. Die Kontaktlinse 28 (7-8): 30–35.
Jendrusch G Senner V, Schaff P, Heck H (1999). Vision an Essential Factor for Safety in Skiing: Visual Acuity, Stereoscopic Depth Perception, Effect of Colored Lenses. In: Johnson RJ (ed.). Skiing Trauma and Safety, 12th Volume. ASTM STP 1345, American Society for Testing and Materials, West Conshohocken, PA: pp 23–24
Jendrusch G, Heck H (1999). Bedeutung des visuellen Systems im Zusammenhang mit „Sicherheit im Sport". Sportorthop Sporttraumatolog 15/4: 187–196.
Jendrusch G, Franke C, Heck H, Völker K (2004). Zur Prävention von Augenverletzungen im Squash: Werden Schutzbrillen akzeptiert? In: Institut „Sicher Leben" (ed.). „Mit Sicherheit mehr Sport" Beiträge zum 2. Dreiländerkongress, 26.–27. September 2002 in Wien. Wien, p 141–145.
Jones NP, Tullo AB (1986). Severe eye injuries in cricket. Brit J Sports Med 20 (4): 178-179.
Jones NP (1987). Eye injuries in sport: an increasing problem. Brit J Sports Med 21 (4): 168–170.
Jones NP (1993). Eye injury in sport: incidence, biomechanics, clinical effects and prevention. J Roy Coll Surg Edinburgh 38 (3): 127–133.
Kahle G, Dach Th, Wollensak J (1993). Augenverletzungen beim Squash. Klein Monatsbl Augenheilkd 203: 195–199.
Kirchhoff E, Kroll P (1991). Mit Brille wär' das nicht passiert. TW Sport und Medizin 3: 424–526.

References

Kroll P, Stoll W, Meyer-Rüsenberg H-W (1983). Sportverletzungen am Auge. In: Heck H, Hollmann W, Liesen H, Rost R (eds.). Sport: Leistung und Gesundheit. Dtsch Ärzte-Verlag, Köln, pp 741–746.

Labelle P, Mercier M, Podtetenev M, Trudeau F (1988). Eye injuries in Sports: Results of a five-year study. Physic Sportsmed 16 (5): 126–138.

Lawless M, Porter W, Pountney R, Simpson M (1986). Surfboard-related ocular injuries. Austral New Zeal J Ophthalmol 14 (1): 55–57.

Lingelbach B, Jendrusch G (2005). Contrastenhancing filters in ski sports. Journal of ASTM International 2 (1): 1-8.

Loew T, Zimmermann U, Hummel T, Wildt L (1993). Bungee Jumping. Münch Med Wschr 135 (30/31): 396–399.

MacEwen CJ (1987). Sport-associated eye injury: A casualty department survey. Brit J Ophthalmol 71 (9): 701–705.

MacEwen CJ (1989). Eye injuries: A prospective survey of 5671 cases. Brit J Ophthalmol 73 (11): 888–894.

Maguire JI, Benson WE (1986). Retinal injury and detachment in boxers. Jama 255 (18): 2451–2453.

McWhae J, LaRoche GR (1990). Badminton-related eye injuries. Can J Ophthalmol 25 (3): 170.

Mc Graw MB, Myrtle B. (1935): Growth. A Study of Jonny and Jimmy. New York: Arno Press. In: Winter, R. (1975): Zur Periodisierung der motorischen Ontogenese in der Kindheit und Jugend. Theorie u. Praxis der Körperkultur 24: 39.

Myles WM, Dickinson JD, LaRoche GR (1993). Ice hockey and spectators' eye injuries. New Engl J Med 329 (5): 364

Nelson C (1970). Eye injuries from exploding golf balls. Brit J Ophthalmol 51: 670.

Pashby TJ (1985). Eye injuries in Canadian amateur hockey. Can J Ophthalmol 20 (1): 2–4.

Pashby TJ (1987). Eye injuries in Canadian amateur hockey – still a concern. Can J Ophthalmol 22 (6): 293–295.

Pashby TJ (1988). Ocular injuries in hockey. Internat Ophthalmol Clin 28 (3): 228–231.

Pashby TJ (1989). Eye injuries in sports. J Ophthalmic Nurse Technol 8 (3): 99–101.

Pashby TJ (1992). Eye injuries in Canadian sports and recreational activities. Can J Ophthalmol 27 (5): 226–229.

Pavlidis M, Stupp T, Georgalas I, Georgiadou E, Mosxos M, Thanos S (2004). Intraocular pressure changes during high-altitude acclimatisation. Graefes Arch 04 (07431): 1–22.

Polkinghome PJ Sehmi K, Cross MR, Minassian D, Bird AC (1988). Ocular fundus lesions in divers. Lancet 2 (8625): 1381–1383.

Rapoport I, Romem M, Kinek M, Koval R, Reller J, Belkin M, Yelin N, Yanco L, Savir H (1990). Eye injuries in children in Israel. A nationwide collaborative study. Arch Ophthalmol 108 (3): 376–379.

Reim M (1977). Der Einfluß von Kontaktlinsen auf den Stoffwechsel der Kornea. In: Arbeitskreis Kontaktlinsen des BVA, 4.

Rice R, Allen RC (1986). Yoga in glaucoma. Am J Ophthalmol 100: 738–739.

Rompe G, Rieder H, Klumpp H (1981). Grenzen der Unfallforschung im Schulsport. Dtsch Ztsch Sportmed 32 (8): 222–226.

Scherer K (2005). Persönliche Mitteilung des Fachbereichs Statistik und Epidemiologie des Bundesverbandes der Unfallkassen. Basis: Schülerunfallstatistik.

Schnell D (1987). Verletzungen und andere Affektionen der Augenregion beim Ballsport. Dtsch Zeitschr Sportmed 38 (3): 112–117.

Schnell D (1987). Augenverletzungen, Verletzungsfolgen und andere Affektionen während sportlicher Betätigung. In: Rieckert H (ed.). Sportmedizin Kursbestimmung. Springer, Berlin-Heidelberg.

Schnell DSchnell D (1996). Sehorgan und Sport. In: Bartmus U, Heck H, Schumann H, Tidow G (eds.). Aspekte der Sinnes- und Neurophysiologie im Sport. Verlag Sport und Buch Strauß, pp 175–240.

Schnell D (1997). Das kann ins Auge gehen. Verlag Sport und Buch Strauß, pp 11–90.

Schnell D (2002). Sportophthalmologische Aspekte des Tauchsports. Teil 1. Z Prakt Augenheikd 23: 457–462.

Schnell D (2003). Sportophthalmologische Aspekte des Tauchsports. Teil 2. Z Prakt Augenheikd 23: 27–34.

Schnell D (2003). Sport mit Kontaktlinsen. Z Prakt Augenheikd (ISBN 3-922777-57-0), pp 1–32

Schnell D, Bolsinger A (2009): Augenkrankheiten und organische Einschränkungen beim Sport und Bewegungsunterricht mit Blinden und Sehbehinderten. In: Giese, M. (Hrsg): Sport und Bewegungsunterricht mit Blinden und Sehbehinderten. Band 1: Theoretische Grundlagen und blindenspezifische bzw. adaptierte Sportarten, Schriftenreihe des Behindertensportverbandes NRW „aktiv dabei" Band 1 Meyer und Meyer Verlag (2009) 84–116

Scholz R, Hoffmann H, Duncker G (1991). Reihenuntersuchungen des Blausinnes bei Tauchern mit dem desaturierten Lanthony-15-Hue-Test. Fortschr der Ophthalmol 88 (5): 505–506.

Senner V, Jendrusch G, Schaff P, Heck H (1999). Vision an Essential Factor for Safety in Skiing: Perception, Reaction and Motion Control Aspects. In: Johnson RJ (ed.). Skiing Trauma and Safety, 12th Volume. ASTM STP 1345, American Society for Testing and Materials, West Conshohocken, PA, pp 11–22.

Sherwood DJ (1989). Eye injuries to football players. New Engl J Med 320 (11): 742.

Socks JF (1988). Rigid gas permeable contact lenses in hyperbaric environments. Am J Optom 12.

Toppel L (1972). Augenverletzungen bei Sportunfällen. Med Monatsschr 25 (8): 371–374.

Vinger PF (1990). Prevention of sports injuries. J Ophthal Nurse Technol 9 (5): 210–214.

Vinger PF (1993). Prescribing for contact sports. Optom Clin 3 (1): 129–143.

Wedrich A, Velikay M, Binder S, Radax U, Stolba U, Datlinger P (1993). Ocular findings in asyptomatic amateur boxers. Retina 13 (2): 114–119.

Zagelbaum BM (1993). Sports-related eye trauma. Physic Sportsmed 21 (9): 25–42.

Zagelbaum BM, Hersch PS, Donnenfeld ED, Perry HD, Hochman MA (1994). Ocular trauma in major-league baseball players. New Engl J Med 330 (14): 1021–1023.

Chapter 14

Ears, facial cranium and cervical soft-tissue

Christoph Schlegel-Wagner

14.1 Injuries in the area of the ear

14.1.1 External ear

Auricle

Auricle injuries often occur in **martial arts with body contact**. A blunt trauma already leads to an **othematoma**. In this process, the skin of the anterior auricular surface is sheared off directly from the auricular cartilage below, possibly causing a hemorrhage between these two layers. Othematomas untreated for longer time periods show **cartilage necroses** and also deformations of the auricle afterwards.

> Othematomas need to be decompressed within hours.

Transfixion sutures through the auricle have proven successful in preventing a relapse. Relapsing and untreated othematomas lead to a deformed auricle – the so-called "**cauliflower ear**", e.g. in wrestlers.

An auricle **laceration** or an auricle **avulsion** requires a reconstruction of the auricle within hours in order to protect the exposed cartilage of infections and to induce a cosmetically immaculate wound healing.

External auditory canal

Often only a small contusion mark on the chin is visible in a first examination of the isolated fracture of the auditory canal. At a fall to the chin the jaw condyles are often pushed into the acetabulum of the temporomandibular joint and thus into the osseous parts of the external auditory canal resulting in fracture. Fractures of the auditory canal are also found with **longitudinal fractures of the petrous bone**.

Fractures of the auditory canal are treated by splinting with an ointment strip tamponade. A surgical opening has to be performed if a relevant stenosis persists that leads to the retention of cerumen and repeated otitis externa.

14.1.2 Middle ear

Air in the external auditory canal encased under pressure, e.g. due to a hit to the ear by a ball or a jump into water, leads to a **traumatic tympanic membrane perforation**. Depending on the severity of the trauma, a **dislocation of the auditory ossicles** is also possible. An impalement injury can also lead to a tympanum perforation and a dislocation of the auditory ossicles. Tinnitus and dizziness in addition to a hearing impairment indicates a **stapes dislocation and a perilymphatic fistula**. A perilymphatic fistula has to be sealed up immediately in order to prevent deafness.

Negative pressure in the middle ear, often occurring with a **barotrauma** in diving, can also lead to traumatic tympanic membrane perforation. Insufficient pressure compensation by the auditory tube is the cause for barotraumas of the middle ear. A negative pressure in the middle ear develops here and leads to an exudation from the mucosa and no more than a bleeding into the middle ear. A tympanic membrane perforation is caused by negative pressure occurring very rapidly in very fast submerging and with the stability of the tympanic membrane being exceeded,. Cold water can penetrate into the middle ear and induces a violent **rotatory vertigo** by caloric irritation of the semicircular canals. Panic reactions and emergency ascends endanger the diver of a rupture of the lung or an arterial gas embolism (Klingmann 2004).

Many recent trend sports (paragliding, snowboarding etc.) have led to a important **increase of basal skull fractures** lately. By definition, a **longitudinal fracture of the petrous bone** (➤ Fig. 14.1) runs through the middle ear and leads to conductive hearing impairment. This can either be conditioned by a hematotympanum and/or a dislocation of the auditory ossicles.

A **transverse petrous bone fracture** must be differential-diagnostically distinguished from it. Both fractures can already be differentiated clinically by a simple test with the **tuning fork** (test according to Weber and Rinne) in the emergency examination (➤ Tab. 14.1).

Tab. 14.1 Clinical findings with petrous bone fractures.

	Longitudinal petrous bone fracture	Transverse petrous bone fracture
tympanum	ruptured	often intact
hearing Impairment	conductive hearing impairment	sensorineural hearing impairment
tuning fork: Weber Rinne	in the affected negative	in the healthy ear overhearing into the healthy ear
spontaneous nystagmus	no	into the healthy ear
facial nerve paresis	10–20%	30–40%

> The longitudinal petrous bone fracture runs through the middle ear and leads to a conductive hearing impairment. The transverse petrous bone fracture runs through the internal ear and leads to a sensorineural hearing impairment. Both fractures can be distinguished by means of the tuning-fork test.

In general, the **longitudinal petrous bone fracture** shows:

- overlapping bones in the external auditory canal
- a tympanum perforation and
- a purely sanguineous or liquid-compounded otorrhea (otoliquorrhea).

A **facial nerve paresis** or paralysis develops in 10–20% of the cases.

The tympanic membrane perforation often seals in many cases during the process. Conductive hearing impairment caused by a dislocation of the auditory ossicles can be eliminated by **ossicular chain recontruction**. The clinically suspected persisting CSF leak must be confirmed by identification of β_2 **transferrin or β-trace** in CSF-suspicious secretion. The CSF leak needs to idenfied by high-resolution **computed tomography**.

14.1.3 Internal ear

Barotraumas of the internal ear are less common than those of the middle ear. In general, they are caused by a **forced Valsalva maneuver**. It either leads to a rupture of the round window membrane with perilymphatic fistula or to a bleeding into the labyrinth and to membrane ruptures. The symptoms of an acute **cochleovestibular dysfunction** develop with hearing impairment up to deafness, rotatory vertigo and tinnitus.

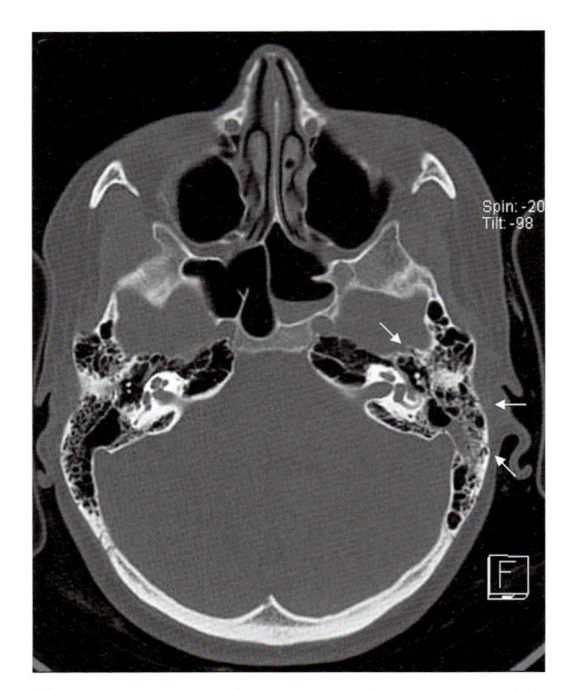

Fig. 14.1 Longitudinal petrous bone fracture left (arrow). Unsuspicious petrous bone right.

14.2 Facial cranium

14.2.1 External soft-tissue

Facial nerve injuries are particular soft-tissue injuries of the face, which should be treated primarily. **Sensory disturbances in the trigeminal area** might also occur, but mostly they have to be seen as an indirect sign for a **midfacial fracture** (Donald 1991).

14.2.2 Midface

Midfacial fractures are caused primarily in team sports (ice hockey, soccer, handball, etc.) as well as in martial arts, and they are classified into central and lateral midfacial fractures.

Central midfacial fractures

Central midfacial fractures range from uncomplicated closed and non-dislocated **nose fractures** to complex **midfacial fractures** with involvement of the frontobasal structures (➤ Tab. 14.2). In addition to the exact external inspection and palpation, an endoscopic exploration is required for all fractures concerning the nose and the paranasal sinuses.

Often, the following is overlooked:
- a septal hematoma
- a septal fracture or
- a rhinoliquorrhea.

It must not be forgotten to test the **sense of smell** in order to register a hyposmia or anosmia. An exact assessment of the fracture process with conventional radiographs is im-

Decompression sickness of the internal ear inducing a sufficient inert gas load of the body and caused by the formation of gas bubbles in the internal ear has to be differentiated in the development mechanism.

A cochleo-vestibular function failure can be caused by a **transverse petrous bone fracture**. At the examination, a sensorineural hearing impairment and a spontaneous nystagmus to the healthy side are found. The tympanum is intact in many cases. A facial nerve paresis or paralysis develops in 30–40% of the cases. A facial nerve paralysis must be considered repeatedly in the course and additionally has to be clarified by means of electroneuronography. If necessary, a surgical decompression or reconstruction of the facial nerve should be considered.

Since a transverse petrous bone fracture runs through the otic capsule (➤ Fig. 14.2), it can heal up **only fibrously**.

> The fracture cleft after a transverse petrous bone fracture never shows an osseous knitting again. There is a life-long danger of otogenic meningitis.

In general, the **safe sealing** by **subtotal petrosectomy** of the due to the transverse fracture already deaf petrous bone the trais recommended in order to prevent the risk of late meningitis (Fisch 1988).

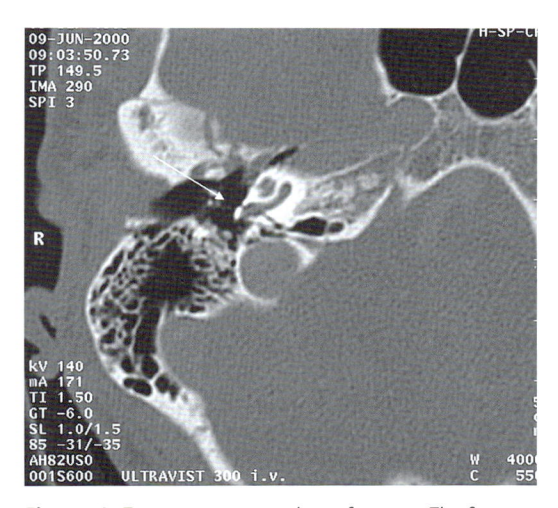

Fig. 14.2 Transverse petrous bone fracture: The fracture is running through the cochlea (arrow).

Tab. 14.2 Midfacial fractures.

Central midfacial fractures	Lateral midfacial fractures
- nasal fractures (without/with septal fracture)	- orbital fractures (isolated/combined)
- naso-ethmoidal fractures	- fractures of the zygomatic bone
- naso-ethmoido-frontal fractures	- fractures of the zygomatic arch
- LeFort's fractures I–III	

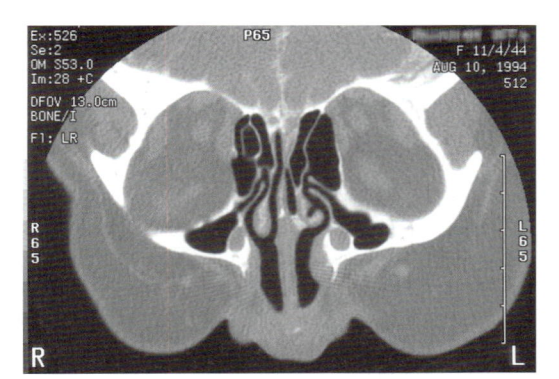

Fig. 14.3 CSF rhinorrhea (left olfactory fissure filled with CSF).

possible in most cases. **Computed tomography** is the imaging of choice. It can be helpful for the diagnosis of suspected **CSF rhinorrhea** at a frontobasal fracture to verify β$_2$ transferrin or β-trace in the nose.

A **CSF leak** can mostly be localized by high-resolution **computed tomography** (➤ Fig. 14.3). For uncertain images, additional examinations by **MRI** (T2 sequence, CISS) or an **intraoperative nose endoscopy** with simultaneous **intrathecal administration of fluorescein** can be helpful (Marshall et al. 1999).

Nose fractures show a wide range of appearances and range from the simple closed or non-dislocated kind to the open comminuted fracture. A nose fracture is primarily diagnosed clinically.

> A typical sign of fracture is the dislocation with tilting or depression of the nasal pyramid.

Overlapping bones can be palpated and a **crepitation** of the fracture fragments can be triggered, at best. Conventional radiographs are only of little significance for the diagnosis and the treatment concept. Complex fractures are examined further by computed tomography (➤ Fig. 14.4).

In addition to the fractures of the osseous nose pyramid, also the **cartilaginous nasal skeleton** must be examined. **Septal fractures** are often missed. With a present caudal nose trauma after a frontal blow to the nose an isolated **caudal septal trauma** is possible. The compressed and fractured cartilaginous septum causes the tip

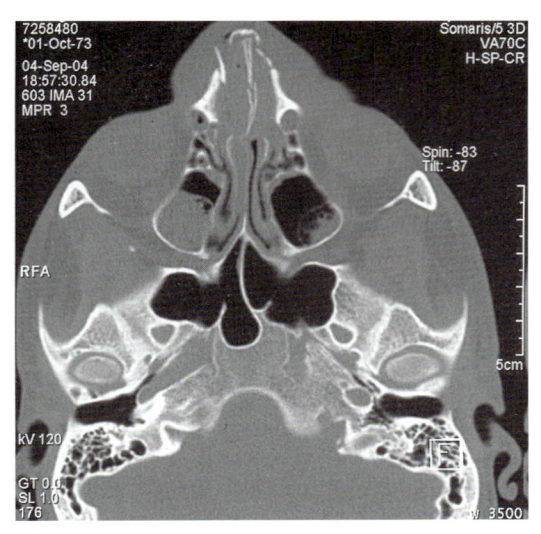

Fig. 14.4 Comminuted nasal fracture (CT in axial sections).

of the nose to lose its support in the long term. This can easily be missed in the first examination, because no fractures exist in the osseous region. A **plunging tip of the nose** is the subsequent result because of the lacking support of the tip of the nose. This ptosis of the tip of the nose leads to a significantly impaired nasal breathing and requires a **surgical restoration**, in which the support of the tip of the nose must be reconstructed by a functional rhinoplasty.

Open nasal fractures and nasal fractures with existence of a **septal hematoma** (➤ Fig. 14.5) must be operated immediately. Otherwise, a septal hematoma can become infected and

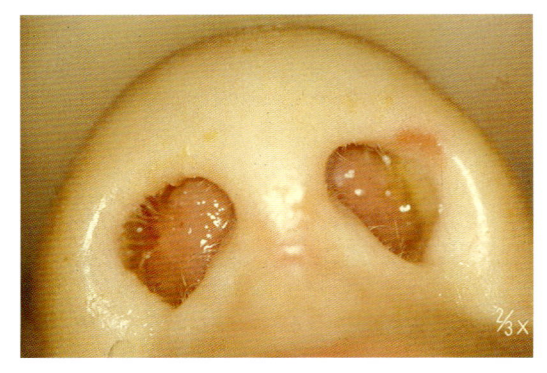

Fig. 14.5 Septal hematoma. The ballooned septum displaces both main nasal cavities.

14.2 Facial cranium

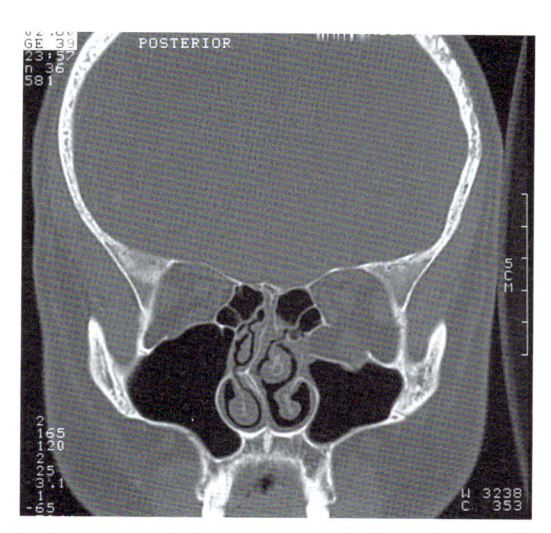

Fig. 14.6 Isolated fracture of the orbital floor, left side (CT scan, coronar section).

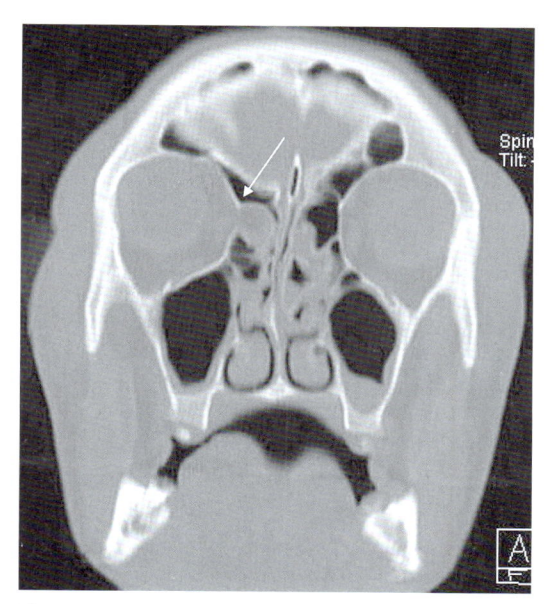

Fig. 14.7 Isolated fracture of the medial orbital wall (lamina papyracea) right-sided with fatty tissue prolapsing into the ethmoid.

lead to a necrosis of the septal cartilage as **septal abscess**. Subsequently, a **saddle nose deformity** develops.

Simple, closed nasal fractures can be reduced ideally in most cases in a detumesced condition, thus 4–5 days after the trauma. A rhinoplasty is carried out secondarily a few months later, nonetheless, with a persisting deformity. **Complex comminuted fractures** will primarily be treated openly with a **rhinoplasty**.

Lateral midfacial fractures

The lateral midfacial fractures apply to the **zygomatic bone**, the **zygomatic arch** and the **orbital cavity** (Rowe 1985).

Clinical indications are:

- asymmetry of the facial contour
- hypesthesia of the infraorbital nerve
- double vision at dysmotility of the eyes
- trismus and
- malocclusions.

Conventional cranial radiographs provide a rough overview and are amended by **computed tomography** in order to be able to diagnose the exact fracture process.

An **isolated fracture of the orbital floor** ("blow-out fracture") develops due to a **collision of a tennis ball with the eye**, for example (➤ Fig. 14.6). Less often, also the **medial orbital wall** can be affected in the area of the lamina papyracea (➤ Fig. 14.7). Today these isolated fractures of the medial orbital wall can be elegantly treated endoscopically (➤ Fig. 14.8 a and b, see page 172).

14.2.3 Lower jaw

Fractures of the lower jaw mainly develop after a direct trauma (blow/fall). Primarily, the main symptoms are the **blocked mouth opening** and the **disturbed occlusion**. Fractures of the lower jaw require **surgery**. **Concomitant injuries of the cervical soft-tissue**, especially laryngeal injuries, must be ruled out because of the severity of the triggering trauma. Fractures of the lower jaw often are combined with laryngeal fractures, especially with injuries triggered by a kick of a horse (Kuttenberger et al. 2004).

Clinical **guiding symptoms** of laryngeal fractures are **stridor, dyspnea and skin emphysemas**.

14.2.4 Oral cavity

In addition to **tooth injuries**, **bite injuries** affect the tongue in the area of the mouth after falls. Sticks (e.g. in ice hockey) can lead to **impalement traumas** in the palatal area.

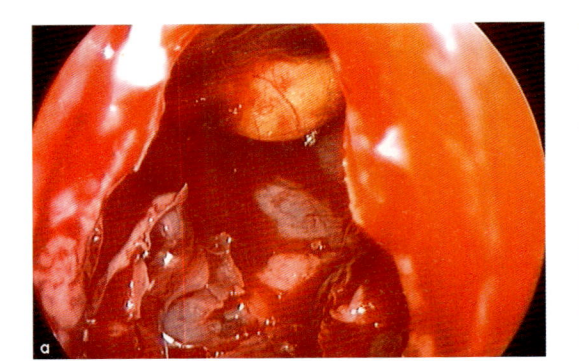

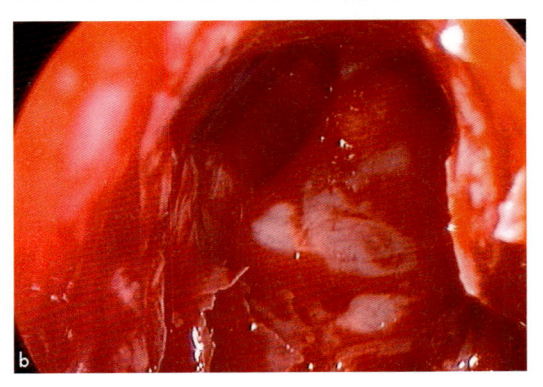

Fig. 14.8 Intraoperative findings of a fracture of the medial orbital wall (lamina papyracea). a: Opened ethmoid with prolapsed orbital fatty tissue. b: Reconstruction of the medial orbital wall with PDS screen after repositioning the prolapsed fatty tissue.

14.3 Cervical soft-tissue

14.3.1 Soft-tissue injuries

In addition to the superficial injuries as well as the **injuries of the cervical vessels**, also caudal **cranial nerves** and nerves of the cervical and brachial plexus can be affected. Special attention has to be paid to lesions of the

- accessory nerve
- the vagus nerve and the recurrent laryngeal nerve and the
- phrenic nerve.

Additionally, **intimal lesions of the carotid artery** (Cox 1986) are feared after stroke trauma (e.g. karate).

14.3.2 Larynx

Comminuted laryngeal fractures (➤ Fig. 14.9) might lead immediately to a dramatic disorder with danger of suffocation, which necessitates an **emergency cricothyrotomy or tracheotomy** (Fuhrmann 1990, Schaefer 1992).

> Even for seemingly negligible laryngeal contusions the risk of an obstructing endolaryngeal swelling – even after hour trauma – must be considered.

An **external laryngeal injury** is suspected because of the following guiding symptoms:

- for light injuries
  - hoarseness
  - dyspnea
  - irritation of the throat
  - odynophagia

- for more serious injuries
  - stridor and dyspnea
  - increasing pain
  - aphonia and
  - hemoptysis.

An external contusion mark or an external soft-tissue injury, a relieve posture of the head and, above all, a **subcutaneous air emphysema** must be looked for in the **clinical examination**. The endolarynx is assessed **fiber optic nasal endoscopy**. **Computer tomography** of the lar-

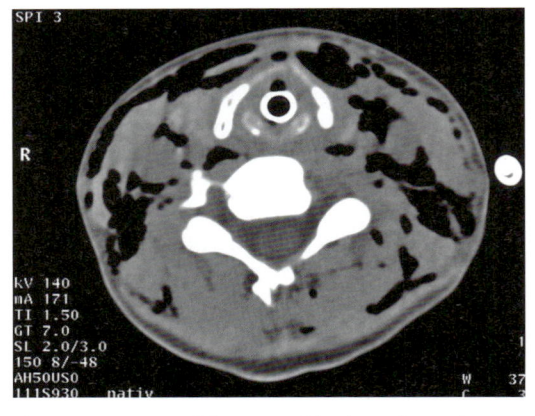

Fig. 14.9 Laryngeal fracture with clear air emphysema of cervical soft tissue.

Tab. 14.3 Classification of the laryngeal trauma according to the degree of severity of the injury (modified according to Fuhrmann and Schaefer).

Degree of severity of the injury	Symptoms
I	■ external contusion mark ■ endolaryngeal mucosal hematoma
II	■ edema ■ hematoma ■ superficial mucosal lesion and/or ■ non-displaced, isolated fracture
III	■ dislocated fracture ■ massive edema ■ mucosal rupture ■ endolaryngeal free cartilage ■ arrest of the vocal folds
IV	■ comminuted laryngeal fracture
V	■ aryngotracheal separation

ynx amends the examination, so that the degree of severity of the laryngeal injury can be defined eventually (➤ Tab. 14.3).

> **Summary**
>
> The most frequent injury of the auricle is the othematoma. A deformity of the auricle is prevented by surgery. A longitudinal fracture of the petrous bone causes a conductive hearing impairment; a transverse fracture of the petrous bone causes a sound-perceiving impairment. These can easily be distinguished clinically by a tuning fork test. In addition, a facial nerve paresis or CSF otorrhea must be considered in petrous bone fractures. In diving, the barotraumas of the middle ear, the barotraumas of the internal ear and the decompression sickness of the internal ear have to be distinguished. Midfacial fractures range from the uncomplicated closed and non-displaced nasal fracture to the complex midfacial fracture with involvement of the frontobasal structure. Although a fracture of the osseous nasal pyramid is clinically evident, a caudal fracture of the nasal septum is often being ignored. A nasal septal hematoma and an open nasal fracture require an immediate surgical treatment. Eye motility disorders and malocclusions must be looked for with midfacial fractures. In general, a CSF rhinorrhea appears with the involvement of the frontobasal structure. In addition, a hyposmia or anosmia is apparent. In a trauma of the cervical soft tissue, a laryngeal injury must be looked for or has to be ruled out, primarily. Additionally, lesions of the caudal cranial nerves and the large cervical vessels can occur.

References

Cox JN (1986). Full-contact et aneurisme dissequant de l'artère carotid interne thrombosée avec ramolissement cerebral. Schweiz Med Wochenschrift 116: 1687–1692.

Donald PJ (1991). The management of soft tissue trauma to face and neck. In: Paparella MM, Shumrick DA, Gluckmann JL, Meyerhoff WL (eds.). Otolaryngoly, 3rd ed., Vol. IV. Saunders, Philadelphia.

Fisch U, Mattox D (1988). Microsurgery of the Skull Base. Thieme, Stuttgart, New York.

Fuhrmann GM, Stieg FH, Buerk CA (1990). Blunt laryngeal trauma: classification and management protocol. J Traumatol 30: 87–92.

Klingmann C, Wallner F (2004). Tauchmedizinische Aspekte in der HNO-Heilkunde. HNO 52: 757–769.

Kuttenberger J, Hardt N, Schlegel C (2004). Diagnosis and initial management of laryngotracheal injuries associated with facial fractures. J Craniomaxillofrac Surg 32: 80–84.

Marshall AH, Jones NS, Robertson IJA (1999). An algorithm for the management of CSF rhinorrhoea illustrated by 36 cases. Rhinology 37: 182–185.

Rowe NL, Williams JL (1985). Maxillofacial injuries. Churchill Livingstone, Edinburgh.

Schaefer SD (1992). The acute management of external laryngeal trauma. Arch Otolaryngol 118: 598–604.

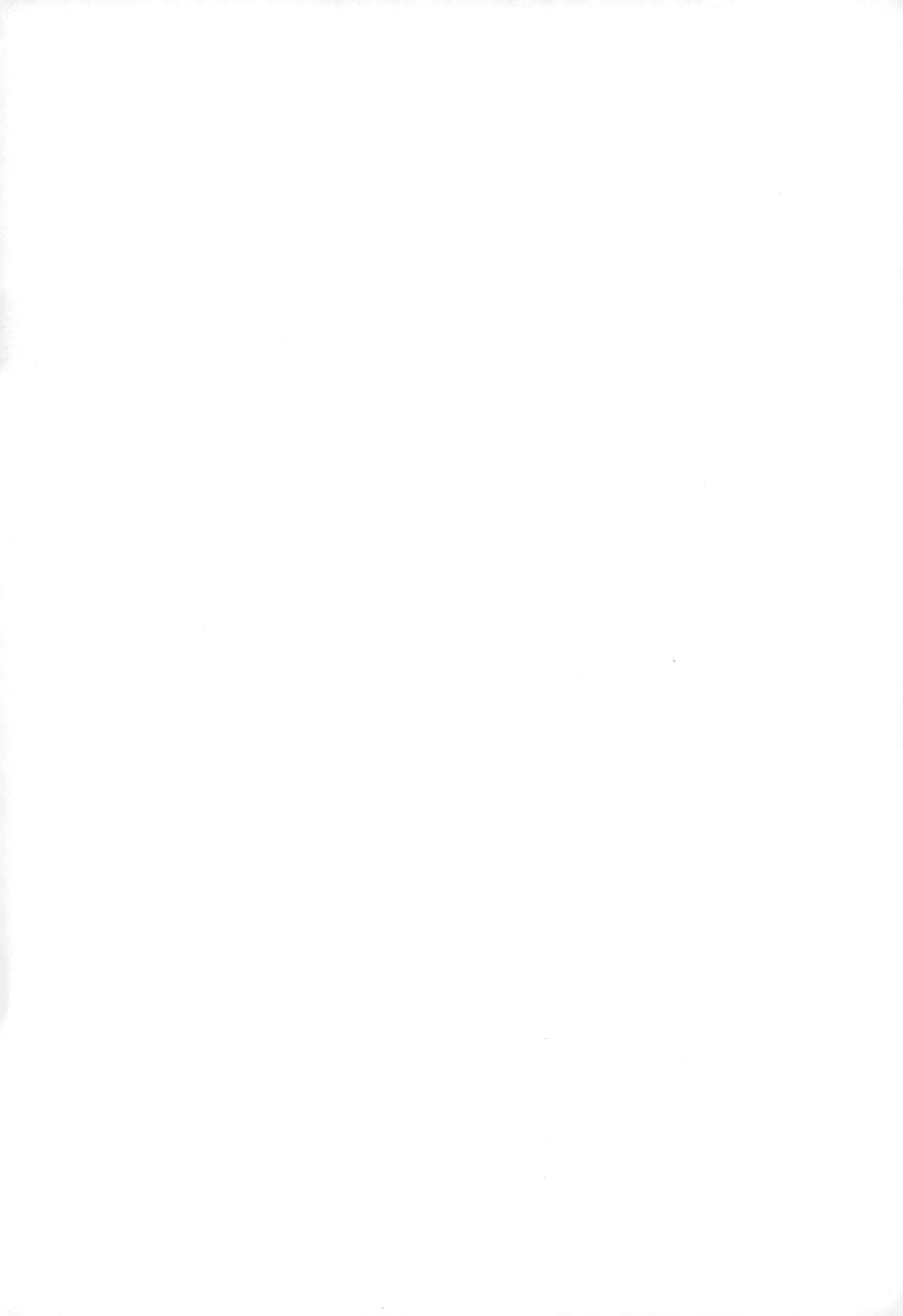

Chapter 15 Shoulder joint

Klaus Dann and Gernot Sperner

15.1 Arthroscopic minimally invasive procedures

Klaus Dann

15.1.1 Epidemiology of shoulder injuries

New sports such as mountain biking, snowboarding, kite- or windsurfing, inline skating, but also the overhead ball-racquet sports or swimming sports especially lead to many acute injuries and chronic medical conditions. 5 to 8% of all acute injuries of the human body affect the shoulder joint; about 3% are overuse impairments (Steinbrück 1999). Primarily active male athletes from puberty to the 45th year of age suffer acute shoulder injuries. 30% of all acute shoulder injuries are dislocations mainly in sport-active men of the age of 35 years and younger. In 95% of the cases, the dislocations are anterior, in 3% they are posterior, and in about 2% of the cases the instabilities are multidirectional.

Concomitant injuries of the rotator cuff in line with dislocations are possible starting with the age of 35 years, and therefore they always must be ruled out. Further 20% of the acute shoulder injuries affect the shoulder joint and the clavicle. Fractures of the humeral head are primarily found in connection with high speed traumas in sports. Fractures of the shoulder blades and injuries of the sternoclavicular joint are rare. Most often, the subacromial impingement is found in diverse forms in older sport-active patients. Instability-associated kinds of impingement and the biceps-tendon pathologies of the SLAP lesion or even the biceps pulley lesion are hard to diagnose clinically.

15.1.2 Shoulder dislocation and instability

The shoulder instability shows an incidence of 2% of the general population and thus represents the classic young persons' injury suffered during sports and recreation (Hovelius 1978 and 1982, Hovelius et al. 1996). Causes of injuries can be the classic external rotation-abduction injuries, direct traumas and also repetitive micro-traumatisms eventually leading to instability.

An exact definition of the injury and classification are important for the treatment and the indication of surgery. In addition to the simplified Anglo-American classification into TUBS (traumatically caused instability) and AMBRII (atraumatically conditioned instability) (Matson et al. 1990), the classification according to Gerber has proved successful in the European area, because the hyperlaxation has been incorporated here (➤ Tab. 15.1; Gerber 1997).

Anamnesis, imaging by radiographs in three layers, sonography and contrast MRI, if required, lead to an exact diagnosis.

Table 15.1 Classification of the instability according to Gerber (Gerber 1997).

type I	hooked dislocation
type II	unidirectional instability without hyperlaxation
type III	unidirectional instability with hyperlaxation
type IV	multidirectional instability without hyperlaxation
type V	multidirectional instability with hyperlaxation
type VI	arbitrary dislocation

Indications and methods of arthroscopic stabilization

Open and arthroscopic procedures are available as surgical techniques: **posttraumatic unidirectional initial dislocations or few relapsing dislocations** are suitable for arthroscopic stabilization.

The ideal patient is young with primarily traumatic initial dislocation with anterior instability, a defined stable labral avulsion identified with athroscopy, missing or only minor ligament, or capsule laxation (Habermeyer 1995, Resch (1) (2) 1995). According to literature, te purely conservative treatment of such young athletes leads to relapse in more than 80-95%, according to literature (Henry and Genung 1982, Wheeler et al. 1989, Norlin 1993, Jakobsen and Sojberg 1996, Sunder and Jakobsen 1997). Therefore, a primary care of this instability would be vindicated, but is not mandatory. Cause of a traumatic instability without hyperlaxation **(type II according to Gerber)** is a trauma with extreme external rotation and abduction injuring the anatomic structures such as IGHL and MGHL (inferior and medial glenohumeral ligaments) as well as the labrum.

The traumatic instability with existing hyperlaxation **(type III according to Gerber)** is mostly caused by external rotation abduction traumas of minor extent. The examination of these patients in lateral comparison often show positive laxation tests and the sulcus sign, but without the classic stability tests such as apprehension and relocation tests being positive. That means, the affected shoulder had been well compensated and stable until the accident. The present injury very often causes re-dislocations. These chronic symptomatic subluxations are very cumbersome for the patients and reduce their capacity especially in overhead sports.

Indications for the arthroscopic stabilization with traumatic instability:

1. Traumatic initial dislocation in patients under 30 years of age with high athletic demands
   - detection of a Hill-Sachs dent
   - detection of a Bankart's Perthes lesion in contrast enhanced MRI
   - elimination of a hyperlaxation
2. Chronic-relapsing traumatic dislocation with and without hyperlaxation with sufficient consistency of the capsule-labrum complex (IGHL and MGHL)
   - no osteochondral limbus impairment or fracture of the socket edge
   - correct socket geometry with retroversion of the socket
3. Symptomatic subluxation.

Contra-indications for arthroscopic stabilization are:

- the large osseous Bankart's defect (Bankart 1932)
- "engaging Hill-Sachs dent" with clasping mechanism
- hypoplasia or missing labrum, destruction of IGHL or MGHL
- HAGL (humeral avulsion injury of the glenohumeral ligaments)
- arbitrary instability (type VI according to Gerber).

The **thread-anchor technique** has clearly established as the method of choice in the last few years because of the rapid development of tearproof, biodegradable thread anchors or even knotless anchors equipped with one or two highly tearproof color-coded threads and according thread-return instruments. The ventral instrumentation and the high tear resistance of the implants with the option of involving the capsule-labrum complex into the stabilization are advantages of this method (➢ Fig. 15.1 a–c; Habermeyer 1995, Dann et al. 2002 and 2004).

The arthroscopic stabilization of the **atraumatic anterior lower instability** is still debatable; the relatively high recurrence rates are the reason. An insufficient IGHL with impaired flexibility and too deep insertion of the IGHL at the scapular neck often accompany this atraumatic instability **(type III according to Gerber)**. This often results in development of a large anterior dislocation pouch. It is congenital with atraumatic instability, while this pouch seems to be acquired by relapsing dislocation in the traumatic instability. The **multidirectional instability (type IV and V according to Gerber)**

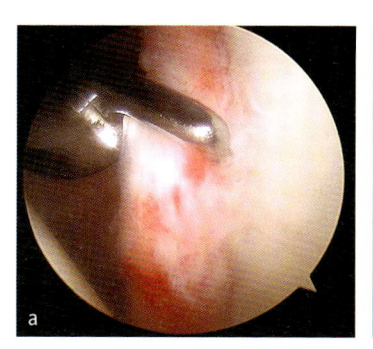

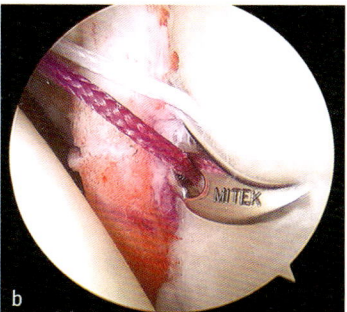

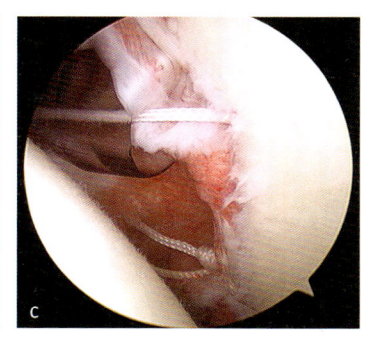

Fig. 15.1 Arthroscopic Bankart surgery with thread anchor technique (image + Lupine Loop anchor system, Mitek company). a: Relocating of the mobile capsule-labrum complex. b: Perforation of the capsule-labrum complex to be refixed by "retrograde" (Sixter) and recirculation of the thread. c: Fixation of the capsule-labrum complex by sliding-knot technique.

with possible dislocations in several directions must be distinguished here. The instability of the opposing side, which can be proved by positive laxation tests, is also important. A strict surgery prohibit exists for the arbitrary multi-directional instability (type VI according to Gerber).

It must be the **aim of arthroscopic stabilization** to remove the dislocation pouch by tightening, to anatomically reconstruct and shorten the IGHL, to elevate it to glenoid level and to refix it at the limbus (concomitant changes such as the rotator interval and the Weitbrecht foramen, but also the posterior capsule laxation should be included into the surgical treatment). The re-fixation technique is mostly carried out by different thread-anchor systems similar to the posttraumatic instability, as described above. A sufficient tightening can be achieved by doubly loaded color-coded thread pairs and mattress and circular sutures.

The **open procedure with capsular shift** (Neer and Foster 1980) and capsular lamination is still applied widely.

Laser and electrothermal methods (capsular shrinking)

High frequency bicoagulation provides clear advantages over laser treatment of the capsular tissue. New temperature controls in these instruments prevent an overheating of the tissue. The electrothermic procedures with high frequency bicoagulators allow a shrinking of the widened capsule by application of heat. Indications for the use of capsular shrinking would be the multidirectional instability with subluxation or instability-associated impingement. However, the problem of those techniques is the exact assessment of the extent of shrinking, which is difficult to acquire subjectively but can only be acquired empirically; therefore, the arthroscopic capsule placation is still preferred by many shoulder surgeons.

After-treatment after stabilizing procedures

Postoperatively, the patients receive a shoulder ligature for 4 weeks, day and night, although the design of the ligature has to be reconsidered(Itoi et al. 2001). Bearing the arm in neutral position seems to be reasonable in the conservative method after trauma as well as after postoperative immobilization (➢ Fig. 15.2).

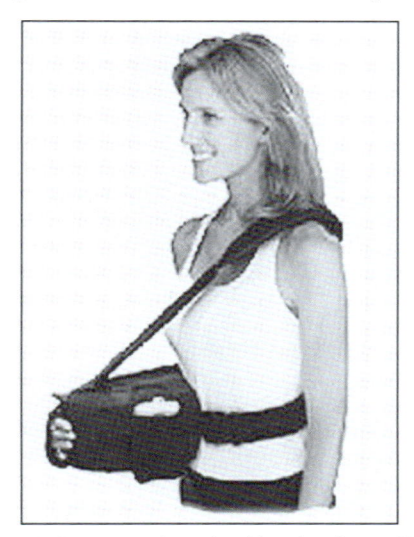

Fig. 15.2 Postoperative shoulder bandage: Neutral Wedge (Breg company).

Active exercises for elbow and wrist, such as swinging exercises beginning with the first postoperative day are permitted. Anteversion up to 60°, retroversion up to 30° and abduction to 60° at most may often be carried out passively until the end of the 4th week. External rotations are strictly forbidden for 6 weeks. Retraction of the shoulder with stretching of the pectoral muscle and strengthening of the scapular fixators is important. A sport prohibition for overhead or contact sports is required for 6 months, for all other sports for 4 months.

15.1.3 Impingement and injuries of the rotator cuff

Rotator cuff rupture and instability impingement

The incidence of rotator cuff ruptures in the individual decades of life has been specified very differently. Degeneration of the cuff startsnat the age of 30 years and successively increases. Particularly the minor perfusion of the tendon tissue close to the insertion promotes the increasing rotator cuff insufficiency. 50% of the ruptures are of atraumatic genesis. The combination of outlet impingement and secondary rupture is frequent.

Ruptures of purely traumatic genesis are rare and occur in only 8% of the cases, according to literature, often combined with dislocations in patients of 40 years and older. The subscapular rupture is caused by a trauma in 70% and is not recognized primarily in 50% of the cases. More often, a trauma at a degeneratively pre-damaged cuff leads to the rupture of the supra- and/or infra-spinal tendon. The "suspension bridge" model of S. Burkhart describes very well the function of the rotator cuff and why some ruptures have hardly any effect on the shoulder function (1993).

Classification of rotator cuff ruptures:

The classification is done by

- localization: a – particulate, b – bursa-sided, c – complex
- size: specification in cm
- number of involved tendons
- retraction degree of the tendon.

Often a **combination of instability with subacromial impingement** is found in overhead sports.

The **classification** of Jobe and Kvitne (1989) provides the following classification of the painful shoulder injuries in overhead sports:

- group 1: primary outlet impingement, caused by the subacromial bow
- group 2: primary instability – secondary impingement, caused by relapsing micro-traumas
- group 3: primary instability – secondary impingement, caused by general hyperlaxation
- group 4: instability caused by macro-trauma, no impingement

Indications for the surgical treatment of rotator cuff ruptures are clearly defined:

- absolute indication:
  - traumatic isolated subscapular rupture (acute case must be treated within 4 weeks)
  - traumatic rotator cuff rupture without pre-damage with functional failure of the shoulder
  - rotator cuff rupture after shoulder dislocation at employable age with good compliance
- relative indication:
  - acute rotator cuff rupture with degenerative pre-damage
  - deep joint-sided supraspinal rupture.

The **surgical treatment** can be carried out as open technique, as mini-open repair or as arthroscopic repair. The open technique has been replaced by mini-open repair technique almost completely; an open procedure is only necessary with tendon transfer surgeries. It is possible to sufficiently carry out rotator cuff sutures increasingly by endoscope due to improvement of thread anchor, thread material and knotting techniques with the double-row fixation called "suture bridging" and especially the instruments. In addition, intraoperative criteria such as size of the tear, shape of the tear, solid stable edge, easily mobilizable and retractable tendon determine the proceeding. Furthermore, the factors of surgical experi-

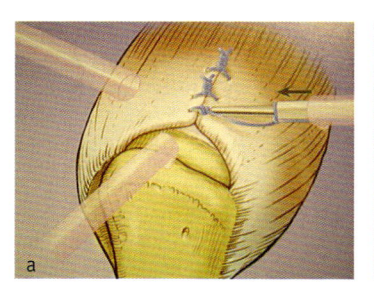

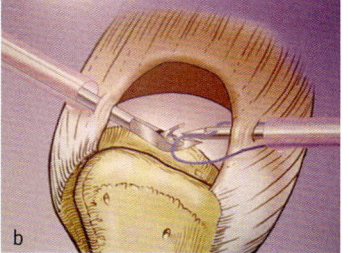

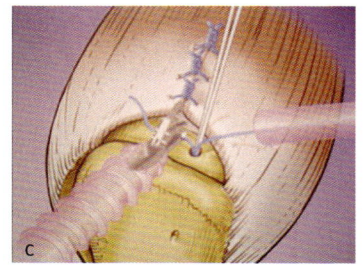

Fig. 15.3 Arthroscopic treatment of the rotator cuff. a: Arthroscopic RM suture technique. b: Arthroscopic RM side-to-side sutures. c: Arthroscopic RM sutures thread anchor technique.

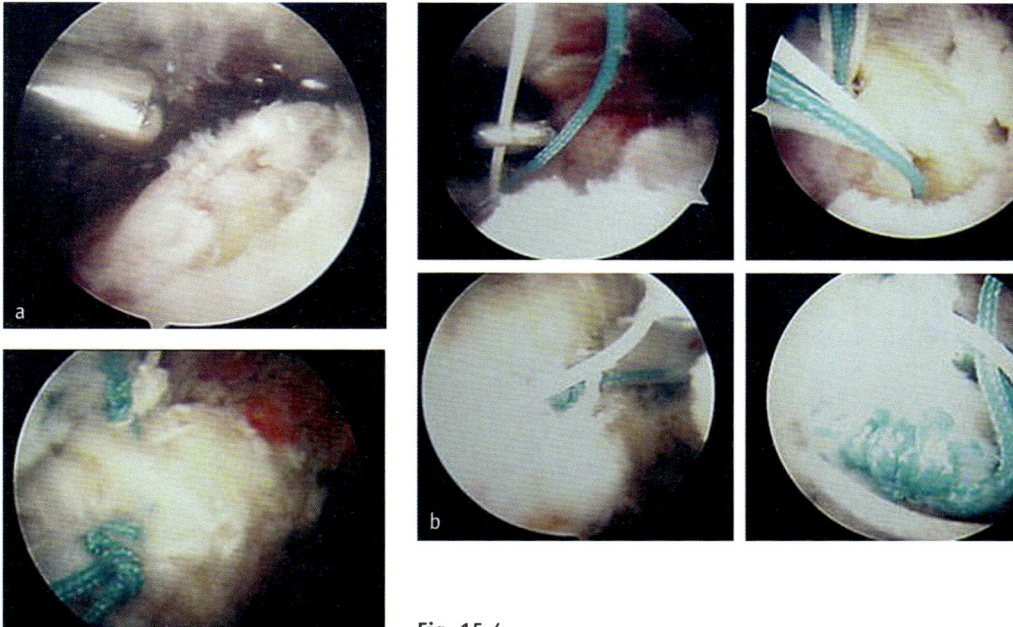

Fig. 15.4 Arthroscopic thread-anchor technique from the arthroscopic view.

ence, time, expenses and set-up in the operating room play a major role (➤ Fig. 15.3 a–d and ➤ Fig. 15.4 a–c).

Without these conditions being fulfilled, the mini-open repair is the preferred method.

The torn rotator cuff should be reinserted; the bursa does not play a role and is remoed in the open techniques as well as in the endoscopic procedures. The less the deltoid muscle is disturbed, the better the shoulder works; a tension-free closure is the condition for the healing. Tendon transfer surgeries are extra-anatomic compromises in order to replace non-reconstructable cuffs;, and should not be applied in athletes. Acromioplasty can be necessary – either isolated or combined with the closure of the tendon defect. With pronounced deforming painful arthroses of the acromioclavicular joint, a resection of both joint surfaces must be done at the same time as a planing of the lower contour, a so-call coplaning. A sole ASD (arthroscopic subacromial decompression) is strongly contra-indicated for instability-associated types of impingement as it does not remove the cause of the medical condition.

Post-treatment, the arm is immobilized in neutral position with a shoulder-arm bandage at an abduction of 15° and an anteversion of 15°. On the 3rd day, passively led movements out of the bandage can be performed. The extent is increased step by step with the aim of achieving a passive elevation of 120° between the 3rd and 6th week, depending on the reinsertion technique. After the 6th week, the arm is released for active mobilization. Without reconstruction of the cuff, the shoulder mobilization increases rapidly.

Functional internal impingement

With the **posterosuperior impingement** (Walch et al. 1992), hyperlax athletes show an increased translation of the humeral head in rotation movements to anteroinferior. As a result, a close contact of the rotator cuff with the glenoid is caused posterosuperiorly in forced external rotation. In further consequence, this leads to a joint-sided impairment of the rotator cuff or to a cartilage and capsule-labrum lesion in the sense of an internal posterosuperior impingement.

With the **anterosuperior impingement** (Burkhart and Morgan 1998), the external rotation position required of overhead athletes in throwing movements additionally leads to a shortening of the posterior parts of the capsule and therefore to an anterosuperior translation of the humeral head. This leads to an impairment of the rotator interval below the coracoacromial bow. The rotator interval is formed of the edge of the subscapularis tendon, the supraspinatus tendon, the superior glenohumeral ligament, the coracohumeral ligament and the long biceps tendon. Therefore, this intraarticular part of the long biceps tendon is lead to the osseous sulcus in a sling; it is also called a biceps pulley.

Not every acutely occurring shoulder pain caused by a relative instability or a lesion of the rotator cuff requires a surgical therapy. Rather, **conservative measures** are indicated – initially by a local antiphlogistic and drug-induced therapy, later by movement exercises and muscle increase. A harmonization of the movement process consisting of an activation of the depressors of the humeral head on the one hand and the rotator cuff on the other hand for the elevation must be restored. Additionally, the synergy between rotator cuff and the deltoid muscle tomuld be exercised. The stretching of the posterior capsular parts and the strengthening of the capsular fixators are of major importance.

Differential diagnoses must not be neglected. A lower cervical syndrome caused by an extradural space-consuming lesion in the C4/C5 area of the cervical spine, shoulder pain with internal diseases or polymyalgia rheumatic have to be thought of as reasons for therapy resistance.

15.1.4 Lesions of the upper labrum-biceps-tendon complex

Andrews lesion

This injury mostly occurring in young overhead throwers shows a **traumatic detachment of the anterosuperior labrum** (Andrews et al. 1985). Because of repeated traction loads at the long biceps tendon, a detachment of the labrum that is less vascularized at this point occurs at the maximum lunge movement. This injury with the symptoms of anterosuperior instability should be taken seriously in young athletes, and it requires surgical stabilization by arthroscopy with refixation of the labrum by thread-anchor technique.

The anatomic norm variants, such as the "sublabral hole" in the 1:00 position and the Buford complex with the labrum missing in the same position and the LGHM inserting directly at the biceps anchor or osseously at the glenoid, respectively, have to be distinguished from this.

SLAP lesion

These **"superior labrum anterior to posterior" lesions** appear with an incidence of 3.9–10% in shoulder arthroscopies (Snyder et al. 1990). Possible reason is heterotopic trauma with fall on the extended arm or flexed elbow with compression or cranial subluxation of the humeral head or an external rotation abduction trauma in combination with a classic Bankart lesion. The SLAP lesion is an overuse disorder in throwers due to traction and shearing forces. Torsion forces at the long biceps tendon can also lead to a posterior SLAP lesion by transferring to posterosuperior.

In addition to an exact anamnesis, clinical tests such as the specific O'Brian's test, the speed-up test and the Yergason test indicate this lesion. The posterosuperior impingement can be detected by relocation test. The arthro-MRI is a highly relevant imaging procedure for the examination of the upper labral pathologies. Still, arthroscopy gives information about the exact lesion type.

The most common classification is the one according to S. Snyder (➤Tab. 15.2; Snyder et al. 1990).

Surgical treatment of the lesions of the upper labral complex, such as the biceps anchor, can only be carried out as arthroscopic technique, where special ventro- and dorsocranial accesses are necessary in order to refix the biceps anchor in the front and in the back with thread anchors or tacs, respectively. We prefer thread anchors for this technique exclusively. The knotting and thread-anchor technique is carried out the same way as in stabilization surgery (➤ Fig. 15.5 a–d).

Table 15.2 Classification of SLAP lesions according to Snyder et al. (1990).

type I	fraying of the superior labrum + biceps anchor without detachment
type II	detachment of the superior labrum-biceps complex to cranial
type III	superior part of the labrum with intact biceps anchor, folded into the joint like a bucket-handle
type IV	Longitudinal fission of the biceps tendon with dislocation of a labrum-biceps part into the joint

An immobilization for three weeks in a shoulder bandage follows postoperatively. Active flexion in the elbow against resistance and supination should be avoided for 6 weeks. Depending on the discipline, sport is allowed only after 3 or after 6 months for contact sports respectively.

15.1.5 Dislocations of the acromioclavicular joint

Injuries of the acromioclavicular joint (AC joint) primarily develop due to a fall to the extended arm held in front as well as due to direct impact traumas, typically suffered in falls from the bicycle.

The **injury** is **classified of** by the extent of the ligament injury in **Tossy degree I–III** and according to **Rockwood I–VI** with involvement of the muscle insertions and the rare kinds of posterior dislocation of the lateral clavicula as well as the theoretical option of a subacromial one.

The **indications for surgery** must be discussed individually with the athlete. In general, surgical treatment is indicated with a lesion of Tossy III and higher (relative indication) or Rockwood IV (dorsal dislocation of the clavicula) and V (additional avulsion of the muscle sling of deltoid and trapezius muscle with consecutive horizontal and vertical instability). We prefer the mini-open repair technique with a small pulley system into the base of the coracoid process and transosseous refixation of the clavicula as well as augmentation of the ligaments by tear-proof thread material. This technique can be carried out with endoscopical assistance now using new tear-proof threads; it is very

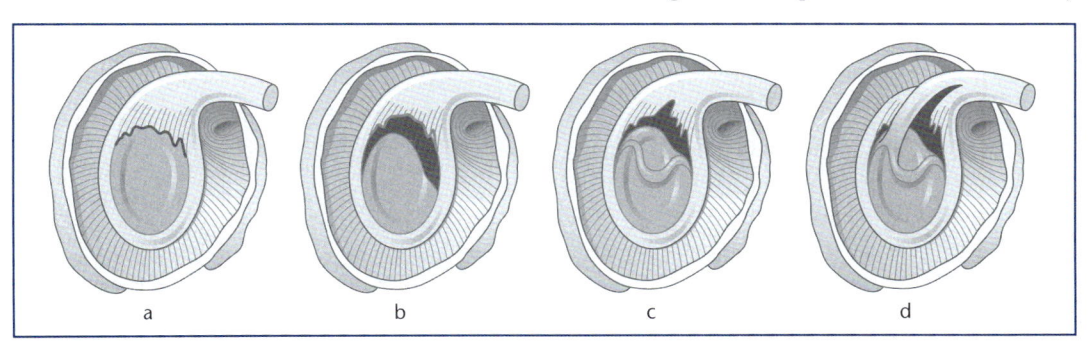

Fig. 15.5 Arthroscopic treatment of an SLAP-II lesion. a: 0-debridement. b: Refixation. c: Resection of the flap. d: Refixation and resection (according to Snyder et al. 1990).

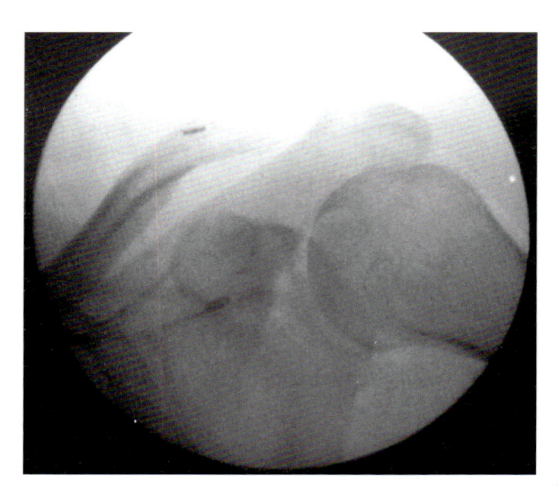

Fig. 15.6 Minimally invasive stabilization of the AC joint by pulley system.

time-consuming and difficult, though (➢ Fig. 15.6).

15.1.6 Fractures of the proximal humerus

5% of all extremity fractures are fractures of the humeral head. Mostly, high speed traumas are the cause for these fractures in athletes younger than 45 years. Trivial falls often lead to multi-fragment fractures (osteoporosis) in the over-60-year-olds. The dislocated multi-fragment fractures of active employed persons engaging in sport activities are a therapeutic challenge. The vitality of the humeral head depends on the supply via both tubercula, because there is no central vessel. The risk of a necrosis of the head increases with the number of dislocated fragments. This was also considered in the classification of the fractures of the humeral head according to Habermeyer, a combination of Neer and AO classification. A four-fragment fracture therefore presents a primarily avascular fracture; it must be treated extremely carefully and the soft-tissue must be protected as much as possible.

With the indication for **surgical stabilization** and therefore for early functional after-treatment, the fractures must be treated as early as possible. Generally all fractures that involve rejections of the contour of the humeral head or the actual joint surface are treated surgically.

Subcapital fractures without gomphosis at the transition to the shaft are also treated surgically, because a conservative therapy would require an immobilization for 6–8 weeks. The repositioning and screw connections of isolated avulsions of the tubercula are technically challenging, but may be carried out in many cases covered and minimally invasive (➢ Fig. 15.7 a–d).

With fractures in the collum chirurgicum, but also with reconstructive osteosyntheses of multi-fragment fractures, the angle-solid proximal humeral plate that has been developed for these problem fractures especially is employed here (➢ Fig. 15.7 e–i).

Today, the indication for **conservatively immobilizing procedures** is set rather tightly, because the glenohumeral joint tends to become stiff very quickly. Fractures with the contour of the humeral head and the position of the tubercula allowing a humeroscapular slipping without impingement syndrome can be treated conservatively. Furthermore, the fractures must be firm enough for a conservative therapy, so that an exercise treatment can begin after recession of the first pain phase. The non-displaced fractures of the tuberculum majus belong to this indication, as well.

The **after-treatments** after conservative and surgical therapy are similar. During the first pain phase, the shoulder joint is immobilized by a shoulder-arm bandage; in addition to ice-onlays, analgetics are given. The exercise treatment of physiotherapy starts on the 3rd day and takes weeks to months for all proximal humerus fractures.

Summary

As in the knee joint, the minimally invasive technique has gained acceptance for the shoulder. The endoscopic procedure for the treatment of the instability, the biceps tendon pathologies and the rotator cuff ruptures as well as covered repositioning and osteosynthesis with the new angle-solid implants have added fundamentally to the rapid return of patients to sports.

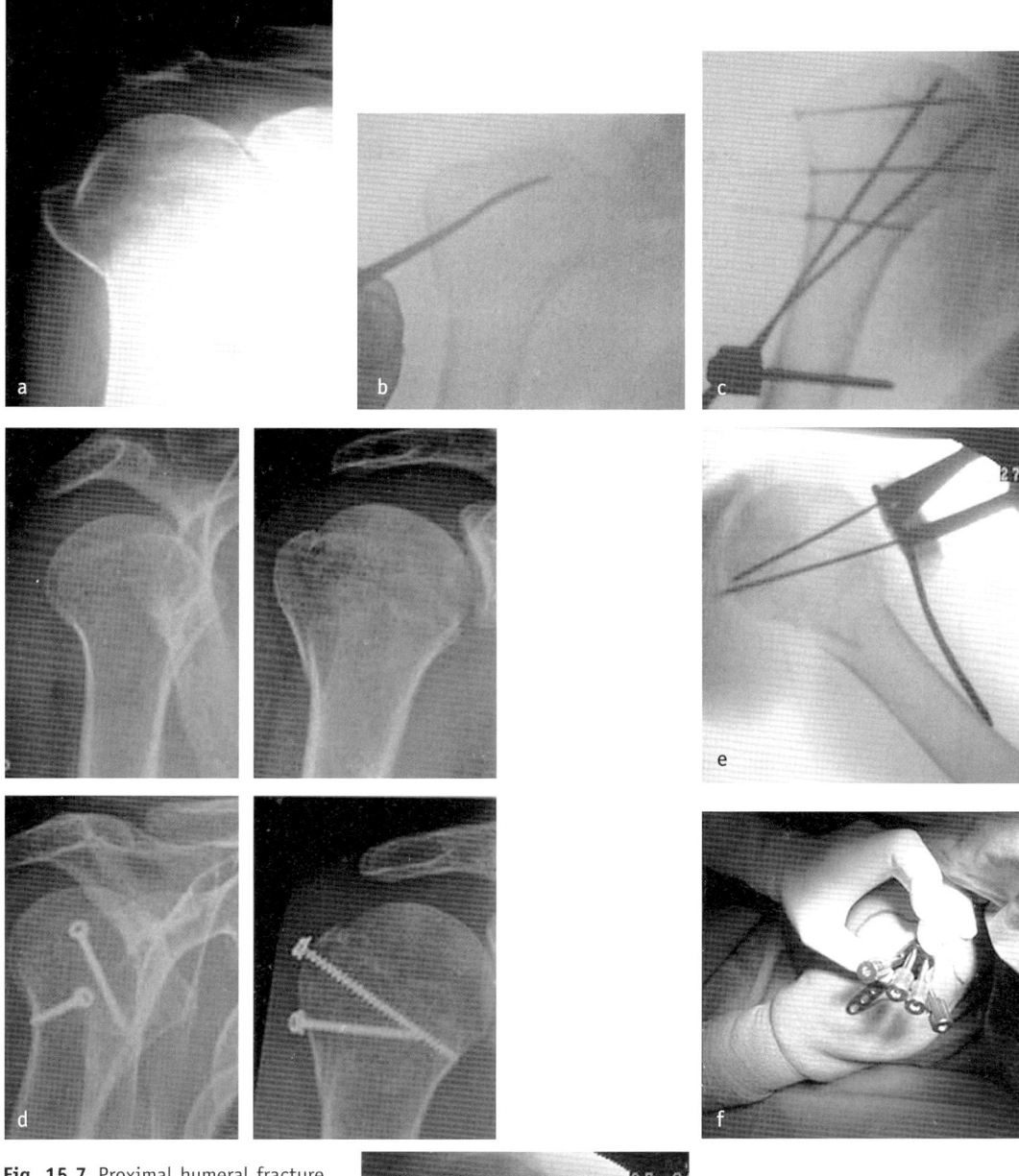

Fig. 15.7 Proximal humeral fracture. a–d: Minimally invasive treatment by percutaneous wiring or by screws. e–i: Half-open treatment with fixed-angle humeral plate of the type Philos.

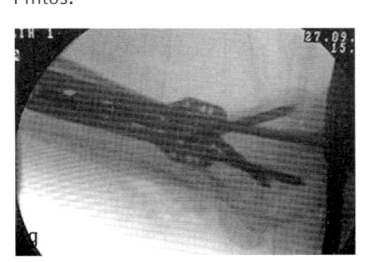

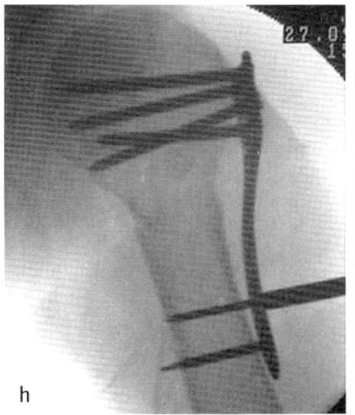

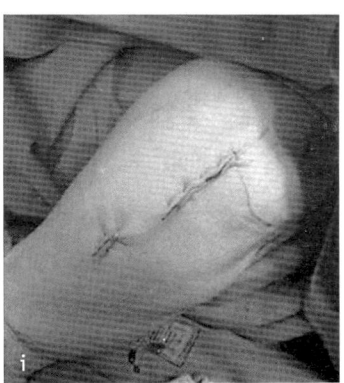

References

Andrews JR, Carson WG, McLeod WD (1985). Glenoid labrum tears related to the long head of the biceps. Am Sports Med 13: 337.

Bankart ASB (1932). Recurrent or habitual dislocation of the shoulder joint. Br Med J 2: 1132.

Burkhart SS, Morgan CD (1998). The peel back mechanism: its role in producing and extending posterior type II SLAP-lesions and its effect on SLAP repairs rehabilitation.

Burkhart SS, Esch JC, Jolson RS (1993). The Rotator crescent and the rotator cable: an anatomic description of the shoulder's "suspension bridge". Arthroscopy 9: 611–616.

Dann K, Wahler G, Huber M, Tschabitscher M (2002). Arthroskopische Bankart-Operation mit biodegradierbaren Fadenankern und retrograder Technik. Arthroskopie 15: 5–10.

Dann K, Wahler G, Wagner M, Rüter A (2004). Chapter 67. In: Rüter, Trentz, Wagner (eds.). Unfallchirurgie, 2nd ed. Urban & Fischer Verlag, Munich-Jena, pp 1177–1208.

Gerber C (1997). Observations on the classification of instability. In: Warner JP, Jeannette JP, Gerber C (eds.). Complex and Revision Problems in Shoulder Surgery. Lippincott Raven, Philadelphia, pp 99–119.

Habermeyer P (1995). In: Habermeyer P, Schweiberer (eds.). Schulterchirurgie. 2nd ed. Urban & Schwarzenberg, Munich-Vienna-Baltimore, p 285.

Henry JH, Genung JA (1982). Natural history of glenohumeral dislocation revisited. Am J Spots Med 10: 135–137.

Hovelius L (1978). Shoulder dislocation in Swedish ice hockey players. Am J Sports Med 6: 373–377.

Hovelius L (1982). Incidence of shoulder dislocation in Sweden. Clin Orthop Rel Res 166: 127–131.

Hovelius L, Augustini BG, Fredin H, Johanson O, Norlin R, Thorling J (1996). Primary anterior dislocation of the shoulder in young patients. J Bone Joint Surg (am) 78: 1677–1684.

Itoi E, Sashi R, Minagawa H, Shimizu T, Wakabayashi L, Sato K (2001). Position of immobilization after dislocation of the glenohumeral joint. A study with use of magnetic resonance imaging. JBJS 83-A (5): 661–667.

Jakobsen BW, Sojberg JO (1996). Primary repair after traumatic anterior dislocation of the shoulder joint. A prospective randomized study comparing open Bankart procedure and non-operative treatment. J Shoulder Elbow Surg 6: 28 (abstract).

Jobe FW, Kvitne RS (1989). Shoulder pain in the overhand or throwing athletes. Orthop Rev 18: 963–975.

Matson FA III., Thomas SC, Rockwood Jr C (1990). Anterior glenohumeral instability. In: Rockwood CA Jr, Matson FA III. (eds.). The Shoulder. Saunders, Philadelphia, p 526.

Neer CS II., Foster CR (1980). Interior capsular shift for involuntary inferior and multidirectional instability of the shoulder: a preliminary report. J Bone Joint Surg (Am) 62: 897.

Norlin R (1993). Interarticular pathology in acute, first-time anterior shoulder dislocation: an arthroscopic study. Arthroscopy 9: 546–549.

Resch H (1995a). Klassifikation und Pathomorphologie der vorderen Schulterinstabilität. Arthroskopie 8: 156.

Resch H (1995b). OP-Strategien bei Luxationen, Knorpel- und Sehnenverletzungen: Auffrischkurs. Sportverletz Sportschaden 13: 45.

Snyder SJ, Karzel RP, Del-Pizzo W, Ferkel RD, Friedmann MJ (1990). Slap lesions of the shoulder. Arthroscopy 6 (4): 274–279.

Sunder PA, Jakobsen BW (1997). Results of conservative treatment of traumatic primary anterior shoulder dislocation correlated to initial arthroscopic findings. L Shoulder Elbow Surg 6: 213 (abstract).

Watch G, Boileau P, Noel E, Donell ST (1992). Impingement of the deep surface of the supraspinatus tendon on the posteriosuperior glenoid rim; an arthroscopic study. J Shoulder Elbow Surg 1: 238.

Wheeler JH, Ryan JB, Arciero RA, Molinari RN (1989). Arthroscopy versus non-operative treatment of acute shoulder dislocations in young athletes. Arthroscopy V: 213–217.

Williams MM, Snyder SJ, Buford D Jr (1994). The Buford complex – the "cord-like" middle glenohumeral ligament and absent anterosuperior labrum complex. A normal anatomic capsulabral variant. Arthroscopy 10 (3): 241–247.

15.2 Open surgery procedures

Gernot Sperner

15.2.1 Anterior instability of the shoulder

The arthroscopic stabilization of an unstable shoulder has gained in importance during recent years and has therefore partially superseded open procedures (Cole and Warner 2000). Instability makes an open treatment necessary in many cases and is far more likely after arthroscopy (Walch et al. 1995).

Large osseous defects of the edge of the socket or classic multidirectional instabilities are only treatable by arthroscopy in exceptional cases.

Therefore, an exact preoperative diagnosis is absolutely essential and should also include an arthro-CT or an arthro-MRI examination in addition to the clinical, plain radiological and sonographic clarification.

Primarily, the remediation of the anterior labrum-capsule complex or the socket edge, respectively, is the aim of the surgical treatment; the Hill-Sachs dent, which is always present with posttraumatic dislocations, mostly will not be worthy of treatment. A simultaneous diagnostic arthroscopy is useful also with preoperatively planned open stabilization techniques, because possible additional pathologies in some cases can be verified only by arthroscopy despite exact radiographic clarification.

Surgery according to Bankart

Surgery according to Bankart still is considered a classical open procedure for post-traumatic shoulder dislocation. This method, already described in 1923, shows a very low rate of post-operative relapse (Bankart 1923) and aims for the reconstruction of the anterior labrum-capsule complex. The reinsertion is considered challenging, because modifications of this surgical method have been described repeatedly in the past.

Surgical technique: The patient is positioned in so-called half-sitting beach-chair position. In this process, the head lies firmly fixed in a half-shell. The arm receives a mobile cover.

The skin incision is effected according to the anterior access and starts scarcely distal of the coracoid process pulling into the direction of the anterior axillary fold. The pectoral deltoid sulcus is widened bluntly, the cephalic vein is held away laterally. The common tendon at the coracoids can be laterally notched slightly, if required. The subscapularis muscle below is found and the transition between muscle and tendon is represented by external rotation. Two retaining threads are set; afterwards the tendon is cleared off sharply lengthwise. An injury of the capsule lying underneath must be avoided here, by all means.

In further consequence, the joint capsule is indicated crosswise and so the joint is being opened. A Hohmann elevator is inserted at the medial socket edge and a dislocation spoon holds away the humeral head laterally. At the height of the glenoid notch, the glenoid labrum mostly destroyed is cut crosswise then together with the medial joint capsule and the periost and is shifted to medial-caudallly. The socket edge is roughened by a small fraise or by other comparable instruments in order to achieve subcortical hemorrhages. This step is of great importance, because a successive solid healing of the refixed labrum-capsule complex is made possible by micro-hemorrhages.

In the classic Bankart technique, lateral boreholes are applied, which are armed with non-resorbable suture material. The capsule or the remaining labrum is collected by the threads, thus creating U-sutures. After the tying, the knot must lay intraaricularly and the refixed labrum-capsule complex must be pressed to the socket edge. This method is technically highly advanced, because the small bone canals can easily break out in very sclerotic bones or in re-operations after failed first surgeries. In recent years, a modification with use of diverse expansion plugs or suture anchors has become prevalent increasingly for that reason. The procedure is practically identical, anchors with non-resorbable suture material are inserted into the socket edge instead of the bore holes (➢ Fig. 15.8 a and b). The use of resorbable implants is recommended (➢ Fig. 15.8 c and d).

After the removal of the dislocation elevator, the quality of the refixation can be tested under careful external rotation. At good stability

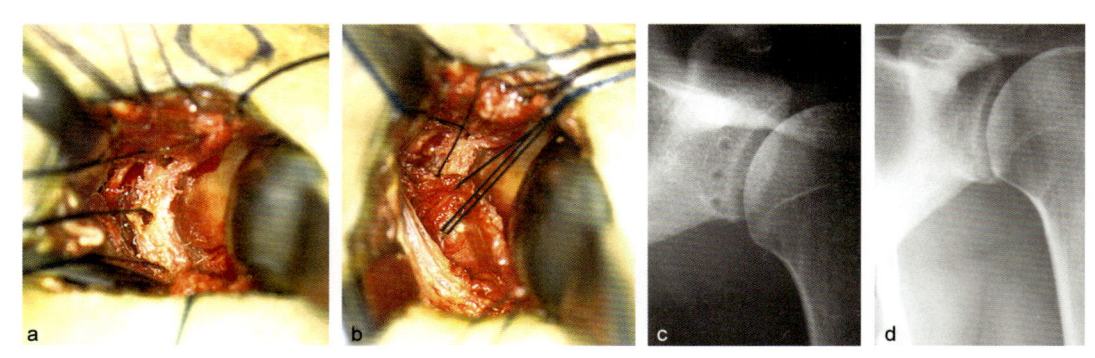

Fig. 15.8 a, b: Open Bankart surgery. c, d: Radiographic examination of the left shoulder after Bankart surgery. a: Left shoulder: view into the joint socket, three thread anchors with non-absorbable suture material, drilled into the anterior socket rim. b: The joint capsule is being looped to the medial side by U-sutures; after the knotting of the threads, the head lies extraarticularly. c: Adequately visible position of the absorbable thread anchors 6 weeks after surgery. d: Drilling hole is not visible anymore 8 months after surgery.

without substantial limitation of the external rotation, the previously opened transverse limb of the capsule is closed with resorbable suture material. Here the external rotation is tested again, as well. With a very wide joint capsule, an additional condensing of the lower capsule part to cranial can occur. After the closure of the capsule, the detached subscapularis muscle is refixed without shortening.

Post-treatment: The arm is fixed in a shoulder bandage; lymph drainage starts on the 1st postoperative day. The immobilization lasts 3 weeks. Beginning with the 4th week after surgery, the shoulder strap is removed and active movement exercises are initiated under therapeutic support. The patient must not flex or abduct the operated extremity to approx. 100° for 3 more weeks. The external rotation is limited to 0°, though. Only after 3 more weeks (i.e. 6 weeks post-operatively), the flexibility on all levels is being approved, and the active external rotation is going to be allowed. Overhead activities should not be carried out within the first 3 postoperative months; shoulder-wearing sports or contact sports are not allowed during the first 6 postoperative months.

J-chip plastic (according to Resch)

With defects of the anterior osseous socket edge, this procedure is recommended for the extensive reconstruction of the glenoid (Sperner and Resch 1988). No osseous abutment against the dislocation is intended, but an anatomic reconstruction of the former socket edge. Therefore, a difference to other mostly extraarticular chip plastics must be made.

Surgical technique: Positioning, access, opening of the joint capsule, adjustment and representation of the socket edge are carried out in the same way as in the surgery according to Bankart. A fold of a length of approx. 2 cm is driven into the bone about 5 mm medially of the cartilage-bone border by a chisel of a breadth of approx. 1 cm after the exposure of the socket edge. Here it is important that the position of the chisel is aimed slightly dorsomedially, in order to cause an iatrogenic fracture of the socket edge. The depth of the notch averages 1.5 cm. The socket edge is lightly abducted laterally; this prepares the bed for the chip to be studded in.

The chip is taken out of the junction between the anterior and medial third of the crista iliaca. In this area, the chip can be taken best from the iliac wing, because here the junction to the external cortical substance of the bone is mostly shaped very edged. A wedge of about 2×2 cm is taken out by the oscillating saw, taking along the external crista and the external cortical substance of the bone (➤ Fig. 15.9 a). Subsequently, the chip is being shaped into a J by milling off the spongiosa at the inner surface by pulling movements with the oscillating saw. The thickness of the side to be folded in depends on the intended raise of the socket edge. The length on the inner surface amounts to 10–12 mm (➤ Fig. 15.9 b).

15.2 Open surgery procedures

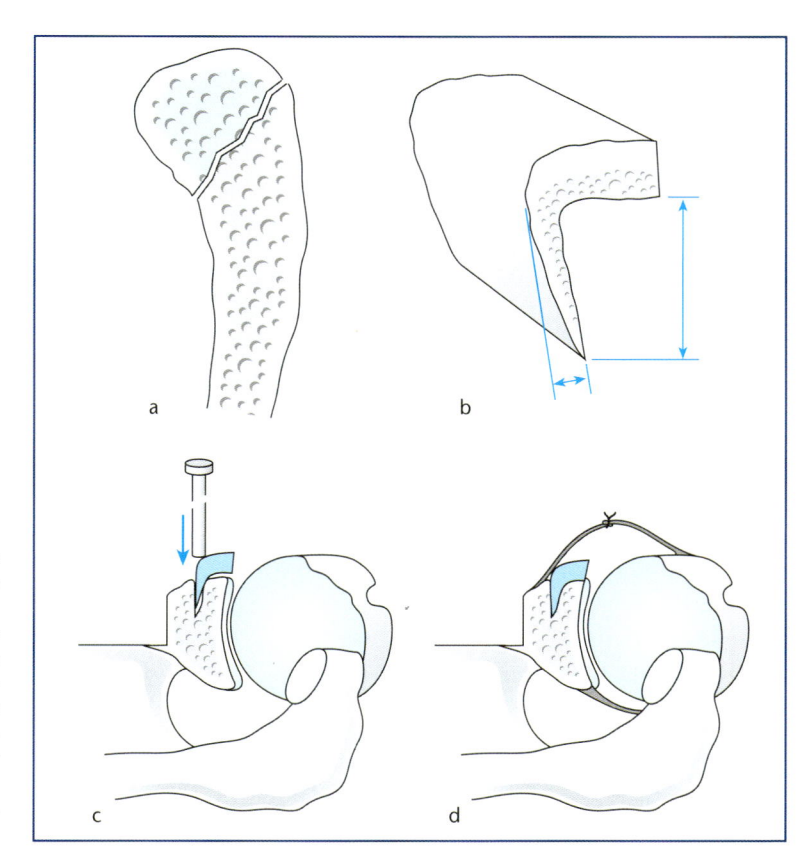

Fig. 15.9 J-chip plastic according to Resch. a: Corticospongiose block removal from the external portion of the iliac crest. b: Finished J-chip ready for the insertion into the edge of the socket. c: The chip is driven into the preformed folding at the anterior glenoidal edge. d: Finished chip in situ; the position is completely intraarticular.

After the refining of the osseous socket edge, the chip with its wedge-shaped sides is driven into the previously prepared notch now. Due to the external rounding of the chip, the striking with a regular pestle is mostly very difficult because of the danger of slipping off, but it can be accomplished easily by a small tip being attached laterally to the impaction armamentarium (➤ Fig. 15.9 c). After driving it in, the settle of the chip is mostly firm enough for the fine adaption of the socket-widening part of the chip to be carried out in situ by a small olive fraise. The internal surface of the chip facing the joint is adjusted homogeneously to the socket shape and curve. A too small curve radius and the associated ventral hook-shaped protrusion of the chip must be avoided by all means in order to prevent the development of early arthroses. The continuity of the joint surface crossing over steplessly into the one of the chip provides an exact positioning. The correct curve can easily be tested with a meniscal touch hook.

The joint capsule is sutured end-to-end above the chip then, causing it to lie entirely intraarticularly (➤ Fig. 15.9 d).

Post-treatment: The treated extremity is immobilized by a shoulder strap postoperatively. The further treatment is the same as after a Bankart surgery.

Glenoid reconstruction according to Eden-Hybinette

Principally, non-anatomic bone block operations are afflicted with a higher risk of arthroses. With extended socket edge defects, an extensive reconstruction is only possible with accumulated bone blocks, though, in order to guarantee an adequate supporting function of the socket edge. The indication for such techniques is only given by missing osseous support of at least a fourth of the anterior lower glenoidal area.

The post-operative treatment is carried out in the same way as with the J-chip plastic or the Bankart surgery.

Coracoid transfer according to Bristow-Latarjet

With extensive osseous defects, a transposition of the osteotomized coracoid tip can also be applicable for the sanitation of the anterior glenoid area.

In the after-treatment, the treated extremity is immobilized for 2–3 weeks in a shoulder strap; forced activities of the biceps must be avoided for 4–6 weeks. The osseous knitting must be controlled radiologically or by CT.

Ventral capsule plastic according to Neer

Predominantly, this technique is used for the classic multidirectional instabilities type IV and V according to Gerber (Schneeberger et al. 1997). However, it can also be used for uni-directional instabilities with concurrent hyperlaxation in combination with a Bankart surgery. The condensing process of a too wide joint capsule is the aim of this procedure, which does not represent an adequate form of therapy for fractures of the socket edge (Neer and Foster 1989).

Surgical technique: Positioning and access correspond to the procedure described above. After separating the subscapularis muscle, the joint capsule is displayed. It is opened in terms of a lying T. There is the horizontal capsule incision between the medial and the lower glenohumeral ligament. A longitudinal incision is conducted in the height of the anatomical neck. Thereby, two triangular capsular flaps can be won that can be shifted against one another. The flap below is mobilized far to dorsal-caudal; attention must be paid to position and course of the axillaris nerve.

Successively, this flap is pulled cranially and laterally. A small notch is shaped by a fraise at the anatomical neck. The distal capsular flap is re-fixed via transosseous bore holes or by help of suture anchors (also a direct end-to-end suture can be carried out with sufficient lateral capsular protrusion in good soft tissue quality). Analogously, the proximal flap is stretched to distal and sutured above the lower one. Corresponding to the size of the capsule, a doubling of the lateral capsular parts develops under substantial elimination of the lower recess.

Post-treatment: A post-operative immobilization is necessary in order to allow an according healing of the refixed capsular parts. At the suggestion of Neer, this should be carried out in an internal rotation of about 20° (this corresponds widely to the physiological null rotation of the humeral head). The fixation remains for 6 weeks, careful movement exercises follow afterwards. Isometric exercises for the strengthening of the musculature of the shoulder girdle start after 8 weeks. Maximum physical exercise, including sports stressing the shoulders, is not recommended earlier than nine months post-operatively.

Subcapital derotation according to Weber

Traumatic dislocations often lead to differently sized Hill-Sachs lesions depending on the force of violence. In rare, very pronounced cases, the dent placed dorsocranially at the humeral head may "snap in" of at the anterior socket edge in moderate external rotation movements of abduction already, which involves the danger of redislocation (Bankart lesion; ➢ Fig. 15.10). In these exceptional cases, a derotation according to Weber can make sense in addition to the reconstruction of the anterior socket edge (surgery according to Bankart or J-chip, respectively; Weber 1969).

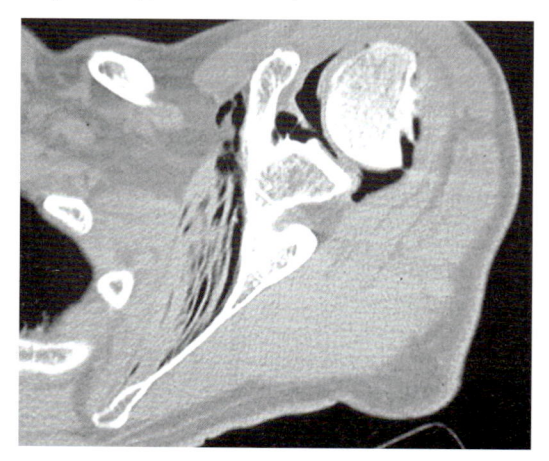

Fig. 15.10 Extensive Hill-Sachs lesion in the arthro CT – an indication for a derotation according to Weber.

Primarily, the **post-treatment** is determined by the surgery carried out additionally at the socket edge. Weber recommends a Gilchrist's bandage for the first 10 postoperative days. Active flexibility within the pain threshold is allowed after 15 days. With correct implementation, the osteotomy is reconstructed after 8 weeks.

15.2.2 Posterior instability of the shoulder

With an incidence of 2–3% of all shoulder instabilities, the posterior instability is much rarer than the anterior one. Principally, a posttraumatic dislocation or a caught sprain has to be distinguished from a posterior instability. The relocation of a posterior posttraumatic sprain mostly is only successful using general anesthesia; in general, depressed fractures at the humeral head (reversed Hill-Sachs dent) are far more impressive than in anterior sprains and frequently require a surgical reconstruction, as well. The therapy of the posterior instability is primarily conservative with the aim of the muscular strengthening of the external rotators. Surgical measures are only indicated for remaining limitations with corresponding psychological stress.

Dorsal capsule plastic according to Neer

As with the anterior capsular plastic, a reduction of the overlarge capsule volume is to be achieved in this procedure.

Surgical technique: The patient is in a lateral recumbent position, the injured arm receives a mobile cover; the posterior shoulder girdle is exposable. The incision takes place two fingers beneath the posterior soft spot (arthroscopic access) and stretches caudally into the direction of the posterior axillary fold. The deltoid muscle is split in the direction of the fibers after opening. The procedure goes in deeper between the lower margin of the infraspinatus muscle and the upper margin of the teres minor muscle. The capsule is displayed; the upper and lower edges of the socket are palpated. Two Hohmann elevators are inserted carefully (cave: proximal-medial suprascapularis nerve and caudal axillary nerve). The capsule is opened identically as in the anterior plastic in terms of a lying T-leg. The two obtained triangular flaps are mobilized and refixed laterally.

In the original work, the refixation of the upper flap is described first. In succession, the lower part is pulled laterally upwards and is sutured in part onto the first one.

Post-treatment: The immobilization is carried out in neutral or slightly external rotational position for 3-4 weeks.

Dorsal chip plastic

With the presence of an osseous posterior defect of the socket edge, the correction by help of a bone block is appropriate analogously to the anterior instability. This bone block is taken off the iliac crest and fixed in terms of a J-chip or a screwed block to the posterior glenoid part.

Postoperatively, the immobilization is done by a shoulder strap in neutral position for 3 weeks. Internal rotations are not allowed for 6 weeks. External rotations may be carried out.

15.2.3 Rupture of the rotator cuff

The rupture of the rotator cuff appears predominantly in the second half of life. It is caused by **mostly degenerative changes of the tendon structure**. An inferior blood flow, especially in the insertion area of the tendon, increases the progressive quality degradation of the tissue (Neer 1983). Mechanical irritations – mostly caused by osteophytary protrusions at the anterior lower margin of the acromion – affect a chronically irritated bursa subacromialis and a primary acromial-sided partial rupture (Uhthoff and Sakar 1991). With continuing mechanical impulse, the complete picture of a complete tear appears in further succession. The osseous changes are mostly traction osteophytes formed by chronic pressure and traction stress of the coracoacromial ligament in its area of irradiation at the lower acromial margin. These osteophytes impose as dash-shaped sclerosings also clearly visible on scout film in the a.p. standard radiograph at the lower margin of the acromion.

Ruptures mostly appear in the area of the supraspinatus tendon and can expand successively dorsally into the infraspinatus as well as ventrally into the subscapularis. Isolated ruptures of the infraspinatus tendon have not been described, but solitary tears of the scapularis tendon have been known very well. These patients cannot perform active internal rotations; the development is mostly conditioned traumatically. There is no healing in a conservative way; surgical treatment is considered the therapy of choice.

Especially in oblique movements of the arm, there are shearing movements inside the tendon because of the different stresses of the acromial and joint-sided parts of the rotator cuff. With according degenerative pre-existing defects, an **intratendinous partial rupture** can develop thus.

Articular partial ruptures mostly have a degenerative-traumatic cause and develop as a consequence of falls to the elbow or at the retaining of a fall by the wrist. The humeral head is pushed cranially then, whereby a previously impaired tendon can tear.

The true **traumatic tendon rupture** of young patients is rare, but it requires a surgical reconstruction in any case.

The **indication for surgery** is given basically for extreme pain conditions or after failed attempt of conservative therapy, respectively. The age of the patient, his expectations, and his functional limitations as well are also important parameters (Cofield et al. 2001).

In general, similar facts apply to the surgery of the rupture of the rotator cuff as for the shoulder instability: arthroscopic treatment techniques receive increasingly more priority because of the continuing development of better implants, resorbable suture anchors and special forcepses and perforation appliances (Thomazeau et al. 2000). In general, it has to be remarked that these procedures are mostly very difficult in correct execution and presume an according arthroscopic basic experience of the surgeon and also of the assistants. Many ruptures are not convenient for an arthroscopic reinsertion or only convenient for the arthroscopic reinsertion by an experienced surgeon because of their expanse, their localization and the tendon quality (Duralde and Bair 2005). A sufficient frequency must be given in the patient's treatment in order to keep the learning curve as short as possible. Considering these criteria, open techniques are still justified in many cases (Lam and Mok 2004).

Tendon reconstruction

A primary closure of the defect is aspired in younger active patients.

Surgical technique: The patient is set in a beach-chair position. The access is superoanterior with the skin cut beginning succinctly ventral of the acromion and expanding about 5–7 cm in a shape of a curve distal-laterally. The subcutis is split, and both skin flaps are kept away by retaining sutures. The deltoid muscle is spread in fiber direction in terms of a muscle splitting. Approximately 6–7 cm below the anterior acromial edge, a safety suture is applied through the deltoid muscle, in order to prevent a caudal tearing of the muscle fibers. This serves the protection of the axillary nerve, which could be impaired by pushing the muscle fibers too forcefully apart.

The fascia subdeltoidea is split longitudinally in order to see the bursa subdeltoidea lying beneath it. The inflammatory parts are removed and the tendinous defect is displayed. The deltoid muscle is notched a little at the anterior margin of the acromion for better subacromial inspection. The coracoacromial ligament is separated; the ramus acromialis of the thoracoacromial artery must be coagulated afterwards, in order to prevent hemorrhages. An acromion plastic according to Neer follows. Thereby, the palpable spur at the lower anterior margin of the acromion is skimmed and removed by a chisel (➤ Fig. 15.11 a). The lower margin is filed by an oscillating file until a sufficiently wide acromial space has developed palpatorically at a smooth bone undersurface.

The tendon is gripped by tendon alligator forceps or looped by a retaining suture and is mobilized by a raspatory (➤ Fig. 15.11 b). A widely tension-free closure is apired. The tuberculum majus is freshened by a chisel or oscillating file at the planned insertion point until subcortical hemorrhages occur. Thereby the tendon end comes to lie on well vascularizing spongy bone and can heal better this way. Afterwards, the tendon is sparingly freshened in the area of the rupture. Without the possibility of a tension-free closure, a so-called juxta-bicipital arthrotomy is an option for further mobilization. Thereby, the joint capsule is perforated sharply by scissors or a raspatory above the biceps tendon anchor. A gain of a length of about 1 cm is thus achieved. Increased caution

15.2 Open surgery procedures

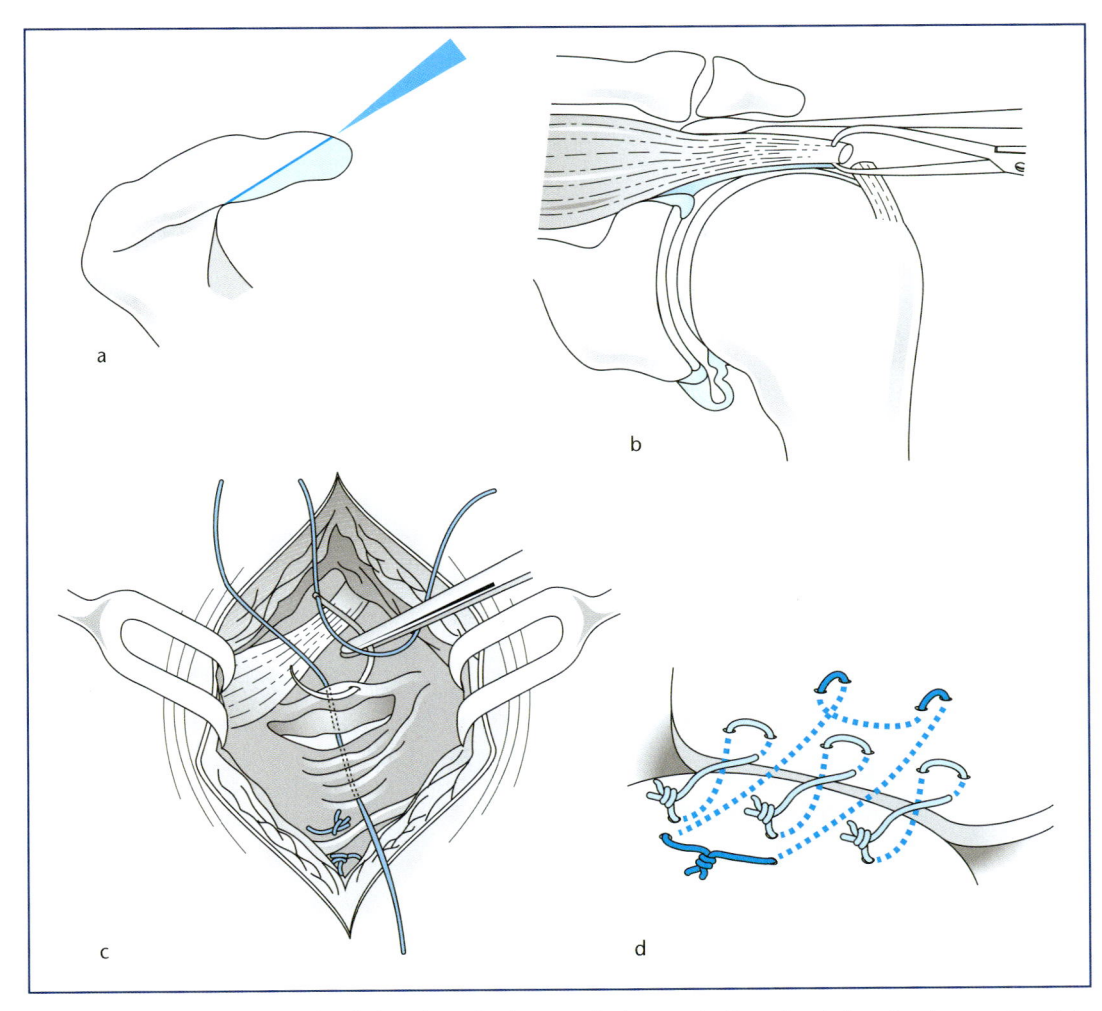

Fig. 15.11 Tendon reconstruction (scheme). a: In the acromioplasty, only the osteophyt or the downwards pointy anterior acromial rim are removed. b: The tendon is grabbed at its ruptured point by vise grip pliers; adhesions are dissolved carefully by the raspatory. c: Placing of the sutures, the heads lie laterally at the humeral head in tractive direction. d: Sewing technique: modified U-suture with non-absorbable thread (dark blue), several pushed-in transosseous sutures with absorbable threads (light blue).

is advisable for this maneuver, though, in order to protect the suprascapular nerves.

Transosseous bore canals are set into the spongy bone from lateral at the tuberculum majus. The tendon is gripped by non-resorbable suture material in terms of an interlaced U-suture and is knotted transosseously. The knois located laterally at the cortical substance of the bone (➤ Fig. 15.11 c). Additional in-pushing sutures are also set transosseously with resorbable suture material (➤ Fig. 15.11 d).

A careful passive moving of the arm follows and is expected to give some indication of the quality of the reinsertion that has been carried out.

Post-treatment: The extremity is immobilized by a shoulder strap for 3 weeks. During this time, no active movement exercises are allowed. The Redon drainage is removed at the first postoperative day; lymphatic drainages are induced for the reduction of the swelling. Physical therapeutic treatments follow, although only passive exercises will be carried out in the first 3 weeks after surgery. Forced rotating movements are being avoided; the mobilization is mainly done on the scapular level. With small tears closed without tension, an underwater therapy follows after suture removal (it is postponed to the 4th postoperative week for larger ruptures and moderate tendon quality). The shoulder strap is removed 4 weeks after surgery; active movements are being allowed increasingly then.

Infraspinatus transfer according to Neviaser

A tension-reduced closure is mostly possible for transverse-oval ruptures without pronounced retraction of the tendon tissue. A stable transosseous reinsertion is often far more difficult for longitudinal-oval ruptures. The place of rupture can be brought close to the tuberculum majus mostly under substantial tension only; in addition, tendinous protrusion appears in the anterior and posterior area of the rupture, imposing as "dog ears". These kinds of rupture can be treated with reduced tension by a so-called infraspinatus shift.

Post-treatment: The positioning is carried out in a shoulder strap with the elbow being supported additionally by a small cushion. The light abduction of approx. 20° in the shoulder joint reduces the tension to the reinserted tendon tissue. Apart from that, the kind of after-treatment is mainly the same as the one described in the previous section.

Latissimus-dorsi transfer according to Gerber

This procedure is carried out primarily in patients younger than 65 years with reconstructable ruptures of supra- and infraspinatus tendon (➤ Fig. 15.12 a). An intact tendon of the subscapularis muscle is the precondition for a successful surgery, though. No complete closure of the defect, but a compensation of balance between internal and external rotators is aspired by this technique. The reconstruction in terms of an equatorial reconstruction reduces the cranial migration of the head and compensates the dysbalance between ventral

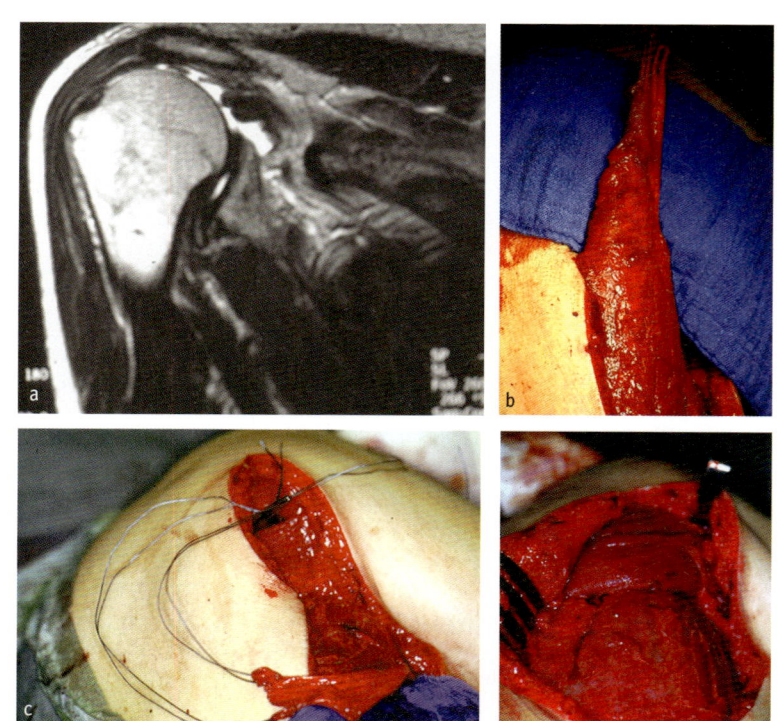

Fig. 15.12 Expanded, non-reconstructable rupture of the supraspinal and infraspinal tendon in a 45-year-old patient (MRI). b, c, d: Latissimus dorsi transfer. b: Latissimus dorsi muscle detached from the insertion point and attached to the tendon. c: Repositioning of the latissimus dorsi from vetral-lateral between the deltoid muscle and the infraspinal muscle. d: Site after accomplished translocation.

15.2 Open surgery procedures

(intact subscapularis) and dorsal (missing infraspinatus) forces.

At the same time, the external rotation, severely reduced by of the missing infraspinatus tendon, is being at least partly restored by repositioning the latissimus dorsi (➤ Fig. 15.12 b to d; Gerber et al. 1988 and 1992).

Post-treatment: The arm is positioned in the shoulder strap with additional small abduction cushions. Physical therapy is carried out solely passively on the scapular level in the first 4 postoperative weeks. Internal rotations must be prevented by all means during this time in order not to create additional tension to the transposed tendon tissue. The strap can be removed after the 5th postoperative week, active movement exercises with additional underwater therapy follow.

Pectoralis major transfer according to Resch

The patients are limited seriously in their external rotation with present ruptures of the subscapularis tendon. The transfer of the pectoralis major presents the method of choice for non-reconstructable ruptures. Thereby, the cranial part of the pectoralis major muscle is being detached and used as subscapularis substitute (➤ Fig. 15.13 a and b; Resch et al. 2000).

Post-treatment: Immobilization in the shoulder strap for 4 weeks, passive movement exercises after the 1st postoperative day with avoidance of external rotations in order not to overstretch the muscle. Underwater therapy after suture removal, active exercises can be performed after the removal of the strap 4 weeks later.

15.2.4 Acromioclavicular joint

Separations of the AC joint are very frequent injuries, mostly conditioned by direct collision traumas or by fall to the extended arm. Depending on the athletic aspiration of the patients and their expectations, a surgical treatment is given for Tossy-III (relative indication) as well as for Rockwood-IV and -V lesions.

A stable reconstruction of the dislocated joint is the aim of all procedures.

Surgical technique: After positioning in the beach-chair position, access is gained by saber cut incision of a length of about 5 cm above the dislocated joint. The fascia or the tendon, respectively, above acromion and lateral clavicula are split longitudinally – in expansive sprains, these soft-tissue structures are often traumatically ruptured. The ruptured coracoclavicular ligaments are looped with resorbable suture material. The ruptured intraarticular disk is removed. A Kirschner wire (2 or 2.2 mm thick) is drilled in transarticularly from lateral through the acromion after digital repositioning of the lateral clavicular end. The exact position of the pin is to be examined via the image converter.

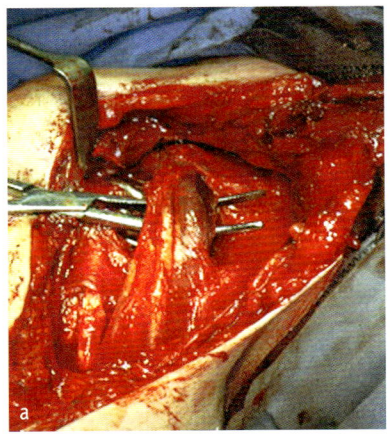

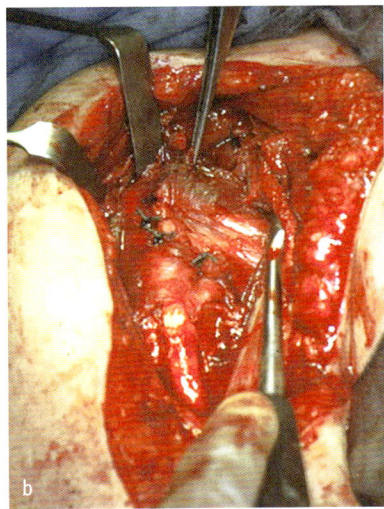

Fig. 15.13 Transfer of pectoralis major. a: Preparation of a connective tissue gap medially of the coracobrachialis muscle for the passage of the removed deltoid muscle portion. b: Detached and cranially-laterally transposed proximal portion of the pectoralis major muscle.

A transverse bore hole of a size of 2 mm is set through the clavicula, about 3 cm medially of the AC joint, and a strong, non-resorbable cord (e.g. cervical cerglage) is pulled through. The cord is looped around the pin and knotted. This way, an additional tension band effect is formed. The Kirschner wire is bent laterally, clipped off and calibrated medially.

Post-treatment: Fixation in the shoulder strap for 3 weeks, careful movements up to a flexion and abduction of approx. 70° are allowed. The pin is removed 6–7 weeks later, the cerclage remains.

Alternatives are the following surgical procedures:

- **Hooked plate according to Dreithaler:** Advantage: very firm fixation; disadvantage: relatively complex second operation for the metal removal.

- **Screw connection according to Bosworth:** Screw fixation through lateral clavicula and coracoids. Advantage: minor soft-tissue detachment; disadvantage: frequent occurrence of broken screws.

References

Bankart ASB (1923). Recurrent or habitual dislocation of the shoulder joint. Brit Med J 2: 1132–1133.

Cofield RH, Pavizi J, Hoffmeyer PJ, Lanzer WL, Ilstrup DM, Rowland CM (2001). Surgical repair of chronic rotator cuff tears. A prospective long term study. J Bone Joint Surg 83A: 71–77.

Cole BJ, Warner JJ (2000). Arthroscopic versus open Bankart repair for traumatic anterior shoulder instability. Clin Orthop 19: 19–48.

Duralde XA, Bair B (2005). Massive rotator cuff tears: The results of partial rotator cuff repair. J Shoulder Elbow Surg 14: 121–127.

Gerber C, Vinh TS, Hertel R, Hess CW (1988). Latissimus dorsi transfer for the treatment of massive tears of the rotator cuff. Clin Orthop Relat Res 232: 51–61.

Gerber C (1992). Latissimus dorsi transfer of irreparable tears of the rotator cuff. Clin Orthop Relat Res 275: 152–160.

Lam F, Mok D (2004). Open repair of massive rotator cuff tears in patients aged sixty-five years or over: is it worth while? J Shoulder Elbow Surg 13: 517–521.

Latarjat M (1954). A propos du traitement des luxations récidivantes de l'epaule. Lyons Chir 49: 994–1003.

Neer CS (1983). Impingement lesions. Clin Orthop 173: 70–77.

Neer CS, Foster CR (1989). Inferior capsular shift for involuntary inferior and multidirectional instability of the shoulder. J Bone Joint Surg 62A: 897–908.

Resch H, Povasz P, Ritter E (2000). Transfer of the pectoralis muscle for the treatment of irreparable rupture of the subscapularis tendon. J Bone Joint Surg 82A: 372–382.

Schneeberger AG, Herrsche O, Gerber C (1997). Die instabile Schulter. Klassifikation und Therapie. Orthopädie 26: 909–914.

Sperner G, Resch H (1988). Die vordere Instabilität des Schultergelenkes. In: Resch H, Beck E. Praktische Chirurgie des Schultergelenkes. Fronweiler, Innsbruck, 71–92.

Thomazeau H, Gleyze P, Lafosse L, Walch G, Kelberine F, Coudane H (2000). Arthroscopic assessment of full-thickness rotator cuff tears. Arthroscopy 16: 367–372.

Uhthoff HK, Sakar K (1991). Surgical repair of rotator cuff ruptures: the importance of the subacromial bursa. J Bone Joint Surg 73B: 399–401.

Walch G, Boileau P, Levigne C, , Mandrino A, Neyret P, Donnell S (1995). Arthroscopic stabilization for recurrent anterior shoulder dislocation: results in 59 cases. Arthroscopy 11: 173–179.

Weber BG (1969). Operative treatment of recurrent dislocation of the shoulder. Injury 1: 107–109.

16 Elbow and forearm

Hans-Gerd Pieper

Compared to shoulder, knee, or ankle joints, sports injuries and overuse syndromes of the elbow region are less common. An analysis of 34,742 sports injuries over a time period of 25 years showed the elbow region to be affected in only 2 % of the cases (Steinbrück und Krzycki 2005). The incidence is **age-dependent**; however, the distribution of injuries varies in different athletic disciplines. In **baseball pitchers, javelin throwers** or **tennis players** the incidence of elbow injuries is relatively high (Tullos und King 1973, Andrews und Timmermann 1995, Raschka et al. 1995, Steinbrück und Krzycki 2005).

16.1 Sports injuries

16.1.1 Elbow dislocation

Injury mechanism

Dislocations of the elbow joint may occur as the result of a **fall on the bended or outstretched elbow**. The direction of the dislocation is mainly dorsal, often in combination with a **fracture**.

Diagnosis

The injury can easily be recognized by mere **inspection**, because the physiologic bone constellation (**Hueter's triangle**, formed by the two epicondyles and the tip of the olecranon) is no longer present. The interpretation of X-rays (➤ Fig. 16.1 a–c) can be difficult, because superpositions might occur if the radiographs are not taken in the exact axial planes.

Treatment

After initial search for neurovascular lesions, treatment of an elbow dislocation consist of the **earliest possible reduction** of the dislocation. This may be achieved non-surgically by gentle traction with the elbow held in 30° of flexion or under anaesthesia (Collins 1985). In case of **interposition** (fracture of the coronoid process) or **extensive soft-tissue injury** with instability, the reduction has to be carried out **surgically**.

Following reduction and short immobilization – depending on the severity of the soft-tissue injury or the extent of the instability – **functional treatment** should be started early (out of a splint after 3–4 days) or after immobilization of 3–4 weeks at the most (Collins 1985).

Since dislocations always lead to injuries of the medial and lateral capsulo-ligamentous complex, in spite of immediate reduction **secondary impairments** might remain, such as instabilities (Kolb und Holz 1999, Mehta und Bain 2004) or permanent contractures in case of extended immobilization. **Neurovascular damage** can also be a primary consequence of the injury.

16.1.2 Forearm fracture

Injury mechanism

Fractures of the forearm are rather common, amounting to 17.9 % of all fractures caused by sports accidents. Children are clearly affected more frequently than adults (Steinbrück 1987). Generally, both radius and ulna are fractured. This kind of injury mainly occurs due to direct force striking the forearm, like an oppo-

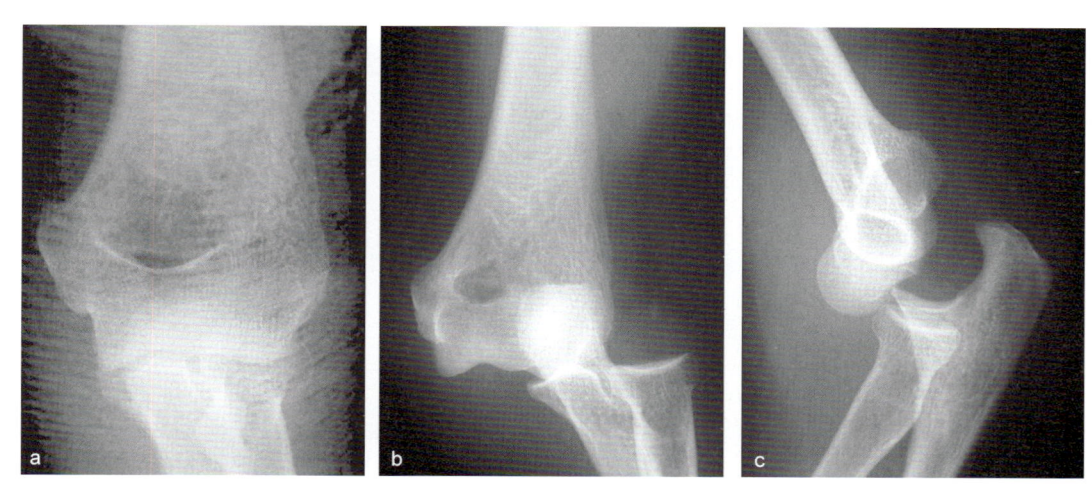

Fig. 16.1 Dislocation of the elbow joint in anterior-posterior (a), oblique lateral (b) and lateral (c) projection.

nent falling onto the arm of the injured athlete in American football or rugby, or as a result of a fall on the outstretched arm in contact sports such as soccer or team handball.

In case of using the forearm to block a strike, an **isolated fracture of the ulna (parry fracture)** may also occur.

A fracture of the ulna in combination with a dislocation of the radial head but without simultaneous fracture of the radius is called Monteggia's fracture. Due to the obvious injury of the ulna, the dislocation of the radial head is prone to being overlooked.

> That is why the elbow joint itself should always be X-rayed in case of ulna fractures.

Treatment

Generally, fractures of the forearm should be treated **conservatively through prompt anatomical reduction** of ulna and radius or of the radial head respectively in case of Monteggia's fracture, followed by **immobilization** in a cast or splint for 4–6 weeks, depending on the severity of the bone injury and the age of the injured athlete (Küster und Rompe 1983, Wirth 2001). If closed anatomical reduction cannot be achieved, **surgical treatment** should be carried out through internal fixation or open reduction of the radial head and reconstruction of the anular ligament.

In case of additional injuries to the radiohumeral joint and thus danger of recurrent instability, in adult patients **removal of the radial head** is often preferred to a reduction (Collins 1985, Wirth 2001). During childhood, however, a resection is contraindicated due to the growth-related axial malposition and deformity of the elbow to be expected at the end of growth.

16.1.3 Distal biceps tendon rupture

Causes and injury mechanism

Tears of the distal biceps tendon are extremely rare and make up only 3 % of all biceps tendon ruptures (Gilcreest 1925). As is true for tears of the long head of biceps tendon, they usually develop **spontaneously** without adequate trauma mostly in athletes aged 50 years or older, mainly due to pre-existing degenerative conditions

Typically, the tear occurs in **abrupt everyday movements** (mostly eccentric contraction). This fact and the typical localization close to the tendon insertion at the radial tuberosity within the hypovascular area suggest that it is a matter of tendon degeneration, possibly impaired additionally by a mechanical impingement in this particular area (Seiler et al. 1995). **Smoking** is said to be increasing the risk of a distal biceps tendon tear by the factor 7.5

(Safran und Graham 2002). Spontaneous ruptures have also been described following **abuse of anabolic steroids** by athletes, especially in **body-building** (Visuri und Lindholm 1994, Wirth 2001). Tears of the distal biceps tendon in younger athletes due to adequate trauma are extremely rare (Williams et al. 1996).

Diagnosis

The affected patients describe **sudden pain with transposition of the muscle belly** upwards (➢ Fig. 16.2). **Physical examination** will reveal a swelling in the crook of the arm caused by hematoma in addition to a marked weakness of elbow flexion and supination of the forearm. **Ultrasound** examination can often demonstrate the tendon stump in the antecubital fossa. Documentation by MRI should only be restricted to cases of doubt.

Treatment

Surgical therapy will be the treatment of choice due to the considerable loss of strength as far as supination is concerned when treating conservatively. Surgery consists of **tendon refixation** at the anatomical insertion at the radial tubercle. The so-called **looping operation** (transosseous fixation of one half of the tendon through a bone canal in the radius) has proven sucessful (Hegelmaier und Schramm 1992). As an alternative, fixation techniques using suture anchors have been described. These means, however, do not achieve the primary fixation strength as compared to the fixation in an osseous tunnel (Pereira et al. 2002, Kelly et al. 2003,).

Post-operatve treatment will be carried out partially functional out of a full-arm splint with a temporary limitation of range of motion for 6 weeks. Afterwards full active range of motion is allowed, aiming for normal range of activity after about 3 months.

16.2 Overuse syndromes

16.2.1 Stress reactions/stress fractures

Epidemiology

Stress reactions or stress fractures respectively are bound to occur in case of imbalances between load and load-bearing capacity at **unfamiliar or excessive strain** (Orava et al. 1978, ➢ Chapter 23). The **lower extremities** are hereby affected in more than 95% of all cases, while only individual observations have been made of stress reactions concerning the upper

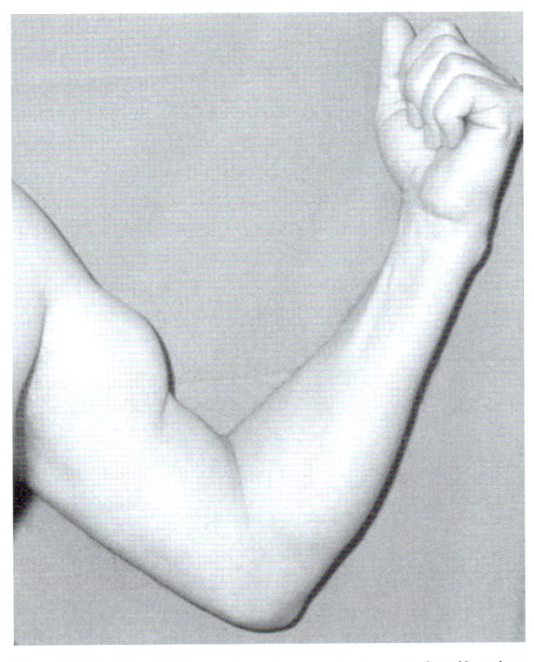

Fig. 16.2 Distal biceps tendon rupture: proximalization of the muscle belly.

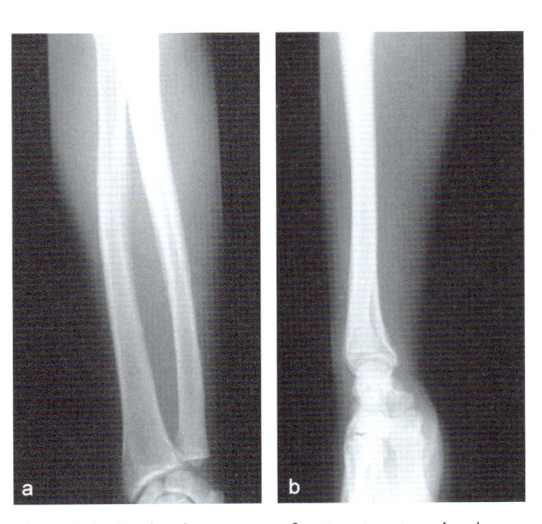

Fig. 16.3 Predominant arm of a top-ten tennis player: no radiological changes in the anterior-posterior (a) and lateral (b) projection.

extremities. With regard to the elbow and forearm region, in the literature stress reactions of the olecranon in baseball pitchers (Bennett 1959, Nuber und Diment 1992), tennis players (Pieper et al. 1997) and javelin throwers (Waris 1946, Miller 1960) as well as stress reactions at the distal radius or the distal ulna respectively in tennis players (Bell 1986, Loosli 1991) have been described.

In case of chronic conditions of the elbow or forearm in throwing or racket sports without radiological correlation, stress reactions should always be considered, and further diagnostic procedures should be started.

Diagnosis

Among our patients, a stress reaction of the proximal ulna was found in a top-ten tennis player complaining about therapy-resistant discomforts during sport-specific strain (Pieper et al. 1997). Physical examination presented diffuse pressure sensitivity upon the proximal ulna at free range of motion of the elbow joint. At the time of the final diagnosis, no radiological abnormality could be demonstrated (➢ Fig. 16.3 a and b), while the final diagnosis was confirmed by bone scintigraphy (➢ Fig. 16.4 a and b).

Treatment

Conservative treatment by avoiding sport-specific local strain for 6 to 8 weeks is the therapy of choice followed by controlled slow increase of specific loads. Only in rare cases, immobilization may be necessary, especially if the athlete does not seem to be fully compliant. Full sport-specific capacity will be restored after approximately 3 months.

16.2.2 Medial and lateral epicondylitis

Causes

In 1873, Runge was the first to describe an overuse strain of the hand and finger extensor tendons as a functional overload reaction, using the term **"graphospasm"**. Nowadays more commonly the term "tennis elbow" is used for this clinical condition. This term, however, does not meet the facts, because non-athletes are affected more often than tennis players,

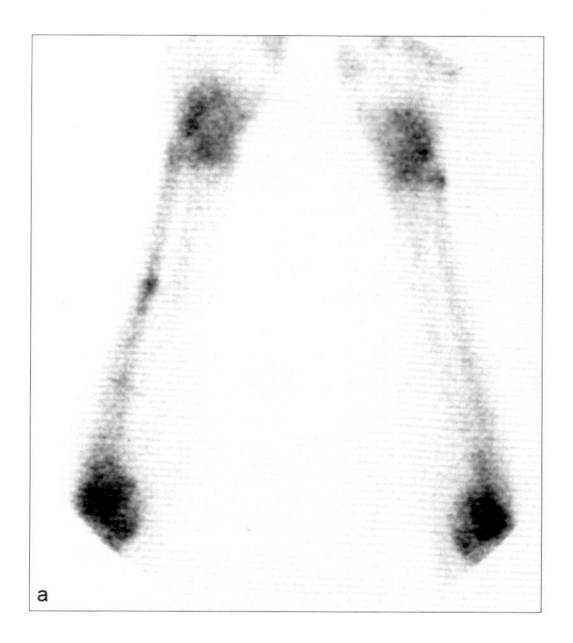

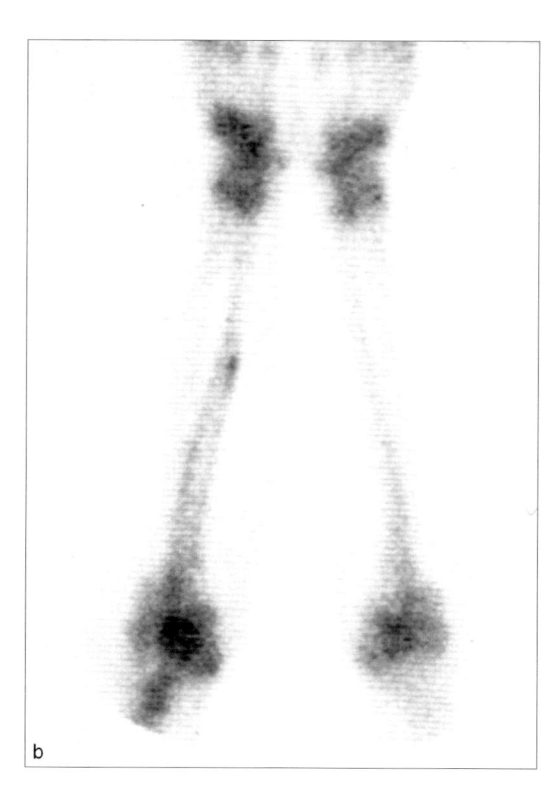

Fig. 16.4 Presentation of the stress reaction in scintigram of the same athlete as in ➢ Fig. 16.3.

and among those, professionals are affected less frequently than recreational athletes (Biener 1982, Krahl et al. 1997).

Medial or ulnar epicondylitis is often referred to as "thrower's" or "golfer's elbow", respectively. This is also not appropriate either, because especially in throwers presenting ulnar-sided elbow symptoms the specific tendon insertions are only partially affected while the main cause of the discomforts originates in the medial capsulo-ligamentous complex and the elbow joint itself (see below).

> Epicondylitis is defined as functional overload of the hand and finger extensor and flexor tendons respectively.

In lateral or radial epicondylitis mainly the **extensor carpi radialis muscle** is affected, occupational or athletic strain with **degenerative changes of the tendon insertions** (intratendinous necroses) being the cause (Kraushaar und Nirschl 1999). Lateral epicondylitis occurs about 5 to 10 times more often than medial epicondylitis.

Symptoms

In the case of **lateral or radial epicondylitis**, the athlete complains of tenderness over the lateral epicondyle of the elbow especially when closing the fist, being unable to grasp firmly. These conditions can appear at small strain like picking up a coffee cup, turning a doorknob, or even shaking hands. Occasionally an inhibition of hand or finger extension (pain-related) can be found.

Medial or ulnar epicondylitis presents local pain on the medial side of the elbow during pronation or supination of the forearm or when spreading the fingers.

Diagnosis

On physical examination there is **local tenderness to palpation** over the respective epicondyle of the humerus, frequently induration and hypertonus of the hand and finger extensors or flexors, pain when stretching hand and finger flexors **(Thomsen's test)**, a positive **chair test** (lifting a chair when forearm is pronated) or overextension of the wrist.

Radiographs are usually negative. Rarely traction osteophytes may be noted in the area of tendon insertion.

Differential diagnosis

Regarding possible **differential diagnosis**, the following must be considered

- synovitis of the elbow joint
- a synovial plica (Kim et al. 2006, Ruch et al. 2006)
- a blockage or a cartilage degeneration of the radial head
- loose bodies
- supinator syndrome (local irritation of the deep branches of the radial nerve)
- a compression syndrome of the ulnar nerve.

Occasionally, **degenerative changes in the region of the 5th and 6th cervical vertebrae** accompanied by radicular irritation can be the cause (Peterson und Renström 2002).

Treatment

Conservative

Conservative treatment will lead to success rates of up to 90% (Nirschl 1995 a und b). In the acute condition, **antiinflammatory medication**, local ice application, and rest from specific strain is helpful until the symptoms fade. Additionally, local **infiltration of steroids** can be applied. However, more than 2 to 3 cortisone injections should be avoided (Peterson und Renström 2002). After the acute symptoms subside (appr. 1–2 weeks), active rehabilitation should be started to restore strength, endurance, and flexibility.

Physiotherapy particularly involves stretching of the appropriate muscles, deep friction, application of ice, heat treatment if appropriate, as well as electrotherapy including ultrasound (Trudel et al. 2004, Rosemeyer 2005). **Short-term immobilization in a cast** may sometimes be helpful, however, it should only be applied embedding hand and fingers to prevent extension strain.

> To avoid harm through immobilization, the elbow joint itself should not be immobilized. Thus, local treatment despite a cast could be administered!

The effect of an **epicondylitis brace** is to influence the direction of tendon tension by means of applying pressure upon the tendon insertion. Likewise shock wave therapy (Haupt 1997), acupuncture (Trinh et al. 2004) or injections of botulinum toxin (Wong et al. 2005) have been reported to be successful. Long-term results of these treatment methods remain to be demonstrated.

In **racket sports**, a **specific training** should be carried out simultaneously to improve stroke technique and grip. Complete rehabilitation treatment will take approximately 4 months (Nirschl 1995a). Sports-specific training at higher loads should not be resumed unless full strength and flexibility have been restored and the athlete is free of pain, if the success of the treatment should not be put to a risk (Peterson und Renström 2002).

Surgical

Surgical treatment will only be necessary, if all non-operative treatment options have been carried out with patience (Nirschl 1995b). The most common surgical method is **Hohmann's tendon incision technique**, which is frequently carried out in combination with the denervation technique first described by Wilhelm. Less frequently local excision of pathological angiofibroplastic tendon tissue, mainly within the extensor carpi radialis brevis tendon, is performed (Nirschl 1995b). The **period of rehabilitation** following surgical treatment will last up to 6 months (Nirschl 1995b).

16.2.3 Thrower's elbow

Causes

Irrespective of the less common overload syndromes at the tendon insertions of the hand and finger extensors at the ulnar or medial epicondyle, **throwing athletes** such as baseball pitchers or javelin throwers more frequently suffer from chronic pain in the **medial capsule and ligaments** of the elbow joint.

An **extremely high valgus stress** is applied to the elbow in throwing. Throwing velocity of up to 39.6 m/s in 18-year-old high school pitchers (Cooper und Glassow 1976) and discharge speeds of more than 100 km/h by javelin throwers (Steinbrück und Krzycki 2005) with repetitions from 8,000 to more than 10,000 per year are observed. This jerky valgus stress will lead to **repetitive microtrauma** with increasing loosening of the medial capsulo-ligamentous structures (Mirowitz und London 1992, Werner et al. 2002). Exophytic spurs may grow as a consequence of the progressive instability. Especially on the postero-medial side of the fossa olecrani, osteophytes may develop leading to an increasing limitation of extension range.

Treatment

For surgical treatment, various stabilizing procedures are used. In the early phase, anatomical reconstruction of the original capsulo-ligamentous structures may be possible. For chronic instability, complex ligament replacement procedures using free tendon transfers have been described. Return to the same level of athletic performance, however, can only be achieved in one half or at a maximum two thirds of the cases (Bell und Hawkins 1986, Conway et al. 1992).

In young athletes, whose growth plates have not closed yet, repetitive valgus stress may occasionally lead to overuse conditions with separation of the medial epicondyle as a result of constant traction on the open medial epicondylar epiphysis, popularly termed **"Little Leaguer's Elbow"** (➤ Fig. 16.5) (Hang et al. 2004). At the

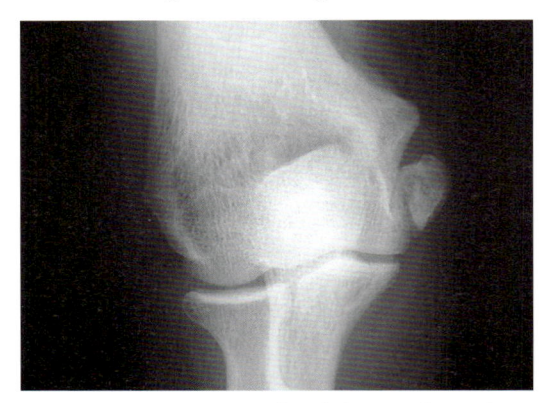

Fig. 16.5 "Little leaguer's elbow": late condition after a typical stress reaction by repeated valgus stress at the age of growth with separation of the ulnar epicondyle.

occurrence of the slightest discomfort, especially these adolescent athletes should be taken off throwing strain immediately. These cases in particular require rapid and good diagnostic effort in order to prevent injuries and stress reactions of the growth plates.

Summary

Injuries and overload syndromes of the elbow joint are relatively rare in sports. They are encountered mainly in baseball pitchers, javelin throwers, tennis players and wrestlers. Elbow dislocations, forearm fractures, and ruptures of the distal biceps tendon are the most significant injuries. Insertion tendinopathies (medial and lateral epicondylitis as well as thrower's elbow) and stress fractures are the prevailing overuse syndromes.

References

Andrews JR, Timmermann LA (1995) Outcome of elbow surgery in professional baseball players. Am J Sports Med 23: 407–413.

Bell RH, Hawkins RJ (1986) Stress fracture of the distal ulna. A case report. Clin Orthop 209: 169–171.

Bennett GE (1959) Elbow and shoulder lesions of baseball players. Am J Surg 98: 484–492.

Biener K (1982) Sportunfälle. Epidemiologie und Prävention, Lehre, Forschung, Verhütung. 2. Aufl. Huber, Bern-Göttingen-Toronto.

Collins HR (1985) The treatment of shoulder and elbow trauma in the athlete. In: Schneider RC, Kennedy JC, Plant ML (Hrsg): Sports Injuries. Mechanisms, Prevention, and Treatment. Williams & Wilkins, Baltimore-London-Sydney.

Conway JE, Jobe FW, Glousman RE, Pink M (1992) Medial instability of the elbow in throwing athletes. Treatment by repair or reconstruction of the ulnar collateral ligament. J Bone Joint Surg 74 A: 67–83.

Cooper JM, Glassow RB (1976) Kinesiology. 4th ed. Mosby, St. Louis.

Gilcreest EL (1925) Rupture of muscles and tendons particularly subcutaneous rupture of the biceps flexor cubiti. JAMA 84: 1819–1822.

Hang DW, Chao CM, Hang YS (2004) A clinical and roentgenographic study of little leaguer's elbow. Am J Sports Med 32: 79–84.

Haupt G (1997) Use of extracorporeal shock waves in the treatment of pseudoarthrosis, tendinopathy and other orthopaedic diseases. J Urol 158: 4–11.

Hegelmaier C, Schramm W (1992) Die Umschlingungsoperation zur Wiederherstellung der distal rupturierten Bizepssehne. Operat Orthop Traumatol 4: 185–193.

Hohmann G (1933) Das Wesen und die Behandlung des sogenannten Tennisellenbogens. Münch Med Wochenschr 80: 250–252.

Kelly EW, Steinmann S, O'Driscoll SW (2003) Surgical treatment of partial distal biceps tendon ruptures through a single posterior incision. J Shoulder Elbow Surg 12: 456–461.

Kim DH, Gambardella RA, ElAttrache NS, Yocum LA, Jobe FW (2006) Arthroscopic treatment of posterolateral elbow impingement from lateral synovial plicae in throwing athletes and golfers. Am J Sports Med 34: 438–444.

Kolb K, Holz U (1999) Das instabile Ellenbogengelenk. Unfallchirurg 102: 554–571.

Krahl H, Maibaum S, Braun M (1997) Tennis. In: Engelhardt M, Hintermann B, Segesser B (Hrsg.): GOTS-Manual der Sporttraumatologie. Huber, Bern.

Kraushaar BS, Nirschl RP (1999) Tendinosis of the elbow (tennis elbow). Clinical features and findings of histological, immunohistochemical, and electron microscopy studies. J Bone Joint Surg 81 A: 259–278.

Küster HH, Rompe G (1983) Die Monteggia-Verletzung im Sport. Unfallmechanismus Diagnostik Therapie. Dtsch Z Sportmed 34: 78–86.

Loosli AR, Leslie M (1991) Stress fractures of the distal radius. A case report. Am J Sports Med 19: 523–524.

Mehta JA, Bain GI (2004) Posterolateral rotatory instability of the elbow. J Am Acad Orthop Surg 12: 405–415.

Miller JE (1960) Javelin thrower's elbow. J Bone Joint Surg 42-B: 788–792.

Mirowitz SA, London SL (1992) Ulnar collateral ligament injury in baseball pitchers: MR imaging evaluation. Radiology 185: 573–576.

Nirschl RP (1995a) Tennis elbow tendinosis. Pathoanatomy and non-operative treatment. In: Krahl H, Pieper HG, Kibler, WB, Renström PA (Hrsg.): Tennis: Sports Medicine and Science. Rau, Düsseldorf.

Nirschl RP (1995b) Surgical management of medial and lateral tennis elbow tendinosis. In: Krahl H, Pieper HG, Kibler, WB, Renström PA (Hrsg.): Tennis: Sports Medicine and Science. Rau, Düsseldorf.

Nuber GW, Diment MT (1992) Olecranon stress fractures in throwers. Clin Orthop 278: 58–61.

Orava S, Puranen J, Ala-Ketola L (1978) Stress fractures caused by physical exercise. Acta Orthop Scand 49: 19–27.

Pereira DS, Kvitne RS, Liang M, Giacobetti FB, Ebramzadeh E (2002) Surgical repair of distal biceps tendon ruptures. Am J Sports Med 30: 432–436.

Peterson L, Renström P (2002) Verletzungen im Sport. Prävention und Behandlung. 3. Aufl. Deutscher Ärzte-Verlag, Köln.

Pieper HG, Radas CB, Krahl H, Montag M (1997) Die Streßfraktur der Ulnadiaphyse und des Olekranon beim Tennisspieler eine seltene Differenzialdiagnose des Tennisellenbogens. Literaturüberblick und zwei Fallbeispiele. Dtsch Z Sportmed 48: 110–118.

Raschka C, Gläser H, de Marées H (1995) Unfallhergangstypen im Volleyball und Vorschläge zu ihrer Prävention. Dtsch Z Sportmed 46: 366–371.

Rosemeyer B (2005) Golf. In: Engelhardt M, Krüger-Franke M, Pieper HG, Siebert CH (Hrsg.): Sportverletzungen Sportschäden. Thieme, Stuttgart-New York.

Ruch DS, Papadonikolakis A, Campolattaro RM (2006) The posterolateral plica: a cause of refractory lateral elbow pain. J Shoulder Elbow Surg 15: 367–370.

Runge F (1873) Zur Genese und Behandlung des Schreibekrampfes. Berl Klin Wochenschr 10: 245–248.

Safran MR, Graham SM (2002) Distal biceps tendon ruptures: incidence, demographics and the effect of smoking. Clin Orthop 404: 275–283.

Seiler III JG, Parker LM, Chamberland PCD, Sherbourne GM, Carpenter WA (1995) The distal biceps tendon. J Shoulder Elbow Surg 4: 149–156.

Steinbrück K (1987) Epidemiologie von Sportverletzungen. 15-Jahres-Analyse einer sportorthopädischen Ambulanz. Sportverl Sportschad 1: 2–12.

Steinbrück K, Krzycki J (2005) Epicondylopathia humeri ulnaris der Werfer- oder Golferellenbogen. Dtsch Z Sportmed 56: 90–95.

Trinh KV, Phillips SD, Ho E, Damsma K (2004) Acupuncture for the alleviation of lateral epicondyle pain: a systematic review. Rheumatology 43: 1085–1090.

Trudel D, Duley J, Zastrow I, Kerr EW, Davidson R, MacDermid JC (2004) Rehabilitation for patients with lateral epicondylitis: a systematic review. J Hand Ther 17: 243–266.

Tullos HS, King JW (1973) Throwing mechanism in sports. Orthop Clin North Am 4: 709–720.

Visuri T, Lindholm H (1994) Bilateral distal biceps tendon avulsions with use of anabolic steroids. Med Science Sports Exerc 26: 941–944.

Waris W (1946) Elbow injuries of javelin-throwers. Acta Chir Scand 93: 563–575.

Werner SL, Murray TA, Hawkins RJ, Gill TJ (2002) Relationship between throwing mechanics and elbow valgus in professional baseball pitchers. J Shoulder Elbow Surg 2: 151–155.

Wilhelm A (1989) Therapieresistente Epicondylitis humeri radialis und Denervationsoperation. Operat Orthop Traumatol 1: 25–34.

Williams JS, Hang DW, Bach BR (1996) Distal biceps rupture in a snowboarder. Phys Sportsmed 24: 66–70.

Wirth CJ (2001) Ellenbogengelenk. In: Wirth CJ (Hrsg.): Praxis der Orthopädie Bd. II: Operative Orthopädie. 3. Aufl. Thieme, Stuttgart.

Wong SM, Hui ACF, Tong PY, Poon DWF, Yu E, Wong LKS (2005) Treatment of lateral epicondylitis with botulinum toxin. A randomized, double-blind, placebo-controlled trial. Ann Intern Med 143: 793–797.

17 Hand and wrist joint

Andreas Englert and Bernhard Lukas

Wrist joint and hand define the endpoint of the upper extremity. Forces coming from the shoulder, the humerus, the elbow and the forearm are transmitted to the piece of sports equipment in some sports (e.g. javelin throwing, shotput, ice hockey, tennis, etc.). In contrast, forces working from the outside have to be intercepted by hand and wrist in some sports (e.g. downhill mountain biking, floor exercises, weight lifting, etc.).

Concerning the volume, the wrist is a very "weak" joint, in comparison with other joints. Only its complex anatomy makes it an extremely functional, firm and thus "strong" joint.

17.1 Anatomy and kinematics

Hand and wrist – excluding both bones of the forearm – consist of 29 bones altogether:
- eight carpal bones:
  - proximal row: os scaphoideum, os lunatum, os triquetrum, os pisiforme
  - distal row: os trapezium, os trapezoideum, os capitatum, os hamatum
- five metacarpal bones (MC I to V)
- twelve phalanges of the fingers II to V
- two phalanges of the thumbs
- two sesamoid bones at the metacarpophalangeal joint of the thumb.

The **wrist joint** consists of several components:
- the distal radioulnar joint with the ulnocarpal complex (triangular fibro-cartilage complex, TFCC; Taleisnik 1985)
- the proximal wrist, divided into a radiocarpal and an ulnocarpal compartment with an altogether large movement amplitude on all levels
- the distal wrist joint or mediocarpal wrist joint with an altogether lesser movement extent.

The proximal carpal row stands out due to an extensive mobility of the carpal bones among one another and is thus particularly interference-prone. In contrast, the distal carpal row can be considered as firm, solid monolith.

The **stability of the carpal bone** is provided by a system consisting of three layers (Kuhlmann 1982):
- the superficial layer of flexor and extensor tendon retinacula
- the medial layer of joint capsule and extrinsic ligament system between carpal bone, radius and ulna
- the deep layer, consisting of the intrinsic ligaments, with the scapholunar (SL) and the lunotriquetral (LT) ligaments being the best known and most important.

The carpometacarpal joints (CMC) of the fingers I–IV only show a very low measure of movement.

The CMC I or **saddle joint of the thumb** is a special form. It does not only allow flexion and extension, but also abduction and adduction as well as rotation movements, and thus is functionally comparable to a spheroid joint.

The **metacarpophalangeal joints** (MCP) are spheroid joints and also allow a multidimensional mobility, while the proximal and distal **interphalangeal joints** (PIP and DIP) are hinge joints and only allow a one-dimensional mobility (extension/flexion).

The joint capsules of the MCP and the PIP joints are stabilized by collateral ligaments; the so-called palmar plate serves these joints as protection against hyperextension on the flexor side.

Two **sesamoid bones** functioning as passive stabilizers and preventing the overextension of the joint are located palmarly at the MCP joint of the thumb.

A large number of **tendons, muscles and ligaments** are set at the bones, and the intrinsic muscles additionally originate from the metacarpal bones.

The interaction of the bony skeleton with muscles, tendons and ligaments is **controlled centrally** and receives the necessary impulses via the peripheral nerve pathways. Due to this filigree netting, we can perform finest movements or movement processes using our hands and wrists with dosed strength and highest precision. Otherwise, a controlled, accurate placing of a tennis or golf ball or the catching of a football at full run would not be possible.

A disorder of this complex system by injuries therefore has negative impacts on many sports requiring the use of our hands.

> The anatomy and kinematics of the wrist and the whole hand are extremely complex. Injuries have a direct influence on kinematics and can throw the complex interaction between bones, ligaments, muscles and tendons out of the natural balance and can thus severely impair the function of hand and wrist. The exact knowledge of anatomy and kinematics is the precondition for correct diagnoses and adequate therapy.

17.2 Epidemiology and etiology

Very different data regarding the frequency of sports injuries of hand and wrist are given in literature. While some authors speak of 3–9% (Lee et al. 2002, Rettig 2003), others report 20–30% (Hursh 1967, Thiebault 1980). Whichever of these numbers are brought up, a relatively high number of unknown cases must be assumed.

Sports injuries at hand and wrist can be segmented into traumatic and chronic or overstress impairments.

Fractures, ligament injuries and dislocations as are often found in contact sports, martial arts or as consequences of falls are **traumatic injuries**. **Overstress syndromes** are found rather in sports with the use of racquets (tennis, golf, etc.), in gymnastics or in endurance sports.

Mixed forms with chronic overstress by fresh trauma becoming symptomatic are not uncommon, either.

> Injuries at wrist or hand are of traumatic or chronic-degenerative genesis. The rate of injuries is often underestimated and is probably much higher than stated in literature.

17.3 Fractures

Fractures are almost exclusively **traumatic lesions**. Stress fractures, like they are known in the metatarsal bones of runners, are extremely rare at hand and wrist joint.

In literature, statistics are found (Hame et al. 2004) according to which fractures of the hands of **college athletes** of different sports are **in the first place** of all fractures and the frequency of wrist fractures also remains in the upper third.

17.3.1 Fractures of the carpal bones

Fractures of the carpal bones are in the second place of the fractures of the upper extremity behind the distal radius fracture (Green et al. 2005).

As in the distal radius fracture, the pathomechanism is the **fall to the extended wrist joint** here as well. According to the position of the wrist, different fractures develop. Dependent on the degree of the dorsal extension and the axial position of the wrist joint at the collision, either a **fracture** of the carpal bones or a **rupture** of ligament structures appears.

By far the most frequent fracture in the region of the carpal bones is the **scaphoid fracture** with 60–80%, followed by triquetrum fractures with 10–15%. The **most severe kind** of injury is the **perilunar dislocation** or **dislocation frac-**

ture. All other fractures are extremely rare and require a surgical treatment only in exceptional cases.

> A fall to the extended wrist joint can cause a fracture of the distal radius and also a fracture of carpal bones.

Scaphoid fracture

This fracture is very often found in American football, basketball, hockey, snowboarding and in falls off the bike.

In several respects, this is considered a **problem fracture**:

- It is often unnoticed.
- The fracture line is often not determinable in conventional radiographs of the wrist joint in two layers. Athletes, coaches or physicians often trivialize such injuries as sprains, because swelling and pain recede after a relatively short time.
- The scaphoid has a poor blood circulation.

Especially the **blood supply of the proximal pole** is problematic. This entails, that proximal fractures without surgery or immobilization cannot fully heal and a **pseudoarthrosis** can hereby develop (10-15%) (Topper et al. 1998).

Diagnosis

The **radiographical examination** of the wrist joint on two levels is standard procedure in addition to the **clinical examination** often showing a swelling and pain in the area of the tabatière. A **Stecher radiograph** (posterior-anterior beam projection, clenched fist and wrist in maximum ulnaduction) should be taken additionally, because it shows the scaphoid at full length.

The diagnosis must be continued even without a fracture being detectable but with an existing anamnestic and clinical suspicion.

Primarily, **MRI** plays only a minor role for scaphoid fractures. It is indicated at a pseudoarthrosis for the assessment of the blood supply of the fragments.

CT examination has proved of value as continuative diagnosis because of its high local resolution. Here it is important to make sure that a **thin-layer CT** (layer thickness <1 mm) is made in the longitudinal axis of the scaphoid.

It should be used in any case – even with a fracture proven in the conventional radiograph – in order to show the expanse of the fracture and to assign it to the according fracture type.

Regarding the type classification, the arrangement according to Herbert has proved of value (➤ Fig. 17.1), in which a division into firm and unstable forms of fracture is made.

Therapy

Solid scaphoid fractures can be treated conservatively; unstable ones should be treated surgically.

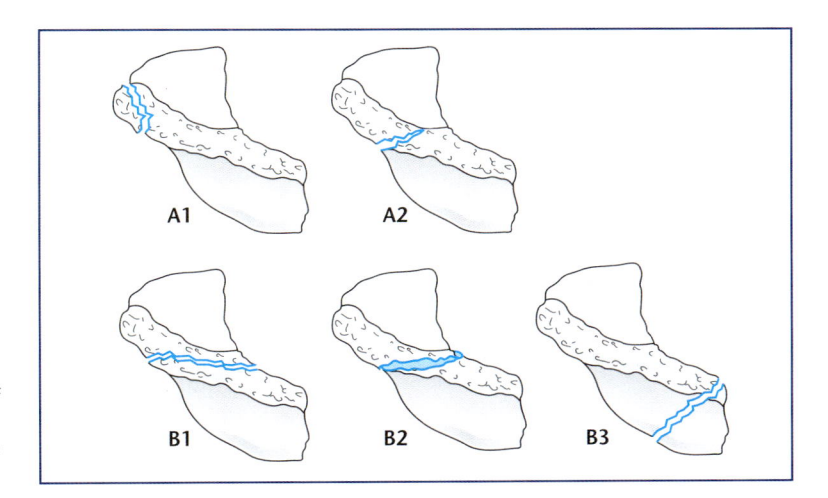

Fig. 17.1 Classification of scaphoid fractures according to Herbert. A: Stable fractures. B: Unstable fractures.

The **conservative therapy** is usually carried out by a forearm cast with thumb embedding for 6 weeks. At the removal of the cast, a radiologic test is applied and may be amended by a CT examination, if required.

Due to the development of the **cannulated Herbert screw**, stable fractures are treated increasingly by **minimally invasive surgeries**, especially in athletes. In addition to the A2 fractures, non-dislocated or only slightly dislocated B1 and B2 fractures are suited for minimally invasive osteosynthesis as well (≻ Fig. 17.2). A guide wire is inserted into the scaphoid under radiographic supervision from palmar to distal via a skin incision of a length of just 1 cm; the bone is trephined via this wire and a cannulated Herbert screw is screwed in. In a similar way, proximal pole fractures can be treated by newly developed, cannulated mini-Herbert screws via mini-incision. These procedures offer the advantage that an **immobilization can be abandoned** and the athlete can be coached quickly again this way.

A **resumption of exercise** is usually possible after 6 weeks. The full osseous knitting must be ascertained by thin-layer CT in sports with extreme stress to the wrists, e.g. gymnastics, boxing, martial arts or weight lifting, before the resumption of the sport-specific workout after 3 months at the earliest.

All strongly **dislocated unstable fractures** are approached openly from palmar (B1 and B2) or from dorsal (B3). A **postoperative immobilization for 2 to 6 weeks**, according to the degree of dislocation, is necessary because of the primary instability and the transection of the joint capsule and stabilizing ligament structures.

An incompletely healed scaphoid fracture leads inevitably to carpal instability and thus to carpal collapse – the so-called SNAC wrist (scaphoid non-union advanced collapse; Krimmer et al. 1997), in further succession.

> With 60–80%, the scaphoid fracture is the most frequent fracture of a carpal bone and at the same time a problem case. Without treatment, it often ends in pseudoarthrosis by reason of the precarious blood supply of the scaphoid and because it is often not recognized radiologically. The least suspicion of a scaphoid fracture must be pursued until it can be ruled out. In athletes, the minimally invasive technique for the therapy of simple fractures has proven of value. In general, exercise can be resumed after 6 weeks; a full workout in sports with according loads to the wrist is possible after 3 months. A fracture that has not been recognized or has "healed out" in a pseudoarthrosis of the scaphoid implicates a carpal collapse (SNAC wrist) and a massive limitation of usability of the wrist in the long run.

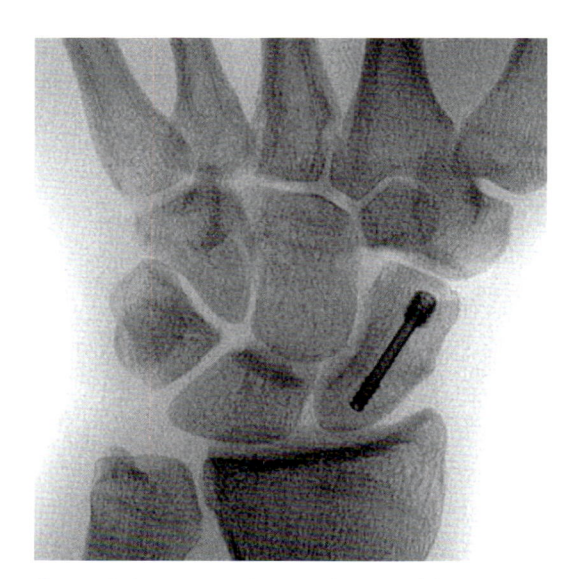

Fig. 17.2 Percutaneously treated scaphoid fracture type B2.

Hamulus fracture of the os hamatum

With an incidence of 2–3% (Rettig 2003), the hamulus fracture belongs to the rather rare but still important fractures in the area of the carpal bones.

It is mainly found in sports using a **racquet**, such as golf, tennis, baseball etc. At gripping the racquet, its handle comes to lie directly at the os hamatum. A fracture can be caused by direct, uncontrolled force effect via the ligamentous insertions.

The hamulus of the os hamatum is located in projection to the center of the hypothenar. The carpi transversus ligament and the pisohamatum ligament insert here. Parts of the flexor digiti minimi brevis muscle, the abductor digiti minimi muscle and the opponens digiti minimi muscle originate here. Furthermore, the deep branch of the **ulnar nerve** passes the basis of the hamulus.

A **fracture** in the region of the hamulus always involves the danger of an impairment of these closely adjacent structures.

Athletes, who use a racquet in their sport and experience **ulnar hand or wrist pain**, should always be examined for a hamulus fracture.

A **typical clinical sign** is the pressure pain directly distal of the os pisiforme. Failures in the area of the ulnar nerve, pain in flexion, abduction or opposition of the little finger are possible, as well, because of the anatomic conditions described above.

Radiologically, the carpal tunnel image is standard. In case of doubt, a CT examination must follow (➤ Fig. 17.3).

The **options of therapy** range from immobilization to refixation up to removal of the hamulus (Stark et al. 1977). In immobilization, there is the great **danger of pseudoarthrosis development** and thus the secondary resection. The **open refixation** (e.g. by a mini-Herbert screw) is to be aspired because of the number of inserting structures. In any case, a **longer incapacity of sport** (4–10 weeks) is to be expected.

> The hamulus fracture of the hamatum is altogether very rare and mainly found in sports with racquet use. The fracture of the hamulus can lead to clear functional conditions and limitations, because some important structures insert here or pass it directly. A hamulus fracture should always be thought of with ulnar hand and wrist pain of athletes of according sports, and this suspicion has to be followed up. Only a fresh hamulus fracture can be refixed adequately; for older hamulus fractures, there is only the choice of hamulus resection.

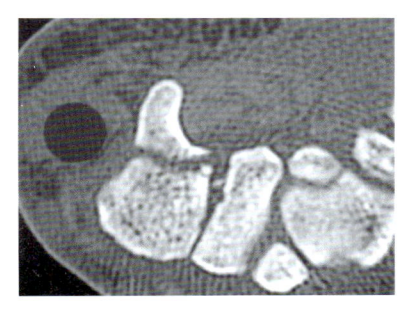

Fig. 17.3 CT image of a hamulus fracture (golf player).

17.3.2 Metacarpal and phalangeal fractures

In nearly all sports – in contact sports, (hand)ball sports and martial arts to a high degree –, fractures in the area of the metacarpal bones and finger phalanges can appear. These mostly are **stable fractures**. **Dislocated fractures** can often be induced, though, by **high-energy traumas** (motor sports, fall from the piece of sport equipment).

Stable fractures can be treated conservatively by according splints. At the immobilization in the area of the MCP, PIP and DIP joints, an anatomy-respective positioning must be provided (intrinsic-plus position) to avoid joint contractures and thus movement limitations (➤ Fig. 17.4).

Open unstable metacarpal and phalangeal fractures with rotation fault, axial malposition or shortenings should be treated surgically.

Percutane K-wire or open osteosynthesis procedures with screws or plates are used (➤ Fig. 17.5).

A reposition as exact and smooth as possible must be provided especially for fractures with joint involvement (e.g. Bennet fracture). Intraarticular fractures of the intermediate phalanges are particularly problematic. A combination of distraction (fixateur externe) and K-wire osteosynthesis is necessary for them.

A relatively fast return to athletic activity is possible in some sports after osteosynthesis and ergotherapeutic splint supply (Strickland 1992).

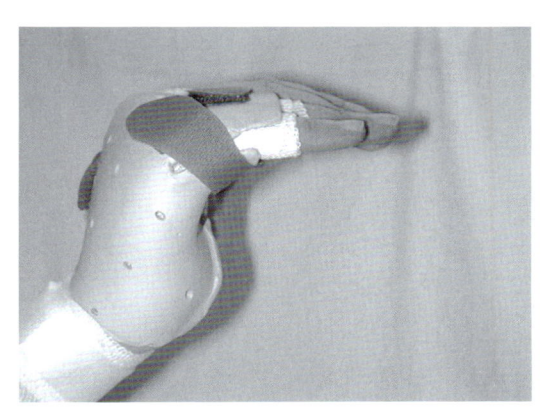

Fig. 17.4 Ergotherapeutic splint in intrinsic-plus position.

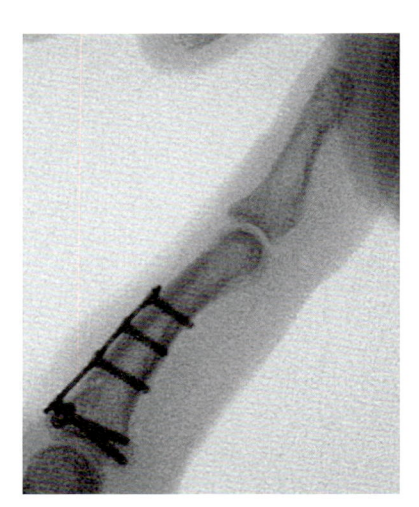

Fig. 17.5 Exercise-stably treated middle phalanx fracture of several fragments.

A metacarpal or phalangeal fracture can be found in virtually every sport. In general, its diagnosis is easy; the therapy has to be considered differently, depending on the form of fracture and the sport. A smooth reposition is important in fractures with joint involvement. A correct position according to anatomy (intrinsic-plus position) must be provided in immobilization in any case. In exceptional cases, an early functional treatment is possible.

17.4 Ligament injuries in the wrist

Ligament injuries in the wrist are as often the consequence of a trauma as fractures are. They are overlooked more often, though; they also lead to carpal instability successively and – without adequate treatment – end in a carpal collapse (Krimmer et al. 1997).

17.4.1 SL ligament lesions

The far most frequent ligament injury in the wrist is the SL ligament lesion (Jones 1988).

Such lesions are caused by force effects to the hyperextended, ulnaduced and mediocarpally supinated wrist joint, as in a fall onto the pronated forearm. The danger of this is found in all **contact sports** or sports involving collisions.

Three segments with different biomechanical functions each are distinguished:
- The dorsal segment ensures the main part of stability.
- The medial segment (fibrocartilaginous membrane) is only of minor significance for the stability.
- The palmar segment allows movements between scaphoid and lunate bone.

In general, **three degrees of severity of SL ligament lesions** are distinguished:
- degree I: partial rupture, mostly of the palmar segment, without instability
- degree II: complete rupture of all segments, including a lesion of the extrinsic apparatus with dynamic rotation instability
- degree III: complete rupture of all segments, including a lesion of the extrinsic apparatus with static instability (flexed scaphoid, dorsally rotated lunatum).

According to the degree of lesion, **conditions** can range from light to severe stress pain. For that reason, such injuries are often dismissed as bagatelles and are disregarded; they may have **serious consequences**, though, because of the instability of the wrist.

A suspected ligament lesion should be examined further at an according anamnesis, pain above the SL ligament, a pain-conditioned movement limitation or "clunk phenomena".

A **complete rupture** shows a painful clunk above the dorsal edge of the radius at pressure from palmar to the easily felt tubercle of the scaphoid bone and simultaneous radial-ulnaduction of the wrist (**Watson test**). Conditioned by the instability, the scaphoid can be subluxated in ulnaduction over the dorsal radial lip. This test often is unfeasible with fresh injuries, though, because of the pain.

The **radiologic standard examination** includes imaging of the wrist in two layers and additionally a clenched-fist image or a ball image (strong clenching of the fist leads to stress to the SL ligament) of both sides for comparison. In the images, attention must be paid to the tilting of the scaphoid to palmar and of the lunate bone to dorsal, the **d**orsal **i**ntercalated **s**egment **i**nstability (**DISI position of the lunate bone**). This rotational malposition is often misconstrued in MRI (Pfirrmann et al. 2002).

17.4 Ligament injuries in the wrist

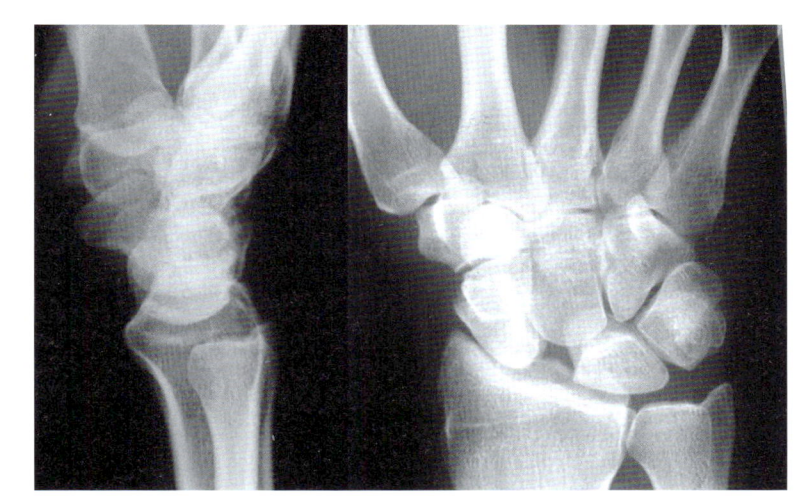

Fig. 17.6 Image of a static lesion of the scapholunate ligament.

Without the complete picture of a static ligament lesion (ring signs of the scaphoid, trapezoid shape of the lunate bone, extended SL fissure, SL angle >65°, ➤ Fig. 17.6), **cinematography** is used for the further diagnosis. Dissociation between scaphoid and lunate bone in ulna-radialduction movements shows in a dynamic instability.

Thanks to the spatial resolution becoming higher and higher, the **MRI** becomes more important in diagnosing SL ligament lesions. The sensitivity and specificity still is to be increased by the **MR arthrography** (Schmitt and Lanz 2004), although it is no part of the routine because of its invasiveness and the considerable amount of time and money.

Arthroscopy is the end point of the diagnosis and at the same time the starting point of therapy. Stage 1 can often only by diagnosed by arthroscopy (➤ Tab. 17.1). In stage 2, it serves the discerning of the extent of the lesion and thus the specifying of further procedures. In stage 3, the possibly already existing degree of arthrosis is assessed by arthroscopy.

The **therapy** of the SL ligament lesion is highly differentiated. According to the stage, the age of the injured person, the degree of tilting of the carpal bones and their restorability, the existence of an arthrosis and the activity of the athlete, the therapeutic options range from **cast immobilization** to ligament suture and augmentation, ligament plastics and up to **rescue operations**, such as limited midcarpal arthrodesis or the removal of the proximal row with serious loss of wrist mobility.

This can even cause sport incapacity, depending on the sport.

> The most frequent ligament injury of the wrist is by far the SL ligament rupture. Its pathomechanism is similar to the one of a fracture of a carpal bone. The conditions in an SL ligament lesion are mostly only minor, so that it often fails to be diagnosed primarily. In addition to clinical

Tab. 17.1 Diagnoses of lesions of the scapholunate ligament.

	Watson's test	Radiographic standard	Radiographic stress	Cinematography	MRI	Arthroscopy
stage 1	pain	normal	normal	normal	positive!?	pathologic
stage 2	snapping	normal	Widened scapholunate cleft	pathologic	positive	pathologic
stage 3	snapping	malposition	not applicable	not applicable	not applicable!?	pathologic

and radiologic standard examinations, cinematography plays a key role in diagnostics. With currently still subordinate significance of MRI, arthroscopy is the diagnostic endpoint and the therapeutic beginning at the same time. Therapy is corresponding to the stage of the ligament lesion and ranges from the simple immobilization to the complex ligament plastic. Similar to a scaphoid pseudoarthrosis, a neglected or not adequately treated SL ligament lesion can lead to carpal collapse (SLAC wrist) and thus to severe functional limitations.

17.4.2 LT ligament lesions

Though rarer than the lesions of the ligament between os scaphoideum and os lunatum, the rupture of the ligament between os lunatum and os triquetrum is serious.

Such ligament injuries are caused by force effect to the hyperextended, radialduced and mediocarpally pronated wrist. In addition to the typical anamnesis (fall onto the extended hand), the athlete reports ulnocarpal **stress pain**, and in extreme cases even a "clunk" in this area.

In the **examination**, pain exists ulnocarpally and especially in a dorsopalmar translation test of the triquetrum against the lunatum (Reagan`s test).

The **radiographs** are mostly normal. Rarely, a step in the connecting line of the proximal carpal row can be recognized. A **tilting** of the lunatum to palmar, the **p**almar **i**ntercalated **s**egment **i**nstability (**PISI** position), is often the result of a lesion of the secondary stabilizers, the ligaments of the extrinsic ligament apparatus.

Cinematography is diagnostically pioneering in LT ligament lesions; the MRI is unreliable (Schmitt and Lanz 2004).

Arthroscopy is also indicated here at an according suspected diagnosis.

In the **fresh stage**, the wrist is immobilized for 4 weeks or a temporary fusion is made with arthroscopical assistance between triquetrum and lunatum by K-wires. In **older lesions**, the immobilization is applied after an arthroscopic debridement. This is the reason for the healing of about 80% of these cases (Cohen 1998).

In addition to symptomatic measures such as NSAR application, local cortisone injections etc., often only the **lunotriquetral arthrodesis** remains for the remaining 20%. It has a **high fail rate**, though, and leads to a movement limitation of the complete wrist.

The LT ligament lesion is less frequent, but almost as serious as the SL ligament lesion. Also in diagnosis, cinematography is pioneering for similar pathomechanism. This therapy is mostly carried out arthroscopically and thereby provides high chances of healing. Without according therapy, the tilting of the lunatum in flexion (PISI position) can appear and thus a change of the kinematics as well as thereby conditioned functional limitations.

17.5 Injuries of the TFCC

Injuries of the triangular disk, also called TFCC (**t**riangular **f**ibro-**c**artilage **c**omplex), are very often found in athletes. The injuries can develop by an **acute trauma** (fall and avulsion trauma) or can lead to **chronic ulnocarpal pain** by repeated traumas/overstress (tennis, gymnastics, etc.).

The TFCC includes the central, relatively avascular ulnocarpal disk and the well vascularized dorsal and palmar ligaments surrounding it, the ulnocarpal meniscus sitting ulnarly and the bottom of the tendon sheath of the extensor carpi ulnaris muscle (➤ Fig. 17.7). About 20%

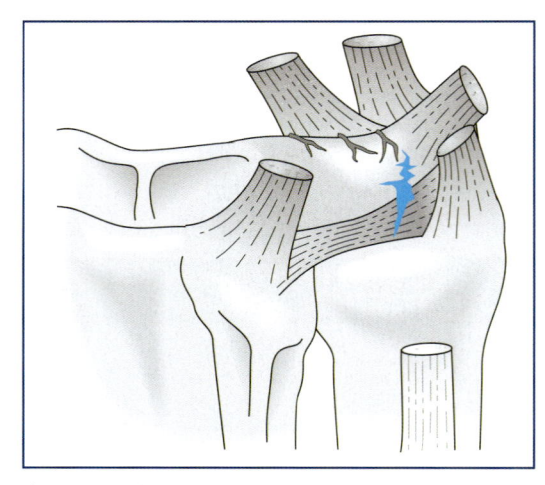

Fig. 17.7 Schematic presentation of the TFCC with ulnar lesion.

of the axial forces of the wrist have to be transmitted by this complex. Especially the well vascularized parts of the TFCC serve the stability of the distal radioulnar joint (DRUG).

The **ulnocarpal pain**, especially in rotational movements, is the main clinical sign of TFCC injuries. It can be increased further by provocation maneuvers.

In **conventional radiographs**, pathologies are mostly imperceptible, but a **widening** of the space between radius and ulna has to be considered as well as avulsion fractures of styloideus ulnae process close to the basis, because the TFCC inserts here.

Similar to SL ligament lesions (see above), the **MRI** becomes more significant in the diagnosis of TFCC lesions. The examination by contrast medium in high-performance equipment (1.5 Tesla) provides good results (➤ Fig. 17.8).

CT is inappropriate for the detection of TFCC lesions; it is indispensable for an existing instability of the distal radioulnar joint in neutral, pronated and supinated position, though.

With clinically and/or radiologically suspected TFCC lesions, the indication for **arthroscopy** is given. A lesion cannot only be diagnosed by this, but it also can be treated therapeutically at the same time. Generally, central lesions caused by repetitive traumas receive debridement; only ulnar avulsions can be refixed because of their good vascularity. Own examinations supplied good and very good results after arthroscopic refixation in 80% of the cases (Bäcker et al. 2004). If instability of the distal radioulnar joint exists additionally, an open refixing of the disk by bone anchor in the folvea of the ulnar head and the reconstruction of the radioulnar ligaments is necessary.

After a debridement, the wrist is being immobilized for 1–2 weeks, light activities can be taken up after 3–4 weeks, and increasing exercises can be carried out after about 6 weeks.

After a refixation, an immobilization of 4 weeks within an above elbow splint and 2 weeks within a forearm splint are necessary, followed by physical therapy and a sports break of 3–4 months.

> Ulnocarpal pain caused by trauma or chric overuse is often the expression of an injury of the triangular disk, also called TFCC. The clinical examination and the MRI by high-performance equipment (12.5 Tesla) are diagnostically pioneering. At the time being, arthroscopy is the "gold standard" of diagnosis with the option of definite therapy in more than 80% of the cases. Because of its sufficiently existing vascularity, ulnar avulsions can be refixed by an arthroscopically arthroscopy assisted technique atesswith a hi being mostly degenerative or conditioned by chronic overstress/inappropriate stress receive debridement. A re-uptake of sport activities with a pure debridement is possible after about 6 weeks, with a refixation after about 3–4 months.

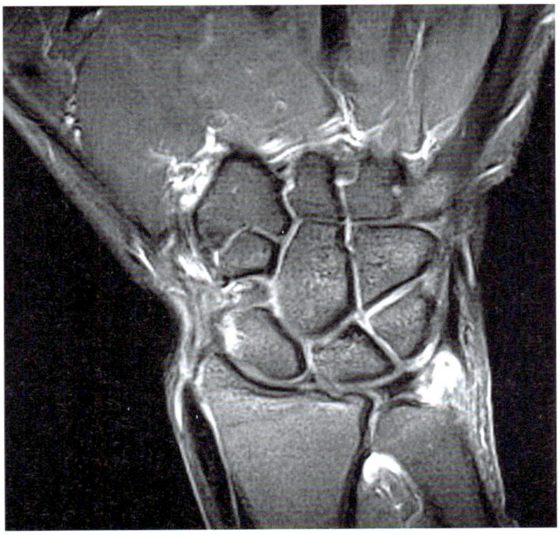

Fig. 17.8 Signal enhancement with ulnar TFCC lesion.

17.6 Injuries of the finger joints

The most frequent injuries of the finger joints affect the proximal interphalangeal joints (PIP) and the metacarpophalangeal joint (MCP) of the thumb. In the **PIP joints**, dislocations and capsule/ligament injuries are frequent; the **thumb** is often affected by injuries of the ulnar collateral ligament at the metacarpophalangeal joint

17.6.1 Injuries of the PIP joint

The most frequently affected joint in sports injuries is the PIP joint of the fingers (Strickland et al. 1992, Rettig 2004).

The joint is stabilized palmarly by the palmar plate, laterally by the collateral ligaments and dorsally by the tractus intermedius of the extensor tendon.

Most injuries are **contusions and sprains** with persistent pain and swellings. These should be sedated only for a short time, and they require a **long symptomatic treatment**.

Complete ruptures of the collateral ligaments are rare. With an early identification and treatment, a splint immobilization for 2-3 weeks is sufficient for injuries of these ligaments. After conclusive mobilization, activities can be started after 6 weeks.

With a **dislocation in the PIP joint**, an **immediate closed reposition** is necessary right on site. This may fail because of soft-tissue parts being interposed. An immediate **open reposition** is indicated then.

Corresponding to the direction of dislocation (palmar, dorsal, lateral), according structures are impaired. Mostly, an immobilization of 2–3 weeks is sufficient here, as well; a primary suture of the ligaments is rarely necessary.

With **injuries of the palmar plate** by dislocation or hyperextension trauma (ball against the finger), a complete extension must be avoided for 10 days by help of according splinting.

The **surgical refixation**, e.g. by a bone anchor, or a plastic, e.g. by a part of the superficial flexor tendon, are indicated for a **chronic instability of the palmar plate**.

An extension deficit after the end of the splint treatment has to be corrected mostly by physical therapy and/or a Howitt finger splint.

> The proximal interphalangeal joint (PIP) of the fingers is the most often affected joint in sports injuries. The according anatomical structures, such as collateral ligaments, palmar plate or the middle rein of the extensor tendon, can be impaired by contusion or sprain or by dislocation, respectively. An adequate therapy is very important for the prevention of a functional limitation by cicatrization in the region of these structures and an insufficient healing with the consequences of instability. Too long immobilization in a false position of the joint leads to the stiffening of this joint. Secondary reconstructions of the capsule/ligament apparatus or arthrolyses are rarely followed by a restitutio ad integrum.

17.6.2 Skier's thumb

Skier's thumb is the most common injury of the upper extremities in skiing sports (Browne et al. 1976), but it can be found in all other sports as well (ball sports).

The accident mechanism consists of a force effect coming from ulnar to the abducted thumb, as for instance in a fall on the skiing stick. For this reason, the **ulnar collateral ligament** of the metacarpophalangeal joint of the thumb becomes subject to stress and is **ruptured**.

After primary radiological diagnosis for the exclusion **of an osseous lesion**, the clinical examination follows.

At the acute stage, this is often difficult because of the distinct local pain and it can be carried out only under local anesthesia or after the pain has eased.

The differentiation between a complete and a partial rupture of the collateral ligament is important for the treatment of the skier's thumb.

The examination is carried out at a flexion of the metacarpophalangeal joint of 30°. A **complete rupture** must be assumed with an increased ability of up-folding by more than 30° in performing a radialduction in lateral comparison.

Incomplete ruptures can be treated by an immobilization of 5 weeks within the skier's thumb splint.

A conservative treatment is unsuccessful with the distally off-torn collateral ligament retracting to proximal and folding around the margin of the adductor pollicis aponeurosis (**Stener lesion**). Such ruptures, confirmed by high-resolution **sonography** or – in case of doubt – by **MRI**, must be treated by a primary, **intraligamentous ligament suture** or the osseous **reinsertion by a bone anchor**.

In an **osseous avulsion** of the collateral ligament, the sole splint immobilization is only indicated for cases without significant dislocation of the fragment. The **surgical refixation** is indicated for a distinct **dislocation**. Very small fragments (<20% of the joint surface) are excised and larger ones are refixed by mini-screws or wires (Lee et al. 2002, Green et al. 2005). The post-operative after-treatment correlates with the one of conservative therapy.

The rupture of the radial collateral ligament is far less common than the one of the ulnar ligament. Nevertheless, the same procedure applies to diagnosis and therapy.

> The so-called skier's thumb does not only occur in skiing, but also primarily in many ball sports. The complete rupture of the ulnar collateral ligament at the metacarpophangeal joint of the thumb must be treated surgically because of the danger of a permanent instability, especially with a present Stener lesion. Incomplete ruptures can be treated conservatively, the same as non-dislocated osseous avulsions. The conservative as well as the postoperative therapy consist of a 5-week immobilization within a skier's thumb splint. An analogous procedure applies to injuries in the area of the radial collateral ligament.

17.7 Tendon injuries

17.7.1 Flexor tendon injuries

Injuries of the flexor tendon in athletes are rather rare and occur mostly with open injuries by sports equipment (e.g. edges in skiing).

An example for subcutaneous ruptures of the flexor tendon is the **"jersey finger"**. Here the deep flexor tendon is ruptured at its insertion on the distal phalanx. This is caused by a sudden, strong extension with maximum flexed DIP joint, as in grabbing the jersey of the opponent. Athletes are especially at this risk in football, rugby, handball, but also players of water polo or judo fighters (Lee 2002, Rettig 2004). A special form is the **osseous avulsion of the flexor tendon**.

The **diagnosis** of open flexor tendon injuries mostly is easy; the closed rupture is often identified late. Both require an **immediate surgical therapy** by tendon suture or osseous refixing with subsequent intensive after-treatment, though.

> Lesions of the flexor tendons are mostly consequences of open injuries, far more rarely of subcutaneous ruptures. Though the diagnosis of open flexor tendon injuries is easy, closed ruptures are often identified late. There is no distinct difference in the kind of therapy, with the rare exception of an osseous avulsion of the flexor tendon.

17.7.2 Extensor tendon injuries

Subcutaneous extensor tendon ruptures at the height of the phalanges are relatively common, contrary to the injuries of the flexor tendons.

Especially in all **ball sports**, such ruptures can be caused by a collision of the ball with the finger. Subcutaneous ruptures above the DIP joint of the finger (zone 1) are the most common. A drooping of the distal phalanx of the finger without active extension is the clinical result. The imbalance of the extensor apparatus developing thus can result in a hyperextension in the PIP joint and thus in a **swan-neck deformity** (Lee et al. 2002).

The **therapy** of the extensor tendon rupture in zone 1 implies an immobilization in a **stack splint** for at least 8 weeks (➤ Fig. 17.9). The **surgical tendon suture** with subsequent immobilization is recommended at a late start of therapy or extreme extension deficit.

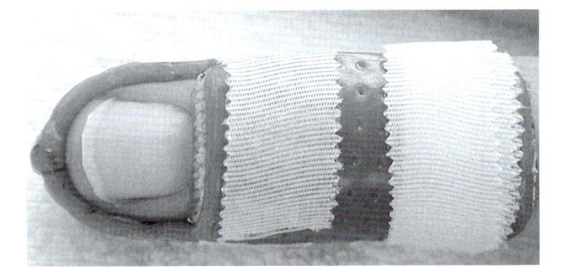

Fig. 17.9 Stack splint with rupture of the extensor tendon zone 1.

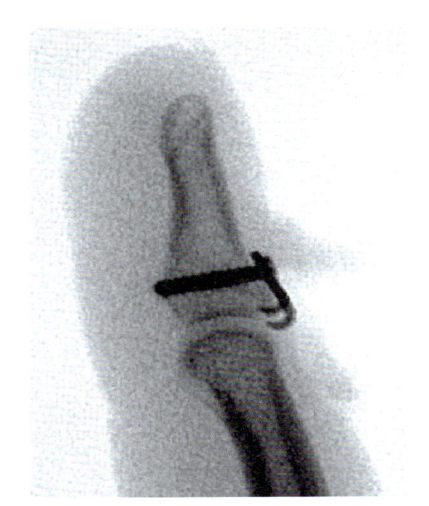

Fig. 17.10 Hook plate for the refixation of an osseous extensor tendon avulsion at the distal phalanx.

A special case is the osseous extensor tendon rupture at the distal phalanx. With a dislocation, it requires a surgical refixation of the fragment (➤ Fig. 17.10).

Injuries at the height of the **PIP joint** (zone 3) due to collision traumas or palmar dislocations are common, as well. They affect the tractus intermedius and lead to an extension deficit in the PIP joint, later additionally to an overextension of the DIP joint by an off-slipping of the tractus lateralis to palmar (**buttonhole deformity**).

Conservative immobilization of the joint in extended position for 6–8 weeks in a finger splint is the therapy of choice for fresh injuries, as well. The **surgical reconstruction** of the tractus intermedius is necessary for older injuries.

Closed lesions of the extensor tendons proximal of the PIP joint are rare and invariably require surgical therapy.

> Axial force effect, e.g. by a ball to the finger, can lead to subcutaneous injuries of the extensor tendon. With the exclusion of an osseous lesion, the therapy of such lesions at the height of the DIP joint (zone 1) and the PIP joint (zone 3) mostly includes an according conservative immobilization. All open injuries and all lesions proximal of the PIP joint require surgical therapy without exception.

17.7.3 Annular ligament injury

The flexor tendons in the area of the fingers are lead by a system of annular and cruciate ligaments. Especially the **A2 and the A4 annular ligament** are of distinctive functional meaning.

In **sports climbing** (➤ Chapter 44), up to 420 N especially bear on the A2 annular ligament according to the method of gripping (e.g. pull-up technique with put up fingers) (Bollen 1990). The closed rupture of the A2 annular ligament is one of the most frequent injuries of the fingers in sports climbers (Schöffl et al. 2002).

At mostly acute events with a **"bang"** (similar to the rupture of the Achilles tendon), a distinct **local pressure pain** is found in addition to a local swelling and – depending on whether one or several annular ligaments are affected – a more or less pronounced **bowstring phenomenon**.

The **radiological examination** serves the exclusion of an osseous lesion. Though the annular ligaments cannot be displayed directly in **MRI**, a broadened space rich of liquid of more than 1 mm between finger bone and the flexor tendon has proven reliable as an indirect sign (Schmitt and Lanz 2004).

Sonography is still superior, though, because dynamic examination can show the bowstring phenomenon directly (Schmitt and Lanz 2004, Kaluser et al. 2005).

At the rupture of **only one annular ligament**, the **conservative therapy** with an immobilization of 2 weeks and subsequent exercising with **annular ligament protection** (thermoplastic ring over the affected annular ligament, ➤ Fig. 17.11) for 3 more weeks has proven sufficient. Sports exercises can be started after 8 weeks, also using the annular ligament protection (tape wrapping). Full sport capacity is reacquired – also for professional climbers – after 3–4 months.

At the rupture of **several annular ligaments**, the **surgical annular ligament plastic** is carried out. For its processing, there are diverse surgical techniques with strips of retinaculum or tendon material (Lin et al. 1989, Schöffl 2002). The postoperative treatment correlates with the conservative therapy. Climbing should be started after 4 months at the earliest. Full sport capacity is only achieved after 6–9 months. For professional sports climbers, the complex annular ligament injury not uncommonly means the end of the professional sports career, because high grades of difficulty cannot be managed anymore.

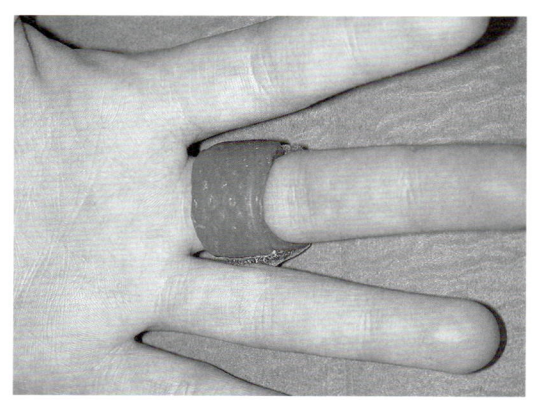

Fig. 17.11 Thermoplastic A2 annular band protection.

The closed rupture of the A2 annular ligament belongs to the most common injuries of the fingers of sports climbers. In addition to the clinical examination, the MRI and the superior high-resolution sonography are diagnostically pioneering. At the rupture of only one annular ligament, conservative therapy is indicated, and so is the surgical annular ligament plastic at the rupture of several annular ligaments. The sport capacity is achieved after 3–4 months at the earliest, in complex cases only after 6–9 months.

17.8 Nerve impairments

Conditioned by posture and the resulting compressive load to the wrists, not only impairments of the **ulnar nerve (cyclist's palsy)** in Guyon's canal, but also in the area of the **medianus nerve** in the carpal canal might appear **in cyclists** (Topper et al. 1998, Patterson et al. 2003). In up to 70%, these symptoms are found in long-distance cyclists (Patterson et al. 2003). This applies to bicycle racers as well as mountain bikers, to amateurs as well as professional cyclists.

Mostly, the **motor symptoms** of the ulnar nerve are in the foreground with weakness, paresis and atrophy of the intrinsic musculature.

The nerve irritation of the medianus nerve manifests itself mostly by **fingers going numb**, and less often by sensory disorders.

For distinctive symptoms, the **therapy** consists of an **immobilization** and an **administration of anti-phlogistics** until the acute symptoms decline. Persistent conditions of the sensory deficits or an atrophy of the musculature possibly indicate a surgical **decompression** for the securing of the localization of the impairment after neurological examination.

Cycling should only be resumed after the normalization of the symptoms.

The best prophylaxis is a sitting position optimally adjusted to the body height, the use of padded gloves (gel pads) and frequent changing of the hand position on the handlebars.

Bicycle racers as well as mountain bikers can suffer from "cyclist's palsy" because of the compressive load to the wrists and to the ulnar nerve, but also the medianus nerve. Conservative therapy is often sufficient; the surgical decompression is only indicated in exceptional cases. Prophylaxis by according material or adjusted sitting position and frequent change of the hand position on the handlebars, respectively, is very important.

17.9 Tendinitides

Tendinitides can occur at practically every tendon in the area of the wrist and the hand. They are the consequence of an acute or persisting overuse or improper load.

17.9.1 Tendovaginitis stenosans de Quervain

This is the most frequent tendovaginitis of athletes (Topper et al. 1998).

The tendon of the abductor pollicis longus muscle (APL) runs together with the tendon of the extensor pollicis brevis muscle (EPB) at the radial distal forearm in the first extensor tendon compartment. The roof of the compartment is shaped by the retinaculum extensorum, the styloideus radii process forms the bottom.

Microtraumas and inflammations of the tendon sheath develop here by continuous load in this region, e.g. in rowing, golf, volleyball or even squash and badminton (Gosheger et al. 2003, Rettig 2004, Rossi et al. 2005).

Clinically, the athlete shows a swelling and pain above the first extensor tendon compartment. In the examination, the pain can be increased by a passive, quick ulnaduction of the hand with maximum flexed thumb (**Finkelstein's test**).

At the acute stage, the **therapy** includes immobilization and the administration of anti-phlogistics. In persistence, an improvement can be achieved by **local corticoid injection**. The repeated injection is highly disputed, because it can lead to impairment or even to the rupture of the tendons.

The **surgical fissuring** of the first extensor tendon case is the measure of choice for chronic conditions. Complete fissuring of the compartment including the additional compartment of the possibly existing EPB tendon has to be taken care of. The sensitive **nerve branch of the radial nerve** running above the extensor tendon case **must be saved categorically**.

Sports incapacity is effective until the completion of the wound healing; afterwards the bearing of loads determined by the medical condition can be started.

> The tendovaginitis of the APL and the EPB tendon in the first extensor tendon compartment at the wrist is the most common localization of a tendovaginitis of an athlete's wrist or hand. Microtraumas caused by continuing overuse or improper loads are the cause. Finkelstein's test is diagnostically pioneering in most cases. The conservative therapy with the potential inclusion of local cortisone therapy is the measure of choice for the acute stage. The surgical fissure of the tendon compartment is measure of choice for the chronic stage.

17.9.2 Intersection syndrome

The intersection syndrome is an **inflammation of the muscle-tendon junctions of the APL and EPB** at their cross point with the ones of the second tendon compartment, the extensor carpi radialis longus and brevis about 4–6 cm proximal of the radiocarpal joint. It is often found in sports with repeated extension/flexion of the wrist against resistance, e.g. rowing or weight lifting (Wood and Dobyns 1986).

A painful swelling at the described cross point shows **clinically**. Sometimes a crepitation can be felt in active extension/flexion.

Usually, convalescence is achieved by **immobilization and administration of anti-phlogistics**. Only in exceptional cases, a surgical therapy by fissuring of the forearm fascia is indicated.

Sports can be exercised again after the regression of the afflictions.

> Inflammations can appear at the cross point of the APL and EPB with the muscles/tendons of the second extensor tendon compartment. Especially those sports with repeated extension/flexion of the wrist are affected. Because conservative measures are mostly sufficient, a surgical therapy is required only in exceptional cases.

17.10 Overstrain syndromes at the wrist joint

Especially in **gymnastics**, wrist conditions might appear very often (Mandelbaum et al. 1989). Chronic wrist conditions have also been known in other sports with the wrist being subject to constantly recurring strong forces in different and extreme positions (e.g. rowing, weight lifting, golf), though.

The **reasons** for these conditions can be manifold; they range from a simple strain of the joint capsule/ligaments to tendinitides, capsule ganglia up to "bone bruises" or impairments of the growths plates in youths.

Overstress syndromes of wrists and hands are **mostly sport-specific** and require analysis and collective clarification between athlete, coach, physiotherapist and hand surgeon. **Trivializing** overuse conditions can have **far-ranging consequences** (the pain becoming chronic, cartilage disorders, arthroses, growth disturbances) and even lead to an early sports incapacity.

> The downplaying of such overstress conditions by the athletes themselves, coaches, managers or also the treating physicians or physiotherapists occurs very often. The cause of such conditions must be gone further investigated. Otherwise severe impairments can develop and lead to early sports incapacity.

References

Bäcker K, Englert A, Lukas B (2004). Die Refixierung des Discus ulnocarpalis bei Läsionen vom Typ 1B nach Palmer. Vortrag beim 45. DAH-Symposium, Bad Neustadt an der Saale.

Bollen SR (1990). Injury to the A2 pulley in rock climbers. J Hand Surg 15B: 268–270.

Browne EZ, Dunn HK, Snyder CC (1976). Ski pole thumb injury. Plast Reconstr Surg 58: 19–23.

Cohen MS (1998). Ligamentous injuries of the wrist in the athlete. Clin Sports Med 17: 53–552.

Gosherger G, Liem D, Ludwig K, Greshake O, Winkelmann W. Injuries and overuse syndromes in golf. Am J Sports Med 31: 438–443.

Green DP, Hotchkiss RN, Pederson WC, Wolfe SW (2005). Green's Operative Hand Surgery. 5th ed. Elsevier, Churchill-Livinstone.

Hame SL, LaFemina JM, McAllister DR, Schaadt GW, Dorey FJ (2004). Fractures in the collegiate athlete. Am J Sports Med 32: 446–451.

Hursh LM (1967). Numbers and types of sport injuries (letter to the editor). JAMA 199: 507.Jones WA (1988). Beware of the sprained wrist: the incidence and diagnosis of scapholunate instability. J Bone Joint Surg 70B: 293–297.

Klausner A, Frauscher F, Gabl M, Smekal V (2005). Hochauflösende Sonographie zur Erkennung von Fingerverletzungen beim Sportklettern. Sportorthopädie Sporttraumatologie 21: 24–30.

Krimmer H, Krapohl B, Sauerbier M, Lanz, U (1997). Der posttraumatische karpale Kollaps (SLAC- und SNAC-Wrist) – Stadieneinteilung und therapeutische Möglichkeiten. Handchir Mikrochir Plast Chir 29: 228–233.

Kuhlmann JN (1982). Experimentelle Untersuchung zur Stabilität und Instabilität des Karpus. In: Nigst H (ed.). Frakturen, Luxationen und Dissoziationen der Karpalknochen. Hipokrates, Stuttgart.

Lee SJ, Montgomery K (2002). Athletic hand injuries. Orthop Clin N Am 33: 547–554.

Lin GT, Amadio PC, An KN, Cooney WP, Chao EY (1989). Biomechanical analysis of finger flexor pulley reconstruction. J Hand Surg 14B: 278–282.

Mandelbaum BR, Bartolozzi AR, Davis CA, Tuerlings L, Bragonier B (1989). Wrist pain syndrome in the gymnast – pathogenetic, diagnostic and therapeutic considerations. Am J Sports Med 17: 305–317.

Patterson JM, Jaggars MM, Boyer MI (2003). Ulnar and median nerve palsy in long-distance cyclists – A prospective study. Am J Sports Med 31: 585–589.

Pfirrmann CWA, Zanetti M, Hodler J (2002). Joint magnetic resonance imaging – normal variants and pitfalls related to sport injuries. Radiol Clin Am 40: 167–180.

Rettig AC (2003). Athletic injuries of the wrist and hand part I: traumatic injuries of the wrist. Am J Sports Med 31: 1038–1048.

Rettig AC (2004). Athletic injuries of the wrist and hand part II: overuse injuries of the wrist and traumatic injuries to the hand. Am J Sports Med 32: 262–273.

Rossi C, Cellocco P, Margaritondo E, Bizzarri F, Constanzo G (2005). De Quervain disease in volleyball players. Am J Sports Med 33: 424–427.

Schmitt R, Lanz U (2004). Bildgebende Diagnostik der Hand. 2nd ed. Thieme, Stuttgart.

Schöffl V, Hochholzer T, Winkelmann HP (2002). Management der geschlossenen Ringbandruptur bei Sportkletterern. Sportorthopädie Sporttraumatologie 18: 79–85.

Stark HH, Jobe FW, Boyes JH, Ashwoth CR (1977). Fractures of the hook of the hamate in athletes. J Bone Joint Surg 59A: 575–582.

Strickland JW, Rettig AC (1992). Hand Injuries in Athletes. W.B. Saunders Company.

Taleisnik J (1985). The Wrist. Elsevier, Churchill-Livingston.

Thiebault J (1980). Le risqué sportif: etude de 43 093 dossier concernant 57 disciplines (sport amateur). Rev Franc Dom Corp 6: 319–352.

Topper SM, Wood MB, Cooney WP (1998). Athletic Injuries of the Wrist. In: Cooney WP (ed.). The Wrist.

Wood MB, Dobyns JH (1986). Sports-related extraarticular wrist syndromes. Clin Orthop 202: 93–102.

Chapter 18 Pelvis and hip joint

Roland Biedert

18.1 Anatomy and biomechanics

The pelvis is formed on each side by the ilium, ischium, and pubis. The acetabulum provides bony coverage of 40% of the femoral head. Both form the hip joint. The two parts of the pubis are anterior connected at the symphysis. At posterior both sacroiliac joints are composed of the bilateral ilium and the sacrum in the centre.

The pelvis represents the central point of complex movement patterns in the upright gait (Biedert and Meyer 1997). With its **posterior part**, it serves especially the direct **transmission of body weight** and forms a functional unit in the lumbosacral junction. The **anterior part** serves as **insertion area of different muscle groups**. All muscle loops influencing our posture insert at the pelvis, some extending to the groin (Segesser 1996).

For the upright gait, the pelvic ring must be able to sustain the complete body weight also in dynamic one-leg standing. The medial and small glutei muscles work as multifunctional abductors and are responsible for the **pelvic balance**.

The inserting muscles at the pelvis ventrally or dorsally influence the **tilt of the pelvis** according to the rotation point of the hip joints. The abdominal musculature in combination with the gluteus maximus and medius muscles as well as the ischiocrural muscles will set the pelvis upright, while the iliopsoas muscle will effect a pelvic tilting to ventral.

18.2 Pelvic injuries

18.2.1 Apophyseal avulsion fractures

Apophyses are bone processes without an independent center of ossification. They are connected to the central skeleton by a **growth plate**. According to their different shapes, the apophyses are called spina, tuber, crista, tuberositas or trochanter.

The resistance of the growth plate decreases at the age of growth caused by increase of endogenous STH production with an expanse of the layer of columnar cartilage. Strong muscle contraction may lead to an **avulsion of the apophyses**, especially in athletes (Steinbrück and Krahl 1985). The **diagnosis** results from the history, the clinical examination as well as radiography, CT or MRI. The **therapy** is mostly **conservative** except for few cases. Soccer, sprinting or gymnastics are the disciplines affected most. **Boys** suffer from these injuries in more than 90% (Biedert et al. 2000).

Anterior superior iliac spine

The tensor fasciae latae muscle and the sartorius muscle insert at this point. The injuries mostly occur in track and field athletics, in running or throwing caused by hyperextension of the trunk or excessive hip extension. Clinically, both active flexion and passive extension of the hip joint are limited by pain. The radiological documentation of an injury may be difficult. The therapy is generally conservative with rest

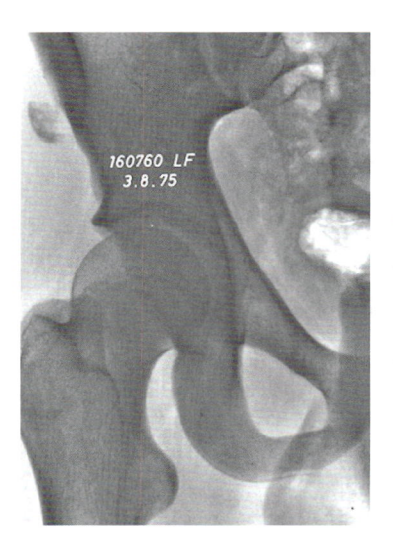

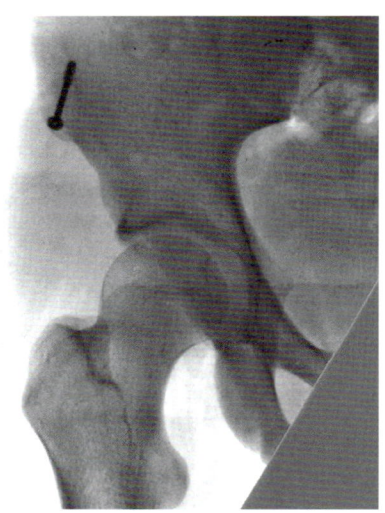

Fig. 18.1 Dislocated avulsion of the anterior superior iliac spine with surgical refixation.

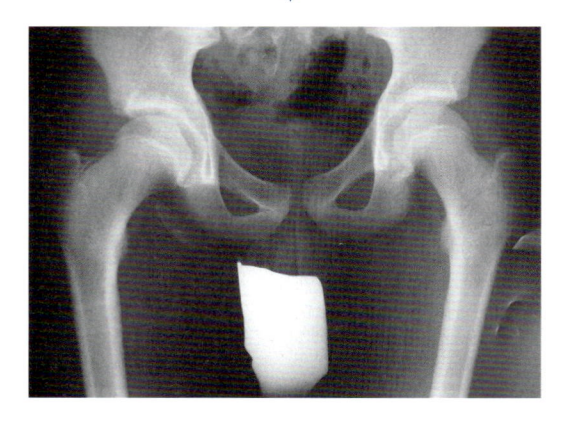

Fig. 18.2 MRT examination with a fresh, large avulsion of the tuber ossis ischii on the right-hand side.

and decreased activity; in specific cases a surgical refixation has to be considered for competitive athletes with significant dislocation of the fragment (➢ Fig. 18.1).

Anterior inferior iliac spine

The rectus femoris muscle inserts at this apophysis. Very strong muscle activation in starting, a sudden fall or excessive kicking in soccer can lead to injuries of this apophysis. A loud noise and a sharp pain are often indicated at the injury. The clinical examination shows swelling or hematoma in the groin and pain when raising the leg. Injuries might only be depicted on **oblique radiographic images**. The **treatment** is mostly conservative and in rare cases surgical. Too early **sports activities may cause new fractures**.

Ischial tuberosity

The half-moon-shaped ischial apophysis closes rather late. The quadratus femoris muscle inserts laterally, the biceps femoris muscle, the semimembranosus muscle and the semitendinosus muscle dorsolaterally – the adductor magnus muscle inserts medially. A strong flexion of the hip joint with simultaneous extension in the knee joint or a sudden tension of the hamstrings will lead to the avulsion of the apophysis (➢ Fig. 18.2). Typical sports activities causing hamstrings injuries or avulsion lesions of the ischial tuberosity are soccer, sprinting and water skiing. A feeling of snapping or rupture in combination with a sharp pain are typical. The suspected **diagnosis** is confirmed by radiographs or MRI.

The classification describes three **progressive types** (Biedert et al. 2000, modified according to Steinbrück):

- In **type I** (the apophysis has not been osseously formed yet), the primary radiological findings are negative and a uniform pseudo-tumor develops, which will have to be distinguished from an osteoblastic tumor.
- **Type II** develops in slightly older adolescents (already developed apophysis). An osteoapophyseal fracture appears in imaging. The fragment can heal after months or

18.2 Pelvic injuries

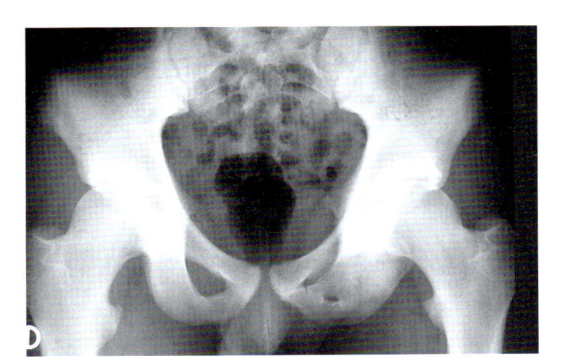

Fig. 18.3 Multiform pseudotumor – tuber ischiadicum on the left-hand side after former avulsion.

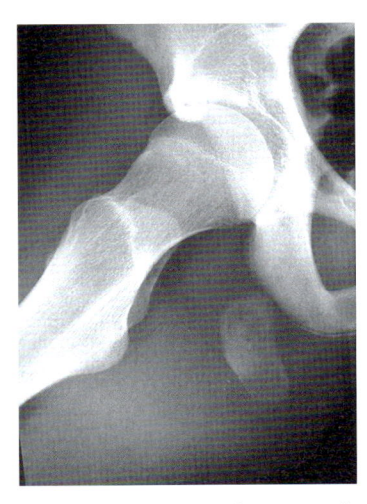

Fig. 18.4 Dislocated osseous fragment after former avulsion of the tuber ossis ischii on the right-hand side.

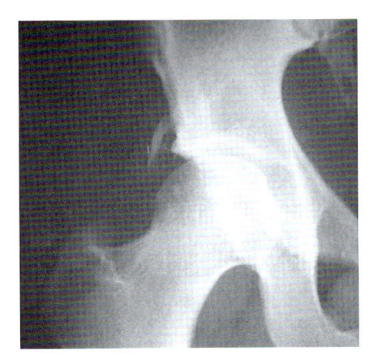

Fig. 18.5 Osseous fragment after former avulsion of the reflected head of of the rectus femoris muscle.

years and a multiform pseudotumor develops (➤ Fig. 18.3).
- In **type III** (the apophysis is fully developed), an osteoapophyseal avulsion fracture appears, in which the osseous consolidation fails. The fragment keeps growing isolatedly and severe deformities of the ischium can appear (➤ Fig. 18.4). Only in exceptional cases, surgical interventions will be considered (extreme sitting problems, very large dislocated apophysis).

Reflected head of the rectus femoris muscle

The quadriceps muscle consists of four muscles: rectus femoris muscle, vastus lateralis muscle, vastus intermedius muscle and vastus medialis muscle. Distally, it inserts as quadriceps tendon (four layers) at the proximal pole of the patella and further down as part of the galea aponeurotica above patella and patellar tendon at the tuberosity. The proximal origin of those four muscles is different.. The vastus lateralis, intermedius and medialis muscles have their origin at the (proximal) femur. The rectus femoris muscle inserts with the direct head at the anterior inferior iliac spine and with the second part, the reflected head along the contour of the lateral acetabulum.

Accordingly, all four muscles are involved in the extension of the knee joint, while the rectus femoris muscle as muscle of two joints also flexes in the hip joint. **Isolated avulsions of the reflected part of the rectus femoris muscle** may be caused by a forced stretching of the hip with the knee in extension and simultaneous hip flexion (Biedert 2003). This avulsed insertion can already show an osseous fragment primarily or lead to secondary **ossification** (➤ Fig. 18.5). Clinically, a large osseous fragment may cause pain and limited range of motion. In such cases, **surgical** excision of the fragment is indicated.

18.2.2 Fractures

About 3–5 % of all fractures are pelvic fractures, which mostly develop because of high speeds or falls from great heights (Pohlemann et al. 1996). Despite the low incidence of pelvic fractures, especially regarding sports injuries, these fractures have a great clinical relevance because of the **high mortality rate** (up to 20 % in complex pelvic traumas) (Tscherne and

Pohlemann 1998). The high mortality is explained by the **concomitant soft-tissue injuries**.

Simple pelvic fractures are purely osseous injuries of the anterior or posterior pelvic ring without concomitant soft-tissue injuries. **Complex** pelvic injuries, in contrast, are defined as fractures of the pelvic ring with concomitant soft-tissue damages (nerves, vessels, musculature, and intestines).

According to the degree of severity, the different pelvic fractures require a therapy individually tailored to the exact injury.

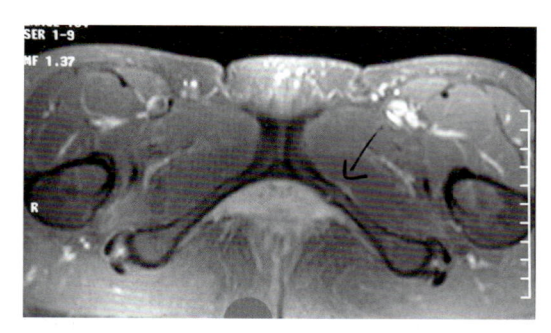

Fig. 18.6 Complete stress fracture of os pubis on the left-hand side with continuous fracture line in MRT.

18.2.3 Stress fractures

Stress fractures of pelvis and hip belong to the classic overuse problems of athletes (➤ Chapter 23). This affects especially **endurance athletes**. Suprapysiologic loading of the affected structure for a longer duration or a unique maximum overload are the etiological factors. For both, muscle fatigue probably plays a decisive role, because the forces affecting the skeleton can become too strong by reduced muscular support.

At anterior, the stress fracture of the **os pubis** is relatively frequent. **MRI examination** (➤ Fig. 18.6) is the best and fastest diagnostic clue for the diagnosis. Bone scintigraphy can also indicate a stress reaction, but is not specific enough. The **therapy** is mostly conservative with stress reduction. Crutches with partial weight bearing are recommended for several weeks until the athlete is completely free of pain.

At the hip joint, stress fractures can appear in the region of the femoral neck and less often between the greater and lesser trochanter (➤ Fig. 18.7). The early diagnosis is relevant because of the possible long-term consequences. Pain is experienced classically on exertion with pain reduction at rest. In most cases, excessive of training or competition activities is found in the history, or at least an unusual accumulation of activities. **During physical examination**, pain can already be induced by lifting the extended leg because of the muscle contraction. Additionally, rotation movements or compressions can also be very painful. With a suspected stress fracture in the region of the hip joint, an **MRI examination**

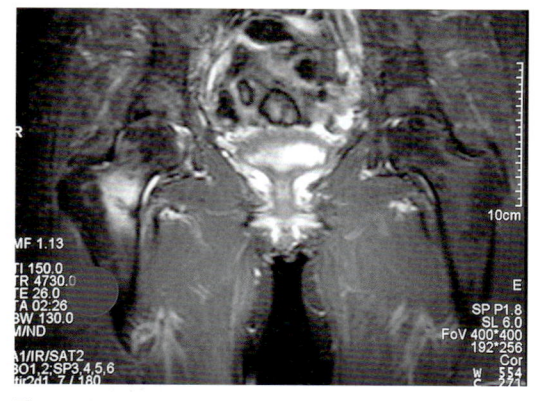

Fig. 18.7 Incomplete posteromedial intertrochanteric stress fracture on the right-hand side in MRT.

should be carried out in any case and as early as possible in order to be able to depict the fracture in an early stage. **Therapeutically**, incomplete fractures can be brought to complete healing mostly by consequent use of crutches for 6 at least weeks. In cases with a complete fracture or even mild dislocation, immediate stabilization (**osteosynthesis**) is indicated.

18.2.4 Anterior ventral pelvic ring instability

The pelvic ring is composed of an anterior and a posterior segment . The **anterior pelvic ring** includes the area of the os pubis and the os ischii up to the height of the acetabulum. The **posterior pelvic ring** includes the sacrum, the SI joint and the os ilium up to the acetabulum.

In sports, fresh fractures of the pelvic ring must be distinguished from the instabilities of the pelvic ring by chronic overuse. At anterior, the

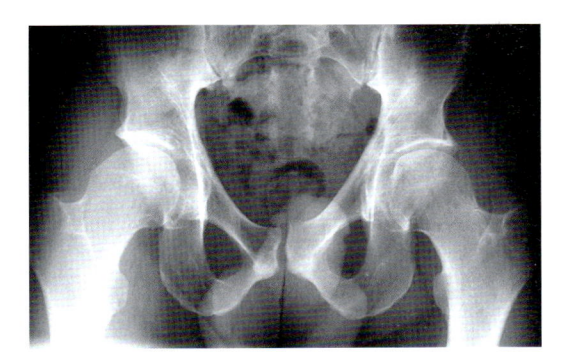

Fig. 18.8 Symphysis instability with ascent of the os pubis on the left-hand side in one-legged standing.

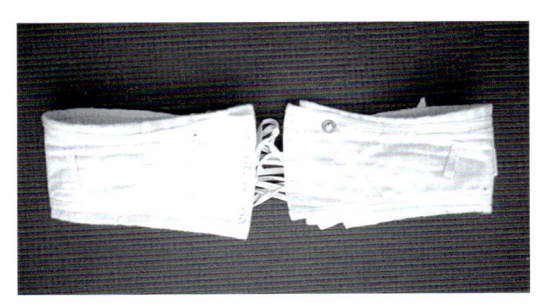

Fig. 18.9 Pelvic restraint for the treatment of the ventral instability of the pelvic ring.

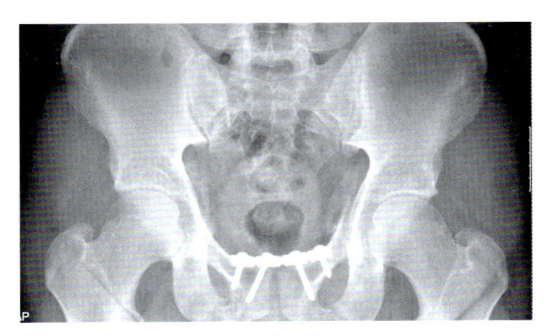

Fig. 18.10 Symphysis stabilization with plate.

The **diagnosis** of a ventral instability of the pelvic ring is made performing radiographs of the pelvis with one leg standing pictures, left and right. An instability shows an elevation of the os pubis of one side (➢ Fig. 18.8).

Therapeutically, a **conservative treatment** is the first joice including improvement of the stabilizing musculature. At the same time, a **pelvic belt** can be helpful, in order to be able to perform the necessary training and exercises (➢ Fig. 18.9). Unsuccessful conservative long-term treatment, may lead to surgical stabilization with temporary fixation of the symphysis by a plate (➢ Fig. 18.10).

18.3 Hip injuries

18.3.1 Dislocations

Isolated dislocations of the hip in sports are rare, but clinically very important, as they represent an **emergency situation. Anterior (10%) and posterior (90%) dislocations of the hip are differentiated**, which will be decisive for an early reposition. **Standard radiographs of the pelvis** are taken **before reposition** in order to eliminate concomitant fractures (femoral head or neck) whenever possible. A **femoral head avascular necrosis** must be expected in up to 10% of the isolated dislocations because of the critical blood supply of the femoral head, mainly by the circumflexa femoris medialis artery.

The **central forms of dislocation** have to be distinguished from the isolated dislocations. The rate of head necroses lies between 20 and 25% here, and also the danger of a **posttraumatic arthritis** is clearly increased.

18.3.2 Fractures

Traumatic fractures of the proximal femur are more frequent in sports than the dislocations and also present an **emergency situation**. Fractures of the femoral head will be distinguished from fractures of the femoral neck as well as from pertrochanteric, intertrochanteric and subtrochanteric fractures. In most cases, an emergency **reposition and osteosynthesis** will be necessary. Only with this, the present dan-

symphysis, consists of hyaline cartilage, the interpubic disk and reinforcing ligaments. The major demands to the symphysis occur by pressure in lying, by traction in standing and by shearing in running. All sports with high shearing forces affecting the symphyis can lead to **anterior instability of the pelvic ring**. Soccer, ice hockey, horse riding or track and field athletics (hurdling) belong to these sports.

ger of a **necrosis of the femoral head** can be reduced. A rather immense **posttraumatic loss of blood** must be considered, as well.

18.3.3 Acetabular labrum lesions

Although the first rupture of the acetabular labrum after a hip dislocation had been described about 50 years ago (Paterson 1957), labrum lesions have only been included into the differential diagnosis of groin and hip pain increasingly within the last 10 years. **Magnet resonance arthrography** (MRA) studies have shown a prevalence of more than 20% of labrum lesions in athletes with groin problems (Narvani et al. 2003).

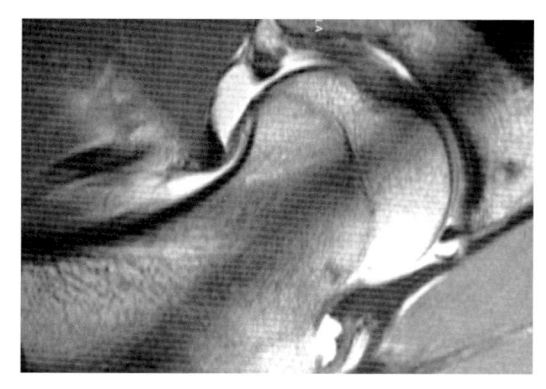

Fig. 18.11 Anterosuperior labrum ruptures with intralabral ganglion on the right-hand side in the MRA in an 18-year-old soccer player.

Anatomy and histology

The labrum is a fibrocartilaginous rim which encompasses the circumference of the acetabulum, effectively deepening the socket. Shape, size and thickness vary. The labrum has three surfaces: an internal articular surface, an external surface with connection to the joint capsule, and a basal surface attached to the acetabular bone and transverse ligaments (Narvani et al. 2003). The distal edge is free and forms the lateral border of the acetabulum. The anterior shape of the labrum is rather triangular in radial section; the posterior is more bulbous and lip like.

In the main part, the labrum consists of collagen fiber bundles type I. At the junction to the joint surface, it merges with the articular hyaline cartilage on a length of 1–2 mm. It is supplied with blood (Seldes et al. 2001), but only in the range of the exterior third towards the capsule at a depth of 0.5 mm, and thus is **not vascularized for the most part** (Narvani et al. 2003). Free nerve endings are present in all parts, forming a **nociceptive and proprioceptive system** (Kim and Azuma 1995).

Function

The acetabular labrum deepens the hip socket, and therefore improves the stability of the hip joint not only mechanically, but also by the negative intraarticular pressure. Additionally, the sealing function of the labrum enhances a fluid film lubrication (Narvani et al. 2003). It also limits the contact of the joint surfaces, and distributes the applied force more evenly across the articular surface. However, no major significance could be demonstrated for the weight transmission after the resection of the labrum (Konrath et al. 1998).

Causes

Most labral lesions are combined with acute posterior hip dislocations, dysplastic hips, degenerative processes. Also a direct traumatic correlation has been described as a result of sports activities (Ikeda et al. 1998) as well as in femoroacetabular impingement (Biedert and Netzer 2005).

Imaging and classification

An exact diagnosis and classification of the labrum lesion is only possible by **MRA** (Czerny et al. 1996), (➤ Fig. 18.11). Changes of shape, swellings, changes of signal intensity, and the separation of the complete labrum can be shown here in addition to obvious tears. The classification of labrum lesions is given in ➤ Table 18.1.

Clinical features

In most cases range of motion is not limited, but **painful** at the extremes. Snapping, clicking, locking, or episodes of sharp pain associated with pivoting or twisting are typical clinical issues. A number of different clinical tests is available, which will indicate the localization of

18.3 Hip injuries

Tab. 18.1 Classification of labral tears in MRA (modified according to Czerny 1996).

Stage	Findings
0	■ homogenous signal of the labrum, triangular, deep signal intensity ■ continuous attachment to the acetabulum ■ normal recessus between joint capsule and labrum
1A	■ increased signal intensity in the middle of the labrum ■ surface/undersurface intact, triangular ■ continuous attachment, normal recessus
1B	■ as in stage 1A, but with swollen labrum and mising recessus
2A	■ contrast material through a tear into the labrum, no detachment from the acetabulum ■ triangular, normal recessus
2B	■ as in stage 2A, but with swollen labrum and missing recessus
3A	■ labrum detached from the acetabulum, triangular
3B	■ labrum thickened and detached from the acetabulum

Tab. 18.2 Clinical tests with provocation of pain (Klaue et al. 1991, Fitzgerald 1995, Leunig et al. 1997, Narvani 2003a).

Movements in the hip joint	Affected labral portion
■ flexion, adduction, internal rotation	anterosuperior rupture
■ passive hyperextension, abduction, external rotation	posterior rupture
■ acute hip flexion with external rotation and full abduction, followed by extension, abduction and internal rotation	anterior rupture
■ extension, abduction and external rotation, followed by flexion, adduction and internal rotation	posterior rupture

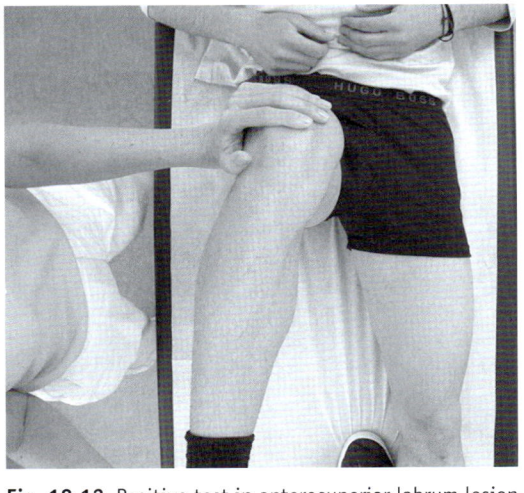

Fig. 18.12 Positive test in anterosuperior labrum lesion and femoroacetabular impingement: significant and painful limitation of the internal rotation by reduced femoroacetabular offset on the right-hand side.

A click phenomenon in correlation with hip pain is virtually proving a labral tear (Narvani et al. 2003b).

Treatment

The therapy of labrum lesions is determined by the underlying pathology (isolated lesion or combined with hip pathologies), the localization and degree of severity of the lesion, the patient's complaints as well as the technical possibilities. Therefore, therapy ranges from **load adaptation** and adjustment of the athletic activities to a physical therapy, an arthroscopic therapy (➤ segment 18.3.4) to the **open hip revision**.

18.3.4 Femoroacetabular impingement

In recent years, new concepts of etiologies of early osteoarthritis (OA) have been described and mechanical factors have been distinguished from nonmechanical factors (Ganz et al. 2003).

The **mechanical etiologies** include the dysplasia, the different types of femoroacetabular impingement **(FAI)**, Legg-Calvé-Perthe disease, and post traumatic. The **nonmechanical etiologies** include inflammatory, biochemical,

the labrum lesion (➤ Tab. 18.2). A reproducible pain can be provoked by hip flexion, internal rotation and slight adduction (➤ Fig. 18.12).

Tab. 18.3 Pathomorphologic features of femoroacetabular impingement.

Acetabular	Femoral
■ insufficient lateral and ventral covering ■ acetabular retroversion ■ decreased acetabular anteversion ■ protrusion	■ aspherical femoral head ■ lessened or missing offset-retro-tilt of the head opposed to the neck (e.g. epiphysiolysis capitis femoris) ■ reduced antetorsion of the femoral neck ■ short femoral neck ■ low CCD angle

vascular, and genetic factors leading to osteoarthritis of the hip.

A high number of early degenerative hip diseases is caused by the collision of the head and neck junction of the proximal femur with the acetabular components, a **FAI**.

The different acetabular or femoral morphologic etiologies for an impingement are listed in ➤ Table 18.3. According to the underlying pathomorphology, two different types of femoroacetabular impingement can be distinguished: **cam impingement** and **pincer impingement** (Ganz et al. 2003, Ito et al. 2001).

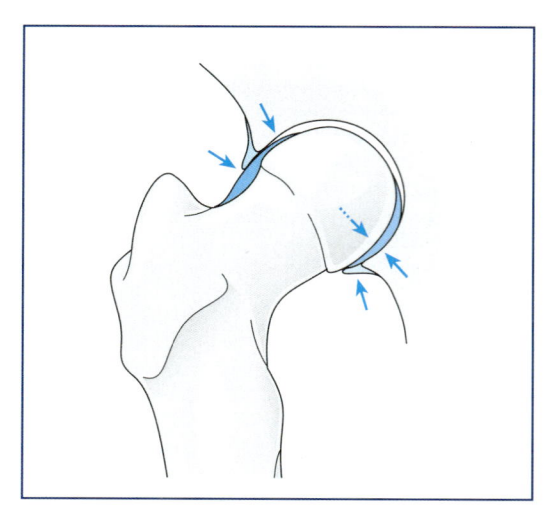

Fig. 18.13 Schematic presentation of the principle of cam impingement with reduced offset by cam (darkly shaded), cartilage lesion cranial-ventral and secondary labral lesion (subluxation of the head to dorsal; Biedert and Netzer 2005).

Cam impingement

The cam impingement is caused by jamming of an a nonspherical (aspherical) femoral head with increasing radius into the acetabulum during forceful motion, especially flexion (➤ Fig. 18.13, ➤ Fig. 18.14). The resulting shear forces produce outside-in abrasion of the acetabular cartilage and/or its avulsion from the labrum and the subchondral bone in the anterosuperior rim area. The cartilage of the femoral head remains normal for a long time. The **degeneration** of the labrum is a secondary consequence of the cartilage detachment in the socket. The causing hip movement – internal rotation with flexion – leads to a **subluxation** of the head to dorsal with corresponding secondary cartilage destruction and labrum lesions in the dorsal part.

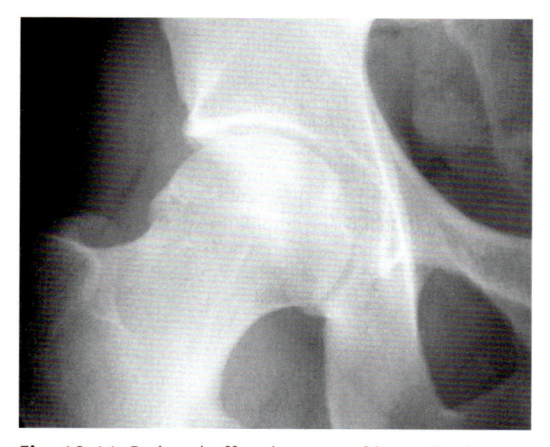

Fig. 18.14 Reduced offset because of bump in the area of the femoral neck.

Pincer impingement

The pincer impingement is the result of linear contact between the acetabulum rim and the femoral head-neck junction (➤ Fig. 18.15). The femoral head may have normal morphologic features. The first structure to fail is the acetabular labrum. Continued impact will often lead to degenerations of a deformed labrum and **formation of ganglia** in the labral substance. It can also lead to **mucoid dysplasia** of the labrum or **ossifications**. **Reactive bone**

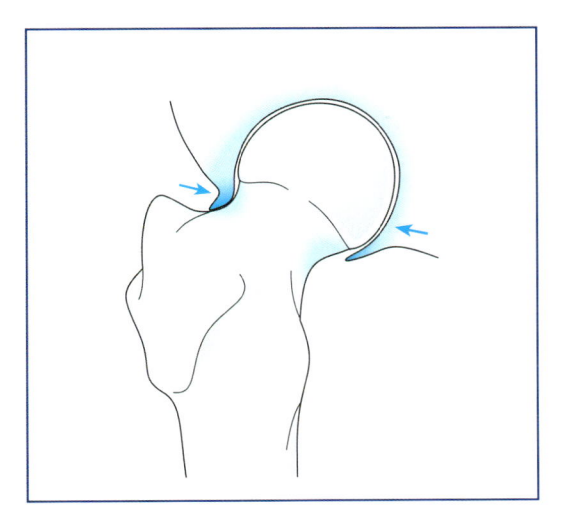

Fig. 18.15 Principle of the pincer impingement. The primary impairment will affect the anterior labrum (Biedert and Netzer 2005).

appositions of the socket edge are found early **in MRI**, and those push the labrum forward until thinning.

In this type of impingement, the cartilage of the spherical femoral head remains normal for a long time. The cartilage destruction by pincer impingement proceeds more slowly and is less expanded than in cam impingement.

Pure cam or pincer hips are rare; **mixed forms** are found more frequently. Pincer impingement is seen more frequently in middleaged women, and cam impingement in young and athletic males.

Treatment concepts

Conservative treatment is performed as long as possible. This only applies to impingement types with mild or moderate morphological pathology. In case of severe pathomorphology and at young age, surgical treatment is recommended.

Conservative therapy

The conservative treatment includes different **medications**, which have disease-modifying (glucosamine sulfate, hyaluronic acid, interleukin-1 receptor antagonist, chondroitin sulfate), antiphlogistic or analgetic effects. This drug therapy supports by load adaptation. In addition, active as well as passive forms of therapy are carried out. The **active therapy** primarily includes an improvement of coordination and balance. In **passive therapy**, myofascial techniques as well as diverse forms of injections are applied.

Arthroscopic hip surgery

Arthroscopic hip surgery has improved in the recent years (➤ Chapter 9). But it still remains a **highly demanding surgical intervention with long operating time** and requires an **optimal infrastructure** (positioning, traction, distraction control with image converter, etc.). Indications in athletes are different forms of labrum lesions, cartilage treatments (smoothing, microfracturing), injuries of the capitis femoris ligament as well as anterior types of the femoroacetabular impingement (cam) (➤ Fig. 18.16 a and b; Bachelier et al. 2003).

Major cartilage destruction, massive movement limitations, tense joint capsules with limited distraction, lateral deformities, and pincer impingement (➤ Tab. 18.4) form the **limits of arthroscopic treatment**.

Open hip revision

An indication for open hip revision is given with severe, clearly documented (radiographs, arthro-MRI, perhaps intraarticular local anesthesia) pathology. The younger the patient is,

Tab. 18.4 Arthroscopic hip surgery in athletes (Bachelier et al. 2003, Biedert et al. 2005).

Indication	Limitations	Advantages
■ labrum lesions ■ cartilaginous lesions (degenerative, traumatic, osteochondrosis dissecans, Perthes' disease) ■ cam impingement ■ loose bodies ■ lesions of the head of femur ■ "indistinct hip pain"	■ restricted limitation of movement (distraction!) ■ advanced cartilage damages ■ pincer impingement ■ lateral deformity (cam) ■ osteophytes	■ minimally invasive ■ outpatient/day-bed ■ fast rehabilitation ■ superior diagnostics ■ no damage before other surgeries

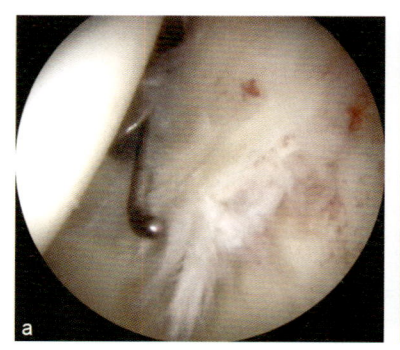

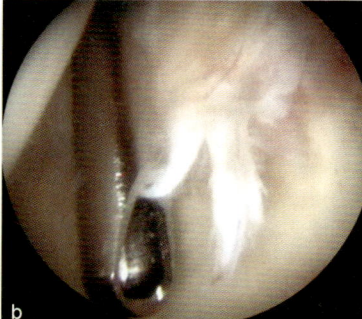

Fig. 18.16 Arthroscopic findings in a labrum lesion. b: Arthroscopic resection by the shaver (figures with permission by M. Dienst, Homburg/Saar).

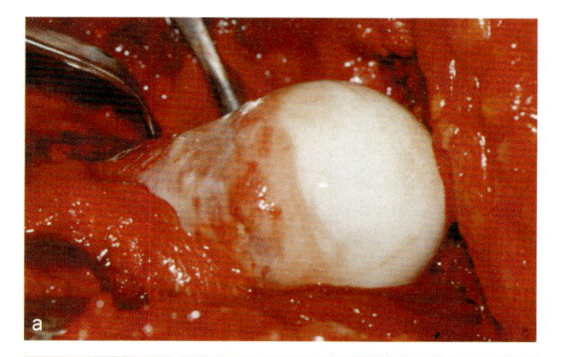

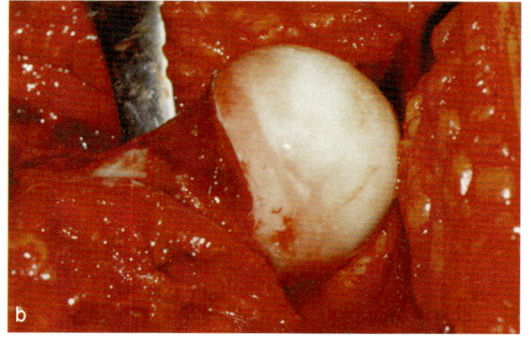

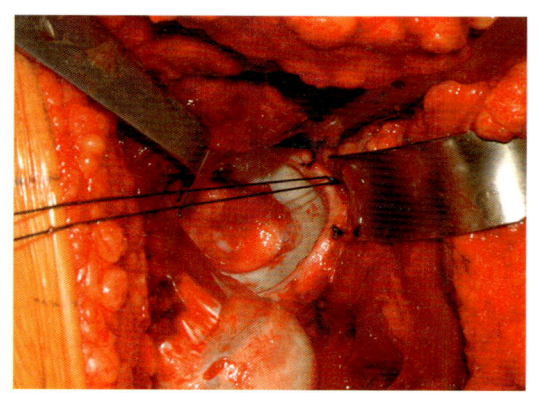

Fig. 18.18 Intraoperative view after an open refixation of the labrum (figures with permission by H. Nötzli, Bern).

Fig. 18.17 a: Proximal femur with reduced offset. b: view after bone removal and formation of an offset (figures with permission by H. Nötzli, Bern).

the further the indication can be made here. A **surgical limit** for the open revision lies at the age of about 40 years.

Open surgical revision primarily serves to **improve the mechanics** of the hip joint (abrasion of bones and osteophytes; ➤ Fig. 18.17), and to **revise the labrum.** In 90% of the cases, a refixation of the labrum is performed, to restore its important function as sealing ring, and to improve centering of the femoral head (➤ Fig. 18.18). Simultaneously, unstable cartilage parts can be removed and a mini-fracturing can be possibly performed. In an open revision, the **cartilage destruction at the femoral head**, not at the acetabulum, determines the further mid to long-term outcome. Normalization of the range of motion of the hip without impingement is the aim of all surgical interventions.

Other surgical forms of therapy

Other forms of therapy can be necessary especially in young patients. An epiphysiolysis capitis femoris, for example, can lead to a reduced or missing offset of the femoral neck and thus to a cam impingement. The surgical correction includes an osteotomy for the removal of the impingement and formation of the offset. An osteotomy can also be necessary in **latent detachment of the epiphysis** ("tilt deformity"), which often appears during **growth**.

18.3.5 Rehabilitation

After open hip revision, the rehabilitation of top athletes includes an extensive program by steps and thus more time and complexity than the one for recreational athletes.

Principally, **six phases** can be distinguished after surgical hip dislocation and revision:

- The first postoperative phase lasts **2 months**. It aims at providing enough time for the tissue to heal. The patient will walk with partial weight-bearing using forearm crutches. In physical therapy, measures supporting the healing will be applied (ultrasound, lymphatic drainage, isometric muscle training, etc.).
- From the **9th postoperative week** (second phase), the acquired abilities (isometric and isotronic contraction) stabilize and eventually the loads can be enhanced progressively.
- The third phase starts with the **4th postoperative month**. Sport-specific movement processes are practiced. Strength and endurance are in the foreground.
- Subsequently, i.e. **from the 19th week**, velocity and reactivity will be encouraged and thus further growth of strength will be achieved. This phase lasts up to 6 weeks.
- If top athletes reach 90% of their preoperative performance, this will lead them to the next phase, the **return to sport**, i.e. the athletes return to the playing field (ice, lawn, court, etc.). Specific movement patterns are practiced, at first slowly and controlled, then fast and finally explosively.
- If the professional athletes have achieved their **full capacity** (physical and mental) compared to the preoperative condition, they will be **approved for the game**. The last phase, the reintegration of top athletes into their professional environment, concludes the phase of physiotherapeutic rehabilitation.

Especially in combined surgeries (bone resection at the femur and socket edge ablation with refixation of the labrum), the healing including rehabilitation can take up 9 to 12 months. With bilateral pathology, the continuation of the career must be discussed. Most appropriately, too serious burdens are often renounced and adjustment to given conditions takes place.

18.3.6 Osteoarthritis of the hip joint

Osteoarthritis (degenerative change of the hip joint) is an important clinical problem in athletes of **middle and higher age**. In contrast to the degenerations caused by a FAI, the "classic coxarthrosis" develops **within the joint** by a concentric or eccentric **overload**. The underlying deformity leads to excessive overload of the socket edge with destruction of the labral complex. Thus, the femoral head will be destabilized and in general moves to anterolateral. The deteriorating congruency in the hip joint increases the critical stress and leads to rapid destruction of the joint (➤ Fig. 18.19).

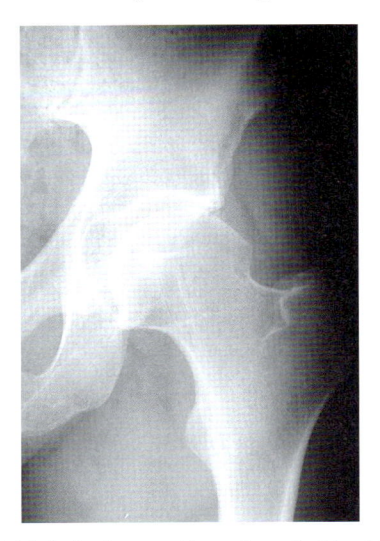

Fig. 18.19 Early degenerative osteoarthritis of the hip in a 37-year-old patient.

Clinically, groin pain is typically found, often emanating into the knee joint on the same side. This pain is present in getting up from sitting as well as in walking. Night-time pain can be observed as a first symptom.

> Osteoarthritis of the hip joint is a significant differential diagnosis of groin pain.

The **therapy** of osteoarthritis of the hip joint is primarily **conservative**. With disabling pain and exhaustion of the options of conservative therapy, a **total hip joint replacement** can become necessary in relatively young patients already.

References

Bachelier F, Seil R Kohn D, Dienst M (2003). Erkrankungen und Verletzungen des Hüftgelenks im Sport – Untersuchungsalgorhitmus und Indikationsstellung zur Hüftarthroskopie. Sportorthopädie Sporttraumatologie 19: 185–195.

Biedert R, Meyer S (1997). Das Symphysensyndrom beim Sportler. Schweiz Z Sportmed Sporttraumatol 45: 57–60.

Biedert R, Hintermann B, Hoppeler H, Meyer ST, Schori R, Spring H, Steinbruck K (2000). Leistenbeschwerden beim Sportler. Sportorthopädie Sporttraumatologie 16: 119–125.

Biedert RM (2003). Leistenbeschwerden. Abstract. 18. Jahreskongress der GOTS, Munich.

Biedert RM, Netzer P (2005). Femoroazetabuläres Impingement beim Sportler. Sportorthopädie Sporttraumatologie 21: 195–200.

Czerny C, Hofmann S, Neuhold A (1996): Lesions of the acetabular labrum: accuracy of MR arthrography in detection and staging. Radiology 200: 225–239.

Fitzgerald RH (1995). Acetabular labrum tears. Diagnosis and treatment. Clin Orthop 311: 60–68.

Ganz R, Parvizi J, Beck M, Leunig M, Nötli H, Siebenrock K (2003). Femoroacetabular impingement. Clin Orthop (rel res) 717: 112–120.

Ikeda T, Awaya G, Suzuki S, Okada Y, Tada H (1998). Torn acetabular labrum in young patients: arthroscopic diagnosis and management. J Bone Joint Surg 70 Br: 13–16.

Ito K, Minka II MA, Leunig M (2001). Femoroacetabular impingement and the cam-effect: A MRI-based quantitative study of the femoral head-neck offset. J Bone Joint Surg 83B: 171–176.

Kim YK, Azuma H (1995). The nerve endings of the acetabular labrum. Clin Orthop 320: 176–181.

Klaue K, Durnin CW, Ganz R (1991). The acetabular rim syndrome: a clinical representation of dysplasia of the hip. J Bone Joint Surg 73 Br: 423–429.

Konrath GA, Hamel AJ, Olsen SA (1998). The role of the acetabular labrum and the transverse acetabular ligament in load transmission in hip. J Bone Joint Surge 80A: 1781–1787.

Leunig M, Werlen S, Ungersbock A (1997). Evaluation of the acetabulum lanrum by MR arthrography. J Bone Joint Surg 79 Br: 230–234.

Narvani AA, Tsirdis E, Kendall S, Chaudhuri R, Thomas P (2003a). A preliminary report on prevalence of acetabular labrum tears in sports patients with groin pain. Knee Surg Sports Traumatol Arthrosc 11: 403–408.

Narvani AA, Tsirdis E, Kendall S, Chaudhuri R, Thomas P (2003b). Acetabular labrum and its tears. Br J Sports Med 37: 207–211.

Paterson I (1957). The torn acetabular labrum: a block to reduction of a dislocated hip. J Bone Joint Surg 39 Br: 306–309.

Pohlemann T, Tscherne H, Baumgärtel F, Egbers HJ, Euler E, Maurer T, Fell M, Mayr E, Quirini W, Schlickewei W, Weinberg A (1996). Beckenverletzungen: Epidemiologie, Therapie und Langzeitverlauf. Unfallchirurg 99: 160–167.

Seldes RM, Tan V, Hunt J (2001). Anatomy, histological features, and vascularity of the adult acetabular labrum. Clin Orthop 382: 232–240.

Segesser B (1996). Leiste. GOTS Manual Sporttraumatologie. Verlag Hans Huber, Bern-Göttingen-Toronto-Seattle.

Tscherne H, Pohlemann T (eds.) (1998). Becken und Azetabulum. Springer, Berlin-Heidelberg-New York.

Steinbrück K, Krahl H (1985). Apophysäre Frakturen am Becken beim Jugendlichen. In: Pförringer W, Rosemeyer B, Bär HW (eds.). Sport Trauma und Belastung. Perimed, Erlangen, pp 545–560.

Chapter 19 Groin

Roland Biedert

Groin injuries belongs with 10–60% of all sports injuries to the most frequent problems (Biedert and Meyer 1997). Different sports such as **soccer, ice hockey or track and field athletics** are especially affected (Biedert 1987 and 1996, Biedert and Meyer 1997). Groin injuries have most often multifactorial conditions with often overlapping etiology and pathology, and can therefore not directly ssigned to a defined individual structure.

In addition to the anatomical region of the "groin", the ventral and dorsal **pelvic ring**, the spine with the lumbosacral junction, the **sacroiliac joint** (SI joint), the **hip joint**, and the **adductor groups** have to be assessed in **differential diagnosis** (➢ Tab. 19.1; ➢ Fig. 19.1). Groin problems can be caused by fresh injuries, chronic overuse, degenerative changes, inflammatory processes, or neurological factors.

Tab. 19.1 Differential diagnosis with groin complaints.

Differential diagnosis
■ inguinal hernia (direct, indirect)
■ soft groin
■ abdominal wall hernia (spigelian hernia)
■ femoral hernia
■ injury aponeurosis of the external oblique muscle
■ insertion tendinosis of the rectus abdominis muscle – entrapment syndrome – genitofemoral nerve – ilioinguinal nerve – femoral nerve – lateral femoral cutaneous nerve – obturator nerve
■ psoas syndrome
■ bursitis iliopectinea
■ symphysis instability, instability of the pelvic ring
■ pelvic-torso instability
■ herniated disk
■ spondylolysis, spondylolisthesis
■ spondylogenic pain – iliosacral joints – blocking (partial, complete) – hypermobility – rheumatologic disease
■ avulsion fractures – apophyses (SIAS, SIAI, tuber ossis ischii, trochanter major and minor) – epiphyses (epiphysiolysis capitis femoris and lenta)
■ stress fractures
■ femoroacetabular impingement
■ labrum lesions
■ coxarthrosis
■ internistic diseases
■ urologic diseases – epididymitis – hydrocele – prostatitis

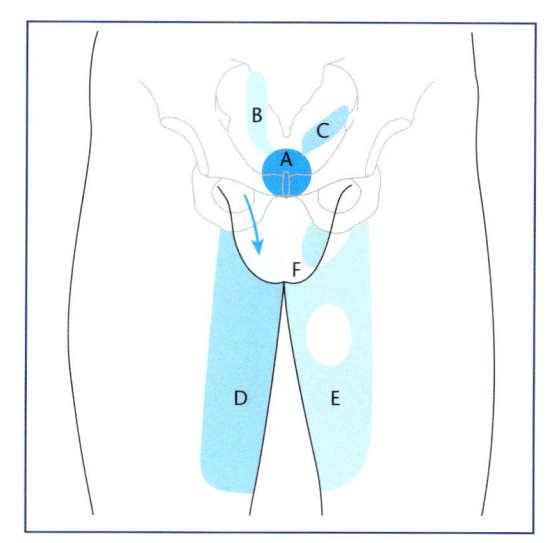

Fig. 19.1 Different pain localizations with groin complaints: (A) symphysis and os pubis; (B) lateral rim of the rectus abdominis muscle; (C) external inguinal ring; (D) radiating pain inner thigh (obturator nerve); (E) adductor musculature with myogeloses; (F) adductor insertion at the pelvis; (↓) scrotum.

19.1 Biomechanics

The **typical sports specific movement patterns** leading to groin problems are one leg standing with flexion in hip and knee joint, external rotation and simultaneous abduction (➤ Fig. 19.2). Here the adductors are the most important stabilizers with extreme load peaks in the standing phase as well as in the free-leg phase. Because the abdominal musculature is diagonally contracted in combination with the contraction of the adductors against a resistance (e.g. ball), the close functional **interaction of these muscle groups** is decisive for the positioning of the pelvis. Accordingly, the complete movement unit has to be assessed diagnostically and, if necessary, be approached therapeutically.

19.2 Hernias

The different types of hernias have to be taken into account for differential diagnosis. Hernia is the term for the extravasation of visceral parts into an abnormal protrusion of the peritoneal sac (Siewert 2001). The **surgical treatment** of the hernia with persisting complaints is carried out either open or by laparoscopy.

19.2.1 Inguinal hernia

Inguinal hernias are the **most frequent hernias**, and are classified into **direct** (localizations above the inguinal and medial ligaments of the epigastric vessels) and **indirect** (above the inguinal ligament and lateral of the epigastric vessels). **Men** are affected in more than 90%.

19.2.2 Femoral hernia

The femoral hernia is to be distinguished from the inguinal hernias. It is localized **below the inguinal ligament** and medial of the femoral vessels in the region of the lacuna vasorum. It occurs only rarely in sports.

19.2.3 Spieghel hernia

The Spieghel hernia is a rather rare external hernia. The **hernia orifice** with protrusion through the abdominal wall lies at the lateral cross point of linea semilunaris and linea semicircularis (Siewert 2001). Mostly this form of hernia is **not be visible from the outside** and the definitive diagnosis is often only made during surgery.

19.2.4 Weak groin

The weak groin is a typical and relatively frequent **sport-specific problem** and is distinguished from the common hernias. The weak groin (➤ Fig. 19.3) is an **anatomical, mostly bilateral weak point of men** in the lower ventral abdominal region (Biedert et al. 2000 and 2003). The weak groin represents a deficiency of the posterior inguinal wall with clinical signs of hernia (Biedert et al. 2003). This area is defined medially by the lateral edge of the rectus abdominis muscle and the aponeurosis of obliquus externus abdominis muscle (**crus mediale**), proximally by the aponeurosis and the muscle belly of the obliquus internus abdominis muscle, laterally by the aponeurosis of the obliquus externus abdominis muscle (**crus laterale**) and the inguinal ligament and distally by the os pubis as well as the reflexum ligament (Biedert et al. 1997 and 2003).

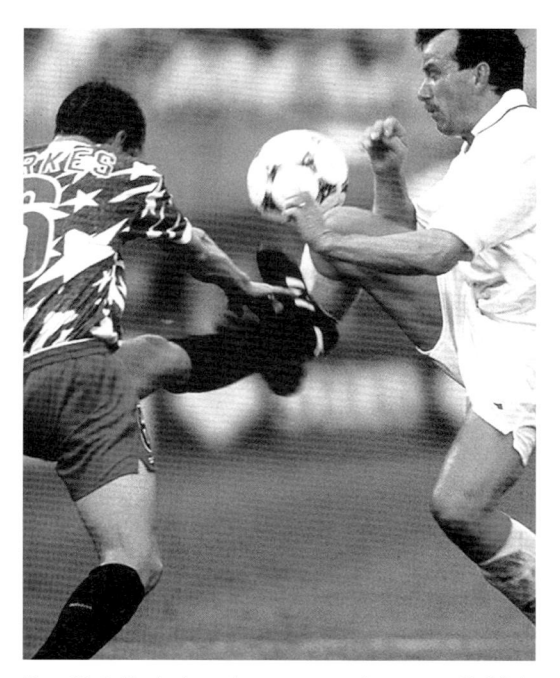

Fig. 19.2 Typical motion sequence in soccer. Multiple forces affect the pelvis being in the center and the groin region.

Fig. 19.3 Schematic illustration of the soft groin (Biedert et al. 2003, modified according to Skandalakis et al. 1989).

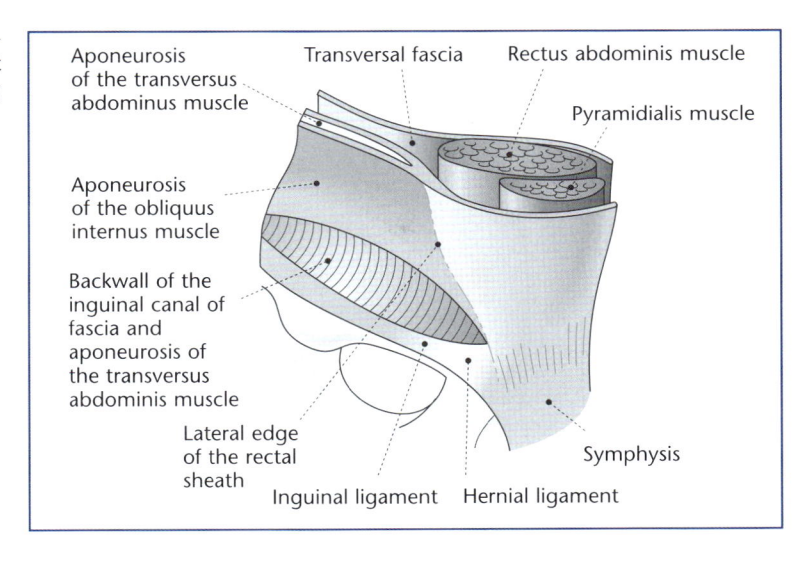

This area itself consists of the peritoneum (inside) and the transversal fascia (outside) and includes the **inguinal canal** with the **funiculus spermaticus**. The funiculus spermaticus traverses the abdominal wall to the outside through the annulus inguinalis profundus or superficialis.

Only athletes of certain sports suffer from weak groin problems. Therefore sport-specific movement patterns must be responsible for the occurrence of these complaints. In **soccer and ice hockey**, the control of rotation, adduction, and flexion of the thigh in respect to hip and pelvis always is activated together with the abdominal muscles, gluteus muscles, and hamstrings. To achieve a permanent control of the rotation of the pelvis and the position of the lumbosacral connection, these muscles must work together as a functional unit. Extraordinary stress to this zone is known by the continuous tension of the abdominal musculature to stabilize the pelvis (especially in the one-leg standing) and the high intraabdominal pressure. The peritoneum and also the parts of the aponeuroses of the transversus abdominis muscle, the obliquus internus and externus have to hold against this high pressure from the outside.

Chronic overuse or a laceration into the external aponeurosis can lead to an increased open and thus painful external groin ring (Hess and Huberty 1985, Fried and Lloyd 1992, Biedert and Meyer 1997, 2000, 2003). An **inguinal hernia** has to be distinguished in **differential diagnosis**.

The presence of **abnormalities of the rectus abdominis muscle** (small insertion area) enlarges the local weak zone. A **small insertion area** of the rectus abdominis muscle at the pubis increases the local tension forces and creates a chronic overload of this area with pain. In contrast to the normal anatomic situation, the small muscle belly does not cover the weak groin. Additionally, the presence of a high **proximal ending internal oblique muscle** enlarges this area of weakness (Biedert et al. 2003) and is known as the second anatomical variant. (➤ Fig. 19.4). The external (lateral) border of the rectus abdominis muscle goes less far towards lateral-distal and cannot cover

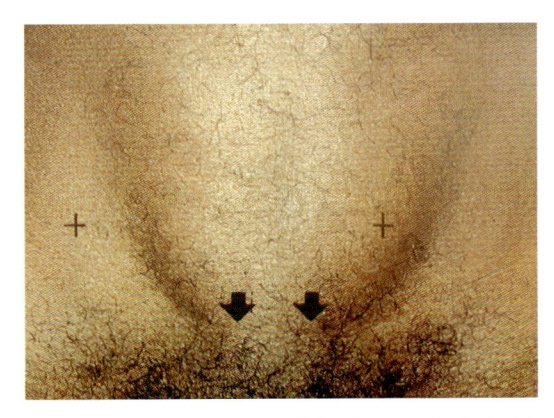

Fig. 19.4 Very strong rectus abdominis muscle, but with small insertion zone at the os pubis (↓) and accordingly high local traction forces, (+) protruding weak spots of the soft groin on both sides.

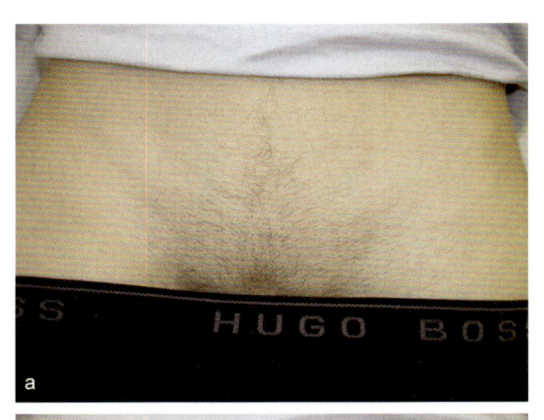

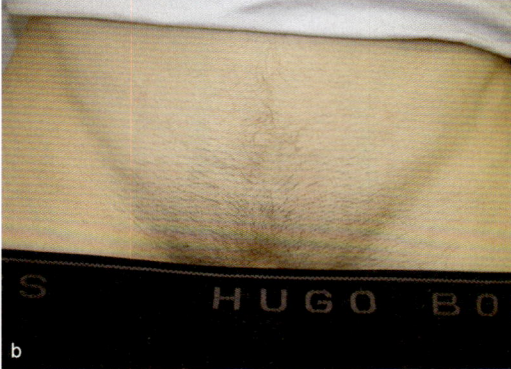

Fig. 19.5 Soft groin on both sides. a: No protrusion without pressing. b: Strong protrusion on both sides by pressing with increase of the intraabdominal pressure.

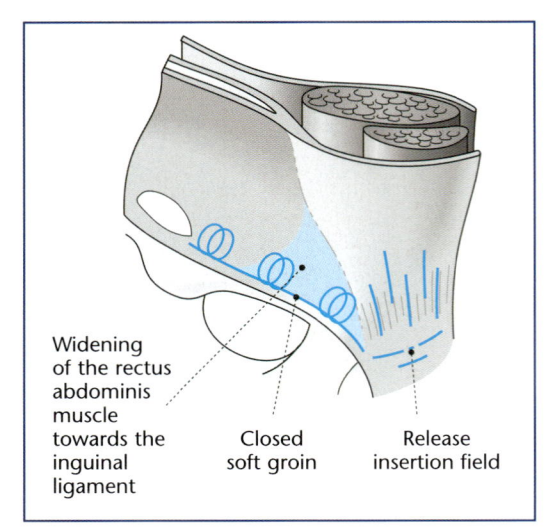

Fig. 19.6 Schematic illustration of the condition after the closing of a soft groin.

the weak point sufficiently, especially medially. A palpation pain is found clinically in both abnormalities at the lateral border of the sheath of the rectus abdominis muscle as well as above the part of the aponeuroses and the external inguinal ring The exquisite painful palpation is often combined with a visible **protrusion** of the weak involved zone (➢ Fig. 19.5 a and b).

Surgical treatment

The surgical therapy especially for active athletes is indicated if conservative therapy (load adjustment, optimization of the musculature) remains without success. Different techniques will be applied here.

Open technique

The surgical intervention aims to **close the weak soft groin** and to **enlarge the insertion of the rectus abdominis muscle** (➢ Fig. 19.6; Biedert et al. 2003). With this, the traction forces at the os pubis are reduced and the insertion tendinosis can heal simultaneously. At the intervention, the lateral border of the sheath of the rectus abdominis muscle together with the aponeuroses of the transversus abdominis muscle and the internal oblique muscle will be fixed to the inguinal ligament (➢ Fig. 19.7 a and b).

The postoperative rehabilitation includes 2 weeks of rest, enhanced activation of the abdominal muscles from the 3rd week on, running training beginning with the 4th week and full athletic activity after about 8 weeks.

Laparoscopic technique

The principle of this method is based on the **strengthening of the abdominal wall** with the coverage of possible hernia orifices. An almost painless surgery and a quick recovery are intended.

According to the localization, an **indirect hernia** (widening of the internal groin ring) is distinguished from a beginning **direct hernia** (widening of the transversial fascia). From a laparoscopic point of view, a special anatomy ap-

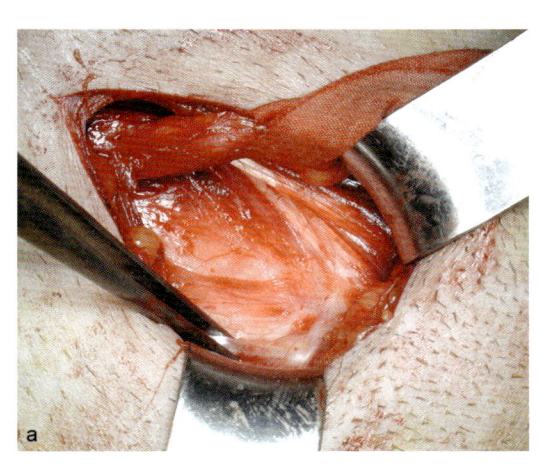

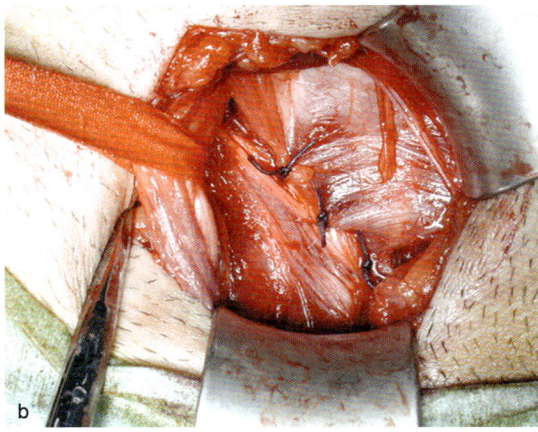

Fig. 19.7 a: Large weak spot with soft groin on the right-hand side with insufficient back wall; lateral rim of rectus abdominis muscle (upper right); inguinal ligament (in pincers). Funiculus spermaticus kept away by a band. b: Situation after closure.

pears at seeing from the back onto the abdominal wall. The groin region is well visible at one look after surgical removal of the peritoneum and it shows especially all possible hernia orifices at the same time. In endoscopic therapy, a **net** can be deposited either as **transabdominal preperitoneal** (TAPP) or **total extraperitoneal** (TEP). These methods (TAPP and TEP) require three injection sites. After the insertion of the net, it will be fixed with glue or staples. An **intraperitoneal appliance** of a synthetic net (IPOM technique) is possible, as well (Siewert 2001). In recent times, increasingly lighter nets with bio-resorbable staples or even without staples have been used. The future will show whether they will sustain especially for the high demands of young athletes. A secondary shift seems to be possible, at least, theoretically. An important advantage of these methods is the fact that all **possible hernia orifices** are covered **at the same time** in the laparoscopic and endoscopic technique. The postoperative phase is relatively pain-free; the patient can take loads quickly and exercise sport after 2–3 weeks.

Previous **long-term results** (30 years with polypropylene nets) mostly show a **good acceptance of the synthetic nets**, but we partly observed indurations in the area of the nets caused by strong fibrosing. In addition, a widening of the rectus abdominis muscle will not be possible.

19.3 Psoas syndrome

The iliopsoas muscle is formed of three muscles: psoas major muscle, psoas minor muscle (insertions L2–L5) and the iliacus muscle (insertion at the inside of the os ilium). Together they insert at the trochanter minor. In the middle region, the iliopsoas muscle runs over the ventral socket edge of the hip joint and is redirected there.

Both **hypertrophy** or **shortening of the iliopsoas muscle** is clinically important. Both conditions can cause diffuse, deep-set pain in the groin region. A hypertrophy or a shortening often cause also conditions in the lower area of the lumbar spine by increased traction forces.

In few cases, a hypertrophy can also cause an **entrapment syndrome** of the femoral nerve with a pain from the hip to the knee joint down to the lower leg. The shortening of the iliopsoas muscle can lead to a limited hip extension with a secondary ventral tilting of the pelvis and according **formation of a lumbar lordosis**. A combined hypertrophy with shortening of the iliopsoas muscle will often be found and is typical in **soccer players**.

The **diagnosis** of a psoas syndrome will be given by history and clinical examination. The functional testing of the iliopsoas muscle is carried out in **dorsal position:** one leg will be flexed to a maximum in the hip and knee joints. In addition, the head will be slightly elevated by a cushion (correction of a possible lumbar malposition). In a shortened iliopsoas muscle, the femur of the tested side will be lifted, the hip stays lightly flexed. The strength of the iliopsoas muscle will be tested in sitting with hip and knee flexed to 90° (Segesser 1996).

The **treatment** of the psoas syndrome is in most cases **conservatively**. **Stretching** of the muscles is the most important and effective therapy. It can be done by the patient himself after instruction or, with distinctive shortening, additionally by the physical therapist. Often, an additional mobilization of the lumbosacral region might be necessary. Other simultaneously shortened muscle groups (especially adductors) should be treated at the same time.

19.4 Iliopectinea bursa

The pathology of the iliopectinal bursa is a rare problem, which still must be included into differential diagnosis. An irritation of the iliopectinal bursa can develop because of the **friction of the iliopsoas muscle** at the anterior socket edge at the hip joint. The bursa can be on palpation in front of the osseous part of the pelvis with flexed hip and relaxed iliopsoas muscle. A local anesthesia into the bursa is often helpful for the exact diagnosis. If otherwise resistance to conservative therapy (stretching, infiltration) is given, the **surgical sectioning** of fibrosed parts of the iliopsoas muscle presents a form of therapy, in which the friction at the ventral pelvic edge can be reduced (Segesser 1996).

19.5 Entrapment syndrome

Different entrapment syndromes of the groin region and the peripheral nerves must be considered in differential diagnosis (> Fig. 19.8). The genitofemoral nerve (Rischbeith 1986), the ilioinguinal nerve (Kopell and Thompson 1960), the iliohypogastric nerve, the femoral nerve (Mumenthaler and Mattle 2002), the cutaneus femoris lateralis nerve as well as the **obturator nerve** (Bradshaw and McCrory 1997), which is also clinically important, will be affected.

19.5.1 Genitofemoral nerve and ilioinguinal nerve

The genitofemoral nerve and the ilioinguinal nerve (L1–L2) proceed as combined nerves partly through the iliopsoas muscle towards the outside of the groin. A lesion leads to local pain in the groin region (ilioinguinal syndrome) with **losses of sensitivity** in the affected regions of the skin. In men, the **cremasteric reflex** can also be missing.

Etiologically, secondary problems after revision of the groin are most frequent which contingently can make a local surgical revision necessary for remaining complaints.

19.5.2 Cutaneus femoris lateralis nerve

The absolutely sensitive cutaneus femoris lateralis nerve (L2–L3) runs through the three layers of the abdominal wall and meets the fascia of the thigh about 2–4 cm medially from the anterior superior iliac spina passing through the inguinal ligament (Mumenthaler and Mattle 2002). It sensitively sustains a palm-sized area of the skin at the anterior outside of the thigh.

The classic entrapment syndrome develops at the **passage through the inguinal ligament**. This neuropathy is clinically known as **meralgia paraesthetica** (nocturna) with **burning dysesthesias** in the sustained region of the nerve. These paresthesias can be increased by an overstretching of the leg in the hip joint and can be decreased by a flexion of the hip. The passage point of the nerve through the inguinal ligament is often pressure sensitive.

A gain of weight or a pregnancy can be responsible **etiologically**. Complications after a groin surgery are also possible. With remaining conditions, the surgical enlargement of the point of passage of the nerve in the inguinal ligament will be possible.

19.5.3 Femoral nerve

The femoral nerve (L1–L4) provides the motor supply of the hip flexors (major psoas muscle, iliacus muscle) as well as the quadriceps femoris muscle (Mumenthaler and Mattle 2002). It sensitively innervates the anterior side of the thigh as well as the inner part of the

Fig. 19.8 Frequently affected nerves in entrapment syndromes (modified according to Mumenthaler 2002).

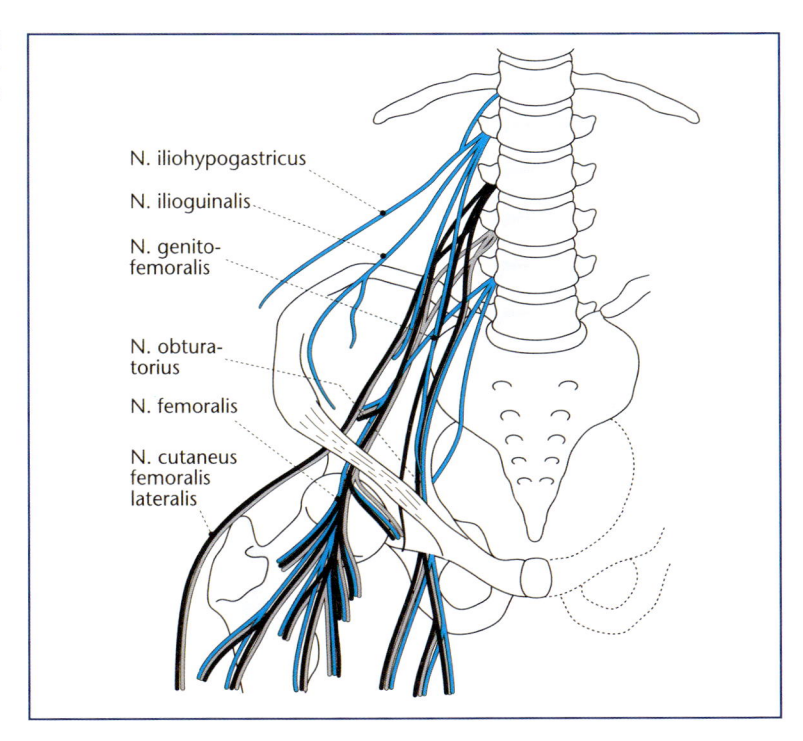

N. iliohypogastricus
N. ilioguinalis
N. genitofemoralis
N. obturatorius
N. femoralis
N. cutaneus femoralis lateralis

anterior side of the lower leg via the saphenous nerve. Anatomically, it runs through the iliopsoas muscle, leaves the groin region via the lacuna vasorum and enters the thigh region.

With a lesion of the femoral nerve, **hip flexion** and **knee extension**, as well, will be clinically impaired. Therefore, the hip flexors will be tested in a sitting position, the knee extensors will be tested in dorsal position. It will be typical for the **patellar tendon reflex to be missing**. In standing patients, a patella infera can possibly be observed. Climbing stairs can be troublesome or even impossible; the knee joint will be held overextended in walking. According to the lesion, the skin sensitivity in the sustained region will be disturbed.

In sports, the femoral nerve can be compressed by a **hypertrophy of the iliopsoas muscle**. A large **hematoma in the psoas sheath** can cause the same symptoms. Injuries of the femoral nerve can also appear traumatically or as a complication of surgical revision.

Therapeutically, the repair of causes (conservative or surgical) is to be discussed.

19.5.4 Obturator nerve

The obturator nerve (L2–L4) leaves the pelvic region through the foramen obturatorium and proceeds with its ventral branch above the obturator exterius muscle on the abductor brevis muscle and below the abductor longus muscle. It will be covered by the pectineus muscle. The anterior branch sustains the adductors longus and brevis muscles, the gracilis muscle and occasionally the pectineus muscle. Further distal, it forms the skin branch, which will sustain the skin and fascia of the distal two thirds of the medial thigh along the abductor canal (Bradshaw and McCrory 1997).

In the obturatorius entrapment syndrome, the **pain** is typically specified as occuring **deep and burning** in the insert region of the adductors. At the inside of the thigh, it often relocates to distal. Not uncommonly, it occurs intermittently and can cause a stress-dependent weakening of the affected leg. A chronic-relapsing compartment syndrome with an irritated condition of the obturatorius nerve must be considered with such symptoms as well as with relapsing myogeloses in the adductor region (Segesser 1996, Bradshaw and McCrory 1997).

The radiographic examination is mostly normal, and beginning muscle atrophy is shown in lateral comparison in **MRI** only after long lasting complaints. **Electrophysiologically**, a chronic denervation of the adductor longus and brevis muscles can be shown under the use of a fine-needle EMG. The **block of the obturator nerve** is diagnostically the most valuable under nerve stimulating control. The pain should disappear after local anesthesia and a potential feeling of weakness, as possibly observed anamnestically by the patient, can appear.

The conservative therapy will mostly be unsuccessful (stretching and ice). The **surgical treatment** involves a longitudinal incision of the fascia above the obturatorius nerve, which is located behind the adductor longus muscle and the pectineus muscle. The nerve has to be freed up to the formanen obturatorium. An opening of the adductor compartment will be necessary here.

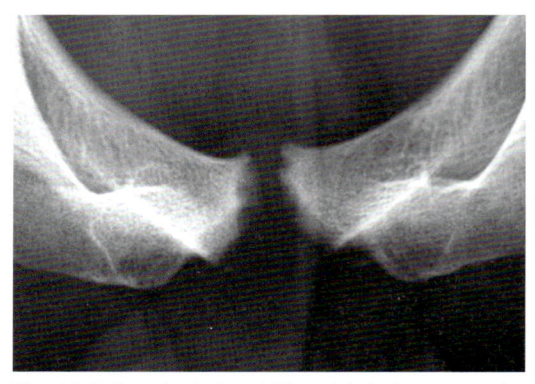

Fig. 19.9 Symphysis instability with lysis zones, sclerosings and osteophytes as etiology of chronic adductor complaints.

19.6 Adductor syndrome

Adductor problems can develop either by **acute injuries** (strain, torn muscle fiber) or by **chronic overload**. Especially unbalanced loads and overloads lead to inflammations of the tendon insertions at the os pubis via myogeloses (insertion tendinoses). Overloads develop by badly tolerated training or competition units, which present a high challenge to the stabilizing of the pelvis in one-leg standing. An optimal example is playing soccer on deep, wet ground.

In comparison, **improper loads** often occur because of a changed mobility of the pelvic parts, e.g. locking of the SI joint, hypermobility of the SI joint, symphysis loosening or instability, respectively, or pelvic malrotations. In clinical examinations, the exquisite **pain on palpation** at the tendon insertion to the os pubis, a myogelosis or the painful exertion of the adductors against a resistance is found. The adductor longus muscle and the gracilis muscle are affected the most. The etiologies can be gathered by additional examinations (mobility of the SI joint, radiographs of stress in one-leg standing, testing the stabilization of pelvis and trunk).

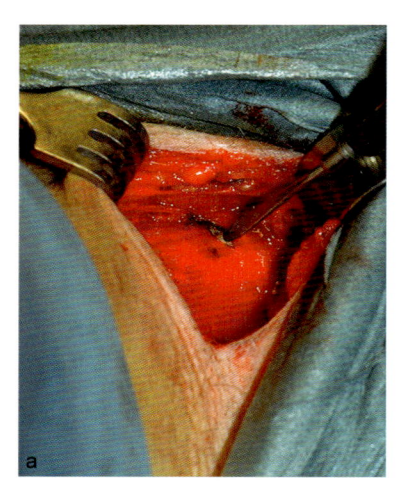

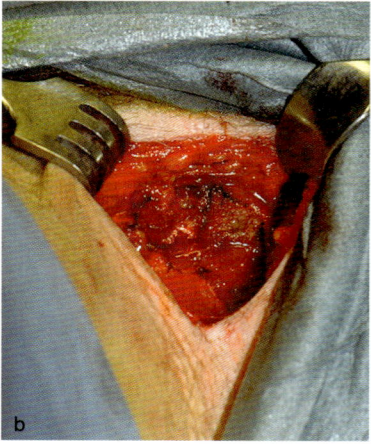

Fig. 19.10 a: Specific cutting of septes with electrocautery in the muscle-tendon junction in order to lessen the tension (right gracilis muscle). b: Intraoperative findings after the release.

Either lysis zones with reactive sclerosis (➤ Fig. 19.9), osseous protrusions, or unstable parts of the symphysis in alternating one-leg stand are found **radiologically**. At first, the cause must be removed **therapeutically** (e.g. SI joint treatment, attachment of a pelvic restraint with instability). Important **conservative measures** are the retrieval of the muscular balance, improvement of the stabilization of the lumbosacral unit as well as anti-phlogistic therapy (Biedert and Meyer 1997).

If the therapy remains unsuccessful and pain is chronic and relapsing, a **surgical intervention** will be indicated. This mostly involves a release near the insertion (no tenotomy) of the septa in the muscle junction of the gracilis muscle and the adductor longus muscle for the reduction of tension (➤ Fig. 19.10 a and b; Biedert 1987, Biedert et al. 2003).

References

Biedert R (1987). Insertionstendinosen im Beckenbereich beim Fußballer. Dtsch Z Sportmed 38: 452–458.

Biedert R (1996). Sportartspezifische Traumatologie Fußball. GOTS-Manual Sporttraumatologie. Hans-Huber-Verlag, Bern-Göttingen-Toronto-Seattle, pp 298–302.

Biedert R, Meyer S (1997). Das Symphysensyndrom beim Sportler. Schweiz Z Sportmed Sporttraumatol 45: 57–60.

Biedert R, Hintermann B, Hoppeler H, Meyer ST, Schori R, Spring H, Steinbruck K (2000). Leistenbeschwerden beim Sportler. Sportorthopädie Sporttraumatologie 16: 119–125.

Biedert R, Warnke K, Meyer ST (2003). Symphysis syndrome in athletes' surgical treatment for chronic lower abdominal, groin, and adductor pain in athletes. Clin J Sports Med 13: 278–284.

Bradshaw C, McCrory P (1997). Obturator nerve entrapment. A cause of groin pain in athletes. Am J Sports Med 25: 402–408.

Fried T, Lloyd GJ (1992). An overview of common soccer injuries. Sports Med 14: 269–275.

Hess H, Huberty R (1985). Soccer Injuries. In: Schneider RC, Kennedy JC, Plant ML (eds.). Sport Injuries, Mechanisms, Prevention and Treatment. Williams & Wilkins, Baltimore-London-Sydney, pp 163–177.

Kopell HP, Thompson W (1960). Peripheral entrapment neuropathies of the lower extremity. N Eng J Med 262: 5.

Mumenthaler M, Mattle H (2002). Grundkurs Neurologie. Thieme, Stuttgart-New York.

Rischbeith RH (1986). Genitofemoral neuropathy. Clin Exp Neurol 22: 145–147.

Segesser B (1996). Leiste. In: Engelhardt M, Hintermann B, Segesser B (eds.). GOTS-Manual Sporttraumatologie. Huber, Bern, pp 118–123.

Siewert JR (2001). Chirurgie. Springer, Berlin-Heidelberg-New York.

Skandalakis JE, Gray SW, Skandalakis LJ (1989). Surgical anatomy of the inguinal area. World J Surg 13: 490–498.

Chapter 20 Knee joint

Michael Krüger-Franke

The knee joint is the largest joint of the human body and exhibits a complex structure with the strongest ligaments and the biomechanics of a rolling-sliding movement. In addition, it is one of the most often injured joints among 2 million sports injuries registered every year. Knee joint injuries often lead to sports invalidity of top athletes and competitive athletes. The top sport capacity cannot always be recovered despite great progress in diagnosis and therapy of sport injuries of the knee joint. In Europe, soccer and alpine skiing are the sports leading most often to injuries of the knee joint, but all contact sports with opponent contact and high rotator stress bear the danger of knee injuries. The impulse to the joint eventually decides whether a meniscal, ligamentous or osseous/cartilagineous injury occurs.

20.1 Anatomy

The knee joint is formed by femur, tibia and patella, which are connected with each other by a complex formation of ligament and capsule structures. The knee can be divided into two joints: the tibiofemoral and the femoropatellar joint. The **collateral ligaments** stabilize the joint against varus and valgus stress. The medial collateral ligament is integrated in several layers into the medial capsule and extending from the epicondylus femoris medialis to the medial tibia. The lateral collaeral ligament runs extracapsular from the epicondylus lateralis femoris to the end of the fibula.

In addition, the medial collateral ligament with the fibers of its deep layer extends to the medial meniscus and increases its stability by meniscofemoral and meniscotibial fibers, but also its vulnerability. The collateral ligaments have a different tension in extension and flexion, and stabilize the joint the most in maximum extension. The **cruciate ligaments** are located within the fossa intercondylaris and form the central column of the knee joint. The anterior cruciate ligament, comprising an anteromedial and posteromedial bundle, extends from the area intercondylaris to the medial surface of the condylus lateralis of the femur. In extension, the anterior cruciate ligament runs steeply and the anteromedial bundle stabilizes. In flexion, it runs nearly horizontally and the posterolateral bundle tenses up. This is important for the use of the examining hook in arthroscopic diagnosis. The posterior cruciate ligament extends from the dorsal tibial edge below the joint line to the lateral surface of the condylus medialis of the femur. It more or less runs to the femur in a right angle and is stronger than the anterior cruciate ligament. It consists of an anterolateral bundle stabilizing more in flexion and a posteromedial bundle tensing more in extension.

The **menisci** are transportable joint surfaces. They compensate the incongruence of the joint partners femur and tibia in addition to a buffer function and contribute to a homogeneous pressure transmission in the knee joint. They are mobile and migrate on the tibial plateau from dorsal to ventral in flexion and extension (➤ Fig. 20.1 a and b). They consist of fibrous cartilage arranged in layers and a complexly interweaved structure. They subsist by diffusion from synovial liquid and by blood supply out of the capsular attachment (➤ Fig. 20.2). This can only sustain a part of the meniscal corpus, though. Therefore, the three zones of the meniscus are distinguished according to the blood supply and the option of repair by

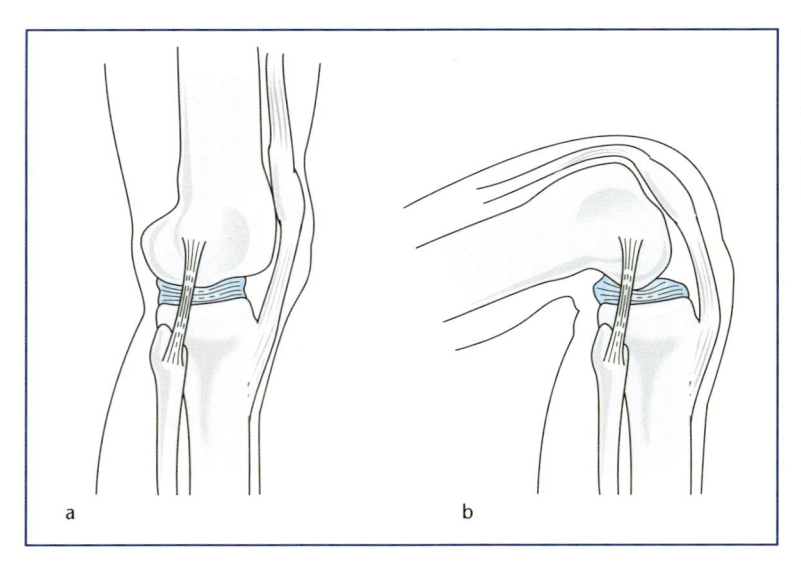

Fig. 20.1 Knee joint, view from lateral. a: Position of the menisci in extension. b: Position of the menisci in flexion (Sobotta, Atlas der Anatomie des Menschen, vol. 2, 21st ed, Urban & Fischer Verlag, 2000).

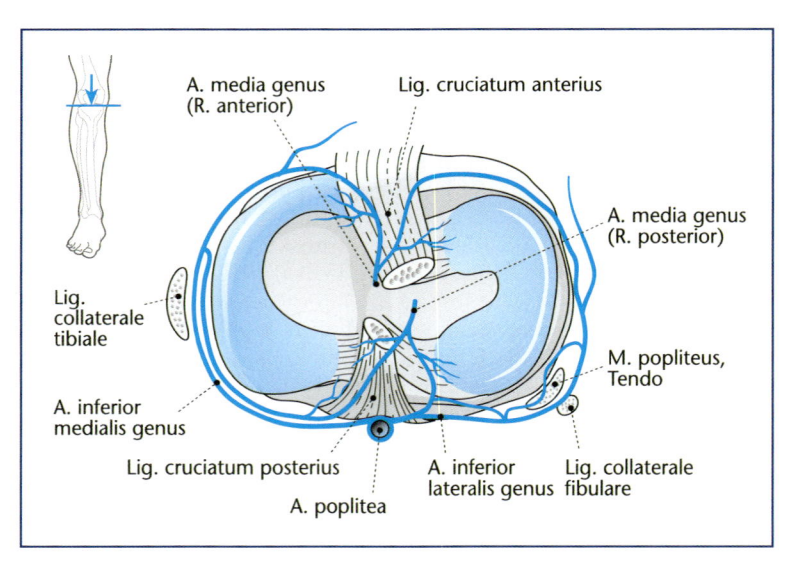

Fig. 20.2 Arterial treatment of the menisci, view from proximal (Sobotta, Atlas der Anatomie des Menschen, vol. 2, 21st ed, Urban & Fischer Verlag, 2000).

refixation in meniscus surgery: the red, capsular zone, the white-red, medial zone with healing potential, but only suboptimal conditions in this respect, and the white, free zone, which does not show any blood supply and cannot heal.

20.2 Biomechanics

Functionally, the knee joint is a **trocho-ginglymoid joint**: there are flexion and extension around the transversal axis and rotation around the vertical axis. In contrast to other joints with nearly congruent heads and sockets, the femurcondyle and the tibial plateau only have punctiform contact with each other in the knee joint, where the roll-slide process extrapolates. Therefore, the convex femur in flexion also migrates to dorsal on the concave tibial plateau. Additionally, there is a translation movement of the femur against the tibia, pathologically increased in ruptures of the cruciate ligaments.

20.3 Injuries

20.3.1 Meniscus injuries

Meniscus injuries belong to the most frequent sports injuries of the knee joint; their therapy has significantly changed in the past years. The conservation of the meniscus is now the primary goal. Meniscus injuries are distinguished by **localization (anterior horn, pars intermedia and posterior horn)** and **type of rupture**. These are divided into **longitudinal, radial and horizontal tears** leading to basket handle tears or lobe tears (➤ Fig. 20.3). These tears can emerge on a degenerative basis or can be purely traumatic; the chance of healing in a reconstruction is only given for purely traumatic tears. The diagnosis of meniscal lesions is primarily clinical, although imaging procedures are reasonable for diagnosis, the indication of surgery, for an according surgery planning (refixation) and for informing the patient. MRT is indispensable for the diagnosis of meniscus lesions. The interpretation of the findings represents a point of discussion between radiologists and clinicians. However, every surgeon must judge the MRT images himself/herself and must not solely rely on radiology reports.

Partial meniscus resection

A complete meniscectomy is obsolete nowadays (Kesenheimer et al. 1990). Nevertheless, it can be necessary for distinct complex meniscus impairments; a meniscus replacement or a meniscus transplant should be considered. Degenerative changes can be expected after a partial meniscectomy (Krüger-Franke et al. 1999). Expanded meniscus resections will result in osteoarthritis.

> In order to avoid postoperative arthritis, the following rule applies to the partial meniscectomy: resect as much as necessary, but as little as possible. A solid resection edge with fluent junctions to the healthy residual tissue must be the goal.

The degeneration is often located centrally, especially with degenerative menisci after partial resection. The radiologist diagnoses a horizontal rupture by MRT, which is only feigned by the "sandwich-like" meniscus structure with central degeneration. A similar problem is degree 2 lesions with horizontal tears without surface contact (Reicher et al. 1986). An intact meniscus surface by arthroscopy "undulates" at the examining hook test, but does not show a rupture. The best results are achieved in cases of symptomatic degree 2 lesions with a partial resection under protection of the meniscus basis. Pure "meniscus scarification" or horizontal suture attempts are not recommended.

The technique of partial meniscus resection should protect the joint cartilage and form a stable resection edge. Therefore, multiple changes of optics, instrument accesses, and use

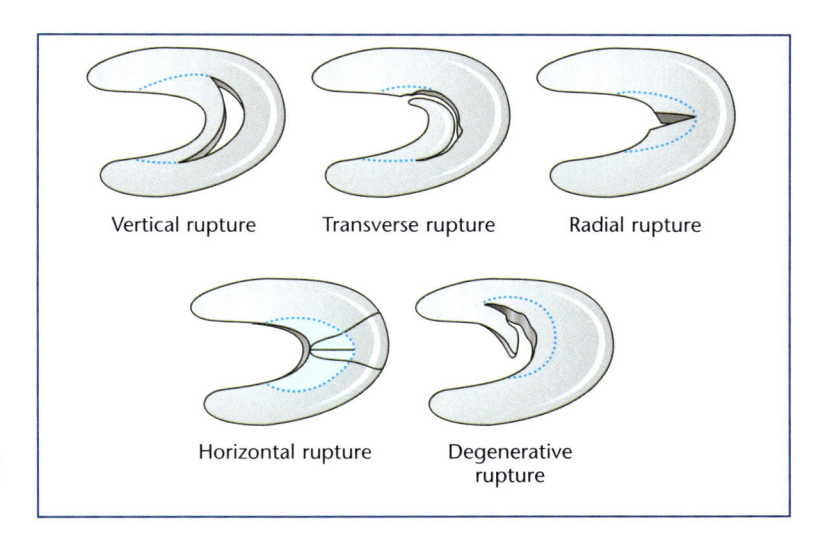

Fig. 20.3 Meniscus shapes and recommended resection (Miller 2004).

of swages are necessary (> Fig. 20.4). Motor-controlled shaver systems for the removal of resected fragments and the smoothing of edges are useful.

The **rehabilitation** after partial meniscus resections is early functional and allows pain and swelling-adapted, full weight bearing in free mobility.

Meniscus refixation

Meniscus refixation requires 3–6 sports-free months. Therefore, the individual situation of the injured athlete must be considered in addition to the localization, type and extent of the rupture and the state of the joint are important decision factors that need to be balanced. After a partial resection, the exercising of the sport at a return to high-level sports is possible after 2–4 weeks. Furthermore, sports exposing the knee joint like wrestling or soccer show a high rate of re-rupturing for meniscus refixations, especially in top sports. Therefore, the 50% risk of a re-rupture and thus a re-surgery must be explained to the athlete. The danger of a long-term damage in form of uni-compartment osteoarthritis is high, but the option chosen by most athletes.

The refixation is indicated for longitudinal ruptures in the red-red or in the red-white zones of the internal and external meniscus (Galla and Lobenhoffer 2005). Basic requirement is a preparation of the rupture edges and the synovial environment of the meniscus to improve the blood supply. The refixation itself can be by sutures. Different fixation systems lead to very different procedures:

The **refixation by sutures** can be carried out by open surgery or arthroscopy. There is the inside-out or the outside-in technique for the arthroscopic suture and also the superior inside-in technique in the region of the posterior horn. The protection of neurovascular structures is important medially and laterally. Therefore, an additional incision and the use of according retractors are highly recommended. The sutures can be arranged horizontally or vertically, they can be at the surface or subsurface of the meniscus and can also achieve solid refixations. Resorbable as well as non-resorbable suture material has been described (> Fig. 20.5).

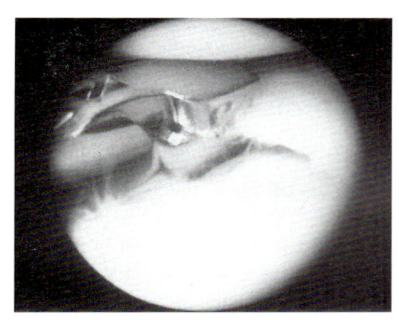

Fig. 20.4 Meniscus swage at the arthroscopic partial resection of the medial meniscus.

Tab. 20.1 Advantages and disadvantages of the meniscus fixation systems.

Advantages	Disadvantages
fast implantation	expensive
good accessibility in the posterior horn	less stable than sutures
no additional incisions	foreign body in the knee joint
no neurovascular complications	secondary cartilage damages by protrusion or dislocation

Different advantages and disadvantages have been described (> Tab. 20.1) for the use of the numerous different **fixation systems** (> Fig. 20.6) offered by industry. The stability of the meniscus must be the purpose of every refixation. Nevertheless, the fixation to the capsule especially in the posterior horn of the external meniscus must not be too rigid to preserve the physiologic mobility and kinematics. The re-rupture rate after meniscus refixation depends significantly on the stability of the fixation. Many studies show that the meniscus sutures with simultaneous reconstruction of the cruciate ligaments provide the best results. Meniscus refixations in unstable joints are contraindicated, because a re-rupture is herepredictable.

The **rehabilitation** after meniscus refixations is discussed controversially. Many authors recommend a brace with F/E 90-10-0° for 6 weeks under full weight exposure of the leg. Others treat small ruptures without braces. This is only possible with according compliance of

Fig. 20.5 Arthroscopic meniscus refixation at the internal meniscus with non-absorbable suture material in the inside-out technique.

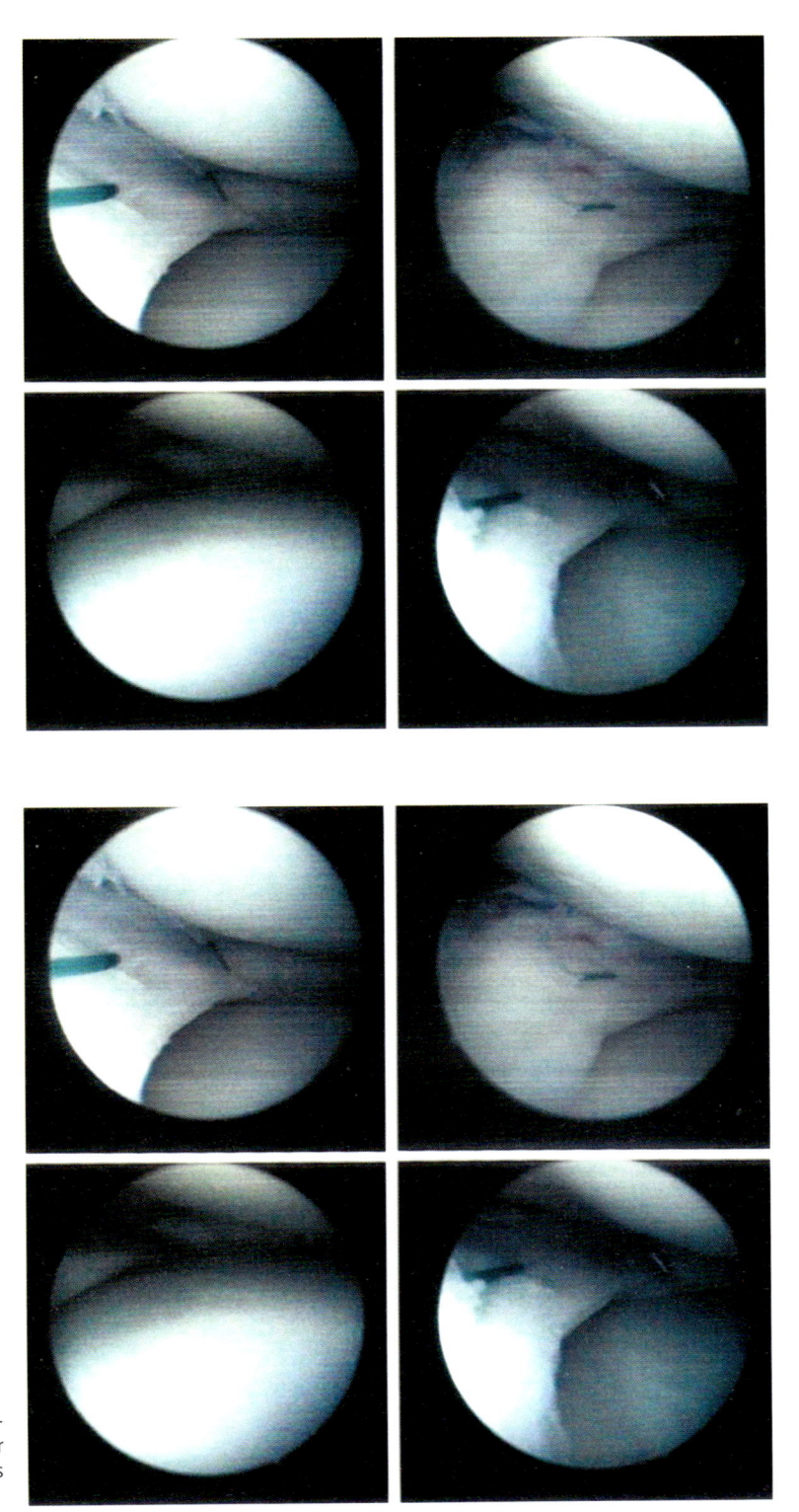

Fig. 20.6 Arthroscopic meniscus refixation in the posterior horn of the external meniscus by the T-fix system.

the patient, though. The return to sport is possible step by step; full sport capacity in competitive sports can only be regained after 6 months.

Meniscus replacement

The replacement of the meniscus for the prevention of uni-compartmental osteoarthritis has to be discussed for young patients with total meniscectomy and for patients with medial or lateral knee-joint problems after subtotal meniscectomy. For 15 years, meniscus transplants have been carried out; the results – depending on the used transplant – are very different. The transplantation of meniscus allografts has been successful in about 50% of the cases (Noyes et al. 1998). The attempt of meniscus replacement by stripes of the quadriceps tendon is only useful in selected cases (Verdonk et al. 2005). To achieve stable results, the transosseous fixation of the meniscus transplant in the region of the posterior or anterior horn is necessary.

> The European Meniscal Transplantation Group principle states: There is nothing better than the human meniscal transplant.

The collagenous meniscal implant (CMI) has not fulfilled the expectations yet. The implants loose substance and can therefore replace the own meniscus biomechanics only incompletely in patients with partial meniscectomy. The implant is overloaded in a total meniscectomy joint.

20.3.2 Capsule-ligament injuries

Collateral ligament injuries

Medial collateral ligament injuries are often a consequence of a valgus trauma in the knee joint, sometimes combined with a rupture of the cruciate ligament. The **clinical examination ranks first** in the diagnosis of the medial collateral ligament rupture: The medial instability in 0° and 30° of flexion shows very sensitively the presence of a rupture. In the clinical examination, there is still the classification in- to I to III (Engelhardt et al. 1997) according to a instability of 5 mm (+), 10 mm (++) or >10 mm (+++). If a instability is marked to +++ and not painful, this indicates a complete rupture. Radiographic diagnostics is important for the exclusion of osseous avulsion fractures or for the diagnosis of an old injury with the presence of Stieda-Pellegrini sign. The rupture can be diagnosed by ultrasound as well as by MRT, but the question whether the medial meniscus is damaged can only be answered by MRT.

> The medial ligament rupture is conservatively treated, with the exception of the complete distal rupture and the osseous avulsions at the femoral condyle. They require surgery.

The conservative therapy is a functional treatment using a brace with limited range of motion for 6 weeks under full weight bearing.

The **lateral collateral ligament injuries** are rarerare less frequent than the medial injuries (1:15) (Engelhardt et al. 1997), and thy are never isolated. They are complex injuries of the lateral stabilizers including the tractus iliotibialis, the popliteus muscle, the capsule and the anterior or posterior cruciate ligament. Therefore, a reconstruction of the fresh injury makes sense. Chronic lateral collateral ligament ruptures are difficult to treat and mostly not stabilized to full satisfaction. Often a osseous axis correction is necessary simultaneously for the protection of the ligament reconstruction. Many cases need an additional osteotomy to correct leg axis and protect ligament reconstruction.

> In order to achieve a satisfying result of treatment, the early diagnosis and immediate acute and correct therapy of the lateral instability are very important.

At present, the best reconstruction of a chronic lateral collateral ligament rupture uses the semitendinosus tendon or the gracilis tendon, taken out ipsi-laterally or contra-laterally. The tendons are led through the fibular head, and subsequently fixed isometrically to the insertion at the epicondylus femoris lateralis with a resorbable interference screw.

Anterior cruciate ligament rupture

The anterior cruciate ligament rupture is a very frequent injury of the knee joint and has different injury mechanisms, such as hyperextension, valgus-rotation stress or forced quadriceps tension with flexed knee joint. Due to the loss of function of the anterior cruciate ligament, the central column of the stabilization of the knee joint is destroyed: instability, "giving way" symptoms and painful swellings can be the consequence after these injuries. The cruciate ligament should be reconstructed for symptomatic, i.e. patients who experience such instabilitiy episodes repeatedly. Cartilage and menisci are destroyed progressively by repeated subluxation phenomena and the instability increases by the elongation of other ligament structures.

Reasons for the increase of anterior ligament ruptures in sports are complex. Prevention programs of recent years could definitely decrease the incidence of anterior ligament ruptures, e.g. at women's soccer in the US. Still, large numbers of patients with an anterior ligament rupture are symptomatic. Stabilization is necessary especially in sports such as soccer or alpine skiing.

The operative treatment of a acute rupture of the anterior cruciate ligament had been the state of art for many years. Numerous examinations demonstrated that the cruciate ligament suture is obsolete (Krüger-Franke et al. 1996). They have also shown the treatment with reinsertion and augmentation by e.g. the semitendinosus tendon leading to satisfying results in only few cases of a far femorally localized rupture (Krüger-Franke et al. [2] 1995, Hertel [2] 2005). The intra-ligamentous ruptures cannot be treated by suture and augmentation, here a surgical reconstruction is necessary.

> Cruciate ligament surgery is not applied in the acute state of injury. The delayed treatment has established as state of the art and operation is carried out if the knee joint is not considered „inflammatory" anymore. The requires a flexibility of the knee joint of F/E 90-0-0° without significant effusion, swelling, and pain.

Acute treatment is possible and sensible for treatment-requiring concomitant injuries, especially meniscal basket handle tears or large chondral shear fractures; otherwise the surgery is performed 2–6 weeks post trauma, depending on the condition of the knee joint.

Nowadays, the reconstruction of the anterior cruciate ligament is done by a so-called **minimal invasive surgery**, the tendinous or ligamentous transplant is implanted by arthroscopy. The positioning of the drill holes at tibia and femur is surgically decisive. For that reason, drill jigs guarantee a sufficiently precise insertion. Nevertheless, examination of the position in extension is essential, especially at the tibial insertion. Different authors demand routine intraoperative lateral generoscopic control preventing a notch impingement. In the femoral positioning, it is important to drill through the anteromedial arthroscopic portal. Do not trust the jigs blindly because the insertion is often too far cranial in the 12-o'clock position. The femoral insertion of the anterior cruciate ligament can be seen in this 2-o'clock position at the left knee joint, and in the 10-o'clock position at the right knee joint. It is also important to place the insertion femoral correct in the notch. Otherwise flexion will be limited (➢ Fig. 20.7).

The positioning of the femoral drill hole through the anteromedial arthroscopic portal allows the correct placement of the transplant.

Common transplants are the tendons of the hamstrings, semitendinous or gracilis tendon, a third of the patellar tendon with or without bone block and a part of the quadriceps tendon, which is often used as primary transplant especially in Switzerland. We use this tendon mostly as revision transplant (Miller et al. 2004). In Germany, the allografts do not have the same importance yet as they have reached in the U.S.

The fixation of the cruciate ligament replacement has not been uniform, and it depends on the kind of transplant. The fixation with interference screws – either metallic or resorbable – has prevailed for the patellar tendon. For the hamstring tendons, a variety of fixation procedures are available commercially. In general, fixations close to the joint and far from the

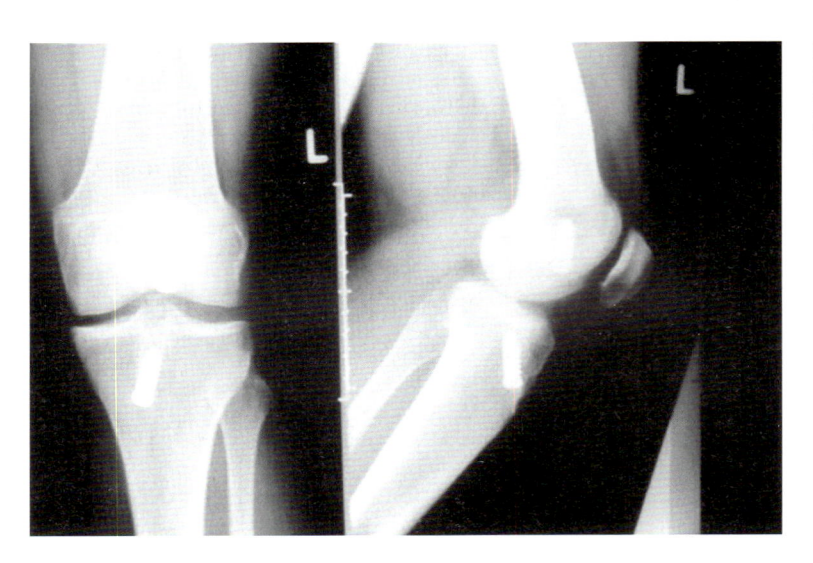

Fig. 20.7 X-ray of a knee after anterior cruciate ligament reconstruction a.p. and lateral view. Femoral tunnel with enough position.

joint are distinguished. Fixation procedures close to the joint are the fixation by interference screws and the procedures for the transverse locking ("rigid fix" and "trans-fix"). Fixation techniques far from the joint are the endo-button, suture-disc or pole screw fixation. The fixation far from the joint causes so-called windshield wiper effects or "bungee" effects due to the inherent elasticity of the transplant, resulting in an a widening of the drill hole and theoretically loosen transplant. However, this loosening could not be detected in several studies. Therefore, the fixation of the cruciate ligament transplant far from the joint and close to the joint line are the treatment choices. The hamstring tendons are used 4-fold as transplant and the third of the patellar tendon as well as the quadriceps tendon stripe as single-fold transplant. The "double bundle" technique proposed during recent years can be used for the hamstring tendons. In this technique, the anteromedial and the posterolateral bundles are replaced separately with the requirement of four drill holes. The fixation of the transplant is done with the same implants as in the conventional single-bundle technique. Nonetheless, both bundles are fixed in different degrees flexions of the knee joint. Biomechanical examinations show a superiority of the double-bundle technique regarding stability, especially rotational stability. Clinical medium-term studies show no significant differences between single- and double-bundle techniques.

The **rehabilitation** of isolated cruciate ligament replacements is functional, with the knee in extension within the first 24–48 hours, and then to improve the flexibility afterwards by CPM (continuous passive motion) treatment, remedial gymnastics and physiotherapy improve flexibility. The weight bearing is increased, adapted to the pain, so that the full weight bearing is achieved after 14 days.

Posterior cruciate ligament rupture

The posterior cruciate ligament rupture is rare. Especially in these cases the concomitant injuries have to be considered, which might determine surgery. An isolated posterior cruciate ligament rupture should be treated conventionally, though a medial and retropatellar osteoarthritis can develop in the mid- or long-term. Therefore, some authors request a replacement surgery also for an isolated posterior cruciate ligament rupture (Galla and Lobenhoffer 2005).

A conservative therapy should be done standard of care for acute isolated posterior cruciate ligament ruptures, which prevents the posterior subluxation of the tibial head by a brace and takes about 8–12 weeks (PCL-Jack brace).

20.3 Injuries

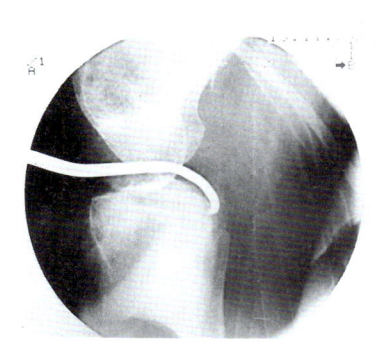

Fig. 20.8 Radiograph of a knee joint (II technique) lateral, inoperative: applying of the tibial target hook at the posterior cruciate ligament plastic.

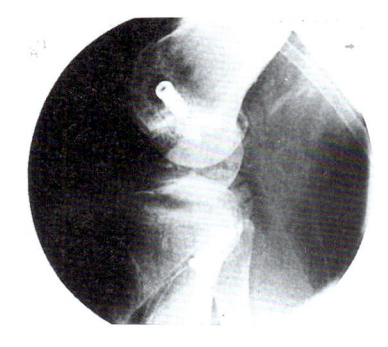

Fig. 20.9 Radiograph of a knee joint lateral, postoperative: posterior cruciate ligament plastic with medium third of the patellar tendon.

With the existence of concomitant injuries of the medial or lateral capsule-ligament complex, the primary replacement surgery of the posterior cruciate ligament combined with a treatment of the capsule-ligament injuries medial and lateral is required. This treatment is done with a patellar tendon transplant (➤ Fig. 20.8) or the hamstring tendons being fixed by endo-button or interference screw implants (➤ Fig. 20.9) known from the anterior cruciate ligament replacement.

The **rehabilitation** is much more restrictive than after anterior cruciate ligament replacement. An orthesis brace is necessary for 9 weeks to prevent a posterior subluxation of the tibial head. Limitation of the flexion to 90° for 6 weeks with partial weight bearing of the operated leg is recommended.

Osseous cruciate ligament injuries

The osseous ligament avulsions are a special type of injury of the anterior and posterior cruciate ligaments. The osseous ligament avulsion is always localized at the tibia. The anterior cruciate ligament avulsions are classified according to Meyers and McKeever (1970). Without dislocation of the fragment, they are treated conservatively. Arthroscopic assisted refixation is indicated for a dislocation of the fragment of the tibial cruciate ligament insertion (Hoffmann 2000). The treatment of osseous cruciate ligament avulsions at the posterior cruciate ligament can also be performed arthroscopically or open in abdominal supine position; a stable fixation by screw osteosynthesis has to be achieved (Benedetto 2000). A rehabilitation with a brace is necessary for fractures of the refixed osseous cruciate ligament avulsion in order to primarily prevent the full extension and the flexion of more than 90°.

Cruciate ligament injuries at open epiphyseal plate

Injuries of the cruciate ligaments become more frequent in young patients. The central problem of the treatment of such injuries is the compromising of the epiphyseal plates. This must be prevented at any time. The fear of growth disorders induced by surgery had been the reason for the conservative treatment of cruciate ligament injuries at the age of childhood and adolescence.

> A premature partial closure of the epiphyseal plate is caused by drill tunnels of cruciate ligaments not completely filled with tendon tissue and the use of bone-tendon-bone transplants (Stadelmaier et al. 1995, Hoffmann 2000).

No premature closure of the plate or a consecutive growth disorder is expected, if the drill hole is filled completely with hamstring tissue and drilled tibially with consideration of the apophysis and epiphyseal plate. As could be demonstrated in long-term studies, children and adolescents with a "chronic" instability develop meniscal and cartilage damages to a high percentage. Thus, a surgical stabilization of the anterior cruciate ligament is necessary by cruciate ligament surgery with 4-fold semitendinosus tendon transplant, regardless of age.

The applying of an brace for 6 weeks is recommended for children and adolescents, in order to reduce the compulsion to move and to protect the transplant.

Patellar instability

The instability of the patella (➤ Fig. 20.10, ➤ Fig. 20.11) is a frequent problem in sports traumatology, the manifest dislocation is a most severe injury of the capsule-ligament apparatus complex with facultative osteochondral concomitant injury. The acute **patellar dislocation** mostly develops on the ground of a patellofemoral dysplasia and involves the rupture of the medial retinaculum or the medial patellofemoral ligament, a chondral and osteochondral lesion at the medial patellar facette and at the lateral femur condyle. The instability is always directed laterally. The extend of the injury depends on the dysplasia and the instability intensity of the trauma.

> An osteochondral concomitant injury with an osteochondral fragment >1 cm² makes the patellar dislocation a true emergency with the indication for immediate surgical refixation.

Apart from these cases with larger osteochondral fragments, the surgical planning follows different criteria: age of the patient, number of dislocations, as well as type of the patellofemoral dysplasia. The **stepwise concept of surgical therapy** consists of a primary reconstruction of the ruptured structures, meaning a suture of the medial retinaculum. This can be carried out arthroscopically in case of midrupture. A reinsertion of the ligament at the femoral condyle is useful for a femorally localized rupture of the MPFL. The MPFL has to be reconstructed, e.g. by a semitendinosus plastic (Schöttle et al. 2005) for an insufficiency of the medial patellar supporting ligaments by multiple dislocations, and the medial retinaculum must be reconstructed as well. We consider the lateral extension release or splitting of the retinaculum (Biedert and Netzer 2005); Dejour and Locatelli (2005) reject it. At the same time it is the recommended therapy together with the medial reconstruction for patients with open epiphyseal plates. Osseous procedures are not allowed at this age.

Osseous correcting procedures are indicated for existing chronic instabilities of the patella with the increased Q-angle and concluded growth of the patient. The transfer of the tuberositas tibiae according to Elmslie or Blauth is the most frequent procedure for prevention of a repeated dislocation when the TT-TG-distance is more than 20 mm. The trochlear dysplasia can be improved by a trochlear plastic in the technique according to Dejour (Dejour and Locatelli 2005). This procedure is indicated rarely and should be used only by experienced surgeons.

The **rehabilitation** after these procedures requires limiting the knee joint mobility to protect the healing of the medial retinaculum complex and the healing of the tuberositas tibiae. The brace is limited to a flexion of F/E 0–40° for 2 weeks, afterwards to 0–60° for another 2 weeks, and to 0–90° for the last 2 weeks.

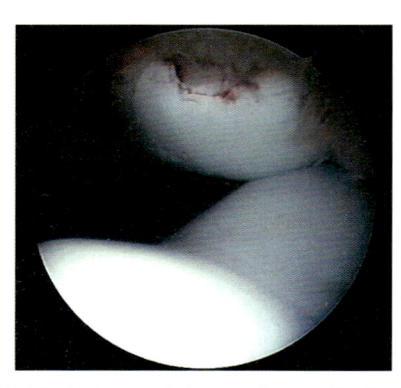

Fig. 20.10 Arthroscopic image of a patellar instability after luxation.

Fig. 20.11 Radiograph of both patellae tangential with left-hand luxation.

20.3 Injuries

Muscle stimulation and CPM in the allowed range of mobility is essential for rehabilitation.

Rupture of the quadriceps tendon

The rupture of the quadriceps tendon develops by an arbitrary maximum tension of the muscles against resistance. Patients older than 40 years mostly experience rupture of the quadriceps tendon. If the extension apparatus is affected, a limitation of the active knee extension develops. If the extension apparatus is preserved, extension is possible despite rupture of the tendon.

The **therapy** is surgical for every complete rupture of the quadriceps tendon. Otherwise the knee joint in extension cannot be stabilized anymore and the affected leg can no longer be used. The rupture is mostly localized near the patella, making the refixation at the patella by transosseous sutures indispensable (Galla and Lobenhoffer 2005, Lobenhoffer and Thermann 2005).

The **rehabilitation** after tendon suture requires a protection of the suture by an a orthesis with limitation of the flexion to 60° for 4 weeks, afterwards to 90° until the 6th week under partial weight bearing of 20 kg for 6 weeks.

Rupture of the patellar tendon

The patellar tendon rupture is very rare and mostly localized at the distal patellar pole. It is a described complication after an anterior cruciate ligament surgery with the medial third of the patellar tendon, but also appears without previous surgery at the patellar tendon. The active extension in the knee joint is not possible anymore with a rupture in the knee extension apparatus. The reconstruction is an absolute urgent indication for surgery. The treatment of the ruptured patellar tendon is carried out by sutures with adaption of the structures and a protective patellotibial cerclage with a wire or a PDS cord for 6–8 weeks (Galla and Lobenhoffer 2005). With a very weak patellar tendon, the augmentation can be done with the semitendinosus tendon (Hertel [1] 2005). During this time, the flexibility of the knee joint has to be limited with a brace to 60°.

20.3.3 Cartilage injuries

Cartilage injuries at the knee joint are hard to diagnose and are a consequence of trauma like cruciate ligament ruptures or patellar dislocations (➢ Fig. 20.12). The differential-diagnostic discrimination is possible by the localization of the traumatic cartilage lesions. The therapy of cartilage injuries is discussed in detail in chapter 24.

> A cartilage injury with large chondral or even osteochondral flake is an absolute emergency indication for surgical treatment as the fragment is macerating by the hemarthrosis. The fragment deforms and fragments further due to the movement in the knee joint. Thus it cannot be refixed anymore.

A refixation by screws in osteochondral fragments or by ethipins or cartilage arrows in chondral fragments always is to be aimed at with adequate localization, size and texture of the fragment. The following principle is applicable for cartilage more than for other kinds of tissue: "Nothing is as good as the original."

Osteochondrosis dissecans

The osteochondrosis dissecans belongs to the antiseptic osteochondronecroses with a partial or complete separation of a chondral or osteochondral fragment of the surrounding cartilage and bone. In the case of a complete separation, it is called a loose body or **joint mouse** with an according defect in the joint surface,

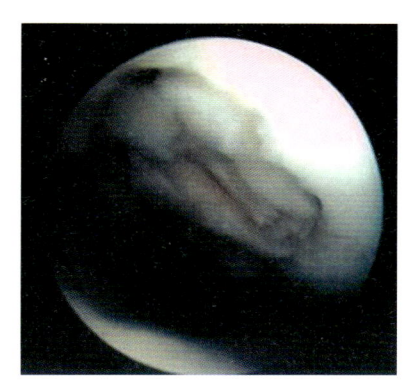

Fig. 20.12 Arthroscopic image of traumatic cartilage damage at the lateral femur condyle after cruciate ligament rupture.

the mouse bed. This disease is the most frequent cause of incarcerations at the knee joint in young patients (Hoffmann 2000). The younger the patient, the better is the prognosis at the age of growth. As long as the epiphyseal plates are still open, spontaneous recoveries have often been described. The osteochondrosis dissecans of the knee joint is localized at the lateral part of the medial femur condyle in 85% of the cases. Unspecific stress-conditioned pain in the knee joint is symptomatic.

Therapy depends on the stage. With intact cartilage of the stages 1–2 (Guhl 1984), a retrograde or anterograde (stage 2) drilling should be applied; in stages 3 and 4, the loose body is refixed after the mouse ground has been refreshed and also been assembled by a spongious plastic. The defect must be filled by a transplantation of an osteochondral cylinder in the case of already massively deformed loose bodies without the chance of refixation (Hoffmann 2000).

The **rehabilitation** is **treatment** according to the surgical procedure. A CPM treatment is sensible for every therapy at the cartilage. The leg has to be relieved for a period of about 6 weeks.

20.3.4 Osseous injuries

Also fractures close to the knee joint are found in sports traumatology of the knee joint primarily fractures of the tibial head and the patella, less often distal femoral fractures. In assessing the fracture, especially the situation of the soft tissue is decisive. The vessel state must be examined for all dislocation fractures of the knee joint, and the accesses must be adapted to the localization and the expanse of the fracture.

Distal femoral fractures

The distal femoral fractures are very difficult injuries of the knee joint demanding high standards of the surgeon and the implant. The **AO classification** is used to categorize into localization A (supracondylar fracture), B (involvement of a condyle) and C (involvement of both condyles) and the degrees of severity 1–3 (Müller et al. 1990). Additional classifications emerge from the course of the fracture.

The treatment of these fractures is usually surgical. Only non-dislocated fissured fractures of the condyles with high remnant stability can be treated conservatively (Lobenhoffer 2000). In addition to the anatomical foundations, the regular axial relation must be considered and reconstructed in every **surgical treatment**. The anatomical axis of the femur forms a valgus angle of 6° to the mechanical leg axis (central point of the femoral head, central point of the ankle joint). The femoral condyles are not parallel to the horizontal, but show a valgus posture of 3° to the ground level. Therefore, the condylar line and the mechanical leg axis form an angle of 87° open to lateral and together with the anatomical axis of the femoral shaft a laterally open angle of 81°. The fixed-angle implants (DCS, condyle plate, LISS) used nowadays in surgical treatment are produced in a way that allows an alignment of the part implanted in the femoral condyle region, parallel to the femoral condyle line. The standard access for the treatment of distal femoral fractures is the posterolateral access. Medial access is only chosen for monocondylar medial fractures (B2). An anterolateral access is sensible for the treatment of complex bicondylar joint fractures with metaphyseal impairment. The plate is attached submuscularly and large exposures of the bone and the joint combined with disturbed blood supply via medial and lateral accesses are avoided (Krettek et al. 1996, Lobenhoffer 2000).

The **rehabilitation** after osteosyntheses of distal femoral fractures is very long. It takes 9–12 weeks until full weight bearing. The full capacity of flexion of the knee joint mostly cannot be achieved anymore.

Tibia head fractures

Diagnosis and therapy of fractures of the tibial head and the tibial plateau are very complex. The reconstruction of the joint surface and of the stability of the joint is the basic precondition for the deceleration of the development of a posttraumatic osteoarthritis. The **classification** of tibial plateau fractures is also carried out according to AO, with A-fractures indicating the extraarticular and eminence avulsions,

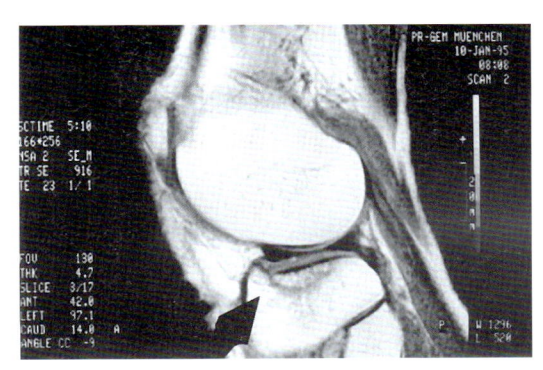

Fig. 20.13 MRI image: lateral depressed fracture of the tibial joint surface.

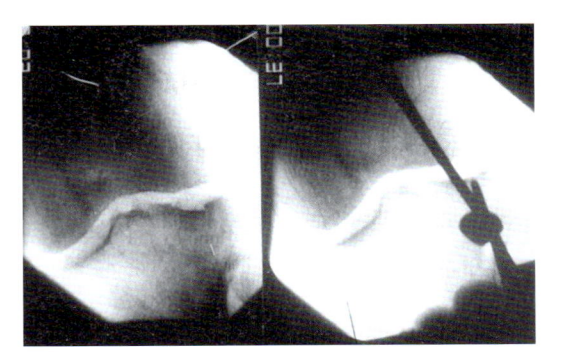

Fig. 20.14 Radiograph (II technique), intraoperative: arthroscopically assisted reposition of a depressed tibial fracture.

B-fractures including the monocondylar and the C-fractures the bicondylar fractures (Müller 1990). Impression fractures and fissured fractures of the lateral tibial plateau are very often found in sport injuries in soccer or skiing, and those are sometimes even missed in conventional X-raying and are only discovered with MRI (➤ Fig. 20.13). An exact diagnosis of the concomitant ligamentous and chondral injuries is necessary.

In our opinion, the **surgical treatment** should be used for every athlete, the treatment of the B-fractures may be carried out with arthroscopic assistance (➤ Fig. 20.14; Krüger-Franke et al. [1] 1995, Trouillier et al. 1995). The external meniscus must be detached and lifted for the correct restoring of the joint surface in the open treatment of lateral tibial plateau fractures. For the stabilization of tibial head fractures, screws are used in arthroscopy. The open reduction and internal fixation of C-fractures has to be implemented by L- or T-plate fixation. Angle-stable implants definitely improve the primary stability in addition to the minimalinvasive percutane application and allow an early functional rehabilitation. Their use is also recommended for the tibial head. In addition, the bone defect of the impression fractures must be lifted up and filled. This can be done out by an autologous bone graft or by bone substitutes or bone bank grafts, respectively.

The partial weight bearing of the operated leg must be ensured for 6–8 weeks under continuous movement therapy and mobilizing of the patella in the **rehabilitation** after an osteosynthesis of a tibial head fracture.

Patellar fractures

The patella is the largest sesamoid bone of the human body and serves the improvement of the muscular strength development of the femoral quadriceps muscle. It is embedded between the quadriceps tendon and the patellar tendon as well as medially and laterally into the retinacula or the so-called reserve extension apparatus of the knee joint. Injuries of the patella are – with the exception of patellar dislocations – consequences of direct collision traumas. These traumas can lead to fractures and pole avulsions. Following **fracture types** are distinguished at the patella:

- transverse fractures
- longitudinal fractures
- comminuted fractures
- avulsion fractures (pole avulsions)
- osteochondral fractures (dislocation consequence).

In all cases, the anatomic knowledge is important. The chance of a so-called patella bipartita or multipartita possibly diagnosed wrongly as a fracture after a collision trauma must be considered (➤ Fig. 20.15).

Therapeutically, the indication for surgical treatment depens on kind and extend of the fracture. The **conservative therapy** is possible for solid longitudinal fractures or non-dislocated, very wide distally placed polar avulsions. The limitation of the maximum flexion by a brace (F/E 90–0–0°), the partial weight bearing with 20 kg of body weight for 4–6 weeks and a physiotherapy belong to this kind of the rehabilitation. Indication for a **surgical stabilization** are dislocation of the fracture or a joint step of >2 mm; a tension band or screw osteosynthesis or a combination of both should be applied (> Fig. 20.16; Galla and Lobenhoffer 2005). A proximal or distal soft tissue irritation by the wires is often disturbing at the tension band osteosyntheses: Too short wires can cause a dislocation; too long wires bother in the flexion of the quadriceps or the patellar tendon.

The ultimate goal is the stable internal fixation with functional **rehabilitation**. The flexion is limited for 2 weeks in a brace of 0–60°, then 0–90° until the 6th week; the weight bearing should start with 20 kg for 2 weeks and should afterwards progress to full weight bearing.

20.4 Overuse impairments of the knee joint

Sport-conditioned overuse injuries of the knee joint are common and can raise serious diagnostic problems.

> Overuse injuries are caused by loads exceeding the capacity of the joint. This can result from the duration of the load or its intensity. While causes are mostly evident for sport injuries, overuse impairments are not in direct timely correlation with the loading and can sometimes be hard to assign to a cause.

For that reason, the attending physician must know the sport and its sport-specific load patterns with overuse conditions in order to make a correct diagnosis and especially to treat the conditions successfully without having to withdraw the athlete from the sport.

The **causes** for overuse conditions are sometimes found in posttraumatic functional disorders of the knee joint after capsule-ligament injuries or surgeries. In addition, the individual physical capacity is subject to changes. The epiphyseal plates and the apophyses are less capable at the age of growth, for example. High tensile stress and hormonally conditioned loosening of the epiphyseal plates can lead to apophyseal loosening, ossifications and even to a lifting of the patella by lengthening of the patellotibial distance (Segesser 1997). Anatomical anomalies can lead to overuse conditions of the knee joint, especially in learning new sports or in an intensification of a sport so far exerted in minor intensity. The patellofemoral joint has to be considered first. Dysplasias of this joint or malpositions of the leg axes by valgus posture or increased tibial torsions and an increased torsion of the femoral neck can lead to a change of the patellofemoral pressure relations and cause overuse conditions.

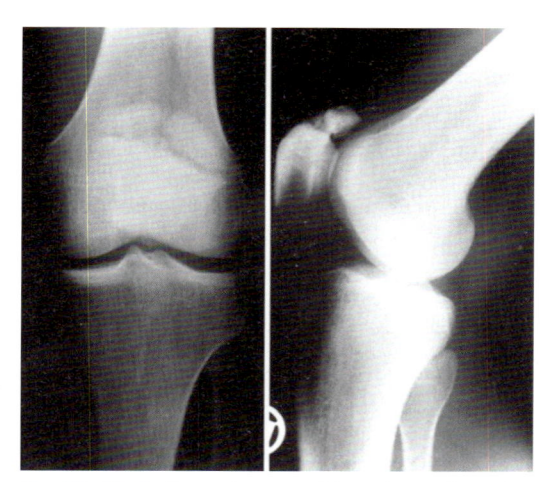

Fig. 20.15 Radiograph a.p. and lateral: patella multipartita.

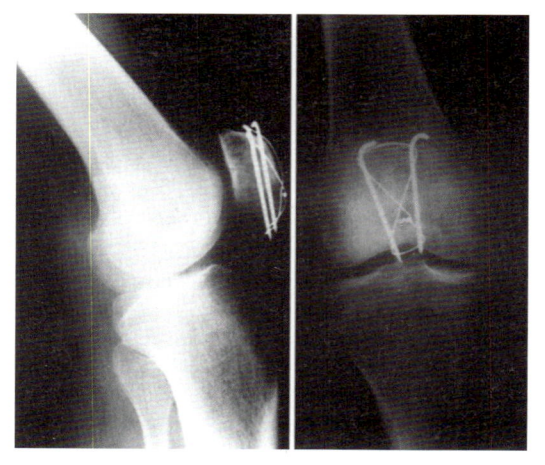

Fig. 20.16 Radiograph a.p. and lateral, postoperative: osteosynthesis of a patellar fracture by tension banding.

Apart from these anatomical causes, **external factors can participate in the development of** the sport impairments. Primarily, the arrangement of training, the athlete's capability to recover and the degree of fatigue as well as the training environment are to be inquired and have to be involved into the diagnosis. Sport shoes are an important factor for knee joint conditions in sports. Shape, function and sport must be considered and the shoe has to be individually adapted to the foot to allow full capacity. A good forefoot damping, for example, and a pronation control within the shoe are necessary with the patellar apex syndrome; a solid hindfoot control is necessary for the tractus syndrome.

Primarily the clinical examination and the history of the problems regarding the conditions and the sport as well as intensity of training are necessary for the **diagnosis** of overuse conditions. The imaging procedures must be geared to the results of the clinical examinations. The sensible use of the different procedures is very important. Bone scan is important in the diagnosis of overuse conditions of the knee joint (Dye 1998).

Anterior knee pain

The anterior knee pain involves many symptoms with pain in the ventral, ventromedial and ventrolateral knee joint in common and has very different reasons. The **femoropatellar pain syndrome** belongs to the classic symptoms. It can show a retropatellar cartilage impairment, a missing centering of the patella with a hypercompression in the lateral trochlear region or even interposing plicae as a cause. Often an anterior knee pain syndrome develops also by a **muscular dysbalance**, e.g. with the mainly tonic musculature as the rectus femoris muscle being shortened and the elasticity of the complete musculotendinous system being disturbed. Thus, the mobility of the joint reduces in flexion at the rectus femoris muscle or in extension at the iliopsoas muscle. This leads to improper load of the knee joint with changed femoropatellar strength conditions and resulting pain (Segesser 1997). The recovery of the muscular balance is essential in all **insertion tendinoses** like patellar apex syndrome or tendinitis of the quadriceps tendon, in order to be able to control the clinical symptoms in the long term (Segesser 1997, Galla and Lobenhoffer 2005).

Chondromalacia patellae

Retropatellar cartilage damages, regardless of their cause, can cause knee pain (➢ Fig. 20.17). The treatment of these conditions must regard the cause of the cartilage lesion first and intervene causally. The treatment of the cartilage lesion can mostly be done by arthroscopy; a required patellar alignment is performed in the same session. The principles of cartilage therapy are to be considered in the arthroscopic **treatment** of the cartilage impairment. A smoothing of cartilage must be done only very sparely, healthy cartilage tissue must be preserved and the thermal treatment of the cartilage has to be dismissed because of its depth effect.

Plica syndrome

Three plicae are to be found in the arthroscopic surgery of the knee joint. They are of different meaning (Landsiedl 2000).

The **plica semilunaris**, localized in the upper recessus, separates the retropatellar joint segment from the suprapatellar parts and has no significance for the anterior knee pain. Occasionally, loose bodies are accumulating above this plica. They cannot be seen in arthroscopy, because the plica represents a complete separation of the joint parts. In such cases, the plica must be resected and the loose bodies have to be extracted.

The **plica infrapetellaris** is also widely insignificant for the pain development, because it only runs tibially as a connection between the ante-

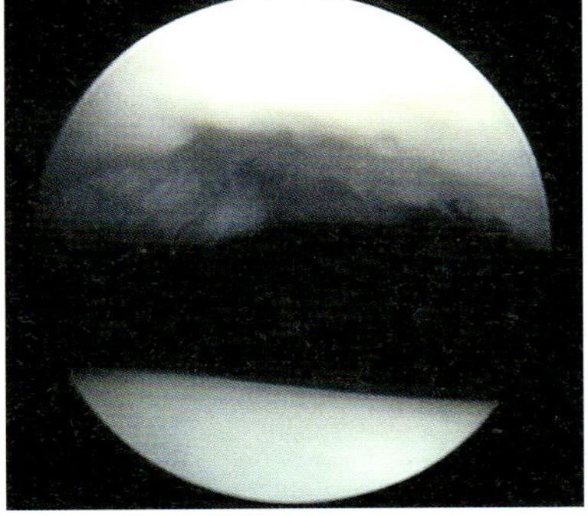

Fig. 20.17 Arthroscopic image of profound cartilage damage (degree 3 according to Outerbridge) in the patellar back surfaces.

rior upper notch roof and the insertion of Hoffa's fat pad. It cannot generate snapping phenomena or cartilage arrosions. Nonetheless, Segesser has described fibrosis of the plica infrapetellaris and of the Hoffa responsible for anterior knee pain. They could be removed permanently by an arthroscopic plica resection (Segesser 1997).

The case is different with the **plica mediopatellaris** (➢ Fig. 20.18). Lying between patella and medial condyle in flexion/extension movements, it can cause pain at the medial knee joint. It also generates arrosions on both joint surfaces or even defects of the cartilaginous surface. These plicae are mostly fibrozed by large flexion/extension excursions, e.g. in cycling, rowing or weight lifting, and then become symptomatic. This can cause contusions with hemorrhages into the plica or by postarthroscopic changes of the plica. The symptoms are medial pain above the condyle in flexion and extension, a palpable snapping phenomenon at this point and possibly a pseudo-blocking. In imaging, this plica can only be shown by MRT or double-contrast CT examination. The arthroscopic resection of the plica is the only therapeutic option. Only the symptomatic plica should be removed, though.

Patellar apex syndrome

The patellar apex syndrome, also called "jumper's knee", is an **insertion tendinosis** of the patellar ligament at the patellar insertion. It can lead even to Sinding-Larsen-Johansson disease at the age of growth. This is interpreted as aseptic necrosis of the patellar apex by increased tension stress or inflammatory changes. The patellar apex syndrome is the most common manifestation of overuse of the extension apparatus of the knee joint and is found especially in sports that generate frequent positive and negative accelerations in the knee joint, like indoor tennis, basketball, volleyball or other jumping sports.

In addition to the radiographic scout film in two layers, especially the sonographic examination of the patellar tendon and MRT are indicated in the diagnosis.

The **conservative measures** are mostly successful in therapy. In addition to local and personal application of antiphlogistic drugs, the physiotherapeutic treatment is in the foreground: transverse friction by ultrasound and stretching of the extension apparatus with recovery of the muscular balance between extensors and flexors of the knee joint (Segesser 1997, Landsiedl 2000). In addition, taping or bandages for the patellar tendon can prevent stress peaks at the insertion of the patellar ligament. **Surgical measures** are required for substantial tendon impairments, such as necroses or partial ruptures. The wedge-shaped excision of the tissue with a drilling of the patellar apex differs from the "reversed plastic" with a healthy strip of ligament with bone block being extracted surgically from the distal insertion of the patellar ligament and being transferred into the diseased area that has been resected previously (Biedert 1995).

The **rehabilitation** of this procedure requires up to 6 months of patience and physiotherapeutic measures. Altogether, the sport break or the temporary change to a sport less stressing to the knee joint is very important.

Osgood-Schlatter disease

The Osgood-Schlatter disease is an **insertion tendinosis** of the patellar ligament at the tibia during the age of growth between the 12th and 14th year of age. It is also called apophysitis. A swelling of the apophysis, an ossification disorder as in the Sinding-Larsen-Johansson disease and a formation of ossicles distally in the patellar tendon can be the consequences. This disease shows clinically already during inspec-

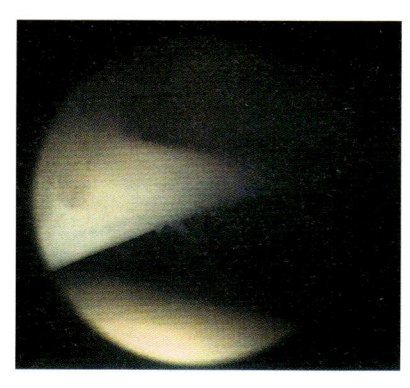

Fig. 20.18 Arthroscopic image of a pica mediopatellaris.

tion. The swelling of the ligament can be displayed by ultrasound and the apophysis is enlarged and fragmented in the X-ray. In **therapy**, the reduction of stress, the recovery of muscular balance and local anti-phlogistic measures are the priority. Surgical intervention is only applied after the conclusion of growth for present ossicles in the distal patellar tendon causing local irritation and pain (Hoffmann 2000).

Bursitis praepatellaris

The bursitis praepatellaris or infrapatellaris can also be cause of anterior knee pain. These bursitides appear after an acute or chronic pressure strain with liquid accumulating in the bursa and an inflammatory swelling of the bursa leaves. This inflammatory swelling can cause pain. Diagnostically, ultrasound is the best method beyond the clinical examination. The treatment mainly includes immobilization of the knee joint in a brace with extension and local as well as peroral antiphlogistic measures. Bursectomy is the only sensible therapy for bacterially inflammable bursitis or for chronic, therapy-resistant abacterial bursitis.

Iliotibial friction syndrome

The so-called tractus-iliotibialis syndrome always has to be considered with overuse conditions in the region of the lateral knee joint in athletes. In this respect, it involves a **bursitis** between the lateral femoral condyle and the tractus iliotibialis occuring most often in runners and cyclists. Athletes with genu varum and increasingly setting down the lateral edge of the foot in running or braking a sideways movement with the extended knee joint are affected especially (Segesser 1997). The running shoe is often responsible for these pain symptoms. The link between heel cap and sole loses its stability in a profound dampening of the shoe. The calcaneus gets in varus position and the pronation movement of the foot cannot be controlled anymore. This implies an optimized shoe supply for **therapy** in addition to the local anti-phlogistic measures. In cyclists, also the non-physiological posture of external rotation of the foot in the pedal can be responsible for the clinical picture.

References

Benedetto KP (2000). Frische Kapsel-Band-Verletzungen des Kniegelenkes. In: Kohn D (ed.). Das Knie. Thieme, Stuttgart-New York, pp. 151–162.

Biedert RM (1995). Chronic jumper's knee: surgical treatment for partial tendon rupture. Amendola A (ed.). Evolving strategies in the diagnosis and treatment of tendinopathy. Isakos Sports Medicine Committee, pp. 46–50.

Biedert RM, Netzer P (2005). Anatomische Betrachtungen der arthroskopischen lateralen Retinakulumspaltung. Arthroskopie 18: 289–292.

Dejour D, Locatelli E (2005). Patellainstabilität bei Erwachsenen. In: Chirurgische Techniken in Orthopädie und Traumatologie. Oberschenkel und Knie. Elsevier-Verlag, pp. 107–115.

Dye S (1998). Use of scintigraphy in assessing patients with anterior knee pain. In: Chan M, Fu F, Maffulli N, Rolf C, Kurosaka M, Liv S (eds.). Controversies in Orthopedic Sports Medicine. Williams & Wilkins, Hongkong.

Engelhardt M, Freiwald J, Leonhardt T, Dann K (1997). Kniegelenk: Kapsel-Band-Verletzungen. In: GOTS-Manual. Verlag Hans Huber, pp. 124–133.

Galla M, Lobenhoffer P (2005). Kniegelenk. In: Engelhardt M, Krüger-Franke M, Pieper HG, Siebert CH (eds.). Sportverletzungen Sportschäden. Thieme, Stuttgart, pp. 65–74.

Guhl J (1984). Osteochondritis dissecans. In: Casscells SW (ed.). Arthroscopy: Diagnostic and Surgical Practice. Lea & Felbiger, Philadelphia.

Hertel P (2005a). Rupturen der Patellarsehne. In: Duparc J (ed.). Chirurgische Techniken in Orthopädie und Traumatologie. Oberschenkel und Knie. Elsevier, pp. 71–75.

Hertel P (2005b). Spezifische Operationstechniken bei frischen Kniebandverletzungen. In: Duparc J (ed.). Chirurgische Techniken in Orthopädie und Traumatologie. Oberschenkel und Knie. Elsevier, pp. 161–172

Hoffmann F (2000). Kniegelenk des Kindes. In: Kohn D (ed.). Das Knie. Thieme, Stuttgart-New York, pp. 120–137.

Kesenheimer E, Kolb M, Rosemeyer B (1990). Spätresultate nach Meniskektomie. Sportverletz Sportschad 4: 79–86.

Krettek C, Schandelmaier P, Tscherne H (1996). Distale Femurfrakturen. Transartikuläre Rekonstruktion, perkutane Plattenosteosynthese und retrograde Nagelung. Unfallchirurg 99 (1): 2–11.

Krüger-Franke M, Trouillier HH, Strähnz C, Rosemeyer B (1995a). Arthroskopisch assistierte Osteosynthese proximaler Tibialgelenkfrakturen. Arthroskopie 8: 35–37.

Krüger-Franke M, Trouillier HH, Kugler A, Schupp A, Rosemeyer B (1995b). Die Reinsertion und Semitendinosusaugmentation frischer proximaler vorderer Kreuzbandrupturen. Sportorthop Sporttraumatol 11 (2): 72–77.

Krüger-Franke M, Buchner M, Brandmaier R, Rosemeyer B (1996). Rerupturen des vorderen Kreuzbandes. Arthroskopie 9: 202–206.

Krüger-Franke M, Kugler A, Trouillier HH, Reischl A, Rosemeyer B (1999). Klinische und radiologische Ergebnisse nach arthroskopischer partieller Innenmeniskusresektion. Unfallchirurg 102: 434–438.

Landsiedl F (2000). Strechapparat. In: Kohn D (ed.). Das Knie. Thieme, Stuttgart-New York, pp. 180–197.

Lobenhoffer P (2000). Frakturen des Kniegelenkes. In: Kohn D (ed.). Das Knie. Thieme, Stuttgart-New York, pp. 278–307.

Lobenhoffer P, Thermann H (2005). Rupturen der Quadrizepssehne. In: Duparc J (ed.). Chirurgische Techniken in Orthopädie und Traumatologie. Oberschenkel und Knie. Elsevier, pp. 65–69.

Meyers MH, McKeever FM (1970). Fracture of the intercondylar eminence of the tibia. J Bone Joint Surg Am 52 (8): 1677–1684.

Miller MD, Howard RF, Plancher KD (2004). Operationsatlas Sportorthopädie-Sporttraumatologie: Vordere Kreuzbandrekonstruktion. Elsevier, pp. 43–59.

Müller ME, Koch P, Nazarian S (1990). The Comprehensive Classification of Fractures of Long Bones. Springer, Heidelberg.

Noyes FR, Barber-Westin SD, Butler DL, Wilkins RM (1998). The role of allografts in repair and reconstruction of knee joint ligaments and menisci. Instruct Course Lect 47: 379–396.

Reicher MA, Hartzmann S, Duckwalter GR, Basset LW, Anderson LJ, Gold RH (1986). Meniscal injuries: detction using MR imaging. Radiology 159: 753–757.

Schöttle PB, Weiler A, Romero J (2005). Rekonstruktion des Lig. patellofemorale mediale bei patellofemoraler Instabilität. Arthroskopie 18: 293–300.

Segesser B (1997). Kniegelenk: Fehlbelastungsfolgen. In: GOTS-Manual. Huber, Bern, pp. 134–139.

Stadelmaier DM, Arnoczky SP, Dodds J, Ross H (1995). The effect of drilling and soft tissue grafting across open growth plates. Am J Sports Med 23: 431–435.

Trouillier HH, Krüger-Franke M, Kugler A, Rosemeyer B (1995). Die Operationstechnik der arthroskopisch assistierten Osteosynthese der Tibiaplateaufraktur. Sportorthop Sporttraumatol 11 (2): 100–104.

Verdonk R, Goble EM, Kohn D (2005). Transplantation eines Meniskusallograft. In: Chirurgische Techniken in Orthopädie und Traumatologie. Oberschenkel und Knie. Elsevier, pp. 97–102.

Chapter 21
Shank, ankle joint and foot

Arno Frigg, Beat Hintermann, Markus Knupp, Geert Pagenstert, Michaela Schneiderbauer and Victor Valderrabano

21.1 Fractures of foot and ankle

Markus Knupp, Beat Hintermann

The foot consists of 26 different bones connected by more than 30 joints, all of which carry the load of walking, jumping, running, and other movements. These forces can amount up to three or four times one's normal body weight, such as in running and can frequently result in foot and ankle fractures (Nachbauer and Nigg 1992).

Foot and upper ankle fractures which commonly occur in sports have been compiled in ➤ Tab. 21.1. Further external forces found in

Tab. 21.1 Overview of the most frequent fractures of the foot and upper ankle joint in athletes.

Type of fracture	Injury mechanism	Symptoms	Sports activities at higher risk
malleolar	pronation/supination, or abduction/adduction, respectively, of the upper ankle joint with dislocation/subluxation of the talus	■ pain ■ swelling above the upper ankle joint	■ soccer ■ indoor sports ■ running/orienteering
talar neck	dorsal flexion of the upper ankle joint, e.g. fall from a great height	■ pain ■ swelling above the upper ankle joint ■ no full weight bearing possible	■ paragliding ■ climbing ■ high jumping
lateralis tali process	dorsal flexion of the upper ankle joint in combination with external rotation	■ pain ■ swelling of the lateral hindfoot	■ snowboarding
corpus and tuber of calcaneus	axial force towards calcaneus, e.g. fall from a great height	■ pain ■ swelling above heel ■ broadened hindfoot silhouette	■ skydiving ■ paragliding ■ climbing
anterior process of calcaneus	adduction/inversion in combination with plantar flexion	■ pain ■ swelling above the lateral midfoot	■ orienteering ■ soccer, rugby
Lisfranc joint	direct force or bending moments with fixed forefoot	■ pressure dolence of the midfoot with swelling and hematoma	■ soccer ■ equestrianism ■ indoor sports
metatarsal bones	direct force towards to the midfoot	■ hematoma ■ swelling ■ pain	■ team sports
Jones fracture	supination trauma	■ hematoma ■ at the lateral edge of the foot	■ indoor sports ■ orienteering
toes (phalangeal fractures)	axial compression forces	■ hematoma ■ swelling ■ pain	■ wrestling ■ soccer

contact sports as well as extreme sports (i.e. soccer, ice hockey, handball, rugby or American football) can also add to the ground reaction force therefore exposing the athletes to a higher risk of injury (Giza et al. 2003). In addition to the mentioned team sports, also other sports such as skiing, gymnastics or horse-riding should be mentioned.

21.1.1 General contemplations

Fractures of the foot must always be taken seriously, especially considering that it is easy to miss the diagnosis of non-dislocated fractures of the hindfoot in patients with concomitant sprain of the ankle joint (Judd and Kim 2002). The delayed diagnosis of these fractures can also lead to permanent limitations requiring long-term therapy.

> In patients presenting ankle sprain the hindfoot fractures should be excluded clinically and (if necessary) radiologically.

Additional concomitant injuries can exist in surrounding soft tissues but only in osseous structures depending on the injury mechanisms. Thus, tendons, ligaments, muscles, nerves, vessels, and skin can be affected and can be of great significance for therapy and prognosis.

The initial diagnosis is often carried out at the location and is based on typical clinical characteristics listed in ➢ Table 21.2. In general, **as little manipulation as possible** should be undertaken in patients possibly presenting with bone fractures. Open wounds and exposed bone ends should be covered with a sterile cloth. The fracture itself should be **stabilized** (splinting) and put into an **elevated position** especially in case of serious injuries.

Tab. 21.2 Typical clinical symptoms of fractures.

Clinical symptoms of fractures
■ swelling
■ hematoma
■ painful manipulation
■ deformation and abnormal flexibility
■ crepitation
■ visible free bone fragments (open fracture)

Tab. 21.3 Imaging diagnostic procedures for the evaluation of the extent of injury.

Imaging diagnostics	
conventional X-rays	■ fracture diagnosis
computed tomography (CT)	■ hidden fractures ■ osteochondrosis dissecans
magnetic resonance imaging (MRI)	■ extraarticular concomitant ■ injuries (e.g. ligamental structures) ■ intraosseous changes (e.g. cysts)
arthroscopy	■ intraarticular diagnostics

Tab. 21.4 Overview of the possible reasons for the failure of surgical fracture treatment.

Reasons for the fracture treatment failure
■ misinterpretation of the injury mechanism and, therefore, of the resulting injury pattern
■ underestimating the osseous injury
■ underestimating the concomitant injuries of the soft tissue
■ insufficient reposition of the fracture elements, which may lead to malposition and instability
■ insufficient fixation of the fracture elements, which may lead to pseudo-arthrosis formation

After this first aid the patient should undergo radiological assessment and computer tomography, if necessary (➢ Tab. 21.3). Understanding the extent of the injury is critical to design a suitable therapeutic program and to make a realistic prognosis of healing. Misinterpretation of accident mechanisms and not proper diagnosis are the main factors in fracture treatment failure (➢ Tab. 21.4).

> An accurate diagnosis of all – main and concomitant – injuries is the key when determining therapy and prognosis.

21.1.2 Fractures of the upper ankle (malleolar fractures)

The malleolar fractures constitute the most frequent fractures in sports related injuries. **30 to 50% of all injuries** affect the upper ankle joint (Weiker 1984). **Injuries of both, bones and ligaments** are frequent since the combination of osseous structures and ligaments create the

21.1 Fractures of foot and ankle

Tab. 21.5 Overview of possible secondary problems after fractures of the upper ankle joint.

Consequences of malleolar fractures
■ non-union
■ malunion
■ axial malposition
■ instability
■ posttraumatic osteoarthritis

congruity and stability of the ankle joint (Inman 1974, Johnson and Markolf 1983, Rassmussen and Tavberg-Jensen1982). The complex biomechanics of the ankle joint explains why patients with ankle fractures (especially athletes) often complain about remaining, long-term pain and functional impairments. Some possible **complications** are listed in ➤ Table 21.5.

Correct diagnosis and appropriate treatment are essential for a more realistic prognosis regarding remaining symptoms and decreased recovery time, respectively (Turco 1977). Considering that the majority of sports activities require extensive movement of ankle joint complex, injuries to this region of the foot must be taken seriously.

21.1.3 Hindfoot

Talus

Injuries of the talus normally result from major trauma and **rarely** occur in athletes due to the sports related injuries. However, associated concomitant injuries often present with other secondary adverse effects resulting in extensively prolonged rehabilitation often combined with **permanent functional limitations**.

Fractures of the talus are commonly found in sports such as soccer, alpine skiing, snowboarding, high jumping, indoor athletics, etc. and are a direct result of **striking the talar neck** against the tibial edge (➤ Fig. 21.1) such as when one falls from a high object and lands in a squatting position.

The healing process of fractures can be complicated considerably by commonly found local **vessel injuries**. **Bone necrosis** is found regularly depending on the severity of the injury and it presents serious complication often resulting

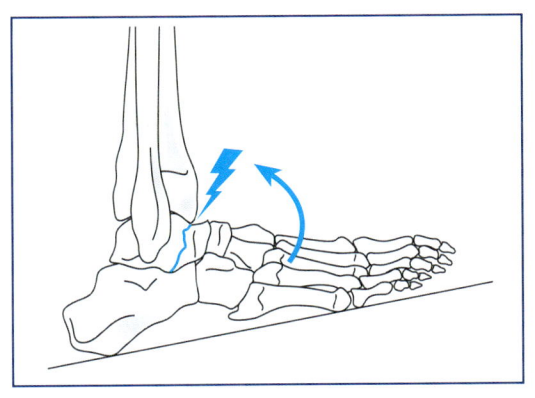

Fig. 21.1 Typical injury mechanism of talus neck fracture: talus neck hitting against the tibial edge at forced dorsal flexion in the upper ankle joint.

in remaining symptoms and functional deficits (Elgafy et al. 2000, Fortin and Balazsy 2001).

A special form of talus fracture is the **avulsion of the processus lateralis tali** or so called "snowboarder's ankle", which is characterized by an axial compression of the loaded lower leg accompanied by an external rotation or eversion (Boon et al. 2001, Kirkpatrick et al. 1998, Valderrabano et al. 2005). This injury is also often mistaken for a severe lateral ankle joint sprain in the acute phase.

> Non-dislocated fractures of talus can often be treated conservatively whereas dislocated fractures mostly require open reduction and internal fixation.

Calcaneus

The most frequent mechanism of injury of the calcaneus is due to a fall from a great height to landing on the heels (Sanders 2000), i.e. skydiving and paragliding accidents (➤ Fig. 21.2, ➤ Fig. 21.3; Schulze et al. 2000). The extent and severity of the injury depends on the height of the fall, hardness of the ground, and the weight of patient. Early diagnosis and therapy are essential due to frequent **concomitant injuries** in conjunction with soft tissue and skin damage that accompany this type of injury. Every calcaneal fracture should be analyzed by **computer tomography** (CT) in addition to the standard radiographs, in order to completely assess the extent of the injury and to determine the adequate therapy.

Fracture of the **anterior process** (➤ Fig. 21.4) is an easily overlooked calcaneal injury that is caused by a forced inversion/plantar flexion (Rosen and Kanat 1993, Trnka et al. 1998). In some patients an osseous avulsion of bifurcatum ligament can be observed. Also this injury should be routinely excluded in patients with severe ankle sprain. Occasionally, small avulsion fractures of the anterior calcaneal process do not consolidate which results in chronic pain.

> In all patients presenting with acute/chronic pain in the midfoot after an inversion/plantar flexion injury mechanism a fracture of calcanei process should be excluded.

Even though **non-dislocated fractures** of the calcaneus can be treated **conservatively** there are clinical reports that suggest that patients who have undergone reconstructive surgery can return to training and sports activities faster (Randle et al. 2000, Tufescu and Buckley 2001). Nevertheless, one should be careful when considering surgical treatment, especially regarding the soft tissue and skin conditions.

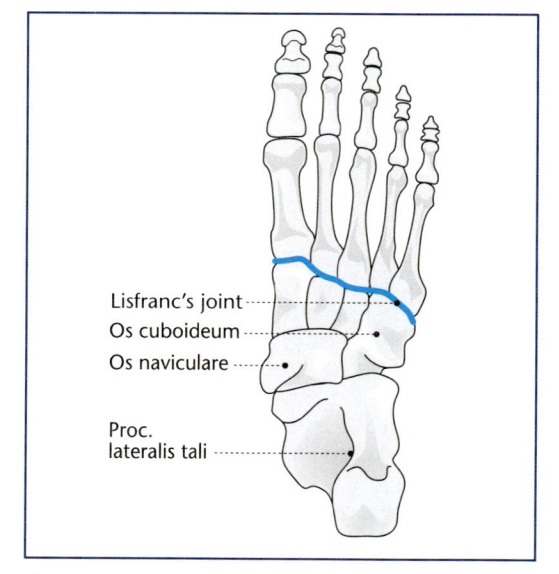

Fig. 21.2 Localization of the processus lateralis tali and the Lisfranc joint line (tarsometatarsal joint).

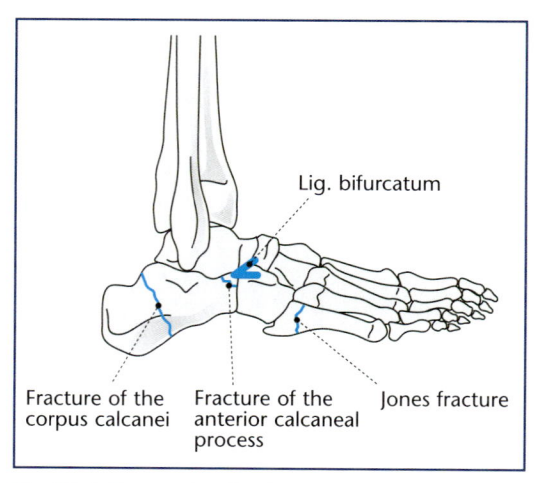

Fig. 21.4 Fracture localization at the calcaneus (corpus fracture and avulsion fracture of proc. anterior) as well as the metatarsal V.

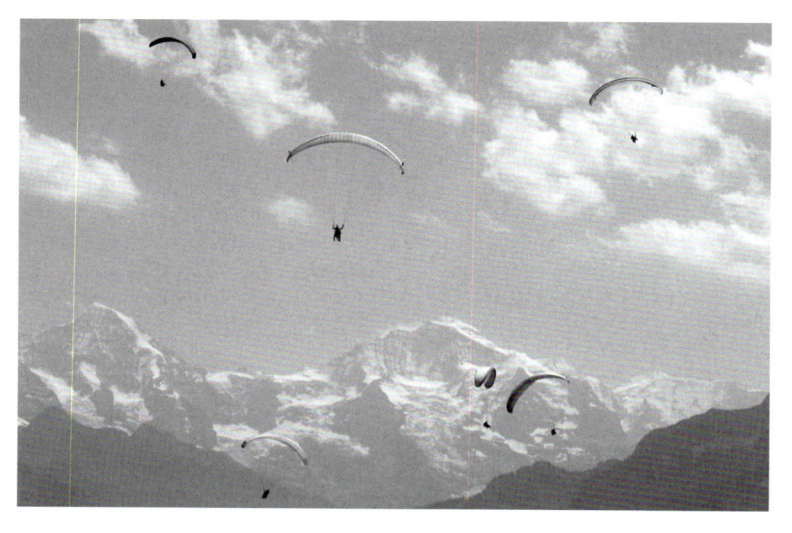

Fig. 21.3 Paragliding: Risky sport for injuries of the foot and the upper ankle joint, with most injuries occurring during landing (photograph: own source).

Calcaneus fracture can increase recovery time due to persisting load-conditioned pain, and **occasionally** results in **permanent limitations**. Many athletes suffer from morning stiffness, sports limitations, and discomfort after running long distances in the area of the former fracture, even years after the initial trauma (Myerson and Quill 1993).

The following concomitant injuries can be ruled out:

- contralateral calcaneal fractures (bilateral fractures in 10%),
- compression fractures of the vertebral bodies (most frequently in the thoracolumbar transition).

21.1.4 Midfoot

Fractures of the os naviculare and the tarsometatarsal joint complex (Lisfranc joint, ➤ Fig. 21.2) often require **surgical stabilization**. Fractures in the region of Lisfranc joint are rare, but they often lead to severe degenerative changes of the joint and the adjacent structures if overlooked.

Os naviculare

Although acute fractures of the os naviculare (➤ Fig. 21.2) are rare, most fractures in this region are **"fatigue fractures"** (➤ Chapter 23).

With **traumatic fractures**, there are compression as well as avulsion mechanisms which are caused by axial compression and/or by an eversion of the forefoot. These injuries often correlate with **cartilage damages**, which extensively deteriorate the diagnosis (Pinney and Sangeorzan 2001). In addition, the patients with this type of injury – the same as in fractures of the ankle joint – are at higher risk for a **posttraumatic necrosis** as a long-term complication. The navicular bone assumes an important function, which can also affect the adjacent bones in the injury because of the central position in the midfoot. For this reason, the early diagnosis and the consequent therapy of these fractures are of great importance.

Os cuboideum

Fractures of the os cuboideum (➤ Fig. 21.2) are rare and in most cases are only found as a concomitant injury in severely injured foot. For that reason, **osseous concomitant injuries** must be considered, particularly at the Lisfranc's joint. In general, these fractures are caused by compression forces/contusions or by a directly affecting force (blow) (Pinney and Sangeorzan 2001).

Fractures in the region of the Lisfranc joint

Dislocation fractures in the region of the Lisfranc joint (➤ Fig. 21.2) are very rare but if missed in the diagnosis can have serious consequences for the athlete and therefore should be considered in athletes with any midfoot trauma (Mantas and Burks 1994).

These fractures can be caused by a direct trauma (contusion/hit) or by indirect forces (flexion/torsion forces) (Chiodo and Myerson 2001). These injuries are often found in **horseback riders**. For example, if the foot is still positioned in the stirrup at a fall, a bending moment in Lisfranc's joint occurs at plantar-flexed ankle joint, dorsal-extended toes and an axial force at the heel. A similar mechanism that affects this joint is found in **soccer players** where the player is hit laterally at the heel by an opponent while the upper ankle joint is flexed, the toes are extended dorsally and the forefoot is fixed to the ground.

> Fractures of the os naviculare and in the region of Lisfranc's joint are rare but if overlooked lead to serious functional limitations.

Midfoot (metatarsalia)

Fractures of the midfoot (metatarsalia) are the **most frequent fractures of the foot**. These injuries are especially found in **team sports** such as ball games, if the players step on each other's feet. A peculiarity is the isolated fracture in the region of the diaphysis of the fifth metatarsal and is called **"dancer's fracture"**. This fracture is caused by an inversion of the plantar-flexed forefoot. Most fractures of the toes and metatarsals can be treated **conservatively** especially if the injury is not multifragmented and the fragments are not dislocated.

Another special case of metatarsal fracture is a fracture on the base of the fifth metatarsal (so called **Jones fracture**, ➤ Fig. 21.4). It is localized at the metaphyseal-diaphyseal junction and lies in a zone of reduced blood supply therefore **non-unions** are a common complication especially in patients with conservative treatment. The fracture is caused by an acute tension at the insertion of the peroneus brevis muscle in line with a supination trauma (Fortin and Balazsy 2001, Weiker 1984). The physiological muscle tension can lead to a dehiscence of the fragments and thus additionally impair the healing. Especially in active athletes this type of injury should be treated surgically (Nunley 2004).

> Most fractures of the metatarsalia can be treated conservatively, especially if no dislocation exists. In most cases, the Jones fracture should be approached surgically, especially in active athletes.

21.1.5 Forefoot

Sesamoid bone fractures

Fractures of the sesamoid bones of the hallux are usually **stress fractures**. Acute fractures are only found in very rare cases, usually in combination with an extensive forefoot trauma.

Toe fractures

Toe fractures (phalangeal fractures) mostly result from axially occurring forces, as are found in **wrestlers**, for example. In most case, these injuries also can be treated **conservatively**.

A surgical treatment should be considered in patients with intraarticular or significantly dislocated fractures especially if the **first toe** is affected (Armagan and Shereff 2001). Tape bandages can easily treat these injuries.

References

Armagan OE, Shereff MJ (2001). Injuries to the toes and metatarsals. Orthop Cln North Am 32: 1–9.

Boon AJ, Smith J, Zobitz ME, Amrami KM (2001). Snowboarder's talus fracture: Mechanism of injury. Am J Sports Med 29: 333–338.

Chiodo CP, Myerson MS (2001). Developments and advances in the diagnosis and treatment of injuries to the tarsometatarsal joint. Orthop Clin North Am 32: 11–20.

Elgafy H, Ebraheim NA, Tile M, Stephen D, Kase J (2000). Fractures of the talus: Experience of two level 1 trauma centers. Foot Ankle Int 21: 1023–1029.

Fortin PT, Balazsy JE (2001). Talus fractures: evaluation and treatment. J Am Acad Orthop Surg 9: 114–127.

Giza E, Fuller C, Junge A, Dvorak J (2003). Mechanisms of foot and ankle injuries in soccer. Am J Sports Med 31 (4): 550–554.

Inman VT (1974). The joints of the ankle. 2nd ed. Williams & Wilkins, Baltimore, pp 31–74.

Johnson EE, Markolf KL (1983). The contribution of the anterior talofibular ligament to the ankle laxity. J Bone Joint Surg Am 65: 81–88.

Judd DB, Kim DH (2002). Foot fractures frequently misdiagnosed as ankle sprains. Am Fam Physician 66 (5): 785–794.

Kirkpatrick DP, Hunter RE, Janes PC, Mastrangelo J, Nicholas RA (1998). The snowboarder's foot and ankle. Am J Sports Med 26 (2): 271–277.

Mantas JP, Burks RT (1994). Lisfranc injuries in the athlete. Clin Sports Med 13 (4): 719–730.

Myerson M, Quill GE Jr (1993). Late complication of fractures of the calcaneus. J Bone Joint Surg Am 75: 331–341.

Nachbauer W, Nigg BM (1992). Effects of arch height of the foot on ground reaction forces in running. Med Sci Sports Exerc 24 (11): 1264–1269.

Nunley JA (2004). Jones Fracture in the Fifth Metatarsal. Advanced Recontruction Foot and Ankle. American Academy of Orthopedic Surgeons, pp 319–322.

Pinney SJ, Sangeotzan BJ (2001). Fractures of the tarsal bones. Orthop Clin North Am 32: 21–33.

Randle JA, Kreder HJ, Stephen D, Williams J, Jaglal S, Hu R (2000). Should calcaneal fractures be treated surgically? A meta-analysis. Clin Orthop 377: 217–227.

Rassmussen O, Tavberg-Jensen I (1982). Mobility of the ankle joint: recording of rotatory movements in the talocrural joint in vitro with and without the lateral collateral ligaments of the ankle. Acta Orthop Scand 53: 155–160.

Roesen HM, Kanat O (1993). Anterior process fracture of the calcaneus. J Foot Ankle Surg 32 (4): 424–429.

Sanders R (2000). Displaced intra-articular fractures of the calcaneus. J Bone Joint Surg Am 82: 225–250.

Schulze W, Hesse B, Blatter G, Schmidtler B, Muhr G (2000). Pattern of injuries and prophylaxis in paragliding. Sportverletz Sportschaden 14 (2): 41–49.

Trinka HJ, Zetti R, Ritschl P (1998). Fracture of the anterior superior process of the calcaneus: an often misdiagnosed fracture. Arch Orthop Trauma Surg 117 (4–5): 300–302.

Tufescu TV, Buckley R (2001). Age, gender, work capability, and worker's compensation in patients with displaced intraarticular calcaneal fracture. J Orthop Trauma 15: 275–279.

Turco VJ (1977). Injuries to the ankle and foot in athletics. Orthop Clin North Am 8 (3): 669–682.

Valderrabano V, Perren T, Ryf C, Rillmann P, Hintermann B (2005). Snowboarder's talus fracture: treatment outcome of 20 cases after 3.5 years. Am J Sports Med 33 (6): 871–880.

Weiker GG (1984). Ankle injuries in the athlete. Prim Care 11 (1): 101–108.

21.2 Stress fractures of shank and foot

Michaela Schneiderbauer and Victor Valderrabano

In contrast to fractures after a direct trauma, stress fractures are a consequence of repeated stress forces. Cyclic stress of the repetitive noxae exceeds the mechanical and maximum biological capacity of the specific bone segment and leads to an incomplete transformative reaction.

Stress fractures develop if the biological osteoclastic activity in the early phase of transformative reaction exceeds the new bone formation by osteoblasts.

The extension of stress conditioning a stress fracture has a high individual variability. The **epiphyseal plates** or **apophyseal cores** of **children and adolescents** are often affected as loci memoris resistentiae. On the other hand, in **adults** stress fractures occur most often at the **lower extremity**. Approximately 70% of stress fractures appear in runners (Matheson et al. 1987).

$\Delta_{individ}$. Capacity (biological + mechanical) − stress intensity (extent, duration, frequency) < 0
⇒ stress fracture

A compilation of extrinsic and intrinsic **risk factors** for stress fractures is presented in ➤ Table 21.6. Monarthritides, infections and tumors should be excluded by **differential diagnosis**, as well as a "female athletic triad" with anorexia, secondary amenorrhea and osteoporosis.

Tab. 21.6 Possible intrinsic and extrinsic risk factors for stress fractures.

Intrinsic factors	Extrinsic factors
demographic characteristics: ■ female gender ■ advanced age ■ white race anatomic factors: ■ hollow foot ■ pes planovalgus (pronation foot) ■ valgus knee ■ increased Q-angle ■ leg length difference bone characteristics: ■ geometry (small diameter, thin cortical substance of the bone) ■ low bone density physical fitness: ■ low aerobic fitness ■ low muscle strength and endurance ■ low flexibility ■ anorectic or adipose type health behavior: ■ lifestyle lacking in physical exercise ■ nicotine abuse ■ no preparations containing estrogen ■ injuries in the medical history	sport: running sports, above all type of exercise: ■ high total load ■ high frequency/intensity/duration equipment: ■ type of shoes ■ type of boots (alpine boots/walking boots) ■ arch supports ground of exercise: ■ asphalt ■ tartan ■ cross country

In general, **high-risk** and **low-risk stress fractures** are distinguished. High-risk stress fractures are fractures of the ventral tibial edge, the malleolus medialis, the os naviculare and the base of the fifth metatarsal, because those have a tendency of retarded fracture healing and dislocation (mal-union or non-union).

Typical localizations combined with the according diagnosis and therapy are listed in ➤ Table 21.7 (further expositions of pathogenesis, diagnosis and therapy ➤ Chapter 23).

21.2.1 Tibia

The tibia represents with 41–55% the most frequent point of stress fractures in the lower extremities (Hulkko and Orava 1987, Matheson et al. 1987, Orava 1978 and 1980, Sullivan et al. 1984). It typically appears with enhanced pronation posture in of foot. Pain is often a combination of a soft-tissue swelling and hyperthermia.

Tab. 21.7 Localization, diagnostic and therapy of stress fractures of the lower extremity.

Bone	Typical localization	Typical sports	Diagnostic	Therapy
tibia	distal diaphysis	■ track and field ■ running sports	■ anamnesis ■ findings ■ radiograph ■ MRT, if required	■ relief ■ osteosynthesis for delayed fracture healing or dislocation
fibula	diaphysis	■ running sports	■ anamnesis ■ findings ■ radiograph ■ MRT, if required	■ relief ■ osteosynthesis for delayed fracture healing or dislocation
talus	corpus	■ running sports ■ recruiting ■ gymnasts	■ anamnesis ■ findings ■ radiograph ■ scintigraphy ■ CT ■ MRT	■ relief ■ osteosynthesis for delayed fracture healing or dislocation
calcaneus	corpus	■ long-distance running ■ sprinting ■ recruiting	■ anamnesis ■ findings ■ radiograph ■ MRT, if required	■ relief or plaster immobilization ■ arch supports (pronation position: medial support)
os naviculare	medium third	■ running sports ■ track and field, especially long jump	■ anamnesis ■ findings ■ radiograph ■ scintigraphy ■ CT ■ MRT	■ stability boot or plaster for 6 weeks ■ arch supports (pronation position: medial support) ■ osteosynthesis for delayed fracture healing or dislocation
metatarsal bones	■ MT I, II ■ Basis MT V (Jones fracture)	■ road racing ■ hiking ■ marching ■ recruiting ■ ballet ■ gymnastics	■ anamnesis ■ findings ■ radiograph ■ MRT, if required	■ conservative for MT II-IV ■ surgery for Jones fracture

According to the characteristics of the injury, the therapeutic spectrum ranges from a few weeks of relief to a formal osteosynthesis. Especially stress fractures at the ventral tibial edge and at the medial malleolus are to be considered as high-risk stress fractures. In these stress fractures, an osteosynthesis should be considered early with an adverse prognosis to avoid the mal-union or non-union, which often requires additional surgery.

21.2.2 Fibula

Altogether, the fibula is definitely less affected by stress fractures than the tibia. Mostly, a sparing for a few weeks is sufficient for the healing of the stress fracture.

21.2.3 Talus

Talar stress fractures are **rare** in sports orthopedics/medicine. Rossi and Dragoni could show an incidence rate of 0.32% of talar stress fractures in a recently published survey carried out on 24,562 female athletes (Rossi and Dragoni 2005). In most cases step-by-step diagnostic approach using advanced imaging (scintigraphy, MRI and CT) is indicated in order to make a reliable diagnosis.

21.2.4 Calcaneus

In the beginning, pain appears mostly 1–2 cm ventrally of the apophysis, and it extends on the whole calcaneus in the process. The stress fracture can be distinguished from these entities by the **more ventral localization** in comparison to the bursitis subachillea and the insertion tendinosis of the Achilles tendon.

The stress fracture is mostly localized in the **corpus of calcaneus**. The stress fractures are associated to an increased **pronation posture** of the foot at the calcaneus as well as in the os naviculare (Weber et al. 2005).

The dominant part of these stress fractures can be treated within 4–6 weeks by **reduced weight bearing** in a stable walker combined with bumper heels for some weeks.

21.2.5 Os naviculare

The os naviculare carries a **high-risk of stress fracture**, which has a disposition of a **pro-**

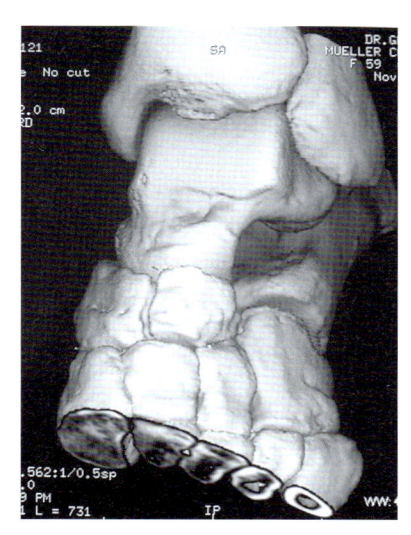

Fig. 21.5 Image of a stress fracture of os naviculare in a CT 3D reconstruction.

longed fracture healing and **secondary dislocation** because of the stress mechanism. Most patients present with diffuse pain across the midfoot. Occasionally, there is tenderness on percussion and compression pain above the dorsal os naviculare.

In addition to an **immobilization** of 6 weeks in a stable walker or below knee cast, a cushion with medial support should be considered for an existing pronated malposition. **Osteosynthesis** should be indicated with persisting symptoms or dislocation of the fragments. It can be carried out percutaneously by two cannulated screws, which cross in the frontal layer of the os naviculare (Coris and Lombardo 2003). ➢ Figure 21.5 shows a three-dimensional CT reconstruction of a stress fracture at the os naviculare.

21.2.6 Metatarsalia

Most patients present with pain in the region of the metatarsalia often combined with swelling. The **metatarsalia II and III** are affected most in the region of the distal diaphysis. Some studies describe a positive correlation between the existence of a pes cavus and the appearance of metatarsal stress fractures (Korpelainen et al. 2001). The fractures of **metatarsalia II–IV** without dislocation can be treat-

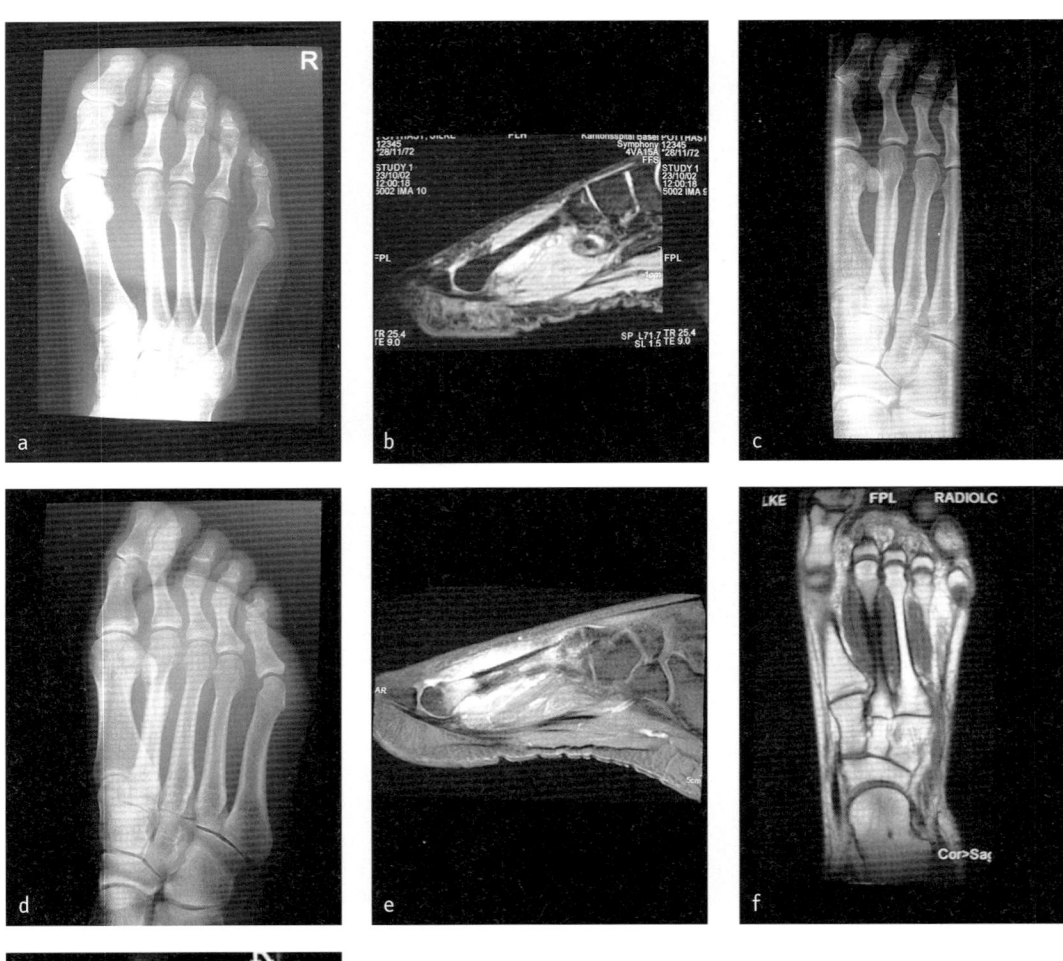

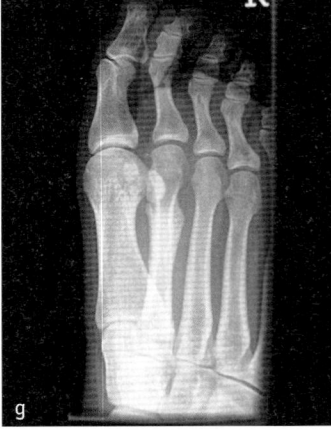

Fig. 21.6 a: X-ray without pathologic findings at the beginning of the symptoms at the metatarsal bone II.
b: MRT few days after the beginning of the symptoms with the image of a soft-tissue reaction around the metatarsal bone II.
c: Cortical thickening at about 4 weeks after the beginning of the symptoms at the metatarsal bone II.
d: Image of the stress fracture, 5 weeks after the beginning of the symptoms at the metatarsal bone II.
e–f: Confirmation of the image of the stress fracture, 5 weeks after the beginning of the symptoms at the metatarsal bone II by MRT.
g: Metatarsal-bone-II fracture 7 weeks after the beginning of the symptoms, in healing with clear callus formation.

ed **conservatively** by mobilization with a rigid sole. Fractures of metatarsalia I and V and especially at the **base of metatarsal V** (Jones fracture, ➢ Chapter 21.1.4) should be stabilized **surgically** (Porter et al. 2005).

In general, it has to be considered in **radiological diagnosis** that positive findings often are found after 1–2 weeks and not yet in the very beginning of the pain symptoms. ➢ Figure 21.6 shows the proceeding of a stress fracture at the metatarsal II as assessed using imaging methods. No pathologic alteration is visible in the initial radiograph (➢ Fig. 21.6 a) while the patient had already symptoms. A soft-tissue reaction is shown in the MRI carried out few days later but no proof of fracture (➢ Fig. 21.6 b). The control X-ray after 4 weeks shows a cortical swelling of metatarsal II retrospectively (➢ Fig. 21.6 c). Five weeks after the beginning of the symptoms, the stress fracture can be recognized easily (➢ Fig. 21.6 d). At the same time, the MRT examination of the fracture is traceable without a doubt (➢ Fig. 21.6 e, f). The X-ray control, carried out 7 weeks later, shows a healing stress fracture with callus formation (➢ Fig. 21.6 g).

> Overuse damages are frequent in sports and present highest diagnostic and therapeutic challenge to sports physicians. Medical treatment of the athlete alone should have the highest priority regarding prophylaxis, treatment, and rehabilitation of overuse damages. Close follow-up by physiotherapists, coaches, and other attendants of the athletes are critical to long-term success of therapy.

References

Coris EE, Lombardo JA (2003). Tarsal navicular stress fractures. Am Fam Physician 67 (1): 85–90.

Hulkko A, Orava S (1987). Stress fractures in athletes. Int J Sports Med 8 (3): 221–226.

Korpelainen R, Orava S, Karpakka J, Siira P, Hulkko A (2001). Risk factors for recurrent stress fractures in athletes. Am J Sports Med 29 (3): 304–310.

Matheson GO, Clement DB, McKenzie DC, Taunton JE, Lloyd-Smith DR, MacIntire JG (1987). Stress fractures in athletes. A study of 320 cases. Am J Sports Med 15 (1): 46–58.

Orava S (1980). Stress fractures. Br J Sports Med 14 (1): 40–44.

Orava S, Puranen J, Ala-Ketola L (1978). Stress fractures caused by physical exercise. Acta Orthop Scand 49 (1): 19–27.

Porter DA, Duncan M, Meyer SJ (2005). Fifth metatarsal Jones fracture fication with a 4.5–mm cannulated stainless steel screw in the competitive and recreational athlete: a clinical and radiographic evaluation. Am J Sports Med 33 (5): 726–733.

Rossi F, Dragoni S (2005). Talar body fatigue stress fractures: three cases observed in elite female gymnasts. Skeletal Radiol 34 (7): 389–394.

Sullivan D, Warren RF, Pavlov H, Kelman G (1984). Stress fractures in 51 runners. Clin Orthop Relat Res (187): 188–192.

Weber JM, Vidt LG, Gehl RS, Montgomery T (2005). Calcaneal stress fractures. Clin Podiatr Med Surg 22 (1): 45–54.

21.3 Tendon injuries of the foot

Arno Frigg and Victor Valderrabano

Tendon injuries at the lower extremities are rare; only 14% of all tendon damages are localized in this region (DeLee and Drez 2003). An **overpronation** or **oversupination** of the foot causes **overstress syndromes** of the long foot tendons (e.g. medial tibial pain syndrome at overpronation) as well as the ligaments and joints. Detailed treatment concepts similar to the tendons of the hand have been developed with profound knowledge of the functions and diseases of foot and ankle tendons.

Tendons are surrounded by loose connective tissue, the peritendineum. Tendon sheaths reduce friction and occur in areas where the tendons are deviated from their straight course or led through osteofibrous canals. Accordingly, the **tendinitis** denominates the inflammation of the tendon, the **tenosynovitis/tendovaginitis** the inflammation of the tendon and tendon sheath. The **peritendinitis** describes an inflammation of the tendon and the surrounding peritendineum of tendons without actual tendon sheath (e.g. Achilles tendon). The **tendinosis** stands for degenerative tendon changes.

All long foot tendons of the extensors and deep flexors have an own tendon sheath, the tendon sheaths of the peroneal tendons com-

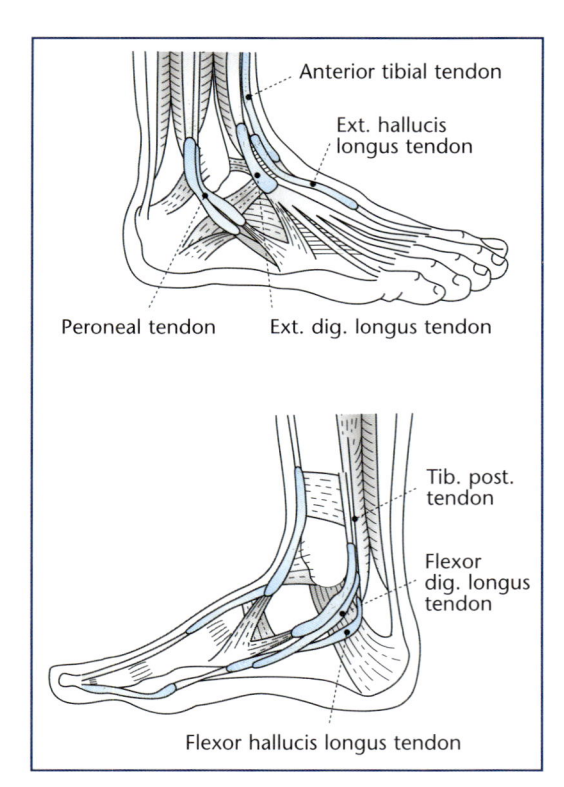

Fig. 21.7 Tendons and tendon sheaths of the foot. Top: view from lateral, bottom: view from medial.

municate with each other (➢ Fig. 21.7). Laterally, the peroneal tendons proceed in a groove dorsally at the distal end of the malleolus lateralis, where they are held by the superior and inferior peroneal retinaculum. Medially, the tarsal tunnel is crossed by the tibialis posterior tendon right, at the front by the flexor digitorum longus tendon (FDL), and dorsally by the flexor hallucis longus tendon (FHL) accompanied by the posterior tibial artery and the tibial nerve. The FHL proceeds in an own sulcus below the sustentaculum tali. It crosses the tibialis posterior tendon (chiasma crurale) at the lower leg and extends along the sole of the foot over the FHL tendon (chiasma plantare).

21.3.1 Peroneal tendons

Peroneal tendinitis

The peroneal tendinitis is a more frequent entity in sports.

In most cases it is the **consequence** of

- an os peroneum
- an old fracture of the os peroneum
- a congenital tendon anomaly
- an instability of the upper ankle joint or a
- a malalignment of the hindfoot

(Zivot et al. 1989, Pierson and Inglis 1992, Trevino and Baumhauer 1992).

With a persisting swelling at the lateral malleolus and retrofibular pain, the **diagnosis** is often made months later, i.e. in the chronic condition.

An accurate diagnosis requires careful clinical examination (pain on palpation, crepitus), conventional radiographs and MRT. Nevertheless, the **MRT** is the diagnostic procedure of choice in imaging, especially for the detection of a rupture or tendon anomaly (Oden 1987).

The therapy implies a sports restriction for several weeks and oral antiphlogistic treatment; occasionally, an immobilization by a cast for the lower leg for 3–4 weeks can be necessary. With symptoms persistence, a synovectomy or release of the tendon sheaths can be carried out open or arthroscopically (Bonnin et al. 1997, Krause and Brodsky 1998, Van Dijk and Kort 1998). In cases with painful os peroneum it should be excised. The possible concomitant instability of the ankle joint should be treated as well (Schneiderbauer et al. 2005).

Dislocation of the peroneal tendon

The tendinitis of the peroneal tendons (➢ Fig. 21.8 a and b) can be the reason for acute or chronic pain in the region of the lateral malleolus. It has been described for soccer, basketball, hockey, ballet and skiing (Oden 1987, Safran et. al. 1999).

The causes for the tendinitis of the peroneal tendons are:

- an anatomic abnormality of the peroneal groove and the retinacula or
- a forced dorsal extension of the upper ankle joint in pronation (Kollias and Ferkel 1997, Safran et al. 1999).

In **acute injury**, the patient usually hears a snapping and feels pain behind the fibula com-

locations in almost all cases (Ferran et al. 2006, Ogawa and Thondarson 2007). Acute dislocations of degree I can be treated with a **cast immobilization in non-athletes** (Selmani et al. 2006). The **chronic dislocation always** must be treated **by surgery** (Safran et al. 1999). The diagnosis of a dislocation of the peroneal tendons is often made with a delay; so the indication for surgery is given in the most cases. Many surgical procedures are described that principally reconstruct and reinforce the retinacula on the one hand and create a deepened sulcus on the other hand (Micheli et al. 1989, Mason and Henderson 1996, Safran et al. 1999).

Peroneal tendon rupture

The rupture of the peroneal tendon is rare and affects especially the **peroneus longus tendon**. The injury of the peroneus brevis is mostly found only in combination with the peroneus longus injury. Rupture as a consequence of an acute trauma is often experienced by soccer players and runners (Kikelly and McHale 1994, Sammarco 1995).

A **sprain of the ankle joint** is described as the event (plantar flexion and supination), in which a tear is felt laterally at the foot. The rupture can also be a consequence of **chronic overuse** at a varus deformity, relapsing supination traumas, lateral instability of the upper ankle joint as well as acute or chronic subluxations.

The area around the malleolus is often swollen and painful, which can also indicate a lateral ligament injury. Therefore, the diagnosis is difficult and often delayed. Pain in active pronation and in palpation along the tendon may be helpful to make an accurate diagnosis. The diagnosis includes **conventional radiographs** for the evaluation and determination of the position of an os perineum, as well as an **MRT**.

After an acute injury, a **cast immobilization** can be used as a first therapeutic step. With chronic pain and dysfunction, the **tendon reconstructive surgery** (end-to-end suture, tenodesis by transfer of longus onto brevis) and possible resection of an os peroneum is indicated (Sobel et al. 1994). Comorbidities, e.g. the hindfoot malalignment and the instability of the upper ankle joint, should be surgically addressed under the same anesthesia.

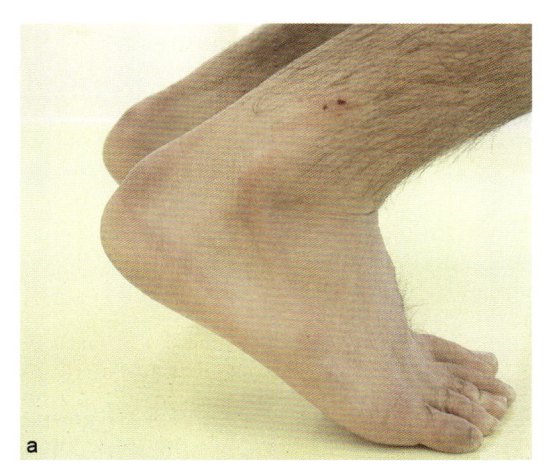

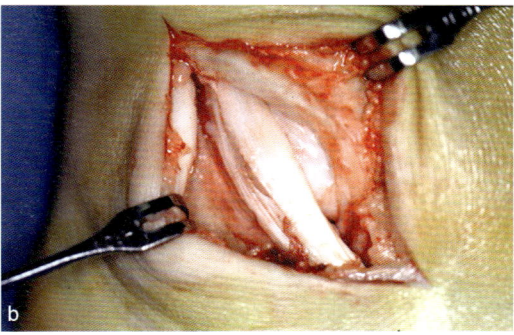

Fig. 21.8 Peroneal tendon dislocation. a: In forced dorsal extension. b: Intraoperative situs with tendon in a position of dislocation and showing degenerative signs already (longitudinal tear, flattening).

bined with a swelling and redness. Since the acute pain passes quickly, **ankle sprain** is often misinterpreted and the diagnosis is only made with chronic conditions (Mason and Henderson 1996). The clinical examination (painful palpation, manual subluxation/dislocation, and dorsal extension-evasion test), radiographic and MRT images are required for the **diagnosis confirmation**. The injury can be classified into **three degrees** according to Eckert and Davis (Eckert and Davis 1976): In degree I, the dislocated tendons are localized between the elevated periost and the bone, under the elevated fibrous edge in degree II, and with an existing osseous avulsion of the retinaculum peroneum superius in degree III.

The **acute dislocation** should be treated **by surgery** in athletes. Results are predictable, while the conservative therapy leads to relapsing dis-

Os peroneum

The os peroneum exists in 5–25% of all feet and is located in the peroneus longus tendon near the cuboid (Wander et al. 1994). Pain in the region of this accessory foot bone is described as POPS (**painful os peroneum syndrome**) and can be conditioned by a fracture or enlargement of the os peroneum as well as by a degenerative tendon rupture.

The os peroneum can be excised and the tendon continuity can be restored surgically. In a fracture, the os peroneum can be sutured directly (Peterson and Stinson 1992, Sobel et al. 1994, Wander et al. 1994). An **os vesalianum**, an ossification of the apophysis, or a basal fracture of fifth metatarsal must be considered as differential-diagnosis.

21.3.2 Tibialis posterior tendon

Tibialis posterior tendon dysfunction and acute rupture

Etiology

The acute rupture or dysfunction of the tibialis posterior tendon is an often missed diagnosis, but not a rare entity in sports (Woods and Leach 1991). It can be caused by **trauma** or **degenerative changes**. The tendon is significantly stressed in sports activities with fast and abrupt changes of direction, such as basketball, tennis, soccer and hockey, but it can be also injured in runners and ballet dancers (Lysholm and Wiklander 1987, Porter et al. 1998). The **incidence** in athletes amounts to about 3% (0.6–6%) (Lysholm and Wiklander 1987, Macintyre et al. 1991).

In general, 40–60 year old women with a standing occupation are at higher risk. A chronic tenosynovitis with a tendon showing **degenerative changes** precedes most ruptures. Dorsal extension and supination are the most common acute injury mechanism. The tendon rupture is usually localized 1–1.5 cm proximally of the insertion at the os naviculare, a hypovascular zone is described 4–5 cm proximal of this, though (Frey et al. 1990).

The closed rupture is **often overlooked** because this entity is not common and does not present with specific symptoms. The diagnosis is often made with a delay of several years (Woods and Leach 1991). The key for a successful treatment is the early diagnosis before the occurrence of a deformity (Valderrabano et al. 2004).

Clinic

The dysfunction of the tibialis posterior tendon can be classified into three stages (Johnson-and-Strom classification, Johnson and Strom 1989):

Stage I: Tenosynovitis

Tenosynovitis can start **without a triggering event** but also after a **sprain of the ankle joint**. Patients usually suffer from medial pain and swelling between the malleolus medialis and the os naviculare. In most cases, **increase in activity** can be observed. Clinically, the palpation shows pain in the tendon process behind the malleolus medialis and at inversion. The force of inversion from maximum abduction and pronation in light plantar flexion is reduced compared to contralateral foot. The tiptoe standing on one foot (**single heel rise test**) is possible, but has to be broken up after about 10 times because of increasing pain. Especially in running sports, the **overpronation** of the foot leads to an overstress with pain in the region of the tibialis posterior and the Achilles tendon, because the posterior tibial muscle and the soleus muscle compensate the pronation. In addition, also the lower tendons (FHL, FDL) and ligaments are stressed and increase the symptoms.

Stage II: Elongated and ruptured tendon with flexible hindfoot deformity

In patients with progressed dysfunction, a painful, mostly one-sided and progressive pes planovalgus et abductus deformity with overstress of the medial ligaments may develop (➤ Fig. 21.9 a and b). The **"too-many-toes sign"** as well as the **single heel rise test** are typical clinical signs. In tiptoe standing, the hindfoot cannot be brought into a stable varus position by the tibialis posterior tendon (due to missing physiological varisation), but remains in the valgus. Furthermore, the patient is not able to lift the heel because of the impaired gastrocnemius function. The subtalar joint has usually a normal range of motion.

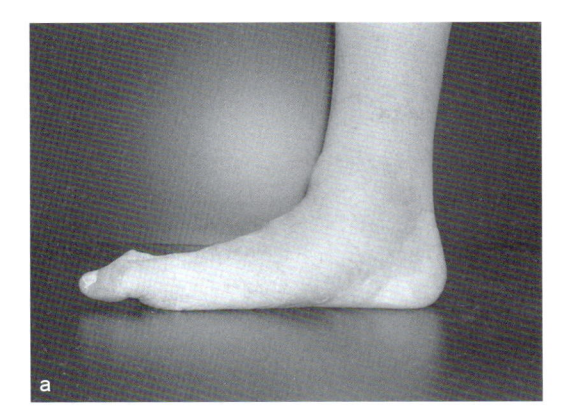

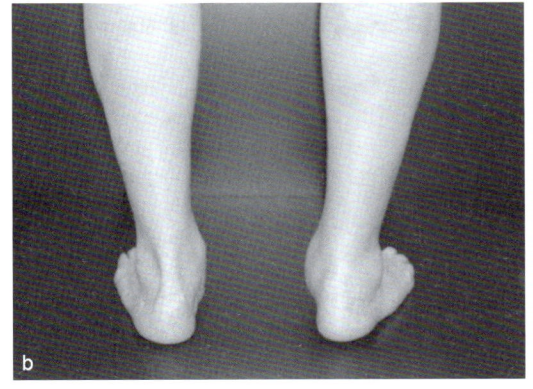

Fig. 21.9 Pes planovalgus et abductus. a: View from medial. b: View from dorsal with "too-many-toe-sign" right.

Stage III: Tendon ruptures with degenerative fixed foot deformity

In stage III a **severe degeneration** of the tendon is observed in combination with progressive and fixed pes planovalgus deformity with abduction of the forefoot of >10°. The single heel rise test is pathological as well as in stage II.

Diagnostics

A deformity can be assessed and quantified by **conventional radiographs** (talo-metatarsal angle normal with <10°). Inflammatory and degenerative changes as well as the rupture can be assessed using **MRI** (Khoury et al. 1996, Feighan et al. 1999). **Sonography** can be also used as a helpful diagnostic tool (Miller et al. 1996). Osteochondral lesions at the talus as well as the lateral ligaments can be assessed differential-diagnostically using MRT.

Therapy

In patients with **stage I** dysfunction, **conservative treatment**, such as the orthopedic insoles with medial support, antiphlogistic medication, and immobilization in a cast or stable walker is recommended. Cortisone injections are prohibited because of risk for increased degenerative changes and possible tendon rupture (Holmes and Mann 1992).

At patients with persisting and/or recurrent symptoms, a release of the tendon sheath, an excision of scar tissue or a partial synovectomy should be performed. For these purposes, the tendoscopy can be performed with satisfying mid-term results (Van Dijk et al. 1997).

In **active patients** with **stage II** dysfunction a **surgical** therapy should be considered (➤ Fig. 21.10). While an elongated tendon is shortened, a ruptured tendon is reconstructed. If the direct end-to-end suture is not possible, a tendon augmentation should be performed (Hintermann et al. 1999). In most cases the FDL tendon or a free transplant (plantaris tendon) can be used for tendon augmentation.

It has been shown, that a sole soft-tissue reconstruction goes along with a high recurrence rate of 50% (Michelson et al. 1992). Therefore, the combination with a lateral lengthening or medial displacement **calcaneal osteotomy** is recommended (Myerson et al. 1995).

The conservative therapy can also be successfully performed in older, less active patients presenting only few symptoms, by shoe inserts or an ankle-foot orthosis.

In **stage III**, the deformity of the foot is fixed so that the posture of the foot cannot be sufficiently corrected by tendon reconstruction sur-

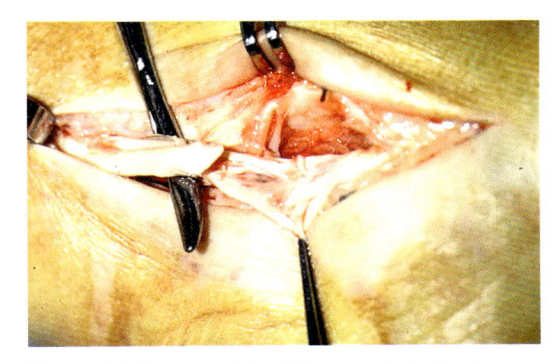

Fig. 21.10 Rupture of the tibialis posterior tendon.

gery alone. The subtalar fusion, as recommended by some authors, may restore the hindfoot malalignment, but not the abduction of the forefoot. Therefore, the triple arthrodesis with involvement of the talonavicular joint is recommended, especially for the existence of degenerative changes in the talonavicular and the calcaneocuboidal joint (DeLee and Drez 2003).

Tibialis posterior tendon dislocation

The dislocation of tibialis posterior tendon (➤ Fig. 21.11) usually occurs in dancers and in patients with sprain of ankle joint (Biedert 1992, Healy et al. 1995, Rolf et al. 1997). The primary therapy is the surgical repair of the retinacula.

Os tibiale externum

In 10–20%, os tibiale externum (➤ Fig. 21.12) can be found in the tibialis posterior tendon (Coughlin and Mann 1999). **Clinically**, it should be considered as differential diagnosis for avulsion fracture of the navicular bone.

21.3.3 Tibialis anterior tendon

Tendon rupture

Etiology

Tibialis anterior ruptures are very rare. Worldwide, only ca. 100 cases have been described (Ouzounian and Anderson 1995, Simonet and Sim 1995, Mankey 1996, Markarian et al. 1998). Those are often **traumatic ruptures** (in such sports activities like cross-country, skiing) or an open injury (e.g. ice hockey).

The rupture is often overlooked in the beginning because the **loss of the dorsal extension** may be interpreted as neurological deficit. Mostly, men with a mean age over 45 years present the rupture of the tibialis anterior tendon, which is **degeneratively** conditioned in the most cases (Ouzounian and Anderson 1995). Other causes are the cortisone injection or a Lisfranc dislocation. The blood supply can also be a factor for a spontaneous rupture: An avascular zone 5–50 mm proximal of the insertion point is described (Peterson et al. 1999), which is conform to the typical place of rupture.

Clinic

The rupture is usually a consequence of a trauma with plantar flexion. Pain without swelling is only present temporarily. Limping gait develops because of the failure of dorsal extension; a pain-free flatfoot and secondarily a contraction of the Achilles tendon are the consequence. The proximal tendon end can show scars with the environment and thus enable a certain dorsal extension. In the examination, a visible and palpable tendinous defect is found (➤ Fig. 21.13 a and b).

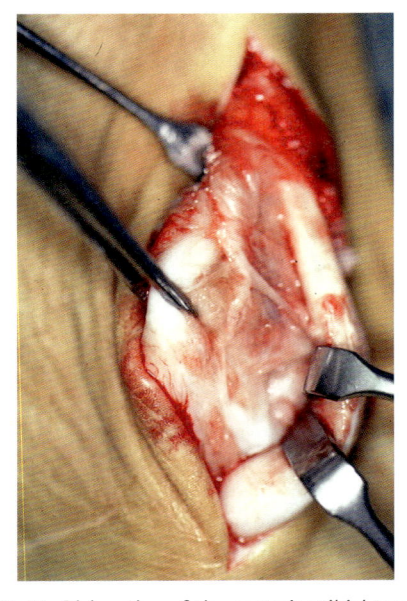

Fig. 21.11 Dislocation of the posterior tibial tendon.

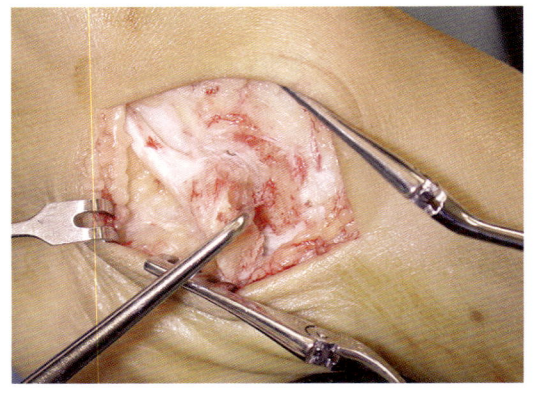

Fig. 21.12 Os tibiale externum.

Fig. 21.13 Rupture of the anterior tibial tendon. a: MRT of complete rupture. b: intraoperative findings with retracted tendon stump.

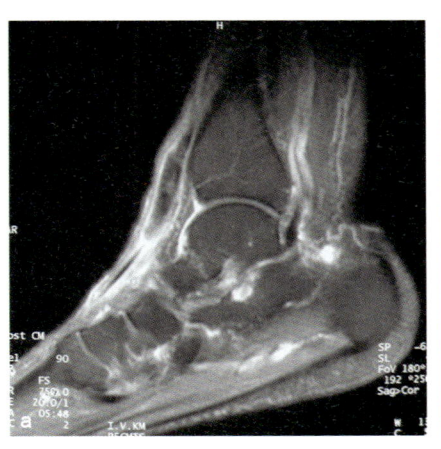

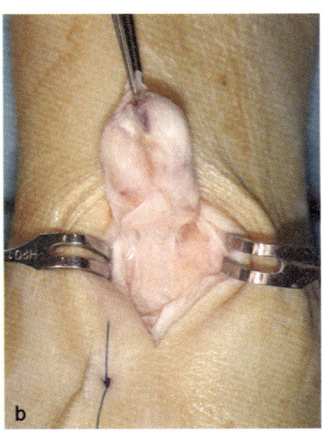

Diagnostics

Conventional radiographs are necessary to exclude avulsion fractures at the medial cuneiforme bone. Ultrasound and MRT can visualize the anterior tibial rupture. Electroneurography is recommended as **differential diagnosis** to exclude possible nerve injury.

Therapy

Acute and subacute injuries (<3 months) should be treated surgically in active patients, independent of the age, to avoid the long-term complications including functional impairments. For this purpose, a direct end-to-end suture or an extensor hallucis longus or extensor digitorum longus transfer with subsequent immobilization in a cast for 6 weeks should be performed. A anterior tibial rupture can also be treated with success **conservatively** in a cast in less active, older patients without sports activities ambitions.

Sesamoid of the anterior tibial tendon

This sesamoid is mostly localized close to the insertion at the cuneiforme bone. It is **without clinical importance**; as differential-diagnosis, a fracture has to be excluded.

21.3.4 Flexor hallucis longus tendon

Flexor hallucis longus tenosynovitis

The tendinitis of the flexor hallucis longus tendon (FHL) is a **typical disease presented in ballet dancers**, but also in runners, soccer players and tennis players (Moorman et al. 1992, Trepman et al. 1995, Theodore et al. 1996). Ballet dancing and here especially the toe dance "en pointe" requires a significantly increased stress of the FHL with secondary narrowing in the fibro-osseous tunnel (Hamilton et al. 1996).

Clinically, medial, swelling and crepitus are found behind the malleolus medialis. All symptoms can be triggered by stress (en pointe, jumping). The flexion of the hallux against resistance is not possible in a plantar-flexed foot in **Hamilton's test**.

As differential-diagnosis, the following entities should be excluded:

- tendinitis of the posterior tibial tendon
- os trigonum
- fracture of the posterior talar process
- Achilles tendinitis or
- osteoarthritis of the upper ankle joint.

An **MRT** can be helpful to ensure an accurate diagnosis.

During the acute phase protection as well as antiphlogistic medication are indicated. Cushioned shoes and the avoidance of hard ground can prevent symptoms in dancers. An **immobilization** for 2–3 weeks in a cast or stable walker is indicated in patients with prolonged symptoms (painful tendinitis for months). A **surgical release** of the fibro-osseous tunnel with removal of possibly existing calcifications and suture of partial ruptures if necessary is indicated in cases with severely persisting tendinitis, which impedes the exercising of the sport.

Flexor hallucis longus tendon rupture

Complete ruptures have been described in the current literature, however a **dysfunction because of lacerations** is more frequent and found especially in dancers, runners, soccer players and tennis players (Thompson et al. 1993, Romash 1994, Inokuchi and Osami 1997). 80% of the FHL ruptures are caused by direct **incised wounds** in going barefooted (Coughlin and Mann 1999).

Clinically, patients present a loss of strength in push-off and not possible spontaneous dorsal extension of the hallux, and flexion. In some cases nerve injuries are often observed as a concomitant injury.

Depending on the localization of the rupture, three zones are distinguished (**zone I:** distal of the sesamoid, **zone II:** distal of the knot of Henry, **zone III:** proximal of the knot of Henry; Coughlin and Mann 1999). A **tendon retraction** is only carried out with a rupture in zone III. At ruptures in zones I and II, the plantar flexion is abolished completely; at a rupture in zone III, a weak flexion in the interphalageal joint is still possible because of the connections to the FDL.

Conventional X-rays as well as **MRT** can help to ensure an accurate diagnosis.

The indication for surgery (direct suture, tenodesis FHL on FDL) is given in athletes needing a forceful push-off as well as in spontaneous dorsal extension. Despite the successful surgery, some studies describe an only minimal possible flexion postoperatively in the interphalangeal joint (Rasmussen and Thyssen 1990). At a laceration, also a tenolysis can be carried out with synovectomy and reconstruction of the tendon.

Os trigonum

The os trigonum is localized at the posterior talar process and is usually asymptomatic. Nevertheless, it can also cause retrocalcaneal pain, which is increased in plantar flexed ankle, in athletes and particularly in dancers. A concomitant **FHL tendinitis** can develop because of its anatomical localization. An activity reduction and antiphlogistic medication usually lead to symptoms relief. In patients with persistent symptoms who cannot be successfully treated by conservative therapy, the os trigonum should be removed using the posterior hindfoot arthroscopy.

21.3.5 Flexor digitorum longus tendon

At the FDL, no spontaneous ruptures have been described (Coughlin and Mann 1999); open cuts cause all injuries. Clinically, the active plantar flexion is significantly reduced and nerve injuries are often observed, as well. The primary suture should be considered as **primary therapy**.

21.3.6 Extensor digitorum longus tendon

An EDL lesion often appears with cuts at the dorsum of the foot. The patients present weakness of the dorsal extension and pronation of the foot. The extension of the toes is not possible anymore. The primary suture should be considered as **primary therapy** and usually result in functional restoration. **Concomitant injuries** of vessels and nerves must be explored and carefully addressed.

21.3.7 Extensor hallucis longus tendon

A rupture of the EHL is very rare; only case reports have been described in the current literature (Menz and Nettle 1989, Poggi and Hall 1995). A sudden snapping as well as a subsequent pain-free swelling and redness have been

Tab. 21.8 Sports related injuries of foot tendons.

Damaged tendon	Sports
peroneal tendon	soccer, basketball, running, hockey, ballet, skiing
posterior tibial tendon	soccer, basketball, running, hockey, ballet, tennis
anterior tibial tendon	hockey, skiing, long-distance running
flexor hallucis longus tendon	soccer, running, ballet, tennis
flexor digitorum longus tendon	cuts
extensor digitorum longus tendon	cuts
extensor hallucis longus tendon	cuts

reported. The dorsal extension of the hallux is not possible anymore. The direct suture should be considered as **primary therapy**; if the tendon is intraoperatively found to be retracted, a tendon transfer with extensor hallucis brevis or peroneus tertius can be carried out as alternative surgical treatment.

Summary

Tendon injuries of the foot appear often in athletes because of the increased use. They are often overlooked because of their rather rare occurrence. In most cases, the diagnosis is made months later while the secondary changes already developed. The careful analysis of the individual clinical symptoms (➤ Tab. 21.8) allows an early diagnosis and can thus prevent deformity, which is especially important in athletes.

References

Biedert R (1992). Dislocation of the tibialis posterior tendon. Am J Sports Med 20: 775–776.

Bonnin M, Tavernier T, Bouysset M (1997). Split lesions of the peroneus brevis tendon in chronic ankle laxity. Am J Sports Med 25: 699–703.

Coughlin MJ, Mann RA (1999). Surgery of the Foot and Ankle. 7th ed. Mosby, St. Louis.

DeLee JC, Drez D (2003). Orthopaedic Sports Medicine. 2nd ed. Saunders, Philadelphia.

Eckert WR, Davis EA Jr (1976). Acute rupture of the peroneal retinaculum. J Bone Joint Surg Am 58: 670–672.

Feighan J, Towers J, Conti S (1999). The use of magnetic resonance imaging in posterior tibial tendon dysfunction. Clin Orthop 365: 23–28.

Ferran NA, Oliva F, Maffuli N (2006). Recurrent subluxation of the peroneal tendons. Sports Med 36: 839–846.

Frey C, Shereff M, Greenidge N (1990). Vascularity of the posterior tibial tendon. J Bone Joint Surg Am 72: 884–888.

Hamilton WG, Geppert MJ, Thompson FM (1996). Pain in the posterior aspect of the ankle in dancers. Differential diagnosis and operative treatment. J Bone Joint Surg Am 78: 1491–1500.

Healy WA III, Starkwether KD, Gruber ME (1995). Chronic dislocation of the posterior tibial tendon. A case report. Am J Sports Med 23: 776–777.

Hintermann B, Valdebarrano V, Kundert HP (1999). Lateral column lengthening by calcaneal osteotomy combined with soft tissue reconstruction for treatment of severe posterior tibial tendon dysfunction. Methods and preliminary results. Orthopäde 9: 760–769.

Holmes GB Jr, Mann RA (1992). Possible epidemiologic factors associated with rupture of the posterior tibial tendon. Foot Ankle 13: 70–79.

Inokuchi S, Usami N (1997). Closed complete rupture of the flexor hallucis longus tendon at the groove of the talus. Foot Ankle Int 18: 47–49.

Johnson KA, Strom DE (1989). Tibialis posterior tendon dysfunction. Clin Orthop 239: 196–206.

Khoury NJ, el Khoury GY, Saltzmann CL, Brandser EA (1996). MR imaging of posterior tibial tendon dysfunction. AJR Am J Roentgenol 167: 675–682.

Kikelly FX, McHale KA (1994). Acute rupture of the peroneal longus tendon in a runner: a case report and review of the literature. Foot Ankle Int 15: 567–569.

Kollias SL, Ferkel RD (1997). Fibular grooving for recurrent peroneal tendon subluxation. Am J Sports Med 25: 329–335.

Krause JO, Brodsky JW (1998). Peroneous brevis tendon tears: Pathophysiology, surgical reconstruction, and clinical results. Foot Ankle Int 19: 271–279.

Lysholm J, Wiklander J (1987). Injuries in runners. Am J Sports Med 15: 168–171.

Macintyre JG, Tunton JE, Clement DB, et al. (1991). Running injuries: a clinical study of 4173 cases. Clin Sports Med 1: 81–87.

Mankey M (1996). Anterior tibial tendon ruptures. Foot Ankle Clin 1: 315–324.

Markaranian G, Kelikian A, Brage M, et al. (1998). Anterior tibial tendon ruptures: an outcome analysis of operative versus nonoperative treatment. Foot Ankle Int 19: 792–802.

Mason RB, Henderson JP (1996). Traumatic peroneal tendon instability. Am J Sports Med 24: 652–658.

Menz P, Nettle W (1989). Closed rupture of the musculotendinous junction of the extensor hallucis longus. Injury 20: 378–381.

Micheli LJ, Waters PM, Sanders DP (1989). Sliding fibular graft repair for chronic dislocation of the peroneal tendons. Am J Sports Med 17: 68–71.

Michelson J, Conti S, Jahss MH (1992). Survivorship analysis of tendon transfer surgery for posterior tibial tendon rupture. Orthop Trans 16: 30–31.

Miller SD, Van Holbeek M, Boruta PM, et al. (1996). Ultrasound in the diagnosis of posterior tibial tendon pathology. Foot Ankle Int 17: 555–558.

Moorman CT III, monto RR, Basett FH III (1992). So-called trigger ankle due to an aberrant flexor hallucis longus muscle in a tennis player. A case report. J Bone Joint Surg Am 74: 294–295.

Myerson MS, Corrigan J, Thompson F, Schon LC (1995). Tendon transfer combined with calcaneal osteotomy for treatment of posterior tibial tendon insufficiency: a radiological investigation. Foot Ankle Int 16: 712–718.

Oden RR (1987). Tendon injuries about the ankle resulting from skiing. Clin Orthop 216: 63–69.

Pierson J, Inglis A (1992). Stenosing tenosynovitis of the peroneus longus tendon. J Bone Joint Surg 74A: 440–442.

Ogawa BK, Thondarson DB (2007). Current concept review: peroneale tendon subluxation and dislocation. Foot Ankle Int 28: 1034–1040.

Ouzounian T, Anderson R (1995). Anterior tibial tendon rupture. Foot Ankle Int 16: 406–410.

Peterson D, Stinson W (1992). Excision of the fracture os perineum: a report on five patients and review of literature. Foot Ankle 13: 277–281.

Petersen W, Stein V, Tillmann B (1999). Blood supply of the tibialis anterior tendon. Arch Orthop Trauma Surg 119: 371–375.

Poggi J, Hall R (1995). Acute rupture of the extensor hallucis longus tendon. Foot Ankle Int 16: 41–43.

Porter DA, Baxter DE, Clanton TO, ezt al. (1998). Posterior tibial tendon tears in young competitive athletes: two case reports. Foot Ankle Int 19: 627–630.

Rasmussen R, Thyssen E (1990). Rupture of the flexor hallucis longus tendon: case report. Foot Ankle 10: 288–289.

Rockett MS, Waitches G, Sudakoff G, Brage M (1998). Use of ultrasonography versus magnetic resonance imaging for tendon abnormalities around the ankle. Foot Ankle Int 19: 604–612.

Rolf C, Guntner P, Ekenman I, Turan I (1997). Dislocation of the tibialis posterior tendon: Diagnosis and treatment. J Foot Ankle Surg 36: 63–65.

Romash MM (1994). Closed rupture of the flexor hallucis longus tendon in a long distance runner: Report of a case and review of the literature. Foot Ankle Int 15: 433–436.

Safran MR, O'Malley D Jr, Fu FH (1999). Peroneal tendon subluxation in athletes: New exam technique, case report, and review. Med Sci Sports Exerc 31: 487–492.

Sammarco GJ (1995). Peroneus longus tendon tears: Acute and chronic. Foot Ankle Int 16: 245–253.

Schneiderbauer M, Frigg A, Valderrabano V, Hintermann B (2005). Arthroskopische Befunde bei der chronischen Sprunggelenksinstabilität. Arthroskopie 18: 104–111.

Selmani E, Gjata V, Gjika E (2006). Current concepts review: peroneal tendon disorders. Foot Ankle Int 27: 221–228.

Simonet W, Sim L (1995). Boot-top tendon lacerations in ice hockey. J Trauma Inj Infect Crit Care 38: 30–31.

Sobel M, Pavlov H, Geppert M, et al. (1994). Painful os perineum syndrome: a spectrum of conditions responsible for plantar lateral foot pain. Foot Ankle 15: 112–124.

Theodore GH, Kolettis GJ, Micheli LJ (1996). Tenosynovitis of the flexor hallucis longus in a long-distance runner. Med Sci Sports Exerc 28: 277–279.

Thompson FM, Snow SW, Hershon SJ (1993). Spontaneous atraumatic rupture of the flexor hallucis longus tendon under the sustenaculum tali: Case report, review of the literature, and treatment options. Foot Ankle 14: 414–417.

Trepman E, Mizel MS, Newberg AH (1995). Spontaneous rupture oft he flexor hallucis longus tendon in a tennis player: A case report. Foot Ankle Int 16: 227–231.

Trevino S, Baumhauer J (1992). Tendon injuries of the foot and ankle. Clin Sports Med 11: 727–739.

Valderrabano V, Hintermann B, Wischer T, Fuhr P, Dick W (2004). Recovery oft he posterior tibial muscle after late reconstruction following tendon rupture. Foot Ankle Int 25: 85–95.

Van Dijk CN, Kort N (1998). Tendoscopy of the peroneal tendons. Arthroscopy 14: 471–478.

Van Dijk CN, Kort N, Scholten PE (1997). Tendoscopy of the posterior tibial tendon. Arthroscopy 14: 471–478.

Wander DS, Galli K, Ludden JW, Mayer DP (1994). Surgical management of a ruptured peroneus longus tendon with a fractured multipartite os perineum. J Foot Ankle Surg 33: 124–128.

Woods L, Leach RE (1991). Posterior tibial tendon rupture in athletic people. Am J Sports Med 19: 495–498.

Zivot M, Pearl S, Pupp G, Pupp J (1989). Stenosing peroneal tenosynovitis. J Foot Surg 28: 20–224.

21.4 Ligament injuries of foot and ankle

Geert Pagestert and Beat Hintermann

21.4.1 Ligament injuries in general

Anamnesis, findings and classification

Foot and ankle injuries are the **most common sport injuries**. The most common **symptoms** are hematomas and painful tenderness at the site of ligament injury, also in combination with a significant joint instability and/or deformity. The accurate diagnosis can be done in most cases by analysis of injury mechanism and a careful clinical investigation. The **conventional radiological assessment** should be done to exclude a fracture. An advanced imaging, e.g. **MRT** is made for the documentation of the injury. The reliability of **ultrasound** depends on the experience of examiner and is less applicable for documentation. **Arthrography** is invasive and has a low specifity.

For ligament injuries, the simple and reliable **classification** of the "American Medical Association" (Rachun 1968) can be used:

- strain (degree 1)
- partial rupture (degree 2) and
- complete rupture (degree 3).

The difference between degree 1 and 2 cannot be always detected by clinical symptoms, which are the following:

- degree 1 = full weight bearing possible, small hematoma
- degree 2 = partial weight bearing possible, extended hematoma
- degree 3 = no weight bearing possible, extended hematoma

The classification of ligament injuries helps to determine the therapeutical steps.

Therapy

In general, in all acute ligamentous injuries a conservative treatment can be successfully performed.

Principles underlying a successful therapy are: stop of sports activities, elevated positioning of the affected lower extremity, avoiding of swelling by cooling, immobilization, compression and non-steroidal antiphlogistics = **RICE** (rest, ice, compression, elevation). A **full weight bearing** is allowed as tolerated.

A partial weight bearing should be recommended in patients with serious injuries of three ligaments, which play a pivotal stabilization role in loaded ankle during the gait:

- deltoid ligament with spring ligament
- syndesmosis
- Lisfranc ligament.

Chronic joint instabilities can be successfully treated non-operatively. The main therapeutic principle is the **physical therapy** for the coordination improvement, proprioception, and active muscular stabilization. In patients with failure of conservative treatment, a surgical therapy should be considered.

Osseous avulsions of ligaments are the special entity of ligamental injuries. In most cases the avulsion fragments are not dislocated and therefore can be treated conservatively while in patients with significant dislocation an open reduction and fixation should be performed. The anatomical reduction and solid fixation may avoid the prolonged osseous healing. Furthermore, in most patients the mobilization can be performed without cast postoperatively. For those reasons the indication for **refixing of osseous avulsion** fractures should be given especially in active athletes.

Rehabilitation, return to sports and prophylaxis

The return to sports should occur successively and with physiotherapeutical support. In patients where the physiotherapy and/or everyday procedures can be absolved without symptoms, sport-specific training should start and be increased to full weight bearing in training, if no symptoms occur. Subsequently, the athlete can be released for competition again.

Stepping back the rehabilitation/physiotherapeutic program is indicated if deterioration of the symptoms occurs. If there is no progress within an expected time limit, the injury must be evaluated again and the therapeutic strategy should be adjusted.

According to the injured ligament, rehabilitation usually takes between 4 to 12 weeks. External stabilizers e.g. braces can increase the intrinsic stability, however, in some cases they may avoid the maximum performance.

21.4.2 Special ligament injuries

Upper ankle joint (UAJ)

The anterior talofibular ligament (ATFL), the calcaneofibular ligament (CFL) and the posterior talofibular ligament (PTFL; ➤ Fig. 21.14) may be involved.

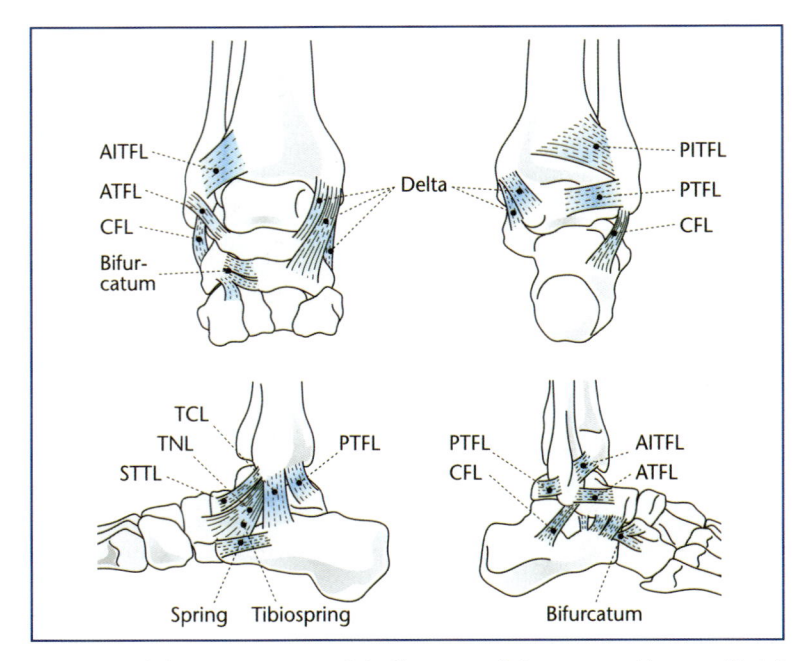

Fig. 21.14 The knowledge of the exact anatomy of the ligaments of the upper and lower ankle joints is a prerequisite for the interpretation of a local pressure dolence (Hintermann et al. 1996 and 2004). This becomes clear in the differentiation of the closely neighboring injuries of the ATFL, the AITFL and the lig. bifurcatum, or of the delta and spring ligaments, respectively. ATFL = anterior tibiofibular lig., PTFL = posterior tibiofibular lig., CFL = calcaneofibular lig., AITFL = anterior-inferior tibiofibular lig., PITFL = posterior-inferior tibiofibular lig., IOL = interosseous lig. Superficial delta ligament: STTL = superficial tibiotalar lig., TNL = tibionavicular lig., TCL = tibiocalcaneal lig., tibio spring lig., (modified according to Hintermann et al. 1999 and 2004, Casillas 2003).

The trauma mechanism is typically a **supination trauma** of the forefoot with inversion of the hindfoot (Hintermann 1996, Hintermann et al. 1992). The following **concomitant injuries** from distal to proximal can occur and should be considered:

- metatarsal V basis avulsion
- rupture of the peroneal tendon
- bifurcatum rupture or avulsion processus anterior calcanei
- lateral fibulotarsal ligament and anterior syndesmosis rupture
- peroneal-tendon-retinaculum rupture with dislocation of the tendon
- fibular and osteochondral talus fractures (Hintermann et al. 2002).

The PTFL is rarely affected and therefore its injury may be initially missed.

Clinical tests for the evaluation of the lateral fibulotarsal ligaments are the talar advance (pathological at the ATFL rupture) and the talus tilt test (pathological at CFL rupture). In acute cases, these clinical tests as well as held radiographs **may not be properly performed** because of pain. They aforementioned tests help to evaluate **chronic instabilities** of the upper ankle joint.

The choice of **therapy** of the acute instability depends on clinical symptoms (e.g. no full weight bearing (➢ Tab. 21.9 and ➢ Fig. 21.15; Jackson et al. 1974).

Chronic lateral instability of the upper ankle joint

Chronic lateral instability of the upper ankle joint may be mainly diagnosed by analysis of previous ankle traumata. Patients typically report feeling unstable while walking on uneven ground in case of **recurrent diversion traumas**. If neurological etiology of instability can be excluded, the chronic lateral instability can be di-

Tab. 21.9 Conservative therapy of ligament injuries of the upper ankle joint (➤ Fig. 21.15).

Degree	Capacity	Injury	Therapy
1	remaining: walking, standing possible	■ distorsion ■ partial rupture	RICE: ■ pneumatic stabilization splint (➤ Fig. 21.15) for 6–8 weeks ■ start of PhysioTx immediately to 1 week ■ starting with sports after about 4–7 days ■ compression stocking intermittent
2	limited: walking, standing only possible for a short time, afterwards pain	■ rupture ATFL ■ possibly anterior syndesmosis	RICE: ■ pneumatic stabilization splint for 12 weeks ■ PhysioTx, then starting sports 1st–2nd week or ■ pneumatic stabilization splint for 4–7 days, then stability boot (Hintermann et al. 1990) for 4–8 weeks ■ start of PhysioTx in the 2nd–4th week ■ additionally, night splint or split soft cast over night for 6 weeks ■ compression stocking intermittent
3	impossible: walking, standing associated with immediate pain	■ rupture of ATFL and CFL ■ anterior syndesmosis **special form:** avulsion fracture (Weber A) of the fibula	RICE: ■ pneumatic stabilization splint or split soft cast and stick relief for 4–7 days ■ PhysioTx, then starting sports from the 2nd–4th week accompanied by pneumatic splint or stabilization boot for about 3–6 months ■ in addition, a night cast or split soft cast over night for 6 weeks ■ compression stocking intermittent **special form:** conservatively in plaster for 6 weeks or, with dislocation, surgical refixation of the osseous ligament tear

vided into two main groups: structural and fuctional instability of the upper ankle joint (Hintermann 1995).

A **structural instability** can be assessed by pathological talar tilt and/or advance tests or of pathological, held images compared to the non-injured contralateral side. The resolution of radiographs does not allow to measure within millimeter range, also remarkable interindividual range of measured values in healthy subjects should be considered (Schafer and Hintermann 1996).

A functional instability should be considered in patients suffering from instability without corresponding structural findings. A **limited muscular stabilization** of the upper ankle joint caused by insufficient proprioception and co-ordination and/or a secondary functional deficit because of previous immobilization, or deficient training may cause a functional instability of the upper ankle joint.

Following therapies are recommended (➤ Fig. 21.16). In all patients the hindfoot alignment should be also assessed clinically and radiographically: the chronic lateral instability of the upper ankle joint may be found with a **varus hindfoot alignment**. In such cases a careful surgical assessment of concomitant hindfoot deformities is necessary. Therefore, a **lateral displacement osteotomy** of the calcaneus in combination with the reconstruction of the ankle ligament should be performed to restore the biomechanics of foot/ankle and to achieve satisfied long-term results (Csizy and Hintermann 1996).

An appropriate **recidive sprain prophylaxis** after acute or at chronic instabilities can be achieved by using of pneumatic stabilization brace during athletic competitions. Permanent stabilization by braces also during training is not recommended because this would decrease the intrinsic ability of ankle stabilizing due to missing proprioception. This ultimately

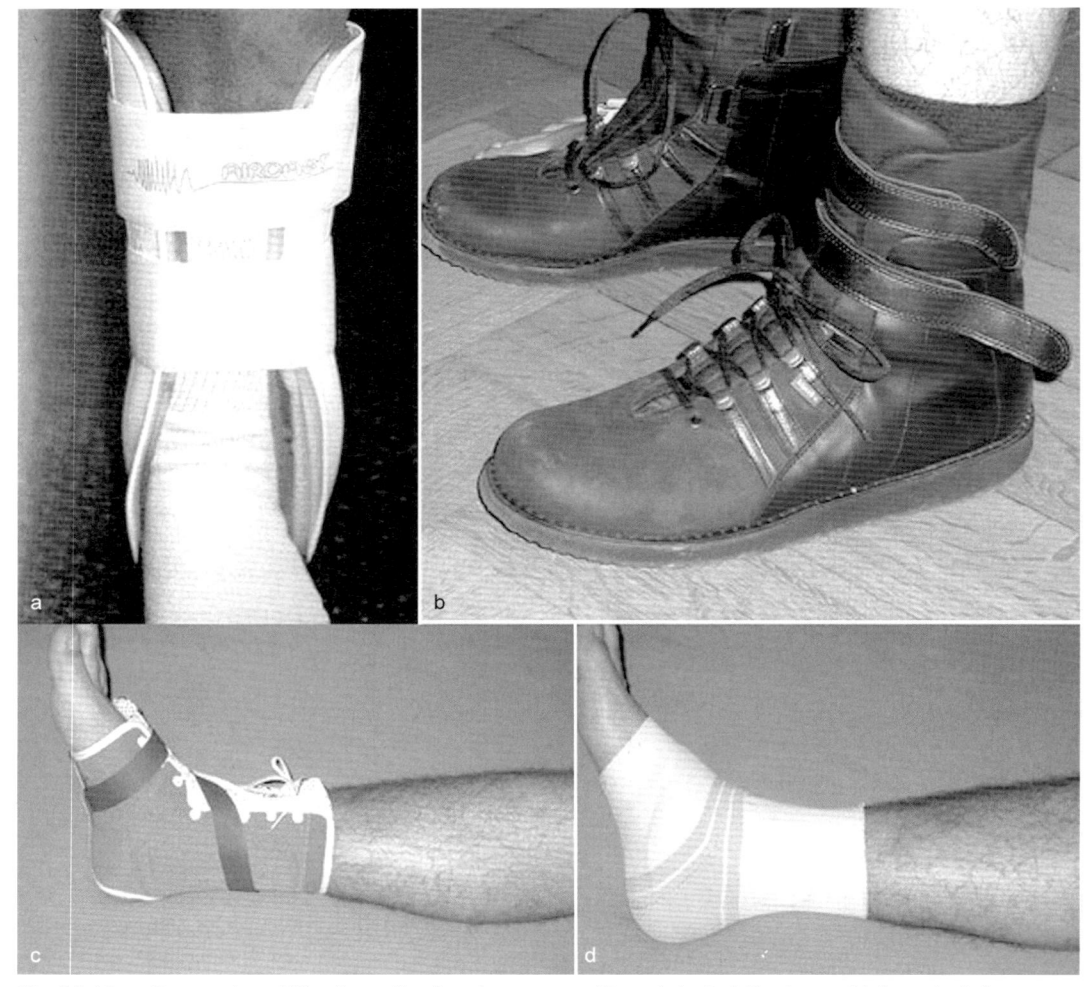

Fig. 21.15 a: Pneumatic stabilization splint (e.g. by company Aircast). b: Stability boot with lateral reinforcements (e.g. by company Künzli). c: Night splint with lateral stabilization and pronation securing (e.g. by company Künzli). d: Elastic stocking.

results in recurrent instability. Using of taping remains controversial because the stability of the tape bandage decreases significantly after its application (Shapiro et al. 1994).

Syndesmosis

The syndesmosis consists of **three ligaments** (➤ Fig. 21.14):

- the anterior-inferior tibiofibular ligament (AITFL)
- the posterior-inferior tibiofibular ligament (PITFL) and
- the interosseous ligament (IOL).

The syndesmosis represents the ligamentous part of the **mortice**, which is responsible for the static stability during axial loads of the upper ankle joint. In cases where any two of three parts of syndesmosis are damages, the syndesmosis usually remains still stable.

Acute injuries usually result from supination, as described above (see lateral upper ankle joint), or from external rotation of the foot in the mortise and/or eversion of the hindfoot. At the injury, first AITFL experiences ruptures, followed by OIL and finally by PITFL If the eversion force continues and exceeds certain individual limits, fibula fracture may occur above

21.4 Ligament injuries of foot and ankle

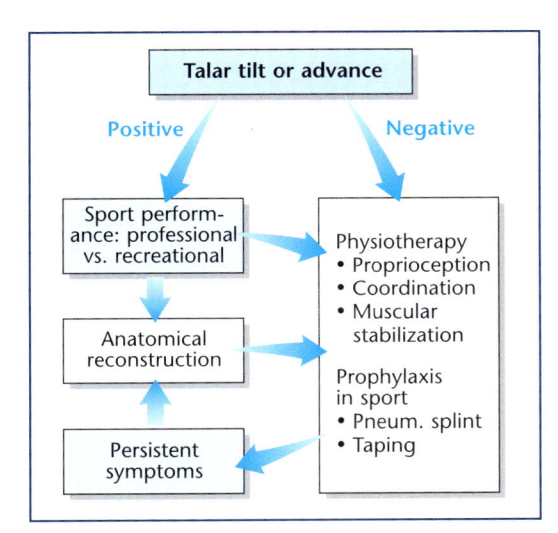

Fig. 21.16 Treatment algorithm of chronic lateral instability of the upper ankle joint: In many cases with functional instability or minimum requirements of the patient, a non-surgical treatment can be successfully performed including training of proprioception, coordination and muscle strength. In case where conservative therapy is unsuccessful, a surgical reconstruction with local tissue should be performed including augmentation with plantaris tendon (Hintermann et al. 1999, Pagenstert et al. 2005) and with extensor retinaculum (Harper 1991). In active athletes a surgical treatment should be considered more generously in order to shorten the rehabilitation time and to reduce the deficiency of training.

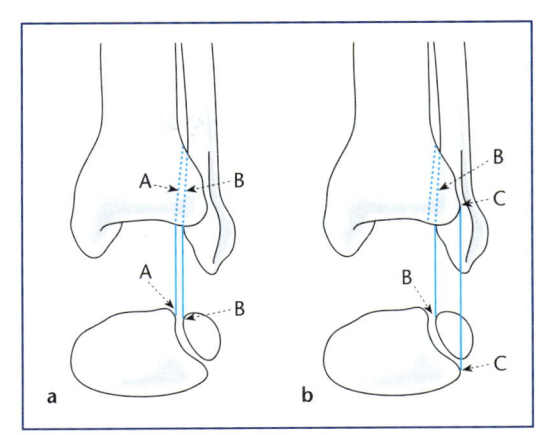

Fig. 21.17 Evaluation of syndesmosis.
a: The distance between tibia and fibula in the distal joint is normally less than 6 mm (distance between A and B < 6 mm = normal).
b: The overlapping of tibia and fibula in a 20° standard a.p. X-ray is normally more than 6 mm (distance between B and C > 6 mm = normal; Casillas 2003).

the syndesmosis. The rupture of IOL is usually found at the height of the fibula fracture.

Special **test procedures** for the assessment of syndesmosis injury may be performed:

- "squeeze test" at the medial lower leg: the fibula is being pushed medially forward against the tibia from posterior-lateral. Positive test localizes pain in the region of the AITFL indicating its injury.
- Enforced external rotation of the foot increases pain in the region of the AITFL.
- Complete fibula should be carefully examined in order not to miss symptoms of a proximal tibiofibular dislocation or a "high" proximal fibular fracture.
- Only subluxations/dislocations of the fibula at the incision are found (➤ Fig. 21.17), which correspond to injuries of the complete syndesmosis. In cases where instability is not obvious, a latent instability with subluxation can occur only under load/stress. For correct diagnosis, weight bearing radiographs should be performed in standing or in held external rotation. If the fibula remains in its anatomic position, complete ruptures of the AITFL and the IOL cannot be excluded. In these cases and in cases where the full weight bearing is not possible because of symptoms, advanced imaging (CT or MRT) should be recommended.
- Injuries of the complete syndesmosis are usually found in combination with injuries of the deltoid ligament. The damaged deltoid ligament can be folded into the joint and thus may prohibit the anatomic reposition of the fibula into the incision.
- The therapy decision should be made based on degree of injury and the loss of mobility (➤ Tab. 21.10).

The **chronic unstable syndesmosis** can be diagnosed by arising of pain in stress and by full weight bearing radiographs, as well as advanced imaging (CT or MRT). Surgical treatment options are the arthroscopic debridement of the scar tissue, ligament reconstructions with free tendon transplants (e.g. plantaris tendon), or as a salvage procedure of the tibiofibular arthrodesis.

Tab. 21.10 Therapy of syndesmosis injury.

Degree	Capacity	Injury	Therapy
1	remaining: walking, standing possible	■ strain ■ partial rupture to complete rupture AITFL	RICE: ■ pneumatic stabilization splint for 6–8 weeks ■ start of PhysioTx immediately to 1 week ■ beginning of sport after ca. 4–7 days ■ surgical stocking intermittently
2	limited: walking, standing only possible for a short time, then painful	■ rupture of the AITFL ■ strain/partial ruptures, other syndesmosis	RICE: ■ pneumatic stabilization splint or split soft cast and relief by canes for 2–3 weeks ■ PhysioTx, the sport beginning in the 2nd–6th week with pneumatic splint or stable boot for ca. 3–6 months ■ Additional night splint or split soft cast over night for 6 weeks ■ Surgical stocking intermittently
3	impossible: walking, standing accompanied by immediate pain	■ rupture of AITFL and IOL ■ with dislocation, syndesmosis also PITFL **special form:** avulsion fracture AITFL (fibula: Wagstaffe fracture; tibia: Tillaux-Chaput fracture)	RICE: ■ incomplete ruptures or latent dislocations: relief by cane in walking cast or split soft cast for 8–10 weeks ■ dislocation: open or closed reposition and fixation by screws of syndesmosis (no traction screw! Set screws through 3–4 corticals), relief by canes until screw removal after 8–12 weeks **special form:** conservatively in a walking cast for 6 weeks or surgical refixation of the osseous ligament avulsion at a dislocation

Medial tibiotarsal ligaments (deltoid ligament)

The deltoid ligament consists of a superficial and a deep layer. The superficial part runs to the calcaneus, talus, navicular bone and spring ligament; the deep part runs to the talus (➤ Fig. 21.14). The ligamental complex biomechanically contributes to the anatomic shape of the medial arch of the foot by the spring ligament and thus contributes to the static stability of the upper ankle joint and the foot.

The deltoid ligament shows a high intrinsic stability, therefore the injuries of the deltoid ligament are usually found in combination with bone fractures, typically resulting from **eversion** and **external rotation injury** mechanism.

Especially at the evaluation of conventional **radiographs**, special attention should be paid to an enlarged distance of the medial malleolus to the talus in comparison to the remaining upper ankle joint – also in combination with syndesmosis injuries.

Also here, the therapy decision should be made based on degree of injury and the loss of mobility (➤ Tab. 21.11).

Chronic medial instability

Chronic medial instability involves a ligament insufficiency of the **ventral deltoid part**: the tibionavicular and tibiospring ligament combined with the spring ligament itself (Hintermann et al. 2004). It becomes evident in **posttraumatic insecurity** on uneven ground, local pressure tenderness at the ventral medial malleolus and hindfoot valgus. The function of the tibialis posterior tendon is usually found to be normal. Apart from that, the medial ligament instability is similar to the ligament instability of tibialis posterior tendon insufficiency.

MRT or arthroscopy confirms the diagnosis. **Conservative therapy options** are only of little success in old ligament injuries. In most cases, we recommend **surgical tightening/suture** of the deltoid and spring ligaments after a debridement of the painful scar tissue. In some cases, a shortening of the tibialis posterior tendon and/or a medial displacement or lateral lengthening calcaneal osteotomy are necessary to restore the biomechanics of the hindfoot. Postoperatively, patients are mobilized with full weight bearing in stable walker or cast for 6

Tab. 21.11 Therapy of injuries of the delta ligament.

Degree	Capacity	Injury	Therapy
1	remaining: walking, standing possible	strain	RICE: ■ pneumatic stabilization splint for 6–8 weeks ■ start of PhysioTx immediately to 1 week ■ beginning of sport after ca. 4–7 days ■ surgical stocking intermittently
2	limited: walking, standing possible only for a short time, then painful	partial rupture	RICE: ■ pneumatic stabilization splint or split soft cast and relief by canes for 2–3 weeks ■ PhysioTx, then sport beginning at the 2nd–6th week with pneumatic splint or stable boot for ca. 3–6 months ■ additional night splint or split soft cast over night for 6 weeks ■ surgical stocking intermittently
3	impossible: walking, standing accompanied by immediate pain	complete rupture **special form:** avulsion fracture of the medial malleolus	RICE: ■ relief by cane in a walking cast or split soft cast for 6 weeks **special form:** conservatively in a walking cast or surgical refixation of the osseous ligament avulsion at a dislocation

weeks (Hintermann et al. 2004; for prophylaxis, see lateral upper ankle joint).

Lower ankle joint

Subtalar joint

Subtalar joint is stabilized by **intrinsic ligaments** (interosseous, cervical, lateral and medial talocalcaneal ligaments) and the **extrinsic ligaments** (deltoid ligament, retinaculum extensorum and CFL) (➤ Fig. 21.14, ➤ Fig. 21.18). A subtalar ligament injury always occurs in combination with an **injury of the upper ankle joint**, or rather: At a larger extent of the distorsion of the upper ankle joint, it follows the rupture of the ligaments of the upper ankle joint.

Clinically, the talus tilt test shows an increased folding of the subtalar joint to medial or lateral. This pathologic finding can be confirmed using radiographs (45° internal rotation to Brodén) as dislocation/subluxation in the subtalar joint is seen and indicates a high-degree injury with medial and/or lateral rupture of the extrinsic and intrinsic ligaments. The **therapy** should primarily address injury of the medial or lateral ligaments of the upper ankle joint (see above).

The special form of subtalar joint injuries is the peritalar dislocation with ruptures of all subtalar ligaments. In this case, joint congruency should be carefully assessed using CT after reposition. In general, treatment of peritalar dislocation is comparable to those of degree-III lesion of the medial ligaments of the upper ankle joint (see above).

> In a peritalar dislocation joint congruency must be carefully restored by closed or open reduction.

The **chronic subtalar instability** is often found in combination with the **chronic lateral instability of the upper ankle joint**. The conservative and surgical therapeutic options are described under "lateral ligament injuries of the upper ankle joint" (➤ Segment 21.4.2). In particular, the augmentation of the lateral ligament reconstruction of the upper ankle joint can be achieved by tightening of the inferior retinaculum extensorum and represents an anatomic reconstruction to treat the lateral subtalar instability (➤ Fig. 21.18). Minor subtalar instabilities (subluxations) are often diagnosed with significant delay when already **degenerative changes of subtalar joint** are present.

Patients with subtalar instability present with following common **symptoms**: feeling unstable during walking on uneven ground, pain beneath the mortise especially in full weight bear-

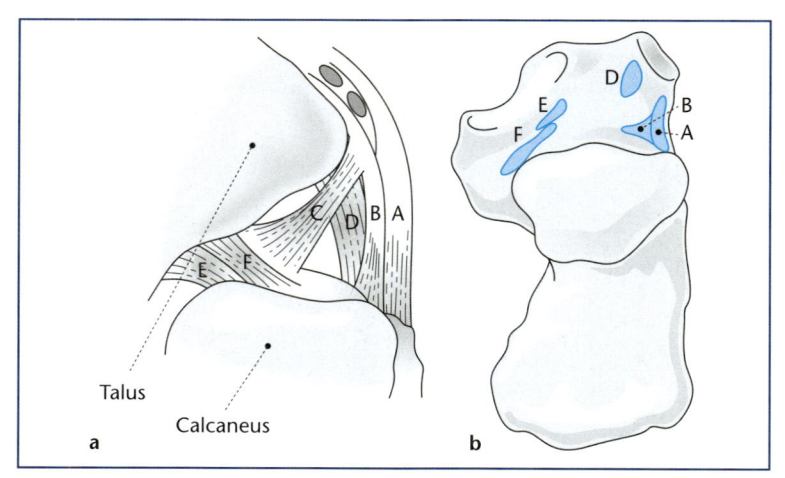

Fig. 21.18 Ligaments of the subtalar joint (taken from Harper 1991). a: view of sinus tarsi. b: view of calcaneus (A–C: insertions of retinaculum extensorum inferior, D: insertion of cervical ligament, E, F: insertion of interosseum ligament).

ing, and a limited flexibility of joint. The conventional radiograph should be carefully analyzed. Advanced imaging (CT) should be used to confirm or to exclude a suspected dislocation/sublocation of subtalar joint. Following **treatment options** should be considered: arthroscopic or open debridement with arthrolysis, reduction of dislocation and ligament reconstruction as well as the subtalar fusion in patients with painful progressive degenerative changes.

Chopart's joint

The talonavicular and the calcaneocuboidal joints may be injured resulting from **distorsion trauma mechanism** with forced plantar flexion and inversion, also ligaments of the upper ankle joint may be found concomitantly injured.

The **spring ligament** (calcaneonavicular ligament) tenses like a spring between calcaneus and navicular bone. As "coxa pedis", the main function of this ligament is to stabilize the medial longitudinal arch of the foot.

In addition, the ventral deltoid ligament with the tibionavicular and the tibiospring parts and the dorsal talonavicular ligament stabilize the **talonavicular joint**. The lateral calcaneocuboidal ligament contributes to stabilization of the **calcaneocuboidal joint**. The bifurcatum ligament has two sides and stabilizes **Chopart's joint** calcaneocuboidally and calcaneonavicularly.

The injury of the ligaments of the lateral upper ankle joint and the bifurcatum should be separately identified. The forefoot is supinated with a stabilized lower leg at first and with fixed calcaneus afterwards. In the first test, pain indicates a ligament injury at the lateral upper ankle joint and an injury of the bifurcatum ligament in the second test.

> The main goal in treatment of injuries of Chopart's joint is to restore the stability and biomechanics of the medial column.

In cases where the deltoid ligament and the spring ligament are found to be injured, treatment options should specifically address all ligamental injuries of the upper ankle joint (see above). If the medial ligament structures are found to be intact, the treatment is the same as for injuries of the lateral ligament apparatus of the upper ankle joint (see above).

Osseous avulsions of the dorsal talonavicular ligament and the bifurcatum ligament present special injury forms. An immobilization of 6 weeks in a walking cast or stable walker with full weight bearing should be recommended in cases with minor dislocations (1–2 mm). Subsequently, patients successfully regained their sports activity level, this with physiotherapeutical support. In patients who undergo the surgical fixation of osseous ligament insertion, a functional rehabilitation without cast and full weight bearing as tolerated can be successfully performed.

Chronic instability of Chopart's may result from non- or malunions of intraarticular fractures of the anterior calcanei process (bifurcatum avulsion fracture). In our experience, surgical refixation should be considered showing superior results in comparison to debridement of the fragment.

Lisfranc joints

The Lisfranc ligament tenses plantarly between the os cuneiforme mediale and the basis of the metatarsal II (MZ II, ➢ Fig. 21.19). **Immense force** applying to the dorsum of the foot or a distorsion at a fixed forefoot may result in injuries of Lisfranc joints.

Clinically, a compression of the transverse arch and/or a forced pronation of the forefoot may provoke pain at the site of ligament injury.

Radiological diagnosis includes conventional foot/ankle radiographs in full weight bearing. Oblique images of foot may be performed to evaluate the Lisfranc joint congruency. However, the reliability of this radiographic method is low. Advanced imaging (CT, scintigraphy) may help to ensure the diagnosis in challenging cases.

The therapy decision should be made based on degree of Lisfranc instability assessed using full weight bearing radiographs (➢ Tab. 21.12; Nunley and Vertullo 2002).

Serious injuries of Lisfranc's ligament may result in the **end of the career of the athlete**. Prophylactic measures preventing the accident mechanism are highly recommended. The individual carbon shoe insole can be used for permanent support for the medial longitudinal arch of the foot and may **prevent** the recurrent injuries.

Toe joints

Hallux

Injuries of the capsule-ligament apparatus (➢ Fig. 21.20) of the metatarsophalangeal joint of the hallux (MTP 1) are rare in Europe. They usually appear in contact sports, such as American football/rugby and martial arts.

Case series in the current literature describe the accident mechanism as axial trauma with hyperextension in the metacarpophalangeal joint of the hallux – mostly on artificial lawn (= "turf"). The firm adhesion of sportshoes on artificial lawn has also been found as a cause for the accidents, which has led to the expression **"turf toe"** in the Anglo-American area (Clanton et al. 1986, Coughlin 2003).

The accurate diagnosis requires careful analysis of injury mechanism and clinical investigation. The positioning of the sesamoid bones towards each other and corresponding to the

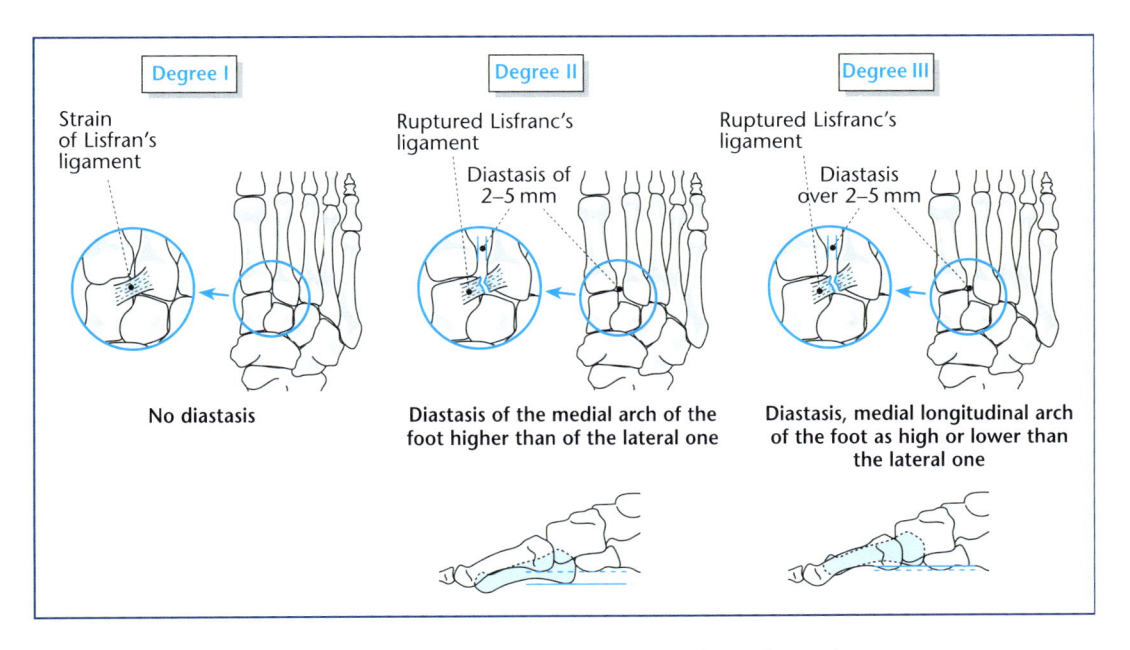

Fig. 21.19 Classification of the Lisfranc ligament instability (Nunley and Vertullo 2002).

Tab. 21.12 Therapy of injuries of the Lisfranc joint.

Degree	Radiograph of the foot a.p.	Lateral radiograph of the foot	Therapy
1	■ distance between MT I and MT II basis: < 2 mm = normal ■ scintigraphy positive	medial longitudinal arch of the foot higher than lateral = normal	RICE: ■ individual carbon stabilization insert for 6–8 weeks ■ start of PhysioTx immediately to 1 week ■ beginning of sport after ca. 4–7 days ■ surgical stocking intermittently
2	■ distance between MT I and MT II basis: 2–5 mm	medial longitudinal arch of the foot higher than lateral = normal	RICE: ■ plaster shoe or individual carbon stabilization insert, with cane relief, if required, for 2–3 weeks ■ PhysioTx, then sport beginning at the 2nd–6th week with individual carbon stabilization insert for ca. 3–6 months ■ surgical stocking intermittently
3	■ distance between MT I and MT II basis: > 5 mm ■ dislocation	medial longitudinal arch of the foot same height as or lower than lateral	■ closed reposition and percutaneous fixation by Kirschner wire ■ relief by cane in a walking cast or split soft cast for 6 weeks ■ afterwards, removal of the wire and progressive loads, sport capacity not before the 12th week (alternatively as for dislocation) ■ at a dislocation: cannulated screws instead of K-wires. Removal after 8th or 24th weeks, depending on the body weight, but 4 weeks before full athletic load

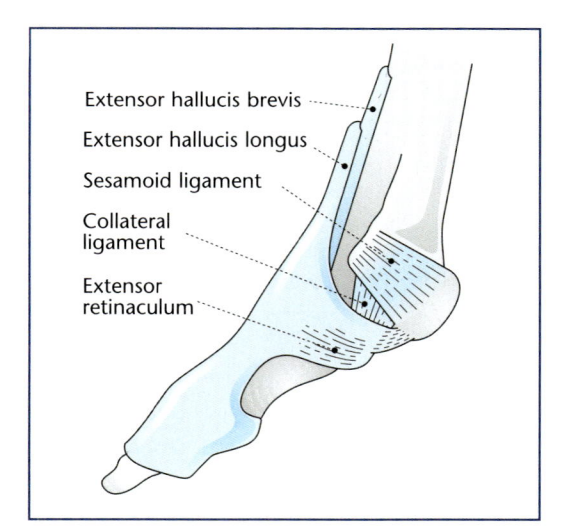

Fig. 21.20 Ligaments and tendons of the hallux metacarpophalangeal joint (Coughlin 2003).

metatarsal head should be evaluated using conventional full weight bearing radiographs. Also MTP joint should be carefully assessed addressing fractures, dislocation, or **osteochondral lesions**. The dislocation of the sesamoid bones or the hallux in high-degree "turf toe" injuries may be sufficiently visualized using conventional radiographs. However, advanced imaging (MRT) should be considered for appropriate assessment of soft tissue injuries.

The **therapy** decision should be made based on degree of injury and the loss of mobility (➤ Tab, 21.13). Generally, the athletes do not see the physician immediately, but only after the loss of capacity, because they underestimate the acute trauma (Clanton et al. 1986).

Chronic instability of the MTP 1 can occur in athletes with hallux valgus. The hallux valgus devormity may increase stress of the sesamoid bone-ligament complex resulting in stress fractures of the medial sesamoid bone. In these cases hallux valgus deformity should be **surgically** corrected followed by osteosynthesis of the sesamoid bone (Pagenstert et al. 2005).

Special sportshoes with stiff soles or inserts with stiffening of the MTP 1 may **prevent** the aforementioned injuries by reducing of mobility of the MTP 1 joint. Especially athletes with limited MTP-1 extension capacity (< 60°) may benefit from this prevention.

Tab. 21.13 Therapy of injuries of the hallux.

Degree	Symptoms	Capacity	Injury	Therapy
1	pressure tenderness	remaining	strain	Symptomatic, sport pause
2	limited mobility	reduced sport capacity 3–14 days	partial rupture	Stable sole for 2–4 weeks or buddy taping
3	advanced symptoms, obvious dislocation	reduced sport capacity 2–6 weeks	complete rupture of: ■ sesamoid/collateral ligaments ■ volar plate ■ adductor/flexor hallucis tendons ■ fracture of the sesamoid bone/avulsion fracture ■ osteochondral lesions	4–6 weeks stable sole or plaster shoe versus early surgical treatment (suture, mini-screw osteosynthesis, debridement, temporary arthrodesis) and stable sole for 4–6 weeks

Small toes

Small toes injuries usually occur in sports without shoes (martial arts, sand sports) and result from axial traumas. Ligamentous injuries of the metatarsophalangeal joints of the small toes should be treated with **buddy taping**.

Chronic instabilities of the MTP joints with consecutive development of hammer and/or claw toes – in some cases in combination with metatarsalgia – are rare, but often combined with **foot deformities**. **Conservative therapeutic options** are retrocapitally supporting inserts for splayfeet, comfort inserts for hollow feet as well as interdigital, redressing ortheses or buddy taping.

Infiltrations with local anesthesia should be performed to exactly localize the source of the pain, but also for short-term treatment of the symptoms.

> Cortisone infiltrations may cause or increase the degenerative changes of the ligamental and capsular joint structures resulting in ruptures of ligaments and tendons.

Surgical treatment options e.g. capsule release and plastics, lengthening of the extensor tendons and transfer of the flexor tendons, arthrodeses and osteotomies at the metatarsalia may be performed especially in a patient who was conservatively treated without success.

Following prophylaxis may prevent injuries and should be recommended: buddy taping in sport, wide shoes and/or interdigital ortheses in everyday routine.

References

Casillas MM (2003). Ligament injuries of the foot and ankle. In: DeLee JC, Drez D, Miller MD (eds.). DeLee & Drez's Sports Medicine, vol. 2. W.B. Saunders Company, Elsevier, Philadelphia.

Clanton TO, Butler JE, Eggert A (1986). Injuries to the metatarsophalangeal joints in athletes. Foot Ankle Int 7: 162–176.

Coughlin MJ (2003). Turf Toe. In: DeLee JC, Drez D, Miller MD (eds.). DeLee & Drez's Sports Medicine, vol. 2. W.B. Saunders Company, Elsevier, Philadelphia.

Csizy M, Hintermann B (1996). Dwyer osteotomy with or without lateral stabilization in calcaneus varus with lateral ligament insufficiency of the upper ankle joint. Sportverletz Sportschaden 10: 100–102.

Harper MC (1991). The lateral ligamentous support of the subtalar joint. Foot Ankle Int 11: 354–358.

Hintermann B, Boss AP, Schaefer D (2002). Arthroscopic findings in patients with chronic ankle instability. Am J Sports Med 30: 402–409.

Hintermann B, Valderrabano V, Boss AP, Trouillier HH, Dick EW (2004). Medial ankle instability – an exploratory prospective study of 52 cases. Am J Sports Med 32: 183–190.

Hintermann B (1995). Biomechanical aspects of muscle-tendon functions. Orthopäde 24: 187–192.

Hintermann B (1996). Biomechanics of the ligaments of the unstable ankle joint. Sportverletz Sportschaden 10: 48–54.

Hintermann B, Holzach P, Matter P (1990). The treatment of fibular ligament lesions using the Ortho-Rehab shoe. Schweiz Z Sportmed 38: 87–93.

Hintermann B, Holzach P, Matter P (1992). Injury pattern of the fibular ligaments. Radiological diagnosis and clinical study. Unfallchirurg 95: 142–147.

Hintermann B, Rengli P (1999). Anatomic reconstruction of the lateral ligaments of the ankle using a plantaris tendon graft in the treatment of chronic ankle joint instability. Orthopäde 28: 778–784.

Jackson DW, Ashley RD, Powell JW (1974). Ankle sprains in young athletes: relation of severity and disability. Clin Orthop 101: 201–215.

Nunley JA, Vertullo CJ (2002). Classification, investigation, and management of midfoot sprains: Lisfranc injuries in athletes. Am J Sports Med 30: 871–879.

Pagenstert GI, Valderrabano V, Hintermann B (2005). Reconstruction of chronic lateral ankle instability using plantaris graft. Tech Foot Ankle Surg 4: 104–112.

Pagenstert GI, Valderrabano V, Hintermann B (2005). Treatment of sesamoid nonunion combined with hallux valgus in athletes. Foot Ankle In (in press).

Rachun A (1968). Standard nomenclature of athletic injuries. American Medical Association, Chicago, pp 99–100.

Schäfer D, Hintermann B (1996). Diagnostic imaging of ankle joint instability. Sportverletz Sportschaden 10: 55–57.

Shapiro MS, Kabo M, Mitchell PW, et al. (1994). Ankle sprain prophylaxis: An analysis of the stabilizing effects of braces and tape. Am J Sports Med 22: 78–82.

Chapter 22 The skeletal muscle

Martin Engelhardt, Matthias Kieb and Olaf Lorbach

The human skeletal muscles constitute about 50 per cent of the body weight; hence, muscle injuries are common. The incidence rate varies in literature between 10 and 55 per cent. Depending on the extent of trauma, a muscle injury may bar an athlete from sport for several months or even end a career, if treated improperly. Only few athletes are aware that an incorrectly treated muscle injury significantly increases the risk of repeated injury.

Today, skeletal muscle is no longer perceived as an isolated issue but as a functional system of muscles, tendon, tendo-osseous transition as well as fascial internal and wrapping structure. The muscle function depends on an intact, proprioceptive activity, motor innervations, mechanical stress, the ability to perform the stretch-shortening cycle and the mobility of a joint.

The skeletal muscle is an organ that can respond in just a few milliseconds because of a direct nervous connection to the joint structures. Due to the high metabolic rate, the time delayed structure-morphological adaptation of the muscles is more pronounced than that of other tissue types, which can be demonstrated by advanced imaging techniques, such as sonography and MRT to determine cross section and volume of the muscle, or by muscle biopsies.

22.1 Structure and control of muscle system

The muscles consist of parallel, elongated, polynuclear muscle fibers. Every muscle fiber consists of numerous parallel myofibrils and the latter of myofilaments. Under the light microscope a longitudinal section the skeletal muscle fibers reveals a cross striation. The latter is created by bright I-bands and dark A-bands. The muscle fibers can be divided into red high mitochondrial type 1 fibers and white low mitochondrial type 2 fibers.

The muscle is controlled centrally by alpha motoneurons and gamma motoneurons. Afferent nerve fibers from the muscle itself, the assigned joints and the skin transmit information on the condition of the biological system from the periphery to the spinal cord and brain. Via polysynaptic connections these afferent nerve fibers influence the central control.

Visceral and vegetative influences and individual psychic factors haven an additional modifying effect.

Mechanical and chemical information is captured by receptors that can be found both in the joint structures (ligaments, menisci, capsules) and in the periarticular tissue (muscles, tendons). The muscle spindles located inside the muscles allow for a differentiated motor control and as a length control system they have a protecting effect on the muscles while the Golgi tendon organs act as a tension control system. Information on pressure, position and movement of joints is registered primarily by Pacini, Ruffini and Golgi organs, in border areas of physiological strength also by free nerve endings (pain perception).

A special position is taken by the free nerve endings. They signal unphysiological states. Multimodal receptors exist along mechanosensitive, thermosensitive and chemosensitive nerve endings. They are capable of responding to substances of the inflammation metabolism, such as bradykinin, carnitine, serotonin and histamine. Part of the free nerve endings is itself capable of releasing substances that reinforce inflammation processes.

22.2 Classification of muscle injuries

Muscle injuries can be classified into acute and chronic injuries. Based on the localization, a more specific allocation is possible (e.g. venter, muscle-tendon transition, tendon and tendon attachment at bone).

Most authors classify muscle injuries into three or four degrees:

- **Degree 1**: Rupture of individual muscle fibers with intact fascia (structure destruction <5% of muscle fibers)
- **Degree 2**: Rupture of several muscle fibers with intact fascia and localized hematoma involving a disruption of continuity of >5% of muscle fibers
- **Degree 3**: Rupture of multiple muscle fibers including partial rupture of the fascia and diffuse hemorrhage at a disruption of continuity of >5% of muscle fibers.
- **Degree 4**: Complete muscle and fascia rupture involving loss of function.

22.3 Mechanisms and causes of injury

Literature reports a range of injury mechanisms. Most muscle injuries are a result of sudden, intense muscle stretches above the tolerance limits and of contusions. Eccentric contractions triggered by sharp acceleration, a sudden stop of acceleration or unexpected change from an eccentric contraction to a concentric, result in an increased tendency of muscle injuries.

> Non load-adapted muscles (insufficient warm-up with an inadequate vascular flow, poor training condition, fatigued or hypothermic muscles) lead to a higher susceptibility to injuries.

Moreover, unhealed injuries, infectious diseases, insufficiently compensated fluid losses including electrolyte disturbances, muscular imbalances, and unsuitable sports equipment increase the risk of muscle injury.

Superficial muscles running over two joints and frequently performing antagonistic functions (e.g. M. rectus femoris, M. semitendinosus and M. gastrocnemius) are especially vulnerable to muscle injuries.

Direct muscle injuries occur upon contact with an opposing player or collision with a hard obstacle. Muscle ruptures caused by overstretching can be primarily found in sports with sprint and jump loads.

In previous muscle injuries the connective tissue forms scars in the muscle structure. The predilection point for a repeated muscle injury is located at the boundary between scar and muscle.

22.4 Pathobiology of muscle healing

After a muscle injury, the healing process progresses **as a repair process in three phases**:

1. Destruction and inflammation phase
2. Reparation phase
3. Remodeling/Repair phase.

Skeletal muscle fibers have postmitotic cell nuclei that have lost their replication capacity. However, the muscle accommodates stem cells (satellite cells) in addition to muscle fibers that have preserved their replicative capacity (Wernig and Irintchev (2001); ➢ Fig. 22.1 and ➢ Fig. 22.2). Wernig demonstrated that muscle fiber sections die after injuries due to noxae of different sort without the muscle fibers causing to perish. While the necrotic fiber sections are engulfed (phagocytosis) by infiltrating macrophages, the basal lamina remains intact in many cases. Surviving satellite cells are activated just a few hours after the injury. These cells, now called myoblasts, reproduce in the subsequent days and eventually merge to become myotubes (➢ Fig. 22.3). However, the complete fiber type differentiation, the achiev-

22.4 Pathology of muscle healing

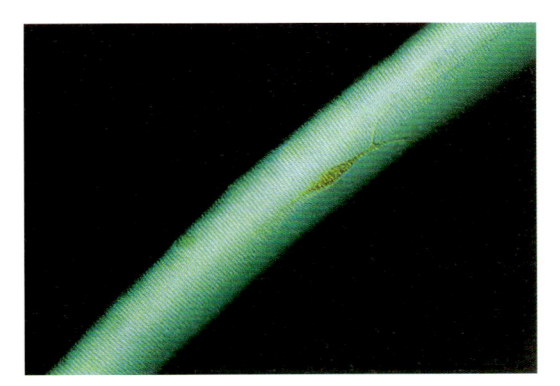

Fig. 22.1 Light microscopical visualization of a satellite cell (brown) on the surface of a single skeletal muscle fibre (reproduced from Wernig and Irintchev 2001)

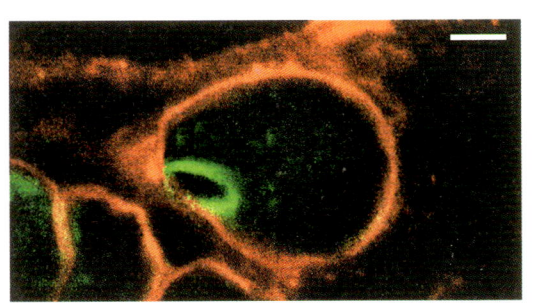

Fig. 22.2 Light microscopical ross-section of a skeletal muscle satellite cell (green) under the basal lamina (reproduced from Wernig and Irintchev 2001)

ing of the normal fiber diameter and the development of normal contraction properties of the muscle require reinnervation.

> Complete healing takes minimum 3 weeks but may even take up to 6 to 13 weeks.

However, limits are set to the muscles' good reparation capacity. After a number of divisions, the muscle cells start ageing, i.e. the cell division comes to a halt eventually.

The entire process of muscle healing is impressively demonstrated in Järvinen's diagram (➤ Fig. 22.4; Järvinen et al. 2005):

1. **Destruction and inflammation phase**: Initially, parts of the muscle fibers die resulting in an inflammatory cell reaction and formation of a hematoma between the ruptured muscle fibers. The healing process is slowed

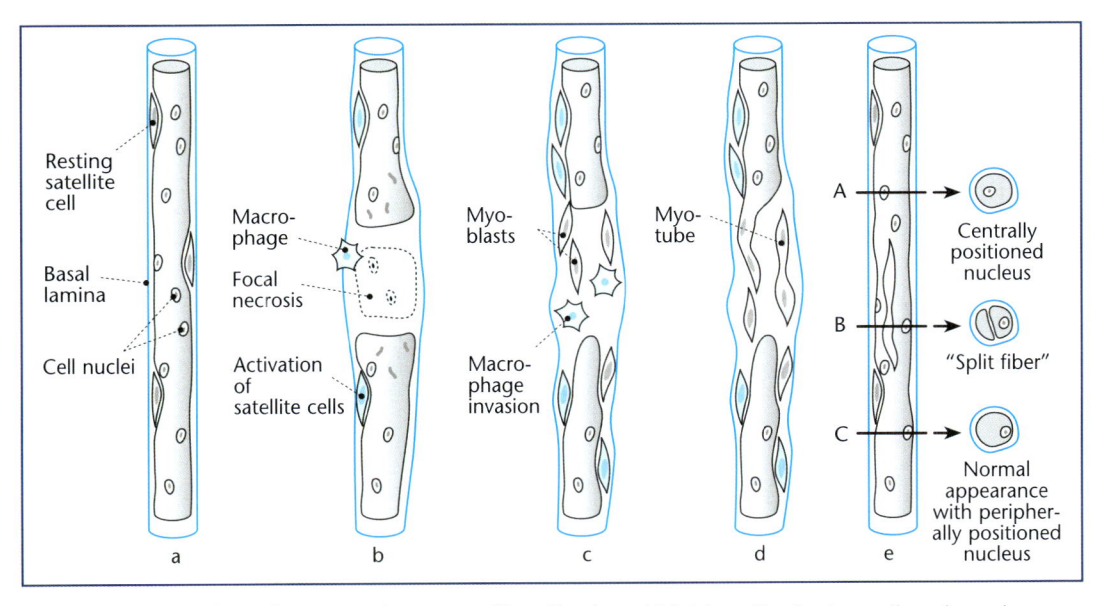

Fig. 22.3 Diagram of muscle regeneration process (from Wernig and Irintchev: Muscle stem cells and muscle regeneration. Sportorthopädie, Sporttraumatologie 2001; 17: 5–10) a: intact skeletal muscle fiber with peripheral nuclei. B: Focal necrosis, macrophage invasion and activation of satellite cells. C: Phagocytosis of cell debris, migration and replication of myoblasts. d: Differentiation and merger of myoblasts. e: Regenerated muscle fiber with regeneration-related structural features: centrally located nucleus (cross section at A) and 'split fiber' (cross section at B); C = normal appearance cross section with a peripheral nucleus.

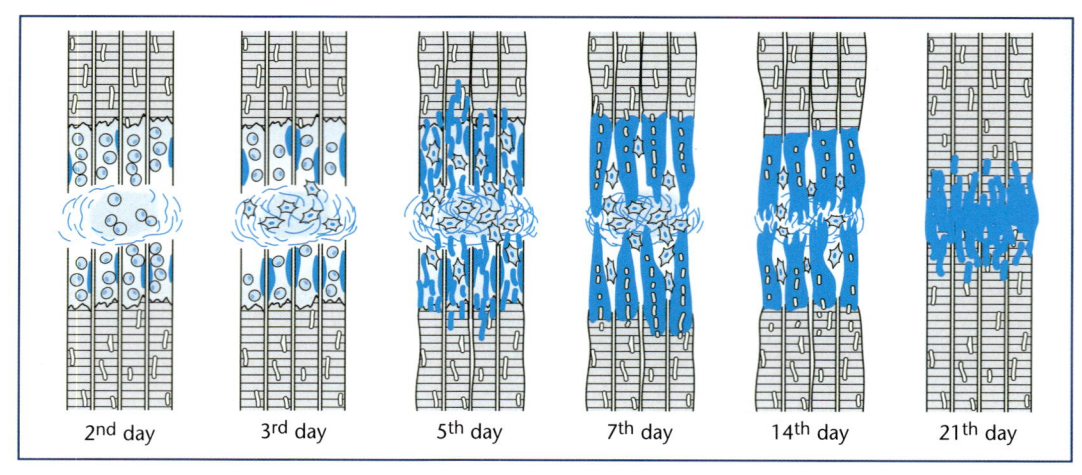

Fig. 22.4 Muscle healing process (from Järvinen et al.: Muscle injuries – biology and treatment. Am J Sports Med 2005 (vol. 33) 5: 745–764)

2nd day   3rd day   5th day   7th day   14th day   21th day

down by the intramuscular or extramuscular hematoma. In addition, the connective tissue forms more and more scars and the fiber regeneration processes is lengthened. The aim of influencing the healing process is therefore, among other things, the avoidance of excessive hematoma formation and a quick removal of hematomas from the injured area.

2. **Reparation phase**: The phagocytosis of the destroyed cell debris by macrophages is followed by a regeneration of muscle fibers as shown in the diagrams ➤ Fig. 22.3 and ➤ Fig. 22.4 by Wernig and Järvinen. In addition, the capillary budding into the injured area sets in, that is why the muscle needs to be optimally supplied with oxygen for the healing process. Muscle fiber regeneration reaches its climax after two weeks; the forming connective tissue scar keeps intensifying up to about 4 weeks after the injury.

3. **Remodeling/Repair phase**: This phase overlaps with the reparation phase. The functional capacity of the muscles is restored, for example by reinnervation (➤ Fig. 22.5).

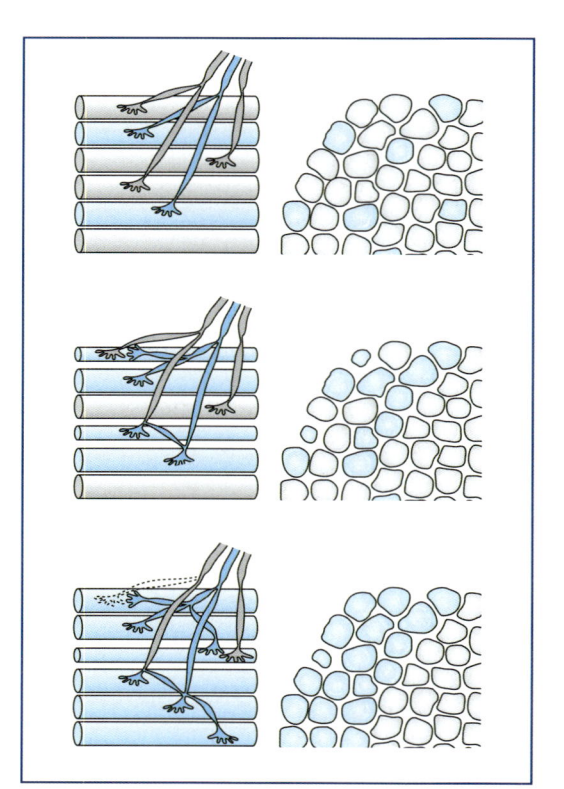

Fig. 22.5 Schematic representation of muscle function repair through innervation-related fiber type conversion in the skeletal muscle upon muscle injury (lateral view and cross section) (from Wernig and Irintchev: Muskelstammzellen und Muskelregeneration. Sportorthopädie Sporttraumatologie 2001; 17: 5–10). Top: Heterogeneous distribution of muscle fibers (blue, blue axon) and rapidly contracting fibers (grey, grey axon). Centre: Axonal budding and synapse formation. Bottom: Fiber type conversion with relevantly changed fiber type distribution triggered by the new additional innervations.

22.5 Diagnostics of muscle injuries

Anamnesis and physical examination

The **anamnesis** reveals the injury mechanism thus giving important information for the diagnosis.

In the **physical examination**, inspection, palpation and functional analysis usually supply the experienced colleague with clear results.

With degree 1 injuries, sometimes also those of the degree 2 and 3, signs of discomfort may be initially absent in the relaxed muscle. In degree 2 and 3 injuries, a disruption of muscle continuity is already sometimes palpable. With degree 4 injuries, the deformation of the injured muscle is verifiable with certainty by the relevant loss of function.

The area surrounding the injury is often swollen and hurts upon contact. After just a few hours, the injured area becomes livid. Muscular cramps can also be palpated in many cases.

Imaging

The ease and availability combined with the high informative value makes sonography a gold standard screening method. Muscle ruptures and intramuscular and extramuscular hematomas can be clearly identified based on the echotexture (➤ Fig. 22.6). Under sonographic control the hematoma can be punctured and injections made at the site of injury, if necessary. One advantage of sonography is that it allows a dynamic assessment of the muscles and tendons during movement. It can supply information on the kind of disorder of the muscle-tendon unit. The results depend very much on the examiner, however, and are not unqualifiedly reproducible. Skills and experience of the colleagues are essential.

Magnetic resonance tomography is an excellent means to display muscle injuries. It is therefore especially suited to diagnose hard-to-reach muscle injuries.

By selecting relevant sequences and administering paramagnetic substances even metabolic information can be obtained.

Conventional X-ray diagnostics has only a limited sensitivity for muscle injuries. Chippings, calcifications (myositis ossificans) and, if necessary, contours of soft tissue shadows can be depicted by a soft tissue X-ray.

Scintigraphy as an excellent method to detect stress fractures can also be used to determine damage to the muscle and the tendo-osseous transition caused by overstressing. The diagnostic significance is limited, however, due to the low specificity and the lack of morphological information.

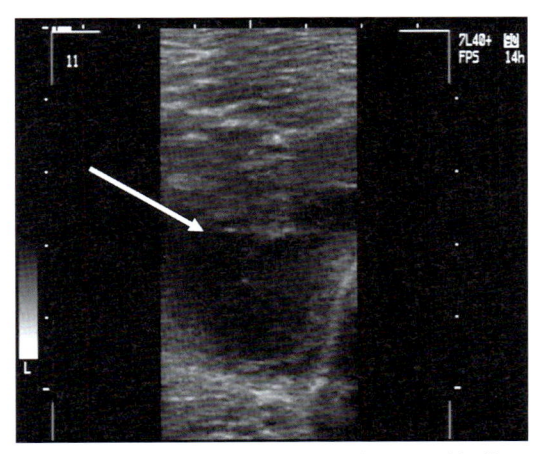

Fig. 22.6 Intramuscular hematoma (sonographic illustration).

22.6 Treatment of acute muscle injuries

22.6.1 Acute treatment

The blood flow in the muscles (resting state 0.8 l/min) may be 18 l/min in physical exercise. In the event of a muscle injury in sports substantial bleeding must therefore be expected at the site of injury. The larger the post-traumatic hematoma the larger will be the connective tissue scar and the more unfavorable the conditions for a repair of the muscle function.

> The main purpose of first treatment is the containment of bleeding after the injury.

The athlete is barred from further sports activities and a compression dressing in form of an elastic bandage or compression cuff is applied. The extremities have to be relieved and rested in an elevated position. Initially cooling is done at regular intervals (minimum 20 min. per hour). Bleeding and edema should be reduced. Therefore, all measures to warm up the injured part of the body and massages should initially be banned. Drugs for muscle relaxation can be administered.

In the first 12 to 24 hours, hematoma formation should come to an end and the extent of injury stabilizes. During this time, the athlete should be under a physician's care. Should the pressure in the soft tissue increase excessively, a surgical intervention (hematoma removal and staunching of bleeding) may become necessary.

After 24 hours the hematoma spreading can be reliably assessed. To reduce the hematoma, puncturing under sonography may be necessary.

In the event the hematoma has assumed a solid state, it can be removed by a small incision. It is also possible to liquefy the solid hematoma again by administering plasminogen activator (Actilyse) and puncture it under sonography. Puncturing is done 12 to 24 hours after medication. Should bleeding relapse, puncturing may become necessary several times every two or three days.

22.6.2 Conservative treatment

Degree 1 injuries and part of the degree 2 and 3 injuries can be treated conservatively. After hematoma removal and completion of the acute-phase treatment an elastic compression bandage is applied in the injured region for two to three weeks. Depending on the kind and extent of injury, treatment through exercise follows after a minimum of five days rest.

The athlete usually expects a quick return to full activity.

> In the event of a muscle injury, the consequences of premature resumption of activities must be explained to the athlete in detail.

Though the kind of treatment always needs to be tailored to the individual athlete and depends on the scope of injury, the biological principles of muscle healing must be taken into account.

The following **timing** for the training program is recommended:

- In the first few days, the training must be limited to static, stress-free exercises.
- Dynamic exercises can be started after one week at the earliest. Scope and intensity of the exercises are limited by the pain.
- Stretching and sensorimotor training should not begin earlier than after two weeks.
- Training with sport equipment (e.g. bicycle ergometer) should start not earlier than three weeks after an injury.
- Training in the specific form of sport usually begins in the 5th week after the injury.

This recommendation should be understood as a model framework program and needs to be tailored to the individual injury. But in any case+ it is strongly advised to avoid any premature uncontrolled physical stress.

As regards **medication,** we recommend muscle relaxants and non-steroidal antiphlogistic agents for the first two weeks after the injury.

According to our experience, massages including muscle stretching elements should start two weeks after the injury at the earliest.

22.6.3 Surgical treatment

Muscle injuries are still conservatively treated in German-speaking countries. International research findings clearly show, however, that major muscle injuries with disruption of continuity have to be treated surgically. In animal tests the best treatment results could be achieved by a surgical muscle suture with a restored maximum contractibility of about 80 per cent compared to the opposing extremity. On the other hand maximum contractibility after conservative early function treatment was 35 per cent compared to the opposing extremity and just 18 per cent in case of immobilization.

An optimum treatment requires a quick decision (at best within 48 hours after the injury) as regards surgical intervention. Surgery is always indicated in cases of **complete muscle rupture and degree 2 and 3 injuries of muscles** that have antagonistic muscles or where existing muscles

22.6 Treatment of acute muscle injuries

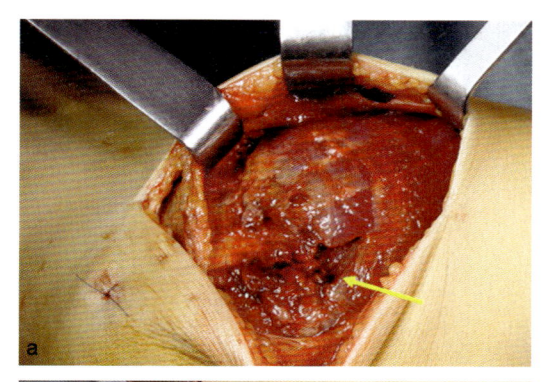

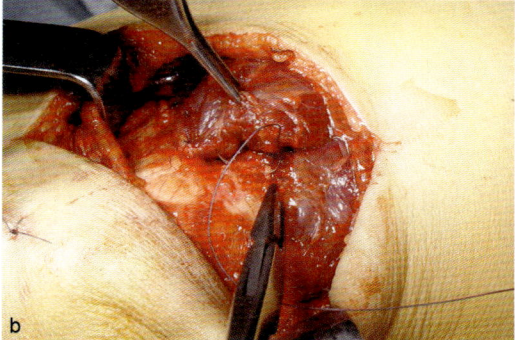

Fig. 22.7 Surgery of a muscle injury
a: Intra-operative site of an abdominal muscle injury (M. adductor longus). b: Surgical tratment to gain functional, optimal results.

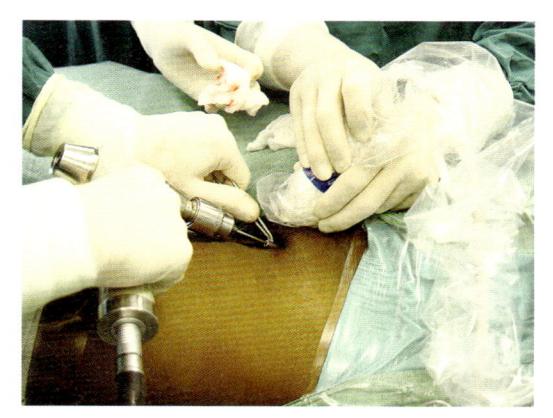

Fig. 22.8 Surgical treatment of a muscle enthesopathy: image guided spot drilling of the pubic bone to stimulate regeneration

are incapable of compensating the work of the injured muscle (➤ Fig. 22.7a and b).

After surgery the extremity should be immobilized and relieved for about 7 days. Subsequent rehabilitation depends on the assessment by sonography of the site of intervention. A rehab program is always tailored to the extent of injury and the function of the muscle concerned.

In cases of **muscle detachment from bone projections or at the tendon attachment**, the indication regarding surgical refixation must be made generously. Especially those muscles should receive adequate surgical treatment that contributes to pelvis stabilization while standing on one leg. It particularly relates to the adductors. This muscle group frequently displays muscle attachment enthesiopathies. In the early stage, the healing process can be stimulated by drilling at the muscle attachment. It can be performed by a stab incision image-intensifier assisted (➤ Fig. 22.8). It is a minimal-invasive surgery in most cases without hospital stay. Generally after three to four weeks, the changes have healed including complete disappearance of discomfort. If the degenerative process has progressed too far, it may be necessary to remove the degenerated tissue from the muscle attachment by surgery.

After the refixation of muscles detached from the bone, the extremity concerned should be saved for three weeks. During this time it is possible for the operated muscle group to do isometric exercises. A mobilization should be done with underarm walkers only. Sonography of the site of surgery is indicated after three weeks. After that further training that includes stretching and increasingly intensive strength exercises begins. Five weeks after surgery it is usually possible to start dynamic exercises.

22.6.4 Influencing the healing process

In the treatment, the pathophysiological principles of muscle healing must always be taken into account. A **quick hematoma removal** reduces the formation of connective tissue scars and accelerates the regeneration processes.

In animal tests, injections of connective tissue growth factors into the site of injury showed a positive effect on muscle healing. Administration of IGF-1 (insulin-like growth factor 1), bFGF (basic fibroblast growth factor) and NGF (nerve growth factor) 2, 5 and 7 days after muscle injuries increased the force of the maximum contractions. The strongest muscle regeneration stimulating effect was detected for IGF-1. Because of the easy availability and low costs, **PDGF** (Platelet-Derived Growth Factor) can be used in clinical practice. PDGF stimulates, for instance, the proliferation of satellite cells. The preparation time for administration is 40 to 60 minutes. According to the authors' experiences the injured muscle tissue heals faster after PDGF administration so that the athlete may resume his/her sports activities 30% earlier.

Research studies also use the preparation **Decorin** to inhibit the formation of connective tissue scars and optimize the muscle regeneration. Decorin is a human proteoglycan acting as an inhibitor of TGF-B1 (transforming growth factor B 1). This preparation is administered 15 days after the muscle injury, i.e. at a time of the healing phase with usually the strongest formation of connective tissue.

22.7 Relapsing/chronic muscle injuries

Insufficient healing of a primary muscle injury and a premature resumption of sports activities may result in a repeat injury. This is usually linked to **new scars formation,** thus limiting the elasticity of the muscle. If the scar formation is too pronounced or adhesions develop between the muscles and the intact muscle fascia, a **scar removal** may be necessary. Scar formations may result in **neuromuscular coordination disorders or cramps.** The impaired contraction behavior of the muscles and the changed elasticity of fascie and gliding layers may trigger pain perceived by the athlete as pressure, cramp or pulling ache.

> Scar formation processes may substantially hamper the athlete's performance.

Chronic muscle injuries also include **intramuscular ossifications,** also called myositis ossificans. It is a calcification of muscle tissue due to metaplasia of histiocytes in osteoblasts. Such dysfunction may occur posttraumatically in the case of pronounced hematoma formation and medical errors (premature massage of the in-

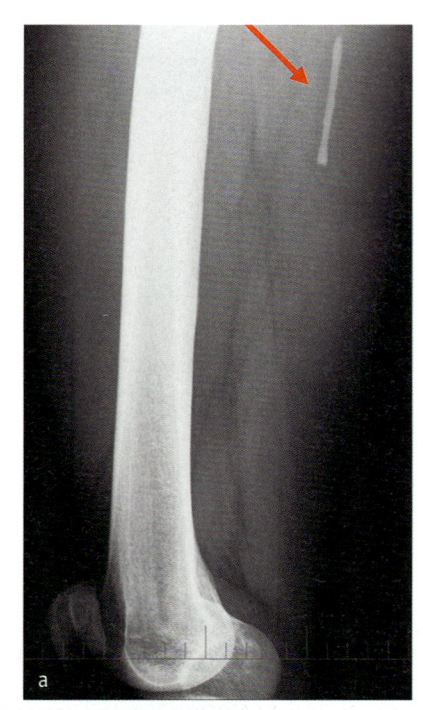

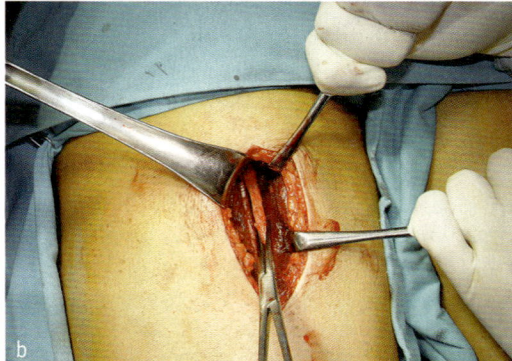

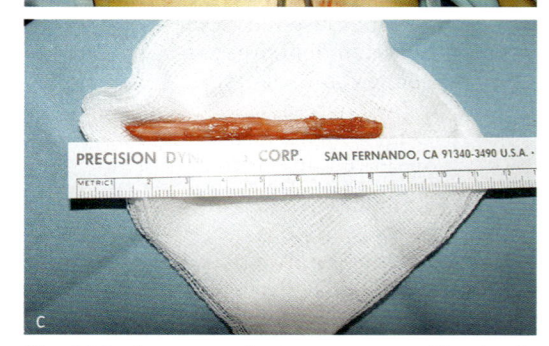

Fig. 22.9 Treatment of extra-osseous ossification in muscles. a: Extra-osseous ossification at the thigh (X-ray); b: Intra-operative site of ossification at the abdomen; c: 7 cm long ossification.

jured site, insufficient immobilization, premature resumption of training neglecting the pain). Also discussed is the presence of a genetic disposition.

Should such ossification affect the athlete's physical capacity, it must be removed by surgery (➤ Fig. 22.9 a–c). The surgery indication should be made with caution and only be opted if the findings are no longer progredient, i.e. the inflammation temperature and the alkaline phosphatase must be falling. Some authors recommend surgery after six months when the inflammation process has come to an end.

22.8 Compartment syndrome

The **acute muscle compartment syndrome** is often a result of a direct trauma or a plaster cast applied too tightly. The trauma damages the soft tissue resulting most frequently in an anterior, lateral and posterior compartment syndrome of the lower extremities.

The clinical symptoms are pain, exacerbation of pain under passive stretch of the muscles affected by the compartment, and sensitive and motor-neurological symptoms. The peripheral pulses can be maintained even with a fully developed compartment syndrome. The pulse may be weakened if the arterial vessel runs through the mainly affected area. Lack of pulse is a rare phenomenon and late sign.

The elevated intracompartmental pressure that can be measured in case of diagnostic doubt, leads to under-oxygenation of the muscles (ischemia) and, if neglected or inadequately treated, to muscle necrosis. Therefore, a quick fasciotomy is indicated in cases of acute muscle compartment syndrome.

Chronic compartment syndromes are a result of overstressing. Massages, stretching, an optimization of the running style, biomechanical corrections of any structure defect, selection of suitable sports shoes with hyperpronation correction, if necessary, and a continuous muscle training can be suitable conservative treatment measures. If conditions persist, fascial split can be indicated.

22.9 Prevention of muscle injuries

Most essential preventive measures are proper warming-up prior to sports activities and post-processing of the physical stress, a targeted muscle training adapted to the individual athlete and correct stretching exercises. Important factors are also a target-oriented balancing of muscular imbalances, general fitness training and optimization of technical movement sequences. Suitable sports equipment and the use of protective equipment are as helpful as the knowledge of the driving mechanisms of muscle injuries. Mention should be made again of the risk of muscle injuries due to malnutrition and fluid loss and training under the influence of infectious diseases and focal infections (teeth, tonsils).

22.10 Muscular dysbalances

Muscular imbalances are blamed both for reduced sporting performance and development and maintenance of locomotor and postural disorders. They are usually detected manually and are defined as follows:

- Comparison between an examined and an assumed value (standard value)
- Comparison of one extremity with the other (right/left, injured/intact)
- Comparison of two antagonistic muscles attached to a joint (flexor/extensor, agonist/antagonist).
- Comparison of synergistic muscles (M. quadriceps femoris with selective weaking of M. vastus medialis).

Setting up muscular standard values has proven to be a difficult effort. Individual factors, such as age, sex, height, weight, form of sport as well as person-related locomotion patterns play a role. The averages of a standard population cannot be used to derive individual training recommendations. In particular, this statement is evident for competitive sports where a one-sided development of basic motor skills areas is required.

Trainers and therapists must differentiate desired, training-related and performance-requiring adjustments of the skeletal muscle (special norm) and undesired changes with pathological causes and potentiality as well as compensatory changes. The boundary between healthy and ill is fluid but not every deviation from normative values in sport should be considered an imbalance.

Considering that the skeletal muscle is controlled by the central nervous system and every change of the muscle is primarily a result of a changed control, the term **neuromuscular imbalance** has been introduced (Engelhardt et al. 1997). In view of the great variety of factors that may cause a neuromuscular imbalance, one-sided treatment approaches do not make sense.

To treat neuromuscular imbalances or influence them through targeted training measures, it is necessary to know the causes. The aspect of muscle control deserves increased attention because morphological changes of the muscles develop in the first place by the specific use or non-use of the same.

> In sports, multi-faceted training must be offered to avoid neuromuscular imbalances.

References

Engelhardt M, Freiwald J, Reuter I (1997). Muskulatur. In: Engelhardt M et al. GOTS-Manual Sporttraumatologie. Verlag Hans Huber, Bern, pp. 161–169.

Fukushima K, Badlani, N, Usas A, Riano F, Fu F, Huard J (2001). The use of antifibrosis agent to improve muscle recovery after laceration. Am J Sports Med 29: 394–402.

Huard J, Li Y, Fu FH (2002). Muscle injuries and repair: current trends in research. J Bone Joint Surg 84A: 822–832.

Järvinen TAH et al. (2005). Muscle injuries-biology and treatment. Am J Sports Med 33(5): 745–764.

Kasemkijwattana C, Menetrey J, Bosch P et al. (2000). Use of growth factors to improve muscle healing after strain injury. Clin Orthop 370: 272–285.

Menetrey J, Kasemkijwattana C, Day CS et al. (2000). Growth factors improve muscle healing in vivo. J Bone Joint Surg 82B: 131–137.

Wernig A, Irintchev A (2001). Muskelstammzellen und Muskelregeneration. Sportorthopädie Sporttraumatologie 17: 5–10.

Zichner L, Engelhardt M, Freiwald J (1994). Die Muskulatur – sensibles integratives und meßbares Organ. Wehr, Ciba-Geigy.

Chapter 23
Stress reactions of the bones

Karlheinz Graff

Not only traumatic events can lead to bone fractures. Also common use or athletic stress without a sudden event can damage the structure of the bone. This type of fracture is called "stress fracture" or "stress reaction", depending on the representation of the morphologic damage in the imaging procedures.

It is difficult to imagine that a solid osseous tissue can fracture only by "simple" physical or athletic stress. Sometimes also physicians consider a stress fracture as the last possibility in the case of disorders. Still, already a "simple" barefoot walk on the beach or a "banal" endurance run can lead to increasing pain or even to stress insufficiency of the foot. After the first mistaken assumption of "overstress" or "tendovaginitis", a stress fracture, e.g. of a midfoot bone, is often diagnosed after consulting of several colleagues.

Already in 1855, the Prussian physician Breithaupt diagnosed the **"march fracture"** in the midfoot of soldiers. These overuse symptoms have been called fatigue fractures for a long time. Nonetheless, the term of "stress" mirrors the **excess of mechanical stimuli** better than "fatigue", which is a physiological phenomenon.

In purely scintigraphic findings or a presentation in an imaging procedure untypical for a fracture, the term "stress fracture" should be substituted by the term **"stress reaction"** (Graff et al. 1987). The normal healing of stress reactions and stress fractures is retarded by late diagnosis and leads to severe training deficiencies in sport.

23.1 Etiology

The same as musculature and tendon, the bone tissue cannot be stressed infinitely. The exceeding of individual stress limits leads to the impairment of the osseous structure (Daffner 1978, Orava and Myllälä 1982, Torg et al. 1982, Wilkerson and Johns 1990). The close connection between types of stress and practice and the localization of the impairment indicates a **mechanical component** in the development (Devas 1958, Krahl et al. 1978, Graff and Krahl 1984, Graff et al. 1985, Graff et al. 1986, Meuermann and Elfving 1980, Orava and Myllälä 1982, Pavlow et al. 1983, Graff and Heinold 1987, Graff 2004).

Stress fractures of the bone are observed almost exclusively in the **lower extremity** in **dynamic sports** with a high ratio of running and jumping stress. Nonetheless, not only excessive or unfamiliar stress leads to "attrition" of the "healthy" bone (**"fatigue fracture"**). "Normal" mechanic use can also damage bone tissue of lesser stability (**"insufficiency fracture"**) (Pecina et al. 1990).

There is the reasonable purpose to recognize an **individually decreased osseous stability** by diagnostic measures especially in sports. Prophylactic treatment would be possible this way, kinds of practice and stress with high demands on the skeleton could be avoided. Individual differences of tissue stability, robustness and training tolerance in athletes can scarcely be found by diagnostic procedures, though. Nonetheless, they do exist.

The correlation between osseous stability and **hormonal constellation** is unquestioned. Polytope stress fractures in short succession without "excessive" stress in female athletes with noticeable hormonal profiles **(reduced osteogenic hormones)** and decreased values of bone density have been described (Wilson and Katz 1969, Krahl and Knebel 1978, Graff and Heinold 1987, Graff 1991). Nonetheless, stress fractures are no "hormonal fractures" (Graff 1991). They also develop in normal hormonal constellation. Their increased appearance especially in large collectives of athletes with a "psychologically" assumed reduction of bone density has not been described so far. This includes the **mass-sport movement of the 40-year-olds and older athletes**. These athletes often expect their bodies to perform stress comparable to high-performance sports. This involves especially the **long-distance running**, in which the quantity of practice and especially the frequency of competition are no less than the ones for high-performance athletes.

The procedures of **measuring the bone density** available by now allow the recognition of a **general decrease of bone density**. A local "weak point" of a bone segment of an athlete at a certain time cannot be recognized yet.

The "fracture" is defined as complete or incomplete **separation of continuity** of the bone (Hilfe 1980, Debrunner 1983). **Traumatic fracture** and **stress "fracture"** differ in the dynamics of their development, in the process of medical conditions and in morphology.

> In contrast to a "traumatic fracture", the separation of continuity is rarely complete in stress fractures in sports.

The conditions lead mostly to stress incapacity even before the occurrence of a fracture.

The kind of circumscribed damage of the bone often is not "fracture-typical".

Defective zones of bone structure fulfilling the criteria of an **osteonecrosis** in the imaging procedures in a stress fracture (Graff et al. 1986, Graff 1987 and 1993) are not uncommon. The **term stress "reaction"** makes more sense in these cases, because the attention of the inexperienced is not necessarily fixed to a fracture gap on the radiograph (Graff and Heinold 1987).

23.2 Diagnostics

23.2.1 Picture of symptoms and clinical findings

The anamnesis and the clinical findings indicate for diagnosis of stress phenomena of the bone. The differentiation into established kinds with typical localizations (region of the midfoot, fibula, and tibia) and typical radiographic image as well as into special kinds cannot be fully perpetuated by the new imaging procedures. Stress impairments with missing or "untypical" representation in the imaging procedures, stress fractures with atypical symptoms and clinical progression as well as uncommon localization (e.g carpus, tarsus, pelvic region; Graff and Heinold 1987) belong to the special kinds.

The increasing **stress incapacity** for dynamic and especially reactive forms of training and stress (e.g. jumps and landings) is indicatory. The **period of time** from the first symptoms to stress incapacity can last hours or even weeks.

The **examination findings** can be very discrete. **Local periosteal swellings** are typical, though not obligatory, and discrete in the beginning (midfoot bone, tibia, and fibula); they are scarcely found in other forms (carpus, tarsus). **Acute forms of progression** with suddenly occurring symptoms or with acute acerbation of present symptoms might occur. The sudden, fierce local pain or a pain-conditioned instability in the motion process with successive stress incapability (e.g. putting down the foot, in jumping or landing) is typical here.

Discrepancies between subjective symptoms, clinical and especially radiological findings can complicate the correct assessment of the picture of symptoms. Too often the correct diagnosis is delayed by the assumption of "overuse symptoms", "periosteal inflammations" and "tendovaginitis".

23.2.1 Imaging procedures

Depending on the localization and on the type of bones (tubular bones, spongiose bones), the radiologic evidence can be difficult or missing.

23.2 Diagnostics

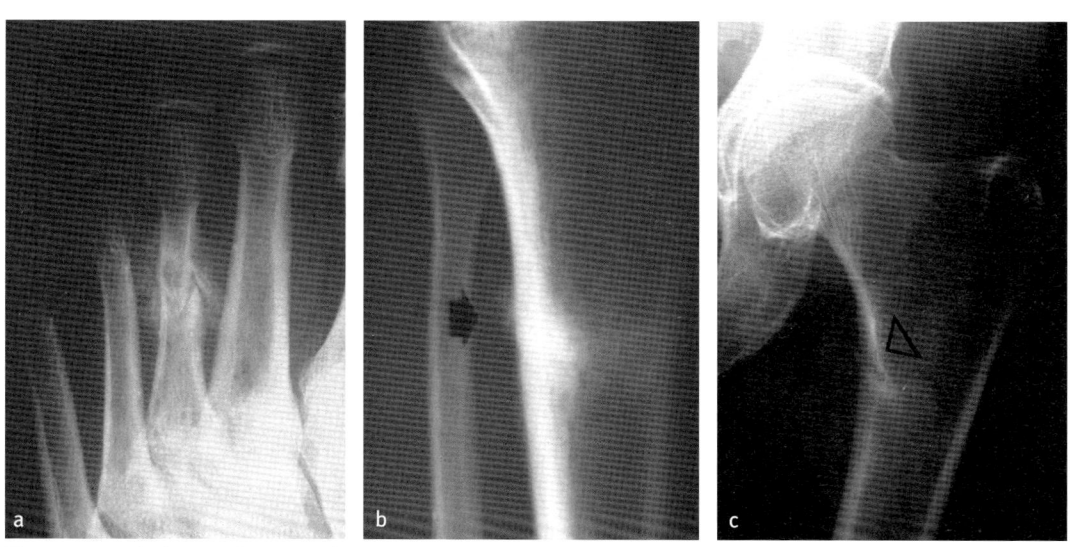

Fig. 23.1 Typical stress fractures of metatarsal (a), tibia (b), and proximal thigh (c). Fracture gap, perifocal callus, endosteal densification.

Radiologic criteria (➤ Fig. 23.1 a–c) are:
- periosteal reactions
- endosteal swellings
- focal sclerosing and
- external callus formations.

Fracture lines are not obligatory. The display on the **radiograph** is influenced significantly by the state of the injury at the time of diagnosis (Daffner 1978). Radiographic spotfilms and radiographic tomograms for rare localizations or questionable findings have been superseded by the use of **magnetic resonance and computer tomography** in further diagnosis (➤ Fig. 23.2 a and b; Towne et al. 1970, Keene and Lash 1992, Breitner and Yousri 1993).

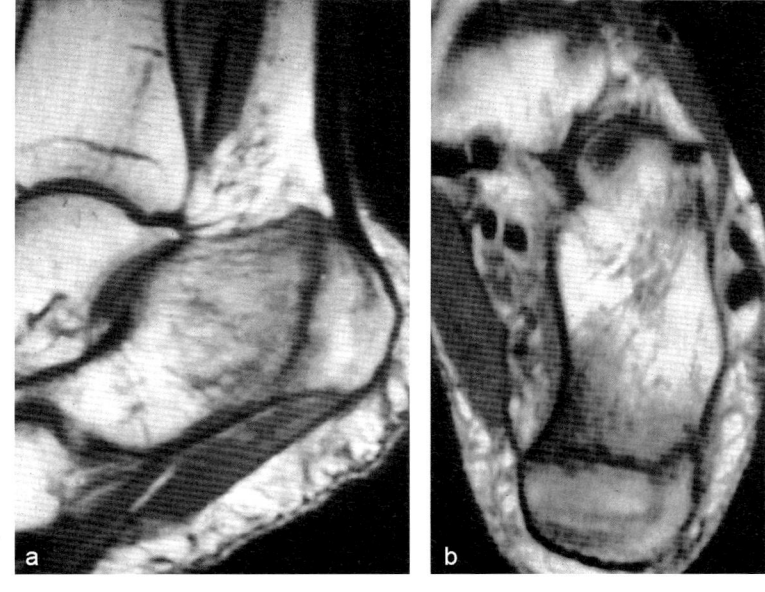

Fig. 23.2 Calcaneal stress fracture.

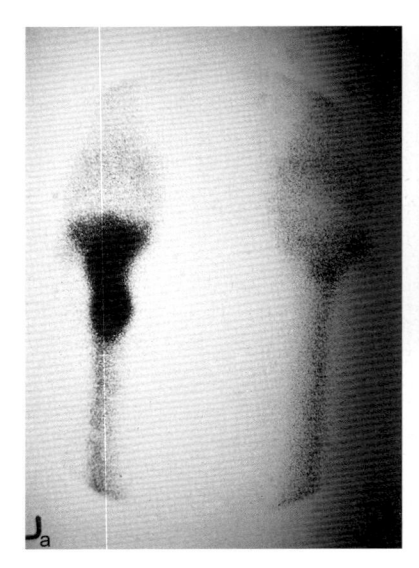

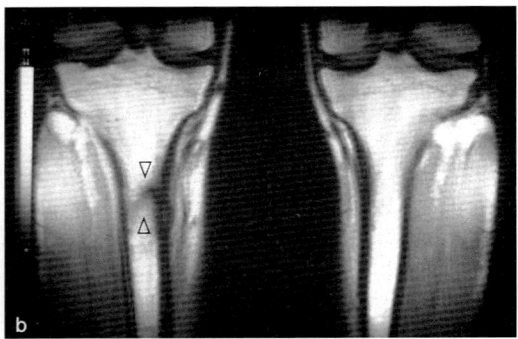

Fig. 23.3 Tibial stress fracture. a: Scintigraphic findings. b: MRI.

The extent and the state of damage as well as the perifocal tissue reaction are displayed incomparably earlier and better in the area of the spongiose bone regions (e.g. carpus, tarsus), and the question of the kind of treatment is facilitated significantly.

Stress fractures and stress reactions are usually found early by **scintigram** (➢ Fig. 23.3 a; Pentcost et al. 1964, Geslien et al. 1976, Graff et al. 1986). Nonetheless, the **MRT** should be preferred for the often young patients, not only for reasons of radiation protection (➢ Fig. 23.3 b). The automatism of X-raying, scintigram, CT or/and MRT does not only have to be questioned for matters of costs. As an unspecific examination procedure (Pentcost et al. 1964, Georgen et al. 1981), it should be limited to **rare cases** and should not replace the exact clinical and sports functional examination as general examination method. The increased enhancement of the radioactive contrast material at a bone segment in the scintigram as an indication of an increased osseous perfusion can lead to a **false positive diagnosis** especially for athletes of disciplines with very dynamic kinds of movement (e.g. jumpers, sprinters). A biopositive increase of perfusion as a consequence of the stress stimulus can be misinterpreted as injury (Graff and Heinold 1987). Scintigraphy can be a justified decision support with pressure of time or localization and procedure being unclear/rare.

23.3 Differential diagnosis

The diagnostic instinct and the **experience of the examiner** are important criteria of the sometimes inconclusive differential-diagnostic assessment and the primary evaluation of the findings (Graff and Heinold 1987). This applies especially to the case of negative radiographic findings, the inconclusive findings of the tomographic images with a positive scintigram at the same time. It also applies to the morphologic special cases, such as congenital sections and separations of skeletal parts without clinical significance (e.g. os naviculare pedis bipartitum [➢ Fig. 23.4 a and b], sesamoid bones of the hallux; Keene and Lash 1992).

The distinction between stress fractures and chronic sclerosing osteomyelitis, the osteogeneous sarcoma, the osteonalacia, the osteoidosteoma (Daffner 1978) as well as the osteonecrosis of the bone (Graff and Heinold 1987), which had been partly difficult before, has become easier by the enhancing quality of tomography imaging (➢ Fig. 23.5 a and b).

Fig. 23.4 Os naviculare pedis: partly difficult to differentiate between congenital compartmentation (a) and stress fracture (b).

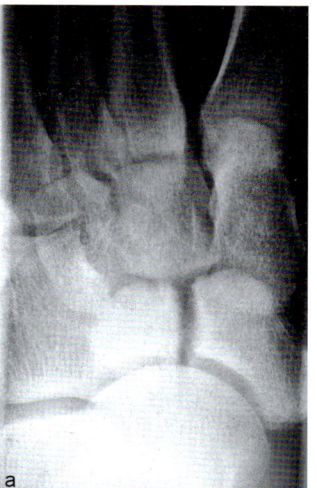

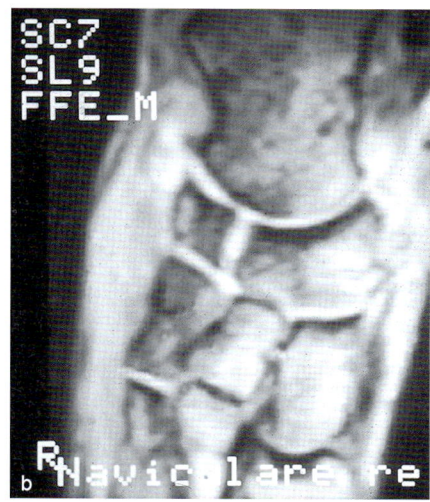

23.4 Therapy

Fractures lead to regular reactions of the local tissue with the purpose to affect a recovery of the bone continuity. A proper healing of osseous fractures requires the intensive contact of the bone fragments, the uninterrupted immobilization and the sufficient local blood supply (Adler 1983).

Stress fractures and stress reactions have a **special status** under these aspects. The intensive contact of the bone fragments exists, with few exceptions. The relative "immobilization" suffices for some forms of stress fractures by normal everyday use with a reduction of training. The **insufficient perfusion** detected by microangiography in the area of the direct structural damage (Torg et al. 1982) is an important factor for the **prolonged healing** to full capacity in some stress fractures. The increased perfusion showing in a scintigram is an indication for the reparative effort of the local, perifocal tissue.

The consideration of stress fractures as therapeutically unproblematic does not imply that all stress fractures and reactions heal out stress-capably for the intended sport. Immobilization by a cast or a plastic sleeve is used rarely. Some special cases may require surgical treatment of complete or incomplete forms (Prather et al. 1977, Orava et al. 1978, Georgen et al. 1981, Torg et al. 1982, Graff et al. 1986, Fullerton and Snowdy 1988, Johansson et al. 1990, Keene and Lash 1992).

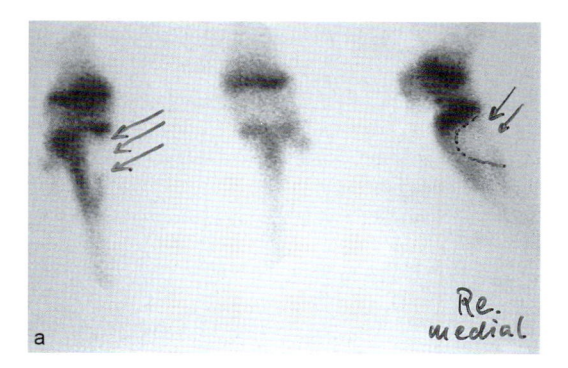

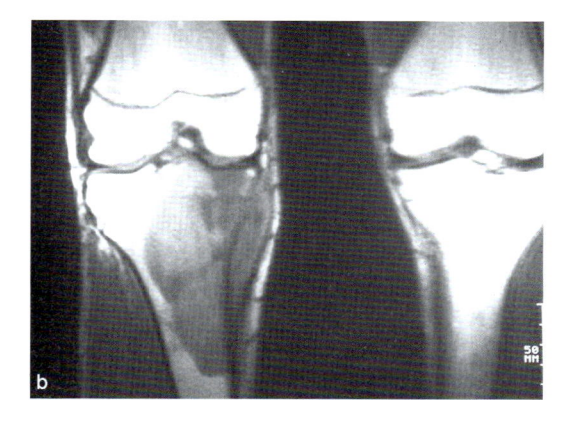

Fig. 23.5 Not a tibial stress fracture! Osteosarcoma in a 16-year-old long jumper.

23.5 Prevention

Prophylaxis of sport injuries and sport impairments is critical. Discrepancies between **general capacity** and **demanded stress** have been discussed as causes for skeletal stress fractures.

The analysis of the, techniques, execution of exercises, and individual training tolerances help to prevent stress fractures (Krahl et al. 1978, Köhler and Zimmer 1982, Graff et al. 1986, Graff and Heinold 1987).

Movement behavior, muscular stabilizing of skeletal and joint segments, technical processing of movement elements, and improvement of the "shoe supply" as well as an individual foot bed can contribute to the prophylaxis. In female athletes with atypical hormonal constellation, the hormonal situation should be discussed with regard to the anti-doping rules especially for polytope stress fractures.

References

Adler CP (1983). Knochenkrankheiten. Thieme, Stuttgart-New York.

Breitner S, Yousri T (1993). Die Stressfrakturen der Tibia im Kernspintomogramm. Sportschaden – Sportverletzung, issue 1. Thieme, Stuttgart-New York.

Daffner H (1978). Stress fractures. Current concepts. Skeletal Radiol 2: 221–229.

Debrunner AM (1983). Orthopädie. Die Störungen des Bewegungsapparates in Klinik und Praxis. Huber, Bern-Stuttgart-Wien.

Devas MB (1958). Stress fracture of the tibia in athletes or "shin soreness". J Bone Joint Surg 40: 227–239.

Fullerton LR, Snowdy HA (1988). Femoral neck stress fractures. Am J Sports Med 16: 365–377.

Geslien GE, Thrall JH, Espinosa JL, et al. (1976). Early detection of stress fractures using 99 TC-polyphosphate. Radiology 121: 683–687.

Georgen TG, et al. (1981). Tarsal navicular stress fractures in runners. Am J Radiol 136: 201–203.

Graff KH, Krahl H (1984). Überlastungsschäden im Fußbereich beim Leichtathleten. Leichtathletik 3: 81–87.

Graff KH, Schoemaecker HJ, Krahl H (1985). Überlastungsreaktionen und -schäden des Fußes. In: Franz IW, Mellerowicz H, Noack W (eds.). Training und Sport zur Prävention und Rehabilitation in der technisierten Umwelt. Springer, Berlin-Heidelberg.

Graff KH, Krahl H, Kirschberger R (1986). Stressfrakturen des Os naviculare pedis. Z Orthop 124: 228–237.

Graff KH (1987). Beurteilung der Sporttauglichkeit aus orthopädischer Sicht. Dtsch Z Sportmed 1: 4–11.

Graff KH, Heinold D (1987). Stressreaktionen am knöchernen Skelett des Athleten. Sportverletzung-Sportschaden 1: 30–52.

Graff KH (1991). Sind Stressfrakturen „Hormonfrakturen"? Zur aktuellen Diskussion über die Ursachen dieses Sportschadens. Sportverletzung-Sportschaden 5: 74–76.

Graff KH (1991). Abschließende Stellungnahme: Sind Stressfrakturen „Hormonfrakturen"? Sportverletzung-Sportschaden 5: 79–80.

Graff KH (1993. Stressfrakturen-Stressreaktionen. In: Wirt HCJ (ed.). Überlastungsschäden im Sport. Thieme, Stuttgart-New York.

Graff KH (2004). Seltene Formen von Stressschäden bei Athleten. (to be published).

Hille E (1980). Dehnungsmesstechnische Untersuchungen am Os naviclare pedis. In: Cotta H, Krahl H, Steinbrück K (eds.). Die Bewegungstoleranz des Haltungs- und Bewegungsapparates. Thieme, Stuttgart.

Johansson C, Ekenmann I, Törnkvist H, Eriksson E (1990). Stress fractures of the femoral neck in athletes. The consequence of a delay in diagnosis. Am J Sports Med 18: 524–528.

Keene JS, Lash EG (1992). Negative bone scan in a femoral neck stress fracture. Am J Sports Med 20: 234–239.

Köhler A, Zimmer EA (1982). Grenzen des Normalen und Anfänge des Pathologischen im Röntgenbild des Skeletts. Thieme, Stuttgart-New York.

Krahl H, Knebel KP, Steinbrück K (1978). Kinematographische Untersuchungen zur Frage der Fußgelenkbelastung und Schuhversorgung des Sportlers. Orthopäd Praxis 11: 821–824.

Krahl H, Knebel KP (1978). Medizinische und trainingsmethodische Aspekte der Absprungphase beim Flop. Leistungssport 6: 501-506.

Meuermann KOA, Elfving S (1980). Stress fractures in soldiers: a multifocal bone disorder. Radiology 134: 483–487.

Orava S, Myllylä T (1982). Stressfrakturen der Sesambeine des ersten Metatarsophalangealgelenkes. Bericht über 5 Fälle bei Sportlern. Med Sport 22: 4–5.

Orava S, Puranen, Ala-Ketola L (1978). Stress fractures caused by physical exercise. Acta Orhop Scand 49: 19–27.

Pavlow H, Torg JS, Freiberger RH (1983). Tarsal navicular stress fractures: radiographic evvaluation. Radiology 148: 641–645.

Pecina M, Bijanic I, Dubravcic S (1990). Stress fractures in figure skaters. Am J Sports Med 18: 277–279.

Pentcost RL, Murray RA, Brindlay HH (1964). Fatigue, insufficiency and pathologic fractures. J Am med Ass 187: 111–114.

Prather JL, Musynovitz ML, Snowdy HA et al. (1977). Scintigraphic findings in stress fractures. J Bone Joint Surg 59: 869–874.

Torg JS, et al. (1982). Stress fractures of the tarsal navicular. J Bone Joint Surge 64A: 700–712.

Towne LC, Blazina ME, Cozen LN (1970). Fatigue fracture of the tarsal naviculare. J Bone Joint Surge 52A: 376–378.

Wilkerson RD, Johns JC (1990). Nonunion of an olecranon stress fracture in an adolescent gymnast. Am J Sports Med 18: 432–434.

Wilson ES. Katz FN (1969). Stress fracture. Radiology 92: 581–486.

24 Cartilage

Stefan Nehrer

Joint cartilage heals only incompletely (Hunter 1743). For decades, very complex tests have been carried out in order to improve the insufficient ability of cartilage to regenerate. **Surgical methods** such as drilling and abrasion arthroplasty for the treatment of cartilage defects can only achieve a **fibrocartilaginous scarring** of the defect with the clinical procedure and the long-term biomechanical capacity remaining unpredictable.

Osteochondral transplantations with cartilage cylinders are technically difficult and are subject to limited graft resources and removal morbidity. Allografts are connected with high logistic expense and have an immunological and infectious risk potential.

The **implantation of cultivated, autologous chondrocytes** at acute and chronic cartilage defects has achieved an improved regeneration of hyaline joint cartilage experimentally as well as in first clinical applications. The introduction of biomaterials in cartilage-cell transplantation has led to the development of the methods of **tissue engineering** improving the prognosis in the treatment of cartilage defects.

24.1 Basics

24.1.1 Composition of joint cartilage

The same as other tissue, cartilage consists of cells, matrix and liquid with dissolved regulators. **Chondrocytes** (cartilage cells) develop from mesenchymal stem cells and form less than 5% of the tissue amount. They have a primarily anaerobe metabolism and mostly show mitotic activity only during growth. Surrounded by matrix of collagen and proteoglycans, they seem isolated and depend on the nutrition by diffusion (➢ Fig. 24.1).

Joint cartilage has **no nourishment by vessels or nerves**, and it is alymphatic.

> The limited proliferation and migration capability of the chondrocytes, the missing hemorrhage and, associated, the missing invasion of pluripotent connective tissue cells limit the healing potency of this tissue.

The **matrix** consists of water (60–80%) and structural macromolecules, such as collagen, proteoglycanes and non-collagen proteins. The swelling capacity of the proteoglycanes and the stable specific fiber structure of the collagen fibrils allow a **"water cushion effect"**, which constitutes the mechanical and functional characteristics of the cartilage.

The cartilage is **arranged in zones** with different amounts of cell and matrix parts. The surface concludes with a thin membrane – the lamina splendens; a zone of calcifying cartilage with lamina limitans is found deep at the junction to the subchondral bone.

Already small changes regarding the composition and architecture are sufficient for the decrease of the resistance and capacity of the tissue and to induce a progressive **degeneration of the joint surface**. A restitutio ad integrum in the cartilage tissue is difficult to achieve, because correct amounts of the cell and matrix components must be present, on the one hand, and the architecture and structure of the whole construction of the joint cartilage must be recovered, on the other hand (Buckwalter et al. 1998).

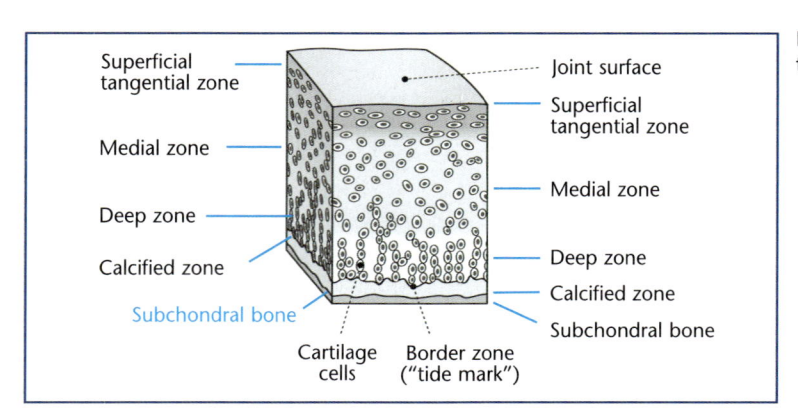

Fig. 24.1 Constitution and histology of joint cartilage.

24.1.2 Exposures and biomechanics of the cartilage

The surface of the joint cartilage serves the **transmission of loads with simultaneous smearing** of the gliding surfaces. The cartilage gains characteristics superior to the friction characteristics of ice on ice (Mankin 1994). The interplay of collagen fibers as frame substance and glucosamine-glycans as water-binding swelling material creates the firm elastic characteristics inducing the **dampening characteristics** with the smearing mechanism by pressing off the interstitial liquid. The **water binding** correlates with the content of proteoglycans and is bound to an intact collagen frame.

Defects on the surface, but also microscopic injuries of the matrix lead to the depletion of these water-binding molecules and thus to a loss of quality of the biomechanical characteristics. **Longer physical exposures** lead to a **decrease in height of the cartilage coating** of up to 5% because of a loss of liquids in certain areas that are subjects to especially high static pressures, e.g. in the femoropatellar joint.

> Joint loads with long-term weight effects can exceed the compensation mechanism of joint cartilage and can lead to persistent damages, especially with the micro-structure of the cartilage being disturbed by traumas.

In addition, the cartilage cell depends on **alternating loads** for the maintaining of the liquid streams in the interstitium, so that sports with cyclic loads and low weight loads, such as cycling, have to be considered positive.

24.1.3 Natural healing process of cartilage defects

Cartilage defects are mostly evaluated morphologically, which includes the different repairing procedures only insufficiently.

Biologically, the following **classification** seems sensible:

- matrix defects without injury of the joint surface
- purely chondral defects without involvement of the subchondral lamella
- osteochondral defects with hemorrhage from the subchondral bone.

Matrix defects include changes of the molecular structure in the course of **blunt traumas and overstress**, with evacuating of proteoglycans and ruptures of the collagen fibrils. Consequentially, the chondrocytes show increased rates of synthesis and try to compensate the loss of matrix components, which can lead to the recovery of full functioning and structure at a limited damage.

In the case of **chondral defects**, **no repairing process** is being induced because of missing formation of blood clots. According to the size and localization of the defects, the lesions of the joint surface either remain unchanged or the bordering cartilage suffers a degeneration of the structures with long-term limitation of the joint function. Short-term attempts of repair by increased synthesis of the bordering chondrocytes and mitotic activity remain insufficient in most cases. Proteoglycans containing keratan (biglycan, dermatan) on the surface of the defection prevent the recovery of a continuous cartilage matrix. The immigration of synovial cells seems to be a possible repair mechanism, but it also leads only to **fibrocartilaginous scarring** of the defect (Buckwalter 1988).

Injuries of the joint cartilage with included **subchondral bone lamella** involve a formation of a **blood clot** that goes along with the hemorrhaging and subsequently is transformed to a fibrocartilaginous scar. While the defect of the subchondral bone is filled completely osseously in most cases, **fibrocartilaginous mixed tissue** develops in the cartilaginous part of the defect. This tissue cannot duplicate the mechanical characteristics of original joint cartilage. According to the size and localization of the defect as well as to the load of the joint, degenerative changes of the structures with consequential **limitation of the joint function** appear.

The relieving mobilization of the joint seems to be decisive for the natural healing of osteochondral defects in order not to endanger the maturing of the cartilage scar. The progressive degeneration of the cartilage and its following change of the intraarticular regulator environment (interleukins) as well as the mechanical insufficiency of repairing tissue often leads to chronic pain of the joint with synovially irritated condition and relapsing effusions, though.

24.1.4 Imaging of cartilage

The cartilage surfaces of large joints could be displayed routinely with the introduction of fat-suppressed gradient echo and fast-spin echo sequences in magnetic resonance. The **3D-gradient-echo sequence** with fat suppression allows an exact assessment of the cartilage thickness and surface.

The **fast-spin echo sequence** can display structural irregularities of the cartilage itself. A relevant image of the joint surface can be obtained with the examination of both sequences. The high-resolution MRT works with surface coil allowing a detailed image of almost all joints.

The assessment of cartilage defects in **MRT** should be carried out by **standardized principles**:

- palpation of the defect
- integration to the bordering cartilage
- surface and cartilage structure
- texture of the subchondral bone
- adhesions and synovitis.

The condition of the cartilage and the complete joint can be described sufficiently because of these criteria (Marlovits 2005).

> **Summary**
>
> Cartilage is short of cells, avascular and alymphatic. Therefore it only has limited healing potential with fibrocartilaginous scar tissue. The main components of cartilage are cartilage cells (5%) and matrix that consists of collagen (type II), glucosaminglycan (GAG) and hyaluronic acid. Cartilage cells are end-differentiated cells that cannot divide anymore in the matrix, but in the Petri dish, where they lose their cartilage-specific characteristics, though. They can get back their cartilage-specific characteristics under three-dimensional culture conditions.

24.2 Cartilage treatment

24.2.1 Conservative treatment

The joint cartilage is subject to high stress in sports and is often endangered by injuries at a young age already.

> Preventive measures of injury prophylaxis and preservation as well as balance of the muscular stabilization and the regulation of weight are of priority.

The **substitution of chondroitin sulfate** (CS) and **glucosaminglycan** (GAG) is offered preventively in the U.S.A. and is available in many preparations as nutritional substitution. Most company-supported studies are promising, but have to be backed up by extensive surveys for a final assessment. Nutritional substitutions often are problematic for the athlete, though, because of possible contaminations with substances of the doping list.

The effectiveness of GAG and CS has been shown for the treatment of **beginning arthritic changes**.

> Combined preparations of GAG and CS with daily doses of about 1,200–1,500 mg are suited best.

Presently, it is hard to judge whether adjuvant oral therapies are sensible after cartilage surgeries. Right now, CS is used in conservative cartilage treatment, because it also has an **antiphlogistic component** and can often be used as a **well-digestible long-term preparation**.

The **intraarticular administration of hyaluronic acid** is a causal principle of treatment of cartilage impairments and incipient arthrosis. Although always discussed critically, meta-analyses show a **clinical effectiveness** of hyaluronic acid exceeding the expected smearing effect. Altogether, these measures improve the clinical symptoms and slow down the progression of cartilage degeneration.

The medicamentous treatment of the symptomatic cartilage damage and the arthrosis includes also the taking of **NSAIDS** or coxiben for the reduction of the inflammatory irritation. These measures can be supported by a number of **physical therapies**.

24.2.2 Conventional surgery methods

Microfracturing

The **direct surgical treatment** of cartilage defects included until now:

- the arthroscopic cartilage smoothing and the debridement
- the cartilage drilling according to Pridie
- the abrasive arthroplasty according to Johnson, and in recent years
- the microfracturing introduced by Steadman.

It is the **aim** of direct surgical methods to induce a **hemorrhage** by opening of the blood vessels of the subchondral lamella, and thus to bring pluripotent stem cells into the defect.

> **All these methods cannot accomplish the complete regeneration of joint cartilage and lead to fibrocartilaginous mixed tissue.**
>
> The abrasive arthroplasty with the shaver leads to distinctive lowering of the bone layer and the drilling is associated with the risk of heat necrosis in drilling and the induction of bone edemas.

The structural formation and mechanical quality of these tissues is not predictable and the

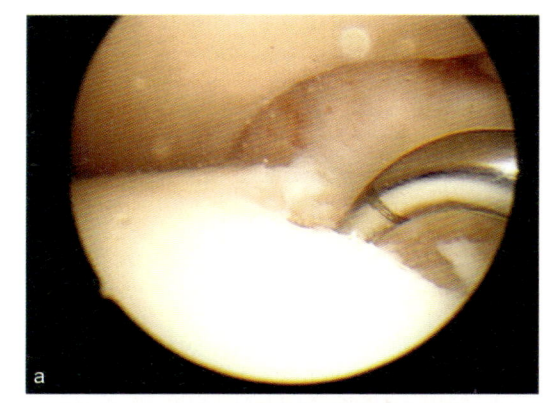

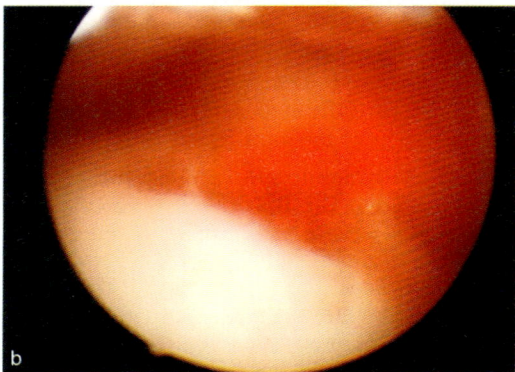

Fig. 24.2 a and b: Micro-fracturing with pointed chisel for the induction of a blood coagulum into the defect.

clinical **prognosis** is therefore insecure (Minas and Nehrer 1997).

In **microfracturing** (➤ Fig. 24.2), the subchondral bone lamella is being perforated by pointed slightly bent chisels after an exact debridement and the cleaning of the defect. It should best be begun at the periphery, perforation should be carried out with a distance of 2–3 mm and the complete defect should be microfractured towards the center. It is crucial to open the **medullary cavity** this way, which is confirmed by the **rise of fat specks** from the bone marrow or small hemorrhages after the opening of the blood barrier. The **bone bridges** between the perforations must be preserved for the prevention of a larger loss of substance of the bone stick.

Cartilage-bone transplantations

Other methods, such as implantations of autologous or allogenic osteochondral trans-

24.2 Cartilage treatment

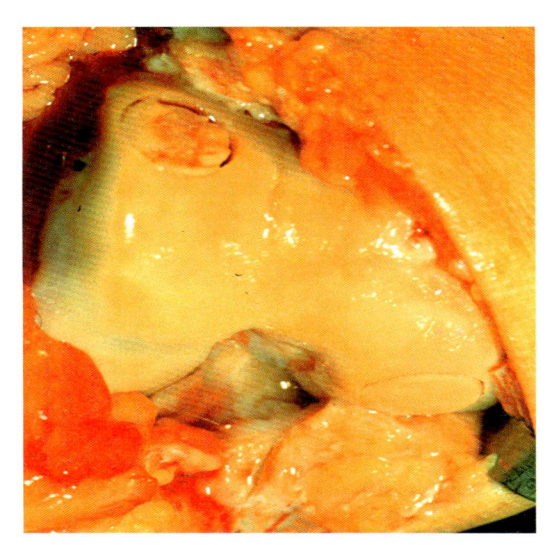

Fig. 24.3 Osteochondral transplantation of a cartilage defect with transfer from the lateral trochlea with DBCS instrumentation at a large osteochondritic center in the exposure zone. The defect cylinder has been used for the filling of the donorsite.

plants (➤ Fig. 24.3), delivered partly good results. The authors Bobic (1996) and Hangody et al. (1996) reported the technique of **mosaic plastic** with osteochondral cylinders being taken from the marginal zones of the knee joint and being transplanted into the defect zone by press-fit procedure. Medium-term results show success rates of more than 90%. Problems at the point of removal are only stated in 5%, although long-term surveys have to be expected. The stability of cylinders not standing on the edge and the reaching of a continuous joint surface seem problematic. Therefore, we recommend implanting of **no more than three cylinders**, which are best to handle surgically with diameters of 6 and 8 mm.

Other authors use fresh **allografts** for large posttraumatic defects. The transplants are only rarely available, associated by a high logistic effort, and are often hard to fix, though. They imply an increased **immunological and infectious risk**. Such procedures seem justified for decreased demands at serious joint destruction after an accident or tumor (Mankin et al. 1976). But they must be seen critically with young, athletic patients.

Healing induction by foreign material

The use of **carbon-fiber implants** for the stimulation of cartilage healing provided different clinical success; only **fibrocartilaginous tissue** is formed here as well. The carbon fibers are available as a net or as pins, with scar tissue growing along the fibers and thus filling the defect with tissue. Many authors see no advantage compared to microfracturing and warn of the **foreign-body reaction** of the carbon fibers (Mortier and Engelhardt 2000).

Adjustment osteotomies

The **indirect methods** of adjusting and correcting osteotomies close to the joint have proven helpful in the treatment of cartilage damages and can often be combined usefully, especially for associated malalignments. The process of cartilage treatments without necessary axial corrections seems obsolete, because the biomechanical overuse ruins all regeneration of tissue.

24.2.3 Cartilage cell transplantation

The enzymatic isolation and **cultivation of chondrocytes ex vivo** allowed the development of new implantation procedures for the treatment of defects of the joint surface. Cartilage cells proliferate in **two-dimensional** cell cultures, but assume a fibroblastic phenotype then and this way lose the ability to produce cartilage-specific type-II collagen and proteoglycan. This characteristic is reactivated under **three-dimensional** culture conditions like agarose gel or spongious matrices.

These observations gave reason to win cartilage cells from **autologous cartilage biopsies** and to implant them in the way of cell suspension into a chondral defect of the joint surface after multiplication in cell culture. Assuming these chondrocytes to produce original cartilaginous matrix, **sufficient cartilage regeneration** can be induced **without the formation of inferior scar tissue**.

Autologous chondrocyte transplantation with the periosteal lobe (ACT)

Autologous cartilage-cell transplantation is a **new approach in the therapy** of cartilage defects. Chondrodrogenic cells are available in the defect because of the contribution of the autologous cultivated cells and they allow cartilage regeneration. Animal experiments gave evidence of a **qualitative and quantitative improvement** of cartilage regeneration during an observation period of 6 months.

The defects treated with periosteal flaps and autologous chondrocytes show a nearly complete filling of the defect with **positive evidence** of collagen type II and cartilage-specific proteoglycans. This significant difference between treated and untreated defects could not be ascertained anymore in the 1-year results, because a degeneration of the newly formed tissue occurred in both groups.

A Swedish work group (Brittberg et al. 1994) reported a significant clinical improvement after autologous cartilage-cell implantation in a relatively small collective of patients. The check-up biopsies after 1 year showed a healing of the periosteal flap by transformation into resistant chondroid tissue. But the results differ, according to the localization of the defect. **Patellar and tibial defects** show a significantly worse result than **femoral defects**.

Currently, a controlled clinical multi-center survey with involvement of arthroscopic biopsies of the regenerated tissue is being carried out to ensure the efficiency of this method. By now, more than 1,000 patients have undergone surgery using this method by the Swedish work group led by Lars Peterson, with the **medium-term success rate** of 92% for isolated defects at the femurcondyle. The success rate amounts to 72 or 85% for multiple defects, combined injuries and in the femoropatellar friction bearing. The **long-term processes** of the first 100 patients also showed a good durability of the results up to 10 years postoperatively (Peterson and Minas 1999).

In ten patients, we found nine good results and one bad result in the 1-year process of a mixed collective with femoral and talar defects. Altogether, an improvement of the clinical findings up to 2 years postoperatively is found in all surveys, which corresponds to the maturing of the regenerated tissue, but there are also reports of considerably lower success rates (Engelhardt et al. 2001). A comparative study of microfracturing and ACT (Knutsen et al. 2004) shows even advantages in the 2-year process in the clinical course of the microfracturation group, although the histology of the biopsies provided a better assessment for the ACT group.

The method is **limited** due to the limited availability of cartilage tissue for cultivation, the limiting of the size of the periosteal flap and the necessity of an arthrotomy. The fixation of periosteal flap and the production of a waterproof compartment are problematic and require some practice.

The cultivation of cartilage cells from biopsies has already been conducted commercially with success by several companies in the U.S.A. and in Europe. The **costs per patient** for the procedure of cell breeding amount to 2,500 or 12,000 €.

Implementation

Small cartilaginous pieces of areas of the joint surface without weight exposure are taken sterilely by arthroscopy off the patient's affected joint. The biopsy is sent in a special container to the cell-culture laboratory, where the preparation of the cartilage cells has to start **within 48 hours**. The chondrocytes (approx. 400,000) are isolated enzymatically and expanded in cell culture.

At the time of implantation, a **cell suspension of 12–20 million cells** is delivered and inserted into the prepared cartilage defect and is covered by the **periosteal flap** sutured in to be water-proof (➤ Fig. 24.4). The periost is taken off

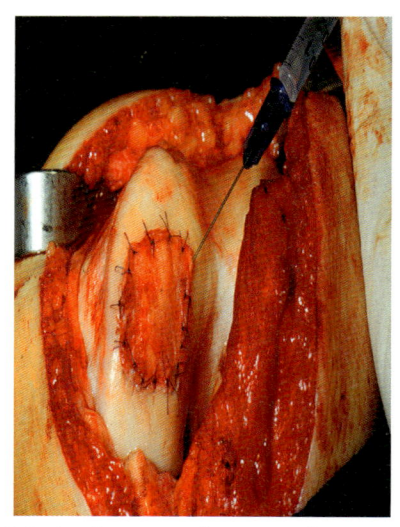

Fig. 24.4 Autologous cartilage transplantation at the time of injection of the cell suspension under the sewn periostal patches.

in an according size via a small skin incision at the anterior tibial edge. The cartilage defect is cut down carefully by a scalpel to achieve an **optimal fixation** of the flap, and the present scar tissue is being removed completely as far as the subchondral lamella. **Hemorrhages definitely have to be avoided**. The edges of the periosteum are sutured with the circumference of the defect by resorbable suture material and are sealed with fibrin to be waterproof.

Rehabilitation by help of a motor splint and relief of the joint for 6–8 weeks becomes effective **postoperatively**.

24.2.4 Biomaterials – tissue engineering

The **matrix-assisted procedures** have shown the advancement of autologous cartilage-cell transplantations, with the cells being implanted into the defect by help of a biomaterial (Nehrer et al. 1998). Numerous experimental approaches brought the collagen fleece and gel, hyaluronate and polyactides to clinical application.

The cartilage cells are isolated and bred as described before and then embedded into the defect together with the biomaterial (Bentley and Green 1971). The used matrices must create a **biologically convenient environment** and must allow the **regeneration of cartilage tissue**.

The **collagen matrix** (Chondro-Gide®) is sutured onto the defect and thus serves as a stable periosteal substitute. The **hyaluronic fleece** (Hyalograft C®, ≻ Fig. 24.5 a–c) can be glued into the defect, which is surgically much easier, allows smaller accesses and this way makes the arthroscopic implantation possible. The stable anchoring of the graft has to be **criticized**, although fibrin glue at the edge of the defect secures the cell-augmented matrix.

At our center more than 60 patients could be treated with the hyaluronic fleece within the last 5 years. First results of the classic indication of the isolated femoral defect are comparable to the ones of classic ACT with the periosteal flap. There are similar reports for collagen fleece (Nehrer et al. 2005). Collagen gel, polyactides and fibrin are in the beginning of the clinical testing and have to prove successful still.

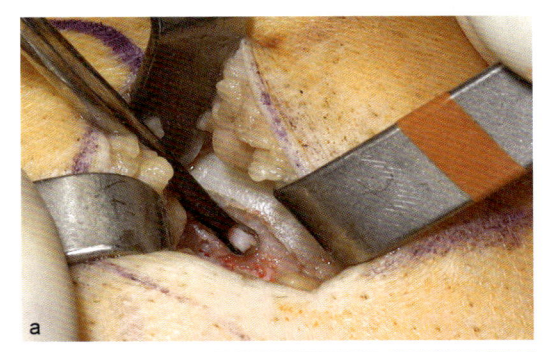

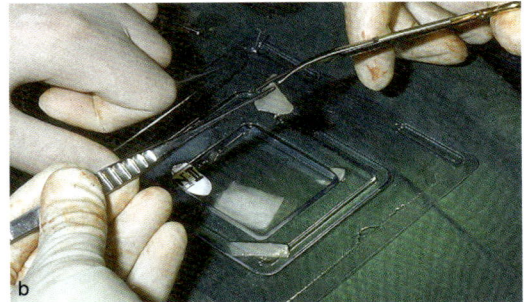

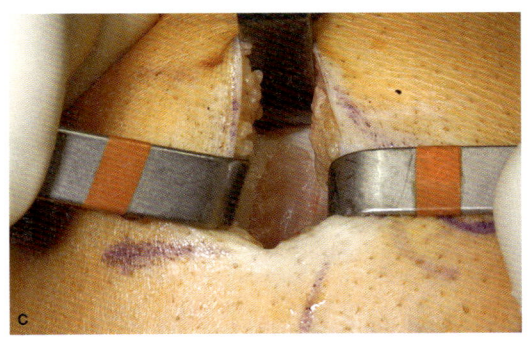

Fig. 24.5 Implantation of a hyaluronic matrix into a cartilage defect at the medial condyle. a: debridement. b: Cutting of the matrix. c: Implantation of the matrix (Hyalograft C®).

The lacking availability of long-term data of any of these matrix techniques is critical; hence, we do not recommend **routine use**. These techniques should be used under exact control and very critically. Long-term studies will show whether the periost can be relinquished and which transport medium is optimal for the cells.

Arthrosis or serious joint deformation is no indication for these procedures.

Attentive, critical and controlled application helps to advance these methods rather than excessive indication and not accomplishable expectations of patients. Altogether, the new methods of tissue engineering seem to open new paths in the treatment of cartilage defects; anyhow, a **paradigm shift from repairing to regeneration** has taken place.

> **Summary**
>
> Techniques of surgical cartilage treatment:
> - microfracturing: inducement of hemorrhages by perforation of the subchondral lamella
> - mosaic plastic: transfer of osteochondral cylinders using pressfit technique
> - ACT: autologous chondrocyte transplantation with the periosteal flap
> - BACT: biomaterial-associated autologous chondrocyte transplantation using collagen fleece or gel, hyaluronic fleece, PLA fleece, and others.

24.3 Strategies of cartilage treatment

With **acute cartilage defects** or osteochondritic lesions broken out freshly, the **preservation** of the cartilage fragment under fixation of the separated cartilage part should be tried at all costs. If this is not successful, a microfracturing follows for defects not bleeding. The intact cartilage of a cartilage flap requiring removal should be sent to **cell breeding**, so that these cells could possibly be implanted at a later point of time; in most procedures, they can be made available for 1 year.

The clinical process has to be given time, especially with **small defects**, because many defects remain asymptomatic and require no further therapies.

> Currently, there is no reliable parameter that allows a prognosis of the process of a defect of the joint surface.

Symptomatic, **chronic defects** that have a diameter of less than 1–2 cm should be treated by **microfracturing** in a first treatment. With the subchondral lamella being affected as well, as in osteochondritis dissecans, a **mosaic plastic** should be carried out already as a primary measure (with 2–3 cylinders with 6–8 mm each at a maximum, if possible). The autologous **cartilage cell transplantation** with periosteal flap or with cell-augmented matrix has to be implemented for more extensive defects or for the case of other methods showing insufficient results (Minas and Nehrer 1997). With changes of the subchondral bone, the osteochondral autologous transplantation is preferred for **smaller defects**. For **larger osseous defects**, a two-timed procedure with cartilage filling and secondary cartilage treatment with cartilage-cell transplantation is the most appropriate.

In a comparison of mosaic plastic and ACT, **ACT** had better results in a study of Bentley et al. (2003) with colagenous membrane being used here. Altogether, it is still too early for a final description, because there are different evaluations (Horas et al. 2003).

The **indication** for the according procedure is decisive: A failed cartilage defect, pre-operated by miocrofracturing surely is an indication for a more complex procedure and large defects are only finitely appropriate for microfracturing. The augmentation of the microfracturing with a collagen membrane without cells has not caused any improvement in experimental studies.

In spite of different studies, the **surgical cartilage treatment has advanced significantly** and the aim of cartilage regeneration has definitely come closer.

References

Bentley G, Green R (1971). Homotransplantation of isolated epiphyseal and articular cartilage chondrocytes into joint surfaces of rabbits. Nature 230: 385–388.

Bentley G, Biant LC, Carrington RWJ, et al. (2003). A prospective randomised comparison of autologous chondrocyte implantation versus mosaicplasty of osteochondral defects in the knee. J Bone Joint Surg Br 85B: 223–230.

Bobic V (1996). Arthroscopic osteochondral autograft transplantation in anterior cruciate ligament reconstruction: a preliminary clinical study. Arthroscopy 3: 262–264.

Brittberg M, et al. (1994). Treatment of deep cartilage defects in the knee with autologous chondrocyte transplantation. N Eng J Med 331: 889–894.

References

Buckwalter J, et al. (1988). Articular cartilage composition and structure. In: Woo S-Y, Buckwlter J (eds.). Injury and Repair of the Musculoskeletal Soft Tissues. AAOS, Park Ridge, Illinois.

Engelhardt M; Mortier J, Mergele T, Leonhard T(2001). Ergebnisse nach autologer Knorpelzelltransplantation am Kniegelenk. Arthritis und Rheuma 21 (5): 279–285.

Hangody L., et al. (1996). Mosaicplasty for the treatment of articular cartilage defects: Application in clinical practice. Orthopedics 21: 751–756.

Horas U, Pelinkovic D, Herr G, Aigner T, Schettler R (2003). Autologous chondrozyte implantation and osteochondral cylinder transplantation in cartilage repair of the knee joint – a prospective, comparative trial. J Bone Joint Surg Am 85A (2): 185–192.

Hunter W (1743). On the structure and disease of articulating cartilage. Philos Trans R Soc Lond 42b: 514–521.

Knutsen G, Engebretsen L, et al. (2004). Autologous chondrocyte implantation compared with minifracture in the knee. A randomized trial. J Bone Joint Surg Am 86A (3): 455–464.

Mankin H, Fogelson F, Trasher A (1976). Massive resection and allograft transplantation in the treatment of malignant bone tumors. N Eng J Med 294: 1247–1255.

Mankin H (1994). Chondrocyte transplantation an answer to an old question. N Eng J Med 331: 940–941.

Marlovits S, Singer P, Zeller P, Mandl I, Haller J, Trattnig S (2005). Magnetic resonance observation of cartilage repair tissue (MOCART) for the evaluation of autologous chondrocyte transplantation. Eur J Radiol 2005, Sep 30.

Minas T, Nehrer S (1997). Current concepts in the treatment of articular cartilage defects. Orthopedics 20: 525–538.

Mortier J, Engelhardt M (2000). Fremdkörperreaktion bei Karbonfaserstiftimplantation im Kniegelenk. Z Orthop 138: 390–394.

Nehrer S, et al. (1998). Chondrocyte-seeded collagen matrices implanted in a chondral defect in a canine model. Biomaterials 19: 2313–2328.

Nehrer S, Domayer S, Dorotka R, Schatz K, Bindreiter U, Kotz R (2005). Three-year clinical outcome after chondrocyte transplantation using a hyaluronan matrix for cartilage repair. Eur J Radiol 2005, Sep 23.

Peterson L, Minas T (1999). Advanced techniques in autologous chondrocyte transplantation. Clin Sports Med 18: 13–44.

25 Tendon injuries

Andreas Gösele and Victor Valderrabano

Injuries and diseases of tendons are a common in sports medicine. The amount of tendon injuries varies significantly and depends on the individual sport. Tendon injuries can be classified in **acute, chronic, or overuse injuries**. Injuries affecting the tendon, the tendon insertion, or origin are considered as **tendon pathologies**. **Differential diagnosis** allows discrimination between **inflammatory diseases** and **degenerative lesions** with partial and total insufficiency such as ruptures. Tendon injuries and diseases in most cases take a **long time** in diagnostics as well as in therapy and require a large amount of experience of the attending physician.

Chronic tendon pathologies have different etiologic factors, which affect diagnosis and therapy. A satisfying therapy is often only achievable with a combination of symptomatic treatment and adjustment or reduction of causal factors.

The **treatment** depends on biomechanical and pathological data. Sport-specific loads, the biomechanics of motion as well as sports equipment (shoes and sports ground) are important factors. Also, anatomy, pathophysiology of inflammation, mechanisms of regeneration and repair, treatment algorithms and surgical techniques need consideration in therapeutic decision-making (Schepsis et al. 2002).

Functional treatment by therapies orientating on shape and function and being least invasive as possible are usually more success-promising than therapy concepts dimensioned for short-term results and invasiveness. After all, the treatment result depends on precise diagnosis, because only exact knowledge of the defect is the base for an according selective therapy. Diagnosis of desperation such as "achillodynia" should be avoided, because they contain more than ten different reasons for pain in the region of the Achilles tendon (Segesser et al. 1995). A partial rupture must be distinguished from a peritendinitis, because the therapeutic consequences are completely different.

25.1 Anatomic-physiological basics

25.1.1 Anatomy

Morphology

Every muscle principally consists of a proximal and distal tendon insertion ensuring the force transmission of the muscle to the bone. The connection between muscle and tendon is called **myotendinous junction**. The healthy tendon is white and shining. The individual tendon bundles are partly visible to the naked eye. Their morphology very much varies, depending on the localization, the size and the exercised condition of the individual.

Dependent on the muscle, the tendon insertion is wide, elongated or short and narrow.

Strong muscles as the quadriceps muscle, for example, have wide short tendon insertions. Muscles responsible for fine motor skills, e.g. the finger flexors, have fine long stretched tendons.

The following anatomical structures are included into the muscle-tendon complex:

- tendon sheaths
- retinaculae
- paratenon and epitenon
- bursa.

Tendon sheaths

The two-leaved tendon sheaths serving as gliding layer are found especially in the region of the long tendons of hand and foot. The **external sheet** consists of fibrous connective tissue and is characterized by its resistance. In contrast, the **internal sheet** consists of a parietal and a visceral part. The **synovial liquid** produced by the internal sheet is similar to the synovial fluid of the joints and ensures an improvement of the gliding and the tendon nutrition. Three different cell types are distinguished (type A, type B, type C), which produce the important hyaluronic acid and glucosaminoglycanes in addition to lysozyme and alpha-1 antitrypsin.

Paratenon and epitenon

Only few tendons have the classic structure of tendons and multi-leaved tendon sheath. These structures are characteristic for zones of increased mechanical loads (retromalleolarly, carpal tunnel). The far larger number of the tendons is surrounded by a layer of connective tissue called **paratenon**. The major components of the paratenon are collagen type I and type III as well as synovial cells. The function of this tendon cover is clearly designed for protection (fibrils) and nutrition (synovia).

The **epitenon** is found directly attached to the sleeve and covering the tendon. The result is a certain state of being two-leaved, similar to the actual classic tendon sheath. This state is often called **peritendineum**. The **endotenon** extends inwards. It consists of connective tissue and surrounds or separates primary, secondary and tertiary bundles of the tendons (➤ Fig. 25.1). The most important function of the endotenon is the nutrition of the tendon and also the securing of gliding mechanism.

Bursa

Another important structure belonging to the muscle-tendon complex is the bursa. **Bursae** are located at points where tendons meet **prominent bone points** (bursa subachillea, bursa trochanterica). They do not only form a gliding layer there, but additionally have a certain buffer function.

Tendon architecture

Although the theory of tendon fibrils having a purely longitudinal direction had held for many decades, especially electron microscopic examinations show the arrangement of the fibrils being far more complex and rich of variants than assumed. In addition to the linear and longitudinal direction, a downright net of transversal and also horizontal fibrils defining a **three-dimensional network geared to tensile, compressive and shearing forces** is found.

Tendons consist of collagen (especially type I) and elastin embedded in a proteoglycan-water matrix and they are produced by tenoblasts and tenocytes. The **myotendinous junction** is a highly specialized anatomical region, the same as the tendon insertion. It is responsible for the **stress-resistant** connection of different types of tissue. In addition to the pure tendon and bone tissue, the tendon insertion also shows interposed, intermediate anatomical zones like **fibrous cartilage** connected to each other by a fibrous net of collagen fibrils and matrix and thus ensuring **mechanical resistance**.

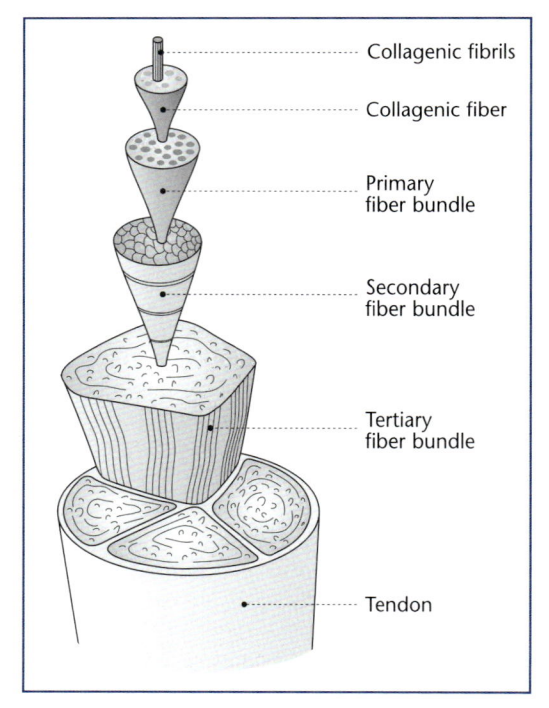

Fig. 25.1 Classic structure of tendons with tendon bundle and connective tissue (according to László G. Józsa and Pekka Kannus, Human Tendons).

25.1.2 Tendon perfusion/tendon nutrition

Until 18th century, the opinion of tendons being avascular, anatomical structures persisted. Three different ways of **blood supply of the tendon** are known nowadays:

- blood vessels from skeletal muscles
- blood vessels from bone and periosteum
- vessels sprouting in through the paratenon and the endotenon.

Compared to the muscle, the tendon is still a poorly circulated tissue. The major part of **tendinous nutrition** is performed through the tissue **surrounding the tendons (diffusion processes)**, but not from the region of the insertion or origin of the tendons. For example, there are zones at the Achilles tendon with more and such with less circulation. The smallest capillary density is found about 3–6 cm above the insertion at the calcaneus, i.e. exactly at the point of the highest rupture rate.

The "peritendinous blood supply" is generally performed via existing tendon sheaths or the paratenon continuing into the endotenon. Not only a **different capillary density** shows here regarding the **localization**, but a certain **age correlation** also seems to be present. Physical activity can significantly influence the capillary density and thus the nutrition of the tendon positively, while chronic overuse and inactivity can have negative effects (Kjaer et al. 2000).

25.1.3 Biomechanics

The most important function of the tendon is **force transmission** from the muscle to the bone. Therefore, tendons should have a balanced relation of elasticity and stiffness and a high mechanical strength. The force transmission should be possible without great losses of mechanical energy.

This mixture of elastic abilities and also a high mechanical resistance must be guaranteed by the tendon and even more so by the whole complex (tendon insertion, myotendinous junction). This is ensured by a unique combination of macromolecular materials and cells.

Not only linear forces, but also **combinations of different force directions** have to be transferred to the bone here.

> The cross-section of the tendon directly relates to its capacity and depends on the load and the stimulus.

Minor loads therefore mean minor cross-section of the tendon. The tendinous cross-section can only be changed very slowly. This can often take months or years, which should be considered in the planning of training and load, especially for sport beginners.

In the early 1970s already, a phenomenon providing an additional load capacity for the tendon has been described for the first time: the **tendon rotation**. The Achilles tendon shows a wringing in its distal part about 2–5 cm above the insertion at the calcaneus, which leads to an additional stiffening and increase of the mechanical capacity, but also to an increased susceptibility for injuries. This **vulnerability** is most extensive in these zones, because the circulation is the least here, but the shear forces are the highest.

The tendon has a certain **own elasticity**. It finds expression in the fact that tendons in a relaxed condition show a slightly wavy shape. This phenomenon can be observed under the microscope with load and thus lengthening of approx. 2%. In case of tension release, the wavy shape returns. With a moderate load up to 4% of deformation, the tendon is always able to move back to its normal shape. At the exceeding of the critical limit, though, structural changes appear in the sense of a partial lesion or even complete **rupture** (➤ Fig. 25.2). Load

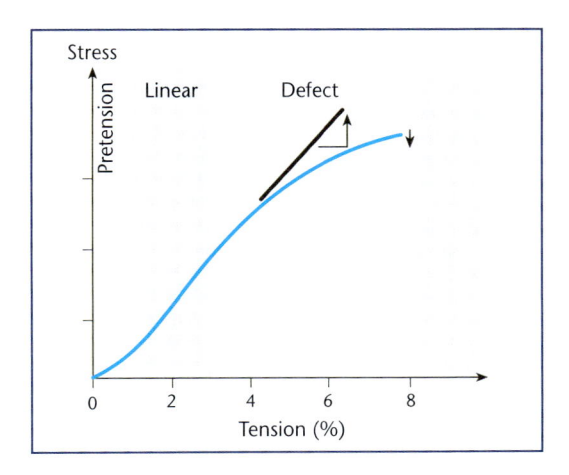

Fig. 25.2 Stress curve of tendons.

values of up to 9,000 N or the 20-fold of the body weight are found in sports and are tolerated by accordingly exercised organisms.

25.2 Tendon diseases

Generally, acute injuries have to be distinguished from overuse damages. In the **acute injuries**, we distinguish ruptures, partial ruptures and a special form, the intratendinous partial rupture.

Tendinoses, endotenonitis and peritendinoses and a number of **concomitant affections**, such as bursitis or tendon dislocation, are found in the **overuse damages** and **chronic injuries** (Jarvinen et al. 2001).

25.2.1 Causes

For a long time, inflammation of the tendon had been postulated as cause of injuries. In current years, it could be shown that especially **degenerative processes** are responsible for tendon injuries, though (Kader et al. 2002). Combinations of degeneration, overuse, insufficient regeneration and reduced blood circulation can influence each other and can increase the risk of injuries.

In degenerative processes, tendon fibrils become separated. The collagen swells and the physiological direction of the fibrils can be lost. The quality of the proteoglycans changes, inflammation cells immigrate and a capillary proliferation appears (Alfredson et al. 2003). The endotenon increases in thickness, the cellular environment changes and **microruptures** can develop. Especially regions with high mechanical loads or a minor blood circulation in the first place, as for example the **Achilles tendon** in the area 3–5 cm above the insertion at the calcaneus, can be affected by this.

Mechanical and biomechanical factors play a major role here, because they can lead to repetitive, **asymmetric exposure** of the tendon. An increased pronation, for example, causes an enhancement of the asymmetric stress forces to the Achilles tendon. The zone of increased stress coincides with the zone of physiological minor blood circulation, which then again coincides with the zone of highest torsion of the tendon. It is obvious that just this region is exactly the zone (3–6 cm above the insertion), where about 90% of the tendon ruptures appear.

But also **extrinsic factors** such as influences in training with a sudden increase of amount and intensity, insufficient regeneration, hard training ground, insufficient material (running shoes) or new techniques (forefoot running) can provoke injuries and diseases of the tendon complex. Not least, **intrinsic factors** like muscular dysbalances with shortening and also disproportion of agonists and antagonists lead to tendon injuries.

25.2.2 Tendon ruptures

Complete tendon ruptures

The complete tendon rupture is caused by **direct force effects** (➤ Fig. 25.3). The load exceeds the stress limit of the tendon and it comes to a rupture. Concentric force can be the reason, but **excentric force maxima** mostly lead to tendon ruptures. A healthy tendon can rupture as well with according force peaks. Nevertheless, ruptures appear in most cases at already degenerative, **pre-damaged tendons** (Segesser et al. 1995, Leppilahti and Orava 1998, Maffulli et al. 2003, Maffulli and Wong 2003).

Sport beginners or returners are endangered most. Although the adjustment of the energy metabolism and musculature in regular training is rather quick, the adaption mechanisms of the tendon apparatus are comparably slow. The tendon "drags behind" the rest of the or-

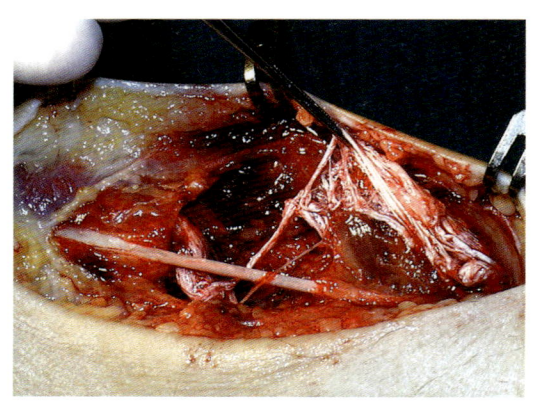

Fig. 25.3 Complete rupture of the Achilles tendon.

ganism. Especially sports with additional eccentric loads, such as ball sports (soccer and tennis), are often affected.

Tendon ruptures are characteristic events. The example of the **Achilles tendon** shows a **whip-like bang** not only perceived by the affected person but also by the environment. Immediate pain, swelling and especially the functional damage are indicatory for diagnosis. Still, about 20% of all fresh ruptures of the Achilles tendon are primarily overlooked. Typically, a disruption of continuity is found in many cases (➤ Fig. 25.4). The **classic clinical examination** with the request of tip-toe standing can be **false positive** here, because approximately 30% of the torsion moment of the upper ankle joint is carried out by the deep toe flexors, thus feigning a fully functional Achilles tendon. A better way is the so-called **"hanging-foot sign"** with the patient in prone position showing a significant lowering of the foot in lateral comparison.

The following tendons are affected most often by complete ruptures:

- Achilles tendon
- supraspinatus tendon
- biceps tendon and
- patellar tendon.

With a clinically suspected tendon rupture, diagnostics have to be pushed on until it is either ensured or can be rejected.

> The treatment of the complete tendon rupture orientates at the age, the athletic activity and the therapeutic options.

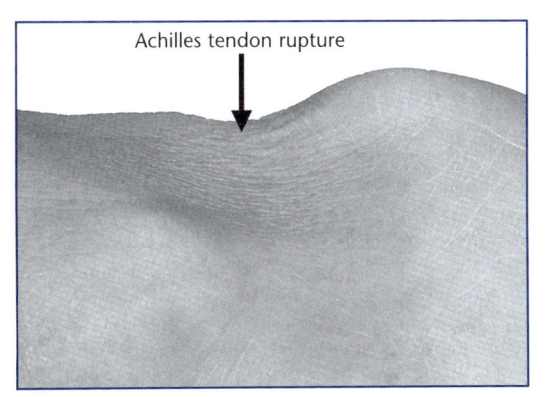

Fig. 25.4 Rupture of the Achilles tendon with typical continuity disruption (dent).

Previously, the opinion had been valid that tendons require surgical treatment within 8 hours, but now experience has shown that also **post-primary surgeries** within 10 days can lead to good or very good results. The **treatment spectrum** ranges from conservative treatment to minimally invasive surgical techniques to open technique (Jarvinen et al. 2001).

The following **principles** apply to all of these techniques: The rehabilitation

- takes a long time
- should be carried out functionally
- must be monitored continuously
- aims at the recovery of the function.

Only this way, a controlled rehabilitation can be carried out individually and possible complications, such as tendon elongations with corresponding decrease of function, can be avoided or detected early.

Partial lesions

In addition to the inflammatory and overstress-conditioned tendinoses as well as the complete rupture, there is a whole range of intermediate forms that can be called partial lesions. Partial lesions of **one or several primary bundles** – either acute or chronical – are distinguished (Segesser et al. 1995).

A special form is the **intra-tendinous partial lesion of the secondary bundles** that can lead to a mostly clear **elongation of the tendon**. Especially the **Achilles tendon** as the largest human tendon shows all variants of lesions; those are partly combined lesions of partial lesions with and without elongation.

Pain in the sense of start-up and stress pain, swelling and thickening and a more or less distinct partial insufficiency according to the force transmission are primary **symptoms**. Especially at the Achilles tendon, this is often expressed in an uncorrectable and untrainable atrophy of the triceps surae and especially the soleus muscle. In addition to the anamnesis, the clinical and functional examination is the most important part of **diagnostics** with the indicatory criteria of strength asymmetries, muscle atrophies and contour differences. These can be supported and confirmed by **imaging procedures** (ultrasound and MRT). Determining the dimension of the damage is important for the planning of the therapy concept.

The etiologic factors of the lesion as well as the severity of the injury, the age and athletic demand of the patient have to be considered in **therapy planning**. **Partial lesions of the Achilles tendon** are **treated surgically** in top athletes with lesions exceeding 7–10%; in recreational sports, on the other hand, they are treated conservatively. Generally, lesions of more than 30% of the full cross-section also receive surgery in recreational sports. Surgery is applied to non-athletes, as well, at an expanse of 50%. According to the extent, either a revision with suture or reinforcement plastic is carried out. Surgery provides the therapeutic foundation by reconstructing the anatomy.

The **interaction** of diagnosis, surgery and rehabilitation is crucial for the success, though. A therapy respecting the function is most important for an appropriate outcome especially in the field of rehabilitation. The rehabilitation, which can take months, should be continuously accompanied clinically and also biomechanically. The challenge of the treatment of top athletes is often of advantage for all patients in sports medicine.

25.2.3 Tendinopathies

Tendinoses and peritendinoses are the **most frequent causes of pain** in the region of the tendons. Tendinoses and peritendinoses can appear alone or accompanied by each other. The amount of the clinical symptoms usually depends on the duration of the disease, but also on the triggering factors. Parts of tendons as well as complete tendinous cross-sections can be affected. Concomitant partial lesions with cyst formation as well as isolated forms have been found.

The tendon typically is **swollen and painful**. In most cases, an **initial pain** after sitting or lying is reported by the patient. At rest and relaxation, the inflammatory endotendineum carrying sensitive nerval endings expands and is compressed by the tertiary bundles under stress. It is thus being irritated painfully. After few steps, the pain mostly vanishes, but reappears under higher loads.

Peritendinitis is completely different. Mostly, a **persistent pain** is found here and also partially the feeling of hyperthermia as well as crepitation in individual cases. In addition to pain under load, a partially rounded or fusiform swelling with distinct pressure pain (clamping pain) is caused in most cases. Different options are considered as **etiological factors**. The spectrum ranges from local irritations – for example, by shoes – to static-dynamic disturbances with asymmetric tensile loadings of the tendon. **Combinations** of increased loads, insufficient regeneration, muscular imbalances (asymmetries and contractions), but also insufficient tension band by the ligament apparatus can cause according overstress impairments of tendons.

Increased tibial rotation in hyperpronation combined with repetitive excentric loads can be considered the **main reason for the tendinosis of the patellar ligament**. The same applies to the **Achilles tendon. Asymmetric tensile loading**, shear forces and possibly an increased intratendinous friction and pressure of the tertiary bundles can lead to a **chronic inflammatory** reaction here as well.

The often used term of "tendinitis" is to be considered wrong, because no tenocytes are inflammatory, but the endotenon and the peritendineum are. Therefore it is not surprising that the tendinous tissue often appears like onion skins in MRT and the individual tendon bundles are pushed apart by the swollen endotenon. The complete scope of the inflammation can often only be seen in MRT, because the fusiform swelling is located in the deep, unpalpable tendon parts. In recent studies, the combination of ultrasound and color doppler examination could show the presence of so-called neo vessels (Alfredson 2003).

The **therapy of endotenonitis and peritendinitis** depends on numerous factors. In addition to the symptomatic treatment of the inflammation, the **etiologic factors** should be determined, if possible, and included into the therapeutic concept. **Intrinsic factors** such as ligament instability, muscular dysbalances, age, gender, overweight and metabolic diseases (diabetes, gout) must be considered the same like the **extrinsic factors** such as mistakes in training, insufficient regeneration and bad sport equipment, but also use of medication. A long-term improvement can only be achieved by the treatment of the etiologic factors and the cause

25.2 Tendon diseases

for further problems might be eliminated at the same time.

Interdisciplinary cooperation between physicians, biomechanics, coaches, physiotherapists and orthopedic technicians is often the basis of an integral treatment, because the conservative way of therapy is to be exhausted to the full extent, whenever possible, and surgery has to be avoided as far as possible. Local and systemic **antiphlogistics** have the same effect as physiotherapeutic and physical measures. **Correcting insoles** for the reduction or prevention of hyperpronation and an enhanced tibial rotation are just as important as a specific home program with **strengthening (excentric strength training)** and **stretching**. This way, surgery is only seldom necessary. Consistency and patience are **decisive** in the treatment of overuse injuries of the tendons. An early increase of the load, compromises in the movement strategy and the injection of steroids only meant for short-term improvement are counterproductive in the long run. The sclerosing therapy with polidocanol seems to be a promising approach of treatment of neovascularizations, though long-term results are still missing (Knobloch 2008).

25.2.4 Other tendon diseases and injuries

Bursitis

In general, bursae serve as damping shift layer at mechanically stressed points. They are found in the classic anatomical regions such as elbow and patella, but also subachillary (➤ Fig. 25.5) and subacromially. Bursae can develop in practically all regions of the body that are subject to increased mechanical loads.

With a **chronic overstress**, the otherwise bland but important and meaningful bursa can inflame and lead to a bursitis. With a bacterial population, we call it an **infected** and otherwise an **aseptic** bursitis. In general, the **treatment** of a bursitis is **conservative**. Local and systemic antiphlogistic therapies are effective the same as cooling compression bandages and punctures. An **infected bursitis** is treated by immobilization and **administration of antibiotics**. A surgical therapy with an excision of the bursa is only necessary in few cases.

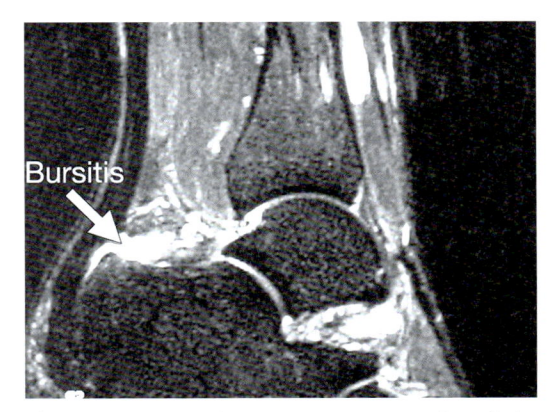

Fig. 25.5 Magnetic resonance tomography of the Achilles tendon with bursitis subachillea.

The **bursa subachillea** is a **special case**. A mostly prominent posterior calcanei process causes increased pressure load between tendon and bone, and the otherwise discretely developed bursa can enlarge inflammatorily to a great extent. A pure bursectomy is not sufficient here; in these cases, the prominent posterior calcanei process as the triggering factor is rather removed as well,

Luxation

Tendons at points of redirection in the area of bones and joints are often protected of changes in position by a relatively rough connective-tissue band (**retinaculum**). With **ruptures** of these retinaculae caused by traumas, so-called tendinous dislocations are the consequence. The dislocation of the peroneal tendon is a typical example.

In addition to the soft-tissue conduction, the **osseous friction bearing** in insufficient development can lead to a tendinous lesion or at least encourage it.

References

Alfredson H, Ohberg L, Forsgren S (2003). Is vasculoneural ingrowth the cause of pain in chronic Achilles tendinosis? An investigation using ultrasonography and colour Doppler, immunohistochemistry, and diagnostic injections. Knee Surg Sports Traumatol Arthrosc 11 (5): 334–338.

Almekinders LC, Temple JD (1998). Etiology, diagnosis and treatment of tendonitis: an analysis of the literature. Med Sci Sports Exerc 30 (8): 1183–1190.

Jarvinen TA, Kannus T, Paavola M, Jarvinen TL, Jozsa L, Jarvinen M (2001). Achilles tendon injuries. Curr Opin Rheumatol 13 (2): 150–155.

Kader D, Saxena A, Movin T, Maffulli N (2002). Achilles tendinopathy: some aspects of basic science and clinical management. Br J Sports Med 36 (4): 239–249.

Kjaer M, Langberg H, Skovgaard D, et al. (2000). In vivo studies of peritendinous tissue in exercise. Scan J Med Sci Sports 10 (6): 326–331.

Knobloch K (2008). Sclerosing polidocanol injections in Achilles tendinopathy in high level athletes. Knee Surg Sports Traumatol Arthrosc 2008 Sep 13 [Epub ahead of print].

Leppilati J, Orava S (1998). Total Achilles tendon rupture. A review. Sports Med 25 (2): 79–100.

Mafulli N, Wong J (2003). Rupture of the Achilles and patellar tendons. Clin Sports Med 22 (4): 761–776.

Mafulli N, Wong J, Almekinders LC (2003). Types and epidemiology of tendinopathy. Clin Sports Med 22 (4): 675–692.

Nigg BM (2001). The role of impact forces and foot pronation: a new paradigm. Clin J Sports Med 11(1): 2–9.

Schepsis AA, Jones H, Haas AL (2002). Achilles tendon disorders in athletes. Am J Sports Med 30 (2): 287–305.

Segesser B, Goesele A, Renggli P (1995). The Achilles tendon in sports. Orthopäde 24 (3): 252–267.

IV Sport-specific injuries

Endurance sports
26	Biathlon	361
27	Short track speed skating	365
28	Canoeing	369
29	Running	375
30	Orienteering	381
31	Cycling	387
32	Rowing	391
33	Swimming	399
34	Cross-country skiing	403
35	Triathlon	407

Strengths sports and power sports
36	Bobsleigh	413
37	Bodybuilding	417
38	Olympic Weightlifting	421
39	Athletics (Jump and Throw)	425
40	Luge	431
41	Skeleton	437
42	Carving	441
43	Ski jumping	447
44	Sport- and Rock Climbing	451

Martial arts
45	Aikido	455
46	Boxing	461
47	Fencing	467
48	Judo	471
49	Karate	477
50	Wrestling	481
51	Sumo	487
52	Taekwondo	491

Contact sports
53	American football	495
54	Baseball	499
55	Basketball	507

56	Beach soccer	515
57	Ice hockey	519
58	Soccer	525
59	Handball	531
60	Field hockey	537
61	Rugby	543

Non-contact sports

62	Badminton	549
63	Beach volleyball	555
64	Squash	561
65	Tennis	565
66	Table tennis	573
67	Volleyball	577

Technical acrobatic sports

68	Ballet	585
69	Figure skating	591
70	Artistic gymnastics	597
71	Rhythmic gymnastics	607
72	Dance	611
73	High diving	615

Trend sports

74	Inline skating	619
75	Kitesurfing	625
76	Mountain biking	631
77	Paragliding	637
78	Snowboarding	643

Other sports

79	Golf	653
80	Motorsports	659
81	Equestrianism	665
82	Shooting sports	671
83	Sailing	675
84	Sport diving	679

26 Biathlon

Alexander Disch

Biathlon (Greek for "two tests") is the **Olympic winter competition** of **cross-country skiing** (since 1985 skating technique only) and **rifle shooting**. Special bore rifles (5.6 mm) with open sight and without automatic loading are used for shooting at five targets from a distance of 50 m. In a lying position, the athletes targets a circular **metal surface** with a 45 mm diameter; targets used in standing position have a diameter of 115 mm.

The **origin of the combination of skiing and shooting** goes back to hunters and gatherers, when wild animals were hunted on ski-like objects and by bow and arrow. **Historic findings of Stone Age arctic arts** show a skiing bowman, dating from the 2nd millennium B.C. First written records of **skiing for the purpose of hunting** are known from Roman, Greek and Chinese history. The Roman poet **Vergil** described hunting on skis 400 B.C.

A second aspect in the development of this sport is its long **tradition in military skiing**. Scandinavia and Russia had independent ski regiments since **1550** and they spread in Central Europe later.

At the 43rd convention of the International Olympic Committee in Rome in 1949, the Swedish proposal to acknowledge the combination of cross-country skiing and shooting as individual Olympic competition had been accepted. The **Olympic premiere** took place in **1960 in Squaw Valley** at the VIII Winter Olympic Games. Since **1992, female biathletes** have also been allowed to win medals at the Winter Olympics (Nitzsche 1998).

26.1 Sport-specific injuries

The collective of athletes is recruited from **professional and semi-professional active athletes** mostly with long-term experiences in biathlon or cross-country skiing. Patterns of injuries and conditions are similar to cross-country skiing.

Compared to other sports **acute traumas** are **rare** events. Incidence rates vary between 0.5 and 5.5 in 1,000 athletes by day of cross-country skiing (Renstrom and Johnson 1989, Smith et al. 1996). This results from the **low risk potential** and from the **missing characteristics of mass sports** with injuries of active, inexperienced athletes.

Over the decades, **individual cases** of **shooting injuries** have been reported. Despite the small firearm caliber, injuries **with fatal outcomes** occurred. **Security standards** have been intensified, which reduced the risk of injury.

Injuries on skis are far less frequent than injuries during preparation **beyond winter season**. Athletes typically train off-season by foot, road or mountain bikes, and roller skis, which are the main training equipment. Roller skis carry a similar injury risk as inline skating.

During training and competition mostly **downfall-conditioned injury** such as contusions and distortions with internal joint disorders of the **hands, the upper ankle joints** and the **knee joints** occur (Butcher et al. 1998, Ueland and Kopjar 1998). **Fractures** of extremities, spine and thorax are **rare** (➤ Tab. 26.1). **Intensive training** carries a considerably higher **risk of**

Tab. 26.1 Acute injuries and their ranking regarding frequency of occurrence.

Type of injury	Localization
avulsions and contusions	1) knee/lower leg 2) ankle joints/foot 3) forearm/hand 4) shoulder girdle 5) skull
fractures	1) forearm/hand 2) ankle joints/foot 3) thorax 4) shoulder girdle

muscle injuries with strains and fibrous ruptures.

The **therapy** of the named injuries includes **physical therapy** with additional balneophysical therapy, ortheses treatment and interventional palliative care in addition to the full spectrum of traumatologic **acute care**. **Surgical treatment** needs to **minimize time out**.

> Low overall risk of acute injuries. Multi-modal, continuous sport-traumatologic treatment.

26.2 Sport-specific overstress conditions

Imbalances of the musculoskeletal system lead to

- acute and chronic muscle dystonias
- insertion tendinopathies
- tendinitis and tendovaginitis as well as
- periosteal irritations (Renstrom and Johnson 1989, Morris and Hoffmann 1999).

Inhomogeneously spread **patterns of medical conditions** are found in the region of:

- the upper extremity with hand and shoulder girdle
- the spine in the region of the lumbosacral junction
- the lower extremity with knee and ankle joints and
- the foot (➤ Tab. 26.2).

In biathlon, the alternation of **static effort** in the course of shooting exercises and en-

Tab. 26.2 Overuse injuries and their manifestations.

Localization	Manifestation
lumbar spine and lumbosacral junction with sacroiliac joint	■ myogeloses ■ blockades ■ nucleus pulposus prolapsed ■ intervertebral osteochondrosis ■ arthroses of the facet joint
knee joint	■ femoropatellar chondropathies ■ ligamentous instabilities ■ meniscus degeneration ■ gonarthrosis
upper ankle joint	■ chronic ligament instability ■ arthrosis
foot	■ deformity of the forefoot with metatarsalgias ■ arthroses
shoulder girdle	■ subacromial bottleneck syndromes ■ arthosis of the AC joint

durance performance results in tonus changes, disorders and functional limitations of the **shoulder and back muscles** (Rundell and Bacharach 1995). To **move** effectively, the **upper body** is flexed against the lower body and straights into a **hyperextended position** (Perrey et al. 1998). The developing force correlates with the flexion/extension cycle (Holmberg et al. 2005). This movement **will lead to an increasedincreases force effect onto the lumbar spine** and the lumbosacral junction (Renstrom and Johnson 1989). Acute conditions as well as **chronic degenerative changes** are typical (Lindsay et al. 1993, Mahlamaki et al. 1998, Bahr et al. 2004).

Skating reduces the relapsing load peaks of the lumbar spine by reducing the active extension and flexion (Rundell and Bacharach 1998). The compensating movements of the pelvis reduces **load of the lumbar spine and hip joints** (Alricson and Werner 2004). A lower frequency of disorders and long-term damages can be expected in biathlon as compared to cross-country skiing, where competition is carried out in the classic running style, which is more stressing for the lumbar spine.

A typical overuse damage at the lower extremity is the chronic compartment syndrome of the lower leg. Repetitive contractions cause minor perfusion with consecutive edema, which leads to an increased intramuscular and intracompartmental pressure Additionally, the persistent load causes microtraumatization of the microfibrils and sarcomeres, which reduces contractibility. The smaller muscular compartment volume chronically increases tissue pressure and results in a contractile condition. This leads to a progressive perfusion reduction and reduced oxygen supply, which results in a vicious circle. Chronic lower leg pain appears and in severe cases can even damage permanently musculatures, vessels and nerves (Gertsch et al. 1987, Lawson et al. 1992). In therapy, the symptom-orientated surgical intervention with compartment relief should be considered especially if conservative pressure reduction failed.

The key treatment concept focuses on prevention and instruction for athletes and coaches in the sport-medical eligibility examination. An early intervention with conservative therapy is stringently required to prevent chronic disease. Treatment in sport-orthopedic surgical centers should be considered if therapy fails.

> Multilocular appearance of overstress conditions. Early conservative and surgical therapy for the minimization of downtimes.

References

Alricsson M, Werner S (2004). The effect of pre-season dance training on physical indices and back pain in elite cross-country skiers. Br J Sports Med 38: 149–153.

Bahr R, Anderse SO, Loken S, Fossan B, Hansen T, Holme E (2004). Low back pain among endurance athletes with and without specific back loading. Spine 28 (4): 449–454.

Butcher JD, Brannen SJ (1998). Comparison of injuries in classic and skating Nordic techniques. Clin J Sport Med 8 (2): 88–91.

Gertsch P, Borgeat A, Walli T (1987). New cross-country skiing technique and compartment syndrome. Am J Sports Med 15 (6): 612–613.

Holmberg H-C, Lindinger S, Stöggl T, Eitzlmair E, Müller E (2005). Biomechanical analysis of double-poling in elite cross-country skiing. Med Sci Sports Exer.

Lawson SK, Reid DC, Wiley JP (1992). Anterior compartment pressures in cross-country skiers. Am J Sports Med 20 (6): 750–753.

Lindsay DM, Meeuwisse WH, Vyse A, Mooney ME, Summersides J (1993). Lumbosacral dysfunctions in elite cross-country skiers. J Orthop Sport Phys Ther 18 (5): 580–585.

Mahlamaki S, Soimakallio S, Michelsson JE (1988). Radiological findings in the lumbar spine of 39 young cross-country skiers with low back pain. Int J Sports Med 9 (3): 196–197.

Morris PJ, Hoffman DF (1999). Injuries in cross-country skiing. Postgrad Med 105 (1): 89–101.

Nitzsche K (1998). Leistung Training Wettkampf. 1st ed. Verlag Limpert, Wiesbaden.

Perrey S, Millet GY, Candau R, Rouillon JD (1998). Stretch shortening cycle in roller ski skating: effects of technique. Int J Sports Med 19 (8): 513–520.

Renstrom P, Johnson RJ (1989). Cross-country skiing injuries and biomechanics. Sports Med 8 (6): 346–370.

Rundell KW, Bacharach DW (1995). Physiological characteristics and performance of top U.S. biathletes. Med Sci Sports Exerc 27 (9): 1302–1310.

Rundell KW, Szmedra L (1998). Energy cost of rifle carriage in biathlon. Med Sci Sports Exerc 30 (4): 570–576.

Smith M, Matheson GO, Meeuwisse WH (1996). Injuries in cross-country skiing. Sports Med 21 (3): 239–250.

Ueland O, Kopjar B (1998). Occurrence and trends in ski injuries in Norway. Br J Sports Med 32: 299–303.

Chapter 27 Short track speed skating

Volker Smasal

More than 3,000 years ago in Northern Europe, animal bones tied up under feet indicated first, historic movement on ice. Wooden shoes with iron blades point to early skating activity in the Netherlands from the 13th century on. First competitions in speed skating were carried out in England in the 18th century. After foundation of the **International Skating Union** (ISU) in 1892, speed skating became Olympic discipline in 1924. Short track, the competition on the short distance, has been added as Olympic sport in 1992. While speed skating is a national sport in the Netherlands, only about 1,000 people perform this sport competitively in Germany. There are about 250 active short-track skaters in Germany and is more popular in Korea, China and Canada.

27.1 Characteristics

Speed-skating competitions are carried out on the 400-m track with distances between 500 m and 5,000 m for women or 10,000 m for men in Olympic Games, with two skaters racing each other on separate lanes and changing lanes at every round. The team races with three had its Olympic premiere at the 2006 Winter Olympics in Turin, with the men skating 6 rounds and the women 8 rounds. Similar to cyclists, a team starts at the finishing straight, and the other team will start at the counter straight. Because the teams only race on the inner lane, the distances will amount to just 2,300 m for women and 3,100 m for men.

The short-track lane is an oval of a length of 111.12 m marked on an ice-hockey field. Individual distances between 500 m and 1.500 m are raced with up to six starters at the same time. Four teams are on the lane for relay races of 3,000 m for women or 5,000 m for men, with four racers replaced in each or every second round.

27.2 Equipment

Speed skaters wear individually adapted **shoes** of carbon or leather, light metals are used for the clasp; the blade is made of steel. The **speed-**

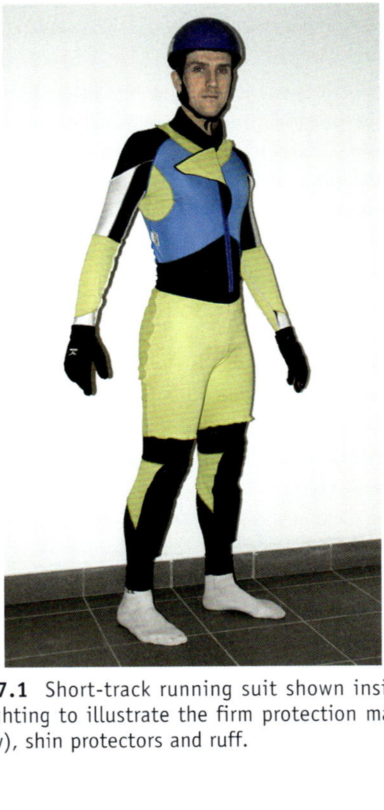

Fig. 27.1 Short-track running suit shown inside-out highlighting to illustrate the firm protection materials (yellow), shin protectors and ruff.

skating suits are made of special, thin fabrics and aim to improve aero-dynamics and stabilize f the body.

Security equipment is required for **short track ice skating** (➢ Fig. 27.1). A helmet, neck protection, gloves, suits with long sleeves and legs, shin pads and knee protection of cut-resistant materials are obligatory. Goggles protect the eye. The shoes are made of hard carbonic shells, partially with a leather coating; the ends of the blades must be rounded; clap skates as in speed skating are not permitted.

27.3 Overuse symptoms

Overuse damages in speed skating are more common than acute injuries; it is reversed in short track. The spectrum is similar, with a focus on spine, knee and ankle joints (➢ Tab. 27.1).

The upper body's permanent forward leaning, simultaneous hyperlordosis, and torsion stresses the lower lumbar spine. Frequent blockades of the iliosacral joints, protrusion and prolapse of the intervertebral disks L4/5 and L5/S1 are the consequence.

The strong femoropatellar contact pressure, which is irregular in the curved running, cumulatively leads to retropatellar cartilage disorders and chondropathic conditions at the knee joints. Insertion tendopathies, especially the patellar apex syndrome, are additional consequences of overuse.

Tab. 27.1 Overuse damages in speed skating and short track.

Lumbar spine	■ Blocking of lumbar spine and iliosacral joints ■ Facet syndrome ■ Bulging and herniation of intervertebral disks L4/S and L5/S1
Knee and ankle joints	■ Chondropathic conditions ■ Retropatellar cartilage damages ■ Unfastening of the capsule-ligament structures of the ankle joint ■ Bursitides at foot and ankle
Insertion tendinopathies	■ Patellar apex syndrome, above all

The typical interaction of pronation and supination and frequent distortions loosen the ankle joint capsule-ligament structures. Typical for ice skates are bursitides at foot and ankle caused by pressure and friction.

27.4 Accident causes and injuries

Falls caused by personal errors explain acute injury in speed skating whereas most cases in short track are caused by collisions with the op-

Tab. 27.2 Spectrum of injuries in speed skating and short track.

Speed skating and short track	
■ Contusions of shoulder, back, pelvis and skull ■ Distortions of the cervical spine, primarily ■ Capsule-ligament injuries in ankle and knee joints, hand, elbow, and shoulder ■ Shoulder dislocations	
Mainly speed skating	**Mainly short track**
■ Strains, torn fibers, (partial) ruptures of the musculature, primarily of the adductors ■ Incisions at the calf and Achilles tendon	■ Fractures ■ Serious spinal injuries ■ Abrasions, lacerations or incisions

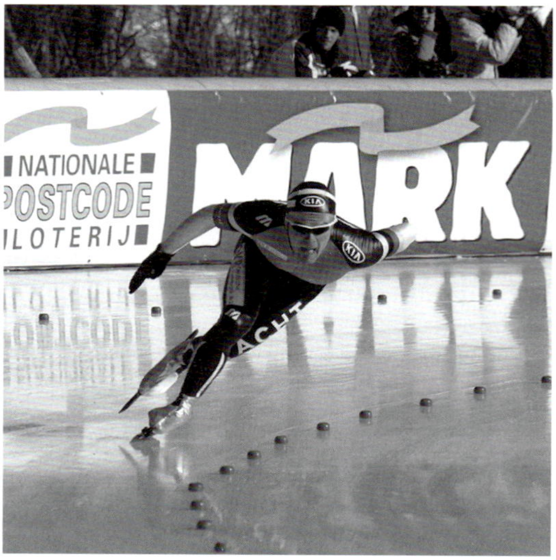

Fig. 27.2 Extreme sloping position and load on skates in dynamic running posture.

Fig. 27.3 Running position in short track with enormous sloping position. Load on the blades and securing of the balance with the left hand.

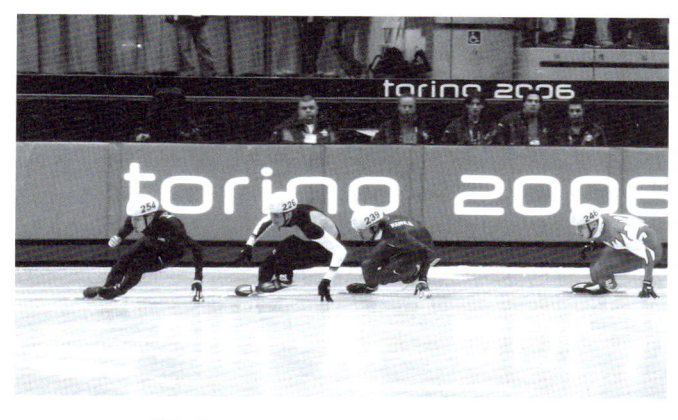

ponent. The **spectrum of injuries** on the 400-m track in speed skating is similar to the one of short track. Injuries in short track are more frequent and more serious (➤ Tab. 27.2).

Since the first use of clap skates for competition in 1997, speeds of about 60 km/h (37 miles/h) have been achieved on the 400-m track. Centrifugal forces at a strong sloping position in the curves cause more frequent falls in high skating speeds (➤ Fig. 27.2). Additionally, the clap mechanism increases instability at the front part of the ice skate. The modern lubricated racing suits intensify the collision speed with walls or opponents.

In short track, the running rail is bent for the permanent running of small curves. Maximum speeds of 50 km/h (31 miles/h) can be reached. Especially the narrow curves with sloping positions of 38 or 40° of the body carry the risk of body contact. The bent and sharp blades increase the risk of injuries (➤ Fig. 27.3).

Falls and collisions lead to **contusions** of shoulders, back, pelvis and cranium. Upper extremity **fractures** – especially of the wrist – are typical as in inline skating. Fallen skaters try to get into a sitting position to establish a high body tension and soften the collision with the padded boards by a rotation of back and shoulder. Nevertheless, the high collision speeds and adverse contact angles often lead to distortions of the cervical spine. Falls in training without the obligatory wall protection mats led to serious spinal injuries, even paraplegias.

Opponents and their sharp blades, the ice and walls cause abrasions, ruptures, incised wounds, or lacerations. The protective clothing in short track skating (➤ Fig. 27.1) reduces the

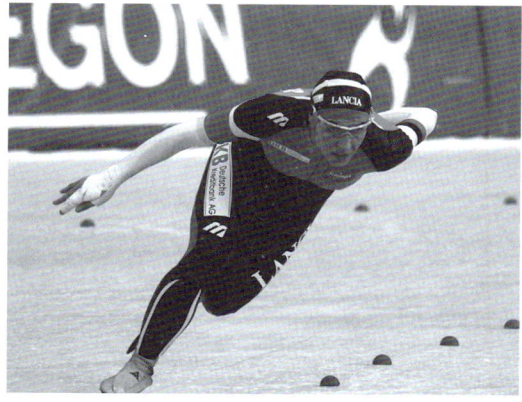

Fig. 27.4 World Cup 2005 over 1,500 m with tape bandage at the right hand after a fall of 2 days before and rupture of the volar plate of the medial joint and distortion of the metacarpophalageal joint of the second finger.

frequency of serious injuries. Capsule-ligament injuries of the knee joints and ankle joints are triggered the torsion of the body and joints, which develop when falling over each other or sliding of the foot under the surrounding walls. Similar injuries happen at hand, elbow and shoulder, if the arm gets caught under the protection mats (➤ Fig. 27.4). The **shoulder dislocations** increase with falls on the 400-m track.

Strains, fibrous ruptures, and complete **ruptures** of the muscles mainly affect the adductors. Major causes are the enormous force at the explosive start, especially at the sprints in speed skating. Self-induced, incised wounds at calf and Achilles tendon come from the sharpened skate blades, especially at the start (➤ Fig. 27.5).

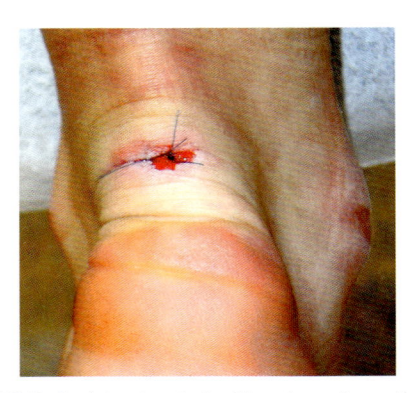

Fig. 27.5 Incision treated with suture above the left Achilles tendon caused by sliding over the own opposing shoe at start of training.

27.5 Therapy and prevention

Acute measures are required during the competition season. Often only manual examination is possible and needs to consider potential long-term damages; hence, care must be taken with the necessary sport-specific experience. Further diagnosis and therapy at the earliest possible time is imperative and requires confirmation. Treatment is performed according to standard practice in competitive sports. **Acute therapies** include but are not limited to joint repositioning, chiropractic manipulations, injections, functional tape bandages and many more. The **pharmacological treatment** requires an exact knowledge of the current anti-doping restrictions with regard to possible obligations and prohibitions.

Follow-up by a **physiotherapist** familiar with the sport is essential. Rehabilitation training is often necessary in particular because of the intense spine load.

Preventively, falls should be exercised early in training. Strength and endurance are prerequisites for competitive performance of speed skating. In addition to training at the gym, cycling and inline skating at high altitude are part of the training program.

Individually shaped ice skates, an exactly fitting running suit with protective equipment in short track, and the wearing of running goggles are material preconditions for prevention and reduction of overuse damages and injuries.

References

Allinger TL, van den Bogert AJ (1996). Skating technique for the straights, based on the optimization of a simulation model. Med Sci Sports Exerc 29: 179–186.

De Groot G, Hollander AP, Sargeant AJ, van Ingen Schenau GJ, De Boer RW (1987). Applied physiology of speed skating. Journal of Sports Science 5: 249–259.

Gemser H, de Koning J, van Ingen Schenau GJ (1999). Handbook of Competitive Speed Skating. ISU, Lausanne

Smasal V, Zeilberger K (2005). Eisschnelllauf. In: Engelhardt et al. Sportverletzungen Sportschäden. Thieme Verlag, Stuttgart.

Smasal V (1994). Muskuloskeletale Verletzungen und Überlastungsschäden bei Eisschnelläufern. Ursachen, Therapie und Prophylaxe. Prakt Sporttraumatol Sportsmed 10: 148–153.

Smasal V (2001). Eisschnelllauf. In: Clasing D, Siegfried I (eds.). Sportärztliche Untersuchung und Beratung. 3rd revised ed. Spitta, Balingen: 294-297.

van Ingen Schenau GJ, De Groot G, Scheurs AW, Meester H, De Koning JJ (1996). A new skate allowing powerful plantar flexions improves performance. Med Sci Sports Exerc 28: 531–535.

28 Canoeing

Roland Eisele

The oldest verifiable canoe has been found in a more than 6,000-year-old grave of a Sumerian king. Around 1830, The Scottish lawyer MacGregor became the father of **modern canoeing**. In 1914, the **German Canoeing Association** was founded, counting more than 114,000 members nowadays.

Folding canoes for racing had been introduced first at the **Olympic Games** in 1936.

Canoe racing and canoe slalom are current Olympic disciplines. Other competitive disciplines with official **world championships** are whitewater racing and sprint, canoe marathon, dragon boat and canoe polo, as well as freestyle (rodeo) and rafting (➤ Tab. 28.1).

Hobby canoeing has shown an unbelievable boom in recent years because of its many-faceted options. The number of canoeists in

Tab. 28.1 Disciplines in the International Canoe Federation (ICF). Duration of competition of the Olympic Games (OG) and the World Championships (WC).

Canoe disciplines	Description of the discipline	Length of competition in meters (m) or minutes (min)	Olympic Games (OG), World Cup (WC)
Flat water racing	1–4 athletes Kayak and canoe in tracks on flat water	200 m, 500 m, 1,000 m	OG, WC
Slalom racing	1–2 athletes Kayak and canoe whitewater through 25 gates, max.	2× approx. 1:30 min	OG, WC
Whitewater racing	1–2 athletes Kayak and canoe whitewater approx. 4 km	approx. 10–20 min	WC
Dragon boat racing	20 athletes with blade paddles	200 m, 500 m, 1,000 m	WC
Canoe polo	5 players to goals	2 × 10 min	WC
Rafting	6 athletes Canoe, rubber raft Whitewater	Slalom: 3–4 min + Sprint: approx. 2 min + Endurance: 20–60 min	WC
Freestyle (rodeo)	1 athlete kayak or canoe Acrobatics on a river feature (rollers)	2 × 0:45 min	WC
Marathon	1–4 athletes Kayak and canoe for even more than 42 km	up to several hours on several days	WC

Tab. 28.2 Acute injuries and chronic overuse damages in percent in whitewater canoeing.

Injury localization	Whitewater kayak	Whitewater canoe
Acute	**60–75%**	**85–90%**
Hand/wrist	20%	20%
Forearm/elbow	10%	5%
Face	5–10%	25–35%
Shoulder	30–35%	5–10%
Foot	10%	10–15%
Knee	5–10%	15%
Chronic	**25–40%**	**10–15%**
Hand/wrist	35%	5%
Forearm/elbow	20%	30%
Shoulder	25–30%	20–45%
Back	15%	30%

the United States and Europe has increased by 15% each year. There are no reliable data for canoe tripping and canoe sailing. Whitewater sport is performed as individual adventurous sport in a kayak by about 2–3 million people; rafting (rubber rafts), mostly offered commercially as group sport, is performed by about 10 million people (Fiore 2003).

In general, two different kinds of canoe are used:

- Canadian canoe: The original forms are mostly open boat forms (Indians, inhabitants of the South Seas) and will be pushed on by a single-bladed paddle, the **canoe paddle**. The seat is positioned at **hip level**.
- Kayaks: Even today, they are used by Eskimos as means of transport and for hunting with the **double paddle**. In the sitting position, **knee joints** are **above the hip level**.

The most frequent injuries and overload damages (Shepard 1987) are deduced from the different competitive disciplines and the boat types (➤ Tab. 28.2).

28.1 Competition disciplines

- **Canoe racing:** on stagnant water in marked straight lanes with up to nine boats. The one who crosses the target line first wins the race. Internationally prevailing **distances** are 200, 500 and 1,000 m. **Boat classes** are single, double and four-seated kayaks (women and men) and Canadians (men only).
- **Canoe slalom:** on a blocked wild river or an artificially created whitewater lane with 18 to 25 gates being maneuvered through by the athletes, partially against the current, as fast as possible. Penalty seconds are assigned for touching the gate poles or missing a gate. The distances mostly have a length of ca. 300–350 m. The athlete using the least time in two runs wins. The **competitive classes** are single kayak (women and men) as well as single and double Canadian (men only).
- **Whitewater racing:** on fast, wild rivers, on a classic distance of 3–7 km or for some years now in sprint over about 500 m. Races start typically every minute. During the 10 and 20 minutes long competition, the athlete must navigate between rocks, waves and barrels. The **competing classes** are identical to canoe slalom.
- **Dragon boat:** boats decorated with a dragon head and tail, with up to 20 paddlers pushing them rhythmically forwards in Canadian style under drum beats and cheers. International **distances of competition** are 250, 500 and 1,000 m.
- **Canoe polo: team sport** in canoe sports. Two teams with five players each face each other on a field of 23 × 35 m. It is the aim to throw the ball into one of the two goals of the size 1 × 1.5 m that are attached to the ends of the playing field at a height of 2 m. One game lasts 2 × 10 minutes.

Safety precautions: Helmets and life vests are obligatory in canoe slalom, whitewater racing and canoe polo.

28.2 Injury and overload damages

Fatal accidents are as frequent as in other adventure sports (mountain hiking, underwater diving, parachuting): approximately 5 lives are lost in 1 million days of exercising this sport. The **injury rates** for whitewater are stated as

3–6 in 100,000 canoeing days in kayaking and 0.26–2.1 in 100,000 canoeing days in rafting.

In **kayaking**, the injuries are mainly caused by capsizing, and in rafting often by collisions of occupants of the boat or with the material in rafting (Fiore 2003). 87% of the injuries of kayakers happen in the boat, with the upper extremities naturally affected most often.

Most frequent **accident causes** are:
- Collision injuries (44%)
- Capsizing (25%) and
- Overstress (25%).

The **acute injury patterns** split up as follows:
- Abrasions 20–25%
- Tendinitis 25%
- Contusions and distortions 25%
- Dislocations 5–15% and
- Fractures >10%.

In **rafting**, 51% occur in the boat, 40% at capsizing and 8% of the injuries happen ashore (Whisman and Holenhorst 1999).

In **racing**, the injuries split up as follows:
- Shoulder 53%
- Back 20%
- Hand and wrist 13%
- Abdominal muscles and fingers 7% (Edwards 1993).

28.2.1 Arms

Tendon sheaths of the wrist joint are especially vulnerable in canoe racing. The dominant hand is definitely more affected (70%). It fixes the paddle while the paddle shaft is rotated in the non-dominant hand. The **tendovaginitis of the wrist joint** is with an average of 23% the most frequent overload damage in marathon regattas. Canoeists with more than 100 km of training per week showed significantly less medical conditions in long-distance competitions than non-exercised persons.

A **hyperextension in the wrist joint** is the most frequent technical mistake in paddling. The stabilization of the boat with a strong muscle-strong trunk and a good capability of balance prevent technical mistakes in paddling (du Troit et al. 1999). An inelastic paddle shaft leads to more frequent medical problems in less exercised persons.

> Tendovaginitis of the wrist joints: long-distance competitions in kayak > Canadian, dominant hand > rotating hand.
>
> Prophylaxis:
> - Aimed technical training (no hyperextension in the wrist joint)
> - Stress preparation by adequately structured training
> - Stress follow-up by adequate stretching
> - Checking of the material conditions of the paddle

28.2.2 Shoulders

The **anterior shoulder luxation** is the most serious injury in canoe slalom, whitewater racing and canoe polo, which is triggered by the capsizing movement.

The tilting movement of the boat is intercepted by the deeper sitting position, the rotated, abducted arm and double paddle of kayakers. Canadian canoeists use mostly internally rotated, adducted arms. Therefore, kayakers (➤ Fig. 28.1) suffer from more shoulder luxations as Canadian canoeists (➤ Fig. 28.2; current national squad 10 vs. 3%).

The shoulder is central in the force transmission between paddle and boat. Overload condi-

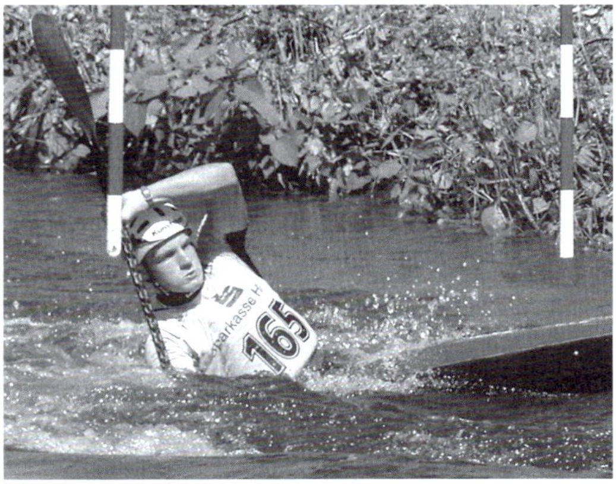

Fig. 28.1 Shoulder stress in canoeing. Solo kayak (third place European championship 2005, Erik Pfannmöller).

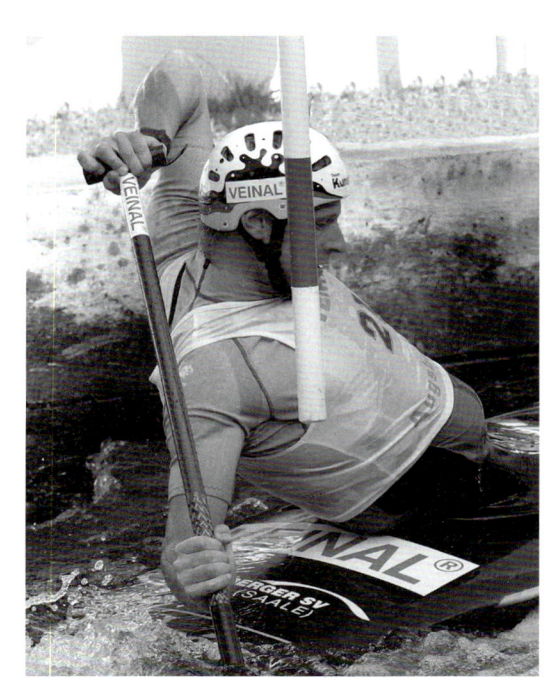

Fig. 28.1 Shoulder stress in canoeing. Solo canoe (Olympic third in canoe slalom in Athens 2004, Stefan Pfannmöller).

tions occur most often at the **rotator cuff**. Lesions of the rotator cuffs due to overload with secondary impingement are found in marathon kayakers twice as often as in sprint paddlers.

Small surveys of racers show **shoulder lesions** in the anamnesis of more than half of the athletes. These divide into:

- Bursitis 14%
- Tendinitis of the biceps tendon 20% and
- Tears of the rotator cuffs 20% (Edwards 1993).

In Canadian canoeing (➢ Fig. 28.2), the one-sided elevation over the level of 90° and the internal rotation with impingement on the side of the paddle stud in the pressure face supervene (Pelham et al. 1995).

An acromioclavicular hypertrophy is a frequent radiologic finding in marathon paddlers (Hagemann et al. 2004).

The shoulder luxation should be treated with immediate surgical stabilization. The relaxation is significantly lower than in a conservative immobilization therapy (Kirkley et al. 2005).

> Lesions of the rotator cuffs and shoulder dislocations: marathon and whitewater canoeing.
> Prophylaxis:
> - Exercises for shoulder stabilization (body blade)
> - Technical training (Canadian support also in kayaking, backwards Eskimo roll)

28.2.3 Spine

Roughly 15% suffer from spinal problems (Schoen and Stano 2002). **Overload** of the spinal middle and caudal region are due to the rotation axis of the trunk. Functional disorders are described more often in Canadian canoeists than in kayakers because of the sideways tilting. Problems of the **cranial** spinal segments are also found more often in these athletes. Due to the sitting position in kayak **These will be localized more often in the caudal** spinal segments are more often affected.

> Spinal conditions: in Canadians more frequent than in kayaks.
> Prophylaxis: muscular stabilization of the spine and modification of the sitting position.

28.1 Conclusion

Canoeing sport is extremely faceted. The sport injuries naturally concentrate to the upper extremities and the trunk. In addition to an adequate **muscular preparation**, appropriate **equipment**, a good **technique** and the reasonable assessment of the own capabilities are the most important preconditions to avoid damages.

References

Du Troit P, Sole G, Bowerbank P, Noakes TD (1999). Incidence and causes of tendosynovitis of wrist extensors in long distance paddle canoeists. Br J Sports Med 33: 105–109.

Edwards A (1993). Injuries in kayaking. Sport Health 11: 8–11.

Fiore DC (2003). Injuries associated with whitewater rafting and kayaking. Wilderness Environ Med 14: 255–250.

Fiore DC, Houston JD (2001). Injuries in whitewater kayaking. Br J Sports Med 35: 977–984.

Hagemann G, Rijke AM, Mars M (2004). Shoulder pathoanatomy in marathon kayakers. Br J Sports Med 38: 413–417.

Kirkeley A, Werstine R, Ratjek A, Griffin S (2005). Prospective randomized clinical trail comparing the effectiveness of immediate arthroscopic stabilization versus immobilization and rehabilitation in first traumatic anterior dislocation of the shoulder: long-term evaluation. Arthroscopy 21: 55–63.

Pelham TW, Holt LE, Stalker RE (1995). The etiology of paddlers shoulders. Aust J Sci Med Sport 27: 43–47.

Schoen RG, Stano MJ (2002). Year 2000 whitewater injury survey. Wilderness Environ Med 13: 119–124.

Shepard RJ (1987). Science and medicine of canoeing and kayaking. Sports Med 4: 19–33.

Whisman SA, Hollenhorst SJ (1999). Injuries in commercial whitewater rafting. Clin J Sports Med 9: 18–23.

www.kanu.de

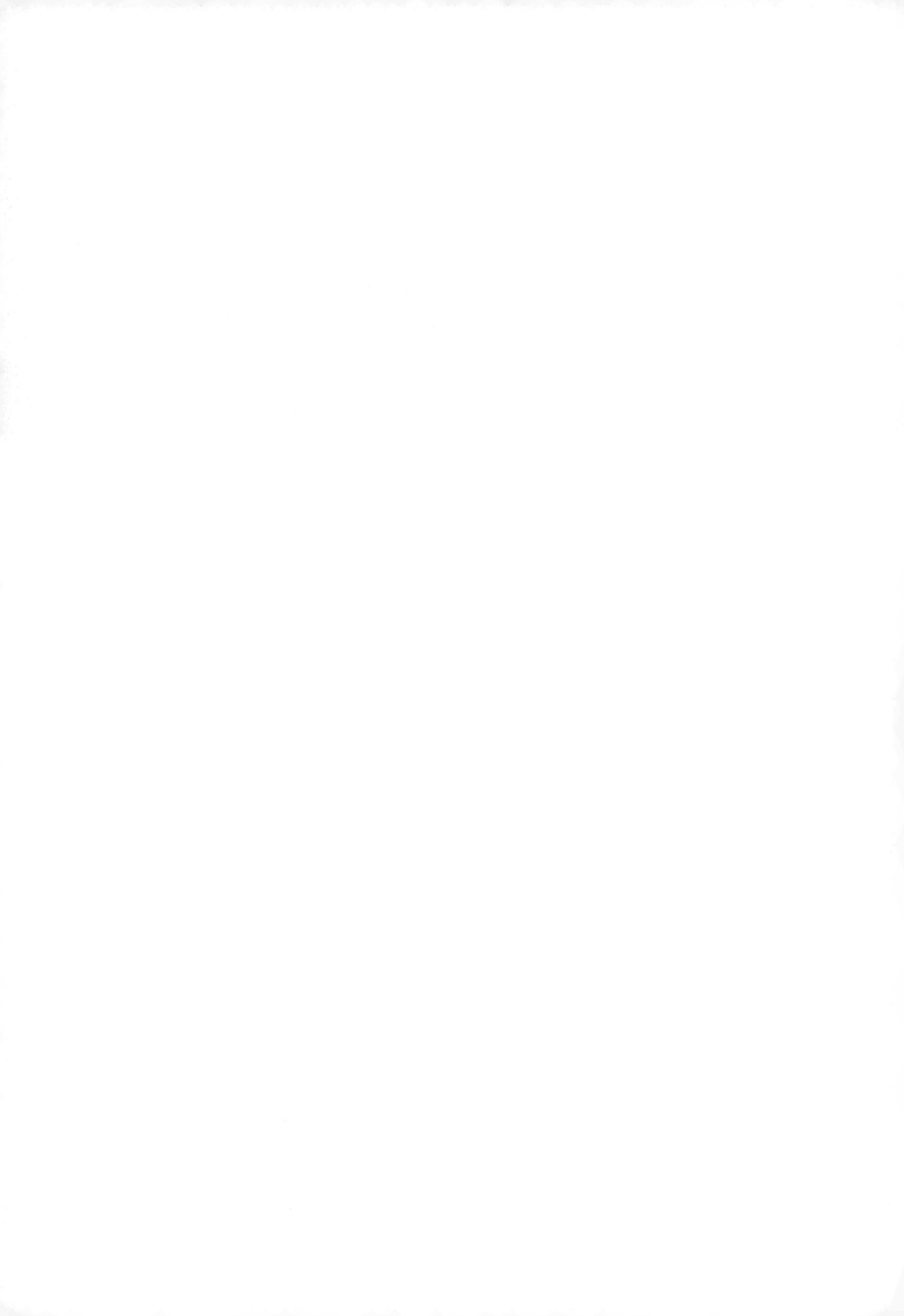

Chapter 29 Running

Martin Engelhardt, Iris Reuter and Casper Grim

Running is one of the most popular sports in Germany, where the first running competition took place in 1880 on the racecourse in Hamburg. Marathon has been part of the Olympic programme since 1896 for men and since 1984 for women. Since the 1960ies, leisure and high-performance running has gained popularity all over the world. In Germany, the number of recreational runners is estimated at about ten million.

29.1 Characteristics of running

Running sets the body mass into motion without external sports equipment thus, it is one of the most strenuous, high energy consuming sports (Stromme and Ingier 1982). Running has a favourable benefit-risk-ratio and prevents cardiovascular diseases (Wilmore and Costill 1999). Positive impacts of running have also been documented in the treatment of depression and headaches (Clement et al. 1981).

The impact on muscles, tendons and ligaments, cartilage and the bones of the lower extremities can, however, cause running injuries of the musculoskeletal system (van Mechelen 1992, Reuter 2005, Walther et al. 2005).

Running is a **sport with a cyclic movement** pattern and a constant repetition of the same sequence of movements. Running technique, axial malalignment, fatigue, and pathological alterations of the muscular system affect the load peaks during running and may lead to certain injury patterns or overload-induced damages.

29.2 Running technique

Forefoot running increases the stress on the calf muscles, the metatarsophalangeal joints, and the metatarsal bones. The more common form of **hindfoot running** entails a stronger distension of the calf muscles and a higher muscular effort of the anterior shinbone muscles in order to absorb the ground reaction forces of the foot.

A minor **step length** results in lower compression forces, but, in the long term, evokes a shortening of the groin muscles and a weakening of the hip extensors, involving an anterior tilt of the pelvis with increased lumbar lordosis that may cause back and knee pain. An increased step length leads to a greater impact on the knee extensors and the calf muscles in the beginning of the support phase.

29.3 Axial malalignment

According to statistics, axial malalignments do not account for increased injury rates in running (Walther et al. 2004). Biomechanical abnormities in the lower extremity can yet trigger an earlier degenerative cartilage wear due to the increased load peaks. Extreme varus or valgus deformities of in the lower extremity are a contraindication for continuous high-performance endurance running.

Hyperpronation

Hyperpronation leads to strong reaction forces in the **medial** foot area. This may cause pain in the first metatarsophalangeal joint and the sesamoid bones and facilitates the emergence of a hallux valgus and the development of exostoses. The formation of calluses in the region of the first metatarsophalangeal joint can be very painful. Hyperpronation also promotes the subsidence of the longitudinal arch of the foot and the occurrence of **plantar fasciitis**. The increased pronation of the foot leads to higher stress on the M. tibialis posterior and the M. soleus, which might cause Achilles' tendon problems and pain of the tendon of the M. tibialis posterior. Moreover, the increased load may cause shin splints. Hyperpronation facilitates **patello-femoral joint dysfunction** with a tendency towards lateral patella hypercompression or subluxation. Pain in the patella tendon and the iliotibial band occur frequently. Another implication of foot malalignment may be the occurrence of stress fractures of the metatarsal bones, the sesamoid bones, and tibia or fibula.

Hypersupination

Factors promoting hypersupination are a valgus position of the forefoot, weak peroneal muscles, or hyperactivity of the M. tibialis posterior, M. gastrocnemius or M. soleus. The foot is less flexible and can not absorb the impact adequately, which leads to increased forces to the **lateral aspect** of the foot with a higher risk of stress fractures for the metatarsal bones IV and V; also pain at iliotibial band and bursitis at the lateral femoral condyl can occur.

Abnormal hip movement

Weak hip-stabilisers (M. iliopsoas, M. gluteus, abdominal muscles) and weak core muscles accentuate the hip movement and may provoke an abnormal load distribution while running. Most often, such muscle insufficiency causes a pelvic tilt, leading to a shortening of the hip flexors. The external rotators of the hip are shortened in the course of compensating the function of the too weak gluteal muscles. Thus, the emerging slight abduction of the leg can with simultaneous weakness of the abdominal muscles, trigger a lumbar hyperlordosis possibly accompanied with pain in the sacroilical area.

An imbalance between the hip abductors and hip adductors may result in a swinging pelvic movement, resulting in increased stress to the lateral hip and knee structures. The increased pelvic tilt leads to a stronger knee flexion that, again, puts additional stress on the patello-femoral joint.

29.4 Running injuries

According to literature, the incidence of running-related injuries is 24–77% (Engelhardt et al. 2003, Walther et al. 2005) and 2.5–5.8 injuries per 1000 hours of running (van Mechelen (1992);

Tab. 29.1 Distribution of running-related injuries and overuse injuries in various publications (in %).

	Clement 1980	Macintyre 1991	Taunton 2002	Taunton 2003
N	1819	4173	2002	844
Study design	retrospective	retrospective	retrospective	retrospective
Knee	34	35	42	34
Lower leg	11	16	13	16
Foot/ankle joint	19	10	17	23
Achilles' tendon	8	4	6	10
Hip/pelvis	2	5	11	8
Back	2	n. m.	4	6
Hamstrings	1	2	n. m.	2
Upper leg	1	1	5	1

n. m. = not mentioned

Knee pain is the most common complaint of runners reaching up to 40% reported until the mid-1990ies (Clement et al. 1981, Walther et al. 2005) (> Tab. 29.1). More recent publications (Mayer et al. 2000), however, report a dominance of Achilles' tendon affections.

In 80% of the cases running injuries concern the **lower extremity**. Acute injuries are rare. There are muscle-tendon-injuries (in sprinters and medium-distance runners mainly on the hamstring side, in long-distance runners predominantly in the calf muscles), ankle joint distorsion (up to ruptures of the fibular capsule-ligament complex), and skin injuries (abrasions, blisters).

29.5 Consequences of overuse

80% of the complaints occurring in the context of running result from a disproportion between the general capacity of the conjunctive and supporting tissue and the actual strain evoked by the sport, most commonly induced by a too fast increase of running load, by omitted warming-up, insufficient regeneration after illnesses or injuries, exertion during infection, inadequate footwear, and malalignment (Engelhardt et al. 2003). The runner perceives the improper strain as muscle pain, soreness of the tendon insertion, the periosteum or joint pain. Complaints and results from repetitive microtrauma are usually reversible if they are correctly diagnosed, treated and if the causing factors are eliminated.

Apart from the exact examination, **anamnesis** is of great importance in the case of runners' complaints:

- How extensive is the training programme? To what extent was it increased lately?
- On what kind of training surface?
- Change of running shoe? What does the running shoe look like?
- How is the workout composed? What was the training speed?
- Are there signs of infection?
- Were there illnesses/injuries in the past?

Typical consequences of overuse to be diagnosed are:

- Patella-femoral pain syndrome
- Inflammation of the Hoffa's fat pad
- Pain below the medial knee joint line (bursitis or tendinosis of the pes anserinus)
- Affection of the Achilles' Tendon (tendinopathy, peritendinitis, bursitis)
- Back pain (sciatic complaints, SI joint affections)
- Stress fractures (predominantly metatarsals II III, calcaneus, tibia, fibula)
- Chronic compartment syndrome
- Plantar fasciits

Depending on the cause of complaints, there are various treatment options at hand:

- Running pause, workout in another sport (swimming, aqua jogging, cycling, cross-country skiing)
- Physical therapy (cooling, electrotherapy, massage/deep frictions, physiotherapy (excentric muscle-training)
- Oral and local antiphlogistics, local injections, acupuncture
- Functional support bandages, insoles, shoe adjustment, bandages
- Surgical measures (debridment, release, bursektomie, axial corrections etc.)

29.6 Limitations of running ability

Orthopedic disorders:

- congenital hip dislocation and dysplastic hip joints
- Profound structural birth defects or abnormalities of the extremities (particularly gross axial malalignment of the lower extremity)
- Pre-existing articular cartilage defects
- Spondylolisthesis over 5 mm or bilateral spondylolysis
- Distinct scoliosis and kyphosis
- Not fully healed OCD
- aseptic bone necrosis with improper healing and persisting complaints

Internal disorders:

- valve defects with hemodynamic consequences
- Acute and chronic myocarditis
- Hypertrophic cardiomyopathy
- Pathologic cardial arrhythmia
- Fixed high blood pressure (> 169/95 mmHg)
- Fixed asthma bronchialis with limited lung function
- Chronic renal diseases
- Disorders of the endocrine system
- Blood diseases with impaired oxygen transport and clotting
- Diabetes mellitus type I

Further health-related reasons:

- Recurrent seizures (epilepsy) and brain damages
- Chronic inflammation of the paranasal sinuses
- Profound obesity

29.7 Prevention

Before starting running sports physician should be consulted to assess possible risks (➤ Tab. 29.2). In particular, "limitations of ability" that should be checked. In the case of contraindications, high-performance running is not recommended.

Injury-proneness can be reduced by means of common general-workout, stretching and the **compensation of muscular imbalances** (Freiwald and Greiwing 2003). This particularly concerns the muscles of the abdomen, back and pelvis and also includes stretching of the M. rectus femoris. The extent of joint mobility can be improved by means of **active and passive mobilization**. This accounts particularly for the ankle joint, which is prone to limited dorsi flexion, and the hip joint with its limited extension. **Instructions** of different running styles improve muscle strength and proprioception on uneven ground. The **training schedule** should include the necessary alternation between work load and recovery, adequate time for regeneration, and a diversified training. A relaxed warm-down supports regeneration and is superior to all other measures including stretching.

Running is contraindicated during infections. For running **appropriate footwear** (which requires periodic replacement) and sportswear is necessary (➤ Chapters 88 and 89).

Healthy food, sufficient fluid intake (particularly during long runs at high temperatures and humidity), an adequate supply with carbohydrates on long runs, and sufficient sleep are basic conditions to maintain a good health.

In cases where higher training loads and increased performance are targeted, the load should be increased stepwise in order to let the bones, cartilage and ligaments adapt to the new demands. An accompanying muscle and core-stability training is advisable.

Children can start with running already at an early age but the workout should be playful. From the age of three on, given motivation, distances up to 1000 m are feasible. Children under nine years should not compete in races exceeding 3000 m. At the age of nine to eleven, distances up to 5000 m can be targeted, and from 12 years on up to 10 km. From 15 years

Tab. 29.2 Risk factors of running-related injuries and overload reactions.

Factors with significant relation to injury	Factors without significant relation to injury	Factors with indeterminate relation to injury or with indifferent results reported in the literature
Earlier injury Competitive sport High workout extent Missing running experience Profound axial malalignments Quick increase of workout intensity	Age Sex BMI Running ground Recreational sport Foot shape	Stretching Warming-up Workout frequency Running shoes Mountain jogs

on, children can run the half marathon, and from 18 years on they can go full marathon distances. Especially for children, a varied and diversified workout including a basic athletic training is essential.

For older runners it is important to know that age for it self does not contain an increased risk of injury. Even at an advanced age and with slight overweight, the positive aspects of running come into effect. However with advancing age muscles need more time to recover.

References

Clement DB, Taunton JE, Smart GE, McNicol KL (1981). A survey of runner's overuse injuries. Phys Sportsmed 9: 47–58.

Engelhardt M, Reuter I, Neumann G (2003). Verletzungen und Fehlbelastungsfolgen beim Laufen. Sportorthop Sporttraumatol 19: 73–77.

Freiwald J, Greiwing A (2003). Prävention von Verletzungen und Fehlbelastungen beim Laufen. Sportorthop Sporttraumatol 19: 79–83.

Mayer F et al. (2000). Achillessehnenbeschwerden im Laufsport – eine aktuelle Übersicht. Dtsch Z Sportmed 51: 161–167.

Reuter I (2005). Laufen. In: Engelhardt M, Krüger-Franke M, Pieper HG, Siebert CH (eds.) Grifka J (editorial director). Sportverletzungen – Sportschäden. Thieme, Stuttgart, pp. 105–114.

Stromme SB, Ingier F (1982). The effect of regular physical training on the cardiovascular system. Scan J Soc Med 29 (Suppl.): 37–45.

van Mechelen W (1992). Running injuries. A Review of the epidemiological literature. Sports Med 14: 320–335.

Walther M, Reuter I, Leonhard T, Engelhardt M (2005). Verletzungen und Überlastungsreaktionen im Laufsport. Orthopädie 34: 399–404.

Wilmore JH, Costill DL (eds.) (1999). Physiology of sports and exercise. 2nd ed. Human Kinetics, Champain.

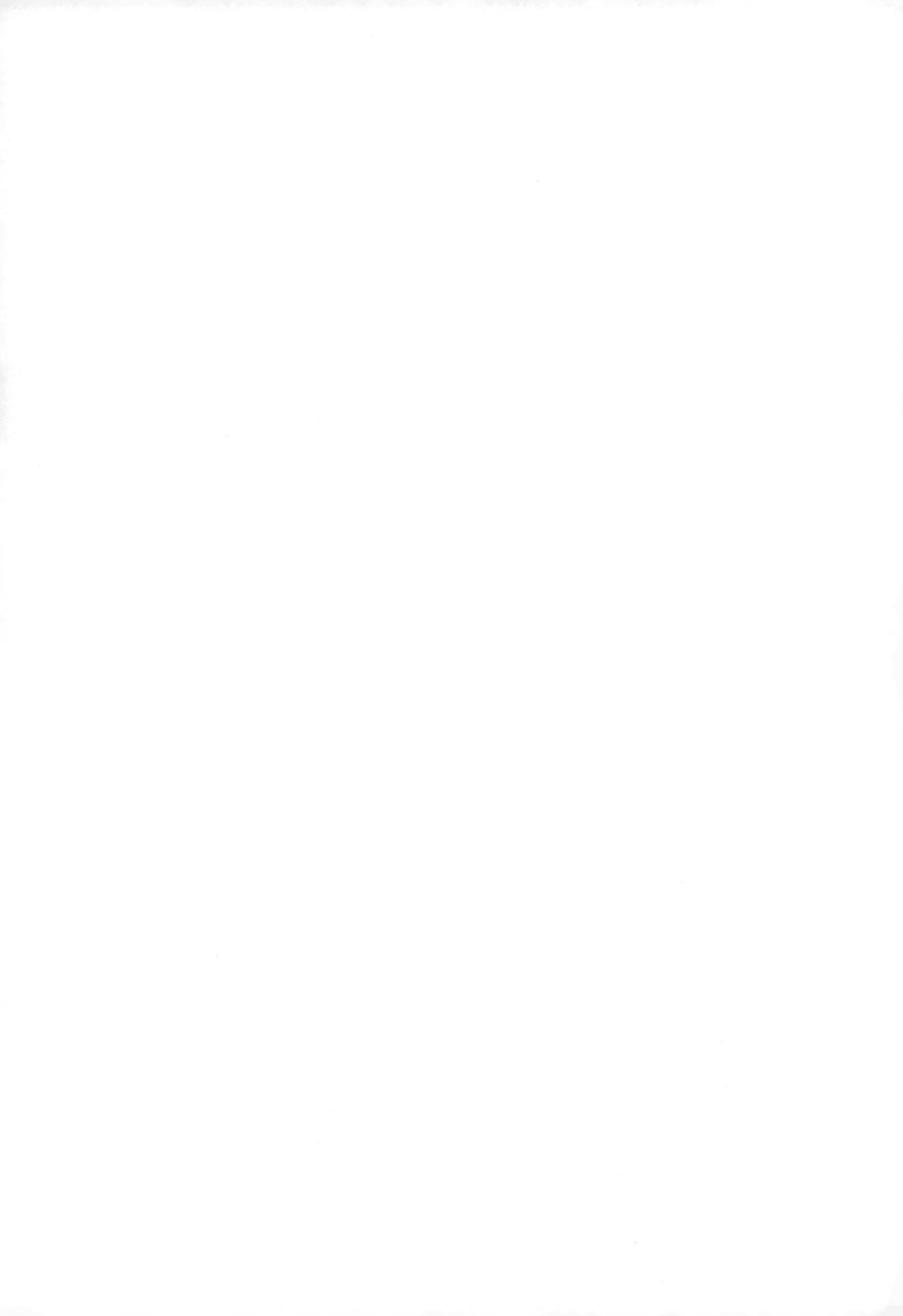

30 Orienteering

André Leumann, Victor Valderrabano and Beat Hintermann

30.1 Characteristics

Orienteering is a sport combining physical and cognitive capabilities. The athlete's target is to reach unknown controls as fast as possible points in a given order. The area is unknown and the track between control points has to be decided by the athlete. The only help is of a special orienteering map (scales of 1:10,000 or 1:15,000) (➤ Fig. 30.1). The choice of the course between the control points is free. Orienteering takes place outdoor, mainly in woods or alpine regions and nowadays even in cities.

Physically, a strong endurance capacity is required combined with strength and coordination in order to move quickly even on difficult grounds. Technically, well skilled map reading is as important as the tactical capability of planning and changing routes (Dresel et al. 1989). Elite athletes are able to read their maps while running at full speed (➤ Fig. 30.2).

Competitions are arranged in different **disciplines**, primarily as individual competitions such as sprint (winning time about 12 minutes), medium distance (winning time about 35 minutes) and long distance (winning time about 100 minutes). Relay, team, nighttime, bike, and (cross-country) ski are related orienteering competitions.

Orienteering is usually known as a **family sport**. In competitions, there are different categories according to different age groups. The groups range from under 10-year-old competitors with focus on playful moving through the countryside to more than 75-year-olds. In Scandinavia, where the orienteering sport has originated more than 100 years ago, even categories for the over 90-year-olds are offered. The International Orienteering Federation (IOF) currently counts 67 member countries altogether, and there is the effort to carry out orienteering

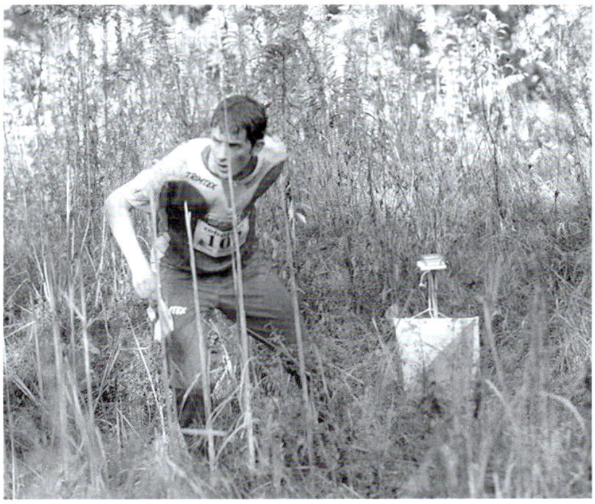

Fig. 30.1 An orienteering athlete while stamping at a control instead of post.

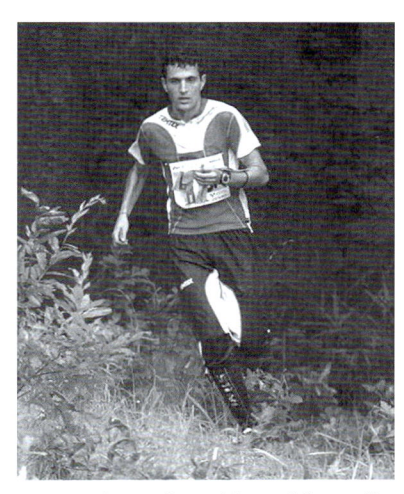

Fig. 30.2 An orienteering athlete while reading a map in running.

competitions at the Olympic Games. The biggest event in orienteering so far is the yearly Swedish 5-day orienteering with more than 15,000 participants.

30.2 Injury types and patterns

Orienteering is a **sport with few injuries** (Dresel et al. 1989). The injuries in orienteering can directly be deduced from the characteristics of orienteering (➢ Tab. 30.1).

2.5% of the athletes in competitions haunt the first-aid center. Only in individual cases further diagnosis on emergency stations is required.

Mostly **wounds, scratches, abrasions, and blisters** occur. According to literature, these "trivial injuries" represent far more than 50% of the first aid in orienteering although the majority of these lesions probably are not even recorded (Linde 1986, Ekstrand et al. 1990, McLean 1990, Hintermann and Hintermann 1992a, Linko et al 1997). However, one third of the athletes have an insufficient **tetanus vaccination** (Hintermann and Hintermann 1992b).

Frequency and severity of injury are closely connected with the type of terrain, vegetation, and weather conditions. Overall, up to 90% of the injuries affect the **lower extremities**. Additionally, mostly **downfall injuries affecting hands and arms** as well as **eye injuries** (corneal erosions) have been reported.

The most frequent and serious injury is the **acute sprain trauma** of the upper ankle joint, mostly affecting the lateral ligament apparatus as a supination trauma. The medial ligament apparatus is affected in pronation trauma or even the syndesmosis can occur in forced dorsal extension-external rotations. In terms of the "ankle activity score" by Halasi et al. (2004), orienteering belongs to the category with the most intensive use of the ankle joint – exceeded by team sports and contact sports. In addition, **sprains** of other joints, **contusions, hematoma, and muscle sprains** have been reported and keep the competition-attending physician busy. Falls will only rarely lead to fractures or dislocations.

C. Johansson (1986) observed 89 Swedish elite runners prospectively for 12 months. During this time, 66 injuries had been recorded. 93.6% of those injuries have affected the lower extremity. 43% have been **acute traumas** whereas 57.1% of those were ankle joint sprains. 57% involved **overuse injuries** such as tendinitis and periostitis and two stress fractures. On average the absence from training caused by injuries amounted to 20 days. In a second study, the author found no correlation of the amount of training and the incidence of injuries (Johansson 1988). In both studies, absence from training ranged between 2.6 and 4.5 injuries/1,000 hours of training. The overuse injuries primarily appeared during the intense winter training, when high amounts of training had been exercised whereas the traumatic injuries occurred mainly in competitions. The distribution of knee and ankle joint injuries is reversed in comparison with other long-distance runners because of a high concentration of injuries of foot and ankle joint injuries prevailing in orienteering (Creagh and Reilly 1998).

Newer data partly show a higher injury incidence of up to 13.6/1,000 hours of sport exer-

Tab. 30.1 Injuries in orienteering.

Type of injury	McLean 1990	Ekstrand et al. 1990	Hintermann and Hintermann (2) 1992	Linko et al. 1997
wounds/blisters	55.9	71	59.6	61.1
contusions/strains	8.7	1.2	13.2	5.7
ankle joint distortion	24.7	7.2	23.7	24.6
fracture/dislocation	1.3	2.7	3.3	0.8
others	9.4	17.9	0	7.8

All data given in percent. The surveys consider competitions ranging from 9,724 to 77,369 participants.

cise (Parkkari et al. 2004). A positive influence on injury incidence by an **individually designed training** could be demonstrated (Johansson 1986).

The fact that orienteering can be practiced at **every** age group leads to a broad spectrum of medical problems. Athletes older than 50 years showed a two-fold increased incidence of injuries (Korpi et al. 1087). The risk of falls in orienteering is clearly present and the increased fracture susceptibility with increasing age is obvious. So far, no data is available that shows an influence of orienteering on endoprothetically treated joints. In the future, sports physicians will besides elite athletes probably also focus on senior athletes who often perform their sport just as intensive as elite athletes. This is particularly the case in orienteering.

Severe injuries are rarely found in orienteering. Individual fatal cases during competitions are mainly of cardiac origin (myocardial infarction). Cases of death that are either caused by exsanguinations after a fall, falling trees, or fall on rocks in athletes treated with oral anticoagulation remain anecdotes.

Acute sprain and chronic instability of the ankle joint

All published studies showed that the most frequent injury is an acute sprain of the ankle joint (up to 25%) (➢ Tab. 30.2). During the Swiss 6-day orienteering event in 1991 out of 36 acute sprains (23.8% of all injuries), eleven cases (31%) were considered first-time sprains and 25 cases (69%) recurrent sprains (Hintermann and Hintermann 1992b). Most of the time earlier sprains had not been treated adequately and 36% (nine cases) had not been treated at all. Besides chronic instability, other overuse injuries, such as Achilles peritendinitis, chondropathia patellae, iliotibial friction syndrome, medial tibial shin splint syndrome and tendinitis of the pes anserinus have been reported. On the basis of an examination of the Swiss National Team in Orienteering, the authors were able to show that in the national orienteering team 86% of the athletes reported a history of acute sprains (Leumann et al. 2006). 73% of the athletes showed at least on one of both ankles signs of a mechanical and/or functional chronic instability at least

Tab. 30.2 Studies that have been published so far about acute ankle joint distortions and chronic instability in orienteering.

Authors	Date	Country	Acute distortions[a]	Chronic instability[b]
Folan	1982	Ireland	13%	no data
Linde	1986	United Kingdom	37%	no data
Johansson (1986a)	1986	Sweden	24%	no data
Johansson	1988	Sweden	52.5%/57.5%	50% relapse of distortion in 3 months
McLean	1990	Scotland	14.5–19.4%	no data
Ekstrand et al.	1990	Sweden	23.9%	no data
Knobloch et al.	1990	Switzerland	no data	60%
Hintermann and Hintermann (1992b)	1992	Switzerland	23.8%	no data
Hintermann and Hintermann (1992a)	1992	Switzerland	30.6% first-time distortion	69.4% relapsing distortions
Kujala et al.	1995	Finland	28.7%	no data
Linko et al.	1997	Finland	25%	no data
Leumann et al.	2006	Switzerland	86%	73%

[a] Percentage of acute ankle distortions in relation to all injuries
[b] Incidence of chronic instability
[c] Percentage considers all injuries of the ankle; distortions have not been considered in isolation
[d] Distortion prevalence by means of a retrospectively collected anamnesis

on one of both ankles. Knobloch et al. (1990) found similarly high values, which were significantly higher in comparison to long-distance runners.

The influence of **chronic instability** on performance is widely unclear. However, reports suggest that the chronic instability may be a long-term predisposing factor of ankle joint osteoarthritis (Harrington 1979, Knobloch et al. 1990). Orienteering runners have an increased neuromuscular stabilization potential and are able to functionally stabilize the hindfoot, which may explain the lacking correlation between osteoarthritis and number of instabilities (Leumann et al. 2006).

The high amount of insufficiently treated sprains and the high rate of chronic instabilities should trigger sport physicians' attention to orienteering athletes.

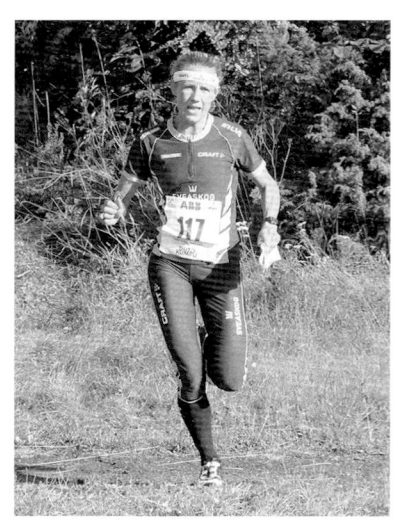

Fig. 30.3 An orienteering athlete on her way through the area.

30.3 Prophylaxis

Many injuries can already be avoided by adequate **equipment**. Long running clothes protect of scratches and abrasions as well as of ticks. Shin guards prevent a sharp penetration of wood or stone. Running shoes with a good profile (there are special competition shoes with deep profile and blunt metal pins available) can help to avoid downfalls (➤ Fig. 30.3). Furthermore, goggles can protect of eye injuries.

A **refreshed vaccination status** is recommended, especially with regard to tetanus, and TBE (tick-borne encephalitis). **Regular training**, sufficient **regenerative measures** (e.g. massage, stretching), and recovery time (e.g. sleep) belong to the prophylaxis of injuries. **Warm-up**, cooling down, and the **right nutrition** before, during, and after competitions are equally important.

Many runners **tape** the ankle joint or they use **external stabilizers** such as bandages, both measures have shown good protection (Sharpe et al. 1997). Mechanical limitation of instability (Müller and Hintermann 1996) and also proprioceptive stimulation of the postural system via skin receptors (Robbins et al. 1995) have been discussed as mechanisms of action. With a regular gymnastic training of the foot, chronic periarticular muscle atrophies due to relief of stabilizers can be avoided (Nigg et al. 1999). The therapy with external stabilization, which especially limits the rotation, combined with early functional neuro-muscular stabilization training has shown good results as a prophylaxis of chronic instability of the ankle joints after acute sprains (Hintermann and Valderrabano 2001). The regular integration of proprioceptive neuromuscular elements into training can definitely be recommended (Tropp et al. 1985).

References

Creagh U, Reilly T (1998). Training and injuries amongst elite female orienteers. J Sports Med Phys Fitness 38: 75–79.

Dresel U, Fach HH, Seiler R (1989). Orientierungslauf-Training. Habegger Verlag, Derendingen.

Ekstrand J, Roos H, Tropp H (1990). The incidence of ankle sprain in orienteering. Sci J Orienteering 6: 3–9.

Folan JM (1982). Orienteering Injuries. Br J Sports Med 16: 236–240.

Halasy T, Kynsburg A, Tallay A, Berkes I (2004). Development of a new activity score for the evaluation of ankle instability. Am J Sports Med 32: 899–908.

Harrington KD (1979). Degenerative arthritis of the ankle secondary to longstanding lateral ligament instability. JBJS Am 61: 354–361.

Hintermann B and Hintermann M (1992a). Ankle sprains in orienteering – a simple injury? Sci J Orienteering 8: 79–86.

Hintermann B and Hintermann M (1992b). Injuries in orienteering. A study of the 1991 Swiss 6-day orienteering event. Sci J Orienteering 8: 72–77.

Hintermann B, Valderrabano V (2001). The effectiveness of rotational stabilization in the conservative treatment of severe ankle sprains: a long-term investigation. Foot & Ankle Surg 7: 235–239.

Johansson C (1986a). Injuries in elite orienteers. Am J Sports Med 14: 410–415.

Johansson C (1986b). Profiling and individually programmed training in prevention of injuries in elite orienteer. Sci J Orienteering 2: 19–24.

Johansson C (1988). Training injury and disease in senior and junior elite orienteers. Sci J Orienteering 4: 3–13.

Knobloch M, Marti B, Biedert R, Howald H (1990). Zur Arthrosegefährdung des oberen Sprunggelenkes bei Langstreckenläufern: Kontrollierte Nachuntersuchung ehemaliger Eliteathleten. Sportverl Sportsch 5: 175–179.

Korpi J, Haapanen A, Svahn T (1987). Frequency, location and types of orienteering injuries. Scand J Sport Sci 9: 53–56.

Kujala U, Nylund T, Taimela S (1995). Acute injuries in orienteers. Int J Sports Med 16: 122–125.

Leumann A, Valderrabano V. Hintermann B, Marti B, Züst P, Clenin G (2006). Die chronische Sprunggelenksinstabilität im Schweizer Orientierungslaufnationalkader. Dissertation. Orthopädische Universitätsklinik Basel. Universität, Basel.

Linde F (1986). Injuries in orienteering. Br J Sports Med 20: 125–127.

Linko PE, Blomberg HK, Frilander HM (1997). Orienteering competition injuries: injuries incurred in the Finnish Jukola and Venla Relay Competitions. Br J Sports Med 31: 205–208.

McLean I (1990). First aid for orienteering in Scotland. Sci J Orienteer 6: 55–63.

Müller CC, Hintermann B (1996). Die Wirkung von äußeren Stabilisierungshilfen auf die Rotationsstabilität der Sprunggelenke. Sportverl Sportsch 20: 84–87.

Nigg BM, Nurse MA, Stefanyshyn DJ (1990). Shoe inserts and orthotics for sport and physical activities. Med Sci Sports Exerc 31: 421–428.

Pakkari J, Kannus P, Natri A, Lapinleimu I, Palvanen M, Heiskanen M, Vuori I, Järvinen M (2004). Active living and injury risk. Int J Sports Med 25: 209–216.

Robbins S, Waked E, Rappel R (1995). Ankle taping improves proprioception before and after exercise in young men. Br J Sports Med 29: 242–247.

Sharpe SR, Knapik J, Jones B (1997). Ankle braces effectively reduce recurrence of ankle sprains in female soccer players. J Athl Train 32: 21–24.

Tropp H, Askling C, Gillquist J (1985). Prevention of ankle sprain. Am J Sports Med 13: 250–262.

Chapter 31 Cycling

Carsten Temme

The sitting position and rotating, 15–30° movement have a low impact on the lower extremities. Hence, cycling is often used as rehabilitation.

These beneficial effects are outweighed with an increased load on the ischial tuberosities, the perineum, and the palms of the hands. The flexed position does not allow a full extension in the knee and hip joints, which leads to lumbar spine delordosis and hyperlodosis of the cervical spine. Hence, these areas are prone to **and thus promotes overstressoveruse**.

Acute injuries are common and occur typically in falls and collisions. The type of injuries varies with the speed and type of accident.

31.1 Overload damages

31.1.1 Spine

The bent forward position triggers **hyperlordosis of the cervical spine**, which is accompanied by tensions and ailments in the neck. Serious troubles or long-term disorders are rare. The discomfort is often eased after adjusting the sitting position. Degenerative predispositions may require a straighter sitting position, which dampens the hyperlodosis.

The thoracic and lumbar spine has different patterns of medical conditions. Back pain is typical for increased muscle activity at uphill climbs, which is combined with increased tension at the handle (cumulatively in mountain bikers). The **paravertebral muscles of the thoracic spine** are mostly affected. The enduring static position, however, often triggers **lumbar spine ailments** due to weakly developed truncal muscles.

The main **therapy** of thoracic and lumbar spine disorders is training and hypertonia of truncal muscles combined with stretching of the hip extensors and flexors. Additionally, adjustment of the sitting position may be necessary.

31.1.2 Upper extremities

Feelings of numbness can appear at the **ulnar nerve** innervations, which are triggered by the grasping pressure at the handle and tremors of the bike. Long tours or races may result in hypoesthesias lasting for several days. Adapting **the gripping position** or improving **the springing** may be required (Patterson et al. 2003).

31.1.3 Lower extremities

Muscle indurations and **tendinoses** are promoted by contraction of the flexor knee and hip muscles. **Post-traumatic conditions** are typical. A swelling of the peritendineum is often found diagnostically, mostly at the Achilles tendon or at the peroneal tendons. Tendons close to the knee, quadriceps tendon, or knee flexors are rarely affected. A localized **pressure pain** is characteristic. Meniscal injuries or femoropatellar problems are often misdiagnosed.

The sitting position and the shoe/pedal system should integral part of tendinoses and muscle indurations **therapy**; simple sitting position adjustments can resolve the problem. A break or **reduced training load** can be necessary depending on the cause and characteristics of the disorder. A combination of ointments (e.g. diclofenac gel, ointment or gel containing Ichthyol®), stretching exercises, and electrotherapy (iontophoresis) have been used successfully. The **ointments** are particularly efficient in slim

Tab. 31.1 Orthopedic examination of the cyclist.

Part of the body	Clinical examination
cervical spine	■ Mobility? ■ Degenerative changes?
thoracic spine	■ Hyper-kyphosis?
lumbar spine	■ Form of paravertebral musculature? ■ Abdominal muscles?
lower extremities	■ Contracted muscles? ■ Perfusion after stress? ■ Peripatellar pressure pain? ■ Radiation of pain? ■ Arch of foot? ■ Leg length discrepancy?
upper extremities	■ Sufficient musculature of the shoulder girdle? ■ Elbow slightly flexed in sitting position?

Tab. 31.2 Frequency of injuries in cycling (Temme et al. 2003, Davidson 2005).

Localization	Number of injurie
supper extremities/shoulder girdle	42–64%
lower extremities	20–24%
head	13.6–23%
thorax/torso	0–24.2%

cyclists. Non-steroid antiphlogistic may be prescribed in addition. If the medical condition does not improve, local corticoid injections may be necessary (Temme 2005, Wanich et al. 2007).

Circulatory disorders can be an atypical condition of the lower extremities. In recent years, the strong bending in the hip joint can trigger **lack of perfusion**. In particular, **bending of the iliaca externa artery** may result in almost complete **vascular occlusions** (Schumacher et al. 2005).

The differential-diagnostic considerations for overuse conditions in cycling are listed in ➤ Table 31.1.

31.2 Injuries

31.2.1 Frequent injuries

The most frequent injuries in cycling are **contusion and skin lesions** ranging from superficial abrasions to tear wounds and deep, contaminated lacerations caused by collision and sliding on the ground or obstacles. **Clavicular fractures and destruction of the acromioclavicular joint**, triggered by direct collision at side fall, are typical cycling injuries. If the rider has time to react and takes his hands off the hand-le, **olecranon fractures and wrist fractures in the area of the wrist joint** occur (➤ Tab. 31.2).

Collision on the trochanter and side falls often result in **fractures of the femoral neck**.

Traumatic brain injury appears in most fatal accidents (without helmets) (Thompson and Rivara 2001, Rosenkranz and Sheridan 2003). Calotte and **midfacial injuries** are typical (Exadaktylos et al. 2004, Lee and Chou 2008). Depending on the collision, skull-base fractures occur with according poor prognosis.

Diverse injuries and **polytrauma** are typical for high speeds at downhill courses.

31.3.2 Therapy

The direct measures are compiled in ➤ Table 31.3.

Abrasions should be cleaned instantly to avoid contamination and disturbed wound healing. Surgical wound debridement may be necessary to remove necrotic tissue and broad contaminations. After the cleaning and suture of deeper injuries, a disinfecting bandage for 12–24 hours is recommended.

First care of **fractures** is correcting bone positions, immobilizations, and pain medication. After transport and final diagnosis, surgery may be indicated. Medium- or long-term sport capacity needs to be balanced with benefits of surgery.

Moderate misalignment after **clavicular fractures and AC joint destruction** will not impair the cyclist. Primary goal is to free the cyclist of **pain**. Hence, decision for surgery at small dislocations depends on the individual pain.

Mid-third clavicula fractures are treated with figure of eight dressing, plate osteosynthesis, or intramedullar nail. A figure of eight dressing is less helpful for **lateral clavicular fractures**; a li-

31.2 Injuries

Tab. 31.3 Primary treatment at accidents in cycling.

Primary treatment at the accident	
1) protection of the injured cyclist	■ parking the racing physician's car behind the cyclist for protection of following automobiles, or ■ recovering the patient at once to a secure place away from the race track
2) accident mechanism	■ Only slid away or serious crash? ■ Injuries to be expected?
3) contacting	■ Conscious? ■ Pain?
4) primary examination	■ Loss of sensitvity? ■ Mobility of the extremities? ■ palpation (shoulder girdle, elbows, hands, thorax, liver, spleen, spinous process of vertebrae, iliac wings, trochanters) ■ Continuing of the ride possible?
5) acute therapy	■ ascertain vital functions ■ immobilization (stiff neck, splints), if necessary ■ wound care (H_2O_2, bandages)
6) evacuationonly, if necessary	■ request another emergency physician/helicopter, or ■ Ambulance sufficient?
7) Race physician should keep on monitoring the competition.	■ Race physician should only accompany the injured if several physicians are on site (treatment of other athletes guaranteed), or ■ aborting the competition

mitation of the abduction and flexion is sufficient for small dislocations. Alternatively, hook plate surgery or stabilization of the lateral clavicula by an arthroscopic thread system between lateral clavicula and coracoid is helpful. After falls, the acromioclavicular joint should be examined in a sitting position to diagnose possible **separation of the AC joint.** The degree of severity is determined according to Rockwood (X-rays in standing/sitting with weight bearing at the wrists). Type I and II injuries are usually treated conservatively by rest; type III to VI are treated by surgery, preferably arthroscopy given the short recovery period. The surgical treatment should be carried out in the first few days after the injury; later a stable healing of the acromioclavicular ligaments is unlikely (➤ Fig. 31.1 a, b and c). **Augmentation or a plastic of the plantaris tendon** is an option for belated surgery; this can be carried out by arthroscopy as well.

> The removal of hamstring tendons is not recommended in cyclists since cyclists use the knee flexors much more than any other athletes.

Fracture treatment requires an exercise/load-stable, post-surgery period (Temme and Riepenhof 2005).

31.2.3 Prevention

Helmets reduce considerably reduce the risk of fatal injuries. Only the midface remains a weak point. Otherwise, only limitation of partici-

Fig. 31.1 a: Five radiographs in a standing posture (with weight load of the arm, at best) have to be taken with an injury of the AC joint, and attention must be paid to the increase of the distance between coracoids and clavicula (secondary findings: old clavicula fracture). b: Arthroscopic treatment: pre-drilling for the thread sling by a spot-film device. c: Post-operative radiographic check. The reduction of the coracoclavicular distance and the position of the titanium pads, on which the thread sling is being hung, can be seen here.

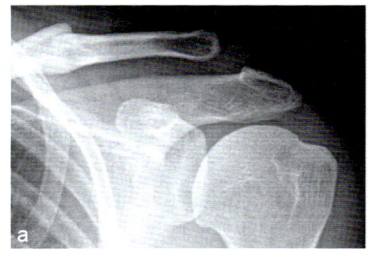

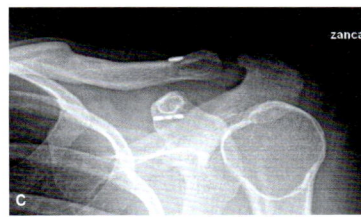

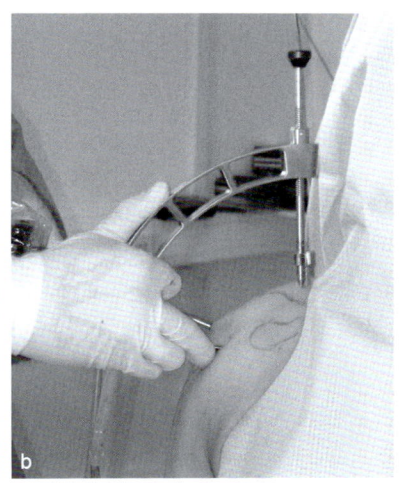

pants (mass falls are almost unavoidable with more than 160 participants) and avoiding obstacles at the end is important to prevent injuries. Time measurement at about 6 miles before the target line can help to prevent overcrowded finish lines.

31.2.4 Rehabilitation

Casual cycling training, starting at an ergometer, can be restarted quickly after most injuries. Misplacements on the bicycle reduce force transmission and/or trigger secondary overuse reactions. Further physical therapy for the treatment of muscular problems and movement control are important, post-traumatic long-term follow-up measures.

References

Davidson JA (2005). Epidemiology and outcome of bicycle injuries presenting to an emergency department in the United Kingdom. Eur J Emerg Med 12 (1): 24–29.

Exadaktylos AK, Eggensperger NM, Eggli S, Smolka KM, Zimmermann H, Izuka T (2004). Sports-related maxillofacial injuries: the first maxillofacial trauma database in Switzerland. Br J Sports Med 38 (6): 750–753.

Lee KH, Chou HJ (2008). Facial fractures in road cyclists. Aust Dent J 53 (3): 246–249.

Patterson JM, Jaggars MM, Boyers MI (2003). Ulnar and median nerve palsy in long-distance cyclists. A prospective study. Am J Sports Med 31 (4): 585–589.

Rosenkranz KM, Sheridan RL (2003). Trauma to adult bicyclists: a growing problem in the urban environment. Injury 34 (11): 825–829.

Schumacher YO, Vogt S, Sandrock M, Pottgießer T, Schmid A (2005). Funktionelle Gefäßobstruktionen bei Hochleistungsradsportlern. Sportorthopädie-Sporttraumatologie 21: 87–93.

Temme C (2005). Radfahren. In: Grifka J (ed.). Praxiswissen Halte- und Bewegungsorgane, Sportverletzungen-Sportschäden. Thieme Verlag, Stuttgart.

Temme C, Riepenhof H, Henche HH (2003). Injuries and overuse syndromes in professional cycling. ISAKOS Congress, Abstracts. 4.90 #204.

Temme C, Riepenhof H (2005). Orthopädische und traumatologische Betreuung im Radsport. Sportorthopädie-Sporttraumatologie 21: 73–77.

Thompson MJ, Rivara FP (2001). Bicycle-related injuries. Am Fam Physic 63 (10): 2007–2014.

Wanich T, Hodgkins C, Columbier JA, Muraski E, Kennedy JG (2007). Cycling injuries of the lower extremity. J Am Acad Orthop Surg Dec 15 (2): 748–756.

Chapter 32

Rowing

Christian Nührenbörger, Nicolien van Giffen and Axel Urhausen

The American College of Sports Medicine (Mitchell et al. 2005) categorizes rowing as one of the **most demanding competitive sports with the highest dynamic and static cardiovascular** strain on the human body. Furthermore, rowing is an effective, well-controlled strength and endurance sport with a low risk of injury, and, is therefore, considered to be beneficial as a recreational sport for increasing overall general health. The International Rowing Federation (FISA) currently has 128 active member states.

32.1 Competition and equipment

The official rowing distance is 2 km (1.2 miles). In addition, long-distance races include distances up to 20 km (12.4 miles) in the eight-man skull while sprint races cover 500 m (0.3 miles). The world championships comprise 22 able-bodied boat classes, from which 14 are part of the Olympic program and 4 adaptive boat classes. Open and lightweight rowing categories exist. In the latter, the maximum body weight of women must not exceed 57 kg (126 lbs, mean value of the crew) or 59 kg (130 lbs, mean value of the crew) and that of men 70 kg (154 lbs, mean value of the crew) or 72.5 kg (160 lbs, individually). The coxes should not exceed a maximum body weight of 50 kg (110 lbs for women) or 55 kg (121 lbs for men), with weighing taking place two hours prior to the race.

Rowers use one-sided oars, 3.81 m in length, with both hands (starboard or port), while in sculling two oars (ca. 2.98 m in length) are used one in each hand. Most athletes are specialized either in sweep rowing or in sculling. Competition boats are made of synthetic materials, the singles have a length of approx. 8.2 m (26 ft) with a weight of approx. 14 kg (30 lbs), and the eights have a length of approx. 19.9 m (65 ft) with a weight of approx. 96 kg (211 lbs). Where rowing is considered as a recreational sport gig boats are more stable and widespread.

Rowing has been part of the Olympic program since the beginning of the modern Olympic Games in 1896, and, in Peking in 2008, rowing became part of the Paralympics for the first time.

Rowing ergometers (wind wheels) are primarily used for performance diagnosis and for training purposes but are also used in indoor-competitions.

Knowledge of exercise physiology and orthopedic load in rowing competition is important for the medical attendance at regattas. A change of a boat crew member at an international regatta, who has already raced, is only allowed with a clear medical indication. In case of any health problem before the of the race, the team physician has to exclude an acute health risk and judge the ability of the athlete to race.

The individual assessment "on-site" must carefully be considered in selection to the exchange by a substitute as a performance decline or failure of a boat member cannot be compensated during the race.

32.2 Physiological criteria

Rowing is known as a classic **strength-endurance sport**. The movement of rowing involves a cyclical use of the femoral and gluteal muscles due to the pressure of the feet fixed to the footrest as well as of the arm, shoulder and back muscles during the pulling of the oar blades. A typical rowing competition takes 5:30 to 8:00 minutes, depending on weather conditions and the boat class. During the competition the performance will be close to the individual maximum oxygen uptake and the energy is supplied up to 80% through the aerobic pathway. This involves high demands on the endurance capacity and world class rowers perform high training loads of up to 5,000–7,000 km (3,100–4,300 miles) per year.

Additionally, an adequate anaerobic mobilization is necessary in top rowing. Maximum anaerobic lactic capacity is challenged as very high concentrations of blood lactate of 15 to 20 mmol/l or more are measured after racing (Steinacker 1993, Hagerman 1994, Urhausen and Kindermann 1994). Resistance training with focus on strength endurance is also a key method in rowing training and is exercised for most of the year (Guellich et al. 2009).

Performance in competitions on a high level requires exceptionally high lever arm ratios. For example, the average body size in the German men's eight who competed in Athens in 2004 was 1.98 m (6'5") and 1.84 m (6'0") in the women's eight. Technical skills allowing an effective and accommodating rowing technique under different weather conditions (wind, waves, current) are equally important.

32.3 Traumatic and overuse injuries

Relatively few injuries occur in the sport of rowing. In a prospective study, the average injury rate was 3.67 per 1,000 exposure hours and the mean number of injuries sustained per athlete was 2.2 over one year. Half of these injuries involved the spine (Wilson et al. 2010). These figures were confirmed in the medical survey of the Beijing Olympic Games 2008, which only showed an incidence of 1.8% for new traumatic or overuse musculoskeletal complaints due to competition or training amongst the rowers (Junge et al. 2009).

32.3.1 Acute injuries

> Rowing has a low risk of acute injuries.

Most of the serious injuries in rowing are attributed to **accidents in compensation training** (soccer, cycling) and falls at the landing stage. If the blade of the oar is not fully out of the water after the drawing and is pressed further forward (so-called **rowing crab**), the oar can cause serious **contusions of the thorax with possible rib fractures** and abdominal **internal organ damages**. Further serious injuries such as blunt abdominal trauma, fractures or muscle-, tendon- and soft-tissue-injuries occur during boat collisions with other rowing boats or inland vessels (Reifschneider 1997).

Contused wounds and abrasions of the fingers in beginners result in minor injuries caused by technical errors with impact and chafing at the board walls. Other chafing points concern the thorax, the groin and the intergluteal cleft as well as by protruding ends of the runway in extending the legs and the calves. Occasionally, distinct development of blisters on the fingers and palms appear at the start of the training season.

32.3.2 Overuse injuries

> The most frequent overuse injuries affect the spine, the thorax, and the tendons of the upper extremities and knee joints.

Thorax and spine

Lower back pain is a common complaint among rowers (Teitz et al. 2002, Teitz et al. 2003, Bahr et al. 2004, McNally et al. 2005, Rumball et al. 2005, Smoljanovic et al. 2009).

The following disorders are common:

- muscular tensions
- segmental and iliosacral functional disorders
- damages of the intervertebral discs with and without radiculopathies
- spondylolysis and osteochondroses.

The increased incidence of Scheuermann's disease in rowers is not yet fully understood. However, during growth of the human body periodical changes of the spine and structural spinal damages can be induced especially in the presence of hereditary constitutional predisposition (Dalichau et al. 2002).

Excessive lumbar flexion and high compressive forces to the lumbar spine during rowing are also responsible for structural spinal damages (Reid and McNair 2000, Soler and Calseron 2000, Caldwell et al. 2003). The fatigue of the erector spinae muscle can lead to an increased lumbar flexion during long exercise sessions (Holt et al. 2003).

Exceptional stress to the lumbar spine with shearing and compressive forces up to 7 times the body weight is reached during the sweeping of the rowing blades. This may induce the spinal damages to corpses (Horsea et al. 1989, Adams and Hutton 1988, Dalichau et al. 2002). Acute conditions can also occur at the landing stage when removing or placing the boat on the water; this is caused by the spinal rotation required by this movement. However, lumbar disorders are not conditioned by muscular weakness. In fact, muscles of rowers with back pain are described to be more developed than in rowers who are free from such pain (McGregor et al. 2002). Further negative influences to the spine include:

- leg length differences >5 mm that will lead to non-physiological pelvic wringing
- contracted ischiocrural musculature causes non-physiological pelvic tilting and increased lumbar flexion with lumbosacral overstress at push off,
- high swell will require an additional balancing by the trunk,
- slight rotation of the lumbar spine at the final draw of the oar (Reifschneider 1997).

Tensions of the trunk musculature and inflammatory kidney diseases can also be noticed during rough weather conditions or when the rower is splashed by water when the ore is incorrectly placed into the water at the catching position.

Scintigraphy, CT or MRT often detect **fatigue fractures of the ribs** (➤ Fig. 32.1) (Christiansen and Kanstrup 1997, Galilee-Belfer and

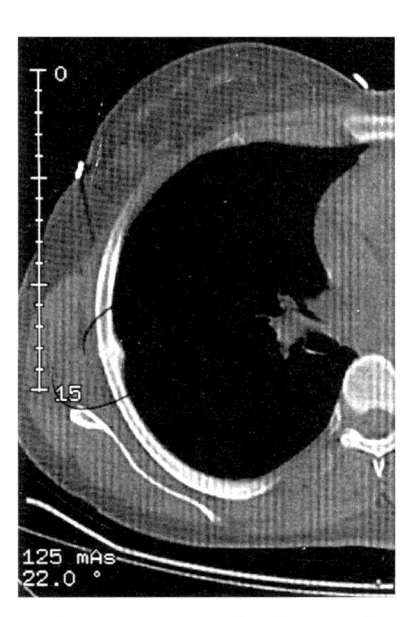

Fig. 32.1 Computer tomography of a stress fracture of the 5th rib laterally in a 20-year old squad light-weight rower (see black circle).

Guskiewicz 2000, Gregory et al. 2002, Davis and Finoff 2003, Iwamoto and Takeda 2003, Vinther et al. 2005, Vinther et al. 2006, Dragoni et al. 2007, Smoljanovic et al. 2007). They are caused by high flexion stress due to strong contractions of the serratus anterior muscle and the rhomboidei muscles during the sweeping phase. They are mostly localized at the posterolateral parts of ribs IV–VIII. They often appear in young female rowers after intensive exercise sessions shortly before competition season (Holden and Jackson 1985, Karlson 1998, Warden et al. 2002).

Stress fractures of the clavicula, the ulna, the fourth metacarpus as well as the tibia and the fibula have been described in the literature (Hickey et al. 1998, Abbot and Hannafin 2001, Losito et al. 2003, Parsons et al. 2005). A reduced bone mass and menstrual disorders in the anamnesis, eating disorders and muscle weakness are considered as risk factors for the development of stress fractures in young female athletes (➤ Chapter 23; Galilee-Belfer and Guskiewicz 2000, Matter et al. 2002, Vinther et al. 2005).

Other causes of chest pain include an avulsion injury of the anterior serratus muscle as well as intercostal muscle lesions, a costovertebral subluxation or costochondritis (Gaffney 1997, Rumball et al. 2005).

Finally, in the differential diagnosis of adolescent rowers with rib pain tumors must be excluded as shown in the case of an Ewing sarcoma in a 13-year-old rower (Smoljanovic and Bojanic 2007).

> Stress fractures of the ribs must be excluded in the case of thoracic pain in rowers!

Upper extremities

The tenosynovitis of the hand extensors (**"rower's wrist"**) is a common overuse injury of the upper extremities. Rower's wrist occurs in cold weather and at beginning of the training season when changing from indoor ergometer rowing to outdoor water training. This is often caused by an incorrect rowing technique during the rotator movement of the wrist and the rowing blade plunging into and emerging from the water (Boland and Hosea 1997, Hickey et al. 1998, McNally et al. 2005).

In addition, a **transitory carpal tunnel syndrome** has been described. This is a condition caused by the compression of the medianus nerve during maximum tension of the forearm or tendinous irritations in the carpal tunnel as a result of the bending of the wrist at the drawing and lifting of the rowing blade (Hertel 1982).

In a few cases, a functional compartment syndrome of the extensor compartments exists and is diagnosed by pressure measuring (Rumball et al. 2005).

Lower extremities

Femoropatellar pain appears more frequently in the knee joints especially in strength training (squats with weight, leg press). These mostly occur in rowers with an increased anteversion of the femur and/or a malposition of the patella as well as with increased valgus or varus malpositions (Boland and Holsea 1997). The **distal iliotibial band friction syndrome** is caused by an increased friction of the tractus iliotibialis at the lateral femur condyle in epicondylus during repeated flexion and extension movements.

Furthermore, regular painful muscle indurations can appear at the trunk as well as at the lower and upper extremities as a result of unilateral permanent load, incorrect grabbing technique, too large of a handle size on the ore, and wrong foot spar angle.

32.4 Therapeutic procedures

Acute injuries and complaints of such injuries mostly require a limitation or interruption of rowing. The spinal injuries should be first treated by **conservative therapeutic measures** with localized warmth applied to the injured area, manual and physiotherapy, non-steroid anti-inflammatory drugs (NSAIDS), muscular relaxants and local infiltrations.

Conservative therapeutic measures for stress fractures of the ribs, the metacarpals and the clavicula include 6 to 8 week interruption of rowing, short-term NSAID, physical measures and compensation training, e.g. on a bicycle ergometer. Affected female athletes should have checked their bone mass by DXA, the parameters of bone metabolism, and the hormonal balance for the exclusion of further risk factors. In particular, young female athletes with stress fractures risk never reaching their normal peak bone mass due to insufficient nutrition and the retarded and reduced pubertal hormonal situation, and, therefore, may have life-long reduced bone mass density (Matter et al. 2002).

Tenosynovitis of the hand extensors mostly requires an immobilization of the forearm, local cryotherapy and application of antiphlogistics, physical therapy and, if necessary, local infiltrations into the tendon sheaths.

Problems with the knee joints are addressed with short-term NSAID, physiotherapy, or intraarticular infiltrations of local anesthetics, corticoids or hyaluronic acid. An extracorporeal shockwave therapy and treatment with bandages can additionally be used in case of the patellar apex syndrome.

The oral and infiltrative drug applications must be undertaken with consideration of the current **anti-doping regulations**. FISA, in its recently revised Bye-Laws to the Rules of Racing, has adapted a "no needles policy".

32.5 Preventive measures

The prevention or therapy of abrasions or chafing requires regular care of the friction surfaces at hands and buttocks with gradual adaption to increased load amounts. Application of hand cream after rowing, sterile punction of blisters and removal of calluses is indicated (➤ Fig. 32.2).

Rowers should only drink from their own drinking bottle for the prophylaxis against infections (Urhausen and Kindermann 1994). Skull and oar handles as well as free weights should be kept clean and rowing clothes should be washed regularly.

Head protection, sunglasses and sun lotion with high sun-protection factor should be used during very hot weather conditions, especially with high UV levels.

The wearing of a life vest is necessary in open waters when there is no direct accompaniment by motorboats. A boat escort is essential in very cold waters, e.g. at high altitude. The literature illustrates that in cases of capsized rowers on cold lakes careful manipulation in rescuing a hypothermic person should be acknowledged and proper procedure observed otherwise death may result due to hypothermic shock (Giesbrecht and Hayward 2006). Special indications regarding security measures in rowing with **disabled athletes** are described in the "Canadian Adaptive Rowing Manual" (National Committee on Adaptive Rowing 2005).

A regular program of exercises with a stretching of the ischiocrural and lumbosacral muscles and **training of coordination and flexibility** should be carried out for the prevention of muscular contractions, dysbalances and insufficiencies in the spinal region. Prolonged exercise sessions on the rowing ergometer will require short breaks every 30 minutes with relief exercises for the lumbosacral junction.

Functional and warm clothes with lumbar and kidney protection are recommended for the protection against splash water and cooling in wet and cold training conditions such as winter and spring, early morning as well as at high altitudes. In addition, leg length differences of more than 5 mm should be compensated at the footrest.

Stress fractures of the ribs, although hardly realizable in competitive sport, may be avoided by a change of technique with a smaller range, pulling power and spinal dorsal position during long distances (Karlson 1998). In order to prevent such fractures a special physiotherapeutic exercise program is recommended for the strengthening of the serratus anterior muscle (Pinciotti et al. 2005).

A **good rowing technique** with adequate handle diameter and correct blade and skull movement is important for the prevention of tendosynovitis at the wrist extensors and transitory carpal tunnel syndrome. The forearms should always be kept warm and dry and regular stretching and strengthening of the forearm muscles should be maintained.

Strengthening and stretching programs of the knee joint muscles (vastus medialis muscle, quadriceps femoris muscle, tractus iliotibialis) are suggested for knee-related problems. In addition, corrections of the sitting position and the foot position with insoles, if required, are recommended.

The therapy and prevention of muscular contractures of the extremities and of the trunk include use of the sauna, relaxation massages, reduction of exercise load, local warmth applications, compensation training with regular stretching and corrections of the rowing technique.

A **preventive sport-medical examination** should uncover relative **contraindications** that

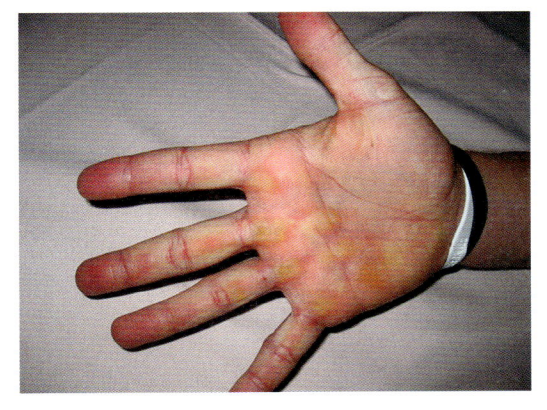

Fig. 32.2 Calluses at the right hand of an athlete of the national squad during the competitive season.

may affect performance during competitive rowing.

From an orthopedic perspective these include:
- known damages of the intervertebral discs
- a florid Scheuermann disease
- a significant spondylolisthesis starting with degree II according to Meyerding
- a femoropatellar cartilage damage (Boland and Hosea 1997).

In case of back pain, rowing might induce a decrease of the complaints (O'Kane et al. 2001). Especially in patients with knee joint instabilities, the led flexion and extension movement of the knee joints in rowing can also be a good alternative to team sports.

From an internist-cardiologic perspective, the same contraindications apply as in other sports with high-level dynamic and static cardiovascular demands (Urhausen et al. 2002, Mitchell et al. 2005).

References

Abbot AE, Hannafin JA (2001). Stress fracture of the clavicle in a female light-weight rower: a case report and review of the literature. Am J Sports Med 29: 370–372.

Adams MA, Hutton WC (1988). Mechanism of the intervertebral disk. In: Gosh P (ed.). The biology of the intervertebral disk. Vol. 2. CRS press, Florida, pp 39–72.

Bahr R, Anderson SO, Loken S, Fossan B, Hansen T, Holme I (2004). Low back pain among athletes with and without specific back loading – a cross-sectional survey of cross-country skiers, rowers, orienteerers and nonathletic controls. Spine 29: 449–454.

Boland AL, Hosea TM (1997). Verletzungen und Überlastungsschäden im Rudern. In: Renström PAFH (ed.). Sportverletzungen und Überlastungsschäden. Prävention, Therapie, Rehabilitation. Enzyklopädie der Sportmedizin. Deutscher Ärzteverlag, Köln, pp 531–539.

Caldwell JS, McNair PJ, Williams M (2003). The effects of repetitive motion on lumbar flexion and erector spinae muscle activity in rowers. Clin Biomech 18: 704–711.

Christiansen E, Kanstrup IL (1997). Increased risk of stress fractures of the ribs in elite rowers. Scand J Med Sci Sports 7: 49–52.

Dalichau S, Scheele K, Buhlmann J (2002). Die motorischen Anforderungen im Leistungsrudern und ihre Bedeutung für die Entwicklung der Wirbelsäulenform. Leistungssport 32: 29–33.

Davis BA, Finnoff JT (2003). Diagnosis and management of thoracic and rib pain in rowers. Curr Sports Med Rep 2: 281–287.

Dragoni S, Giombini A, Di Cesara A, Ripani M, Magliani G (2007). Stress fractures of the ribs in elite competitive rowers: a report of nine cases. Skeletal Radiol 36: 951–054.

Gaffney KM (1997). Avulsion injury of the serratus anterior: a case history. Clin J Sport Med 7: 134–136.

Galilee-Beffer A, Guskiewicz KM (2000). Stress fracture of the eighth rib in a female collegiate rower: a case report. J Athl Train 35: 445–449.

Giesbrecht GG, Hayward JS (2006). Problems and complications with cold-water rescue. Wilderness Environ Med 17: 26–30.

Gregory PL, Biswas AC, Batt ME (2002). Musculoskeletal problems of the chest wall in athletes. Sports Med 32: 235–250.

Guellich A, Seiler S, Emrich E (2009) Training methods and intensity distribution of young world-class rowers. Int J Sports Physiol Perform 4: 448–460.

Hagerman FC (1994). Physiology and nutrition for rowing. In: Lamb D, Knuttgen H, Murray R (eds.). Perspectives in Exercise Sciences. Cooper Publishing, Carmel/U.S.A. pp 221–299.

Hertel P (1982). Rudern. In: Pförringer B (ed.). Sporttraumatologie. Perimed, Erlangen.

Hickey GJ, Fricker PA, McDonald WA (1998). Injuries to elite rowers over a 10-yr period. Med Sci Sports Exerc 12: 1567–1572.

Holden OL, Jackson DW (1985). Stress fractures in the ribs of female rowers. Am J Sports Med 13: 342–348.

Hosea TM, Boland AL, McCarthy K, Kennedy T (1989). Rowing injuries. Post-grad Adv Sports Med 3: 1–16.

Holt BJ, Pull AM, Cashman PM, McGregor AH (2003). Kinematics of spinal motion during prolonged rowing. Int J Sports Med 24: 597–602.

Iwamoto J, Takeda T (2003). Stress fractures in athletes: review of 196 cases. J Orthop Sci 8: 273–278.

Junge A, Engebretsen L, Mountjoy ML, Alonso JM, Renström PAFH, Aubry MJ, Dvorak J (2009) Sports Injuries During the Summer Olympic Games 2008. Am J Sports Med 37: 2165–2172.

Karlson KA (1998). Rib stress fractures in elite rowers, a case series and proposed mechanism. Am J Sports Med 26: 516–519.

Chapter 33 Swimming

Andreas Marka

In population studies' swimming is named the most frequently practiced sport. It is recommended by physicians as therapeutic measure against medical conditions of the supporting ligaments and the locomotor apparatus.

In general, swimming is considered a sport with only few injuries. Opponent impact is only present in training; usually, opponent contact at swimming competitions can be ruled out.

33.1 Sport-specific injuries

Swimmers are mostly hurt outside the pool. Carelessness running on wet tiles often leads to falls or injuries of the extremities caused by the pool edges. **Fractures** or even **craniocerebral traumas** have been described.

Jumps into shallow water and exercise racing dives into exercise pools involve the risk of **cranial and spinal injuries**.

> The most frequent injuries in swimming are found at hands and arms, especially due to clumsy touching at turn and touch or due to missing the pool edge in backstroke.

Foot injuries can also develop at heedless flip turns. Injuries of **fingers and hands** appear more often at the contact with the wave-killer ropes, which are also common in training nowadays (➤ Fig. 33.1).

Since swimmers usually have to share lanes with other swimmers in training, diverse injuries appear triggered by contact with co-swimmers. **Injuries of the eye lids and the orbita** can develop because of kicks or hits to the swimming goggles (➤ Fig. 33.2); **injuries of fingers, metacarpi, arms or head** can be caused by the impact of the swimming paddles of co-swimmers.

Because the amount of dry training in the training of sport swimmers has grown, cases of injuries, e.g. running have increased as well. **Injuries of the ankle joints** such as distortions of the upper ankle joint or fibular ligament ruptures appear more often during dry training. Ankle joint instabilities result from the sport-

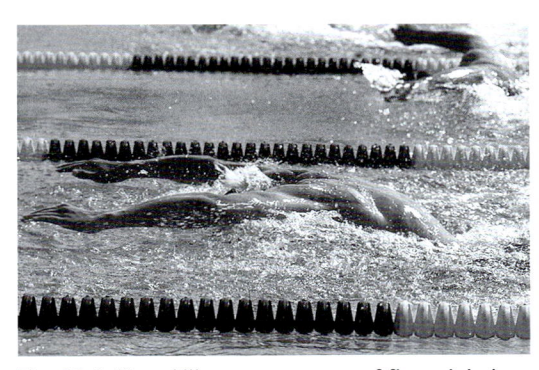

Fig. 33.1 Wave-killer ropes as cause of finger injuries.

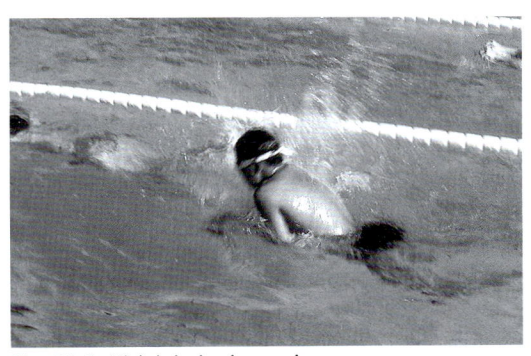

Fig. 33.2 Kick injuries in passing.

specific flexibility necessary for the execution of an optimal leg stroke.

Additionally, **strength training** in the swimming pools becomes more important. Therefore, all injuries specific for strength training are possible e.g. **muscle or joint injuries** (biceps tendon strains during barbell training).

33.2 Injury patterns

A **retrospective study** of 50 competitive swimmers of the age of 15–29 years questioning their sport-conditioned injuries and consequences of inappropriate loads within the last 4 years has shown the following result (Engelhardt et al. 1993):

- An injury frequency of 0.12 injuries/athlete/year has been observed for the average amount of training of 14 hours/week, which is a very low value, compared to sports like triathlon (0.27) and decathlon (0.97).
- During the time of the survey, 44% of the surveyed athletes got hurt during training or competition. 34% of the injuries happened in the swimming pool.
- 50% of the swimmers saw a doctor because of the suffered injury; only 10% of the injuries required a sport break of more than 2 weeks.
- 29% of the registered conditions of the swimmers could be classified as acute injuries and 71% as consequences of inappropriate loads.
- The most serious registered injury was a metacarpal fracture caused by wrong touching.
- A seasonal accumulation of injuries could not be found.
- Compensatory sports or running training caused 16% of all injuries.

The injuries indicated by the 50 surveyed athletes during the period from 1989 to 1993 are listed in ➢ Table 33.1.

Tab. 33.1 Injury patterns of 50 surveyed athletes in the time period from 1989 to 1993.

Type of injury	Number in percent	Injury	Injuries in swimming	Injuries in strength training	Injuries in running training/ recreational sport
Skin injuries	8	Abrasions/tears	×	–	–
	4	Injuries of the eyelid	×	–	–
Capsule-ligament injuries	4	Fibular ligament rupture	–	–	×
	12	Distortion of the upper ankle joint	–	–	×
	4	Distortion of the wrist	×	–	–
Fractures	4	Metacarpus fracture	×	–	–
	2	Toe fracture	×	–	–
Muscle injuries	16	Adductor distortion	×	–	–
	18	Distortion of the shoulder muscle	–	×	–
	2	Distortion of the breast muscle	–	×	–
	4	Distortion of the biceps tendon	–	×	–
	4	Quadriceps distorsion	×	–	–
Other injuries	2	Corneal rupture	×	–	–
	2	Eardrum rupture	×	–	–
	2	Tooth injury	×	–	–

Swimming is a sport with only very few injuries. The number or injuries can even be reduced further by the following measures:

- reduction of the number of swimmers exercising on one lane for the reduction of contact injuries
- consequent warm-up and correct execution of the exercises in the field of strength training
- no running training in darkness
- proprioceptive training of foot and leg muscles for the prevention of injuries of the upper ankle joint.

References

Braumann K-M (1993). Schwimmen. Dtsch Z Sportmed 44 (5): 203–206.

Engelhardt M, Marka A, Wentz S (1993). Verletzungsarten und Verletzungshäufigkeit ausgewählter Ausdauer- und Mehrkampfsportarten – Rückschlüsse für preventives Handeln. Deutscher Sportärztekongress, Paderborn.

Fiedler KM (1982). Schwimmsport – vom Badespaß zum Weltrekord. 1st ed. Sportverlag, Berlin (East).

Marka A (1999). Orthopädische Betreuung im Triathlonsport. In: Engelhardt M, Franz B, Neumann G, Pfützner A (eds.). 14. Internationales Triathlon-Symposium, Xanten, 1999. Czwalina-Verlag, Hamburg.

Marka A (2005). Schwimmen. In: Engelhardt M, Krüger-Franke M, Pieper H-G, Siebert CH (eds.). Sportverletzungen-Sportschäden. Praxiswissen Halte- und Bewegungsorgane. Thieme-Verlag, Stuttgart.

Steinbach K (1997). Schwimmen. In: Engelhardt M, Hintermann B, Segesser B (eds.). GOTS-Manual Sporttraumatologie. Huber-Verlag, Bern.

Steinbach K (1993). Schwimmen aus orthopädischer Sicht. TW Sport und Medizin 5: 33–40.

34 Cross-country skiing

Ludwig Geiger

According to **petroglyphs** and **archeological findings of skis** in Northern Europe and Asia, the invention of skis as means of movement on snow dates back more than **10,000 years**. Only in late 18th century, the so-called **cross-country skiing** established as a popular sport in **Scandinavia**. The cross-country ski has advanced from pure means of movement to sport equipment. The so-called **classic cross-country skiing technique** with its waxed skis and sticks has spread quickly to the Alps, Eastern Europe and North America.

Approximately since 1980, a new technique has revolutionized the cross-country sport: the **skating step**, nowadays called **free technique**. Distinctly faster running times are achieved on skis only primed with glide wax, used in the skating-step technique with symmetric arm work, than with the former diagonal pushing-off technique and impression waxes. All world championship medals of 1985 in Seefeld have been won by the same technique. The initial skepticism also in mass sport has made way for a broad acceptance, which has led to a double-tracked exertion of both techniques in racing and mass sport. Nowadays, cross-country skiing belongs to the most important snow sports in Germany with a yearly number of more than 3 million actives (ASU – evaluation office for skiing accidents).

50 km for **men** as well as for the short sprint, hunt and pursuit races. It is also the most important precondition for a good performance in **biathlon** (free technique, shooting) and in **Nordic combined** (free technique, ski jumping).

The **maximum oxygen absorption**, the gross criterion of endurance capacity, is averagely about 10% higher in the **classic technique** than in the free technique. Free technique requires higher strength endurance. Altogether, top cross-country skiers show the highest maximum values of oxygen absorption of all endurance sports!

> Cross-country skiing has a high health value for prevention and therapy of cardiovascular and metabolic diseases because of the high oxygen conversion in legs and arms.

The increased **strength endurance** in the **free technique** has led to an intensified athletic training of the shoulder girdle and arms. This equally applies to the classic technique, which promotes the propulsion by an increased use of the sticks. **Beginners** are suggested to start with the classic cross-country skiing technique first, because here the technical demands are lower and the running speeds can be dosed better, e.g. for hills. Situations of overload for patients with a latent coronary risk are less likely.

34.1 Sport-specific requirement profile

Endurance is for both amateur and professional cross-country skiing. Very good endurance is imperative for the competition-specific standard distances of 10-30 km for **women** and 15-

34.2 Sports equipment

Classic skis and skating skis differ essentially. While the **classic ski** equipped with a wax or scale zone ("kick zone"), requires an exact correlation of body weight/ski stiffness in order to fulfill its function (push-off and gliding), the averagely 10 cm shorter **skating ski** is more similar to an alpine ski with an even contact face. Consultation of a sports dealer or skiing school is recommended at the first shopping.

The following rules-of-thumb apply to the determination of the stick length:

- ski stick for classic technique: body size minus 15%
- ski stick for free technique: body size minus 10%.

Modern waxing technology has displaced big wax cases with wax types for different temperatures and conditions. Alternatively, also no-wax skis can be used, mostly with a light loss of speed. The glide surfaces of both ski types can be glide-waxed without problems.

The **binding systems** differ by a stronger return spring at the skating ski. Presently, security bindings have not been on the market yet, because the norm systems do not show a strict fixing for technical reasons, but they are responsible for 30% of injuries, which are located at the lower extremity!

34.3   Typical injuries

At the comparison of reported injuries, the **injury relation of alpine skiing to cross-country skiing is 100:1** according to registries of insurance German insurance (ARAG evaluation office for skiing accidents/SIS). The incidence measured by the full number of skiers lies at 0.4%.

Personal observation **localizes** injuries to (➤ Tab. 34.1):

- the **upper extremity** in about **50%**, with the injury pictures of radius fracture, skier's thumb, humeral fracture and dislocation of the shoulder joint

- the **lower extremity** in about **30%**, with ankle fractures, capsule/ligament lesions of the upper ankle joint and the knee joint
- the **trunk** in about **15%**, with rib fractures and blunt abdominal traumas
- the **head** in about **5%**, with cranial contusions and commotio cerebri.

These numbers comply with the literature data of Sutter 1993 and Ruther 2002 (DSV-Lehrbrief 5).

The **causes for the injuries** are mainly **downfalls** because of insufficient downhill and brake technique, using a cross-country ski run in the wrong direction with a risk of collision and increasingly faster material.

34.4   Overuse symptoms/sport damages

Rule of thumb: injuries are rare in amateur athletes but more frequent in professional athletes.

The pattern of overuse symptoms (personal observation German squad athletes, public skiers and participants at senior championships) is summarized in ➤ Table 34.2.

Damages or **damage mechanisms**:

- chondropathia patellae by malposture of the knee axis due to genu valgum and/or overpronation
- lumbar syndrome resulting from an iliopsoas contraction or "wrong" impression of the classic technique
- tibial pain triggered by technical problems (free technique) or development of splay feet
- epicondylopathy by inappropriate pole technique, blunt pole ends with slipping on the

Tab. 34.1 Injury localization and injury pictures (Geiger, examinations 1989–1998, n = 740).

Upper extremity (59%)	Lower extremity (30%)	Trunk (15%)	Head (5%)
- radius fracture - skier's thumb - humerus fracture - dislocation of the shoulder joint	- ankle fracture - capsule ligament lesions of the upper ankle joint - ligament lesion knee joint (collateral ligaments, anterior cruciate ligament)	- hyper-fracture - blunt stomach trauma	- commotio cerebri - skull contusion

Tab. 34.2 Overload damages in competitive athletes (Geiger, examination of squad athletes of DSV/BSV, public skiers and participants of senior championships of the years 1989–1998, n = 740).

Overload damages	Frequency
chondropathia patellae	18%
lumbar syndrome	9%
tibial pain conditions	5%
epicondylopathia	3%
other damages ■ sulcus ulnaris syndrome ■ supraspinatus tendon impingement ■ radicular irritation of the cervicular spine	5%

asphalt in summer-time ski-roller training or "power handle" (special pole handle with horizontal handle equipment, hardly used nowadays).

34.5 Treatments

Injuries in cross-country skiing do not differ from regular injury pictures requiring an orthopedic-traumatologic therapy. Therefore, the regular standards shall not be explained further here.

34.6 Preventive methods

Most injuries and overstress damages in cross-country skiing are **avoidable**, because sport-specifically there is no increased risk disposition.

- Good **summer-time endurance training** is important – especially in mass sports. In competitive sports, it is a necessary precondition anyway, because central and peripheral **fatigue leads to coordinative problems** and to misjudgements, e.g. at steep downhill runs.
- **Strength endurance training** for the shoulder girdle, arm and trunk muscles prevents overload damages.
- The **compensation of wrong statics** with passive insoles of foam material at genu valgum and overpronation is important – in running shoes (summer training) as well as in the cross-country skiing boots. For years, we have successfully used so-called **skating insoles** in order to improve the biomechanical impression relations.
- Respect **rules of cross-country ski runs** to avoid collision accidents.
- A **competent consultation** at the material acquisition will help to avoid overuse symptoms (stick length, kick zone, push-off support, waxes, etc.).

34.7 Internal aspects

From the point of mass and health sports, cross-country skiing especially the classic technique is a **preventive winter sport**. Cross-country skiing is characterized by excellent positive cardiovascular and metabolic effects and stimulates the immune system. The joints are preserved due to the round movements without significant shock loads, and increasingly adapt to stress. Therefore, cross-country skiing can be applied in **internal and orthopedic rehabilitation**.

In **top sports**, a contrary phenomenon can appear due to maximum demands and **over-exercising**: the **immunosuppression**. IgA decrease in the saliva and lymphocyte and killer cell activity is reduced with the consequence of **additional infections**, especially of the upper respiratory tracts (additional exposition to coldness). Change of the training regime, demand-orientated nutrition with additional use of maltodextrin beverages and facultative application of immunomodulatory medication can resolve the problem.

References

ASU-Auswertungsstelle für Skiunfälle, issues SIS, series until 2000/2001 (about "Freunde des Ski-sports im DSV").

DSV-Lehrbrief issue 5, Schriftenreihe des Deutschen Skiverbandes 2002; www.ski-online.de.

Geiger L (1997). Überlastungsschäden im Sport. BLV-Sportwissen.

Geiger L (1998). Vortrag Internationaler Sportärzte-kongress, Garmischpatenkirchen.

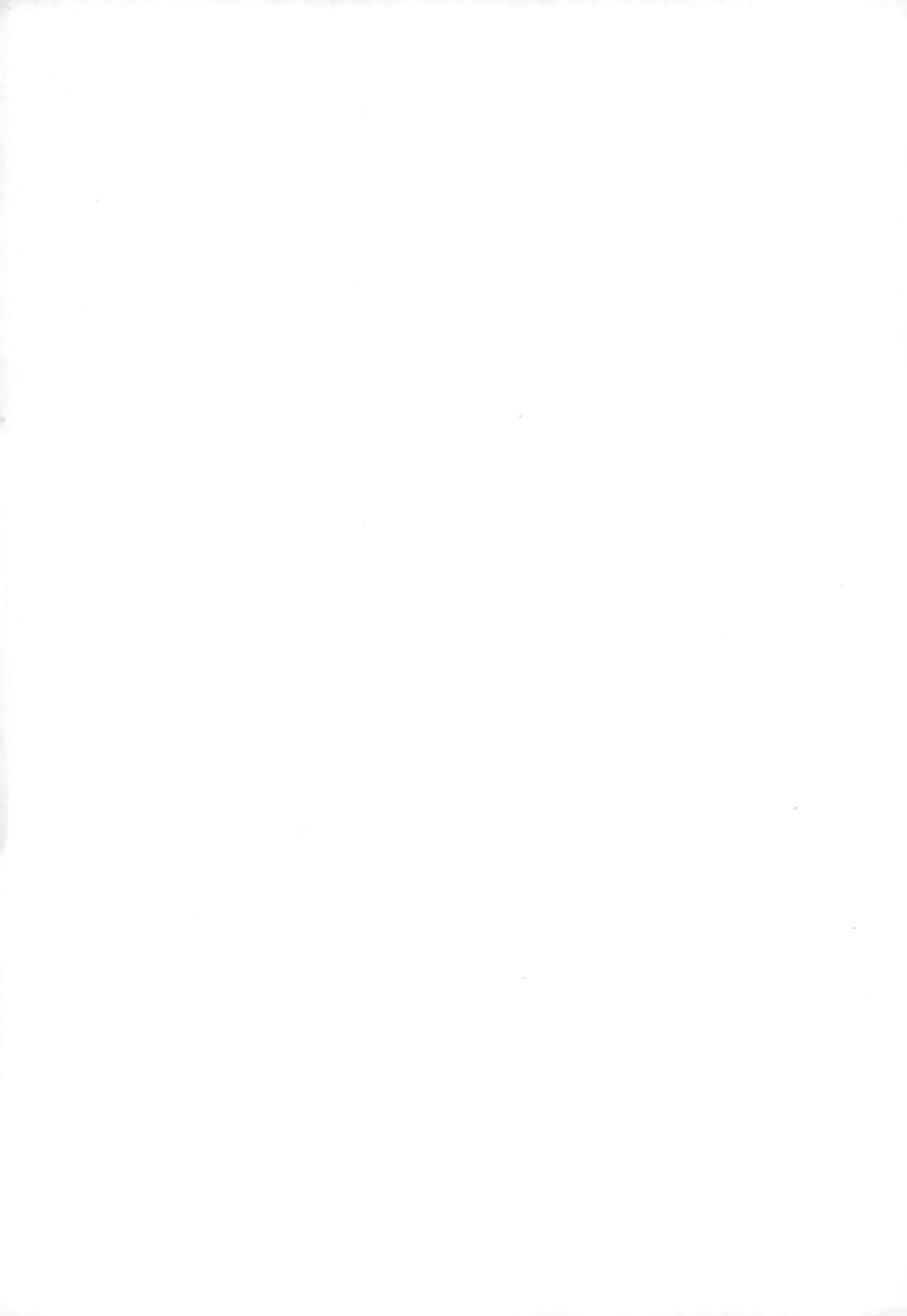

Chapter 35

Triathlon

Martin Engelhardt and Casper Grim

The increasing health awareness of the past 30 years boosted the interest in active, recreational sports as people start to understand that long-term physical wellbeing is only rarely possible without athletic training. Sport, a balanced way of life, and positive environmental conditions are key to healthy life. Amongst other sports disciplines endurance sports are particularly popular and endurance is primarily achieved with training in swimming, biking and running, which are the disciplines of triathlon. In Europe, the triathlon events have an outstanding importance both in amateur as well as in professional sports. ➢ Table 35.1 provides a historical overview of triathlon development.

The combination of the three endurance sports swimming, biking and running allow to push the limits of the endurance capability to completely new dimensions. Press clips from the early days of triathlon with statements like "Big Supermen Show", "Craziness Cubed" or "The Complete Madness" now belong to history. In the course of the recent years, triathlon has turned in a worldwide phenomenon inspiring millions of people. In Germany alone, around 180,000 people per year are active in triathlon, and the high profile of this young sport is constantly growing. Out of respect for the performance, triathletes are often referred to the "true" athletes.

35.1 Characteristics

Triathlon is a non-stop endurance sport in swimming, biking and running. The competition time is taken without interruption, starting with the swim and ends when the triathlete is crossing the run finish line (➢ Table 35.2).

Triathlon is said to be a fancy, innovative and extreme sport. However, triathlon is proven both psychologically as well as physically to be less stressful than marathon. The hormonal as well as the metabolic stress is lower and no other endurance sport is training the muscular system, the metabolism, and the cardiovascular system as thoroughly as triathlon. In professional triathlon, training input (up to 1,600 training hours per year with a non-unusual physical load in the dimension of 30km swimming, 900 km biking and 130 km running per week) lead to extreme requirements on the supporting apparatus as well as the musculoskeletal system.

In the Olympic triathlon the performance structure of swimming is determined by the free water swimming. Competition-specific skills and other parameters such as finding an ideal starting position, a high starting speed, position fights during start and swim course, orientation and as well as effective passing of the buoys are critical components of success.

Since drafting has been allowed in Olympic triathlon, biking changed towards a true bike competition. Training concentrates on speed muscular endurance, development and coordination of physical abilities and capabilities (cadence attitude, short intervals of high-speed training).

Running is a critical factor of success in competition. High intensities and race-speed specific endurance training on the basis of a stable aerobic endurance are central to triathlon training.

Switching between the partial disciplines is more and more important as many athletes stay in the same transition area after swimming

Tab. 35.1 Triathlon – Historical Overview.

1975	First triathlon event in San Diego
02/18/1978	1st Hawaii triathlon (15 starters, 12 finishers)
01/10/1980	ABC broadcasts the 3rd Hawaii Ironman which increases the world-wide popularity of the Hawaii triathlon.
06/21/1980	1st triathlon in Europe in the former USSR
09/15/1981	1st long-distance triathlon in Europe in Den Haag. The first television broadcasting in the Federal Republic of Germany piques the interest of the German endurance athletes.
1983	Manuel Debus is founding the German Triathlon Association (DTV – Deutscher Triathlon-Verband) with a tendency to professional sports. Günter Kissler is founding the German Triathlon Federation (DTriB – Deutscher Triathlon-Bund) with a tendency to amateur sports.
1984	The European Triathlon Union (ETU – Europäische Triathlon Union) is founded on a European level.
02/23/1985	Fusion of DTV and DTriB to incorporate the German Triathlon Union (DTU – Deutsche Triathlon Union). 1st official European Championships (1,3 km/60 km/12 km) in Immenstadt/Allgäu, Germany.
12/05/1987	Admission of the DTU to the German Sports Federation (DSB – Deutscher Sportbund).
04/01/1989	Foundation of the International Triathlon Union (ITU).
08/06/1989	1st official World Championships in Avignon/France (1,5 km/40 km/10 km) with 42 participating nations.
2000	With the opening competition "Triathlon Women" (1,5 km/40 km/10 km) in Sydney triathlon is becoming part of the Olympic program for the first time.

Table 35.2 Triathlon (Engelhardt 2001).

	Distance Swim / Bike / Run
Olympic-Distance Triathlon	1.5 (±10%) km/40 (±10%) km/10 (±5%) km
Half-Ironman Triathlon	2.0 (±5%) km/80 (±5%) km/20 (±5%) km
Ironman/Long-Distance Triathlon	3.8 km/180 km/42.195 km

due to similar performance levels. Thus, automatic procedures in the transition area are a critical performance factor, which requires training change or brick workout.

35.2 Participation requirements

Triathlon is a high physical strain to the organism of the athlete who needs to be 100% healthy before race start. Internal medicine and orthopedic check-up done before the start of any triathlon training are recommended.

Beginners with no contraindication of triathlon training should start with an adaptation training to the physiological strains of triathlon. The initial training duration should not exceed 30 minutes. The first goal is to do the respective sport continuously and with a constant rhythm. In the beginning proper training techniques have priority, it is particularly important to learn how to drive safely on the bike. Training should be done in small gears and with a cadence of 80 to 100 RPM on roads with little traffic. Only after the body adapted to the strain, the distance and length of the training should be increased by 10 minutes intervals until total training length reaches 1 to 1.5 hours.

35.3 Injuries and results of improper biomechanical stress

35.3.1 Swimming

Injuries

- Abrasion by wet suit (axilla, neck)
- Muscle injuries (shoulder)
- Eyelid injuries (kick/hit on the goggles)
- Sunburn (➤ Fig. 35.1)

Injuries during the swim race of triathlon often result from position fights and diving, which is necessary at start and/or the passing of the buoys.

35.3 Injuries and results of improper biomechanical stress

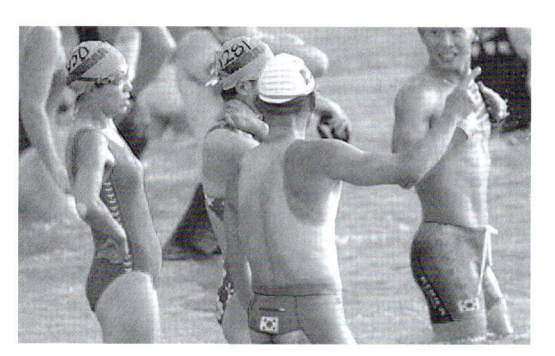

Fig. 35.1 Typical sun burn after exposition to the sun without sun blocker

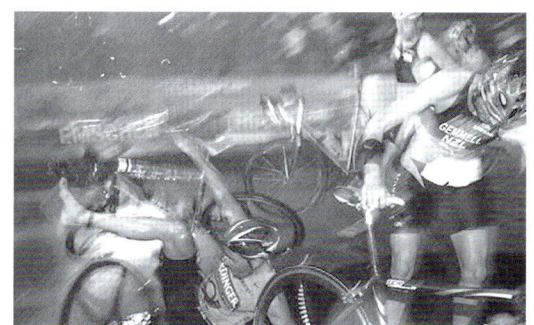

Fig. 35.2 Increased risk of a fracture after spectacular bike crashs on wet ground

Results of Improper Biomechanical Stress

- Tendinitis of the rotator cuff
- Recurrent subacromial bursitis
- Secondary impingement syndrome due to shoulder instability
- Muscular dysbalance of the shoulder girdle.

Prevention of Swim-Specific Problems

- Vaseline/bag balm
- Training of a fast swim start in order to avoid contact injuries
- Training of buoy swim techniques
- No shoulder-damaging warm-up techniques
- No use of paddles at the beginning of the season and during warm-ups
- Muscular balancing of shoulder/neck/back by stretching the contracted muscles
- Strengthening of the rotator cuff

35.3.2 Bike

Injuries

- Abrasions
- Contusions
- Clavicle fracture
- Acromio-clavicular joint dislocation
- Forearm fracture
- Cranio-cerebral injury (CCI)
- Muscle injury of the lower extremity.

The crash-induced injuries during the common drafting races often occur during turns in

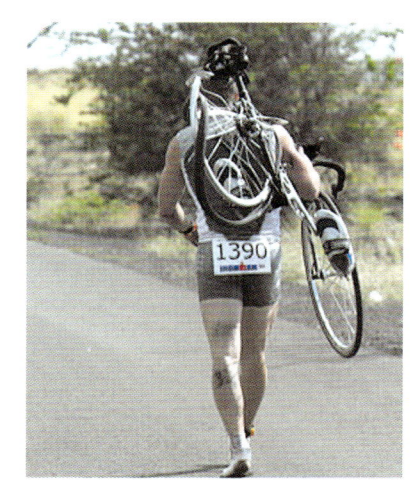

Fig. 35.3 Consequences of a bike crash; bruise and abrasions at body and bike

a group where the athletes riding at the outer side of the curve and are pushed further aside (danger of collision). Cranio-cerebral injury can usually be prevented by obligatory helmets (➢ Fig. 33.2, ➢ Fig. 33.3).

Results of Improper Biomechanical Stress

- Tendinopathy (knee, spine, foot)
- Myalgia/muscular pain in the area of shoulder and neck.

Prevention of Bike-Specific Problems

- Wearing a helmet
- Technical training with cycling specialists

- Improvement of the riding position
- Lumbar spine training/core stability
- Riding in groups.

35.3.3 Running

Injuries

- Muscular injuries
- Capsule-ligament injuries at the upper ankle
- Soft tissue hematoma (➤ Fig. 35.4).

Results of Improper Biomechanical Stress

- Stress fractures (metatarsals, tibia, fibula, calcaneus, femur, pelvis)
- Tendinitis and peritendinitis of the achilles tendon
- Bursitis
- Plantar heel pain, plantar fasciitis
- Tendopathy of the pes anserinus
- Friction syndrom of the ilio-tibial band
- Retropatellar chondropathia/jumpers knee
- shint splints
- Mucscular dysbalance of the lumbar spine.

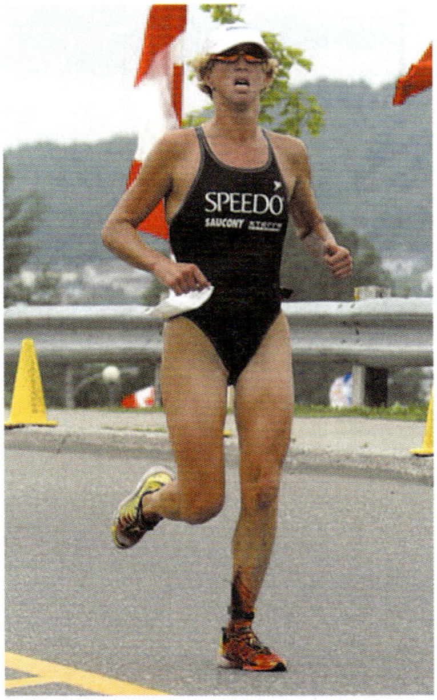

Fig. 35.4 Bloody feet – signs of overstrain (Photo: spomedis GmbH).

Prevention of Running-Specific Problems

- Specific clinical diagnostics of lower extremity and spine static
- Compensation of leg length or provision of insoles, where applicable
- Muscular compensation and improvement of flexibility
- Training camps in warmer countries
- Slow increase of training dimensions
- Nutritional/Hormonal status
- Manual or chiropractic therapy for joint dysfunctions
- Consideration of intensity, previous injury, anatomy, equipment, training territory, body weight.

35.4 Qualification Drawbacks

The below mentioned conditions do not disqualify categorically someone from triathlon, however, they definitely constrain him/her. The potential medical/health risks for the person in question should be weighed carefully. In addition, the permanent development of new operative and therapeutic measures puts the qualification drawbacks into an individual perspective.

Orthopedics

- Spondylolisthesis exceeding 5 mm
- Double-sided spondylolysis
- Fixed scoliosis (exceeding 20° axial variance) and distinctive kyphosis
- Non-resolved juvenile osteochondrosis
- Congenital hip dislocation
- Different types of aseptic bone necrosis
- Profound malformations or aberration at the extremities (with distinct functional restrictions)
- Conditions after muscle, tendon or articular injuries currently cured which lead to significant functional restrictions

Internal medicine

- Heart malformations/valve-disorders with hemodynamic restriction

- Acute and chronic myocarditis
- Hypertrophic cardiomyopathy
- Pathologic cardiac arrhythmia (e.g. WPW syndrome)
- Fixed hypertension (exceeding 160/95 mm Hg)
- Fixed bronchial asthma with restricted lung function
- Chronic renal disorder
- Juvenile-onset diabetes (insulin-dependent)
- Affection of the hormonal system
- Blood diseases with affection of the oxygen transport and the blood coagulation

Other disorders

- Seizure disorders (e.g. epilepsia) and brain damage
- Chronic inflammation of the paranasal sinus

35.5 Recommendations for triathletes

Please see > Table 35.3.

Tab. 35.3 Rules of Conduct for Triathletes (Engelhardt 2001).

> - Always wear a bike helmet, also during training sessions!
> - During triathlons in southern countries or in Hawaii sweat in the amount of up to 6–10 liters in three hours can easily be produced. Drink constantly during the activity and add 1g of salt per liter. If the loss of fluid is not compensated sufficiently, life-threatening, dehydration situations are the result. The following rules of behavior are to be followed during triathlon events at high temperature:
>   – Make sure to be sufficiently acclimatized!
>   – Drink sufficiently before, during and after the competition!
>   – During the competition watch for critical signs of overheating like beating head pressure, giddiness, extreme muscular weakness, goose bumps!
>   – If so, reduce your competition speed!
>   – No medical manipulation!
>   – Do not start without being adequately trained!
>   – Permanently try to cool your head and neck area as well as the legs with water!

References

Engelhardt M et al. (1993). Verletzungsarten und Verletzungshäufigkeiten ausgewählter Ausdauer- und Mehrkampfsportarten. Deutscher Sportärztekongress, Paderborn.

Engelhardt M et al. (1993). Triathlon. Dtsch Z Sportmed 10: 493–500.

Engelhardt M, Reuter I, Neumann G (2004). Triathlon. Sport Orthop Traumatol 20: 239–245.

Ireland ML, Micheli LI (1987). Triathletes: biographic data, training and injury patterns. Ann Sports Med 3: 117–120.

Levy CM, Kolin E, Berson BL (1986). Cross training: risk or benefit? An evaluation of injuries in four athlete populations. Sport Med Clin Forum 3: 1–8.

Levy CM, Kolin E, Berson BL (1986). The effect of cross training on injury incidence, duration and severity (part 2). Sports Med Clin Forum 3: 1–8.

Massimino FA et al. (1988). Common triathlon injuries: special considerations for multisport training. Ann Sports Med 4: 82–86.

Mortier S (1996). Verletzungen und Fehlbelastungsfolgen im Triathlon. Dissertation. Frankfurt/M.

O'Toole ML et al. (1989). Overuse injuries in ultra-endurance triathletes. Am J Sports Med 17: 514–518.

O'Toole ML, Sisk TD (1994). Triathlon. In: Fu FH, Stone DA (eds.). Sport Injuries. Williams and Wilkins, Baltimore, pp. 679–687.

Wiewiorski M et al. (2008). Triathlon. In: Valderrabano V et al. (eds.). Fuß- und Sprunggelenk und Sport. Deutscher Ärzteverlag, Cologne, pp. 319–323.

Important web contact addresses regarding triathlon

International Triathlon Union (ITU): www.triathlon.org

German Triathlon Union (DTU) (Link to the 16 state associations): www.-infor.de

Running-Laufmagazin: www.running-magazin.de

Database Triathlon: www.triathlondata.org

Database of sport-scientific internet sources: www.sponet.de

Triathlon: www.tri-mag.de

Triathlon online: www.triathlon-online.de

International Medical Triathlon Association: www.imta.de

NADA (Bonn) doping list, test procedure: www.nada-bonn.de (e-mail: nada@nada-bonn.de)

WADA (Montreal, Canada), doping regulations (English): www.wada-ama.org

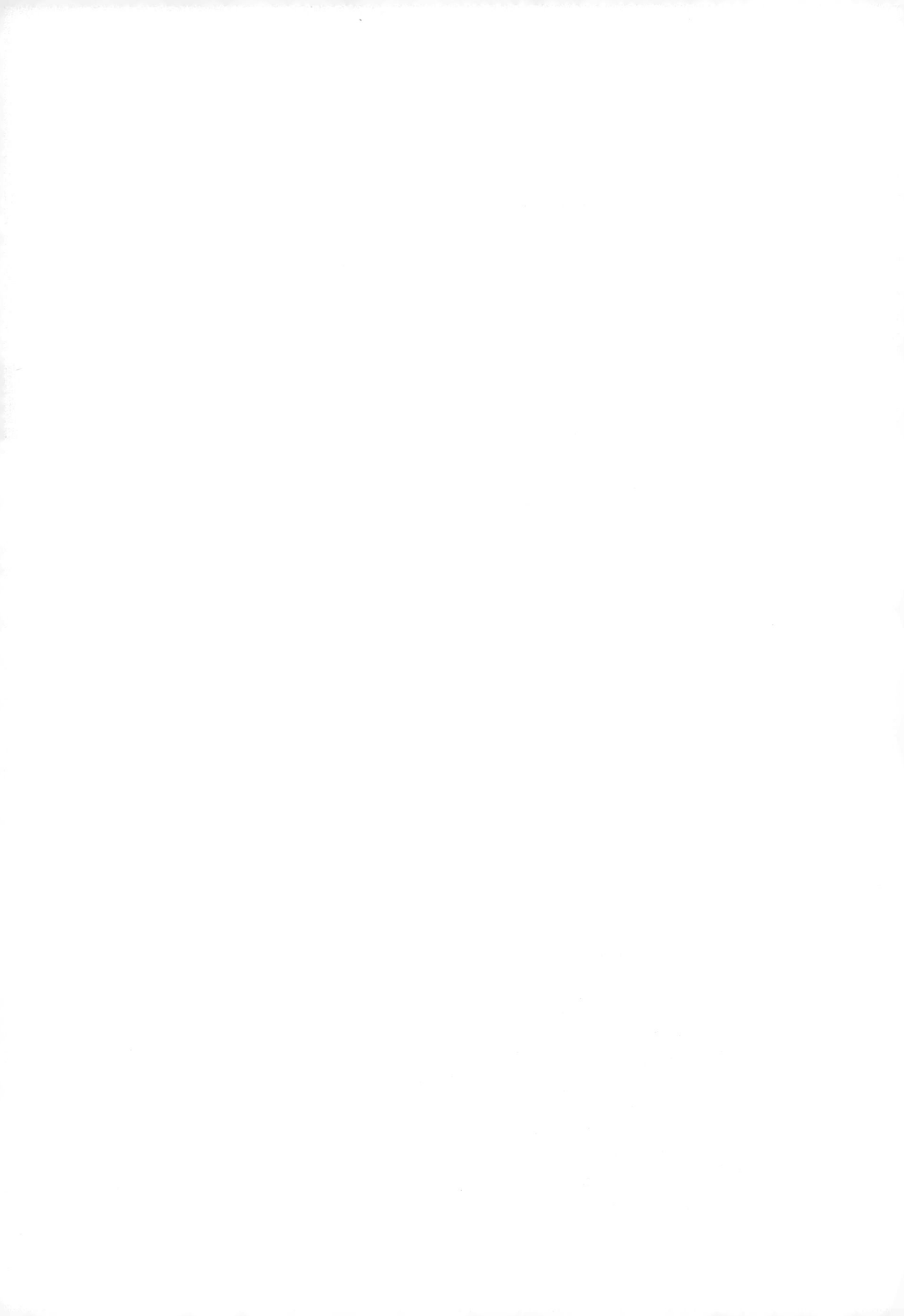

36 Bobsleigh

Christian Schneider

Who does not dream about racing through the ice canal with 120 km/h [75 mph] being protected only by a bobsled and feeling the gravitational pressure on your body? The Formula 1 of the winter sports presents challenges to athletes, technology, logistics and also the field of sports medicine. At the World Cup Races, World Championships and Olympic Games, the BSD squat competes as a national team and the past successes are to be defended (> Fig. 36.1).

36.1 History

It is not exactly known who built the first bobsled. It consisted of two skeleton sleds with a seat board. However, the beginnings of the bobsled lie in St. Moritz where smith Christian Mathis built the first real bobsled back in 1889. The first race took place in 1892 and a first track was also built in St. Moritz in 1903. Bobsleigh rapidly gained popularity in Germany which led to the building of the first German track in Oberhof in 1907 and the founding of the BSD (Bob- und Schlittenverband für Deutschland, German Bobsleigh Association) in 1911.

Since 1924 bobsleigh has been part of the Olympic programme. Since 1930 the World Championships utilized the 4-man bob and since 1931 the 2-man bob. Within competitions, bobsleds were only driven by men; however, since the Winter Olympics in 2002 in Salt Lake City, women also race through the ice canal.

36.2 Equipment

The bobsled is an aerodynamic carriage on four high-grade steel skids made of fibreglass and steel which reaches speeds of up to 150 km/h [93 mph] in the ice canal. It is steered by the pilot with a rope control in the front skid pair. The fitted springs and individually hung skids must be at least 4 mm wide (with the 4-man bob is 6 mm). A two-man bob is up to 2.70 m long and 70 cm wide; a four-seated bob up to 3.85 m long and 87 cm wide.

Because speed decisively depends on the weight – the heavier, the faster – the maximum weight, when occupied, is established in the 2-man bob of 390 kg (ladies 340 kg) and in the 4-man bob of 630 kg. Up to these weights, the bobsled, with firmly linked ballast, may be weighted.

The team with the quickest time after addition of all evaluation runs is the winner. In the World Cup two runs are to be completed, in the World Championships and Olympic Games four runs are required.

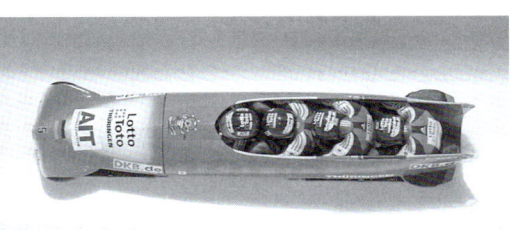

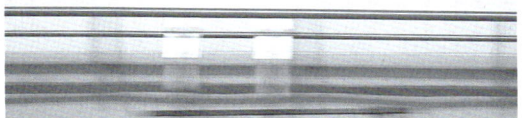

Fig. 36.1 4-man bob on the curve way the ice canal (photo: BSD/Möldner).

A bobsleigh track is an ice track with a length of at least 1200 m [0.75 miles] and a slope between 8 and 15%. It must have at least five strongly banked curves with a radius of 25 m [82 ft] and 5m [16 ft]-high side walls. The curves are calculated with a passing through time of 3 sec, the maximum centrifugal force is not stronger than the fourfold gravitational acceleration (4 g), or with 2 sec passing through time 5 g of centrifugal force.

The athletes wear a tightly fitted textile one-piece suit, gloves, a standardized light-weight helmet with chin protection, sprint shoes and cushions and padding, if necessary.

36.3 Specific features of the bobsleigh

The basis for a good journey in the ice canal is always the start. The team pushes the bobsled as quickly as possible up to 15 m [49 ft] on a 2% slope and the runner jumps into the bobsled. Successful piloting is crucial (➤ Fig. 36.2 a, b and c). Afterwards the start time is measured after 50 m [164 ft] and the pilot tries to steer the bobsled on the ideal line to the finish. Touching the sides or moving off of the ice track can lead to high speed losses. The last athlete (= brakeman) is responsible for the braking of the bobsled with two hand brake levers after crossing the finish line.

Due to the high athletic demands of the crew and brakemen more athletes from athletics are filling these positions. The ideal conditions are combined by specific maximum weight and speed training to obtain quick start times. Then coordination training and improvement of the pushing technique round out the yearly training programme.

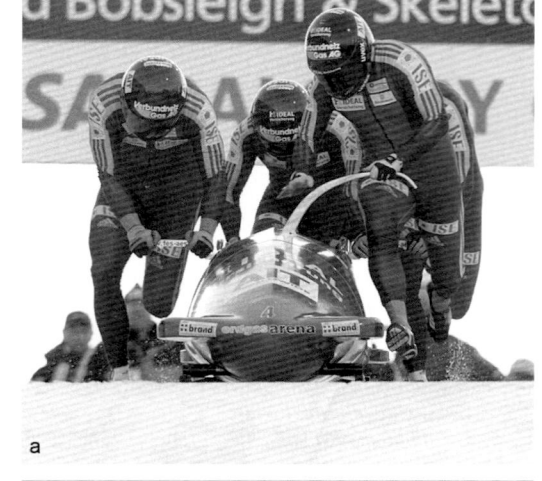

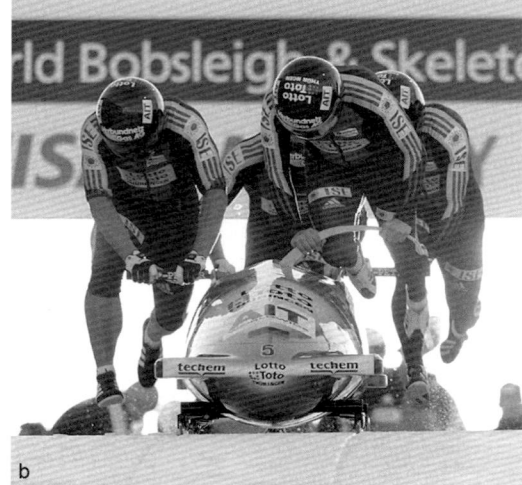

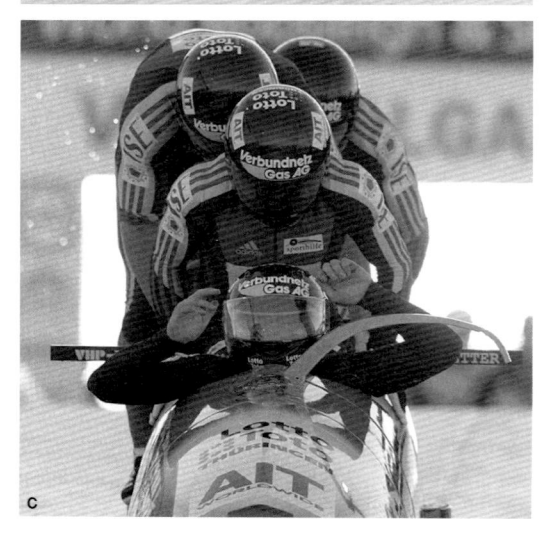

Fig. 36.2 a, b and c start phases with the 4-man bob (photo: BSD/Möldner).

36.4 Injuries and strain damages

The sport in itself is little injury-laden. Often soft tissue injuries occur in the start while getting in the bobsled or by the spikes of the team's members. During the journey the runner "disappear" nearly completely in the bobsled and spends about 60 sec prior to the finish in a sharply forward stooped position. In this position, the whole backbone is subject to strong pressures, which often trigger acute pain attacks. In case of a fall everybody tries to bend lower in the bobsled to protect their heads. Due to the enormously high forces, spinal disc and bone injuries mostly of the cervical vertebra column (➢ Fig. 36.3), compression fractures of the lumbar vertebra column, and concussions can occur.

Now and then the last athlete on the bobsled slips out. He must then leave the track as quickly as possible in order not to sustain further injury. Because of a steady optimisation of the tracks, the bobsleds and specific driving training, deadly injuries are rare.

Nevertheless, most injuries appear in general training. Soccer is often used as coordination training method. Therefore other injury and strain patterns correspond to those of athletics. Overloads of the tendon insertion and the stressed cartilage segments in the knee joints are possible and will have to be diagnosed and treated to full recovery. Because of high stress to the spine, special attention will have to be paid to reoccurring conditions of the cervical and lumbar spine a specific determination of the athletic capability is necessary for the prevention of permanent damages.

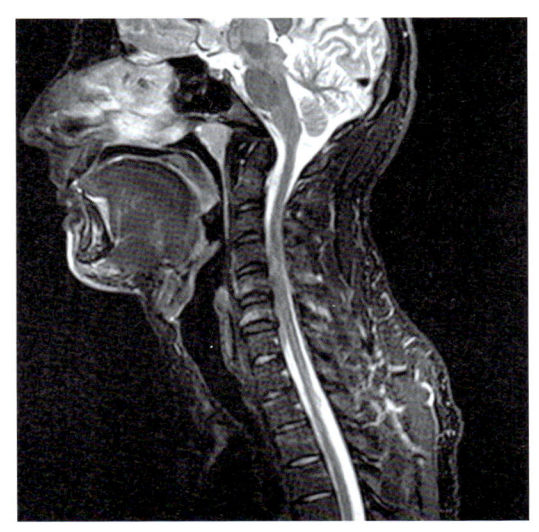

Fig. 36.3 C6 fracture and spinal disc injury C5-7 MRT STIR (Prof. Stäbler, Radiologie München-Harlaching).

Suggestions to the attending physician:
- Knowledge of immunostimulation and adaption to coldness
- Diagnosis and treatment of muscle injuries
- Diagnosis and treatment of spinal injuries
- Knowledge of logistics of the ambulance service on site

37 Bodybuilding
Mathias Ritsch

Bodybuilding is one of the most popular fitness sports. More than 5 million enthusiasts of all age groups practice this sport in Germany alone. About 10 % of those who do bodybuilding are achievement-oriented. This sport has found many new fans especially in Eastern European and Asian countries. It is mostly practiced in commercial fitness studios, and to a lesser extent in sports clubs. The International Federation of Bodybuilders (IFBB) is represented in 173 countries and is recognized by more than 90 national Olympic committees. In Germany, the IFBB is represented by the German Bodybuilding and Fitness Federation (DBFV). The IFBB is a member of the General Association of International Sports Federation (GAISF) and is represented at the World Games. Bodybuilding can be performed up to a high age. The positive effects of specific bodybuilding have been frequently proven, and the risk of injuries is low. In 2005, the number of members in German fitness centers was the lowest it had been for years, counting 4.19 million members, but the numbers have increased since then to 5.25 million members in 2007 (DSSV 2007).

37.1 Characteristics

Weight training with the aim of forming a muscular, proportioned body, concomitantly with a low amount of body fat is the foundation of body building. Bodybuilding is a **presentation sport** classified into different weight classes. It is judged in three different categories. Line-up with compulsory poses is followed by the direct comparison in the seven compulsory poses. After the two physique assessment rounds the free posing routine round is performed to music. In the professional field, there is no weight classification. Men, women and couples are distinguished, as well as bodybuilding and different fitness classes, in which the free exercise routine is evaluated higher. In addition to strength training, **nutrition** is especially decisive for success. The attempt is made to reduce the body fat as low as possible by a **special diet and training cycle** to show the quality of mus-

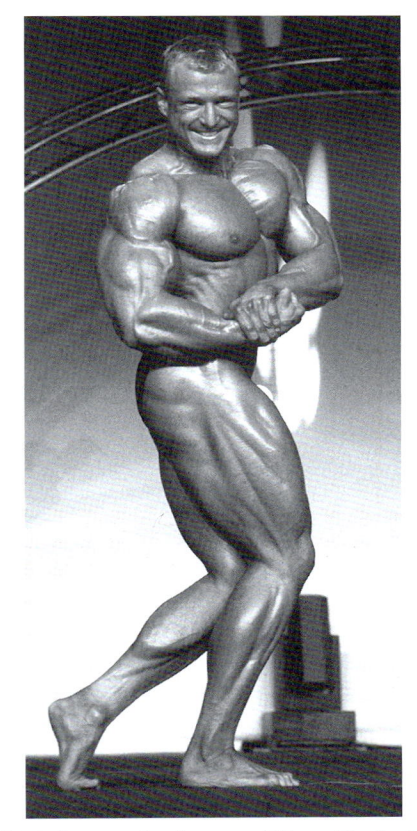

Fig. 37.1 Presentation in competition: side chest pose.

cles – density, separation and definition. In addition to **muscle mass**, the **symmetry** and the **proportions** are especially important at the representation on stage. This can only be achieved to a certain degree and the genetic preconditions play a significant role. Posing pants or a posing bikini are worn at competitions, the body is shaved and tanning lotion and afterwards some oil is applied to the skin (➢ Fig. 37.1).

Muscle training is performed with dumbbells and barbells as well as on different training machines. Classic weight training with barbell and dumbbells is still the basis. Certain muscle groups are exercised in different exercises, which are a combination of sets with one to 15 repetitions. Depending on the frequency of training, circular training or split training are performed whereby the individual muscle groups are trained on different days. This is done as antagonist training or division into flexing and extending muscle groups.

37.2 Equipment

Special equipment, as for many other sports, is not required. Functional clothing and appropriate shoes are sensible. The training machines have reached a high standard by now and can be ideally adjusted to the individual athlete. The free weight training should be performed on special surfaces and requires the support of training partners for the maximum range. Different bandages and also the power lifting belt have proven of value for higher weights.

37.3 Most frequent injuries and strain conditions

In general, there should be no axial deformity of a higher degree, internal capacity should exist and no serious neurologic disorders such as epilepsy are found. Regarding the facts stated above, bodybuilding is possible until high age. The maximum strength training should only be carried out by athletes aged 16 years and older.

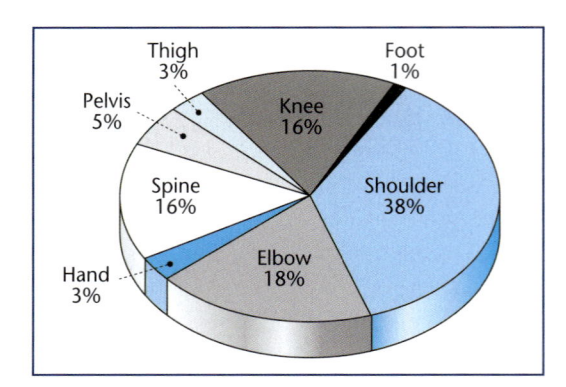

Fig. 37.2 Injury profile of 600 Bodybuilding injuries (Ritsch 2005).

Bodybuilding is one of the **sports with low injury rates**. In the statistics of sport injuries by Steinbrück (1999), bodybuilding constitutes 0.5% of all injuries. Risser (1990) states an incidence of 0.082% injuries by person and year in strength training. Injuries in bodybuilding competitions do usually not occur.

Shoulder and **elbow** are the most common injuries and damage caused by strain in bodybuilding (➢ Fig. 37.2). Two thirds of all damages appear in the region of **tendons and muscles**, osseous injuries usually do not occur. The **injuries caused by strain** are significantly more frequent than real injuries. Based on 600 strength-sport injuries, the following aspects become obvious (Ritsch 2005): The most frequent diagnoses are the rotator cuff impingement, lateral epicondylitis and the femoropatellar pain syndrome (➢ Tab. 37.1). The rupture of the pectoralis major and the atraumatic osteolysis of the distal clavicle are bodybuilding-specific injuries and overload damages.

> Strains and muscle and tendon ruptures are the most frequent injuries in bodybuilding. Insertion tendinitis especially at the elbow, the impingement syndrome at the shoulder and the arthritis of the acromioclavicular joint are the primary typical overload damages.

The **diagnosis** of the soft-tissue injuries, which represent the main part of injuries, should always include ultrasound examination, because the severity of the injury is often misunderstood clinically. Sometimes ultrasound can be even superior to MRI because the real extent of a stretched muscle or tendon injury shows up

Tab. 37.1 Most frequent injuries in Bodybuilding (n = 600, Ritsch 2005).

Injury types	n	Frequency
rotator cuff impingement	69	11.5
lateral epicondylitis	42	7.0
femoropatellar pain syndrome	36	6.0
patellar tendinitis	27	4.5
triceps tendinitis	26	4.3
AC joint arthritis	24	4.0
instability impingement	23	3.8
low back pain	21	3.5
pectoralis major rupture	17	2.8
quadriceps tendinitis	16	2.7
distal biceps tendinitis	16	2.7
atraumatic osteolysis of the distal clavicle	15	2.5

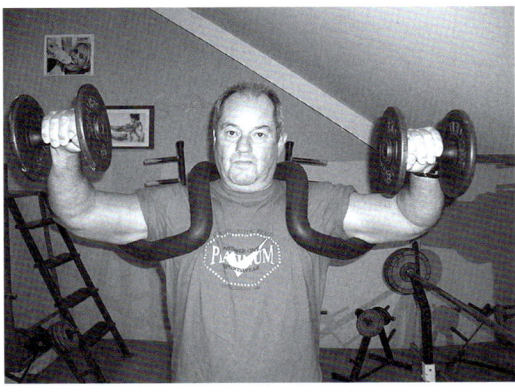

Fig. 37.3 Training of the external rotators with the shoulder horn (Hans Wagner, former world champion in ski bob).

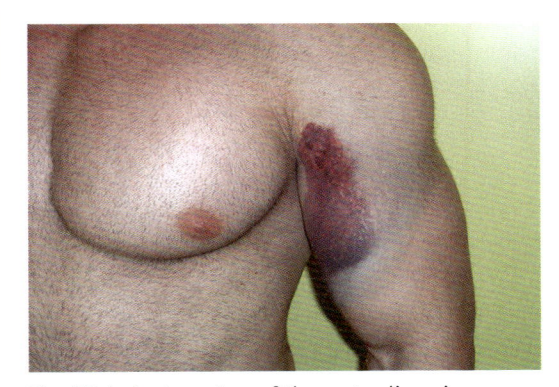

Fig. 37.4 Acute rupture of the pectoralis major.

much better in the dynamic examination. Most injuries and overload damages do not cause difficulties in the orthopedic diagnosis.

The general patterns of treatment are implemented in **therapy**. Usually, no interruption of training will be necessary, because exercises can be performed around most injuries by **adjusting the training**. Tendinitis reacts positively to changes of the joint posture and the grip span; frequent relapses can be prevented. Subacromial syndromes require an adjustment of training. The triggering exercises such as shoulder press behind the head or lat pulldown behind the head should generally be carried out in front of the head. Special exercises for the training of the external rotators at the shoulder have proven valuable because of the increase of imbalance of the internal rotators to the external rotators common in strength sport. The so-called shoulder horn to train the external rotators is accepted very well by many athletes (➢ Fig. 37.3).

> The most important therapy in addition to the known therapy standards is the specified adjustment of training.

In addition to strains, the most frequent muscle injuries are **ruptures of the pectoralis major** (➢ Fig. 37.4). Unlike described in literature (Aarimaa et al. 2004, Petilon et al. 2005), most ruptures are not complete and affect the myotendinous junction rather than the osseous insertion (Ritsch 2010).

Generally, the early therapy is surgery. Secondary reconstructions have clearly worse prospects. The conservative therapy, on the other hand, will always lead to unsatisfactory results.

Tendon ruptures affect the **distal and proximal biceps tendon**, the **rotator cuff**, the **triceps** and the **quadriceps** (Ritsch 2005, Sollender 1998). The rupture of the triceps tendon is a typical injury in weight training ➢ Fig. 37.5). In contrast to the rupture of the proximal long biceps tendon, this injury as well as the rupture of the distal biceps tendon requires always surgical therapy. The rupture of the rotator cuff is although a primary indication for surgery.

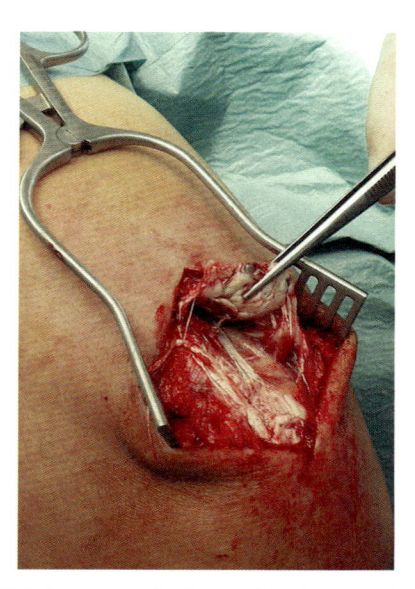

Fig. 37.5 Intraoperative image of a triceps tendon rupture.

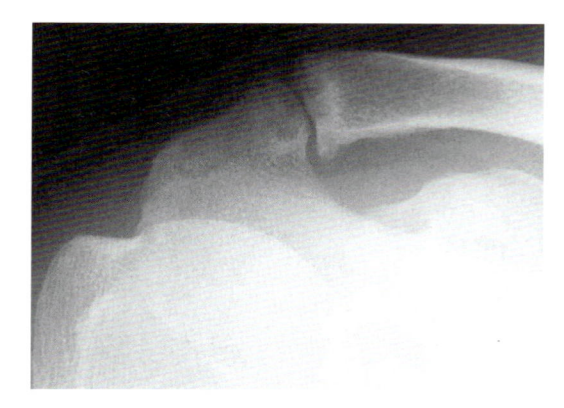

Fig. 37.6 Atraumatic osteolysis of the distal clavicle.

Quadriceps ruptures needs always anatomical refixation.

> Generally, an early surgical therapy is required for muscle and tendon ruptures.

The **atraumatic osteolysis of the distal clavicle** presents an injury typical for this sport (➢ Fig. 37.6). Chronic irritations caused by strain of the AC joint can result in an osteolysis of the lateral clavicle as a consequence (Auge and Fischer 1998). If the therapy by intra-articular cortisone infiltrations is exhausted, only the surgical resection of the lateral clavicle achieves freedom from symptoms.

Provided the exercises are done correctly and the exercise weights are chosen properly, injuries are very unlikely even in high-performance bodybuilding.

References

Aarimaa V, Rantanen J, Heikkila J, Helttula I, Orava S (2004). Rupture of the pectoralis major muscle. Am J Sports Med 32: 1256–1262.

Auge WK, Fischer RA (1998). Arthroscopic distal clavicle resection for isolated atraumatic osteolysis in weight lifters. Am J Sports Med 26: 189–192.

DSSV (2008). Eckdaten 2007. Fitness Management International 76: 28–30.

Petilon J, Carr DR, Sekiya JK, Unger DV (2005). Pectoralis major muscle injuries: evaluation and management. J Am Acad Orthop Surg 13: 59–68.

Risser WL (1990). Musculoskeletal injuries caused by weight training. Clin Pediatrics 29: 305–310.

Ritsch M (2010). Evaluierung und Management der M.-pectoralis-major-Ruptur. Obere Extrem. 5: 179–185.

Ritsch M (2005). Bodybuilding. In: Engelhardt M, Krüger-Franke M, Pieper HG, Siebert CH (eds.). Praxiswissen Halte- und Bewegungsorgane – Sport. Thieme-Verlag, Stuttgart.

Sollender JL, Ryan GM, Barden GA (1998). Triceps tendon rupture in weight lifters. JSES 7: 151–153.

Steinbrück K (1999). Epidemiologie von Sportverletzungen – 25-Jahre-Analyse einer sportorthopädisch-traumatologischen Ambulanz. Sportverl Sportschad 13: 38–52

Chapter 38 Olympic Weightlifting

Dominik Doerr

Weightlifting is one of the oldest Olympic sports. Individual exercises were already developed 4,000 years ago in Egypt and China. The presence of Milos of Kroton in the Olympic winner lists of 540 B.C. is considered a historical proof. Since the modern ear of Olympic Games in 1896, weightlifting has continuously being present. Today, weightlifting is spread worldwide, the umbrella organization, international weightlifting federation (IWF) counts 178 member states. International championships in women's weightlifting have been carried out since 1987; women's weightlifting is an Olympic sport since the Olympic Games in 2000.

38.1 Sport-specific equipment

The sport equipment is a **handlebar** of a length of 2.20 m and a weight of 20 kg (men) or 15 kg (women). It will be equipped on both sides with **disks** with a metal core and a rubber coating on rotatable collars. The handle surfaces are roughened to provide a firm, safe grip. The disks start with a weight of 0.5 kg and are followed by weights of 1 kg, 2 kg, 5 kg, 10 kg, 15 kg, 20 kg and 25 kg.

The lifting will be performed on a wooden platform of a size of 4 × 4 m, mostly with integrated rubber surfaces. The **sports dress** consists of a tricot/one-piece suit. The weightlifting shoes are half-height shoes with a solidly worked sole. Bandages at knee and hand joints as well as a belt are permitted.

38.2 Procedure of competition

Snatch and clean and jerk are the two Olympic disciplines.

- **Snatch:** The weight is pulled with a wide grip – mostly in the squatting technique – to the locked arms overhead (➤ Fig. 38.1).
- **Clean and jerk:** The weight is grasped at shoulder width and will pulled from the floor to a racked position across deltoids and clavicles. After a short gain of momentum by flexion of the knees (sidestep or

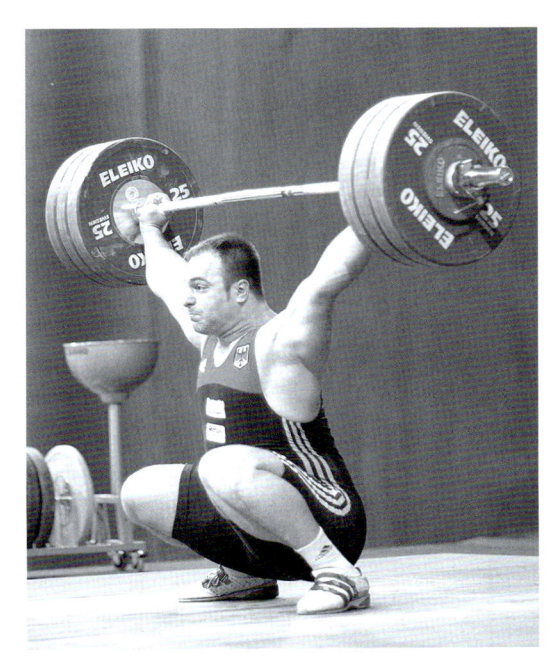

Fig. 38.1 Snatch.

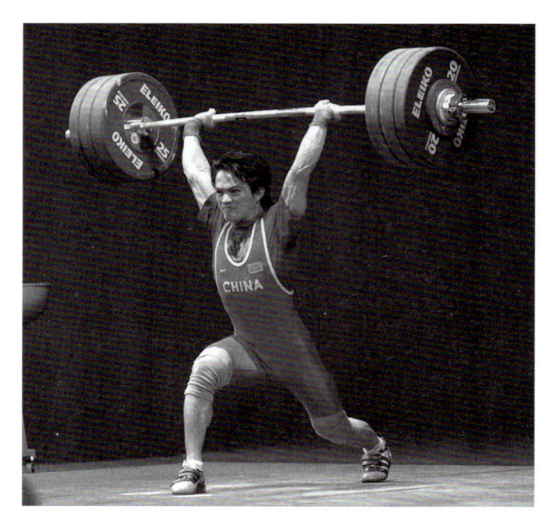

Fig. 38.2 Clean and jerk.

squatting technique) weights are pushed overhead onto the extended arms (➢ Fig. 38.2).

Each lifter has **three attempts per discipline**, in which he or she has to achieve their best performance; each highest achieved weight counts. If two lifters lift the same weight, the lower body weight determines the winner. Judges rate the correct performance of the individual attempts. At the Olympic Games, only the sum of both disciplines is judged, the individual disciplines as well as their sum are judged separately at world championships and continental championships.

The lifting is performed in **different bodyweight categories** – eight classes for men and seven classes for women (➢ Tab. 38.1).

Tab. 38.1 Weight classes for men and women.

Men	Women
–56 kg	–48 kg
–62 kg	–53 kg
–69 kg	–58 kg
–77 kg	–63 kg
–85 kg	–69 kg
–94 kg	–75 kg
–105 kg	75 kg+
105 kg+	

There are two disciplines in weightlifting: the Snatch and Clean and Jerk, each in different bodyweight categories. The athlete always has three attempts for each discipline, but the highest load counts. At the same loads, the lower body weight determines the winner.

38.3 General sport-medical aspects

Weightlifting promotes the development of a good muscle corset and strengthens muscles and supporting ligaments. A special training increases maximum strength and flexibility with a focus on speed-strength and coordination. This explains why weightlifting training now penetrates more and more other sports that also need these capabilities. Additionally, increase in muscular strength and flexibility helps to prevent injuries.

Weightlifting advances maximum strength and speed-strength as well as coordination and flexibility.

Contraindications to the performance of weightlifting are listed in ➢ Table 38.2.

For historical reasons, there have always been several **prejudices** against weightlifting ranging from **damaging the spine** to the development of varicose veins (Steinbrück 1978). The IWF Medical Commission intervened at the Olympic Games in 1972 in Munich, which abandoned the former third discipline of clean and press. In this discipline, the weight had been pushed above the head by a sudden dorsal flexion of the upper body, which increased the risk of spondylolysis. Consequently, injury rate in weightlifting sank rapidly after abandoning this discipline and ranks in the lower third of the injury statistics (Dörr 1997). In today's weightlifting the well-developed back muscles protects the spine.

Tab. 38.2 Contraindications of weightlifting.

distinctive scoliosis
distinctive hollow-/humpback
spondylolisthesis
florid Scheuermann's disease
distinctive patellar dysplasias
stronger axial malpositions of the knee joints
pathologic joint mobility

The weight lifters' technique is recommended as an exemplary back injury prevention technique for the general population.

Weightlifting improves venous function based on its dynamic process (Dörr and Kirchmaier 2004).

The assumption that weightlifting of adolescents **disturbs the epiphyseal plate** requires critical analysis. Growth disturbances of adolescents who have already performed sport-specific training early in their lives are unknown (Zawieja 2005). Additionally, incidence of Osgood-Schlatter disease is observed similar to the average age in the general population (Dörr 1999).

38.4 Special sport-medical aspects

Acute injuries especially in competition are rare in technically experienced athletes. **Overuse conditions** prevail especially in the phase of strength development at the preparation of competitions. Once more, sensible (!) regeneration for the prevention of muscular injuries needs special attention.

Shoulder

Lesions of the rotator cuff are typical sport-specific injuries. Injuries from strains to complete ruptures can appear especially within the scope of a failed attempt to hold the handlebar falling backwards (> Fig. 38.3). The **long biceps tendon** is affected less often. AC joint overuses are effectively non-existent in weightlifting, because there is no training of bench-press.

Elbow

Injuries of the elbow joint are equally rare. A spinning movement at the acceleration of the weight or its repositioning behind the body axis triggers overuse **of the medial ligament structures**. **Dislocations** or **osseous avulsions** have been observed infrequently.

Wrist/palm

The different grabbing postures in snatch and in clean and jerk, the roughened surfaces of

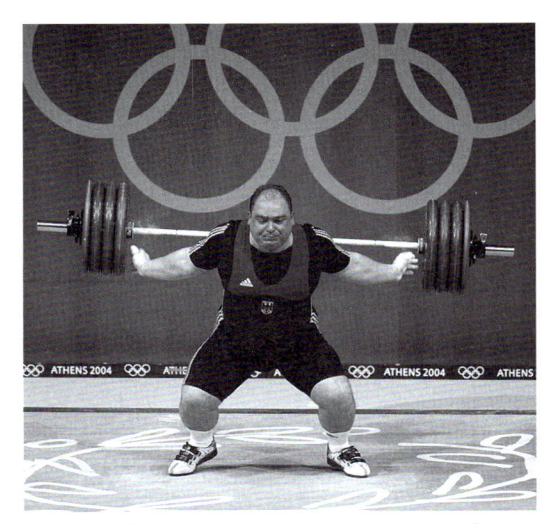

Fig. 38.3 Unsuccessful attempt in snatching with rupture of the rotator cuff.

the handle bar and the partly significant dorsal flexion of the wrist dictate injury patterns. **Cartilage overuse** is the consequence. Straps can be used but they will not be allowed in competition. Typical problems especially in competition are **lacerations of the palm** and the fingers. The enormous tension and shear forces in connection with the rough surfaces of the handlebar trigger these injuries. Already present calluses increase injury risk, hence, their preventive removal is key in weightlifting.

Knee joint/tibia

Overuse of the knee is a critical point in weightlifting. **Retropatellar chondropathies**, upper and lower **patellar apex syndrome** and insertion **tendopathies of the tuberositas tibiae** are often observed. Excoriations of the anterior tibial surface due to scratching with the handlebar in lifting especially with the roughened handles are typical problems in competition. Acute **quadriceps and patellar tendon ruptures** as a result of incompletely healed chronic overload and continued, high-load training are rare.

Hip

Injuries of the hip joint itself have not been observed but **enthesiopathies of the trochanter major** are common.

Back

As described above a good protection of the spine is at the center of an intense, technical training and a good muscular paravertebral development. This makes the spine tolerating to short, high axial stress with a low injury rate. If injuries occur they present as paravertebral myogeloses, insertion tendopathies of the long erector spine muscle, and overload reactions of the vertebral joints. Occasionally, blockades of the thoracic spine and the iliosacral joint and lumbar discopathies appear but are often result of bad technique.

> In weightlifting, overuse syndromes prevail, acute traumas are rare.

References

Dörr B (1997): Gewichthweben [Weightlifiting] In: Engelhardt M, Hintermann B, Segesser B (eds.). GOTS-Manual Sporttraumatologie. Huber-Verlag, Bern, pp 238–242.

Dörr B (1998): Gewichtheben [Olympic Weightlifting] In: Klümper A (ed.). Sporttraumatologie. Ecomed, II-22 1–9, 5. Erg.-Kfg. 12/99.

Dörr D, Kirchmaier CM (2004). Untersuchungen zur Venenfunktion an Unterschenkeln von Gewichthebern mittels Luftplethysmographie. [Examination of weightlifter's lower limbs using airplethysmography] Dt Z Sportmed 55: 12–16.

Steinbrück K (1978). Varikosis und ihre Bedeutung in der Sportmedizin [Varicose veins and her relevance in sports medicine]. Dt Z Sportmed 12: 352–355.

Zawieja M (2005). National Team Coach German Weightlifting Federation (BVDG), personal statement.

39 Athletics (Jump and Throw)

Kirstin Richter

39.1 History

Athletics is one of the core sports of the Olympic Games of modern times. But it has its roots already in the ancient world. Competitions of track and field, especially disciplines of jumping and throwing, have been competitions of the ancient Olympic Games for a long time.

In 19th century, **modern track and field athletics** developed. The first national championships were held in England in 1866. The jump and throw disciplines of track and field have been counted among the sports of the early days at the first Olympic Games of modern times in 1896 in Athens.

At first, track and field was a pure **male domain**. This changed in 1928, when the first **women's competitions** (high jump, discus throw and running competitions, at first) were admitted to the Olympic program. Other disciplines followed.

In recent years, the spectra of disciplines of men and women became more and more similar; most recently added disciplines are pole vault, hammer throw, triple jump and steeplechase over 3,000 m.

39.2 Disciplines

Jump disciplines are:

- long jump
- triple jump
- high jump
- pole vault.

Throw disciplines are:

- javelin throw (600 g for women, 800 g for men)
- shot put (4 kg for women, 7.25 kg for men)
- discus throw (1 kg for women, 2 kg for men)
- hammer throw (4 kg for women, 7.25 kg for men).

Both jump and throw disciplines belong to the technical disciplines, in which the athlete absolves several rounds (usually three qualification rounds and three further final rounds for the eight best athletes). Of all rounds, the best wins. Each athlete has three tries for each performed height in high jump and pole vault.

In addition to the obligatory **spike shoes**, no essential equipment is necessary for **long jump, triple jump and high jump**. **Fiberglass poles** of different stiffness are used additionally for **pole vault**.

Every throw discipline requires **throwing equipment** (discus, shot, javelin, and hammer). With the exception of **javelin throw** performed in **spike shoes**, shoes with even soles – so-called **thrower shoes** – should be used.

The throwing equipment in **hammer throw** as well as in **discus throw** is spun out of a 10-m-high **protective grid** ("cage") into a predefined sector. The use of the equipment requires training and a careful handling, in order not to cause any accidents in spinning and throwing. Even fatal accidents have happened in the past, which were caused by throwing equipment gone astray.

39.3 Sport-specific requirement profile

All track and field disciplines require good **strength**, **velocity**, **flexibility** and **coordination**. The jump disciplines especially require a good **capacity of bounce** and **spring**.

Jumping disciplines

All jump disciplines consist of the following **four phases**: run-up, take-off, flight and landing phase. The competition requirements demand a **one-leg take-off** in all disciplines.

Long jump/triple jump

After an accelerating run-up of 30–50 m at long jump and triple jump the athlete converts the gained speed into a jump and bounces to maximum width.

In triple jump, after the take-off the first landing must be performed by the take-off leg (hop), then a simple jump with landing on the opposite leg will follow (step). Only thereafter the athlete jumps into the jumping pit. This requires major **coordinative and technical capabilities**.

The **primarily affected regions** in long and triple jump are the muscles and the joints of the lower extremities as well as the trunk muscles. Special forms of training for the improvement of reactivity and bounce, e.g. by low jumps or one-legged jumps affect the **spine**.

High jump/pole vault

In both disciplines, a 20–50 m long accelerated run is followed by a rapid take-off. In high jump, the run-up velocity is a little slower. The athlete attempts reaching the optimum run-up velocity, which allows the best conversion of the kinetic energy into bounce and jump height.

In pole vault, the acceleration and bounce is transmitted to the fiberglass pole, which accelerates the body upwards. This movement affects **shoulder**, **trunk muscles**, and **muscles of the lower extremity**.

> Primarily affected regions in the jump disciplines are the lower extremities and the trunk.

39.3.1 Throwing disciplines

Javelin throw

In javelin throw, the body is accelerated in a 20–30 m run-up with the **throwing arm** behind the head in an internal rotation and extension. With an extensive lateral **stemming step** the pelvis and trunk prepare the whip-like throw out of a backwards-bended posture. This lets to a **hyperextension of the lumbar spine**.

Primarily affected regions are the shoulder, trunk (especially the spine), and adductors of the stemming leg.

Shot put/discus/hammer throw

In all three disciplines, different rotation and gliding techniques rotate **the upper body against the pelvis**.

Strongly affected regions are the shoulder and trunk. Especially in **hammer throw**, a well developed musculature of the trunk, **hand and finger flexors** are necessary to hold the hammer, which is extensively accelerated by centrifugal force.

Strength training is indicated for all throwing disciplines. Hence, injuries and overuse symptoms known from strength training can occur.

> The shoulder and trunk are the primarily affected regions in all throw disciplines.

The most frequent injuries in these disciplines of track and field athletics result from movement in jump and throw disciplines with **sprint-like run-ups** and **rapid movements** at take-off and release. **Muscle injuries** (distortions, indurations, partial ruptures/ruptures) are the most frequent injuries (Garrett 1990, Nigg 1991). They often develop because due to neglected warm-up exercises, uncoordinated movements caused by fatigued muscles or technical deficiencies.

Quick movements and jump are required in all technical disciplines of track and field. Accordingly, intensive training focuses on velocity and rapid movement coordination.

> In track and field athletics, most injuries and overuse symptoms appear at muscle-tendon junctions.

39.4 Injuries

➤ Table 39.1 shows typical injuries of jumpers and throwers.

Tab. 39.1 Typical injuries of jumpers and throwers.

Types of injury	Jump disciplines	Throw disciplines
muscle injuries	■ muscular distortion, induration ■ partial rupture: – ischiocrural musculature – musculature of the torso – calf musculature	■ muscular distortion, induration ■ partial rupture/rupture: – muscles of shoulder girdle and arm – trunk muscles – adductors
insertion tendopathies	■ patellar tendon (jumper's knee) ■ Achilles tendon	■ epicondylitis humeri radialis/ulnaris ■ coracoiditis
tendon injuries	■ patellar tendon ■ Achilles tendon	■ rotator cuff ■ impingement symptoms
joints	joints of the lower extremity: knee/upper ankle joint: ■ meniscus injuries (tears, bruises) ■ cartilage contusions ■ ligament injuries ■ arthrosis	■ shoulder joint – instability/dislocation – labrum/SLAP lesions – lesions of the rotator cuff – arthrosis ■ elbow joint – medial instability – distortions – cartilage injuries – arthrosis ■ finger joint dislocations joint capsule injuries
ligament injuries	■ fibular ligament apparatus (OSG distortions) ■ lateral ligament injuries of the knee	■ ulnar lateral ligament
acute osseous injuries: ■ tears of apophyses ■ fractures ■ stress fractures	■ tuberositas tibiae ■ rarely: spinae iliacae ant. sup. et inf., only after accidents (fall beside the pad, breaking of the pole, distortion of the upper ankle joint) ■ ventral tibial edge ■ os naviculare ■ vertebral arch	■ epicondylus humeri radialis/ulnaris rarely: vertebral arch
spine injuries	■ after fall beside the matting or after pole breaking ■ spondylolysis, spondylolisthesis	■ spondylolysis ■ spondylolisthesis
overload damages	■ muscular induration and partial ruptures/ruptures ■ insertion tendinopathies ■ spondylolysis, spondylolisthesis ■ periostitis, stress fractures	■ muscular induration and partial ruptures/ruptures ■ insertion tendinopathies ■ spondylolysis, spondylolisthesis ■ shoulder instabilities, lesions of the rotator cuffs)

39.4.1 Injuries of jumpers

- **Muscle injuries:** Distortions, indurations, partial ruptures/ruptures are triggered by spring movements. Especially affected are:
  - the ischiocrural muscles, because of the sprint-like run-up and the rapid take-off (Nigg 1991) and
  - the muscles of the trunk (abdomen/dorsum), because of the jump movements, the landing and the carrying of the fiberglass pole.
- **Tendon injuries:** especially in the region of the **patellar tendon**, the **Achilles tendon**, because of the short-ranged high local tension forces at take-off. Relapsing microtraumas develop due to repetitive stress that can lead to (partial) ruptures, in case of chronic overuse symptoms (Fredberg and Bolvig 1999).
- **Insertion tendopathies:**
  - Patellar tendon (insertion and origin, **jumper's knee**)
  - Less frequent as Achilles tendon insertion. The pathophysiology is the same as with tendon injuries (Tibesku and Pässler 2005).
- **Meniscus and cartilage damages:** Before the take-off, a stemming phase with minor lowering of the body's center of gravity occurs. If this phase lasts too long (muscular fatigue or inappropriate technique) the braking effect is too strong and compresses the knee and ankle joint with a risk of meniscus and cartilage contusions (Nigg 1991).
- **Ligament injuries:** primarily as supination traumas, e.g. the take-off leg sets down first with the external side of the foot. This can happen in high jump or in the individual jumping sections in triple jump, and at take-off for long and triple jump. The take-off board is marked with a plasticine layer, which is slightly raised. At the step past the foul line and on the plasticine, the risk of a supination trauma with fibular ligament distortions/ruptures or even osseous injuries is very high.
- **Periostitis/stress fractures:** due to chronic stress, alternating ground surfaces in spring/fall as well as exaggerated training with overuse of the ventral tibia relapsing microtraumas occurs. Stress fractures can develop at longer-lasting overuse symptoms. These mainly appear in the region of the **anterior tibial edge** and the **os naviculare**. An interruption of training until pain stops and an adjustment of training with adaption to the individual capacity is indicated (Geyer et al. 1993).
- **Acute osseous injuries:** apophyseal avulsions, e.g. in the area of the tuberositas tibiae or the spinae iliacae anterior superior et inferior, because of the sudden tension of the muscular insertions. Acute non-traumatic tibial fractures have been observed in triple jump. Fractures and dislocations will also appear after the breaking of a pole or a fall beside the pad in **pole vault** (Wolff 2000).
- **Spinal injuries:** Repeated micro-traumas in the region of the pedicles of the vertebral arch can develop because of repetitive overuse symptoms with hyperlordosing of the lumbar spine in high jump. A stress fracture in the region of the pedicles of the vertebral arch with subsequent spondylolysis/spondylolisthesis can develop at longer-lasting overloads and a congenital inferior capacity. In pole vault, it comes to injuries of the back extensors or the spinous processes at hyperlordosing when underrunning the pole at take-off or during take-off. Overload syndromes of the lumbar spine appear also at concomitant strength training (free weights, squats).

39.4.2 Injuries of throwers

- **Muscle injuries:** Distortions, indurations, partial ruptures/ruptures can develop triggered by the powerful spring movements. Especially affected are:
  - muscles of the shoulder
  - muscles of the back extensors and abdominal muscles
  - thigh muscles, especially the adductors.
- **Insertion tendopathies:** primarily in the region of epicondyle humeri ulnaris, but also at the insertion of the adductor longus muscle.
- **Injuries of the shoulder joint:**
  - **anterior instability:** due to relapsing overstretch of the passive shoulder joint stabi-

lizers (labrum, capsule, glenoid) in the acceleration and braking movement at the release. In the long term, it will come to a **laxity** of the capsule or a rupture of the labrum/SLAP lesion.

- **impingement symptoms:** A **bursitis subacromialis** or an "overload tendinitis" with a subsequent calcarea or a **rotator cuff lesion** because of permanent overhead occupation and repeating movements (Altchek and Dines 1995, Schmitt et al. 2001).

■ **Injuries of the elbow joint:** especially in javelin throwers because of a distraction in the area of the medial parts of the elbow joint with increased valgus stress at the release. Injuries of the medial lateral ligament, the epicondyle humeri ulnaris, the medial elbow joint capsule as well as the ulnar nerve are the result (Pincivero et al. 1994).

■ **Spinal injuries:** due to repetitive hyperlordosings in javelin throwers with the risk of a subsequent spondylolysis/spondylolisthesis (Schmitt et al. 2001).

■ **Finger injuries:** Tendon injuries (strains, partial ruptures/ruptures, and osseous avulsions) or injuries of the finger joints (distortion, subluxation/dislocation) can develop caused by the extensive loads and strong tension forces in rotation and release.

References

Altchek DW, Dines DM (1995). Shoulder Injuries. In: The Throwing Athlete. J Am Acad Orthop Surg 3 (3): 159–165.

Fredberg U, Bolvig L (1999). Jumper's knee. Review of the literature. Scand J Med Sci Sports 9: 66–73.

Garett W (1990). Muscle strain injuries. Med Sci Sports Exerc 22: 436–438.

Geyer M, Sander-Beuermann A, Wegner U, Wirth CJ (1993). Stress reactions and stress fractures in the high performance athlete. Causes, diagnosis and therapy. Unfallchirurg 96 (2): 66–74.

Nigg BM (1991). Die leichtathletischen Sprungdisziplinen – Eine Übersicht. Lehre der Leichtathletik 30: 15–18.

Pincivero DM, Heinrichs K, Perrin DH (1994). Medial elbow stability. Clinical implications. Sports Med 18 (2): 141–148.

Schmitt H, Brocai DR, Carstens C (2001). Long-term review of the lumbar spine in javelin throwers. 83 (3): 324–327.

Schmitt H, Hansmann HJ, Brocai DRC, Loew M (2001). Long-term changes of the throwing arm of former elite javelin throwers. Int J Sports Med 22: 275–279.

Schmitt H, Thiele J, Broca DRC, Ewerbeck V (2004). Spätschäden am Bewegungsapparat bei ehemaligen Hochleistungsweit- und -dreispringern. Akt Traumatol 34: 87–91.

Tibesku CO, Pässler HH (2005). Jumper's knee – eine Übersicht. Sportverletzung-Sportschaden 19: 63–71.

Wolff R (2000). Apophysenausrisse Dt Z Sportmed 51 (9): 305–306.

40 Luge

Volker Jägemann

Since 1964, luge is an **Olympic** discipline and since then, German athletes have dominated this sport like no other: the German women (led by Olympic champions Silke Kraushaar, Sylke Otto and Tatjana Huefner) have been undefeated in more than 100 competitions since 1997; the Olympic champions Jens Müller, Felix Loch and the "luge legend" Georg Hackl have made sports history. However, with only 1,000 active athletes it is a fringe sport in Germany.

40.1 Sport-specific stress profile

This sport has three Olympic disciplines: women's single, men's single and the men's double. It is performed either on natural or artificial luge tracks; here we only consider artificial luge tracks.

On the 1,000–1,200 meter track for men and the 800–1,000 meter track for women, athletes reach speeds of up to 140 km/h and experience a pressure load of G4 in the final curves. This pressure load in particular affects the cervical spine, because the athlete's head overlaps beyond the shell of the luge to the back.

Furthermore, **extreme tension and compression loads are applied to the shoulders and the acromioclavicular joints** during the start by the sudden release of the starting handles. A good start time is key for the overall performance and depends on the explosive transition of the extremely kyphosed **lumbar spine** into hyperlordosis. These loads can only be borne by athletes who master the sport-specific technique and have general good core strength to stabilize the execution of the start.

40.2 Equipment

The luge sled for women and men weighs between 21 and 25 kg; the double-seated luge weigh between 25 and 30 kg. To compensate for weight related advantages and disadvantages, it is allowed to wear weight vests. Generally, luge athletes wear textile speed suits, gloves with spikes at the fingertips, ankle-high racing shoes in a slight toe pointed position and a standardized helmet with visor.

Any kind of stabilizing taping and aerodynamic positioning support is forbidden in competitive races. Guards for the protection of arms, legs and feet are allowed, but are only worn during training because of their higher air resistance.

40.3 Causes of accidents

40.3.1 In the luge track

There are frequent incidents of serious contusions caused by contact with the sidewalls of the track at high speeds; the accident consequences are worsened by edges, grooves and noses, i.e. unevenness of the track surface.

Crashing in the track which is almost always attributable to driving errors is much more problematic.

40.3.2 Outside the luge track

As part of the coordination training, indoor soccer plays an important role; accordingly, luge athletes often incur **soccer-typical injuries**. The same applies to injuries pertaining to training modules in volleyball, basketball, jogging and cycling.

40.4 Injury profiles in luge

The injuries listed in Tables 40.1, 40.2 and 40.3 were incurred by a group of 74 members of the German national luge team in the period from 1996 to 2005. Injuries and/or overload damages were only recorded, if a) they had been subject to medical diagnosis and treatment or if b) as a result, the athlete interrupted training or missed competitions.

40.4.1 In the luge track

- Very painful **contusions** at the external side of the upper and lower extremities, often coupled with extensive **hematoma** and partially also with **skin lesions** comparable to burns occur after impact with the walls of the ice canal. Additionally, **fractures of the metatarsal bone V** are observed again and again and must be considered sport-specific because of their frequency. A rapid **osteosynthesis** has proven to be the therapy of choice.

- In addition to serious **contusions** (head, cervical spine, upper and lower extremities), **fractures** of the extremities occur as a result of crashes in the luge track, although no sport-specific pattern emerges here. Spinal fractures affect especially the thoracic spine, but also the lumbar spine. As these fractures are partly unstable, **osteosynthetic** stabilization is required, especially in the region of the thoracic spine. Very rarely, **transverse spinal cord syndromes** occur, but the German luge athletes have been spared this injury. Wearing the mandatory internationally standardized helmet with its predetermined breaking points usually prevents the worst effects of rare craniocerebral traumas.

40.4.2 Outside the luge track

The most frequent injuries outside the ice canal (➢ Tab. 40.3) occur during indoor soccer practice and mostly affect the **upper ankle joint**. They should not be considered sport-specific.

Tab. 40.1 Most frequent injuries by impinging in the ice canal (1996 to 2005, in a collective of 74 squad athletes).

Injuries	Number
fractures of midfoot bone V	7
fractures of toes	3
contusions foot	12
contusions knee (three of them with traumatic prepatellar bursitis)	5
contusions of the upper arm/forearm/elbow	17
traumatic olecranial bursitis	3
contusion hand	6
contusion shoulder	3

Tab. 40.2 Most frequent injuries as a result of crashing in the luge track (1996 to 2005, in a cohort of 74 federal squad athletes).

Injuries	Number
cranial contusion/concussion	5
craniocerebral injury	2
contusion/distortion of the cervical spine	6
fracture of a thoracic vertebral body	5
contusions of thoracic spine	4
fracture of a vertebral body of lumbar vertebral	2
fractures of the clavicula	3
fractures forearm	3
fractures patella	2
ruptures of outside (lateral) aspect of the ankle ligaments	11
fractures metatarsal bone V	8
multiple contusions	20

Tab. 40.3 Most frequent injuries in training outside of the luge track (1996 to 2005, in a cohort of 74 federal squad athletes).

Injuries	Number
ruptures of outside (lateral) aspect of the ankle ligaments (6 surgeries)	16
surgically treated fracture of the lateral malleolus	2
rupture of the anterior cruciate ligament	4
fracture of navicular bone	2
ruptured meniscus	6
ulnar collateral ligament injury, "skier's thumb" (surgery)	2
patellar fracture	3
sprain of outside (lateral) ankle ligaments (without surgery)	10

40.5 Overload damages

Sport-specific overload damages are primarily caused by a) extreme **tension and pressure forces** at the start as well as b) by the **G-forces** in the final curves of the track.

40.5.1 Shoulder and acromioclavicular joint

During the starting procedure, extreme stress is applied to the shoulder and the AC joint because of the **powerful tension** and **pushing off** of the start handles followed by the "paddling".

This leads to

- impingement syndromes of the shoulder joint
- ruptures of the rotator cuffs and
- arthrosis of the acromioclavicular joint. The rapid **resection arthroplast**y of the AC joint is considered the therapy of choice.

40.5.2 Lumbar spine

A perfect start requires the extreme pretension of the lumbar spine in **hyperkyphosing** with subsequent rapid and powerful straightening and conversion into **hyperlordosis.** This explains three surgery-requiring cases of **prolapsed discs** in the lumbosacral region in the cohort of 74 athletes described above.

In addition, **degenerative damages to the intervertebral discs** that represent a clinical lower back pain syndrome with and without nerve root irritation.

40.5.3 Cervical spine

The third extensive problem area of overload damages is the cervical spine. Even consistent training of the neck/nape muscles and the wearing of a so-called neck strap (a permitted strap connecting the helmet to the body and thus preventing a hyperlordosing of the cervical spine due to the high centrifugal force in the final curves), does not prevent significant degenerative damages and **surgery requiring prolapsed discs**. Perhaps the athletes rely too much on the passive support function of the neck strap and therefore neglect the necessary **muscle training** of the neck region.

Chronic Cervical Syndrome, partially with an immense movement limitation of the cervical spine and radicular concomitant symptoms are the consequence; in fact, two Olympic champions had to undergo surgery of the vertebral discs at C5/6 in summer of 2005 in the preparation phase for the Winter Olympics in 2006:

- A female athlete had to undergo surgery because of a prolapsed disc C5/6 (with a sequestrum; ➢ Fig. 40.1 a and b): discectomy with retention of the external posterior segments of the longitudinal ligament with decompression of the spinal canal as well as the spinal nerve C6 left; afterwards, dynamic stabilization of the motion segment with implantation of an intervertebral-disc total-endoprothesis of the type PRODISC C (M/6 mm) via a microsurgical anterolateral access from the right. The athlete resumed full training six weeks after surgery (➢ Fig. 40.2).
- In a second athlete, radiography confirmed serious degeneration with far reaching destruction of the intervertebral discs C5/6/7

Fig. 40.1 Slipped disk in the cervical spine of a female Olympic champion and world champion of luge. a: MRT axial preoperative, b: MRT sagittal preoperative (image by Prof. Dr. Michael Mayer, Munich).

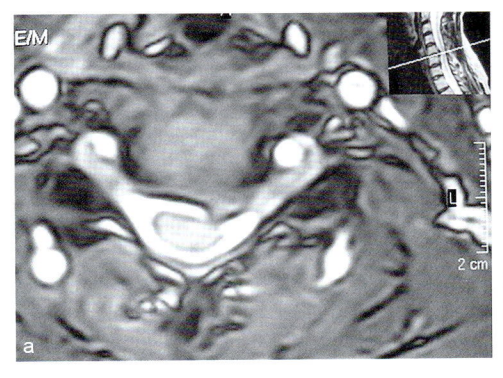

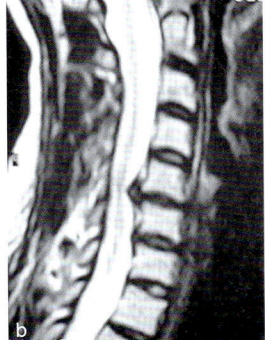

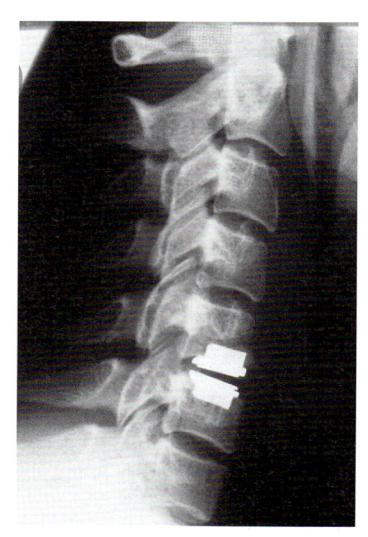

Fig. 40.2 Medical state after implantation of an intervertebral disc prothesis of the same athlete (image by Prof. Dr. Michael Mayer, Munich).

and a prolapsed C5/6 disc (see imgage 40.3 a to c). The sequestrum was microsurgically removed from the dorsal.

Considering that a) a female multiple world champion had to finish her luge career because of a prolapsed disc in the cervical spine and b) two other Olympic champions had to undergo surgery at the cervical spine, it raises the question whether such serious diseases could not be prevented or reduced by changing the rules and regulations. It would be possible, for example, to attach a security head rest which protrudes at the posterior part of the sled and only comes to use in case of an uncontrolled overextension of the cervical spine. Such a solution has been discussed but rejected by the Fédération Internationale de Luge de Course (FIL).

40.5.4 Other overload disorders

In Table 40.4 which lists the most frequently observed overload damages, the frequency of

Tab. 40.4 Most frequent overload damages.

Overload damages	Number
slipped discs of the cervical spine (two of them treated surgically)	6
chronic degenerative disease of the cervical spine	12
slipped disks of the lumbar spine (three of them treated surgically)	4
chronic degenerative disease of the lumbar spine	25
chronic degenerative disease of the thoracic spine	8
AC arthrosis (five of them treated surgically)	9
impingement syndrome of the shoulder joints	24
rupture of the rotator cuff (two surgeries)	4
epicondylitis radialis	13
apicitis patellae	6
patellar chondropathy/ retropatellar arthrosis	9
hallus rigidus	7
achilles tendinitis	3
chronic groin pain	3

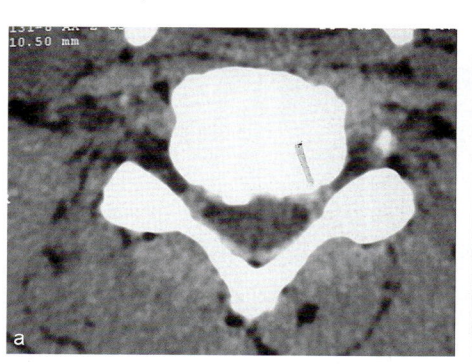

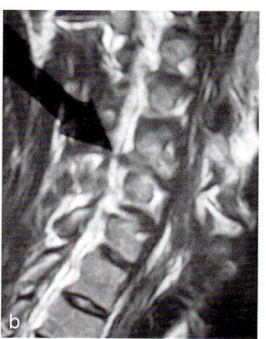

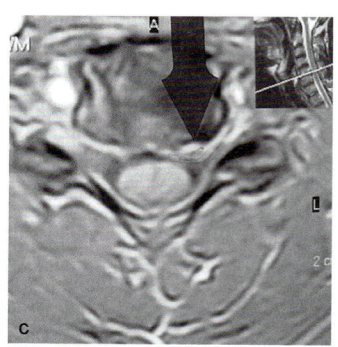

Fig. 40.3 Slipped disc C5/C6 of an Olympic champion. a: CT axial C5/C6 preoperative, b: MRT sagittal preoperative, c: MRI axial preoperative (image by Prof. Dr. Michael Mayer, Munich).

the **epicondylitis radialis**, the **apicitis patellae** and **cartilage damages in the retropatellar joint** is noteworthy; nevertheless, in all probability it cannot be deduced from the sport-specific movement and stress mechanisms that these overload damages are sport-specific. However, the cause for the relatively frequent hallux rigidus could be found in too soft (and therefore inappropriate) shoes worn for the sport-specific (and necessary for luge) indoor soccer training.

Summary

Luge sport remains a fringe sport that in Germany can be performed only on four artificial luge tracks. This sport must be left to well-trained and conditioned athletes because of the sport-specific injuries and overload damages.

References

Jägemann V (2001). Rennrodeln. In: Clasing D, Siegfried I (eds.). Sportärztliche Untersuchung und Beratung. 3rd edition. Spitta-Verlag, Balingen.

Jägemann V (2005). Rennrodeln. In: Engelhardt M, Krüger-Franke M, Pieper H-G, Siebert C (eds.). Sportverletzungen – Spotschäden. ... In: Grifka J (eds.). Praxiswissen Halte- und Bewegungsorgane, 1st edition. Thieme-Verlag, Stuttgart.

Jägemann V (2005). Medizinisches Krisenmanagement vor Ort am Beispiel des Rennrodelns. Sportorthop Sporttraumatol 21: 165–166.

41 Skeleton

Christian Schneider

A ride through the ice canal – lying on the stomach and headfirst – and then reaching speeds of up to 135 km/h is beyond imagination for many people. The rider lies on a heavy skeleton, only a short distance away from the ice (> Fig. 41.1) with his body's center of gravity is below him. This is an explanation for the **scarce appearance of injuries**, with the exception of some bruises and excoriations.

41.1 History

For ages, the sled has been used as means of transport and movement in the snowy countries. In the 18th century, sledging became a leisure activity; the first straight railways of lengths of up to 370 m had just been built in St. Petersburg and Berlin. **English men**, who spent their winter vacations in **St. Moritz**, recognized the athletic potential. In **1883**, the first "international" race was arranged on a post road from Davos to Klosters. In 1887, the first rider rode downhill in a lying, headlong posture – skeleton was born.

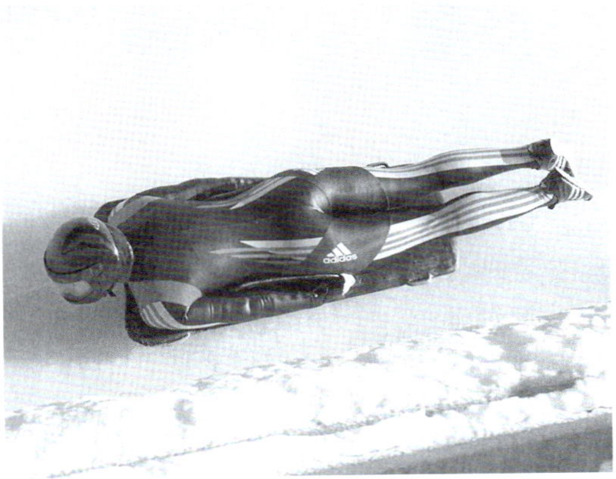

> **Bob sleighing** was invented in 1888 in St. Moritz; the bob consisted of two skeleton sleds, lying one behind the other.

In 1905, the first skeleton race on a natural track was arranged, the **first German championship** was carried out in 1912 in the Harz Mountains, and the **first European championship** took place in Davos in 1914. Skeleton on natural track has almost vanished completely since the time of the Second World War.

Since 1969, the wearing of a diver's suit and a new style with the arms stretched backwards and lying tightly attached to the body has been adapted.

"Bob-track" skeleton spread fast, supported by the newly built artificial ice rinks all over the world. European championships were carried out in Innsbruck in 1981, and the first world championships were carried out in 1982. After 1924 and 1948, skeleton has become a steady part of the **Olympic program** since the Winter Olympics in Salt Lake City in 2002.

41.2 Equipment

Nowadays, the skeleton consists of a massive steel skeleton, where the name of the sport is deduced from. Placed on this is a laterally raised, firm tub with handles and lateral bumpers on the front and back. The steel runners are attached by adjusting screws. Therefore it is possible to adjust the runner form and thus the contact to the ice.

Fig. 41.1 Skeleton in a curve.

According to the regulations, a **minimum weight** of 33 kg and a **maximum weight** of 37 kg for women and 43 kg for men are needed for skeleton. The allowed **combined weight** of sled, athlete and other equipment is regulated as well: 95 kg for women and 115 kg for men, respectively. This will be checked in the target area.

The **measurements** of the skeleton may amount to a length of 80–120 cm and a total height of 8–20 cm.

The athlete wears a tightly fitting textile one-piece suit, gloves, a standardized light-weight helmet with chin protection, sprint shoes with 7-mm spikes and cushions and padding, if necessary.

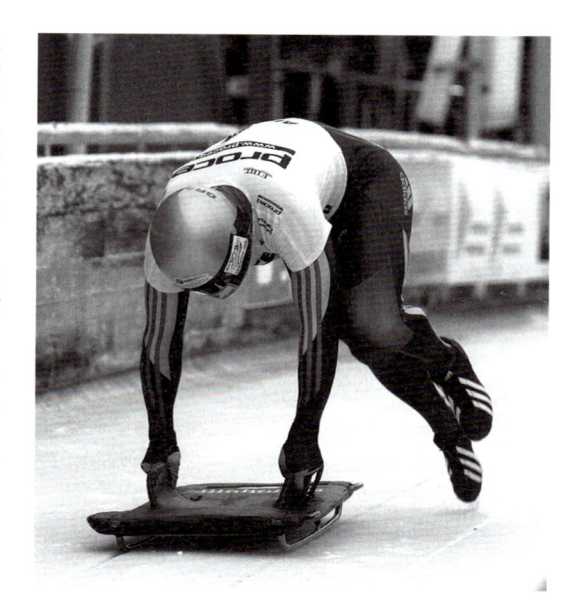

Fig. 41.2 Starting spurt.

41.3 Specialties of the skeleton

A good run through the ice canal depends on the **start**. The skeleton is pushed in the start lane by one or both hands for the sprint in stooped position on a length of approximately 40 m (➢ Fig. 41.2). Afterwards, the athlete jumps (➢ Fig. 41.3) to achieve the correct racing position, which is characterized by an aerodynamically convenient posture.

The **control** of the slide is performed by movements of shoulders and knees, by shifting of the weight and – accompanied by a great loss of speed – by use of the feet on the ice.

Sport-medical demands to the skeleton athlete:
- spurt velocity at the start
- maximum strength and muscle emphasis in the legs
- aerodynamic running position
- optimal muscle coordination
- optimal stabilization of the spine at pressure loads in curves of up to 5 G
- mental strength and even temper
- good immune situation and coldness tolerance

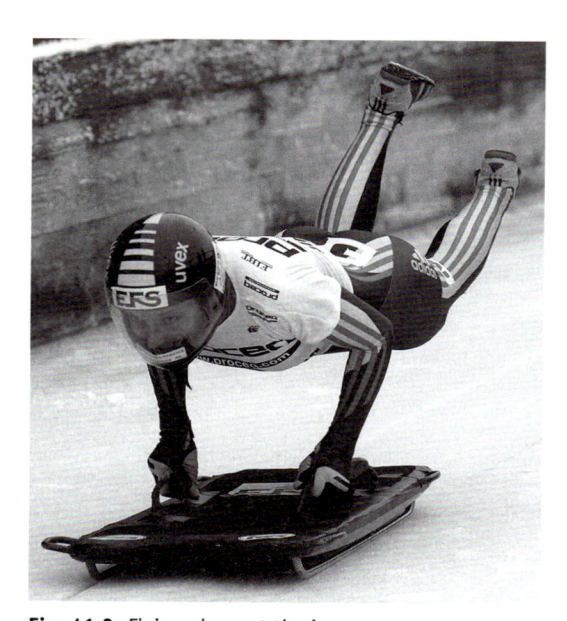

Fig. 41.3 Flying phase at the jump.

41.4 Injuries and overuse damage

In principle, this sport has a low risk of **injuries**. In case of a fall, the athlete tries to hold on to the sled and pull back onto it. If he loses the skeleton, it will just slide down the track and the athlete leaves the track getting off the ice. The ice canal is even and does not show any obstacles that could be hit during the run.

The **typical injuries** are contusions of any kind and minor abrasions – often recognizable by the broken clothing – at shoulders, elbows or thighs. Fractures of the elbows or the metacarpal region can also appear due to very hard collisions with the ice canal. Occasionally, nose bleeding and injuries at chin and nose will occur because of insufficient stabilization of the nape muscles supporting the head. In individual cases, serious injuries after falls to the back will have to be excluded, especially vertebral fractures and cerebral concussions.

Most injuries appear in general training – soccer has a prominent position here. Overuse of the tendon insertion and stressed cartilage segments in the knee joints have to be diagnosed consequently and treated to full recovery. Spinal conditions because of high stress to the spine require special attnetion. A specific determination of the athletic capability is indicated for the prevention of permanent damages.

Suggestions to the attending physician:

- knowledge of immunostimulation and adaption to coldness
- diagnosis and treatment of muscle injuries
- knowledge of logistics of the ambulance service on site.

Photographs

Pictures: BSD (Bob- und Schlittenverband für Deutschland)

Chapter 42 Carving

Hubert Hörterer

Media and industry convey the impression that carving is entirely new. However, Kober and Held consider carving a logical consequence that simply has loomed for years (Kober and Held 1997). The English verb "to carve" defines a form of cutting. For a long time, a "carve turn" has been aspired in ski instruction and in ski racing. In ski racing, skis with a side-cut radius have been used for a long time. Thus, a previously known technique is now pursued using advanced material (Hörterer 1998).

42.1 Material and technique

Carving ski

You will hardly find normal skis on the market and in ski rental. Carving skis are characterized by their **short length** and their larger **side-cut radius**, meaning wider tips and ends of the skis. The result is a different, between 11 and 30 m turn radius.

The initial high number of different carving skis has been reduced to a few basic types. These are: race carver, general carver and freeride carver (➢ Fig. 42.1 a to c).

The following **principles** apply to all carving skis:

- The side-cut radius determines the turn radius in meters.
- Skiing along the edge provides higher speeds in the curves.
- Small radii and high speeds produce large centrifugal forces, which need compensation by the thigh muscles.

Directional stability and running smoothness are decreased due to the shorter skis; thus a closer attention at schuss and steep passages is necessary.

Binding and plate systems

Plate systems significantly influence the control of the skis and the loads on the locomotor apparatus because they lift **the skier**. Studies

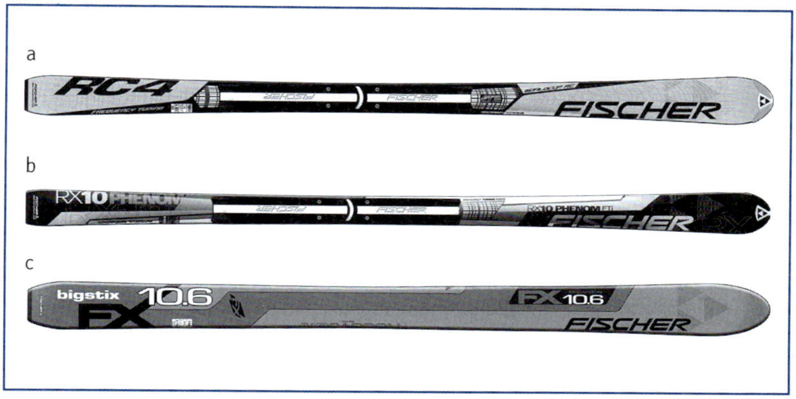

Fig. 42.1 Different carver models with according radiuses. a: race carver, b: general carver, c: freeride carver (photographs: Fischer, Ried).

show that the **stress to the knee** enhances due to the increased height, which is reflected in the changed injury pattern (Niessen and Müller 1999). With increased standing heights, swerves which can break-out the ski are not as easy to avoid. The binding systems have remained unchanged. Regarding the **ski shoe**, no essential requisitions exist with the exception of appropriate side stiffness.

Skiing style

> Carving skis do not principally require a new skiing technique.

Most models have a broadband field of use, allowing short and long, carved and drifted turns. The former confusion to interpret carving only as "cutting" has been overcome by now. The definition of "skiing on the edge" includes all facets from drifting to cutting and allows many skiing and fun variants (Kober and Held 1997). Because the carving ski is a protective ski, it cannot be disconnected by the usual techniques and allows the drifting sideways, so that it will be useable in nearly every technique.

The following **technical characteristics** facilitate the carving:

- open leg posture (➤ Fig. 42.2)
- hardly any vertical movement
- fast change of curves
- elevated stand.

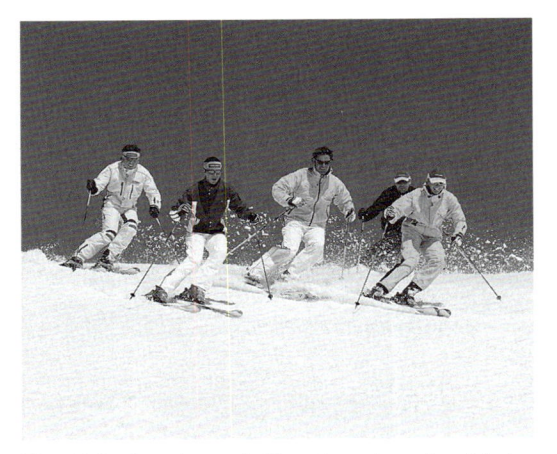

Fig. 42.2 Open leg and ski posture at carving (photograph: Fischer, Ried).

42.2 Sport-specific profile

There will be higher demands to strength, coordination, velocity, flexibility and endurance. Clearly, the **increased strength demand** assumes the first place. Internal turn radii can be controlled purely on the edge because of the stronger side-cut. This way, higher centrifugal forces – at the same speed – are effective and the muscular effort of fixing the skis on the edge will increase. The increased strength demand does not only affect the leg muscles, but also the complete trunk musculature.

The **coordination** is almost as important as the strength. An increased measure of neuromuscular quality is necessary in the carving technique. Since a forward and backward pass that is too intensive will cause crucial mistakes in skiing, a neutral position of the body's center of gravity above the middle of the skis should be kept. Minor adjustments of the center of gravity towards the back or the front can lead to serious mistakes in the run.

Regarding velocity, increased demands to the **speed of reactivity** are the focal point. This will be caused by the faster radial speeds and by the different way of steering the carving skis. **Flexibility** and **endurance** are considered basic preconditions in carving skiing.

42.3 Accident mechanisms and injuries

42.3.1 Accident mechanisms

The analysis of skiing accidents of the 2006/2007 season by the evaluation office for skiing accidents of the ARAG sports insurance (ASU Ski) does not show any significant increase of the injury risk, the same as in previous years. Since the 1993/1994 season, the yearly fluctuations regarding the injury risk have only been minor (➤ Fig. 42.3).

> By now, about 90% of all skiers use carving skis. The introduction of carving skis has not led to an increase of accidents in alpine skiing.

Also considering the total number of skiing accidents, there has been no change compared

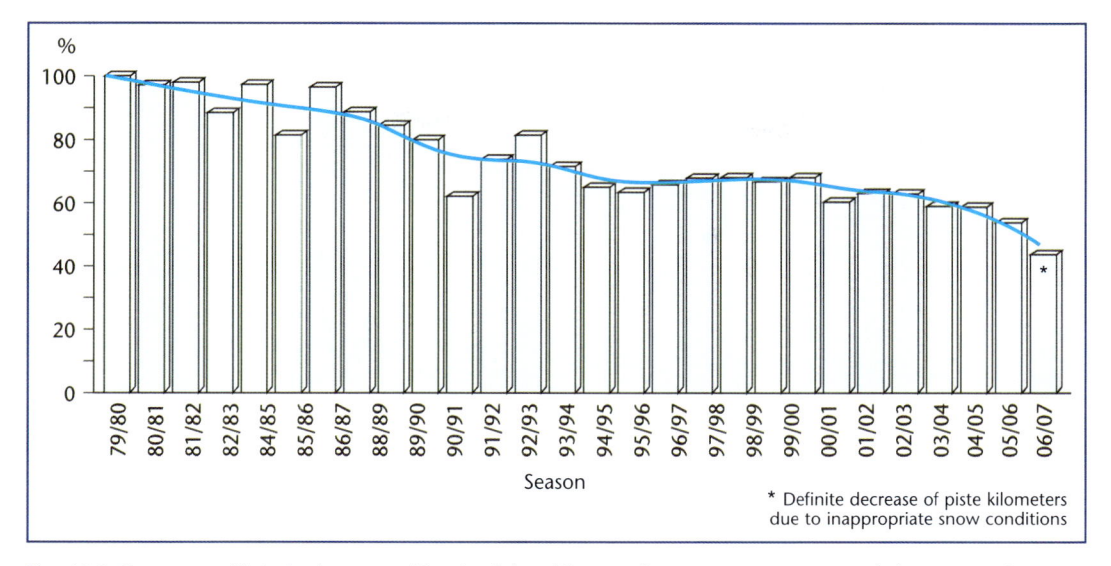

Fig. 42.3 Frequency of injuries by 1,000 skiers in alpine ski-sports from 1979 to 2007, regarded year 1980 (= 100%; Gläser 2007).

* Definite decrease of piste kilometers due to inappropriate snow conditions

to the previous year. The most frequent cause of injury is still the **fall without outside involvement while doing the run**. The average of such accidents in the sample period amounts to 71% of men and even 78% of women. Avoidimg a fall is therefore an important precondition for an absolved skiing season without injuries (Jendrusch et al. 2004).

In alpine ski racing, injuries often occur in **landing after jumps in the downhill race**. Injuries happen almost exclusively at the landing process and not at the subsequent fall. The second most common injuries are caused by **overstress in the momentum**. The stress to the skis and the extensor muscles of the leg is very high due to high skiing speeds and small turn radii. Knee injuries develop because of additional hyperflexion and internal rotation of the knee joint (➢ Fig. 42.4). In addition, the typical turn-off falls will occur because of the high centrifugal force in combination with injuries at upper body and head. The third place in alpine ski racing is taken by injuries due to **break-outs of the skis** – lateral deviation of the ski from the required skiing line per time unit. The likelihood of break-out depends on the standing height, among other things, because a small upstand angle is already sufficient at a major standing height to induce the break-out.

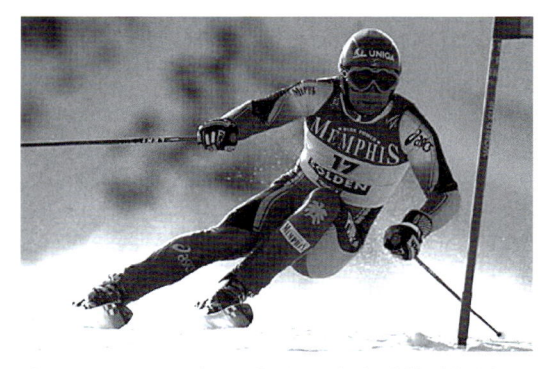

Fig. 42.4 Strong hyperflexion of the hill-sided knee joint in racing (photograph: Atomic).

The intensity depends on the side-cut radius of the ski then (Niessen and Müller 1999).

The **flexion valgus external rotation trauma** is still the most frequent injury mechanism in general skiing. A hyperextension of the knee joint will also lead to according knee injuries. The relatively aggressive artificial snow must neither be underestimated. Enhanced risk disposition, insufficient skiing technique and lack of fitness are also causes for skiing accidents. Several different factors will mostly come together, though.

42.3.2 Injuries and improper loads

Regarding the localization of injuries, definite changes have been found in recent years. In the season of 2006/2007, the knee injuries amounted to 33.1%. For women, those were about half of the injuries, for men and children about a fourth. There has been a percental advance of injuries in the region of shoulder/humerus (23.9%) and trunk (17.4%). The injuries of the head (10.2 %), the lower leg/ankle joint (9.4%) and the forearm/hand (6.0%; ➤ Fig. 42.5; Gläser 2007) have slightly reduced

It is indicated that the topography of injuries in alpine skiing depends on the relative length of the used skis. **The shorter the ski, the further up at the body the according injury will be localized.**

For the normal skier, the carving ski does not present special demands to the movement regulation. The momentum release and control are even facilitated because of the side-cut shape of the ski and will thus reduce the stress to the locomotor apparatus. In a survey of Dingekus and Mang (2001), 61% of all overloads affected the knee joint, followed by the spine (11%), the hip and the foot (6% each). **Irritations of muscles and tendons** (39%) and **cartilage problems** (33%) are in the foreground.

> The knee joint is affected by injuries and overloads most often.

42.4 Treatment measurements

The therapies for consequences of improper loads and overloads do not differ from the ones of other sports. In addition to the different surgical procedures, physiotherapeutic measures are in the foreground. The specific muscular training is of special importance. But also the treatment with insoles in the ski shoes as well as the adjustments of the ski shoes belong to the conservative program. Because the skier does the skiing only at a third of the time and stands at ski-lifts and mountain-railways for two thirds or walks in the ski shoes, the ski shoe must have a conversion mechanism that will correct a permanent flexed position in the knee joint. The consequence will be an essential relief of the retropatellar region.

The treatment of skiing injuries follows the general orthopedic and surgical principles. The surgical treatment of capsule-ligament lesions of the knee joint and their rehabilitation are of special importance.

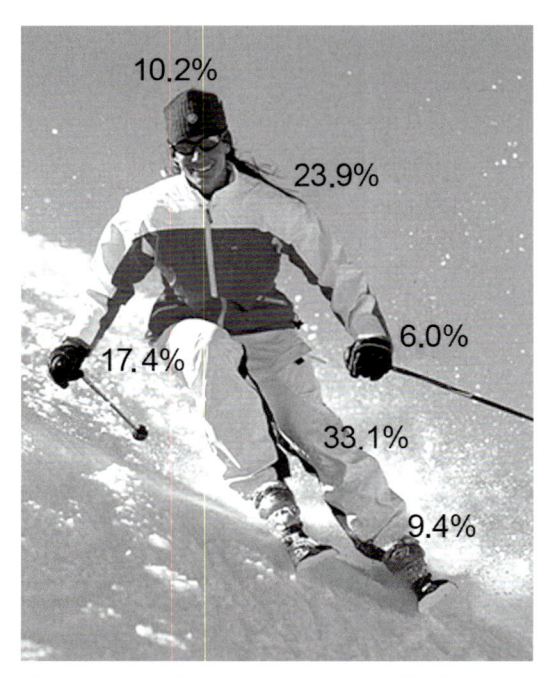

Fig. 42.5 Injury localizations in alpine skiing in percent (Gläser 2007; photograph: Fischer, Ried).

42.5 Preventive measurements

The stress connected to carving skiing can only be compensated by an **athletic whole-year preparation** and **specified skiing gymnastics** in the months before the start of the skiing season. An according **technical training** will additionally help to prevent accidents. Changed skiing tracks with higher speeds and larger radii require better training and more attention.

The correct **choice of appropriate skis** is even more difficult than before, because more factors will depend on the personal style and capabilities. Offered test options should be used. Additional plates and an increase of the standing height will only be necessary for extreme carvers and in ski racing. Standing heights of more than 55 mm have to be declined. A definite reduction below this value must be demanded for the area of children and youth sport (Hörterer and Dingerkus 2001). The binding will have to be adjusted by a specialized dealer before each season.

The **speed** will definitely have to be adjusted to the capability. The skiing day should be finished as early as possible and the ski pass should not be used up, because most accidents happen in the afternoon hours.

> The best injury prophylaxis is to ski with reason and consideration.

References

Dingerkus M, Mang A (2001). Verletzungen und Überlastungen beim Carving. Sportorthop Sporttraumatol 17 (4): 213–218.

Gläser H (2008). Skiunfälle der Saison 2006/2007. Auswertungsstelle für Skiunfälle der ARAG-Sportversicherung (ASU Ski), Düsseldorf.

Hörterer H (1998). Neuer Sport – neue Verletzungen. . Dt Z Sportmed 49 (1): 20–22.

Hörterer H, Dingerkus M (2001). Carving Skiing – Injuries and Prevention. Presentation, Outlines and Abstracts. Isakos Congress: 2.121–2.122.

Jendrusch G, Henke T, Gläser H (2004). Entwicklungen im Ski-Unfallgeschehen im Zeitraum 1997 bis 2002. Auswertungsstelle für Skiunfälle der ARAG-Sportversicherung (ASU Ski), Düsseldorf.

Kober E, Held HJ (1997). Carving erweitert das Skifahren. Sportverletz Sportaschaden 11: 122–123.

Niessen W, Müller E (1999). Carving – biomechanische Aspekte zur Verwendung stark taillierter Skier und erhöhter Standflächen im alpinen Skisport. Leistungssport 29 (1): 17–23.

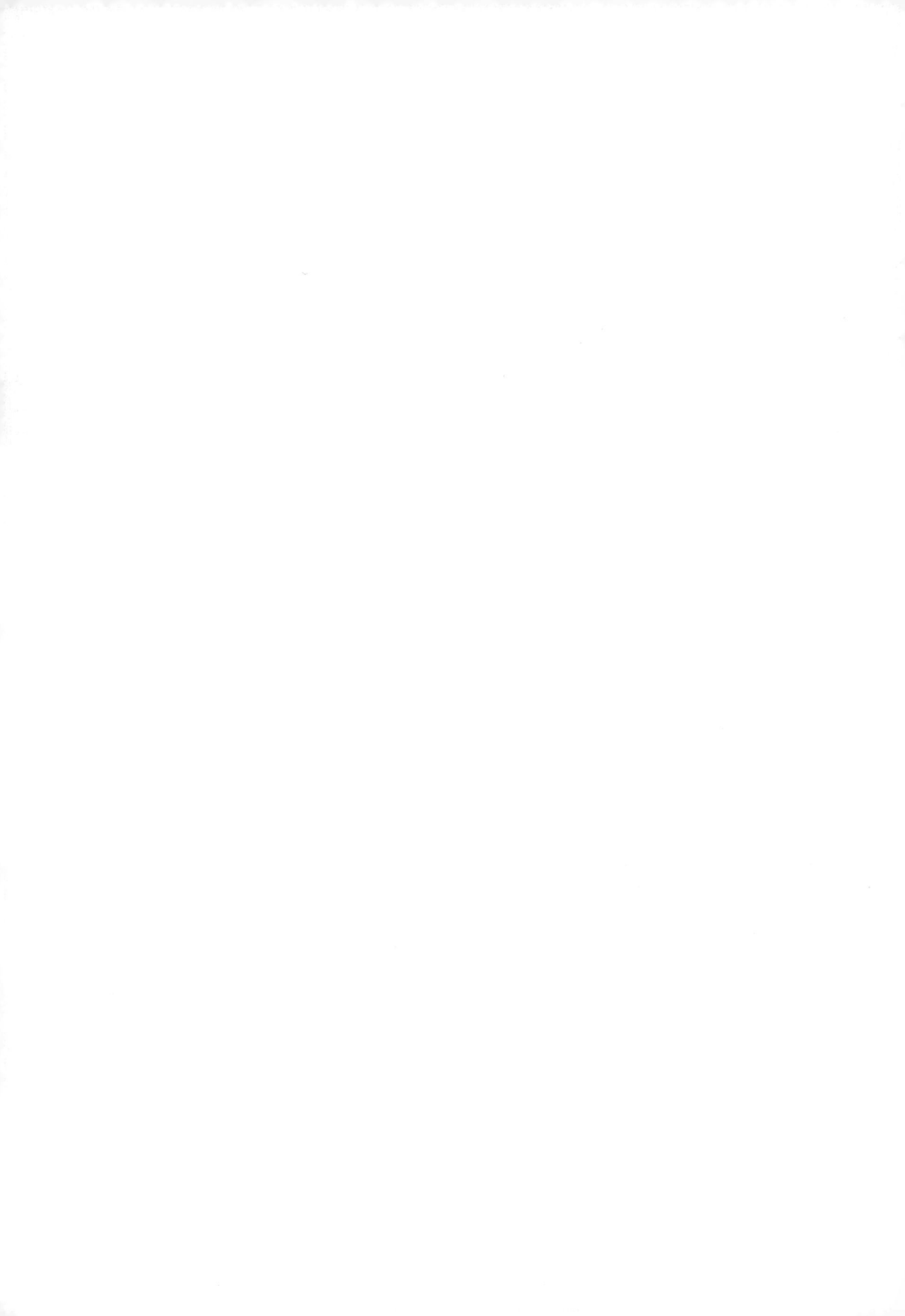

43 Ski jumping

Ludwig Geiger

Since about 1800, ski jumping has emerged and has its origin in **Norway**. First it had been practiced in a "hoppelom", a combination of slalom, downhill and jump. **Natural obstacles** worked as ski jumps, and the width measured about 10 m.

In 1883, ski jumping has become an individual discipline out of the former combined judging of run and jump, which is still practiced with increasing popularity as **Nordic combination**. In 1892, ski jumping started to become popular in Central Europe, as well, at the time of the so-called **Holmenkollen era**.

43.1 Sport-specific demand profile

In general, ski-jumping competitions are carried out in **two sports**:

- **Ski jumpings:** Jumps are classified into **normal hill competitions** (K–90 m), **large hill competitions** (K–120 m) and **sky-flying competitions** (K–185 m), with the current world record in ski-flying (2005) being 239 m. The **K data** consider the so-called critical point; the slope of the hill to jump on will begin to decrease again from the normal 35–37° at this point, from which the hill will be safe again.
- **Nordic combination:** This is a combined competition of ski jumping and cross-country skiing, with K-90 and K-120 jump hills being used for World Cup jumps here. The second discipline is **cross-country skiing** in the free technique with distances of 7.5 km (sprint) and 15 km. Sections of 2.5 km are used for relay competition. The result will be calculated by a combination of cross-country and jumping, with variable regulations being used. In the competition season in winter 2008/2009, a sole new format has been introduced with only one jump and 10 km of freestyle cross-country skiing subsequently.

The overall score in ski jumping involves **style and distance scores**.

43.2 Accident mechanisms

Without a doubt, ski jumping is a **risk sport** that is highly demanding to the body, on the one hand, and to the mind, on the other hand. **Injuries** and **overload defects** as well as **mental overload syndromes** that again can trigger injuries must be considered.

43.2.1 Outside risks

Ski jumping and ski flying are so-called **natural sports**, which always are subject to external influences despite strict regulations.

Especially wind gusts cannot only be decisive for triumph or failure, but can also lead to an unstable flying curve causing an early fall. **Individual mistakes** of the athlete will also contribute to the fall, e.g. an early take-off, adduction of the legs in the air and mistakes in landing. The risk of injuries, especially of the knee joint, at falls with the jump skis of a length of up to 2.85 m could be reduced by the introduction of a **safety binding**. The introduction of the **V-technique** with larger uplift surfaces has also reduced the injury risk. Ski jumping has become definitely safer compared to the parallel ski guidance.

43.2.2 Inner risks

Control regulation

The permanently high stress – especially at an **accumulation of competitions**, e.g. Four Hills Tournament, close World Cup dates and major events – can lead to a non-physiological **increased hormonal rest-stress potential** in individual athletes without sufficient regenerative plateau phases in-between. Even minor stimuli, which are responded to adequately at a normal rest-stress potential, will lead to **psycho-regulative overload** and to **acute** fear reactions in the sense of the fear of failure; they can lead to **chronic** depressive reactions similar to a burn-out syndrome. Additionally, the long-term closeness to underweight by a **catabolic** reaction in the reparative system can enhance the problem and also lead to an **immunosuppression** with a tendency to diseases and overload defects because of the close interconnection of psyche and immune system.

Problem of body weight

Already at the age of childhood, rather slim, small-boned and especially light-weight athletes emerge. This is caused by the **larger flying distance** of light-weight athletes. In terms of figures, the biomechanical aspect of a **weight reduction of 1 kg leading to a distance increase of 1–3 m** at the same aerodynamic preconditions have been added to the philosophy of training. In addition to the common procedures for the promotion of **jumping power and jumping technique**, a drastically reduced **uptake of nutrients** has become a measure. Within the years 1996 to 2003, individual successful athletes have moved on the truly fine line between pathological underweight and success in sport. The dispensable term of **anorexia athletica**, known from women's gymnastics, track-and-field athletics and other sports based on weight, has found a quick alibi-access into ski jumping.

From the medical point of view this neologism is not acceptable but **dangerous**, because it opens the door for the true **anorexia nervosa**, which has already happened in individual cases. The FIS (International Skiing Federation) has begun to implement **counter-regulatory measures** not least by the intervention of the author. These measures ascribe a higher priority again to the athletic values, such as bounce and health, by material adjustments (skis, suit) limitation of the body mass index and education. The present development can be seen as positive.

43.3 Injuries of the locomotor apparatus

In the years of 1998 to 2003, the injuries listed in ➤ Table 43.1 had been found in ski jumpers and Nordic-combination athletes of the German Skiing Federation (A, B, C and D/C squad athletes; n = 136). It should be noted that the **capsule-ligament lesions** of the ankle joint (n = 7) in 5 cases happened in **soccer in the training process** and were caused only twice by a **fall in jumping**.

43.4 Vitally endangering injuries

Independent from the injuries of the locomotor apparatus, the author has observed three **most serious injuries** during the years between 1990 and 2003:

Tab. 43.1 Injuries of the locomotor apparatus of ski-jumpers and combiners (n = 136) during the years from 1998 to 2003.

Injuries	Number	Percentage
Upper extremity		
shoulder joint luxation	2	1.47
fracture of the elbow joint	1	0.74
finger fracture	1	0.74
Lower extremity		
anterior cruciate ligament rupture	2	1.47
patellar fracture	1	0.74
fracture of the ankle joint	1	0.74
capsule-ligament lesions at the ankle joint	7	5.15

- a serious **craniocerebral trauma** with subdural hematoma and coma of 4 weeks with the permanent condition of a persisting motor disorder of speech (fall caused by a wind gust on a K-120 jump hill)
- a two-times **spleen rupture** by the collision of the upper abdomen with the ski binding, and a consecutive partial splenectomy
- a complete **rupture of spleen and left kidney** after a fall on the summer ski jump with massive abdominal compression and consecutive splenectomy and nephrectomy on the left side.

43.5 Overload defects

In the observed period between 1998 and 2003, the overload defects listed in ➢ Table 43.2 have been found, which can be basically traced back to the **sport-specific training** and only to a minor amount to the ski jump itself. The **knee joints** are a preference here.

The second most frequent region of overload defects is the **lumbar spine**; primarily, hypermobilities of the last two lumbar-vertebral segments are found. **Muscular dysbalances** of the muscles leading the spine, which have an effect on health and the sport (starting squat), have **not** been considered as separate clinical pictures.

Tab. 43.2 Number of overload defects at the locomotor apparatus of ski-jumpers and combiners (n = 136) during the years from 1998 to 2003.

Overload defects	Number
Knee joint	
spatellar apex syndrome	15
insertion tendinoses of the tuberositas tibiae	4
Osgood-Schlatter disease	3
internal meniscopathy	4
distal iliotibial band syndrome	3
Lumbar spine	
hyper-mobility	9

43.6 Treatment procedures

The **direct injuries** have been treated according to the current state of orthopedic-traumatological surgery. Those three vitally threatening injuries, which all had occurred abroad (Finland, France, Austria), had been treated optimally there. An optimal treatment system exists thanks to the international contacts and because of the FIS (International Skiing Federation).

The **overload defects** could be treated successfully, as far as possible, by the accompanying physiotherapists of the A and B squats using medical procedures such as injection therapy. The C and C/D squats that had not been accompanied by a physiotherapist had been treated timely at the Olympic bases in Freiburg, Oberhof and Munich or Kolbermoor, respectively. In this respect, **no permanent defects** have **been observed**.

43.7 Preventive procedures

During competition, but not in training, a **wind-measuring system** has been implemented and an accordingly experienced controller has been installed in the area of jump hills for reasons of equal opportunities and to protect the athletes of falls. This instrument informs the jury of FIS representatives and coaches of the current situation at the jump hill, which can even lead to the postponement of the competition or to the discontinuation of the competition.

Regarding the avoidance of overload defects, especially individual **biomechanical improvements** have an effect:

- optimization of training and jump shoes, e.g. by adjustment systems and insoles
- avoidance of muscle imbalances by stretching and strengthening techniques
- regular physiotherapy.

Furthermore, the implementation of **regenerative plateau phases** into the training process will prevent catabolic reactions with immunosuppression and mental overloads. Additionally, we use antioxidant vitamins (vitamin C and E, provitamin A) as well as yeast-bound zinc and selenium for the **support of the repair system**.

References

Geiger L, Schulz A, Teschenmacher H (1998). Beta-Endorphin und Stresshormone beim Skifliegen. Internationaler Sportärztekongress, Garmisch-Patenkirchen.

Schulz A, Geiger L, Teschenmacher H (1999). Propriomelanocortin fragments in the plasma of athletes undergoing aerobic or anaerobic exercise, presentation. 10th European Congress on Sports Medicine, Innsbruck.

Geiger L (1997). Überlastungsschäden im Sport. BLV-Sportwissen.

Useful internet links

www.ski-online.de

www.fis-ski.com

l.geiger@sport-und-gesundheit.de

44 Sport- and Rock Climbing

Volker Schöffl

Climbing and mountaineering changed radically in the early 1970s. Until then, only reaching the top (e.g. the peak of an 8,000er) had been the challenge, and not how to get there. Then the idea of "free climbing" was born. With the skyrocketing of the climbing difficulty levels and the immense participation in this young sport, the need of the climbers to compete under objective criteria has grown. Thus, **competition climbing** was born in the mid-1980s.

Without broad international organization in the beginning, **World and European Championships** have now been carried out **regularly since 1991**, and so have world cups and national competitions. For 15 years, these have been carried out at **artificial climbing walls**, also for reasons of environmental protection. About 200 artificial indoor climbing facilities have arisen within the last 20 years in Germany alone. Sport climbing has developed from an individual sport for extremists to a recreational sport for all age groups, counting more than a million active athletes in the US.

44.1 Terminology

In the terminology of sport and free climbing, a number of terms need correct definition. **Free climbing** means that the rope and the protective devices only serve the securing of the climber and are not to be used as means of movement or rest point. Such a route being climbed in lead climbing as one segment will be called "redpoint".

The solo attempt with roped self belay is called **"soloing"**; the unbelayed solo attempt is called **"free soloing"**. Nevertheless, real free soloing is extremely rare – contrary to the presentation in media. The assessment of the difficulty of a route is shown by different scales of difficulties; most common are the UIAA (Union Internationale des Associations d'Alpinisme, degree 1–11) and the French scale. The ropeless climbing on low height blocs of rocks altitude is called **"bouldering"**.

Although free climbing may still be considered a risk sport in general public, it has proved as a **low-risk** sport with an accident probability of 0.016% per training unit, especially in indoor facilities (Schöffl et al. 2010). Serious accidents have become rare thanks to modern securing techniques and equipment (bolts etc.).

44.2 Equipment

At the beginning of climbing, classic heavy mountaineering boots were worn for climbing in alpine regions as well as in rock faces. Only in the early 1980s, the first real **climbing shoe** with a **friction sole** entered the market. A characteristic that all climbing shoes have in common is the fact that they will have to be worn as tightly as possible (➢ Chapter 88), in order to achieve an optimal contact to the rock, which will often lead to **health problems** (Schöffl and Winkelmann 1999).

The introduction of **bolts** was an important cutting edge for the explosive performance enhancement in climbing. Therefore, falls into the rope are common for sport climbers now. The **climbing harnesses** have also changed essentially. While a combination of chest and sit

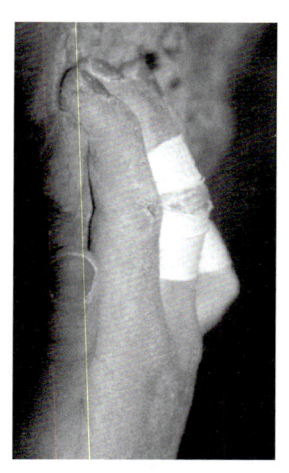

Fig. 44.1 Hanging grip position.

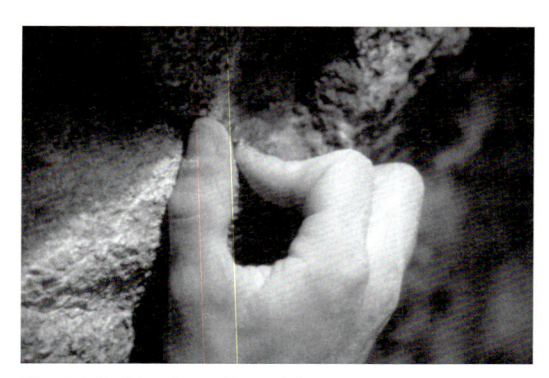

Fig. 44.2 Crimping grip position.

Tab. 44.1 The ten most frequent localizations of climbing-specific diagnoses 1/98–12/01 (n = 604; Schöffl et al. 2003).

Localization	Spreading
fingers	247 (41.0%)
forearm/elbow	81 (13.4%)
foot	55 (9.1%)
hand	47 (7.8%)
spine/torso	43 (7.1%)
skin	42 (6.9%)
shoulder	30 (5.0%)
knee	22 (3.6%)
others	37 (6.1%)
polytraumatic	5 (0.8%)

Tab. 44.2 The ten most frequent injuries and overload signs in the fingers, taken from the complete clientele (n = 604; Schöffl et al. 2003).).

Finger injuries	Spreading
pulley rupture	74
pulley strain	48
tenosynovitis/tendonitis	42
capsular injury	37
osteoarthritis (acute)	13
ganglion	11
tendon strain	7
fracture	7
osteoarthritis (chron.)	5
Dupuytren's contracture	5

harness has been used in traditional mountaineering, a pure **sit harness** is deployed in sport climbing. This will allow an injury-free falling with maximum free movement.

The hanging and the crimping grip position are the most important **hand positions** in holding a climbing hand hold (➢ Fig. 44.1 and ➢ Fig. 44.2).

44.3 Most frequent injuries and over use syndromes

Finger and hand lesions are the most common injuries or overuse syndromes in sport climbers.

In 604 injured sport climbers (1/98–12/01), three of the four most frequent diagnoses applied to the fingers:

- finger pulley injuries 20%
- tenosynovitis 7%
- joint capsular injuries 6.1% (➢ Tab. 44.1, ➢ Tab. 44.2).

> Finger and hand lesions are the most common injuries of sport climbers.

While diagnosis and therapy of most of these injuries do not present a problem for the sport physician, **finger pulley injuries** are a specific entity that is very rare in other sports. The diagnostic process is displayed in ➢ Fig. 44.3; the therapeutic procedure is shown by ➢ Table 44.3.

Fig. 44.3 Diagnostic procedure with injuries of the annular ligaments (pulley) (algorithms by Schöffl et al. 2003).

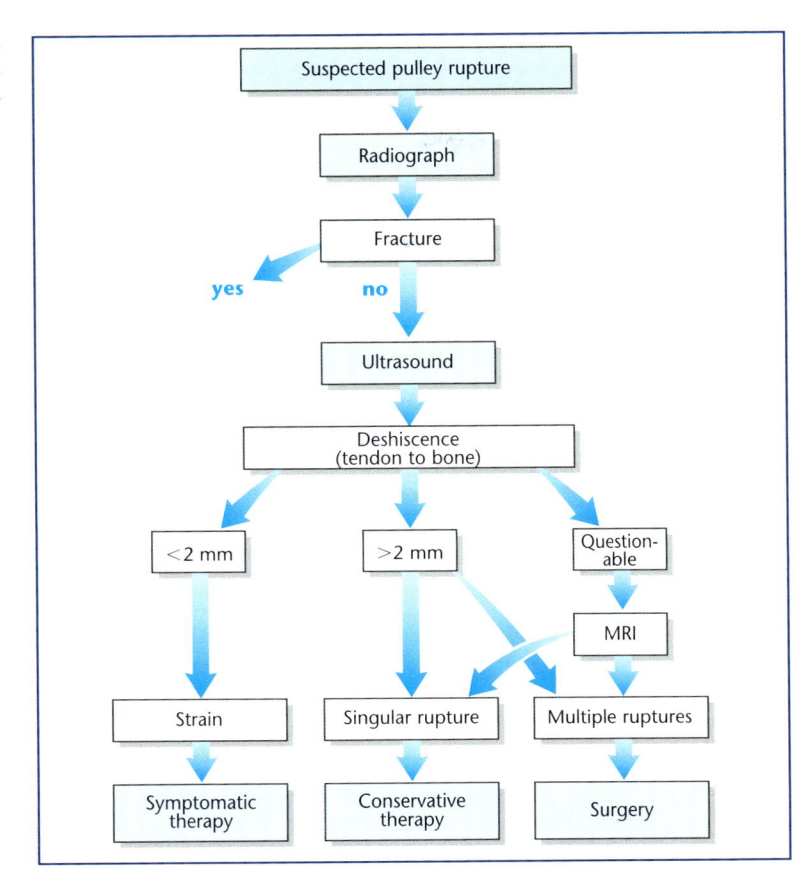

```
Suspected pulley rupture
          ↓
       Radiograph
          ↓
       Fracture
      yes / no
          ↓
       Ultrasound
          ↓
       Deshiscence
      (tendon to bone)
      ↓       ↓        ↓
   <2 mm   >2 mm   Questionable
                          ↓
                         MRI
      ↓       ↓        ↓
    Strain  Singular  Multiple
            rupture   ruptures
      ↓       ↓        ↓
  Symptomatic Conservative Surgery
   therapy    therapy
```

Tab. 44.3 Therapy guidelines with injuries of the annular ligaments (Schöffl et al. 2003).

	Grade I	Grade II	Grade III	Grade IV
Injury	Pulley strain	Complete rupture of A4 or partly rupture of A2 or A3	Complete Rupture A2 or A3	Multiple ruptures, as A2/A3, A2/A3/A4 or single rupture (A2 or A3) combined with Mm. lumbricalis or ligamental trauma
Therapy	Conservative	Conservative	Conservative	Surgical Repair
Immobilisation	None	10 days	10–14 days	Postoperative 14 days
Functional therapy	2–4 weeks	2–4 weeks	4 weeks	4 weeks
Pulley protection	Tape	Tape	Thermo-plastic or soft cast ring	Thermoplastic or soft cast ring
Easy sportspecific activities	after 4 weeks	after 4 weeks	after 6–8 weeks	4 months
Full sportspecific activities	6 weeks	6–8 weeks	3 months	6 months
Taping through climbing	3 months	3 months	6 months	>12 months

Tab. 44.4 Radiographic adoptions of the fingers (modified according to Schöffl et al. 2004).

Parameter	Youth squad 1999–2004	Recreational climbers (adolescents)	Control group (adolescents)	Adults (2–5 YC)	Adults (<10 YC)	Adults (<15 YC)
number	31	18	12	37	74	29
Stress adaption:	19 (61%)	5 (28%)	0	16 (43%)	43 (58%)	20 (69%)
■ cortical thickening	11 (36%)	2 (11%)	0	15 (40%)	41 (51%)	16 (55%)
■ subchondral sclerosing/ epiphysis concentration	11 (36%)	1 (6%)	0	5 (14%)	11 (15%)	4 (14%)
■ insertion calcification (SF/PF tendon)	3 (9.7%)	0	0	4 (11%)	11 (15%)	7 (24%)
■ expansion of the joint base PIP	13 (42%)	5 (28%)	0	11 (30%)	39 (53%)	16 (55%)
■ expansion of the joint base DIP	4 (13%)	0	0	12 (32%)	41 (55%)	18 (62%)
Arthrotic changes:	1 (3.2%)	1 (6%)	0	4 (11%)	15 (20%)	8 (28%)
■ bone spurs PIP	0	0	0	4 (11%)	15 (20%)	8 (28%)
■ bone spurs DIP	0	0	0	4 (11%)	15 (20%)	7 (24%)
■ narrowing of the joint space	0	0	0	0	1	6 (21%)
■ cysts/ decalcifications close to the joint	0	0	0	1	1	4 (14%)
■ epiphyseal injuries	1 (3.2%)	1 (6%)	0	0	0	0

(YC = years of climbing)

> Pulley injuries are the typical injuries, tenosynovitis/ tendonitis is the most frequent overuse syndrome in rock climbers.

Signs of adoptions to highly intensive sport climbing for years in the region of hands and finger, visible in radiographs (➤ Tab. 44.4), have been described and must be distinguished from clear pathologic changes (finger joint osteoarthritis, epiphyseal fractures).

> Radiographic stress reactions need to be distinguished from arthritic deformities.

References

Schöffl V, Morrison A, Schwarz U, Schöffl I, Küpper T (2010). Evaluation of injury and fatality risk in rock and ice climbing. Sports Med 40 (8), 657–679.

Schöffl V, Winkelmann H-P (1999). Fußdeformitäten bei Sportkletterern. Dt Z Sportmed 50: 73–76.

Schöffl V, Hochholzer Th, Winkelmann H-P, Strecker W (2003). Differenzialdiagnose von Fingerschmerzen bei Sportkletterern. Dt Z Sportmed 54: 3–43.

Schöffl V, Hochholzer Th, Winkelmann H-P, Strecker W (2003). Pulley injuries in rock climbers. Wilderness Environ Med 14: 94–100.

Schöffl V, Hochholzer Th, Imhoff A (2004). Radiographic changes in the hands and fingers of young, high-level climbers. Am J Sports Med 32 (7): 1688–1694.

Chapter 45 Aikido

Christoph Raschka

Aikido (Japanese: "way of divine harmony") has similar to judo its origins in the old Japanese martial arts. Therefore, aikido movements are often closely connected to sword techniques, which are expressed in the posture or position as well as the movements of the upper extremities. An observing, passive eluding in finished circular movements is characteristic. The attacker is brought out of balance by absorbing his medium axis in spiral movements. Different from judo, the force of the attacker is not met with resistance. His direction of impact or traction is absorbed in order to break his balance. The Japanese, Morihei Ueshiba (1883–1969), is the father of modern aikido, who emphasized the implementation of a harmonious connection between life and body with nature as well as between mind and ethics in his martial arts.

The repertoire of aikido includes more than 700 techniques, in which primarily the basic techniques (katame waza, see below) as well as throwing techniques (nage waza) are distinguished. "Uke" names the attacker, and the defendant is called "tori" or "nage".

45.1 Sport-specific characteristics

Aikidoka wear **judo suits (Gi)**, which are held together by a **white belt**, and they exercise **barefooted on judo mats**. All kyu grades wear a white belt, different from judo. Black belts are worn from the first dan and additionally also the wide black or blue pants (hakama). **Wooden training weapons** in Aikido are the wooden staff (jo), the sword (bokken) and the wooden knife (tanto; ➤ Fig. 45.1). From the very beginning, the fall training practices the rolling for-

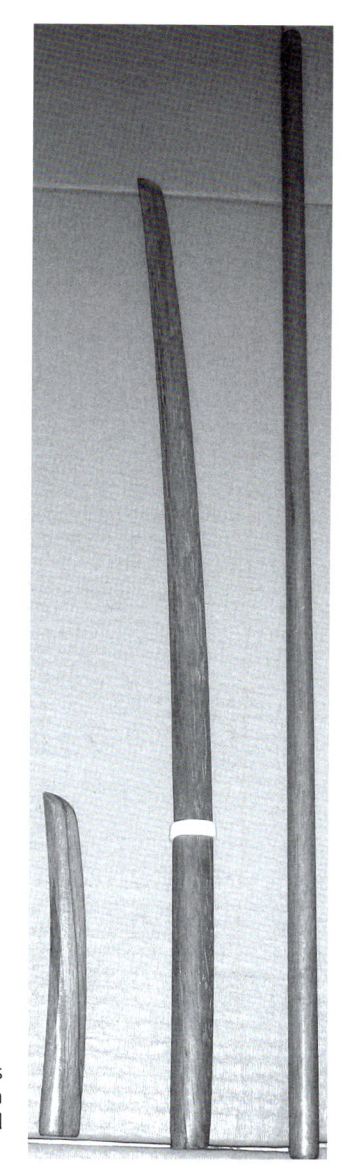

Fig. 45.1 Weapons in aikido – wooden knife, wooden sword and wooden staff.

wards and backwards. Aikido techniques are also performed kneeling.

The techniques basically start with the **freeing from the grip of the opponent**, the **throwing of the opponent** and the **final immobilization by a joint lock**.

There are no official competitions for aikido.

45.2 Sports-physiologic anatomic aspects of the techniques

45.2.1 Ikkyo (First technique)

According to old traditions, the purpose of ikkyo had been aimed to fracture the elbow joint in original martial art. Generally, there are two different variations of application, according to Seitz et al. (1991): on **purely biomechanical fixation of the elbow joint** and **an irritation of the medial nerve of the arm**. If the grip is focused to the right arm, the palm of this arm is turned upwards and the opponent is fixed to the ground by gripping the wrist with the right hand and the elbow with the left hand (➤ Fig. 45.2).

The worst biomechanical result could be a **distortion** at an overstretching of the elbow joint. **Strains of the brachialis muscle or the involved ligaments** could also appear. Pressure can also be put onto the distal, medial humerus end by the front side of the second metacarpophalangeal joint proximally of the medial epicondyle humeri in analogy to yonkyo, according to Seitz et al. (1991), which causes an **irritation of the ulnar nerve** that only has a minor soft-tissue protection here.

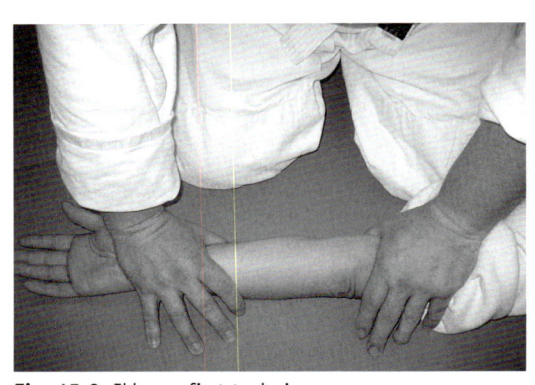

Fig. 45.2 Ikkyo – first technique.

45.2.2 Nikkyo (Second technique)

The leverage above wrist and elbow with the palm gaining full contact to the back of the opponent's hand and radial-sided setting of the little finger is critical (➤ Fig. 45.3). This maneuver gives the opponent's arm a characteristic S-shaped look. The **direct pain** that immediately forces the opponent to his knees is triggered by **a hyperflexion and ulnar deviation of the wrist**. According to Olson and Seitz (1993 and 1994 [2]), the pain (especially of unexercised athletes) is the result of an **over-rotation of the tendinous and muscular structures** of the extensor carpi radialis brevis et longus muscles, the extensor pollicis brevis et longus muscles and the extensor indicis muscle. According to anatomic and radiographic examinations by Eckert and Lee (1993), the pain in nikkyo is a result of the unphysiological **compression of the os pisiforme against the ulna** in exercised athletes, since both bones do not usually articulate with each other. Degenerative changes of the piso-triquetral joint can be the consequence especially at the intensive long-term implementation, according to Eckert and

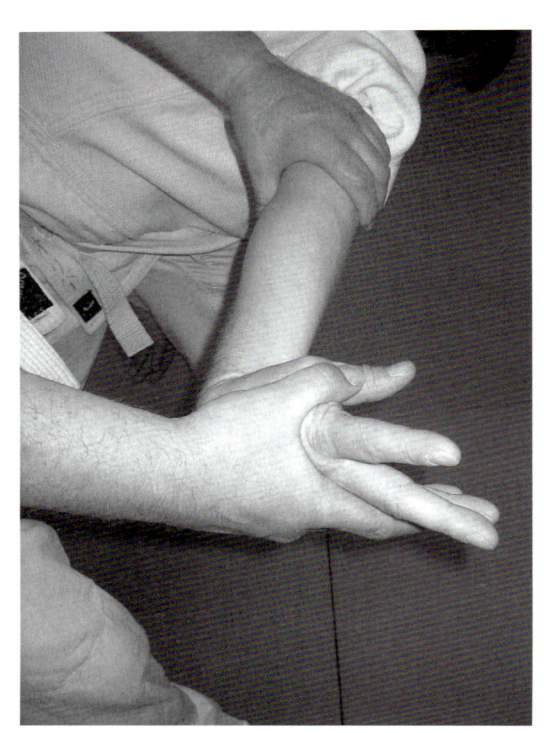

Fig. 45.3 Nikkyo – second technique.

Lee (1993). According to the authors, the immediate pain emanates from the periost.

45.2.3 Sankyo (Third technique)

The opponent's side of the hand is grabbed for the tensioning in the forearm and the palm is kept in full contact to the back of the opponent's hand. The elbow of the opponent is brought forwards (➤ Fig. 45.4). The tension is a result of the external rotation of the wrist. According to Olson and Seitz (1994 [1]), the **pain** results of an extensor digitorum muscle **overextension**, the extensor carpi ulnaris muscle, the extensor carpi radialis longus et brevis muscles, the extensor digiti minimi muscle and the ligamentous structures of the elbow joint as well as the joint capsule in athletes with minor extensibility. Additional pressure by the second metacarpophalangeal joint is applied to the back of the opponent's hand in athletes with higher extensibility, this triggers **periosteal pain** of the third and fourth metacarpal bone.

45.2.4 Yonkyo (Fourth technique)

The forearm of the opponent is held with both hands, while the opponent's elbow is brought forward (➤ Fig. 45.5). According to Rödel (2006), the opponent is controlled by a **pain point at the forearm** in yonkyo. The pain appears, if **pressure** is applied **to the bone by the basis of the metacarpophalangeal joint of the index finger**. According to Olson and Seitz (1990), the mechanism of pain development differs, depending on the yonkyo technique being used from the backside (ura) or the front side (omote). In the **variant of ura**, the pain results of the pressure to the distal end of the radius at the point of heart rate measuring, where the bone is relatively free of protecting soft-tissue coating. Especially the sensitive ramus superficialis of the radial nerve as well as the radial periost are affected most. In the **omote variant**, the medianus nerve, the ramus superficialis of the radial nerve, the tendons of the flexor carpi radialis muscle, the Palmaris longus muscle and the flexor digitorum superficialis muscle are under pressure. The ulnar nerve is not affected.

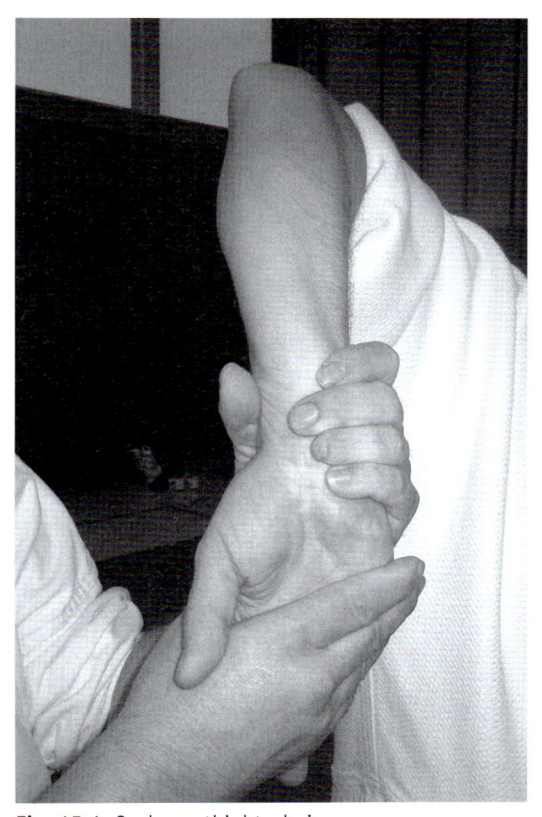

Fig. 45.4 Sankyo – third technique.

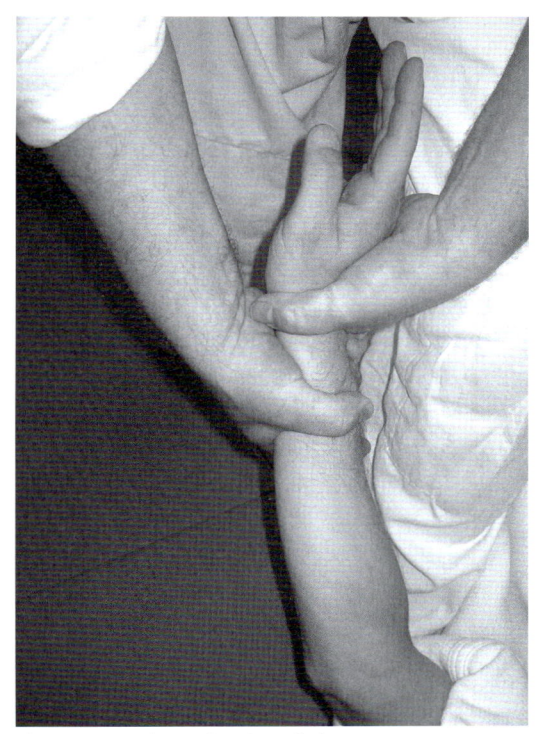

Fig. 45.5 Yonkyo – fourth technique.

45.2.5 Gokyo (Fifth technique)

Gokyo defines the **basic technique against an attack with the knife (tanto)** (Rödel 2005). In contrast to **ikkyo**, the arm of the attacker is not put to the ground completely (➢ Fig. 45.6). The elbow of the attacker is put into overextension. The reflecting countermovement is used to angle the elbow (Rödel 2005). The wrist with the knife is pushed into the direction of the attacker's head. New pressure to the elbow will cause a lever at the wrist of the attacker causing an opening of the fingers and releasing the knife. Especially the **distal wrist with its ligamentous structures** (dorsal-carpometacarpal) are subjected to **maximum extension** in the used technique. The **pain** will be felt most strongly **at the point of the second metacarpal bone** (Olson et al. 1996).

> The effectiveness of the basic aikido techniques is based on the irritation of the periost, minor soft-tissue coating nerves and overextension of tendinous, muscular, ligamentous and capsular structures.

> Beginners of aikido, who cannot adequately assess the effects of each kind of lever with its potential destructive consequences have to be careful.

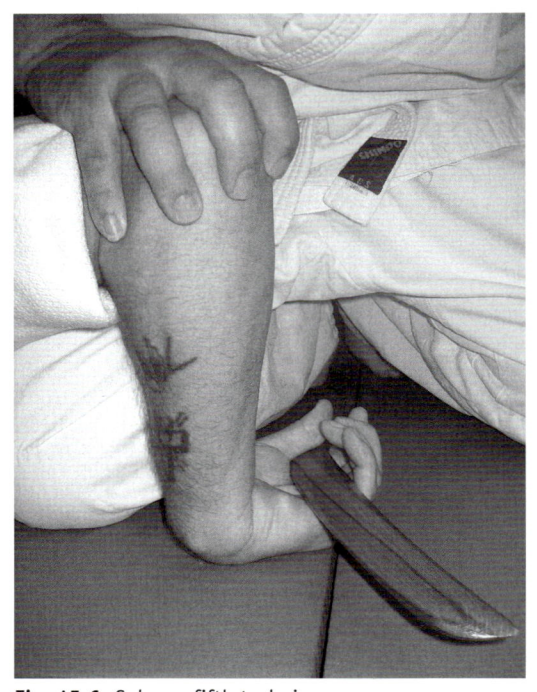

Fig. 45.6 Gokyo – fifth technique.

45.3 Accident rate and kinds of accidents

Based on 136 accidents in martial arts for a survey period of 15 years (1981–1995), a yearly sport accident rate of aikido is 0.11/1,000 aikidoka (Raschka et al. 1999). The accident rate of aikido was definitely lower than taekwondo (0.21/1,000), karate (0.33/1,000), judo (0.21/1,000) or Jujutsu (0.15/1,000).

Zetaruk et al. (2005) compared the accidents of 263 martial arts athletes in a retrospective survey (shotokan karate n = 114, aikido n = 47, taekwondo n = 49, kung fu n = 39, tai chi n = 14). 51% of the aikidoka had been affected by accidents requiring a longer absence from training. Serious injuries affected aikido and taekwondo with 28% and 26%, respectively, as compared to kung fu (18%) and karate (17%). The number of athletes with several traumas reached 50% in taekwondo, followed by aikido with 32%. Karate students suffered significantly fewer soft-tissue injuries than aikido students (25 vs. 51%).

45.4 Injury localization

Aikido injuries were localized in upper extremity (42.6%), lower extremity (34%), groin (6.4%), trunk (25.5%) and head/neck (31.9%). These percentages do not add up to 100%, because in some cases several organs had been affected. According to the authors, head and neck injuries of karateka with a rate of 10% had been very significantly fewer than the 32% of these injuries in akidoka in this comparison of martial arts. In addition, aikido students showed a significantly higher risk for injuries of the upper extremity than karate students did.

> The upper extremity is dominantly affected in aikido.

45.5 Special forms of injury

Aikido foot: This is a neuropraxia of the peroneus profundus nerve and the peroneus superficialis nerve. Naylor and Walsh (1987) reported an 18-year-old athlete, who had developed a partial equinovalgus posture and paresthesias in the area sustained by the peroneus on the right-hand side after a weekend-training of aikido. Two weeks later, the symptoms had completely vanished. The authors ascribed the aikido foot repetitive inversions of the ankle joint during the aikido seminar, because no trauma had occurred. Remarkably enough, the aikido teacher had complained of intermittent paresthesias of the same region (Naylor and Walsh 1987).

Hypothenar-hammer syndrome: The hypothenar-hammer syndrome is a rare form of a secondary Raynaud phenomenon. The hypothenar is used like a hammer in occupational or athletic activity. The hook of the os hamatum meets the superficial palmar branch of the ulnaris artery in the Guyon recess. Marie et al. (2007) have analyzed 47 patients (average age 42.5 years, 44 men, 3 women) with this rare syndrome. Although the cause was occupational in most cases, martial artists were affected in two cases – a karate teacher and an aikido athlete, who had practiced the sport for seven years and with an average weekly training amount of 5 hours. While the cause probably lies in direct hitting and blocking actions in karate, the repetitive exercises of rolling forwards with the rolling being done over the externally rotated side of the hand could perhaps be responsible in aikido. According to Marie et al. (2007), the therapy is be carried out by calcium antagonists and platelet aggregation inhibitors, if no digital ischemia or necrosis is present. The athletic or occupational activity must not be performed anymore.

Stab wounds: Stab wounds by the wooden knife, staff or sword can principally affect every region of the body if handled ineptly. Thus, a participant of aikido training in a town in Lower Franconia recently experienced a stab wound at the lower extremity requiring surgery. In the region of eyes and face, such injuries would be severe, though.

Injuries of the cervical spine, shoulder and elbow can principally appear in unsuccessful throwing and basic techniques, the same as in judo.

Toe lesions can be caused by getting caught in the clothes of the partner in training or in the matting in throwing activities.

Ankle joint distortions and internal knee traumas can generally appear in unsuccessful throws. Viswanath and Rodgers (1999) reported an especially serious knee distortion trauma in aikido in a 20-year-old aikidoka, who not only suffered a complete anterior and posterior cruciate ligament rupture because of the accident, but also an occlusion of the poplitea artery. Fortunately, the leg could be saved by a timely vascular-surgical intervention.

> Typical forms of injury in aikido are the aikido foot, the hypothenar-hammer syndrome, ankle joint distortions, internal knee traumas, stab wounds by wooden training weapons and – as in judo – different lesions of the upper extremity, in general.

45.6 Prevention

Special stretching exercises for the forearm muscles and the **shoulder muscles** are a special attribute of aikido, in addition to the injury prophylaxis also used in other martial arts by **sufficient warm-up, proprioceptive training** and **general stretching exercises** (Planells 2006).

Compared to other sports with special involvement of the upper body (tennis, baseball) or the involvement of the lower extremities (soccer, running), a significantly better goniometrically detectable mobility of all measured joint segments of the upper extremity in aikido after regular training of 3 times 2 hours a week has been reported in a controlled study (Huang et al. 2008).

Complicated exercise demands should not be kept until the end of training. The **correct placement of the matting** always must be checked in order to minimize the risk of getting caught in occurring gaps between the mats. Too long breaks between the exercises and overcrowded mats also have to be avoided.

The use of protection goggles in training with wooden weapons (sword, staff, and knife) should be considered by the federations, because of the risk of eye injuries primary in these exercises cannot be ruled out. In ice hockey, the incidence of eye and midfacial injuries could be clearly reduced by the wearing of helmets with half-visors.

The aikidoka should participate in training again only after full recovery from the overcome injuries.

References

Eckert JW, Lee TK (1993). The anatomy of Nikyo (Aikido's second teaching). Perceptual and Motor Skills 77: 707–715.

Huang CC, Yang YH, Chen CH, Chen TW, Lee CL, Wu CL, Chuang SH, Huang MH (2007). Upper extremities flexibility comparisons of collegiate "soft" martial art practitioners with other athletes. Int J Sports Med 29 (3): 232–237.

Marie I, Hervé F, Primard E, Cailleux N, Levesque H (2007). Long-term follow-up of hypothenar hammer syndrome. A series of 47 patients. Medicine 86 (6): 334–343.

Naylor AR, Walsh ME (1987). "Aikido foot" – a traction injury to the common peroneal nerve. Br J Sports Med 21 (4): 182.

Olson GD, Seitz FC (1990). An examination of Aikido's fourth teaching: an anatomical study of the tissues of the forearm. Perceptual and Motor Skills 71: 1059–1066.

Olson GD, Seitz FC (1993). An anatomical analysis of Aikido's second teaching: an investigation of Nikyo. Perceptual and Motor Skills 77: 123–131.

Olson GD, Seitz FC (1994a). An anatomical analysis of Aikido's third teaching: an investigation of Sankyo. Perceptual and Motor Skills 78: 1347–1352.

Olson GD, Seitz FC (1994b). What's causing the pain? A re-examination of the Aikido Nikyo technique. Perceptual and Motor Skills 79: 1585–1586.

Olson GD, Seitz FC, Guldbrandsen F (1996). An inquiry into application of Gokyo (Aikido's fifth teaching) on human anatomy. Perceptual and Motor Skills 82: 1299–1303.

Planells E (2006) Aikido. Ein Leitfaden zum Vorbeugen und Regenerieren von Verletzungen. Budo International Publ., Madrid.

Raschka C, Parzeller M et al. (1999). 15jährige Versicherungsstatistik zu Inzidenzen und Unfallherangstypen von Kampfsportverletzungen im Landessportbund Rheinland-Pfalz. Sportverletz Sportschad 13: 17–21.

Rödel B (2005). Aikido. Techniken, Angriffe und Bewegungseingänge. BLV Buchverlag, Munich.

Rödel B (2006). Richtig Aikido. BLV Buchverlag, Munich.

Seitz FC, Olson GD, Stenzel TE (1991). A martial arts exploration of elbow anatomy: Ikkyo (Aikido's first teaching). Perceptual and Motor Skills 73: 1227–1234.

Viswanath YK, Rogers IM (1999). A non-contact complete knee dislocation with popliteal artery disruption, a rare martial arts injury. Postgrad Med J 75: 552–553.

Zetaruk MN, Violán MA, Zurakowski D, Micheli LJ (2005). Injuries in martial arts: a comparison of five styles. Br J Sports Med 39: 29–33.

46 Boxing

Holger Schmitt

First records about athletic fist contests are about 7,000 years old and descend from a Sumerian temple. Already in the antique Olympic Games of Greece (688 B.C.), boxing had been one of the disciplines. The modern rules and techniques are ascribed to Jack Broughton. In the Olympic Games of modern times, boxing had been represented for the first time in 1904 in St. Louis.

The number of female athletes in this sport is continuously increasing. So far, no medals have been awarded yet for women's competitions at the Olympic Games.

46.1 Sport-specific characteristics

At present, the fight is carried out in a boxing ring in rounds of 3 min (professionals and amateurs). **Amateur fights** are carried out over three rounds, according to a current change, and the number of scores will decide. In **professional boxing**, the number of rounds is negotiated freely (mostly 12 rounds) and the winner is found by addition of the round scores, if the fight is not broken up early by knockout or technical knockout. The fighting is performed using gloves (10 ounces = 284 g), by which punches are allowed from the front and side against the head, chest and upper abdomen above the waistline.

Internationally, male amateur athletes fight in eleven weight classes (–48, –51, –54, –57, –60, –64, –69, –75, –81, –91, +91 kg). The weight and age classification is shown in ➢ Table 46.1. Physical preconditions for a successful boxing career are velocity, mobility, endurance, reactivity, coordination and strength.

Tab. 46.1 Arrangement of competition times according to age groups and gender in the German boxing federation (www.boxerverband.de).

a) Men					
	Learners	Cadets	Juniors	Youth	Men
age group	AG 10–12	AG 13/14	AG 15/16	AG 17/18	AG 19–30 (37)
competition time	3 × 1 min	3 × 2 min	3 × 2 min	4 × 2 min	3 × 3 min
fights per year	20	20	25	35	without limitation
pause between the fights	5 days	5 days	5 days	4 days	
b) Women					
	Learners	Cadets	Juniors	Youth	Women
age group	AG 10–12	AG 13/14	AG 15/16	AG 17/18	19 years and older
competition time	3 × 1 min	3 × 2 min	3 × 2 min	3 × 2 min	4 × 2 min
fights per year	20	20	25	35	without limitation
pause between the fights	5 days	5 days	5 days	4 days	

46.2 Injuries and overuse symptoms

It is the aim of boxing to strike the opponent with the fist in the area of head and body. Boxing has a characteristic injury pattern, which is different between amateurs and professionals.

In professional boxing, an **injury rate** of 250.6 in 1,000 fights has been reported, in which 90% affected head, neck and face and 7.4% the upper extremity (Zazryn et al. 2003, 2008).

> Sport injuries in boxing primarily affect head, neck and face.

In a study of the German amateur boxing federation, Lemme (1997) could demonstrate that 45.1% of the injuries affect the **skin**. There are lacerations and abrasions in the area of the face and at the eyebrows (so-called cuts), at the back of the nose and in the area of lips and mouth. Massive hematomas appear after direct traumas. Contusions of the inner organs and of the heart are rare. Temporary ventricular repolarization disorders after boxing stress have been observed in individual athletes. Clinical signs of a myocardial defect have not been found (Bianco et al. [1] 2005).

16.2% of the injuries affect the **facial skull**. It has come to fractures of the nasal bone, othematomas, and injuries of the ear drums, teeth and zygomatic arch and also to eye injuries in 2% of the cases. In the control group comparison of 956 boxers and an observed period of 16 years, minor eye injuries (hyposphagmas of the conjunctiva, edemas and degenerations of the retina, partial or total dislocations of the lens) have been found in 40.9% of the cases and serious eye injuries up to retinal detachments have been found in 5.6%, while the tests only showed eye injuries in 3.1% of the cases (Bianco et al. 2005). Eye injuries are seen less often in amateur sport (Llouquet 2008).

> Eye injuries are frequent in professional boxers, affect especially the conjunctiva and retina and can constrain the vision significantly.

Tooth injuries have become rarer because of the obligatory wearing of a mouthpiece. Fractures of the lower jaw can occur with a badly fitting mouth piece and blows to the open mouth.

10.8% of the injuries were **craniocerebral traumas**. Concussions with short-term disturbances of consciousness, possibly combined with a vegetative-hemodynamic dysregulation, are typical. Neurologic deficits with disequilibrium have also been found. In individual cases, acute subdural hematomas with lethal consequence after stress in boxing have been described (Ng'walali et al. 2000). Diffusion adjustments at the brain as an expression of microstructural changes in boxers could be documented by MRT as compared to controls (Zhang et al. 2003). Circulatory disorders have been found in the frontal sections of the brain in 35% of professional boxers and in 29% of amateurs of the cases (Rodriguez et al. 1998). No impairment of cognitive abilities has been found in tournament boxers over a monitored period of one week, with the exception of boxers who had been withdrawn from the fight by the referees (RSC = "referee is stopping the contest") (Moriarity et al. 2004). In a study of Irish boxers, no neuropsychologic abnormalities could be detected in an observation period of 9 years (Porter 2003). The authors of a current systematic analysis of scientific studies came to the conclusion that it has not been sufficiently proved that amateur boxing is associated with a chronic traumatic cerebral defect (Loosemore et al. 2007). Analyses by MRT documented a tendency, but no significant increase of cerebral micro-hemorrhages of amateur boxers in control-group comparison (Hähnel et al. 2008).

27.9% of the injuries of amateur boxers affected the **extremities**. Especially the hand and finger joints of the punch, i.e. the right-hand side in a normal boom, are subject to lesions despite clear improvements of the material of the gloves. Carpal, metacarpal bones and the metacarpophalangeal joints of the long fingers are often affected. Fractures of the metacarpal bones (often at the metacarpal bone V subcapitally = boxer's fracture, ➢ Fig. 46.1) are often found, and additionally also fractures at the 1st beam (e.g. Bennett's fracture). Subcapital fractures of the metacarpal bone V can also be treated conservatively at a correct reposition even with a significant axial deviation and can lead to a resumption of boxing (Statius Müller et al. 2003). A surgical treatment of such injuries by intramedullary splinting provides good results (Winter et al. 2007).

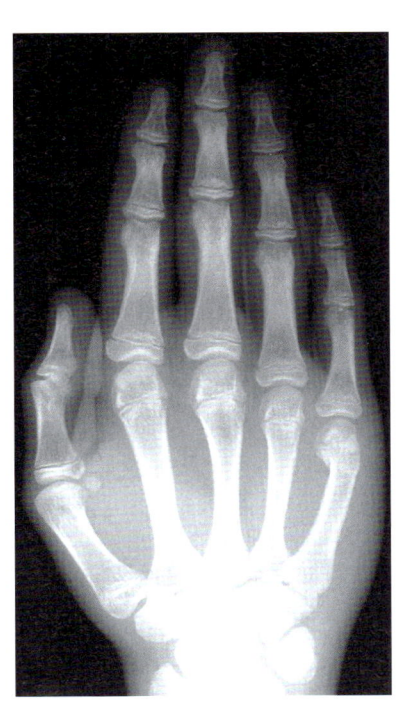

Fig. 46.1 Boxer's fracture: bone V fracture of the subcapital metacarpus.

Tab. 46.2 Overview of injuries and overload defects in boxing.

Head injuries
■ skin lesions (tears or abrasions) in the facial area
■ commotio or contusio cerebri (intracerebral hemorrhages), also in connection with neurologic deficit amnifestations
Viscerocranium injuries
■ fractures of the bridge of nose
■ othematomas, injuries of the eardrum
■ tooth injuries, fractures of the lower jaw
■ fractures and contusions of the zygomatic arch
■ eye injuries
Injuries of the torso
■ rib fractures and contusions
■ contusions of the inner organs and the heart
Injuries of the upper extremity
■ fractures and contusions of fingers, metacarpus and wrist (boxer's fracture, boxer's knuckle)
■ capsule-ligament injuries of the fingers
■ muscle lesions in the area of the shoulder girdle
■ overextension injuries of the elbow with chronic irritations and cartilage damages, posterolateral impingement
Injuries of the lower extremity
■ muscle injuries of thigh and lower leg
■ distorsions of knee and ankle joint with capsule-ligament lesions

The so-called boxer's knuckle is considered sport-specific, which often causes extension-sided avulsions of the capsule as well as the traction apparatus at the 3rd and 5th beam at the height of the metacarpophalangeal joint, which are partly accompanied by subluxations or dislocations of the extensor tendon (Bents et al. 2003, Hame et al. 2000). Surgical reconstructions can become necessary in the region of the metacarpophalangeal joints with chronic conditions and can also lead to sport incapability (Arai et al. 2002).

> Acute hand injuries in boxing affect the metacarpal bones, e.g. in the form of a subcapital metacarpal bone V, the boxer's fracture.

> Chronic overload defects lead to the so-called boxer's knuckle (capsule rupture at the metacarpophalangeal joint and rupture of the traction apparatus with subluxation or dislocation of the extensor tendon) with an accumulation at the 3rd and 5th beam.

A posterolateral impingement can be caused at the elbow by constantly recurring overextensions in the elbow joint, which can lead to an arthroscopic or open osteophyte resection. Instabilities are seldom found in boxers (Valkering 2008).

Injuries of the lower extremity are relatively rare and are found as distortions of the ankle and knee joints with capsule/ligament lesions.

➤ Table 46.2 gives an overview of the different injuries and overload defects of the affected body regions.

46.3 Prevention

The introduction of the **mouthpiece** as well as the use of a **boxing helmet** in amateur sports has reduced the injuries. At first, the introduction of the helmet had been controversial, because its use enlarged the punching surface for the opponent and shearing forces especially affect the skull and the cervical spine. The direct punch force could be intercepted, though, and tear wounds in the area of the face and the eyebrows had been reduced significantly, so that the helmet remains obligatory in amateur sport. The wearing of a mouthpiece and head protection is obligatory for all boxers.

Male boxers have to wear a **jockstrap**. Female boxers can wear a lap and a **chest protector**, but it is not obligatory. Children are only allowed to start participating in competitions with the age of 10 years. Fights of shorter length will be carried out in the youth classes (➢ Tab. 46.1).

Adolescents can only take part in a fight every 5 days and must not do more than 20 fights a year. In the youth classes B and A, fights are stopped after counting down twice in one round because of effective punches or after counting down three times, in the youth class C after the first effective punch.

Competitions and similar training are not allowed at pregnancy.

In individual cases, **fist protection bandages** are used for the reduction of punch stress to the fingers and the metacarpus and are worn in the exercising glove, but are not allowed for competition. A **wrapping of the hands** (tape of a length of 2.5 m at maximum and a width of 5 cm) is obligatory.

Starting with the 30th year of age, competitive activity will only be possible with the permission of the responsible physician of the state association.

> In amateur boxing, head protection and mouthpiece are obligatory. Male boxers will have to wear a jockstrap. Female boxers can wear a lap and a chest protector.

Kittel et al. (2005) could document in the control group comparison how far the sport-specific stress affects functional parameters of the locomotor apparatus: In comparison to the control group, the head and the middle of the shoulder joint of the boxer had often been ventralized, the bilateral position of the shoulder height in boxers had been significantly different and the maximum rotation capability of the boxer had been reduced in comparison to the control group. Concomitant compensation exercises in training have been recommended preventively (Kittel et al. 2005).

46.4 Medical supervision

Once a year, a sport-medical and radiologic examination including the sensory organs is mandatory. The **medical examination of the athletes before and after a fight** is important, especially in order to recognize neurologic abnormalities early. Recommendations are listed in the AIBA Medical Handbook. Differences between professional and amateur sport have been described by Jako (2002).

A fight is not allowed without the attendance of an official physician. All boxers must be examined for their starting ability before the start.

> The ringside physician has to assess the boxers' ability to start before the fight.

A medical treatment during the fight is not allowed in amateur boxing. The ringside physician can only decide whether the fight have to be stopped after an injury or if it can continue.

The competitor have to be medically examined on site after the **head knockout** and after the RSC decision. A medical specialist examination must be carried out within 4 weeks. A safety suspension of 28 days for competition and 21 days for sparring (boxing exercise) is imposed. The protective suspension is 3 months long with a head knockout twice within three months and the sparring suspension last 2 months; with a repeated head knockout within 3 months, the suspension amounts to 1 year and the sparring prohibition will take 9 months. An extensive medical examination is required after the termination of the suspension, which is documented in the start records. Referee and ringside physician together can impose protective suspensions of up to 4 weeks also for serious states of exhaustion and after serious tournament fights. After a knockout, the fighter must be accompanied on the way home and a transfer to the hospital is necessary after longer unconsciousness.

Even though no case of an HIV or hepatitis infection in boxing has been known, but since bleeding injuries can occur the Amateur International Boxing Association (AIBA) has prescribed the following procedure: referees and doctors must use sterile compresses for the examination of bleeding injuries and also have to wear single-use gloves. Splashes of blood should be removed from the body by water and soap and from the ground of the ring by household detergent. The disposal must be done in plastic bags.

References

Arai K, Toh S, Nakahara K, Nishikawa S Harata S (2002). Treatment of soft tissue injuries to the dorsum of the metacarpophalangeal joint (boxer's knuckle). J Hand Surgery 276: 90–95.

Bents RT, Metz JP, Topper SM (2003). Traumatic extensor tendon dislocation in a boxer: a case study. Med Sci Sports Exerc 35: 1645–1647.

Bianco M, Colella F, Pannozzo A, Oradei A, Bucari S, Palmieri V, Zuppi C, Zepilli P (2005a). Boxing and "commotion cordis": ECG and humeral study. Int J Sports Med 26: 151–157.

Bianco M, Vaiano AS, Collela F, Coccimoglio F, Moscetti M, Palmieri V, Focosi F, Zepilli P (2005b). Ocular complications of boxing. Br J Sports Med 39: 70–74.

Jako P (2002). Safety measures in amateur boxing. Br J Sports Med 36: 394–395.

Hähnel S, Stippich C, Weber I, Darm H, Schill T, Jost J, Friedmann B, Heiland S, Blatow M, Meyerding-Lamade U (2008). Prevalence of cerebral microhemorrhages in amateur boxers as detected by 3T MR imaging. Am J Neuroradiol 29: 388–391.

Hame SL, Melone CP Jr (2000). Boxer's knuckle in the professional athlete. Am J Sports Med 28: 879–882.

Kittel R, Misch K, Schmidt M, Ellwanger S, Bittmann F, Badke G (2005). Boxsportartspezifische Auswirkungen auf funktionelle Parameter des Bewegungsapparates. Sportverletz Sportschaden 19: 146–150.

Lemme W (1997). Boxen. In: Engelhardt M, Hintermann B, Segesser B (eds.). GOTS-Manual Sporttraumatologie. Verlag Hans Huber, Bern, pp 258–266.

Loosemore M, Knowles CH, Whyte GP (2007). Amateur boxing and risk of chronic traumatic brain injury: systematic review of observational studies. BMJ 335: 781–782.

Louquet JL (2008). Eye injuries in boxing. www.alba.com

Moriarity J, Collie A, Olson D, Buchanan J, Leary P, McStephen M, McCrory P (2004). A prospective controlled study of cognitive function during an amateur boxing tournament. Neurology 62: 1497–1502.

Ng'walali PM, Muraoka N, HonjyoK, Hamada K, Kibayashi K, Tsunenari S (2000). Medico-legal implications of aute subdural haematoma in boxing. Journal of Clinical Forensic Medicine 7: 153–155.

Porter MD (2003). A 9-year controlled prospective neuropsychologic assessment of amateur boxing. Clin J Sports Med 13: 339–352.

Rodriguez G, Vitali P, Nobili F (1988). Long-term effects of boxing and judo-choking techniques on brain function. Ital J Neurol Sci 19: 367–372.

Statius Muller MG, Poolman RW, van Hoogstraten MJ, Steiler EP (2003). Immediate mobilization gives good results in boxer's fractures with volar angulation up to 70 degrees: a prospective randomized trial comparing immediate mobilization with cast immobilization. Arch Orthop Trauma Surg 123: 534–537.

Valkering KP, van der Hoeven H, Pijnenburg BC (2008). Posterolateral elbow impingement in professional boxers. Am J Sports Med 36: 328–332.

Winter M, Balaguer T, Bessiere C, Carles M, Lebreton E (2007). Surgical treatment of the boxer's fracture: transverse pinning versus intramedullary pinning. J Hand Surg Eur Vol 32: 709–713.

Zazryn TR, Finch CF, McCrory PR (2003). A 16 year study of injuries to professional boxers in the state of Victoria, Australia. Br J Sports Med 37: 321–324.

Zazryn TR, McCrory PR, Cameron PA (2008). Neurologic injuries in boxing and combat sports. Neurol Clin 26: 257–270.

Zhang L, Ravdin LD, Relkin N, Zimmermann RD, Jordan B, Lathan WE, Ulug AM (2003). Increased diffusion in the brain of professional boxers: a preclinical sign of traumatic brain injury? Am J Neuroradiol 24: 52–57.

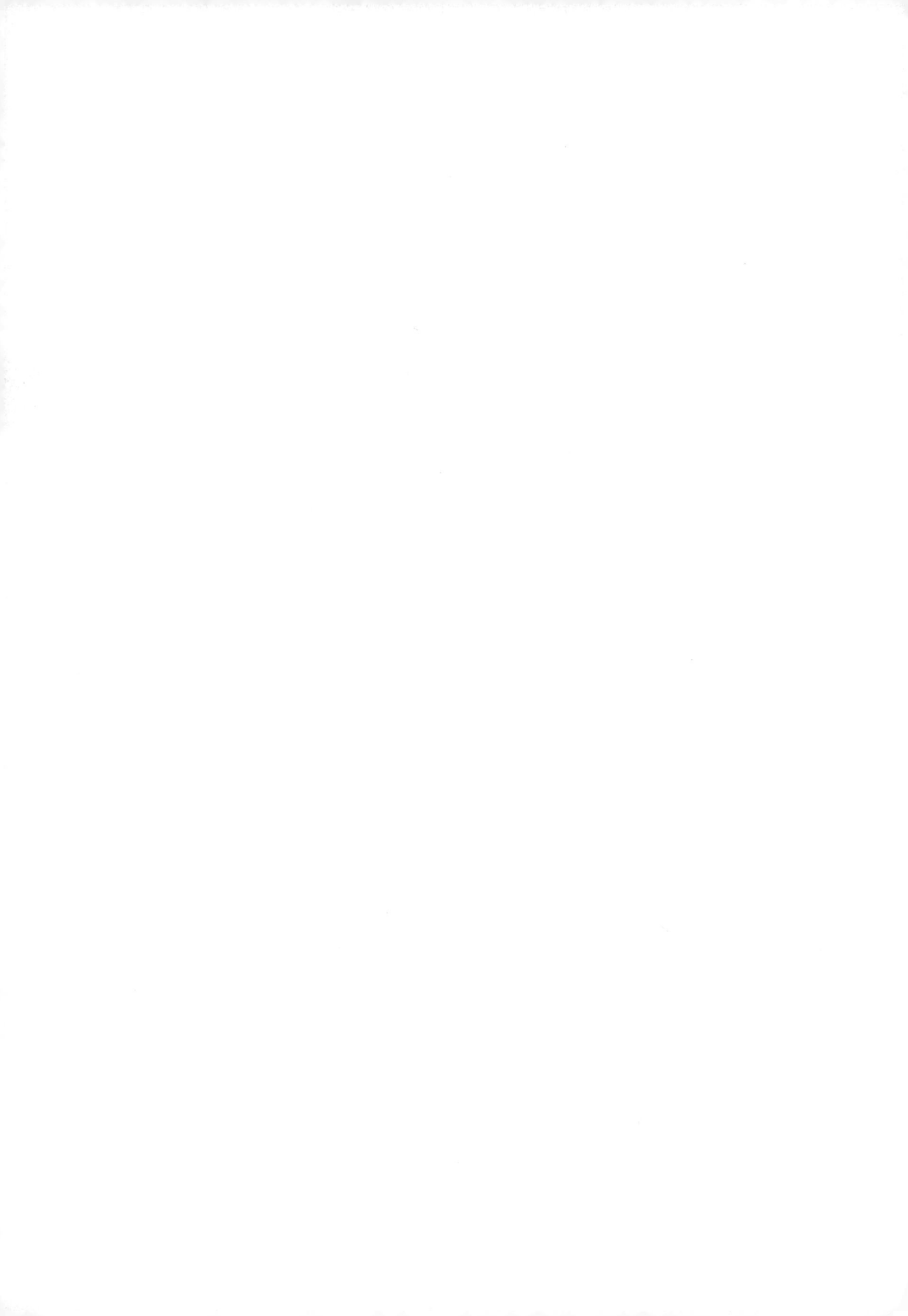

Chapter 47 Fencing

Axel Jäger

Modern sport fencing has developed from ancient self-defense. In the 17th century, the art of fencing was part of the education in military schools and universities. The academic fencing was based on old dueling rules. Spadroon (sabre), heavy sabre and bayonet were used for fencing in a students' duel with a defined distance of the fighters. The posterior foot poised, attack and defense were only carried out with a lunge. Today's academic fencing is still done contrary to sport fencing – in a students' duel.

Within the last 20 years, wheelchair fencing has been established in addition to foot fencing.

47.1 Sport-specific characteristics

In modern fencing (➤ Fig. 47.1), three different weapons are distinguished. **Foil** and **epee** are thrusting weapons; the **sabre** is a cutting weapon. Depending on the weapon, there are differently defined target areas and different rules. In foil as well as in sabre fencing, a fight is carried out by the rule "hitting without getting hit". Here the rule applies to repel an attack first, before the fighter has the right to attack. In foil fencing, the torso is a valid target area; in sabre fencing, only those hits are counted that are set above the waistline. In épée fencing the whole body is a valid target area, and in addition there are double hits, if both fencers place a touch within 40 milliseconds. This leads to other tactic procedures than in sabre and foil fencing.

In **individual tournaments**, the pools are done by 5 or by 15 points in the KO system. **Team competitions** are carried out according to the so-called relay system, in which the fencers alternate after 5 touches or after the expiring of the time of 3 min. The team wins that leads after the given period or that has first reached 45 touches. The **director** (referee) leads the fight and is supported by line judges in large tournaments.

A special training is conducted formed for the improvement of reactivity, the power of con-

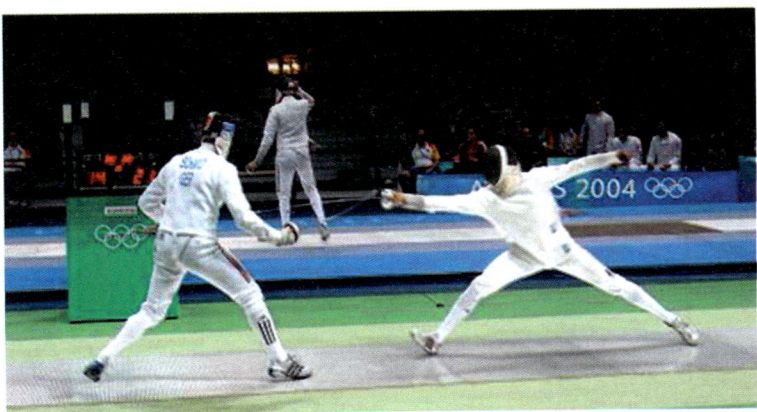

Fig. 47.1 Epée fencers in action.

centration and basic velocity in addition to the fencing-specific training in the way of correct arm and legwork as well as body posture. An important aspect of the training is the springiness and the strength-endurance training. The maximum force training is only of minor importance and will either serve the fast development of atrophied muscles or will be implemented at the start of the first preparation phase of a new fencing season (Hauptmann 2003).

47.2 Equipment

Special clothing is worn in fencing. Those are **protective suits** consisting of Kevlar and **shock-resistant masks**. These have either a complete woven, spot-welded wire grid or a plastic visor (➢ Fig. 47.2). A **special glove** protects the weapon hand. A **vest** is worn underneath the suit, women also wear a **chest protector** and men a **jockstrap**. The personal protection gear of the fencer underlies severe examination. It will only receive the CE sign after fulfilling certain requirements (Haid 2003).

The indication of scores is done electronically by a direct contact between weapon and the valid target area of the opponent. The triggering of the scores is transmitted via corresponding lines, which are led to an annunciator in the weapon and underneath the clothing.

47.3 Injuries and stress symptoms

In the years 1993 to 2000, 886 acute injuries and 584 overload conditions were found in 342 individual fencers at the German Olympic Training Center of fencing in Tauberbischofsheim.

The **foot and ankle joint** take the first place in the list of **acute injuries** (26%; ➢ Fig. 47.3). in particular, external ligament injuries of the ankle joint in the shape of overstretched and ligament ruptures, contusions of the upper ankle joint/foot – especially the anterior foot – as well as the overstretching of the internal ligaments of the upper ankle joint of the posterior foot.

> Foot and ankle joint injuries are the most frequent acute traumas in fencing.

Injuries of the **spine** are in second place (21%), with blockades in all segments, but primarily in the thoracic spine. Injuries of **hands** and **fingers** are in third place. Here the weapon hand is subject to contusion injuries of the metacarpophalangeal joints of the index finger, the wrist as well as the knuckle of the thumb. Distortions of the wrist and contusions of the fingers, capsule-ligament overextensions in the area of the metacarpophalangeal joints D2 and D3 as well as incision wounds of the hands (➢ Fig. 47.4) and forearms are found. In rare cases, fractures occur.

So far, the author has registered six injuries with **lethal consequence** during the period from 1968 to 2005.

In the first place of the detected **overuse symptoms**, overuse of the **knee joints** is found (34%; ➢ Fig. 47.5). In particular, this is a ventral pain of the knee joint, not further distinguishable, often simultaneously with an existing hip flexion contracture and a diminution of the ischiocrural muscles of the anterior leg. Patellar apex syndrome, insertion tendinitis of the patellar ligament and the bursitis infrapatellaris are next.

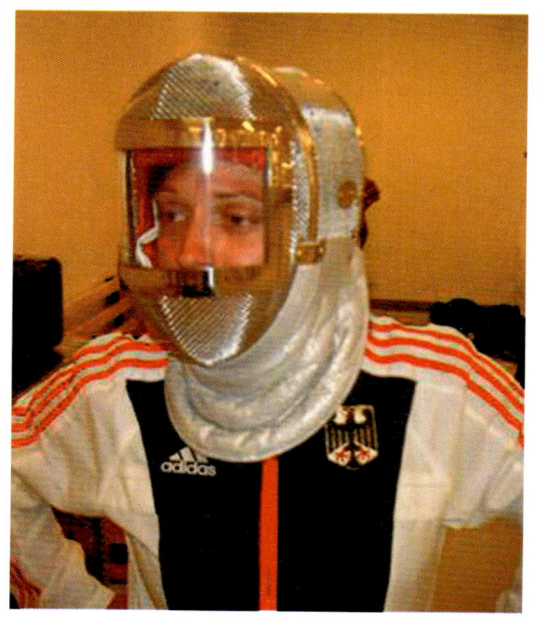

Fig. 47.2 Modern fencing mask.

47.3 Injuries and stress symptoms

Fig. 47.3 Frequency of acute injuries (1993–2000).

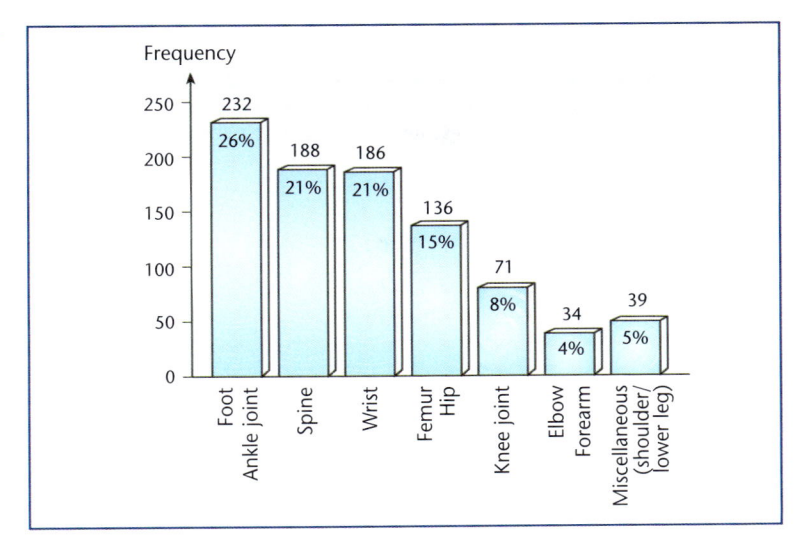

Anterior knee pain is the most frequent one of the overuse conditions of fencing.

In the second place, there are overloads of **foot and ankle joints** (24%) with tendinoses and peritendinoses in the region of the Achilles tendon and the calcaneus as well as metatarsalgias in the area of the forefoot. Intraarticular joint mice of the upper ankle joint of the forefoot are often found in a longer fencing career (➢ Fig. 47.6). Overuse syndromes of the lower leg (11%) follow in the third place with a bilateral medial syndrome of the tibial edge, the tibialis anterior syndrome and the peroneus brevis syndrome. At the **spine** (9%), unspecific lumbagos with muscular dysbalances appear as well as an L4 syndrome with secondary knee pain and inconspicuous radiographic findings of the lumbar spine and the knee joint.

Age-related differences are found in the comparison of the frequency of diagnoses of acute sport injuries between age groups of fencers up to 16 and older than 16 years (Jäger 2003). Injuries of feet and ankle joints (29%) in children and adolescents are in first place, followed by hands/wrists (23%) as well as injuries of the spine. The acute injury of the spine (29%) is in the first place in older athletes, followed by feet and ankle joints (28%) as well as thighs/hip region (15% each). Significant differences between both age groups are also found in the direct comparison of the **overuse signs**. In the younger group, the first place is taken by conditions of the knee joint (41%), followed by conditions of feet/ankle joints (20%) as well as the spine (11%). In the group of the older fencers, the focus lies on overload conditions at the foot or ankle joint (31%), followed by the knee joint (28%) and the shoulder (12%).

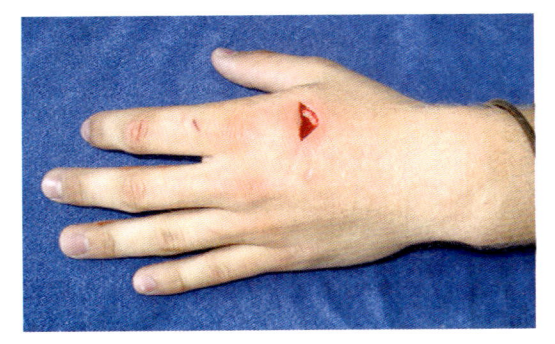

Fig. 47.4 Cut left hand of an olympic fencer.

A different order of frequency of the acute injuries as well as the overload conditions has been found in different age groups.

In order to avoid the frequent injuries and overloads at foot and ankle joints, attention must be paid to an exact performance of the legwork and there should be a consequent

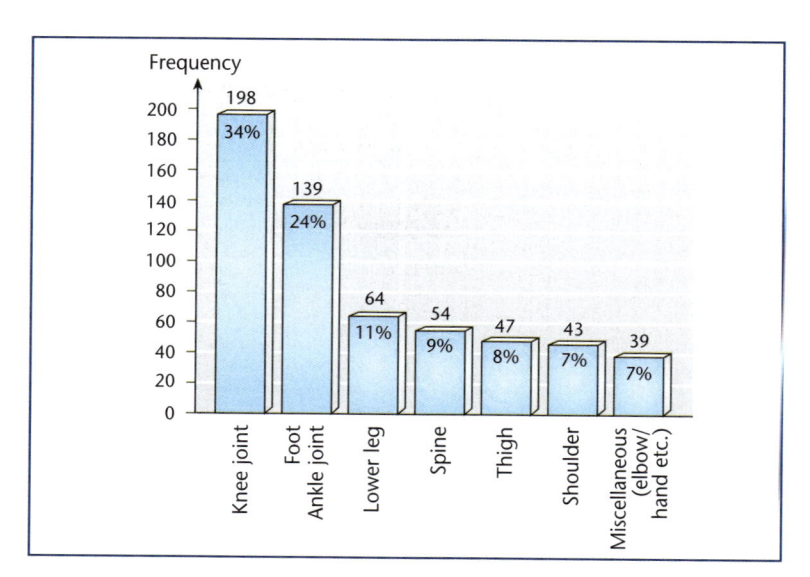

Fig. 47.5 Frequency of overstressed signs (1993–2000).

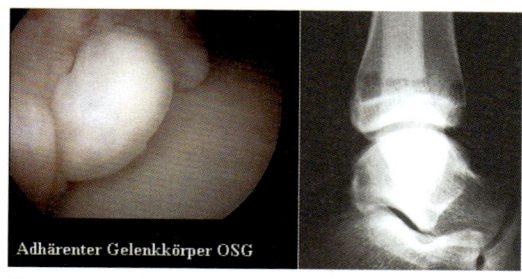

Fig. 47.6 Arthroscopic and radiographic images of an intraarticular joint body in the upper ankle of an olympic fencer.

treatment with insoles. There is a contact pressure of more than 800 Newton at the anterior foot and of more than 900 Newton in the region of the posterior foot (Felder 2003).

Typical muscular dysbalances of trunk and extremities are found because of the distinctive fencing position as well as the ambling (Jäger 1998). A permanent compensatory and early strength trainings are necessary for prevention.

Knowing of the fencing-specific one-sided loads, injuries and overload defects in fencing can be avoided by early compensation training and protective measures.

References

Felder H (2003). Biomechanische Aspekte und leistungsbestimmende Faktoren beim Fechten, dargestellt am Beispiel eines Ausfalls. Orthopädie Traumatologie 4: 263–267.

Haid H (2003). Sichere Ausrüstung im Fechtsport. Orthopädie Traumatologie 4: 281–283.

Hauptmann M (2003). Krafttraining im Fechtsport. Orthopädie Traumatologie 4: 269–271.

Jäger A (1998). Fechtsport. In: Klümper A (ed.). Sporttraumatologie. Ecomed-Verlag, Landsberg, chapter II-19: 1–25.

Jäger A (2003). Sportverletzungen und Schäden beim Fechten unter besonderer Berücksichtigung des Kindes- und Jugendalters. Orthopädie Traumatologie 4: 253–261.

Chapter 48 Judo

Christoph Raschka

Judo (Japanese for "gentle way") derives from the old Japanese martial art. The efficiency of the numerous throws and joint-locks depends on the use of biomechanical knowledge. Judo is practiced barefoot and wearing the traditional jugogi (judo wear). Professor Jigoru Kanu (1860–1938), father of modern judo, withdrew a number of dangerous techniques of Jujutsu from judo, such as strikes, kicks, stabs, finger and wristlocks, but still lock and choke grips seeming dangerous have remained and decide more than 4% of all injuries. Judo is a competitive sport carried out all over the world and has been an Olympic discipline since 1964. Despite this wide spread only one traumatic case of death had been registered in Germany in a 13-year survey (Raschka et al. 1996). The age level of 6 to 14 years has been considered a good training/entering age for judo training by Classing (2002), although competitive training should not be started before the 14th year of age. He states the age of 16–30 as the age of best performance.

48.1 Sport-specific characteristics

Judoka wear white cotton pants and a white jacket on top, fastened by a colored belt. The **belt color** indicates the rank of the judoka. Differentiation is done by belts (kyu ranks, starting with white, continuing with white-yellow, yellow, yellow-orange, orange, orange-green, green, blue to brown) and master belts (dan ranks, 1st–5th dan black, 6th–8th dan red-white, 9th–10th dan red and 11th–12th dan white).

The judoka fight on a square mat of 8 × 8 m; one contest period lasts 5 min for adults. Different scores or penalties can be awarded for the performed actions. An ippon, for example, means a full score.

The following **weight classes** are distinguished: in men –60, –66, –73, –81, –90, –100 and 100 kg+; in women –48, –52, –57, –63, –70, –78 and 78 kg+.

48.2 Sport-physiologic aspects

Regarding the constitution, the judoka is described as heavily-built, muscular and with a special accent on trunk and neck size (Maas 1974). The maximum oxygen uptake of the Canadian national judo team ranges between 34.1 ml/kg/min in heavy-weight athletes to 73.4 ml/kg/min for the light-weight athletes (57.5 ml/kg/min at the average), according to Taylor and Brassard (1981). Degoutte et al. (2003) assume an energy requirement of 50.1 kJ per hour and kg of body weight in judo training.

"Cutting weight" and **"making weight"** in judo indicate short-term reduction of the body mass for a start in a lighter weight class with better prospects of success. In addition to sauna and training in sweat-inducing clothes, diets, laxatives and diuretics are used. According to Braumann and Urhausen (2002), a weight reduction of up to 3% of the body mass in 3–5 days before competition is sustainable.

According to the survey of Scherbaum (1997), there is a direct correlation between the weight difference an athlete is to cut specifically before a competition and the accident rate in judo. Green et al. (2007) could confirm this correlation by a survey of 392 judoka (284 men,

108 women). While there is no significant correlation between accident rate and gender, weight class or rank, a weight loss of more than 5% of the original weight has led to a significant increase of the accident rate.

> Making weight before competitions must not exceed 3% of the body mass! Too intensive weight-making can promote sport accidents in judo.

48.3 The choking maneuver

Significant decreases of the medial systolic flow velocity in the middle cerebral artery and the internal carotid artery with simultaneously low saturation values in the pulse oximetry of the ear could be confirmed in **cross chokes** (juji jime), while the pulse increased by about 20 bpm and the blood pressure fell systolically by ca. 15 mmHg and diastolically by 12 mmHg (Raschka et al. 1998). A short-term decrease of pulse frequency, hypothetically expected because of the irritation of the carotid sinus has not been found for any case, though (Raschka and Koch 2000). It can be assumed that not only the direct compression of the carotids with consecutive cerebral minor perfusion is important in the choke maneuvers, but also the decrease of stroke volume because of the involuntary applied pressure breathing (Valsalva) is of significance (Raschka et al. [1] 1999).

> Caution is advisable for older judoka or participants of self-defense classes because of potential plaque development in the region of the carotid artery or a hypersensitive carotid sinus in exercising chokes (competition, self-defense).

48.4 Accident rate and course of accidents

Menge et al. (1980) and Jansen (1984) give a common **accident rate** for judo and karate of 1.7 or 1.6 accidents per 100 athletes per year.

A yearly sport-accident rate of 2.1/100 judoka (women: 2.2/100, men: 2.1/100) could be measured for judo alone based on 136 martial-arts accidents in an observation period of 15 years (1981–1995). Injuries of women amount to 31.9% of all injuries (Raschka et al. [2] 1999). Mentioned accident rates are based on all athletes performing judo in a club, i.e. mass and top athletes. According to Perren and Biener (1985), there is a much higher accident rate of 15/100 judoka/year for the Swiss competitive sudoka of the national squad, the 1st league and both national leagues (A, B). An especially high accumulation of accidents is found 6 months after entering the club, according to Janssens (1984).

> In German club sport, an average accident rate of 1.6–2.1 accidents per 100 athletes per year is considered for judo in mass and competitive sports together.

Regarding the **accident processes**, unsuccessful throws (36%) dominated over falls (21%), unfortunate hits in ground fight (19%) as well as twisted ankles (15%). 10.6% of the accidents have led to tooth lesions (mostly the front teeth). The athletes had often been hit in the face by the knee of the opponents in ground fights here (Parzeller et al. 1999).

Groove throws (maki-komi), the internal thigh throw (uchi-mata), the pincers (kani-basami) or the head throw (tomoe nage) as well as the shoulder wheel (kata-gurama), for example, have been indicated as exceptionally injury-prone by the judoka in the survey by Perren and Biener (1985).

48.5 Injury localization and kinds of injuries

Injury localization

According to a Swiss survey of 285 judo injuries in 199 men and 43 women of the upper performance classes who had exercised this sport for 9.9 (6.9) years, the lower extremity dominated with 35% in men and with 59% in women, followed by the trunk with 32% or 29% respectively, the upper extremity with 23% or 12% respectively, before the head with 10% (0%) (Perren and Biener 1985).

An analogous survey (Scherbaum 1997) in German high performance centers all over

Germany (primarily national and state squads) of 270 judoka (150 men, 120 women) showed a dominance in men (women) of the upper extremity of 45% (42%) over the lower extremity with 29% (37%), the trunk with 15% (10%) and the head with 10% (9%).

Jansen (1984) determined 39.4% (43.8%) in the shoulder-arm region, 26.1% (23.3%) at the lower extremity, 14% (13.7%) at the head, 4.2% (1.4%) of the thorax, 0.8% (5.5%) at spine and 0.4% (1.4%) at the abdomen and the genitals each in 224 male and 65 female judo accidents for all fields of performance in Schleswig-Holstein.

The survey of Menge et al. (1980) of 51 judoka (brown and black belt) in North Rhine-Westphalia showed a predilection of the shoulder girdle with 20.5% before foot injuries (13.1%), head injuries (13.0%) and also knee and hand with 10.6% each.

> The upper extremity with the shoulder girdle has dominated injury-topographically in judo in Germany.

Kind of injury

According to Perren and Biener (1985), fractures had been found most often in men (women) with 28% (18%), followed by moderate and serious distortions with 24% (35%), contusions with 14% (13%) and dislocations with 12% (4%) in Swiss elite judoka. Fractures mostly affect the ribs, clavicles and toes. According to Scherbaum (1997), distortions had dominated (men 44%, women 35.3%), followed by contusions (men 15.7%, women 14.1%), while fractures had only been in the fourth place of injury frequencies (men 7.2%, women 8.8%).

Steinbrück and Rompe (1980) list distortions in the first place (39.2%), then fractures (17.5%) and Brüggemann (1978) gives distortions (85%) the place before dislocations (15%).

In an analysis of 611 sport accidents with invalidity (Raschka 2005) that had occurred in the states of Berlin and Brandenburg in a period of 4 years, 4.1% have been attributed to judo. Primarily serious knee injuries were in the foreground here.

48.6 Special forms of injury

Judo finger: Clasing (2002) specifies the capsule swellings of the finger joints as typical overload defects in judo. According to Frey and Müller (1984), impaired loads and overloads of the finger joints condition the accumulated development of Heberden's nodes in top judokas as well as Bouchard arthritis, arthritis of the distal and medial phalangeal joints of the fingers caused by the grip attachments at the combat suits. The chronic repetitive micro and macrotraumatizing is essential (Strasser et al. 1997).

Judo elbow: The typical elbow injuries in judo develop in joint locks, which are set too far and with too much force, according to Scherbaum (1997), and this leads the joint to overextension and ligament lesions and can induce bone and cartilage split-offs as well as consecutively degenerations and arthritic changes. Sometimes there is a typical blockade of the elbow joint. Elbow dislocations or distortions in judo often result from the try to gain support in a fall in order to prevent negative judgements.

Separation of the AC joint: According to Scherbaum (1997), dislocations of the AC joint and clavicular fractures often develop if the thrown judoka overturns and cannot land in dorsal, lateral or supine position and only part of the shoulder girdle functions as contact surface.

Lesion of the cervical spine: According to Perren and Biener (1985), cervicobrachial syndromes develop in distortions of the cervical spine.

Toe distortion: According to Seidel (2002), the toes are also subject to high stress in the preparation of throwing techniques and at ground fighting. Toe injuries result from getting caught in the clothes or in the matting at throws or in ground fighting.

Ankle joint distortion: According to Scherbaum (1997), not only unfortunate twist movements, but also getting caught directly in the gaps between the mats is responsible for lesions of the ankle joint

Internal knee trauma: According to Clasing (2002), meniscus lesions, cruciate ligament ruptures or capsule-ligament defects are the result of the twisting for shoulder and hip throws with firmly standing foot. Cartilage defects in

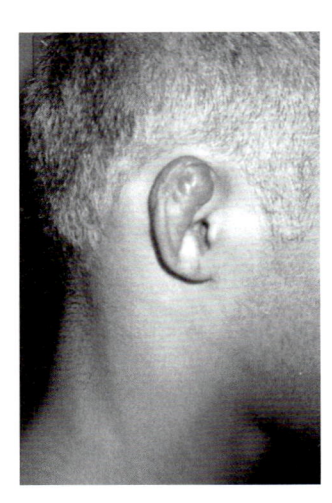

Fig. 48.1 Cauliflower ear of a judoka.

been established in other sports, such as adequate warm-ups (with stretching exercises), intensive body and technique exercises. In part, this is already practiced for youths. He recommends further a comprehensive recording of all techniques leading to injuries in competition, in order to eliminate the ones causing most injuries.

According to Perren and Biener (1985), difficult exercises are not to be done at the end of training. All defective mats have to be removed immediately. Longer training interruptions as well as an overcrowding of the dojo (exercise room) also must be minimized. After an injury or disease, the judoka should only be allowed to participate in the training and competition process again after full recovery.

the knee joint can also be a consequence of repetitive collision traumas at a fall on the mat, according to Scherbaum (1997).

Cauliflower ear: The so-called cauliflower ear is the long-term consequence of an untreated auricle hematoma, which has been caused by the head or knee of the opponent, with the ear being pressed against the petrous bone or also by shear forces. Therefore the hematoma will have to be treated or aspirated immediately.

Scherbaum (1997) found cauliflower ears in 20.7% of the men and in 7.5% of the women in his survey (➤ Fig. 48.1).

> Typical injuries in judo are for example the judo finger, the judo elbow, separations of the acromioclavicular joint, toe distortions and the cauliflower ear.

48.7 Prevention

Scherbaum (1997) recommends the abolishment of health-endangering elements (e.g. joint locks) in judo from active competition events or to judge the correct approach of these techniques as "ippon", if the application of this technique already clearly shows the control over the opponent, in addition to the preventive measures for the minimization of sport injuries and sport defects that have also

References

Braumann KM, Urhausen A (2002). Gewichtmachen. Dt Z Sportmed 53: 254.

Brüggemann G (1978). Sportverletzungen und Sportschäden beim Judo. Orthop Praxis 14: 396–398.

Clasing D (2002). Judo. In: Clasind, Siegfried I (eds.). Sportärztliche Untersuchung und Beratung. Spitta-Verlag, Balingen, pp 257–259.

Degoutte F, Jouanel P, Filaire E (2003). Energy demands during a judo match and recovery. Br J Sports Med 37: 245–249.

Frey A, Müller W (1984). Heberden-Arthrosen bei Judo-Sportlern. Schweiz Med Wschr 114: 40–47.

Green CM, Petrou MJ, Fogarty-Hover ML, Rolf CG (2007). Injuries among judokas during competition. Scand J Med Sci Sports 17 (3): 205–210.

Janssen W (1984). Über Verletzungen beim Judo- und Karatesport. Med Diss, Lübeck.

Maas GD (1974). The physique of athletes. An anthropometric study of 285 top sportsmen from 14 sports in a total of 774 athletes. University Press, Leiden

Menge M, Nick Ch. Niessen P (1980). Sportverletzungen und Sportschäden bei zwei Budo-Sportarten (Judo und Karate). In: Kindermann W, Hort W (eds). Sportmedizin für Breiten- und Leistungssport. Demerter-Verlag, Gräfelfing, pp 449–453.

Parzeller M, Raschka C et al. (1999). Dental injuries in combative sports: a comparison between judo, wrestling and karate. Medicina Sportiva 3: 123–126.

Perren A, Biener K (1985). Jugendsportunfälle – Epidemiologie und Prävention. Dt Z Sportmed 36: 294–300.

Raschka C (2005). Versicherungsmedizinischer Invaliditätsfokus durch Sportunfälle: Das Kniegelenk. Versicherungsmedizin 57 (3): 137–140.

Raschka C, Parzeller M, Gläser H (1996). Todesfälle im Vereinssport in der Bundesrepublik Deutschland. Dt Z Sportmed 47: 17–22.

Raschka C, Rau R, et al. (1998). Assessment of intracerebral blood flow velocity changes during choking (shime-waza) in judo, detected by transcranial Doppler sonography. Int J Sports Cardiola 7: 113–117.

Raschka C, Hölscher A, et al. (1999a). Echocardiographic investigation on the effect of cross-choking (shime-waza) on cardiac action in judo. Int J Sports Cardiol 8: 113–117.

Raschka C, Parzeller M. et al. (1999b). 15jährige Versicherungsstatistik zu Inzidenzen und Unfallhergangstypen von Kampfsportverletzungen im Landessportbund Rheinland-Pfalz. Sportverletz Sportschaden 13: 17–21.

Raschka C, Koch HJ (2000). Analyse der EKG-Funktion unter einem Würgemanöver im Judo. Herz/Kreislauf 32: 253–256.

Scherbaum U (1997). Verletzungen und Schäden im Judo. In: Mosebach U (ed.). Judo – Wurf und Fall. Verlag Karl Hoffmann, Schorndorf, pp 161–179.

Seidel M (2002). Judo. In: Klümper (ed.). Sporttraumatologie. II-26: 1–15. Ecomed, Landsberg.

Steinbrück K, Rompe G (1980). Sportschäden und -verletzungen am Schultergelenk. Dt Ärzteblatt 77: 443–448.

Strasser P, Hauser M, et al. (1997). Traumatische Fingerpolyarthrose bei Judo-Sportlern: Eine Verlaufsuntersuchung. Z Rheumatol 56: 342–350.

Taylor AW, Brassard L (1981). A physiological profile of the Canadian judo team. J Sports Med 21: 160–164.

# Chapter 49 Karate

Holger Schmitt

Karate is a martial art with its origin in the 5th and 6th century A.D. and it is ascribed to Chinese monks of the Chaolin Monastery, who had not been allowed to bear arms and had thus developed a special form of self-defense. Only in the early 20th century, a martial art originated in Japan with own rules. The Far Eastern philosophy is mirrored here even today.

49.1 Sport-specific characteristics

The translation of "karate-do" is "the way of the empty hand" (kara = empty, te = hand, do = way), which means: the karate fighter (karateka) does not have any weapons, the hands are empty. The **development of the own personality by self-control and concentration** is of central importance in karate. 107,227 members had been registered in the German karate federation in 2007.

Strikes by fist and foot are stopped before impacting in training as well as in competition in classic karate. Two competitive disciplines are distinguished: "kumite" and "kata".

The karateka is supposed to try to apply striking, kicking and punching techniques to the opponent on a competition area in **kumite** (free-fighting), while injuries of the opponent should not occur because of the strict rules. In traditional karate, the opponent can be hit at the body, but must not be hit at the head. In contrast, hits to the heads are allowed in full-contact karate. The dueling is performed in different weight classes with an additional open class. A regular bout lasts 2 min, but can also be scheduled to 3 min.

Different offensive and defensive techniques in logic and firm order are performed against imaginary opponents in **kata** as pseudo-fight. The kata in practice is following the synchronic kata by teams of three fighters in team competitions (bunkai).

> Karate injuries occur rather in the kumite competition, in which there is more contact to the opponent, than in the kata competition, in which the offensive and defensive techniques are carried out mainly as pseudo-fight.

The competitors wear a clean, white **karategi**. Metallic objects such as jewelry, watches, hair accessories of or with metal as well as glasses must not be worn. Soft contacts may be worn at one's own risk. Techniques that endanger or injure the opponent are stated in the strict rules and are punished.

49.2 Injuries and overload defects

Traditional karate is one of the sports with relatively low risk of injuries even without the wearing of protection gear because of the fact that striking and punching techniques to the head and neck are to be stopped before impacting the opponent or carried out in a controlled way. The **rate of injuries is especially low** compared to other Asian martial arts (Ngai et al. 2008). The risk of suffering serious injuries with the consequence of absence from training is 3 times as high in taekwondo (Zetaruk et al. 2005). More than half of the injuries in karate occur due to a fist punch, less due to falls (Raschka et al. 1999).

> In karate, more than half of the injuries are caused by fist punches.

Bruises and contusions at head, neck and face are the most frequent (50%), when the movements could not be broken off in time (Arriaza and Leyes 2005). The upper and the lower extremity follow with approximately equal amounts (20%), in which the unprotected **hands and fingers** or **feet and toes** most likely are subject to injuries, and **distortions, capsule-ligament injuries and fractures** are possible.

Tab. 49.1 Localization of injuries (n = 891) in karate, assessed in a prospective survey of 2,837 fights (according to Arriaza and Leyes 2005).

Localization	Frequency
face	646 (72.5%)
head	103 (11.6%)
lower extremity	57 (6.4%)
nape	34 (4%)
upper extremity	28 (3.1%)
thorax	9 (1%)
genitals	7 (0.8%)
abdomen	5 (0.6%)

Tab. 49.2 Overview of injuries and overload defects in karate.

Head injuries	head contusions covered craniocerebral traumas skin lesions in the facial area (tear-crush injuries, abrasions) contusions or fractures of nose and zygomatic bone larynx contusions
Injuries or the torso	thorax and rib contusions rib fractures
Injuries of the upper extremity	contusions and distortions of hand and finger joints dislocations of middle and end joints of the fingers fractures of metacarpus and carpus
Injuries of the lower extremity	muscle distortions and soft-tissue hematomas distortions of the knee joints with injuries of the meniscus and capsule ligaments distortion of the ankle joints with injuries of the external ligament apparatus toe fractures dislocation in the area of the forefoot contusions

The wearing of fist protectors is obligatory at competitions of the DKV and at international competitions, in order to better protect the hands. There are also foot protectors and shin guards. Fractures occur in about 2–3% of the cases, often at the toes (➤ Tab. 49.1 and ➤ Tab. 49.2).

Young and inexperienced karateka are exposed to a higher injury risk (13.5 injuries per 1,000 participants per year) than amateurs and professionals (2.43 or 2.79 injuries per 1,000 participants per year). The youths' injury risk first increases with the training age and afterwards the intensity of stress (Götz and Hörterer 1999, Zetaruk et al. 2000). Injuries that will have to be examined by a physician occur in about every fifth bout of each competition (in about every 3rd bout in the senior range starting with 18 years).

Most injuries are caused by fist punches (up to 40%; Müller-Rath et al. 2000). In amateurs, there is an accumulation of distortions at knee and ankle joint, in professionals rather fractures of the nasal bone, ribs, metacarpal and carpal bones. In a study in Great Britain, it has been found that injuries have led to discontinuation of training for full-contact karateka in 4% of the cases in amateurs and in 5.8% of the cases in professionals (Gartland et al. 2001). In the course of chronic stress situations, stress fractures, e.g. at the forearm, can appear (Steckel et al. 2005).

> In karate, about 50% of the injuries affect head, neck and face (Arriaza and Leyes 2005).

49.3 Prevention

Extensive **rule changes in 2000** have only influenced the injury rate to a minor extent. Every third to fifth athlete has suffered an injury in international competitions. Nonetheless, there have been clear changes regarding the localization, type and cause of the injuries. Facial injuries have occurred definitely less often. Injuries of the lower extremity have appeared more frequently. Bruises and "nosebleeds" have to be treated less often, and the amount of serious injuries could be reduced slightly from 8.3% to 6.3% (Wanke 2008).

The use of a **jockstrap for men** and a **chest protector for women** has proved of value. Both are mandatory, the wearing of a **mouth piece** is highly recommended – it has already been mandatory in DKV, EKF and WKF. The wear of glasses is prohibited. Contacts can be worn at one's own risk. Youths up to 14 years of age can wear sports goggles with the permission of legal guardians in the disciplines jiyu-ippon-kumite and kihon-ippon-kumite.

A **physician on site** (one physician per mat in international competitions; one physician for up to three mats in national competitions, see Medical Rules EKF) must be present in order to be able to medically examine the athlete after impacts to the head and to certify the further fighting capability.

49.4 Medical supervision

The physician is given 3 min for the treatment of injuries during a competition. Subsequently, the referee is informed about the findings and the further capability of the athlete. The attending competition physician informs the referee, if he considers the interruption of the fight sensible. In recent competitions, the physician has to write a protocol.

If **unconsciousness** is caused by a hit to the head, the athlete must not perform any kumite competition for 4 weeks; with a repetition within 3 months, a 3-months recess from competition will follow. After 3 cases of unconsciousness within one year, the karateka must not participate in kumite competitions for 12 months.

Bandages and strapping applied by the team physician because of injuries on the day of competition before competition start will require the approval of the competition team.

References

Arriaza R, Leyes M (2005). Injury profile in competitive karate: prospective analysis of three consecutive World Karate Championship. Knee Surg Sports Traumatol Arthrosc 13: 603–607.

Gartland S, Malik MH, Lovell ME (2001). Injury and injury rates in Muay Thai Kick Boxing. Br J Sports Med 35: 308–313.

Götz U, Hörterer H (1999). Verletzungen be Kindern und Jugendlichen im Karatesport. Sportorthopädie-Sporttraumatologie 15: 180–181.

Müller-Rath R, Bolte S, Petersen P, Mommsen U (2000). Das Verletzungsmuster im modernen Wettkampfkarate. Sportverletz Sportschaden 14: 20–24.

Ngai KM, Levy F, Hsu EB (2008). Injury trends in sanctioned mixed martial arts competition: a five-year review 2002–2007. Br J Sports Med, Mar 4, epub.

Raschka C, Parzeller M, Banzer W (1999). 15jährige Versicherungsstatistik zu Inzidenzen und Unfallhergangstypen von Kampfsportverletzungen im Landessportbund Rheinland-Pfalz. Sportverletzung Sportschaden 13: 17–21.

Steckel H, Oldenburg M, Klinger HM, Schultz W (2005). Tumorartige Knochenalterationen am Unterarm nach Karatetraining. Sportverletz Sportschaden 19: 37–40.

Wanke EM (2008). Verletzungsprävention im Wettkampfkarate am Beispiel von Änderungen im Regelwerk. Z Angew Trainingswissenschaft 15: 142–150.

Zetaruk MN, Violan MA, Zukarowski D, Micheli LJ (2000). Karate injuries in children and adolescents. Accident analysis and prevention 32: 421–425.

Zetaruk MN, Violan MA, Zukarowski D, Micheli LJ (2005). Injuries in martial arts: a comparison of five styles. Br J Sports Med 39: 29–33.

50 Wrestling

Hans-Georg Eisenlauer

Wrestling has a tradition which extends back over thousands of years. A wrestling day was already held in China in 3000 B.C. (Diezemann 1998), and in 708 B.C. wrestling became an Olympic discipline. Karl Schumann won a gold medal in the Greco-Roman style at the first modern Olympics held in 1896 in Athens. Freestyle was included in the Olympic disciplines in 1904. There are now four women's freestyle weight classes, and seven weight classes for men in each style at the Olympic Games.

The German Wrestling Association (DRB), which evolved from the German Heavy Athletics Association, was founded in 1972, and in 2007 comprised 20 state associations with 477 clubs and 17,224 active wrestlers. The DRB is a member of FILA (Fédération Internationale des Luttes Associées), the International Federation of Associated Wrestling Styles.

50.1 Characteristics and Equipment

Wrestling is a hard and dynamic competitive sport. Its aim is to force opponents onto the shoulders or defeat them by points, whereby mutual respect plays an important role.

There are two wrestling styles: **Greco-Roman** and **freestyle**. These two styles are distinguished by fact that the Greco-Roman style forbids holding the opponent below the belt, tripping, grasping the legs or actively using the legs in a hold. This is all permitted in freestyle.

In the German championships women fight freestyle in eight weight classes. Men compete in seven weight classes in each of the two styles. The rounds last 3 × 2 minutes with a break of 30 seconds between each round.

Beach wrestling was officially recognised as a third style in 2005. Beach wrestling is a competition with simple rules which can be held anywhere without any special equipment and which includes elements of traditional wrestling styles. There are two weight categories, light and heavy, and the classification is based on the build of the wrestlers, who are not weighed. A bout lasts a maximum period of 3 minutes and there is only one round.

When a competition is held in a hall, all competitors must wear a one-piece singlet in either red or blue. The shoes must cover the ankles, and heels, loops or other metallic parts are not permitted. If the shoes have laces, these must be secured in place by a bandage or tape, so that they do not become undone during the fight. Ear guards that must be approved by FILA can be worn to protect the ears and also by competitors with long hair (➤ Fig. 50.1).

During beach wrestling competitions men wear a normal pair of swimming trunks and the women a one-piece or two-piece swimsuit. The wrestlers compete barefoot in a sand-filled ring with a diameter of 6 metres.

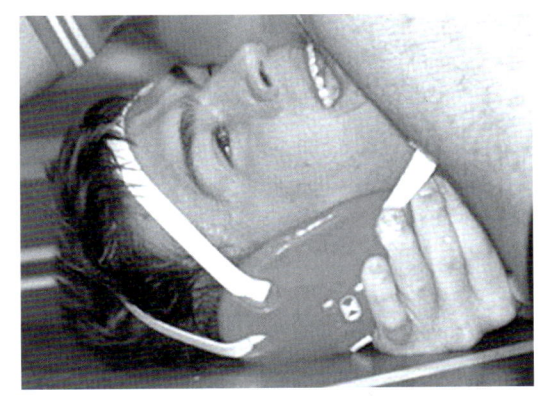

Fig. 50.1 Ear guards.

Wearing knee bandages is permitted if these do not have any metal parts. Corners and edges, even if made of plastic, must be padded. Advertisements are permitted on the thighs or the back of the singlet, except at the Olympic Games. **The following are forbidden:**

- Bandages on the wrists, arms or ankles, unless these are prescribed by a doctor
- Wearing of objects that could injure the opponent such as earrings or finger rings
- Applying greasy or sticky lotions to the body
- Arriving for a competition or incomplete rounds in a perspiring condition (Eisenlauer 2005).

At the beginning of each day of the competition the wrestlers must be either closely-shaven or have a beard of several months' growth.

The competition must be carried out on a FILA-approved mat with a diameter of 9 metres as well as an edge of 1.5 metres with the same thickness as the mat. For reasons of hygiene the mat must be cleaned with a household detergent before every event and with disinfectant if soiled during the fight, for example with blood. The clothes and the skin of the wrestlers as well as the mat must be checked by the referee before each competition, and during international tournaments the skin of the competitors is also checked by the competition doctor.

50.2 Injuries or strains and their treatment

According to records of the Gerling Corporation of the state sport federation of Rhineland-Palatinate (Raschka et al. 1999) the yearly wrestling **accident rate** from 1991 to 1995 totalled 0.71/1,000. Wrestling is therefore statistically in the lower third of this survey when compared with team sports such as handball and volleyball which totalled 29/1,000 and 43/1,000 respectively. The figures recorded at the Olympic Games in Athens in 2004 indicate that these are mainly minor injuries (➢ Table 50.1). As stated in the FILA report of 2005 (Babak 2005), 350 participants in 492 fights suffered 319 injuries during the competition and 29 injuries during training. Three percent

Table 50.1 Characteristics of injuries in wrestling with 350 participants in 492 contests, Athens 2004 (Babak 2005).

Injury types	Frequency	
	absolute	%
Minor	255	73
Moderate	81	24
Serious	12	3
Sum of injuries	**348**	**100**

Tab. 50.2 Diagnoses of n = 348 injuries in 492 contests with 350 participants, Athens 2004 (Babak 2005).

Diagnoses	Frequency in %
Closed skin injury	29
Open skin injury	15
Muscle contusion	14
Torn muscle fibres	11
Nosebleed	8
Ligament injuries	5
Fractures	4
Meniscus injuries	3
Nerve injuries	3
Dislocations	0.5

of these were serious traumas that stopped the competitors continuing in the tournament. The number of moderate injuries requiring diagnosis in the medical centre of the tournament hall or in hospital was 24 percent.

This is also illustrated by the recorded **types of injury** (➢ Table 50.2). Injuries were documented for 261 athletes, as some athletes suffered several injuries at the tournament.

Head

Frequent minor injuries are **nosebleeds, cuts on the head, haematomas**, for example cauliflower ears (➢ Fig. 50.2) which are a typical injury for this type of sport, and also **dental injuries**, all caused by pushing the head across the mat, head-clenching holds or illegal punches or head pushes. Treatment of these injuries is one of the main tasks of the attending team doctor and they are initially treated on the mat, as the contest can only be continued when bleeding has been stilled.

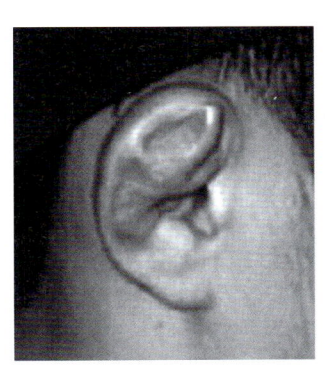

Fig. 50.2 Perichondrial haematoma, also called cauliflower ear.

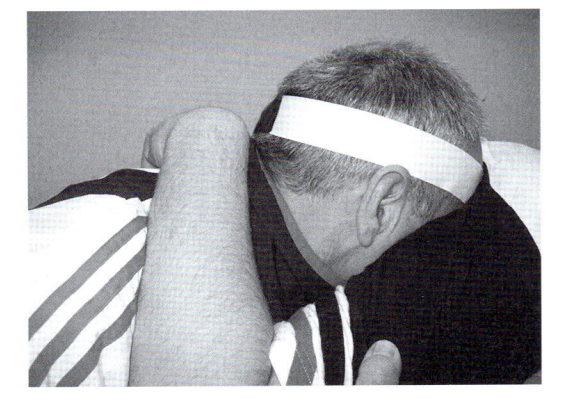

Fig. 50.3 Head cuts, initially treated with tape.

Head cuts are closed by tape strips applied directly onto the skin (➤ Fig. 50.3) and are given proper medical attention after the competition. Haemostatic swabs, dental cotton rolls or a cotton tamponade help to deal with nosebleeds.

Abrasions, which are aggravated by perspiration, are initially treated with tape or a mixture of Vaseline or Suprarenin (Eisenlauer 2005). Abrasions on the rest of the body tend to occur less frequently.

The round is interrupted for an **injury time of two minutes** for the treatment of the bleeding wounds to enable the doctor to treat and wash the athlete and for the mat to be cleaned. This serves to minimise or exclude the risk of an HIV or hepatitis infection. To date no HIV infection resulting from martial arts has been reported in literature (Torree et al. 1990).

After the competition any **othaematoma** is punctured to relieve tension and pain and is also compressed if possible. Unfortunately the actual injury time allowed is insufficient for a resilient scar to form, especially during tournaments, and relapses often occur. If pain tolerance is sufficient, it is sometimes effective to puncture the othaematoma 2–3 days after its development, either for the first or second time. A relapse can generally be avoided by a taking a break from training or competitions or by wearing ear guards during training. If an othaematoma is not treated adequately, deformations of the auricle often occur resulting in a so-called **cauliflower ear** (➤ Fig. 50.2). Deafness is a possible consequence. Unfortunately, no feasible prophylaxis or therapy has been found so far, as generally athletes do not consider a cauliflower ear to be an injury, and it is often even regarded with pride.

The diagnosis, treatment and rehabilitation of the injuries and consequences of undue stress and strain described below are in line with the generally accepted rules of orthodox medicine.

Spine

The cervical and the lumbar spine in particular are at risk when exposed to passive rotation as well as hyperextension – especially the cervical spine during a wrestler's bridge and the lumbar spine during a throw – and also due to hyperflexion during the landing after a throw or during neck holds. Fractures of the transverse processes of the lumbar vertebral bodies, but also extremely serious injuries of the cervical spine with myelopathy have only been rarely recorded. Nevertheless, micro-injuries occur during **distortion of the cervical spine**, which often only become noticeable after finishing the competition in a form of early serious **degenerative changes**, often with restriction of movement of the cervical spine, or irritation of the nerve roots.

Spondylolyses and **spondylolistheses** are observed more often than in normal collectives. Spondylolyses and spondylolistheses were found in six athletes during clinical anamnesis in own examinations of 113 D squad wrestlers with an average age of 18. In radiological examinations Jägermann and Jägermann (1997) found 32 spondylolyses and spondylolistheses in 70 squad athletes – also of the A and B squads – in their collective. An increase in occurrence with advancing age caused specifically by wrestling seems likely.

Injuries and consequences of excess strain and stress on the thoracic spine are rare.

Thorax

The **cartilaginous rib sections** of the thorax are particularly at risk during clenches and at the so-called twisters. The symptom is a piercing pain that is often accompanied by a snapping phenomenon. This injury is extremely painful and the wrestler will often have to finish the competition prematurely, even with the infiltration of a local anaesthetic. A six-week break from competitions is necessary to permit successful healing.

Fractures of the ribs resulting from falls with the involvement of the opponent's body weight often occur and are not problematic from a therapeutic viewpoint.

Shoulder and elbow joint, hand

Movements exceeding the physiological limits in illegal actions with a long joint lock, i.e. for example gripping the forearm, and also active resistance to attacks with a permitted short joint lock, as well as falls on the shoulder and the extended arm can lead to injuries especially of the **acromioclavicular joint** and to **lesions of the glenoid labrum. Shoulder dislocations** occur less frequently than dislocations of the elbow joint. **Dislocation of the elbow joint** without osseous involvement, which occurs in particular in children and adolescents, usually heals after closed repositioning with a short-term immobilisation for a period of two weeks without any consequences. **Fractures** of the upper extremities are rare. **Dislocation of the fingers** is caused by incorrect gripping or by the fingers becoming entangled in the opponent's singlet or by support reactions on the mat. Consequences of excessive strain caused by overextension in a hands and knees position, absorption of the force of falls on an overextended arm or frequent illegal passive extension will often cause premature arthrotic changes when the wrestler has finished active participation in competitions.

Hip joint

Injuries and consequences of excess stress and strain are generally not reported, except for a few individual cases.

A hip dislocation was documented for the first time in 2007.

Knee

The knee joint is subjected to high stresses during wrestling, especially in freestyle wrestling. Frequent maximum legal and illegal flexions and rotations occur which can lead to chronic damage to the menisci, so that inadequate traumas often lead to **meniscus ruptures** as a consequence. 30 percent of internal knee traumas are internal meniscus and 20 percent external meniscus ruptures. Complex internal knee injuries often occur during rotational movements of the upper body when the foot is fixed on the mat, including **rupture of the anterior cruciate ligament** (12 percent). More than one third of all injuries and almost 87 percent of all lesions of the lower extremities affect the knee joint (Jägermann and Jägermann 1997).

Foot

Ruptures of the fibulotalar capsular-ligament are caused on the upper ankle joint by typical sport supination traumas in gaps or at the edge of the mat, and also occur as the result of twisting the ankle during soccer or basketball, often during warm-up. In particular the toes are at risk when playing soccer in soft shoes. **Toe fractures and toe joint dislocations** often occur in this context.

50.3 Prevention

As not only serious injuries or diseases but even minor injuries can have far-reaching consequences for the individual athlete, all possible causes should be prevented as far as possible. The **preventive measures** listed below should therefore be observed for training as well as competitions:

50.3 Prevention

- Thorough diagnosis and therapy before starting selective high-level wrestling training, also as part of team examinations
- Thorough medical diagnosis, therapy and rehabilitation for medical conditions, compliance with prescribed breaks from training and competitions for physiologically necessary therapy and rehabilitation
- Avoidance of stress on the spine, especially during periods of growth, during training of children and adolescents, for example neck bridging.
- Wearing ear guards to prevent a othaematoma, especially during training
- Observing the rules of hygiene in the treatment of bleeding wounds
- Suspension of training and participation in competitions in the event of infectious skin diseases
- A tactical and technical training level suitable for the respective physical condition of the individual athlete, the coordinative, technical and tactical performance level of which should not be impaired by excessive loss of weight
- General warm-ups suitable for the respective sport discipline without soccer or basketball
- Organisation of tournaments and competitions which bring wrestlers of equal performance levels together
- Strict interpretation of the rules by the referee
- Correct placement of the mats with sufficient distance to spectators.

Regular doping tests should also be regarded as part of preventive procedures. During the Olympic Games in Athens, 89 urine tests and two blood tests were performed on wrestlers. One test was positive.

In 2007 the DRB carried out 32 competition tests and 147 training tests. All tests were negative.

References

Babak S (2005). FILA Medical Report. Trainer conference presentation in Ostia/Italy.

Diezemann ED (1998). Wrestling. In: Klümper A (ed.). Sporttraumatologie – Handbuch der Sportarten und ihrer typischen Verletzungen. Ecomed, Landsberg, 2–25.

Eisenlauer H-G (2005). Wrestling. In: Engelhardt M, Krüger-Franke M, Pieper HG, Siebert CH (eds.). Sportverletzungen – Sportschäden. Thieme, Stuttgart/New York, 155–158.

Jägermann V, Jägermann S (1997). Wrestling. In: Engelhardt M, Hintermann B, Segesser B (eds.). GOTS-Manual Sporttraumatologie. Huber, Bern, 272–280.

Raschka C, Parzeller M, Banzer W (1999). 15jährige Versicherungsstatistik zu Inzidenzen und Unfallhergangstypen von Kampfsportverletzungen im Landessportbund Rheinland-Pfalz. Sportverletzung Sportschaden 13: 17–21.

Torre D, Sampietro C, Ferraro G, Zeroli C, Sperenza F (1990). Transmission of HIV-infection via sports injury. Lancet 75: 305–306.

Chapter 51 Sumo

Casper Grim

Sumo is a Japanese style of wrestling and Japan's national sport. Sumo wrestling has simple basic rules: the wrestler (rikishi) who is forced out of the ring or who first touches the ground with any part of his body besides the soles of his feet, loses. Fights take place on an elevated ring. The Sumo ring (dohyo) is a platform of clay and sand, 4.55 meters in diameter (16.26 square meters) and edged by a square of rice straw bales with an inner ring in which the match is fought. At the center of the ring are two white lines (shikirisen), which serve as "startline" behind which the wrestlers position themselves before the bout. From a squat position the opponents take their initial charge (tachiai). The fights usually last only a few seconds, and rarely take longer than a minute.

Sumo's roots lie far back in Japanese history and its origins can be traced back over 2000 years. Many ancient traditions have been preserved in sumo, and even today the sport includes many ritual elements, from the days when sumo was used in the Shinto religion as a performance to entertain and appease the spirits of Shinto.

In the early 20th century emerged as a professional sport and is only practised professionally in Japan. Professional sumo is organized by the Japan Sumo Association.

A professional sumo wrestler leads a highly regimented way of life.

Traditionally sumo wrestlers live in sumo training stables, where all aspects of their daily lives -form what they can eat to what they can wear- are dictated by strict tradition and the stable master. Junior sumo wrestlers enter the sport at the lowest level of its six divisions. They can move up only by performing well in the 6 tournaments held throughout the year (> Tab. 51.1) and, in the same way, their superiors can be pushed down.

Foreigners who wish to train in sumo can be admitted to sumo stables under the regulation of the Japan Sumo Association. The Hawaiian wrestler Chad Rowan, known under the name Akebono, became the first foreign-born competitor to achieve the grand-champion status (yokozuna).

Tab. 51.1

Sumo championship tournaments are held six times a year, rotating among:	
■ Tokyo	January, May and September
■ Osaka	March
■ Nagoya	July
■ Fukuoka	November

A tournament (basho) lasts 15 days. The competition starts at early in the morning with the lowest-ranking. The champions compete last.

51.1 Sportspecific aspects

The Japan Sumo Association is the organisation that regulates and controls professional sumo wrestling in Japan. In professional sumo women are excluded from competitions and ceremonies. Women are not allowed to enter or touch the sumo wrestling ring since this is traditionally considered to be a violation of the purity of the ring.

Examples for traditional sumo rituals as performed in professional bouts:

The wrestlers face the audience and clap their hands. Leg-stomping (shiko) is performed to expel evil spirits from the ring and to intimidate the opponent. Both athletes squat and face each other, clap their hands, then spread them wide to show that they have no weapons. Back in their corners the athletes pick up a handful of salt and toss it onto the ring to purify it. The thick loincloth worn in sumo is called mawashi. The referee (gyoji) will coordinate the bout.

Sumo is also an amateur sport and the International Sumo Federation promotes the development of sumo wrestling worldwide, including international championships. Women are allowed to compete in amateur sumo wrestling. Japan held its first ever Sumo championship for women in 1997.

There are no weight restrictions or classes in professional sumo. Amateur tournaments are divided into weight classes (➤ Tab. 51.2).

Tab. 51.2

- **Men:**
  Lightweight: up to 85 kg
  Middleweight: up to 115 kg
  Heavyweight: 115+ kg
  Open Weight: unrestricted entry

- **Women:**
  Lightweight: up to 65 kg
  Middleweight: up to [80 kg
  Heavyweight: 80+ kg
  Open Weight: unrestricted entry

51.1.1 The bout

There are 70 official winning techniques in Sumo as recognized by the Japan Sumo Association. Some athletes prefer to go straight for the opponent's mawashi (loin cloth) to get a secure grip. Others choose to slap the opponent and push him towards the edge of the ring trying to get him out of balance in order to push him out.

The rikishi loses a match when any part of his body other than the bottoms of his feet touches the bottom of the ring or when he is pushed or thrown outside the ring.

Five judges sit below the ring (dohyo) and around the ring. In a close bout, any of the five judges can dispute the call made by the referee. In this case, a conference is held with the referee (gyoji) and five judges (shinpan) to discuss the match.

The names of the kimarite (winning technique) are usually compound words that combine two or more techniques in order to explain the method used to win.

- oshi: push with elbows bent
- uwate : outer grip on belt
- otoshi: drop
- tsuki: push with elbows locked
- shitate: inner grip on belt
- hineri: twist
- **yori:** lean or force with one's weight
- **taoshi:** knock down to the ring
- kiri: literally to cut, or force out

Example:

yori-taoshi forcing opponent to fall over backwards at the edge of the ring while maintaining a grip on his belt.

Injuries:

It is difficult to obtain a good literature overview and reliable data on sumo wrestling injuries since a lot of publications are written in Japanese und not published internationally.

Due to the squatting position in sumo the ankles are fully dorsi-flexed and the knees are also in a maximum flexed position. The combination of the basic position with the overweighed athletes can lead to anterior ankle-impingement and femoro-patellar joint alterations. Like in judo, skin lacerations and injuries to the first metatarsal joint are very common. Although the most common clinical problem in sumo is the lumbar spine, injuries to the lower leg and knee account for almost half of all injuries in sumo wrestling.

Tsuchiya et al. (2006) evaluated a group of 83 professional wrestlers. Average weight was 150kg with a BMI is 45. He found the most injuries in the leg and knees. Other typical injuries described are lumber disk herniation, shoulder dislocation, contusions, elbow fractures, anterior cruciate ligament ruptures, collateral ligament injury and sprains of the knee and ankle.

Tachiai is the colliding moment at the start of the sumo bout. The westlers bodies sustain very large impact. When the wrestler hits the opponent with his head in tachiai, the mechanical stress on the cervical spine and the neck is very high. This is probably comparable with spear tackling in American football. The wrestlers can have a tachiai-thrust with head or thrust without head. Kuwamori et al. (2002) investigated a series of 96 male collegiate Sumo wrestlers. 55% of the athletes complained of neck pain. In 77% the complaints were typical for a burner syndrome (stretch- or compression-injury to the brachial plexus). Kuwamori concluded that thrusting with the forehead may be a major cause for the burner syndrome.

Training of the neck muscle strength may reduce severe cervical injury.

Fortunately severe cervical injury like spinal cord injuries are rarely reported in sumo wrestling (Nakagawa et al. 1998, 2004)

Since there are no weight restrictions or classes in professional sumo, weight gaining is an essential part of sumo training. Grossly obese athletes develop specific, not directly sports- or competition related problems (Kanehisa 1998). Friction dermatitis, diabetes, altered immune function, left ventricular hypertrophy and high blood pressure are conditions caused by the sumo wrestlers body composition that are described in literature (Inui 2008, Umeda 2008, Kinoshita 2003). The excessive intake of alcohol and calories – which is common – can also lead to liver problems, arthritis and articular gout. Sumo wrestlers are prone to heart attacks.

The mortality rate of sumo wrestlers compared with that of the Japanese male population by Hoshi et al (1995) showed evidence for a higher rate of mortality in sumo wrestlers due to overweight.

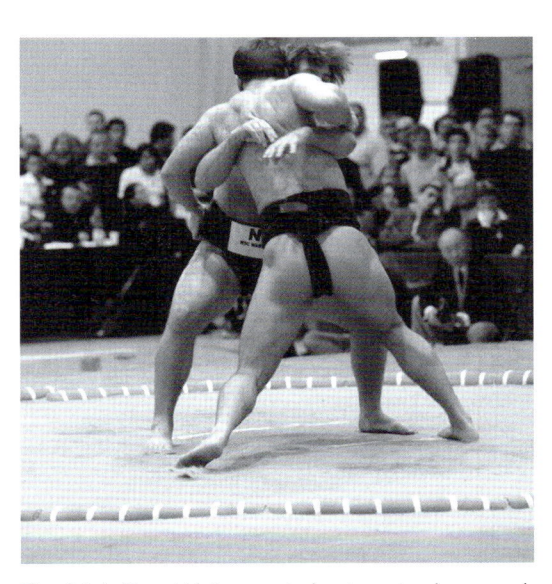

Fig. 51.1 The athletes are trying to get grip on each other in order to bring the opponent out of balance.

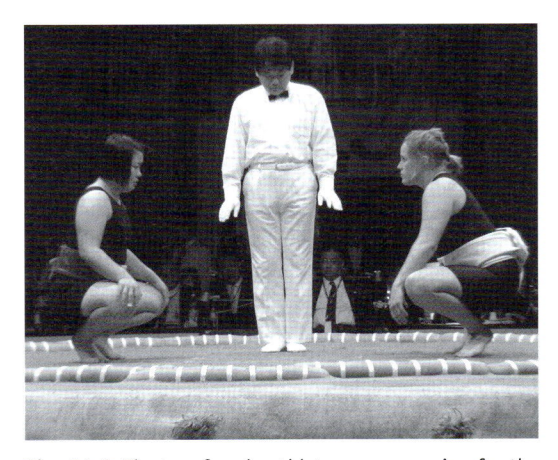

Fig. 51.2 The two female athletes are preparing for the initial charge. Typically with the knees in a highly flexed position.

51.2 Sumo glossary

- **basho:** professional sumo tournament
- **dohyo:** the ring
- **dohyoiri:** ring-entering ceremony
- **heya:** sumo stable; where rishiki live and train
- **gyoij:** referee

- **keiko:** general term for training
- **mawashi:** a canvas or silk belt, garment worn by rishiki
- **ozeki:** champion, second highest rank in sumo
- **rikishi:** *gentleman of strength*; term used for professional sumo wrestlers
- **sekitori:** junior champion, third highest rank in sumo
- **shikiri-sen:** two embedded lines on the dohyo; rikishi crouch behind these in preparation for tachiai; distance from each other is 70 cm
- **shiko:** basic leg stamping exercise which is very characteristical for sumo; rikishi raises his leg high to the side maintaining good posture and keeping his leg as straight as possible, then he stamps his foot on the ground with force and continues to perform the same for the other leg
- **sumotori:** popular but less acurate term used for professional sumo wrestlers, see rikishi
- **tachiai:** initial charge
- **yokozuna:** grand champion, the top rank in sumo

Kanehisa H, Kondo M, Ikegawa S, Fukunaga T (1998). Body composition and isokinetic strength of professional Sumo wrestlers. Eur J Appl Physiol Occup Physiol. 77 (4): 352–359.

Kinoshita N, Onishi S, Yamazaki H, Katsukawa F, Yamada K (2003). Recognition of left ventricular hypertrophy in new recruits of professional sumo wrestling. J Sci Med Sport. 6 (4): 379–386.

Masasuke K, Kazufumi M (2002). Relation between subjective symptoms of cervical injury and neck muscle strength in collegiate Sumo wrestlers International Olympic Committee World Congress on Sport Sciences: Medical Section Award Finalists. Medicine & Science in Sports & Exercise. 34: 5–12.

Nakagawa Y, Miki T, Nakamura T (1998). Atlantoaxial dislocation in a sumo wrestler. Clin J Sport Med. 8 (3): 237–240.

Nakagawa Y, Minami K, Arai T, Okamura Y, Nakamura T (2004). Cervical spinal cord injury in sumo wrestling: a case report. Am J Sports Med. 32 (4): 1054–1058.

Shapiro D, Sumo, A (1995). Pocket Guide Tuttle Pub.

Tsuchiya M, Otani T (2006). Sumo injuries in the top ranked professional sumo wrestlers. Journal of Joint Surgery, (25); 113–118.

Umeda T, Saito K, Matsuzaka M, Nakaji S, Totsuka M, Okumura T, Tsukamoto T, Yaegaki M, Kudoh U, Takahashi I (2008). Effects of a bout of traditional and original sumo training on neutrophil immune function in amateur university sumo wrestlers. Luminescence. 23 (3): 115–120.

References

Benjamin, D (2010). Sumo: A Thinking Fan's Guide to Japan's National Sport, Tuttle Pub.

Hoshi A, Inaba Y (1995). Risk factors for mortality and mortality rate of sumo wrestlers. Nippon Eiseigaku Zasshi. 50 (3): 730–736.

Inui S, Itami S (2008). 2 cases of sumo wrestlers' friction dermatitis. Contact Dermatitis. 58 (6): 374–375.

Websites

International Sumo Federation:
www.amateursumo.com

Japan Sumo Association:
www.sumo.or.jp/eng

Interational World Games Association.
www.worldgames-iwga.org

52 Taekwondo

Holger Schmitt

The origin of taekwondo lies in Korea. Fighting techniques have been shown on wall paintings of the koguryo dynasty (about 37 B.C.), which are still performed in this sport. In 1973, the world federation WTF (World Taekwondo Federation) has been founded officially, and the German taekwondo Union (DTU) in 1981. A little more than 61,000 members have been registered in Germany in 2007. Olympic medals have been awarded for the first time at the Olympic Games in Sydney in 2000 in full-contact competitions in four weight classes.

52.1 Sport-specific characteristics

"Taekwondo" is Korean for "foot-fist way". The most important techniques are kicks (ca. 90%) at the height of the abdomen or head in different variations, i.e. spun or jumped, in part also twice or three-fold. The foot technique most often performed is the **snap kick**. In addition, there are **fist techniques** (10%) and **blocks** for defense. While the most frequent injury situation in women occurs in the own foot offenses, the strike effect after unblocked attacks is in the foreground of the injury causes in men (Jung 2000).

Permitted target surfaces are the torso below the clavicle to above the lower abdomen and the face to the midline of the ears. Although fist and foot techniques are allowed at the torso, the permitted parts of the face must only be reached by foot techniques. Attacks to the back section that is unprotected by the protective vest are not allowed. Grabbing actions, evasive actions, forbidden opposing actions and forbidden/unfair actions can be punished by reprimands (kyong-go) or penalty points (gam-jeon).

One **fight lasts** three bouts of 3 min each with 1-min breaks. The **competition area** is a square of 12 × 12 m and consists of an even surface without protruding markings. The competition surface should be covered by an elastic mat or blanket. The inner part of the competition area with the size of 8 × 8 m is the contest area. The distance between contest and competition area is the safety zone.

The **competition clothes** of the athletes consist of the white taekwondo dobok and the protective clothes.

A classification into the following **weight classes** is done:

- seniors: 18 to 37 years of age
- juniors: 16 to 20 years of age.

The weight is divided into male and female classes. Single and team competitions are carried out.

The weight classes are listed in ➤ Table 52.1.

52.2 Injuries and overuse symptoms

> The injury risk of men is about 3 times higher than the one of women (Kazemi and Pieter 2004). The most frequent injury situation is caused by kicks after unblocked attacks.

Contradictory statements are found for taekwondo in the comparison of injury frequency with other martial arts. Raschka (1999) was able to detect a low injury risk in an injury

Tab. 52.1 Weight classes in single and team competitions of taekwondo sport (8 or 4 weight classes in single competition).

Single competitions				
Description	Weight men	Weight men	Weight women	Weight women
fin weight	54 kg		–47 kg	
flyweight	54–58 kg	–58 kg	47–51 kg	–49 kg
bantamweight	58–62 kg		51–55 kg	
featherweight	62–67 kg	58–68 kg	55–59 kg	49–57 kg
lightweight	67–72 kg		59–63 kg	
welterweight	72–78 kg	68–80 kg	63–67 kg	57–67 kg
middleweight	78–84 kg		67–72 kg	
heavyweight	+84 kg	+80 kg	+72 kg	+67 kg
Team competitions (5 competitors)				
Men			Women	
–54 kg			–47 kg	
54–63 kg			47–54 kg	
63–72 kg			54–61 kg	
72–82 kg			61–68 kg	
+82 kg			+68 kg	
Team competitions may also be carried out in 8 or 4 weight classes.				

analysis of the statistics of sports accidents by an insurance corporation (taekwondo 0.21 injuries per 1,000 hours of exercising the sport compared to karate 0.33/1,000 or wrestling 0.71/1,000). Zetaruk (2005), on the other hand, has found the highest injury risk in taekwondo athletes in a retrospective cohort study of the comparison of the sports taekwondo, aikido, kung-fu, karate and tai-chi. Kazemi (2004) could certify an injury rate of 62.9 per 1,000 hours of exercising the sport in a prospective study on the occasion of the Canadian championships in taekwondo and considers it a moderate injury risk compared to literature of judo or karate. The comparability of the data in present studies is limited because of the different definitions of the injuries.

> The injury risk in taekwondo is classified by ca. 60 injuries per 1,000 hours of exercising the sport.

Considering the **localization of the injuries**, traumas of the lower extremity are in the foreground for men, followed by lesions of head and neck. Spinal injuries are in the third place. Injuries of the lower extremity dominate in women (Kazemi and Pieter 2004). An examination of five German championships by Jung (2000) has shown a similar result, presented in ➤ Table 52.2.

> The most frequent injury is the contusion of the lower leg and the foot.

Taekwondo is performed barefoot. Skin injuries and dislocations occur especially in the forefoot region and at the toes. Open injuries are found, as well (Shin et al. 2008). The knee joint is at risk because of numerous techniques with rotations of the body. In addition to capsule-ligament injuries (mostly medial), menis-

Tab. 52.2 Localization of injuries (n = 312) in taekwondo (according to Jung 2000).

Localization	Percentage
lower extremity	55
upper extremity	17
torso	20
head	8

Tab. 52.3 Overview of injuries and overload defects in taekwondo.

Injury localizaton	Injury type
Head	cranial contusion or commotio cerebri Skin injuries in the facial area (abrasions and lacerations) monocular periorbital hematomas nose and zygomatic bone fractures fractures of the lower jaw
Torso	thorax and rib contusions genital organs: hematomas and tears of the labia, scrotum hematomas blockades of the iliosacral joint
Upper extremity	distortions of hand and finger joints dislocations of the medium and end joints of the fingers metacarpal fractures
Lower extremity	muscle injuries in the area of the adductors (also overload reactions) and of the thigh flexors contusions of lower leg and foot distortions of the knee joints with meniscus injuries, capsule-ligament injuries and patellar dislocations toe fractures, dislocations in the area of the forefoot, (hallux metacarpophalangeal joint and end joints D II–V) skin lesions of the forefoot (blood blisters, tears of the web) insertion tendopathies of the Achilles tendon

cus ruptures, patellar dislocations and also cruciate ligament ruptures can appear. High leg techniques with explosive movements can lead to distortions or even to ruptured muscle bundles in the region of the thigh muscles. Bruises and contusions might also appear at the thigh caused by deep kicks.

The upper body is protected by a protective vest; injuries of the trunk are rare.

The introduction of head protection has led to a reduction of the number of craniocerebral traumas. Still, 17% of the taekwondo athletes participating in competitions reported a cranial contusion or cerebral concussion in the last 12 months (Koh and Cassidy 2004). Injuries in the region of the viscerocranium occur, most frequently caused by unblocked foot kicks, because the facial area is not protected. In addition to the superficial skin lesions, contusions and lacerations, also eye injuries, fractures of the zygomatic arch, injuries of the lower jaw and the teeth have been found.

> 17% of the taekwondo athletes participating in competitions report cranial contusions or cerebral concussions, respectively, during a competing year.

In addition to acute injuries, also **overuse symptoms** are found. The lower extremity is in the foreground here as well. Especially the groin region is at risk because of extremely high leg techniques. Chronic inflammatory reactions appear at the adductors and at the ischiocrural muscle group. Rotatory and explosive overextension loads at the knee joints can lead to irritations of the insertion at the extension apparatus (especially the quadriceps tendon) and to a retropatellar chondropathy and additionally also to meniscus lesion. Jump loads can cause tendopathies of the Achilles tendon at the ankle joint.

➤ Table 52.3 gives a summary of injuries and overload defects in taekwondo.

52.3 Prevention

An **intensive warm-up phase** is necessary for the prevention of injuries and overload defects in taekwondo. Especially the muscle-tendon apparatus of the lower extremity will have to be stretched intensively and prepared for the stress.

In many cases (ca. 90% of the athletes, Kazemi et al. 2005), an excessive weight loss within few days before competition is caused by dietetic measures or endurance loads, because taekwondo is carried out competitively in weight classes. With a substantial weight reduction, the capacity can be reduced significantly by the limitation of endurance capacity on the one hand and the loss of proprioceptive abilities on the other hand.

Protective measures (protection vest, head protection, mouthpiece, jockstraps for men and women. tapes) can minimize the injury risk. The high number of ankle joint and foot injuries can be reduced by the wearing of taekwondo shoes and tapes, at least in training.

> Protective measures, such as protection vest, head protection, mouthpiece and tapes for joint stabilization can reduce the injury risk.

In order to avoid injuries, attention has to be paid that only athletes of the same weight class and with the same level of experience compete.

52.4 Medical treatment

In addition to the treatment of acute injuries in training and competition, also the prevention of injuries and overload defects are in the foreground in the medical treatment of taekwondo athletes. If athletes get hurt by head strikes, the attending physician needs to get an idea of the injury consequences and to deny the sport capability, if necessary. If injuries occur in combination with disturbances of consciousness, analogous criteria will have to be considered as for boxing athletes. After serious head strikes, the fight must only be continued if the competitor has stood up securely until counting to eight and can fix his vision, according to the rules. A suspension from competition for 4 weeks will follow a "knock out". Training and competition stress must only be resumed after medical check-up. The athlete will be suspended for 3 or even 12 months after a renewed "knock out". A competing prohibition will be set up after three "knock outs" within one year.

The use of a mouthpiece should always be checked. Some athletes use a mouth piece only unwillingly, because they fear a limitation of their ability to cry out, which could lead to a loss of points in some techniques.

References

Braun T (1999). Verletzungen bei hochklassigen Taekwon-Do-Turnieren – eine Standortbestimmung. Dt Z Sportmed 7+8: 239–242.

Jung D (2000). Takwondo – neue olympische Disziplin. Sportorthop Traumatol 16: 203–206.

Kazemi M, Pieter W (2004). Injuries at the Canadian National Taek Won Do Championships: a prospective study. BMC Muscoloskelet Disord 5: 22.

Kazemi M, Shearer H, Choung YS (2005). Pre-competition habits and injuries in taekwondo athletes. BMC Muscoloskelet Disord 6: 26.

Koh JO, Cassidy JD (2004). Incidence study of head blows and concussions in competition taekwondo. Clin J Sport Med 14: 72–79.

Raschka C, Parzeller M, Banzer W (1999). 15jährige Versicherungsstatistik zu Inzidenz und Unfallhergangstypen von Kampfsportverletzungen im Landessportbund Rheinland-Pfalz. Sportverl Sportschaden 13: 17–21.

Shin YW, Choi ICH, Rhee NK (2008). Open lateral collateral ligament injury of the interphalangeal joint of the great toe in adolescents during Taekwondo. Am J Sports Med 36: 158–161.

Zetaruk MN, Violan MA, Zurakowski D, Micheli LJ (2005). Injuries in martial arts: a comparison of five styles. Br J Sports Med 39: 29–33.

53 American football

Oliver Miltner and Christian H. Siebert

53.1 Development

Football is a fast-paced, athletic and unpredictable sport. In the course of a game, a fascinating competition develops between power and mathematics, between logic and labor. Football is a tough contact sport, in which even a helmet, shoulder pads and other devices cannot provide absolute protection.

The birth of football is frequently associated with November 6, 1869, when the university teams from Rutgers and Princeton met in New Jersey for the first time and played by the so-called Princeton rules. On August 20, 1920, players from Ohio's industrial centers Akron, Cleveland and Canton founded the National Football League (NFL). After difficult initial years, professional football gained dominance in the early 1940s. As a result stadiums in the U.S. have been sold out for years; about 70% of the Americans refer to football as their favorite sport.

Football was introduced to **Germany** after the Second World War by American occupation forces. The first professional steps were taken in Germany with the founding of the Frankfurt Lions in 1977. Today's boom was possible thanks to the initiative of the NFL, which founded the World League in 1991. In 1995, the NFL Europe further promoted the sport. Unfortunately, operations ceased with the end of the 2007 season. Today, the German Football League (GFL) consists of a North and a South group with six teams each. Arena football is in the early fledling stages.

53.2 The Game

The goal of the game is to gain yardage and improve field position on offense, while preventing the opponent from doing the same on defense. Yardage can be gained by carrying the ball forward or by converting a pass play.

The target is the opponent's end zone **(touchdown)** or to collect points via field goals. A touchdown scores six points. The scoring team receives an attempt at an extra point after a touchdown, which, depending on the level of play, can be executed as a **field goal** (kick) (1 point) or as **conversion** (2 points) by returning the ball into the end zone.

Alternatively, there is the possibility to achieve a field goal (3 points) from the field position achieved by the offense. The defense can also make points by scoring a **safety** (2 points), which describes the stoppage of the offensive player with the ball in his own end zone.

The **field** is 100 yards long, 53.3 yards wide (91.4 × 48.7 m) and has an end zone on each side extending 10 yards with H-shaped goals. The **ball** is egg-shaped, has a longitudinal circumference of 72 cm and a circumference at the center of 54 cm, is 28 cm long and weighs approximately 400 g. Every attacking team (offense) has four attempts (downs) to advance the ball 10 yards by rushing or passing.

If a team fails to advance at least 10 yards in 4 attempts or to score points, the right of offense switches to the opposing team. The net **game** time consists of four 15 min. periods.

53.3 Players

The most prestigious position in football is that of the quarterback. He is responsible for the offense, the plays and, therefore, for putting points on the score board. Next to the quarterback, there is the position of the running back. He will either receive the ball directly by handoff from the quarterback and will try to break his way through the defensive line or he will run short routes in order to catch a pass. In the positions of potential blockers, full and/or half backs can be used.

The **wide receivers** are mostly lined up away from the quarterback near the sideline. They will have to catch the passes, are frequently tall and fast with good jumping ability, but also have exceptional hand-eye coordination.

The so-called offensive line consists of five players **(tackles, center and guards)**, whose task is to protect the quarterback from the defense in a passing situation or to create spaces for the running back. These player are usually large; the offensive line of the Oakland Raiders reported with an average weight of 322.8 pounds in one of the last National Football League seasons.

The defensive line **(ends, tackles)** is positioned right up front on the scrimmage line, and is formed by three to four players, dependant on the formation. They line up in face of the offensive line and their task is to pressure the quarterback during a pass play, so that he cannot release the proper pass or to tackle the quarterback **(sack)**. The linebackers find their place behind the defense line.

The so-called secondary usually consists of four players, two **cornerbacks** with similar degrees of athletic ability as described for the wide receivers. Both have to cover the opposing receivers during pass plays. The second part of the secondary consists of two **safeties**. They are the last line of defense and attempt to prevent touchdowns.

In addition to offensive and defensive squads, there are the so-called **special teams**. The kickoff team brings the ball into play at the beginning of the half and after points have been scored, while the kickreturn team returns the kicked ball. Another task of kickers is the conversion of field goals and extra points. The kicker must be able to calculate the wind and distance exactly, while remaining calm as the defense charges at him.

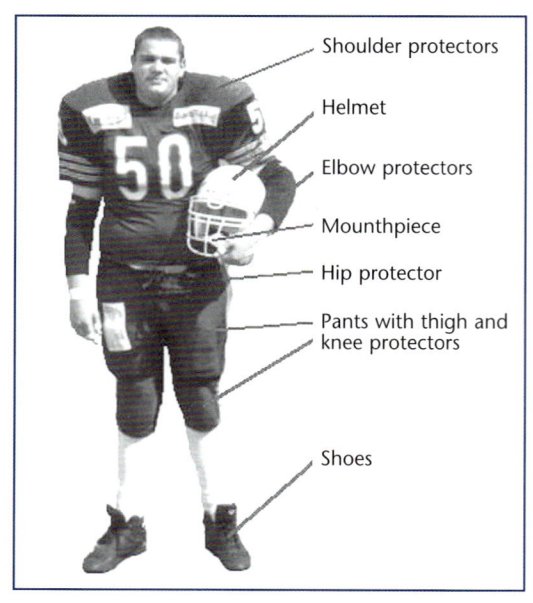

Fig. 53.1 Football equipment.

53.4 Equipment

The equipment necessary for the football is clearly more extensive and specialized than in other sports. A number of pads, plates and protection devices are needed for the body protection alone.

Part of the **standard equipment** are: helmet with face mask, mouthpiece, shoulder and hip protectors, pants with thigh and knee protectors, and shoes.

Depending on the player's position **additional equipment** can be: rib and spine protectors, gloves, humerus and forearm protectors, as well as neck protectors (➢ Fig. 53.1).

53.5 Frequent injuries and overuse syndromes

Insufficient experience of the player, as well as previous injuries are **important risk factors** for the suffering of acute injuries (Tuberville et al. 2003). During football exposures, injury rates of 15.7 to 20.1 per 1000 hours of football per athlete have been reported (Baltzer and Ghadamgahi 1998, Meeuwisse et al. 2000).

> The risk of injury lies between 15 and 20 per 1000 hours of football exposure.

The injuries are distributed follows:
- head/neck injuries 15.9%
- upper extremities 17.9%
- lower extremities 55.2%
- spine/thorax 9.4%
- other 1.6%

(modified according to Meeuwisse et al. 2000).

> The most frequent injuries involve the lower extremities.

53.5.1 Head and neck, upper body

The **most important injuries in the region of head and neck** are:
- the craniocerebral trauma (degree I-III)
- the cervical injury
- the injury of the plexus brachialis (burner syndrome).

The risk of a concussion or Mild Traumaric Brain Injury (MTBI) amounts to 0.41 per game in the NFL. The quarterback, then the wide receiver, tight end and defensive secondary are most at risk. 70% of the concussions occur following contact with the opponent's helmet. Special sport medical **rules of conduct after MTBI** should be observed when caring for a football team (➤ Tab. 53.1). 92% of all players with concussions can resume training and playing activities after less than 7 days (Pellman et al. 2004).

A total of 223 **injuries of the cervical spine** with permanent neurological deficit were reported for American football in the U.S.A. between 1977 and 2001 (Cantu and Mueller 2003). Thankfully, a decreased incidence by 270% has been recorded since 1975. This has been achieved by rule changes, improvement of the neck support and muscular stabilization, as well as by better tackling technique.

It is very important for the attending physician to master the correct **techniques of removing helmet and protectors** (Waninger 2004).

The **brachial plexus injuries or burners** can be caused by an impact to the head, neck or shoulder region leading to lateral flexion of the neck and traction to the shoulder. Clinically, there will be a burning dermatome-spanning pain along the arm. A return to the sport should only be considered after a complete resolution of the symptoms (Vereschagin et al. 1991).

The **shoulder** is clearly in the forefront of injuries in the region of the upper extremity. The largest group (65%) can be described as bruises and contusions. Furthermore, there are injuries of the acromioclavicular joint, dislocations, fractures and ruptures of the rotator cuff. In 83% of the cases shoulder injuries seen in quarterbacks are the result of trauma, while in 14% overuse problems caused by the throwing movement (Kelly et al. 2004) are made responsible.

In the region of the **hands** and **fingers** mostly capsule-ligament injuries, dislocations and fractures are reported. The wearing of gloves, taping of fingers and training of gripping strength should be carried out as prophylactic measures.

53.5.2 Lower extremities

Injuries in the region of the lower extremities are distributed as follows:

Tab. 53.1 Guidelines depending on state of consciousness following head trauma (mod. Siebert et al. 2004).

Grade of Concussion	Treatment	Return to sports
degree 1 no loss of consciousness	Temporary removal from competition, return if clinically unobtrusive	Return to play, if asymptomatic on the same day
	Removal from competition, in case of repeated concussions	after 1 week, if asymptomatic
degree 2 loss of consciousness <5 min.	Removal from competition	after 1 week, if asymptomatic
degree 3 loss of consciousness >5 min.	Hospital evaluation	after 2–4 weeks, if asymptomatic

- knee 26.8%
- thigh 26.1%
- ankle 20.0%
- leg 12.5%
- hip 8%
- foot 6.6%

(modified according to Meeuwisse et al. 2000).

Injuries of the **knee joint** can occur during different phases of the game (running, landing, by contact and fall to the knee). The severity of knee injuries is also influenced by the ground condition of the playing field. There is an increased risk **on artificial turf** in comparison to natural grass (Orchard 2002).

> The most frequent injury in the region of the knee is the rupture of the ACL ligament.

According to the team physicians of the National Football League, the **rupture of the anterior cruciate ligament** should be treated surgically with a patellar tendon graft (Bradley 2002). **Muscle injuries** in the thigh region can be divided into injuries of the muscle fibers, mainly of the ischiocrural musculature and the adductors, and muscle contusions in the area of the quadriceps. In the **ankle joint**, the fibular ligament rupture is the most frequent injury and is influenced in its frequency, as in the knee joint, by the surface, as well as climatic conditions (Orchard and Powell 2003).

> The frequency of injuries of the ankle and knee joint is influenced by the ground and climatic conditions.

Acute injuries of the **lumbar spine** are rare. Chronic low-back pain, degenerative changes of the intervertebral disks and arthroses of the facet joint should be expected (Gerbino and d'Hemecourt 2002). The intensive strength training as well as the forced hyperextension in the region of the lumbar spine can be considered risk factors for these overuse syndromes.

References

Baltzer AWA, Ghadamgahi PD (1998). American-Football-Verletzungen in der Deutschen Bundesliga: Verletzungsrisiko und Verletzungsmuster. Unfallchirurgie 24: 60–65.

Cantu RC, Mueller FO (2003). Catastrophic spine injuries in American Football, 1977–2001. Neurosurgery 53: 358–363.

Bradley JP, Klimkiewicz JJ, Rytel MJ, Powell JW (2002). Anterior cruciate ligament injuries in the National Football League: epidemiology and current treatment trends among team physicians. Arthroscopy 18: 502–509.

Gerbino PG, d'Hemecourt PA (2002). Does football cause an increase in degenerative disease of lumbar spine? Curr Sports Med Rep 1: 47–51.

Kelly BT, Baernes RP, Powell JW, Warren RF (2004). Shoulder injuries to Quarterbacks in the National Football League. Am J Sports Med 32: 328–331.

Meeuwisse WH, Hagel BE, Mohtadi NGH, Butterwick DJ, Fick GH (2000). The distribution of injuries in men's Canada West University football. Am J Sports Med 28: 516–523.

Orchard J (2002). Is there a relationship between ground and climatic conditions and injuries in football? Sports Med 32: 419–432.

Orchard J, Powell JW (2003). Risk of knee and ankle sprain under various weather conditions in American football. Med Sci Sports Exerc 35: 1118–1123.

Pellmann EJ, Powell, JW, Viano DC, Casson IR, Tucker AM, Feuer H, Lovell M, Waecherle JF, Robertson DW (2004). Concussion in professional football: epidemiological features of game injuries and review of the literature. Neurosurgery 54: 81–94.

Siebert CH (2004). Gehirnerschuetterung. In: Siebert CH, Breuer C, Krueger S, Miltner O (eds.). Tipps und Tricks für den Sportmediziner. Thieme-Verlag, Stuttgart.

Tuberville SD, Cowan LD, Owen WL, Asal NR, Andersen MA (2003). Risk factors for injury in high school football players. Am J Sports Med 31: 974–980.

Vereschagin KS, Wiens JJ, Fanton GS (1991). Burners: Don't overlook or underestimate them. Physician Sportsmed 13: 102–114.

Waninger KN (2004). Management of helmeted athlete with suspected cervical spine injury. Am J Sports Med 32: 1331–1349.

Baseball

Hans-Gerd Pieper and Angelika Braun

Even though American Football is often considered to be THE number one American sport, the most popular sport in the USA is actually baseball, even surpassing basketball in popularity.

Various reasons for this have been pointed out (Guttmann 1979, Niedlich 1993).

Baseball has a long tradition in the U.S.A. Today's rules of the game are based on a brochure which was published as early as 1845 by the New York Knickerbockers and authored by Alexander J. Cartwright. They have undergone very little change since then (Waggoner et al. 1990). Baseball thus developed into a national sport long before other sports which are widespread nowadays, such as e.g. soccer, even came into being.

A variant of baseball, i.e. softball, can readily be played even by school children with relatively limited equipment: bats, gloves, and balls. Softball is hence a very popular and widespread school sport.

Baseball lends itself to statistical assessment of player performance – an approach which meets the expectations of the American sports community (Guttmann 1979, Hollander 1989). This has resulted in an abundance of statistical figures extending far beyond the mere game results. For instance, the batting average and the base hits are calculated to the third decimal for each player. Since batter performance is particularly important towards the end of the game, specific batting records starting at the seventh inning are kept (Boeck 2005).

Baseball is among the four most widespread sports in the world and was first recognized as an Olympic discipline in 1988. The first Olympic medals in baseball were awarded in Barcelona in 1992. There are currently about 210 million people worldwide playing baseball or softball.

In Germany, baseball was first introduced on the occasion of the 1936 Olympics as an exhibition event which was attended by more than 100,000 spectators. In the post-war period, Germans perceived baseball primarily as a pastime of the American occupational forces. The first German baseball club, the Frankfurt Juniors, was founded in 1949. Since then, baseball has become popular outside the American military bases, and there is a well-established league structure extending from national to regional level. The number of active members in German baseball and softball clubs has significantly increased during the past 20 years. Whereas there were about 1,000 members enrolled in 30 clubs in 1987, about 28,000 members in 460 clubs were reported in 2008 (DBV homepage 2008).

54.1 Rules of the game

Baseball bears some resemblance to the game of *Schlagball* (rounders) which is well-known in Germany (Niedlich 1993). It is a non-contact sport involving two opposing teams of nine players each. The teams take turns at bat, and the object of the game is to score more runs than the opponent.

In order to score a run, a player has to hit the ball into the field of play and then circle the infield, touching all bases and eventually return to "home base". At the same time, the fielding team tries to prevent this from happening by getting the player "out". This can be achieved by a defensive player catching the ball before it hits the ground or by the defensive player in possession of the ball reaching a base before a runner or by a defensive player touching the runner with the ball.

The infield consists of a diamond with a side length of 27.36 m and a base at each corner. It is bounded by the foul lines (between home base and first and third base) and grass lines (between second base on the one hand and first and third base on the other). The outfield extends beyond the infield, its boundary lines extending beyond first and third base. They have a minimum length of 76 meters and extend up to 98 meters. (➢ Fig. 54.1).

The game consists of nine innings, in which the teams take turns batting (and trying to score runs) and pitching (and defending in the field). The visiting team will generally bat in the first (top) half of an inning. The home team will generally start as the defending team.

Nine player positions are distinguished in the fielding team: pitcher, catcher, first, second, and third baseman, shortstop, left, center and right fielder (outfielders).

The **pitcher** is positioned in the center of the infield on top of a small mound. His task is to throw the ball towards home plate, where the catcher of the fielding team waits to receive it. The pitcher's task is to prevent the batter of the opposing team from scoring a hit (i.e. hitting the ball within the field without being put out) or even a home run (i.e. circling all bases). His pitch has to be inside a certain strike zone in order to give the batter a fair chance to hit the ball. This window is limited horizontally to the area above the home plate (16" wide and reaches from knee height to chest height of the batter. (➢ Fig. 54.2)

Another member of the fielding team, the **catcher**, is located in the so-called catcher's box immediately behind the home plate. The catcher's box measures 11 by 5 feet. His task is to

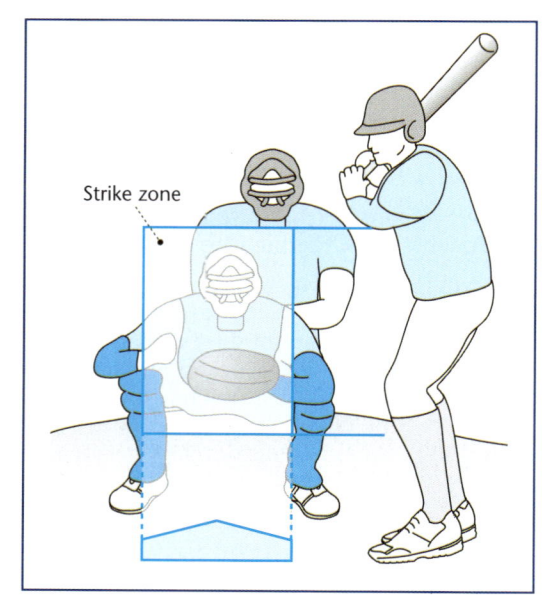

Fig. 54.2 Strike zone, through which the ball has to be thrown.

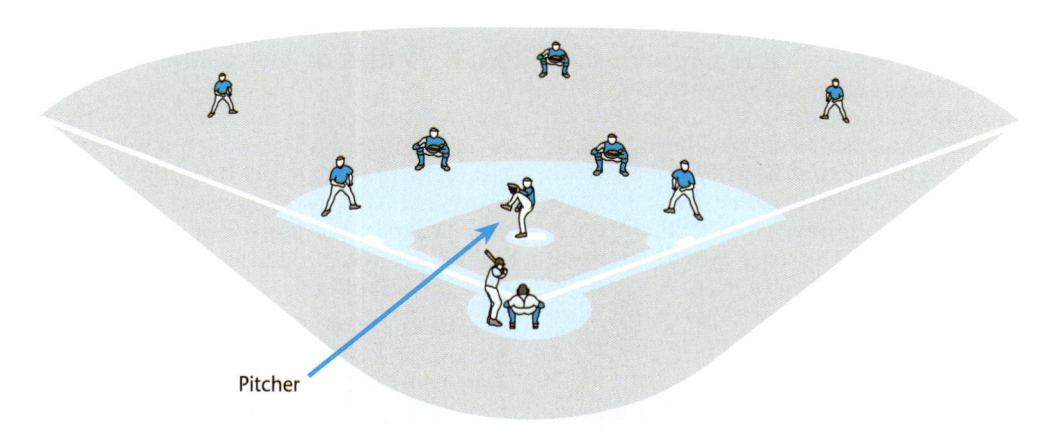

Fig. 54.1 Baseball playing field: positions of the field players in defense and batter.

catch any pitch which is not hit by the batter. As long as he fails to gain control of these balls, base runners will have a chance to advance.

Pitches are delivered until either the batter scores a hit (and becomes a base runner) or the batter misses three pitches which are determined to be inside the strike zone by an umpire, i.e., he strikes out. If, on the other hand, the pitcher fails to place his pitches inside the strike zone four times or hits the batter with his pitch, the batter may advance to first base. This is called a walk. If that base is loaded by another member of the batting team, that team member may advance to second base etc.

Four members of the fielding team cover the infield, one at first, second, and third base each and a shortstop between first and second base. They are called infielders. The outfield is covered by the three remaining players of the fielding team, i.e. the left, center and right fielder.

The goal of the batting team is to score runs. Therefore, the batter will try to hit the ball which has been thrown by the pitcher of the opposing team such that it remains within bounds and is not caught by any player of the fielding team before hitting the ground. If he succeeds, he becomes a base runner whose aim it is to circle the infield, touching all three bases and then to return to home base. The runner needs to reach at least first base in order to stay in the game. He goes on from there when the next batter in line takes his turn. At the same time, the fielding team will try to gain control of the ball and throw it to the respective baseman before the runner reaches that base in order to put him out.

If a batter hits the ball over the outfield boundary yet within the foul lines he will be allowed to circle all four bases and thus score a home run. This implies that all base runners including the batter who has hit the home run will return home and thus score a point each.

From the pitcher's perspective, there are two possibilities: the ball is thrown outside the designated strike zone – in this case a **ball** is called, and the batter is not expected to hit this ball. On the other hand, the pitch may be inside the strike zone, but the batter fails to swing or hit it. This is called a **strike**. The batter has three attempts to hit a ball which is ruled to have been pitched inside the strike zone. If he does not score a hit or if the hit is caught by a member of the receiving team, the batter is put out.

The runners' task is to advance from base to base while the ball is in play, i.e. has been hit by a batter within bounds. If a runner reaches a base before the baseman of the fielding team touches the runner or the base, he is considered safe. If, however, a member of the fielding team touches the runner between bases with the ball, the runner is out. It is important to note in this context that each base can only be occupied by one player, i.e., if a batter is running for first base, his team member occupying first base has to move on to second and so on.

The top of an inning is completed when three members of the batting team have been put out. Subsequently, the bottom of an inning starts with a role reversal, the former receiving team now taking the bat.

The game ends after nine innings have been played or if the home team is ahead after the top of the ninth inning and thus its score can no longer be tied by the visiting team. If the game is tied after nine innings, extra innings are played until one team gains the lead.

54.2 Incidence and pattern of injuries

In recent years the incidence of injuries has increased despite improvements in medical care. Still, baseball is among the sports in which the players are less prone to injuries than others (Conte et al. 2001). Conservative estimates assume about 50000 injuries per year. (Conte et al. 2001). The incidence of injuries per 100 baseball players per year amounts to two in children (Little League) (Hale 1960) and rises to about 58 in the Major League (Garfinkel et al. 1981).

More than half of the injuries (55%) concern the upper extremities (Rowe and Zarins 1981, Collins and Lund 1985, Axe et al. 2001, Conte et al. 2001, Lyman et al. 2002). Shoulder injuries account for 27.8% of all disabled list days in Major League Baseball, followed by elbow injuries (22%; Conte et al. 2001).

When looking at injury patterns it is advisable to consider different player positions separately because they involve different strain patterns and injury risks.

54.2.1 Injuries and overuse syndromes of the pitcher

The pitchers top the injury statistics in all age groups (Axe et al. 2001, Conte et al. 2001, Lyman et al. 2002). A pitcher will carry out about 120 pitches per game at a velocity of up to 170 km/h (Atwater 1979, Collins and Lund 1985, Light 2005, Sain and Andrews 1985). This corresponds to a velocity of about 48 m/s (Elert 2008). In 18 year-old High School pitchers, velocities up to 39.6 m/s were measured (Cooper and Glasgow 1976). The magnitude of the forces exerted on the elbow and shoulder joints will often result in overuse syndromes (➢ Fig. 54.3).

Acute lesions are relatively rare, but they do occur due to the extremely high kinetic energy which may amount to four times the kinetic energy released by throwing a football (Perry 1983). This may result in a spiral fracture of the humeral shaft in adults (Ogawa Yoshida 1998) or a stress reaction of the proximal humeral epiphysial growth plate or a medial epicondylar apophysis (Little Leaguer's Elbow) (Gainor et al. 1980, Collins and Lund 1985, Carson and Gasser 1998).

This high strain in a player's growth years may cause osseous adaptation processes. Thus, an increased retroversion of the humeral head has been observed in the throwing arm of pitchers, resulting in an increased external rotation capacity (Crockett et al. 2002, Osbahr et al. 2002, Reagan et al. 2002). These osseous adaptation processes correspond to those observed in the throwing arm of team handball players (Pieper 1998).

The majority (56%) of the lesions resulting from long periods of overuse are located in the shoulder joint (Barnes and Tullos 1978). However, the so-called "pitcher's shoulder" rarely involves a primary subacromial impingement. Most of the time it consists of a primary instability of the glenohumeral joint which is caused by recurrent microtrauma. This syndrome has likewise been observed in other throwing sports such as javelin or team handball (Pieper et al. 1993, Pieper 1994, Radas et al. 1997). It may cause muscular imbalances and consequently an overstrain of the scapular stabilizers as well as the rotator cuff. The irritation of the rotator cuff is a secondary reaction to muscular overstrain of the infra- and supraspinatus caused by stabilizing the humeral head. The instability may reach a point where a capsulolabral tear takes place (Jobe and Kvitne 1989, Pieper et al. 1994, Andrews et al. 1995, Radas et al. 1997, Pieper 2002).

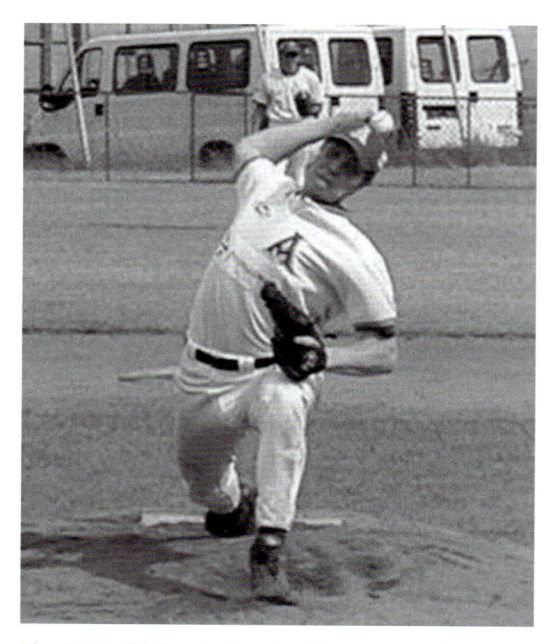

Fig. 54.3 Pitcher during the throw: external rotation of the shoulder and valgus stress of the elbow joint (photograph: Dr. R. Höfel).

Besides the shoulder, the upper arm and the elbow are subject to high acceleration forces during a pitch. In the acceleration stage, the shoulder is jerked forward followed by the upper arm and elbow, while the lower arm and hand stay behind. This involves an enormous valgus strain on the elbow, resulting in an overstrain of the medial elbow muscles (origin of the flexors), the medial collateral ligament, the medial capsule, and the joint itself (Tullos and King 1973, Ellenbecker et al. 1998, Azar et al. 2000, Cain et al. 2003).

This valgus stress presents a problem specifically for young pitchers whose growth plates are not yet ossified. They frequently suffer from a displacement of the medial epicondyle. This syndrome has been termed "Little Leaguer's Elbow" in the medical literature (➤ Chapter 16). In about two thirds of adult professional baseball players posterio-medial osteophytes are found in the olecranon (Azar et al. 2000, Ahmad et al. 2004), and in about one fourth of the cases lesions of the ulnar collateral ligament are observed. About 40% of the players examined showed intraarticular loose bodies (Andrews and Timmermann 1995).

Instabilities of the elbow joint may occur as a consequence of the valgus strain (see above) with recurrent microtrauma (Mirowitz and London 1992) and may eventually result in a valgus deformity (Tulos and King 1973). In 30% of professional pitchers, valgus deformities were observed; more than half of the pitchers studied showed flexion contractures of the elbow joint (King et al. 1069).

54.2.2 Injuries and overuse syndromes of the catcher

The catcher is most prone to injury because his position in the game is close to the batter. By way of protection he wears not only a helmet and facial mask but also protective gear for the chest, groin, and shins. Nonetheless, he may be hit by a foul ball.

The fact that the catcher has to adopt a squatting position for each pitch (i.e. up to 250 times per game) leads to a considerable strain of the extensor system and the patella (➤ Fig. 54.4; Collins and Lund 1985).

The catcher is involved in just about all game actions. That is why physical fitness is particularly important for this game position. He must be able to rise quickly from a squatting position and if necessary even cover first base wearing this protective gear. Extensive sweating may cause dehydration which may, in turn, result in injuries.

54.2.3 Injuries of the fielding team

If two members of the fielding team try to catch a ball, they may collide and thus suffer lesions. Likewise, a baseman may be hurt by a runner who is sliding onto a base (➤ Fig. 54.5).

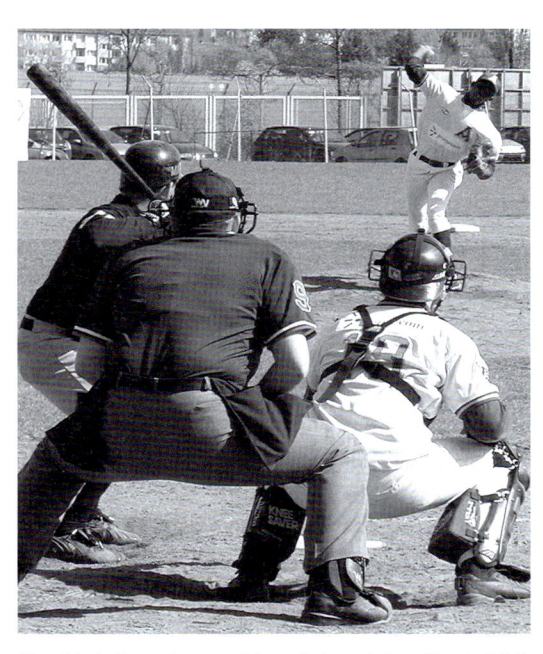

Fig. 54.4 Squatting position of the catcher (front right) during the throw, clothed in heavy protection gear: special strain for patella. Diagonally behind the catcher is the referee, also squatting (umpire of home base).

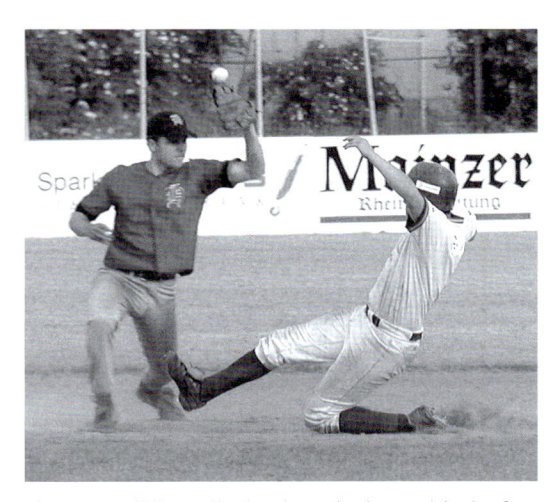

Fig. 54.5 Sliding: slipping into the base with the foot in front: injury risk for the lower extremity of the base man and for knee and ankle joints of the runner (photograph: Dr. R. Höfel).

If the ball to be caught hits the distal interphalangeal joint at high velocity, a tear of the extensor tendons of the fingers may occur. (Gordon 1985).

If an outfielder attempts to catch a ground ball, quick movements or tripping may lead to inversion injury of the ankle or to tears of the hamstrings (Collins and Lund 1985).

54.2.4 Injuries of the batter

If the batter is accidentally hit by a ball pitched at up to 150 km/h, this will, at best, result in contusions and bruises. However, fractures of the hand and lower arm and even mandibular and orbital fractures have also been observed (Johnson 1995).

The batter has to wear a helmet while he is at bat in order to prevent cranial injuries. It may be removed during the run to first base.

54.2.5 Injuries of the runner

In an attempt to make it more difficult to be put out, the runner will seek to present only a small target area when approaching a base. This may involve **sliding** to a base feet-on (**sliding**, ➢ Fig. 54.5) or **diving** towards a base head-on, thus avoiding being touched with the ball by the respective baseman (**diving**, ➢ Fig. 54.6).

Sliding may cause injuries of the ankle or knee joint (McManama and Micheli 1977) irrespective of opposing player contact. **Diving** rather leads to injuries of the **shoulder, neck or head**. The runner's outstretched hand may be **stepped on** as he dives, which constitutes a further cause of injury.

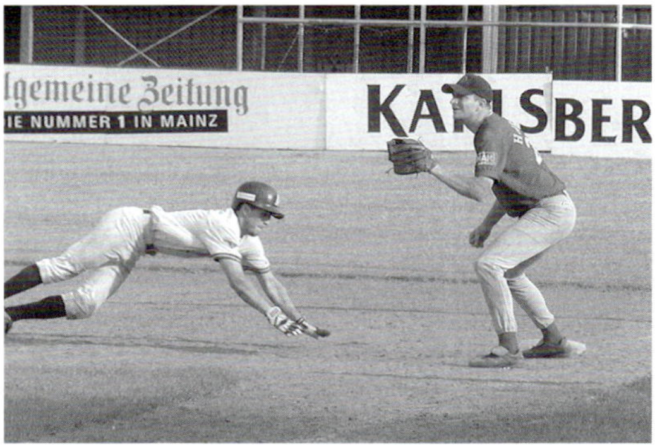

Fig. 54.6 Diving: slipping into the base head or arms first. It is a faster – but also more dangerous – form of gliding with injury risk for head and upper extremities (photograph: Dr. R. Höfel).

54.3 Prevention schemes

Injury prevention is above all achieved by wearing **protective gear**. Helmets are mandatory for the batter and the catcher; the latter must also wear a facial mask, a chest protector, a cup in the athletic support, and shin guards. The fielders wear a cup in the athletic support and a mitt.

Since the focus of the outfielders in particular is entirely on the ball, there is a potential risk that two members of the fielding team may collide or run into the wall/boundary while attempting to catch the ball.

Although a collision with a team mate cannot always be prevented if two players assume responsibility for catching the same ball, it can usually be avoided or at least alleviated by calling out to the team mate. In addition, the distance to the outfield boundary is marked by warning tracks in most ball parks. Hence, collisions with the wall are rare.

Players should try to loosen up well and to keep their musculature warm when not actively engaged in the game. Since the strain on the throwing arm of the pitcher is extreme, it is all the more important to maintain a good pitching technique. This involves a good muscular coordination of the shoulder and elbow joints. In addition, sufficient periods of regeneration between games are of prime importance. In order to achieve this goal there are several pitchers on each team. Thus, they do not have to pitch in each game of the season and usually throw fractions of a game only.

Finally, it would be important to sideline young pitchers whose growth is not complete as soon as they start having problems. Juvenile pitchers should avoid certain types of pitches like curveballs and sliders since they have been found to substantially increase the risk of overuse syndroms in the shoulder and elbow joints (Lyman et al. 2002). Diagnostic measures should include injuries and stress reactions of the growth plates.

References

Ahmad CS, Park MC, El Attrache NS (2004). Elbow medial ulnar collateral ligament insufficiency alters posteromedial olecranon contact. Am J Sports Med 32: 1607–1612.

Andrews JR, Timmermann LA (1995). Outcome of elbow surgery in professional baseball players. Am J Sports Med 23: 407–413.

Andrews JR, Timmermann LA, Wilk KE (1995). Baseball. In: Pettone FA (ed.). Athletic injuries of the shoulder. McGraw-Hill, New York.

Atwater AE (1979). Biomechanics of overarm throwing movements and of throwing injuries. Exerc Sport Sci Rev 7: 43–85.

Axe MJ Wickham R, Snyder-Mackler L (2001). Data-based interval throwing programs for little league, highschool, college, and professional baseball pitchers. Sports Med Arthrosc Rev 9: 24–34.

Azar FM, Andrews JR, Wilk KE, Groh D (2000). Operative treatment of ulnar collateral ligament injuries of the elbow in athletes. Am J Sports Med 28: 16–23.

Barnes DA, Tullos HS (1978). An analysis of 100 symptomatic baseball players. Am J Sports Med 6: 62–67.

Boeck S (2005). New stats are figures of baseball's speech. USA TODAY 09-21-2005: 7C.

Cain EL, Dugas JR, Wolf RS, Andrews JR (2003). Elbow injuries in throwing athletes: a current concepts review. Am J Sports Med 31: 321–635.

Carson WG, Gasser SI (1998). Little leaguer's shoulder. A report of 23 cases. Am J Sports Med 26: 575–580.

Collins HR, Lund D (1985). Baseball injuries. In: Schneider RC, Kennedy JC, Plant ML (eds.). Sports Injuries. Mechanisms, Prevention and Treatment. Williams & Wilkins, Baltimore-London-Sydney.

Collins HR (1985). The treatment of shoulder and elbow trauma in the athlete. In: Schneider RC, Kennedy JC, Plant ML (eds.). Sports Injuries. Mechanisms, Prevention and Treatment. Williams & Wilkins, Baltimore-London-Sydney.

Conte S, Requa RK, Garrick JG (2001). Disability days in major league baseball. Am J Sports Med 29: 431–436,

Cooper JM, Glassow RB (1976). Kinesiology. 4th ed. Mosby, St. Louis.

Crocket HC, Gross LB, Wilk KE, Schwarz ML, Reed J, O'Mara J, Reilly MT, Dugas JR, Meister K, Lyman S, Andrews JR (2002). Osseous adaption and range of motion at the glenohumeral joint in professional baseball pitchers. Am J Sports Med 30: 20–26.

Deutscher Baseball & Softball Verband e.V. (2008). http://www.baseball-softball.de/dbv (state: 08-04-2008).

Elert G (2008). Speed of the fastest pitched baseball. http://hypertextbook.com/facts/2000/LoriGrabel.shtml (state: 08-04-2008).

Ellenbecker TS, Mattalino AJ, Elam EA, Caplinger RA (1998). Medial elbow joint laxity in professional baseball pitchers. A bilateral comparison using stress radiography. Am J Sports Med 26: 420–424.

Gainor BJ, Piotrowski G, Puhl J, Allen WC, Hagen R (1980). The throw: Biomechanics and acute injury. Am J Sports Med 8: 114–118.

Garfinkel D, Talbot AA, Clarizio M, et al. (1981). Medical problems on a professional baseball team. Physician Sportsmed 9: 85–93.

Gordon JC (1985). Baseball. In: Pförringer W, Rosemeyer B, Bär HW (eds.). Sport, Trauma und Belastung. Perimed, Erlangen.

Guttmann A (1979). Vom Ritual zum Rekord. Das Wesen des modernen Sports. Hoffmann Verlag, Schondorf.

Hale CJ (1960). Injuries among 771,810 little league baseball players. J Sports Med Phys Fit 1: 80–83.

Hollander Z (ed.) (1989). The Complete Handbook of Baseball. Signet, New York.

Jobe FW, Kvitne RS (1989). Shoulder pain in the overhand or throwing athlete. The relationship of anterior instability and rotator cuff impingement. Orthop Rev 18: 963–975.

Johnson C (1995). Hard-hitting afternoon. Pucket takes pitch in face; Myers, fan fight. USA TODAY, Sep 29, 1995, 4C.

King JW, Brelsford HJ, Tullos HS (1969). Analysis of the pitching arm of the professional baseball pitcher. Clin Orthop 67: 116–123.

Light JF (2005). The Cultural Encyclopedia of Baseball. 2nd ed. McFarland & Company Inc. Publisher, North Carolina, 312–314.

Lyman S, Fleisig GS, Andrews JR, Osinki ED (2002). Effect of pitch type, pitch count, and pitching mechanics on risk of elbow and shoulder pain in youth baseball pitchers. Am J Sports Med 30: 463–468.

McManama GB, Micheli LJ (1977). The incidence of sport-related epiphyseal injuries in adolescents. Med Sci Sports 9: 57–60.

Mirowitz SA, London SL (1992). Ulnar collateral ligament injury in baseball pitchers: MR imaging evaluation. Radiology 185: 573–576.

Niedlich D (1993). Handbuch für Baseball. Meyer & Meyer, Aachen.

Ogawa K, Yoshida A (1998). Throwing fracture of the humeral shaft. An analysis of 90 patients. Am J Sports Med 26: 242–246.

Osbahr DC, Cannon DL, Speer KP (2002). Retroversion of the humerus in the throwing shoulder of college baseball pitchers. Am J Sports Med 30: 347–353.

Perry J (1983). Anatomy and biomechanics of the shoulder in throwing, swimming, gymnastics, and tennis. Clin Sports Med 2: 247–270.

Pieper HG, Quack G, Krahl H (1993). Impingement of the rotator cuff in athletes caused by instability of the shoulder joint. Knee Surg Sports Traumatol Arthroscopy 1: 97–99.

Pieper HG (1994). Supraspinatussyndrom des Sportlers? Differenzierte Therapieansätze bei chronischen Schulterschmerzen des Überkopfsportlers. In: Jerosch J, Steinbeck J (eds.). Aktuelle Konzepte der Diagnostik und Therapie des instabilen Schultergelenkes. Shaker, Aachen.

Pieper HG, Pöhlmann J, Quack G, Krahl H (1994). Secondary subacromial syndrome in overhead sports caused by instability of the shoulder joint. J Shoulder Elbow Surg 3, Suppl. 32.

Pieper HG (1998). Humeral torsion in the throwing arm of handball players. Am J Sports Med 26: 247–253.

Pieper HG (2002). Überlastungen des Schultergelenks und Fehlbelastungsfolgen am Ellenbogen. Sportorthop Sporttraumatol 18: 241–244.

Radas CB, Pieper HG, Quack G, Krahl H (1997). Schulterengpass-Syndrom des Überkopfsportlers – primäres oder sekundäres Subakromialsyndrom? Dtsch Z Sportmed 48: 379–384.

Reagan KM, Meister K, Horodyski MB, Werner DW, Caruthers C, Wilk K (2002). Humeral retroversion and its relationship to glenohumeral rotation in the shoulder joint of college baseball players. Am J Sports Med 30: 354–360.

Rowe CR, Zarins B (1981). Recurrent transient subluxation of the shoulder. J Bone Joint Surg 63-A: 863–872.

Sain J, Andrews JR (1985). Proper pitching techniques. In: Zarins B, Andrews JR, Carson WG (eds.). Injuries to the Throwing Arm. WB Saunders, Philadelphia.

Tullos HS, King JW (1973). Throwing mechanism in sports. Orthop Clin North Am 4: 709–720.

Waggoner G, Moloney K, Howard H (1990). Baseball by the Rules. New York.

55 Basketball

Christian H. Siebert

55.1 The Game

Since the inception in the U.S., basketball has won friends all over the world. Even in the hidden corners of Asia this sport has it´s fans (Wolff 2002). In 1994, "Newsweek" spoke of "Global Ball" on its cover. Basketball fans can look back on more than 100 years of "hoop history".

Basketball in its modern form was developed by Dr. James Naismith, a teacher at Springfield College, Massachusetts, U.S.A., in **1891**. Senda Berenson adapted the rules and introduced **women's basketball** as early as **1892**. In 1932, the Fédération Internationale de Basketball Amateur (**FIBA**) was founded in Geneva as the world federation for this sport. The first Olympic basketball tournament for men was carried out in Berlin in 1936. Women's basketball was introduced as a discipline during the Olympic Games in Montreal in 1976. Since the Olympic Games of 1992 and the spectacular performances of the first American "Dream Team", basketball has experienced an ongoing boom. Presently, basketball is one of the most common sports in the world with a number of professional leagues of both genders.

The basic concept of basketball reminds of elements dating back to **the Incas and Aztecs**. Two teams compete and try to place the ball in the opponent's basket, while at the same time one´s own basket protecting against the opposing offense. Nowadays, one has to differentiate between the classic **five-against-five basketball**, which is primarily played in gyms and on all-weather courts, **street ball** with three competing against three and **beach basketball**. In addition, **wheelchair basketball** has become very popular.

Basketball places complex demands on the players. The **main motor skills** are to be found in the fields of **endurance, strength, speed** and **coordinative capabilities** (Weineck and Hass 1999). The **main precondition** for a successful player is sound basic basketball skills.

The game is played on a court with a size of 26 × 14 m with a ball weighing 510–650 g, depending on the gender, or of a size of 724–780 mm (circumference). The baskets are placed at the front ends of the court; they consist of a vertical backboard that is equipped with a hoop of 45 cm diameter at the height of 3.05 m above the ground. The backboard is placed into the field, 1.20 m away from the end of the court (DBB 2008).

The foul line is 4.60 m and the three-point arc 6.25 m from the basket (➤ Fig. 55.1). The most important **technical elements** are passing, catching and dribbling of the ball, as well as the shot on basket. The **rapid change between offensive and defensive actions** is characteristic for this team sport.

> Basketball requires endurance, strength, speed and coordinative capabilities.

55.2 Injury patterns

Antiquated theories defining basketball as a non-contact sport have made way for an athletic, fast moving game with a **lot of body contact** and **high injury rates**. The injury rates for children and adolescents, are surprisingly high (Meeuwisse et al. 2003). Despite the development of this sport, there has been no significant change in the injury distribution over the

Tab. 55.1 Literature comparison of injury topography (data in percent).

Author (year of publication)	Head	Upper extremity	Trunk	Lower extremity
Samek (1965)	9.8	24.3	1.3	64.5
Riel and Bernett (1989)	2	22	2	74
Pfeiffer et al. (1992)	11.1	19.8	3.8	65.3
Raschka et al. (1995)	4.7	23.5	1.6	70.4
Gomez et al. (1996)	7	15.5	7	68
Siebert et al. (1997)	9.5	25.3	4.9	60.3
Messina et al. (1999)	11.2	15	7.1	66.1
Meeuwisse et al. (2003)	10.5	13.8	6.7	69
Knobloch et al. (2005) (German school sports)	5.4	65.6	0.7	28.2
Deitch et al. (2006) NBA/WNBA	11.5/10.7	14.8/15.1	8.7/7.4	64.6/65.7
Agel et al. (2007)	14.7	14.1	7.4	60.8

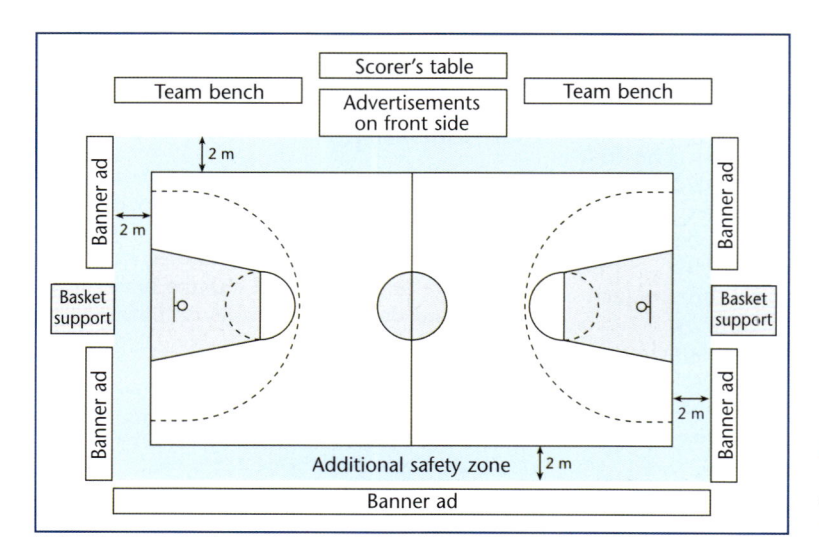

Fig. 55.1 FIBA playing field. Gray area around the basket (⊦○) represents the free-throw area (DBB 2008).

last decades (➤ Tab. 55.1). In various surveys, the injury rate varies between 2.1 and 18.2 injuries per 1000 basketball outings (athlete exposures; Meeuwisse 2003).

Injuries occur primarily under the basket during **rebound work**. Because of the attempt to keep the opponent away from the backboard and thus from rebounding the ball, body contact occurs often, so that a secure landing after jumping for the ball cannot always be guaranteed. Therefore, **most injuries** on the court occur **close to the basket** (in-the-paint; ➤ Fig. 55.1). This also explains the increased risk of injury for the **centers** (Siebert et al. 1997, Meeuwisse et al. 2003, Kotofolis and Kellis 2007).

55.2 Injury patterns

A **frequent cause of injury** is the contact with another player (1.8 injuries in 1000 exposures, 44%; Meeuwisse et al. 2003). In general, most injuries will occur during league games (Siebert et al. 1997, Messina et al. 1999, Rechel et al. 2008), so that the sports medical support should be concentrated here (➢ Fig. 55.2).

Sports injuries have been described mainly as sprains or **capsule/ligament injuries** (62%) by the affected players, while **fractures** represent only approximately 10% of the total amount of injuries. The acute capsule/ligament injuries occurred primarily in the region of the **ankle joint**, followed by the **knee**.

Dislocations were found mainly in the finger and **shoulder joints**. **Fractures** have been localized most often in the region of the **hands**, followed by the foot and nose (Siebert et al. 1997). Though basketball involves many elements that are carried out overhead, injuries of the shoulder region are an exception (Siebert et al. 2006). Compared to other team sports, dental injuries appear quite often with 10.6 per 100 male players in one season (Cohenca et al. 2007).

> Sport injuries in basketball mostly occur in the area of the ankle, while chronic problems are frequently found in the knee joint.

Overuse injuries, on the other hand, occur with more than 50% in the **region of the knee joint** (➢ Fig. 55.3, Siebert 2004). Among the sport-specific impairments, **jumper's knee** – the painful tendinopathy of the proximal or distal patella, deserves a special mention. Up to 55% of all basketball players report a history

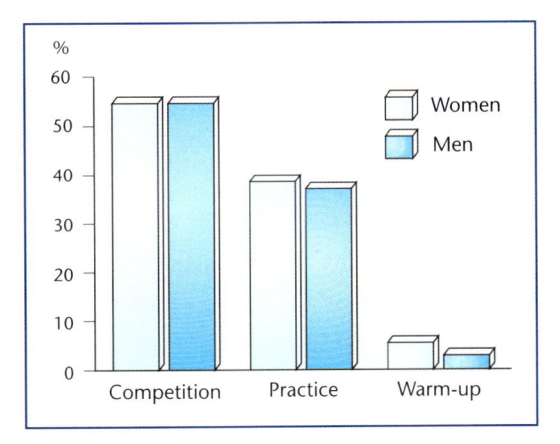

Fig. 55.2 Time of injury in basketball.

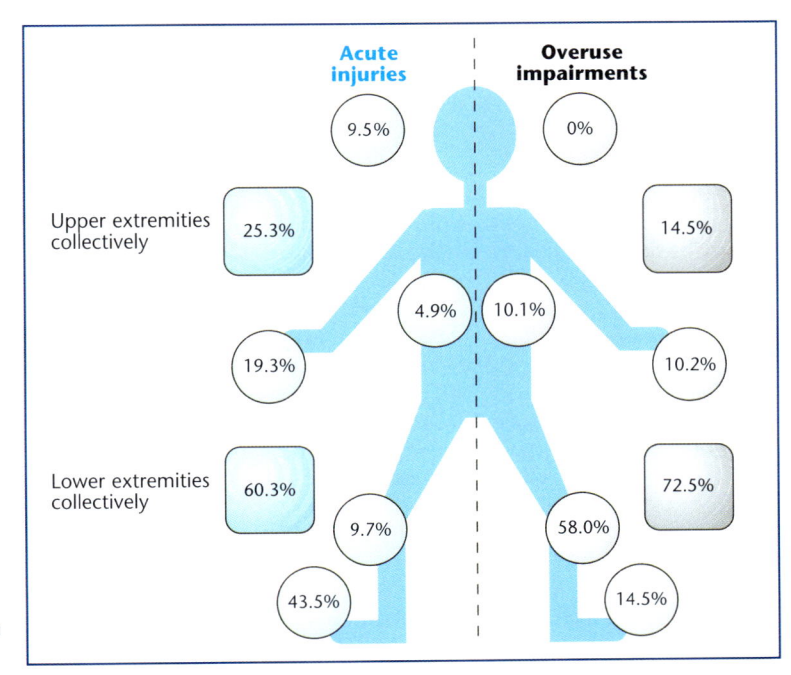

Fig. 55.3 Injury distribution (body regions) in basketball.

and approximately 30% present with clinical symptoms. Men suffer from this knee conditions twice as often as women (Lian et al. 2005). The incidence increases depending on the quality of the playing surface – the harder the ground, the more knee problems will occur (Lian et al. 2005). The high **strain on the patellar tendon** caused by basketball can lead to **structural changes** that can be documented by ultrasound and affect almost every fourth player (Cook et al. 2000). **Fatigue fractures** are primarily found in the region of the foot and prevalently in the area of the fifth metatarsal bone (Guettler et al. 2006, Agel et al. 2007).

> Almost every third player has problems in the region of the patella (jumper's knee), especially if they play on concrete.

Basketball leads the injury statistics in German school sports ahead of soccer with 59.5% of all registered injuries in Lower Saxony. In contrast to other published papers reporting on basketball players, injuries of the upper extremity, especially finger injuries (60.6%), are documented most often in this subpopulation of young players (> Tab. 55.1). In 53% of the cases, deficits during ball handling lead to the injury. Proprioceptive and technical weaknesses of German students, who are still unaccustomed to this sport, are made responsible for this uncommon injury distribution (Knobloch et al. 2005).

An injury risk of 0.4% an hour per athlete or of 49% per season has been reported for high-school basketball players in the U.S.A., and thus is comparable to football (Gomez et al. 1996). An **injury rate for the anterior cruciate ligament** has been documented as one every 952 basketball exposures for men, while such an injury appeared every 247 basketball outings in women. Therefore, the ACL injury rate in female basketball players is four times higher than in the male colleagues, although the general rate of injuries does not show any significant differences (Arendt and Dick 1995, Messina et al. 1999). The comparison of National Basketball Association (NBA) versus Women's NBA (WNBA) players documents differences in the injury frequency (19.3/1000 exposures NBA; 24.9/1000 exposures WNBA) (Deitch et al. 2006). In addition to these gender-specific aspects, a difference between races could also be discovered in the WNBA, with white European-American players being especially at risk of rupturing their anterior cruciate ligament (Trojian and Collins 2006).

> The injury risk in basketball is documented with 0.4% an hour or 2–25 injuries in 1000 basketball exposures.

Abrasions, e.g. after impact on wood surfaces, as well as lacerations, above all in the facial area, and contusions are in the forefront of all **skin and soft-tissue injuries**. Treatment of **hemorrhaging wounds** is required by the rulebook, before play can be continued (sect. 5.6, DBB 2008). **Tetanus vaccination** for the players should to be provided.

Typical sport-specific injuries in basketball

Lower extremity
Hip, thigh/lower leg
- ankle joint (supination trauma with injury of the lateral ligaments)
- muscle injury, primarily thigh ("charley horse")
- knee sprain, internal knee disorders
- anterior knee pain syndrome caused in part by the typical body position on defense
- functional compartment syndrome of the lower leg
- enthesopathies

Foot
- subungual hematomas
- blisters
- fatigue fractures, especially in the area of the midfoot.

Upper extremity
Shoulder, humerus/forearm
- muscle lesions in the region of the shoulder
- tendinitis of the long biceps tendon
- separation of the acromioclavicular joint
- instability impingement
- bursitis

Hand
- finger dislocations, mainly in the area of the DIP and PIP joints of the long fingers
- fractures in the region of the metacarpus and the fingers
- capsule/ligament injuries

Head
- fractures of the nose (mostly caused by the opponent's elbow)
- dental injuries (elbow or head of the opponent)
- lacerations
- commotio cerebri (rare)

Trunk

Spine
- painful limitations of mobility, especially in the region of the thoracolumbar junction and lumbar spine, frequently caused by overuse
- dysfunction of the sacroiliac joint
- contusions.

55.3 Supination injuries of the ankle joint

The supination trauma or sprain of the ankle joint is the most frequent type of sport-specific injury in basketball. Ankle injuries have been described in basketball players (6 times more often than in athletes in general) in rates of up to 89.4% during a 6-year career (Pfeiffer et al. 1992, Raschka et al. 1995). The injury rate in female basketball players is even higher (Ottaviani et al. 2001). A significant gender-specific difference with regard to muscle strength of the ankle evertors and invertors could not be verified after accounting for body weight and size (Ottaviani et al. 2001). Therefore, the accumulation of supination trauma in female basketball players does not seem to be attributed to neuromuscular deficits (Agel et al. 2005).

Ankle injuries occur 3–6.5 times every 1000 basketball exposures; a rate that is up to 6 times higher than in sports in general.

American military cadets suffered 46 ankle joint injuries in the course of 13430 basketball games and practices or 3.4 injuries in 1000 exposures (Sitler et al. 1994). Within the scope of this study, a control group suffered 5.2 injuries of the ankle joint in 1000 exposures, while the **prophylactic use of an ankle orthesis** (Aircast Stirrup®) was able to reduce the rate to 1.6/1000. The orthosis found acceptance by 70% of these players, even though complaints regarding comfort of wear and a limitation in performance were documented (Sitler et al. 1994). Other authors have described frequencies of the 6.5 supination injuries in 1000 games with the use of **tape plus high top shoes** and 33.4 injuries in 1000 basketball games without external stabilizers and with low shoes (Karlsson and Andreasson 1992). The prophylactic efficiency of tape and ortheses seems to be due in part to the **stimulation of the proprioceptors** (Barrett et al. 1993, Shapiro et al. 1994, Ratschka et al. 1995).

In addition, the passive resistance against an inversion movement in the upper ankle joint is increased significantly due to the **use of high-top shoes** in contrast to low sport shoes (Ottaviani 2001). Even though the majority of studies regarding this topic have crucial methodical weaknesses, the high-top seems to improve the efficiency of ortheses and tape (Karlsson and Andreasson 1992, Shapiro et al. 1994, Handoll et al. 2001). Because ortheses have a similar positive influence on the region of the ankle joint as tapes, but are easier to use, can be readjusted and are almost two thirds cheaper over the duration of one season, they are frequently preferred to tape application (Shapiro et al. 1994, Sitler et al. 1994, Olmsted et al. 2004, Kofotolis and Kellis 2007).

The most effective injury prophylaxis is an **improvement of the muscular stabilization** of the ankle joints in form of the so-called **physiological taping** (Raschka et al. 1995, Thacker et al. 1999). **Muscle strengthening** and **proprioceptive training** are recommended, especially during the off-season.

Players with pre-existing injuries of the ankle joint have an increased risk of injury. Muscle strengthening, proprioceptive training and ortheses are sensible prophylactic measures.

Since a **pre-existing ankle joint injury is regarded as a significant risk factor** for a renewed supination trauma, prophylactic measures should be adopted for this subgroup (Thacker et al. 1999, Kofotolis and Kellis 2007). As part of a "need-to-treat" analysis, it was found that 26 athletes with a previously injured ankle joint had to be taped or 18 treated with ortheses in order to prevent one acute supination trauma.

In contrast, 5 or 2 times, respectively, as many basketball players with healthy ankle joints will have to be treated in order to be just as successful (Olmsted et al. 2004).

Therefore, **proprioceptive training** with stretching of the calf muscles, strengthening of the peroneal musculature and **stabilizing measures** using tape, ortheses or high-top shoes are recommended for athletes with impaired ankle joints (Barrett et al. 1993). These measures should be implemented for up to 6 months following an acute sprain (Thacker et al. 1999).

A return to sports following such an injury should be permitted only after a successful rehabilitation. In the course of reintegration of the injured athlete, close attention should be paid to **fatigue**, because it will further increase the risk of injury (Thacker et al. 1999).

55.4 Sport-medical aspects

The medical team should be aware of the **causes of injuries that can be influenced prior to game time**. Almost 10% of the causes can be classified as **environmental** (Siebert et al. 1997). This includes poor playing surfaces, low temperature in the gym, insufficient safety zones, bad equipment and reduced practice times that inhibit the incorporation of a warm-up or cool-down. Season preparation and practice forms need to be scrutinized in order to prevent injuries (Agel et al. 2007). These deficits lie in the responsibility of the organizers and team attendants and are frequently easily corrected. Attention must be paid on behalf of the players to the observance of the safety distance of 5 m to the audience and 2 m to the advertisement boards from the respective sideline (➤ Fig. 55.1; DBB 2008).

The **checking of fingernail length** and the **removal of jewelry**, which is occasionally missed by the referees and during practice, deserves to be pointed out as well. A significant **fluid depletion must be avoided** in the course of basketball exposures, especially since the shooting accuracy is decreased by dehydration (Baker et al. 2007). A sufficient supply of tape and bandaging material should be ensured. **Mouthpieces and sports goggles** should also be discussed as further sport-medical preventive measures (Raschka et al. 1995, Cohenca et al. 2007).

> The support team needs to provide for fluid substitution and the elimination of avoidable causes of injury.

A **warm-up and stretching program** is carried out by the basketball players before the game and during half-time, but is often neglected prior to player substitution. Unplanned, acute substitutions without a proper warm-up phase represent an increased risk of muscle lesions. Space and time must be provided for the warm-up before the game, but also before substitutions.

Shoes with low friction resistance soles and proper ground conditions seem to additionally reduce the number of injuries of the lower extremity (Raschka et al. 1995, Thacker et al. 1999). Torsion stiffness of the sport shoe adapted to the body weight of the player will also provide an advantage (Graumann et al. 2007).

> The prophylaxis for ankle joint injuries can be realized with the help a modified training program combined with an orthesis and appropriate basketball shoes.

References

Agel J, Arendt EA, Bershadsky B (2005). Anterior cruciate ligament injury in national collegiate athletic association basketball and soccer. Am J Sports Med 33: 524–530.

Agel J, Olson DE, Dick R, Arendt EA, Marshall SW, Sikka RS (2007). Descriptive epidemiology of collegiate women's basketball injuries. J Athl Train 42: 202–210.

Arendt E, Dick R (1995). Knee injury patterns among men and women in collegiate basketball and soccer. Am J Sports Med 23: 694–701.

Baker LB, Dougherty KA, Chow M, Kenney WL (2007). Progressive dehydration causes a progressive decline in basketball skills performance. Med Sci Sports Exerc 39: 1114–1123.

Barrett JR, Tanji JL, Drake C, Fuller D, Kawasaki RI, Fenton RM (1993). High- versus low-top shoes for the prevention of ankle sprains in basketball players. Am J Sports Med 21: 582–590.

Cohenca N, Roges RA, Roges R (2007). The incidence and severity of dental trauma in intercollegiate athletes. J Am Dent Assoc 138: 1121–1126.

Cook JL, Khan KM, Kiss ZS, Purdam CR, Griffith L (2000). Prospective imaging study of asymptomatic patellar tendinopathy in elite junior basketball players. J Ultrasound Med 19: 473–79.

Deitch JR, Starkey C, Walters SL, Moseley JB (2006). Injury risk in professional basketball players. Am J Sports Med 34: 1077–1083.

Deutscher Basketball Bund (2008). Offizielle Basketball-Regeln fuer Männer und Frauen – Internationaler Basketballverband (FIBA). Badenia Verlag, Karlsruhe.

Gomez E, DeLee JC, Farney WC (1996). Incidence of injury in Texas girls high school basketball. Am J Sports Med 24: 684–687.

Graumann L, Walther M, Krabbe B, Kleindienst F (2007). Sportverletzungen der unteren Extremitaet im Basketball in Abhaengigkeit von der Torsionssteifigkeit des Sportschuhs. Sportorthop Sporttraumatol 23: 174–177.

Guettler JH, Ruskan GJ, Bytomski JR, Brown CR, Richardson JK, Moorman CT (2006). Fifth metatarsal fractures in elite basketball players. Am J Orthop 35: 532–536.

Handoll HH, Rowe BH, Quinn KM, de Bie R (2001). Interventions for preventing ankle ligament injuries. Cochrane Database Syst Rev 3: CD000018.

Karlsson J, Andreasson GO (1992). The effect of external ankle support in chronic lateral ankle joint instability. Am J Sports Med 20: 257–261.

Knobloch K, Rossner D, Jagodzinski M, Zeichen J, Gössing T, Richter M, Krettek C (2005). Basketballverletzungen im Schulsport. Dtsch Z Sportmed 56: 96–99.

Kofotolis N, Kellis E (2007). Ankle sprain injuries. J Athl Train 42: 388–394.

Lian OB, Engebretsen L, Bahr R (2005). Prevalence of jumper's knee among elite athletes from different sports. Am J Sports Med 33: 561–567.

Mellerowicz H, Matussek J, Wilke S, Leier T, Asamoah V (2000). Sportverletzungen und Sportschäden im Kindes- und Jugendalter. Dtsch Z Sportmed 51: 78–84.

Messina DF, Farney WC, DeLee JC (1999). The incidence of injuries in Texas high school basketball. Am J Sports Med 27: 294–299.

Meeuwisse WH, Sellmer R, Hagel BE (2003). Rates and risks of injury during intercollegiate basketball. Am J Sports Med 31: 379–385.

Olmsted LC, Vela LI, Denegar CR, Hertel J (2004). Prophylactic ankle taping and bracing. J Athl Train 39: 95–100.

Ottaviani RA, Ashton-Miller JA, Wojtys EM (2001). Inversion and eversion strengths in the weight-bearing ankle of young women. Am J Sports Med 29: 219–225.

Pfeiffer JP, Gast W, Pfoerringer W (1992). Traumatologie und Sportschaden im Basketball. Sportverl Sportschaden 6: 91–100.

Raschka C, Glaeser H, de Marees H (1995). Unfallhergangstypen und Vorschläge zu ihrer Prävention im Basketball. Sportverl Sportschaden 9: 84–91.

Rechel JA, Yard EE, Comstock D (2008). An epidemiologic comparison of high school sports injuries sustained in practice and competition. J Athl Train 43: 197–204.

Riel KA, Bernett P (1989). Sportverletzungen und Ueberlastungssyndrome im Frauenbasketball. Prakt Sporttrauma Sportmed 4: 8–13.

Samek L (1965). Unfaelle und Unfallverhuetung im Basketball. Med Sport 5: 160–164.

Shapiro MS, Kabo JM, Mitchell PW, Loren G, Tsenter M (1994). Ankle sprain prophylaxis: an analysis of the stabilizing effects of braces and tape. Am J Sports Med 22: 78–82.

Siebert CH, Bach R, Hansis M (1997). Verletzungsmuster im deutschen Basketball – Gedanken zur Präventivmedizin. Sportorthop Sporttraumatol 13: 168–172.

Siebert CH, Bach R, Miltner O (1999). Injury prevention in German Basketball. Int J Sports Med 20, Suppl 110.

Siebert CH (2004). Orthopaedische Checkliste: Basketball. Sportorthop Sporttraumatol Special Issue (2004): 2–3.

Siebert CH, Philips B, Hagemann L, Behra A, Kaufmann MM (2006). Basketball als Überkopfsportart – Verletzungsmuster im Bereich des Schultergürtels. Sportorthop Sporttraumatol 22: 212–216.

Sitler M, Ryan J, Wheeler B, McBride J, Arceiro R, Anderson J, Horodyski MB (1994). The efficacy of a semirigid ankle stabilizer to reduce acute injuries in basketball. Am J Sports Med 22: 454–461.

Thacker SB, Stroup DF, Branche CM, Gilchrist J, Goodmann RA, Weitman EA (1999). The prevention of ankle sprains in sports. Am J Sports Med 27: 753–757.

Trojian TH, Collins S (2006). The anterior cruciate ligament tear varies by race in professional women's basketball. Am J Sports Med 34: 895–898.

Weineck J, Haas H (1999). Optimales Basketballtraining. Spitta Verlag GmbH, Balingen.

Wolff A (2002). Big game, small world. Warner Books, New York.

Chapter 56 Beach soccer

Thomas Schwamborn and Andreas Gösele-Koppenburg

Beach soccer has been played in official competitions for more than 40 years, especially in South America. This sport experienced a first great boom in 1992 with the introduction of the pro-beach soccer series in the U.S.A. In the following year, the first international large tournament took place in Miami. The U.S.A., Brazil, Argentina and Italy were the participating teams and attracted an audience of more than 10,000 people. Beach soccer has spread all over the world also because of its media attractiveness and has shown double-figure growth rates every year, especially in Europe. In addition to national championships that are directed by the national federations, European and world championships with a qualification mode are carried out every year. Beach soccer has found its place under the roof of the FIFA since 2005. The organization of the world championship is carried out by the world soccer association, which allows an increasing professional and higher level of playing.

The development of beach soccer seen in the example of Switzerland underlines the quick progression. Although the national team had only played five tournaments in foreign countries in 2002, they have already participated in 12 international tournaments in 2008. Likewise, there is an enormous growth regarding the licensed players from 2,500 athletes at first in 2002 to more than 16,000 athletes in 2008. Parallel to this development, the attention of the media all over Europe has increased. Television broadcasts are not only shown by regional or national societies, but also by international cooperating TV stations spread all over the globe.

56.1 Sport-specific characteristics

Beach soccer is marked by **very fast and dynamic, diversified actions with frequent scoring scenes**. On average, a completion is performed every 30 sec. In general, beach soccer and traditional field soccer are only connected by the keynote of two teams competing in playing the ball and the winner being determined by the number of scores. There are immense differences regarding the **frame conditions**, such as field size, ground, and number of players, technical capacities and preconditions of the athletes or even the clothing.

56.1.1 Clothing

The players wear only **sport shorts** and a **tricot**; **shoes are not allowed**. Elastic support and bandages, e.g. ankle guards or tape bandages, are permitted. Shin protectors, as are common in field soccer, are not in use. Only flexible materials are allowed. Though the wearing of stocking-like protectors for the feet is permit-

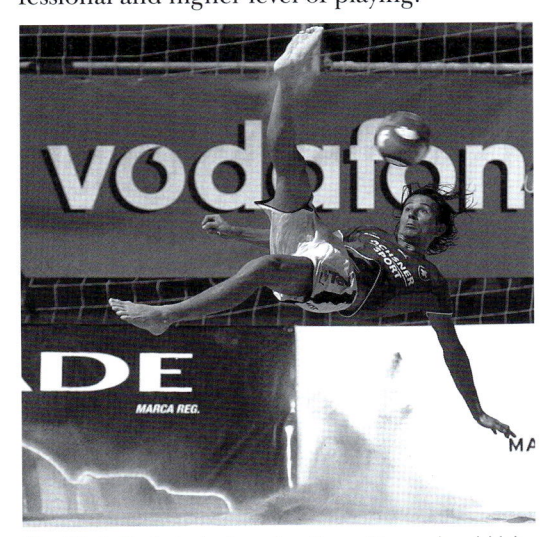

Fig. 56.1 Typical playing situation with overhead kick.

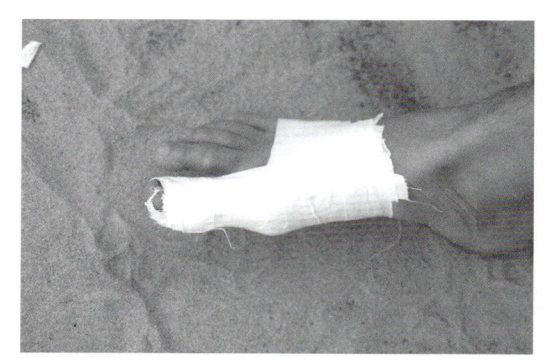

Fig. 56.2 Tape treatment after distortion of the hallux.

ted, these neoprene protectors have not established themselves internationally. They are mainly used temporarily after foot or toe injuries.

Hard or rigid materials, such as plaster casts or ortheses must not be worn because of the potential risk for the opponents. **Face masks or stabilizing splints, for example after fractures of the nasal bone, can be used**. The **goalkeeper** may wear **gloves**, which is used with only few exceptions.

Rings, necklaces or piercings are forbidden in the games and must be removed before the beginning of the game; the referee will check this.

Thus, the players are only sparsely protected, which implies consequences for the frequency and type of injuries.

56.1.2 Special risks

Beach soccer is a typical outdoor sport and is mostly performed in the open at high sun intensity and often combined with high outdoor temperatures. Training or competition is carried out at indoor conditions only in winter. A sufficient sun protection has to be provided because of the partly extreme weather influences. **Burned skin** or **heatstroke** is often found in inexperienced athletes. There is clearly an increased **risk of skin cancer** in outdoor athletes because of the considerable UV exposition (Moehrle 2008). A **sufficient sun protection with waterproof sun lotions** is mandatory. It has to be paid attention to the players remaining in the **shadow** and wearing a **headgear** and **sun glasses** in the game breaks and rests. In addition, there is also an immensely **increased fluid demand** that exceeds the general measurement of other sports. The athletes must be informed about the necessity of the sufficient intake of fluids, especially at tournaments and under midsummer conditions.

Cooling showers and the applying of iced towels in the game breaks as well as between the games are recommended in order to support a fast regeneration.

56.2 Injuries

The sport-specific injury patterns and overstrain impairments differ from soccer on. This has an important influence on the basic training of the athletes, on the one hand, and on the prophylaxis for the minimization of sport-specific injuries and improper loads, on the other hand.

Hitherto, no statistics exist worldwide regarding the injury frequency and injury patterns. Only individual case reports are found in current literature.

56.2.1 Musculature

Muscle injuries in beach soccer often base on a direct traumatizing by **contusions**, but also on indirect force effects with local overstrain of the muscle structures, such as **strains**, fiber lesions or even **complete muscle ruptures**. Injuries of the muscles are the domain of conservative treatment; surgical interventions are only seldom necessary.

In addition to the immediate measures of cooling, compression and analgesia, relaxing measures promoting the resorption of hematomas are recommended. The correct diagnosis with exact determining of the actual extent of the injury is elementary. In addition to the clinical examination, also MRI and especially sonography are of great significance. A composition of loads adapted to the biological healing phases is necessary.

56.2.2 Head and face

Because of the high dueling activity, collisions with the opponent often lead to injuries of the head, as well. Impact on the head occur by hand, elbow, shoulder, foot, triggered by overhead and overhead sidekick. **Contusions** and **contused lacerations** occur, and also **fractures of the nasal bone** and very rarely **fractures of the zygomatic bone** are seen. Despite missing tooth protection – mandatory in martial arts and ice hockey – traumatologic dental problems occur only rarely. The contusio or commotio cerebri is seldom found, compared to field soccer. Serious craniocerebral traumatizing has not been described worldwide.

56.2.3 Back and spine

Frequent acrobatic actions in the sense of overhead kicks, overhead sidekicks and header duels with direct opponent contact repeatedly lead to partly serious **contusions of the back** on the sandy ground. More or less serious bruises are the result, often with reactive **myosclerosis** and/or **blockades of spine segments** requiring treatment. Severe lesions in the sense of disk protrusions or even prolapses have not been described yet and have also not been found in the own group. Fractures of the vertebral bodies and dislocations or even injuries of the nerve trunk have not been known.

The fast local-analgetic treatment and the relaxation of the muscles are important in the case of injuries. Manual-therapeutic techniques are applied as well. The training of "correct falling" is specifically used for prophylaxis. But also the strengthening of the stabilizing dorsal muscles in combination with the abdominal muscle chain is an important point of prevention.

56.2.4 Upper extremities

Treatment-requiring injuries of the **shoulder girdle** as well as the **elbow** and the **hand** are known for field players because of the number of hard landings after air fights or overhead kicks or the high dueling rate, respectively. **Dislocations and fractures of the upper extremity** are **rather rare**, though. Ligament injuries up to dislocations are frequent in goalkeepers; fractures of hands and fingers are rarer. The wearing of appropriate gloves with improved protection of hyperextension injuries has a large influence.

56.2.5 Lower extremities

Knee

Considering the high number of duels with direct opponent contact, it is surprising that capsuloligamentous injuries of the knee joint are rather rare, compared to field soccer. **Strains**, (partial) **lesions** of the **collateral ligaments**, **meniscus ruptures** and very seldom injuries of the central column are found primarily. The most frequent form of injury is the **knee contusion**, which mostly develops in a collision with the opponent, for example knee against knee. The cause of the relatively low number of ligament injuries is seen primarily in the excellent coordination capabilities of the athletes trained in beach soccer. The training on uneven, soft ground with permanently changing stress and pressure moments is an ideal training for the sensorimotor system.

Insertion tendinopathies are the **most frequent overstrain impairments** and affect mostly the patellar tendon, actually stress-conditioned, on the one hand, and predominantly post-traumatic after contusions, on the other hand.

Lower leg

In part, it comes to severe **contusions** of the lower legs, especially the **tibial edge with partly cutaneous degloving** because of the missing protectors and the intensively led duels. These extremely painful injuries immediately will have to be disinfected post-traumatically, covered sterilely and compressed. The direct application of ice for pain and swelling treatment has proved of value. As is known, the healing of cutaneous injuries at the anterior tibial edge is protracted. The necessary care should definitely be applied in the healing of mostly longer duration, because the infection risk is high. An unusual skin disease that has been described in literature is the cutaneous larva migrans population (Veraldi et al. 2006).

Fractures are hardly found. The reason is the prohibition of shoes with hard soles. The necessity of shin protectors is still being discussed. A change of the rules is currently not considered, because of the absence of serious bone injuries.

Foot

The most frequent injury focus is the foot, especially the toes. Primarily, this is caused by the missing the sport shoe. **Tendon distortions or even dislocations**, but also **fractures** (➤ Fig. 56.3), especially of the phalanges, are usually the consequence of unsuccessful ball contacts and ball control, on the one hand, and direct trauma at collision with the opponent, on the other hand.

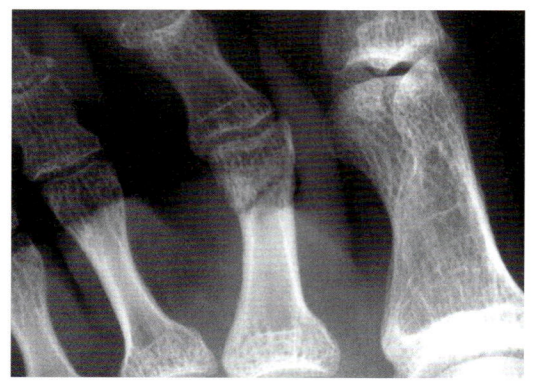

Fig. 56.3 Oblique fracture of the 1st phalanx of digitus II after opponent contact.

Also **contusions of the dorsum of the foot** are often found, caused by direct impact of the foot or the leg of the opponent. Traumatic **osteochondral lesions of the metacarpophalangeal or interphalangeal joints** have been described (Altman et al. 2008). In addition, the formation of an **early arthritis of the metacarpophalangeal joint of the hallux** and the picture of a **hallux rigidus** often occur because of immense strains and microtrauma of the toe joints.

Statements regarding the injury frequency of the foot are not found in literature. Experiences lead to the conclusion that every player on international level shows up to five foot or toe injuries of an extent requiring treatment in each season. Every third player has to expect one dislocation or toe fracture per season. The prophylactic taping as well as the wearing of a neoprene stocking has not gained acceptance for several reasons. An important problem is the subjectively disturbing intrusion of grains of sand into the protective equipment and the possibility of skin lesions. Own experiences with individually made latex coats have been successful, neither, because the material is not sufficient for the high mechanical demands.

56.3 Perspective

Beach soccer is becoming more and more popular. In near future, further studies will be available with more numerical data and will help to better understand and classify the sport-specific features. Even today, beach soccer is increasingly used as additional training for other sports because of its training effects for coordinative abilities and the muscle strengthening (Impellizzeri 2008).

References

Altmann A, Nery C, Sanhudo A, Pinzur MS (2008). Osteochondral injury of the hallux in Beach-Soccer players. Foot Ankle Int 29(9): 919–921.

Impellizzeri FM, Rampnini E, Castagna C, Martino F, Fiorini S, Wisloff U (2008). Effect of plyometric training on sand versus grass on muscle soreness and jumping and sprinting ability in soccer players. Br J Sports Med 42: 42–46.

Moehrle M (2008). Outdoor sports and skin cancer. Clin Dermatol 26(1): 12–15.

Veraldi S, Persico MC (2006). Cutaneus larva migrans in a Beach-Soccer player. Clin J Sport Med 16(5): 430–431.

57 Ice hockey

Bernd Kabelka

Ice hockey is played by both sexes in many countries and has become very popular in Northern America and Europe. It is considered the fastest team sport and is a particularly hard sport, but does not lead the individual injury statistics.

The players run on **sharp blades** and reach **top speeds** of approximately 50 km/h. **Sticks** of wood, carbon or aluminum are used to catapult a **hard rubber disk** to a tempo of up to 160 km/h.

Extremely high start and sprint speeds are reached and speed, sprinting capability and fighting strength on the one hand and opponents, ice surface, boards and equipment on the other hand can lead to very special injury patterns. **Special equipment** is needed to protect the player of his opponents, of the special problems on the ice, the boards, the goal frame, the pucks, sticks and blades, and shall keep him optimally mobile and flexible.

The number of superficial and deep **injuries of the face, eye injuries and dental injuries could be reduced** by improved protection, especially by the use of helmets and facemasks. **Lacerations in the area of head and face** are still the most frequent injuries in all leagues and nations (Ferrara and Schurr 1999).

In the comparison of the North American and the European style of playing, the game in the U.S.A. and Canada is more aggressive and physical than in Europe; in addition, the ice surface in North America with an average size of 1,500 m² is definitely smaller than the European one (1,800 m²), which even increases the injury risk (Watson et al. 1997, Flik et al. 2005).

57.1 Epidemiology of injuries

About 80% of the injuries are caused by an **acute trauma**, 20% are **overstrain impairments**, with 75% of the injuries happening directly in the game and only approx. 25% in training (Daly et al. 1990).

The **offense player** acts on the position that is most often affected by injuries and the **direct collision** with the opponent and/or the boards is the major cause (Groger 2001).

Although different documentation systems exist in North America and Europe, **knee injuries** (especially injuries of the **collateral ligaments**) are the most frequent cause of all playing incapacities (40%), followed by injuries of the **shoulder** (bruises, dislocations, injuries of the AC joint, rotator cuff lesions) with about 20% (Flik et al. 2005; ➤ Fig. 57.1). **Groin injuries** (15%) and **dorsal injuries** (10%) constitute the further causes for playing incapacity (Biasca et al. 1995).

57.2 Injuries

57.2.1 Upper extremities

Falls directly onto the shoulder or the extended, but also the flexed arms, direct **collision to the boards** or "**checking**" **by the opponent** are the most common accident mechanisms. The checking and other collisions with opponent players cause 75% of the shoulder injuries here, 55% of the elbow joint injuries and 45% of the injuries at hand and wrist joint (Moelsae et al. 2003).

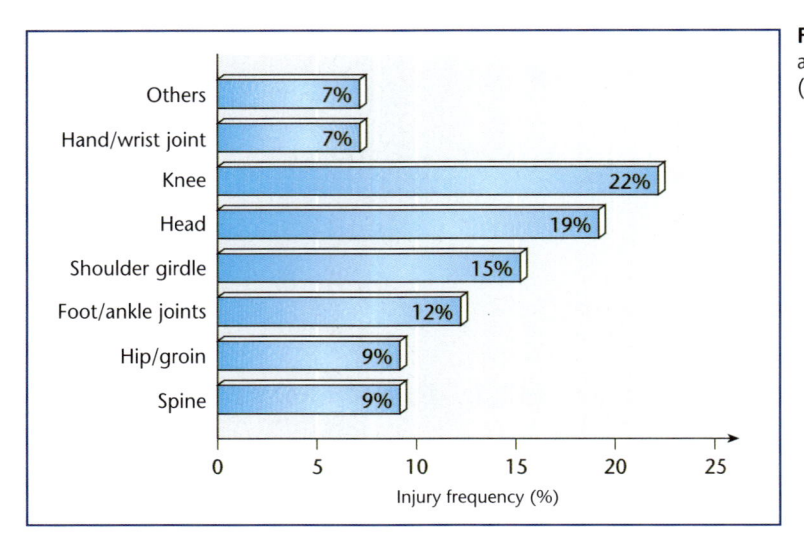

Fig. 57.1 Frequency of injuries according to the body regions (Flik et al. 2005).

- Others: 7%
- Hand/wrist joint: 7%
- Knee: 22%
- Head: 19%
- Shoulder girdle: 15%
- Foot/ankle joints: 12%
- Hip/groin: 9%
- Spine: 9%

Typical shoulder injuries are:

- contusions and strains
- separations of the AC joint and
- shoulder dislocations.

Fractures affect especially the lateral clavicle, but occur rather rarely. The use of new shoulder protectors has significantly reduced the number of these injuries.

Injuries of the elbow joint are mostly **contusions** and/or formations of a **traumatic bursitis olecrani**, especially caused by slipping elbow protection.

Injuries of hand and wrist joint amount to 7% of all injuries (Flik et al. 2005), and 14% of these injuries are caused by direct impacts of the stick or strikes with the puck (Pelletier et al. 1993, Stuart and Smith 1995).

Scaphoid fractures develop seldom, mostly in the course of hyperextensions or flexion traumas of the hand at checks or at the boards. **Capsule and ligament injuries** are often combined with **finger dislocations** ("goal keeper's thumb").

57.2.2 Lower extremities

Especially knee, ankle and hip joint and the groin area are affected in the region of the lower extremity.

By far the most frequent injuries of the lower extremity are ligament injuries of the **knee joint** and here especially the **medial collateral ligament rupture** (Pelletiere et al. 1993). It develops in particular at valgus traumas in the direct duel, but also at falls with contact to the boards. The **preclusion of concomitant injuries** such as cruciate ligament ruptures and meniscus injuries is of great importance for the prognosis. The isolated, medial collateral ligament rupture mostly heals without consequences in **conservative therapy** by stabilizing in an orthesis, while the prophylactic bracing does not offer any secure advantages (Tegner and Lorentzon 1991).

The second-most frequent injuries in the area of the lower extremity affect the **foot** and especially the **upper ankle joint**. Here we find fractures caused by puck impacts, especially in the metatarsal region (Moelsae et al. 2003). **Fibular ligament ruptures and syndesmosis injuries** are the most frequent injuries of the upper ankle joint, while the **prophylactic taping** of the ankle joints can lead to a definite reduction of the injury frequency (Karlsson et al. 1993).

Injuries in the **hip region** and especially **strains in the area of the adductors and the groin** affect especially the goalkeepers, provoked by extremely wide lunges. **Preventive stretching and strengthening programs** are important here, for the time without games as well as integrated into the training program.

57.2 Injuries

Lesions of the **femoral adductors** constitute 10% of all injuries (Emery et al. 1999, Tyler et al. 2001). It has been found that the number of injuries of the adductor muscles and groin strains can be definitely reduced by **special training programs** during pre-season. The relation of the adductors to the abductor strength has proved to be an important indicator for an increased risk of this injury. Thus, a relation of at least 8 : 10 for the adduction compared to the abduction should be aimed at (Tyler et al. 2002).

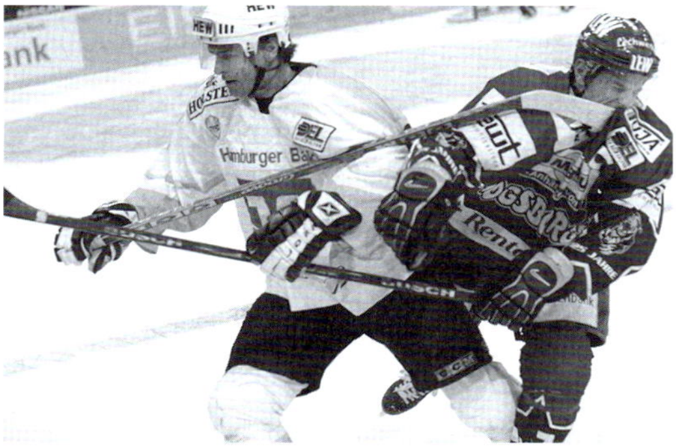

57.2.3 Head and spine

Major localizations of injuries are **face, neck and cranium**, mostly of lacerations, lacerated or incised wounds without osseous involvement, often caused by puck or impacts with the stick (➤ Fig. 57.2). These wounds can mostly be treated on site in order to allow further participation in the game. The number of fractures of the zygomatic bone and midfacial fractures as well as eye injuries can be reduced significantly by wearing **helmets with half-visors**.

Fractures in the facial area affect the upper and the lower jaw with and without dental loss. It has to be remarked, that these injuries can be avoided completely by the use of **grid or full visors**!

Puck impacts in the area of the neck can lead to acute shortness of breath and require an endotracheal intubation or even tracheotomy on the ice (McAlindon 2002, Blanda and Gallo 2003, Butler and Clyne 2003).

> Puck impacts in the neck region causing acute shortness of breath present an absolute emergency situation and require fast emergency-medical treatment.

Injuries of the spine are found in 9% of the cases and **contusions** by player and/or board collisions often occur here in the region of the **thoracic and lumbar spine**.

The very dangerous special injury mechanism of the **cervical spine** is a result of impact on opponent or surrounding walls with hyperflexed cervical spine, which can lead to **fractures and/or dislocations of the vertebral bodies of the cervical spine**, often with **lesions of the cervical medulla**. These catastrophic injuries of the cervical spine with lesions of the cervical medulla occur in ice hockey the same as they do in American football (Banerjee et al. 2004)!

Fig. 57.2 Facial injuries caused by hits with the stick.

Studies in Canadian ice hockey by Tator et al. (1998) between 1966 and 1993 have found 241 serious injuries of the cervical spine with fractures and in more than 50% additional injuries of the cervical medulla with partial or complete palsies of the extremities or even lethal results. The strict observance of the rules for the protection of the players and the prohibition of "checking from behind" has definitely reduced the number of these injuries in recent years (Roberts et al. 1996, Watson et al. 1997, Banerjee et al. 2004).

Concussions

Cranial concussions or even craniocerebral traumas present a special problem in contact sports. About 5% of the players suffer such "concussions" in each season (Johnston et al. 2001).

In addition to an exact classification of the injury, the frequent checking-up and the interdisciplinary diagnostic and therapy of the injured are of special meaning for the prevention of possible late consequences.

Significant progress has been achieved on both international conferences with the topic "Concussion in Sport" in Vienna in 2001 and in Prague in 2004. The introduction of the **SCAT** (sport concussion assessment tool) has proved to be of decisive advantage in diagnostics, therapy and after-treatment of these injuries (Mc Crory et al. 2004).

"Return to play guidelines" (Warren et al. 2000) provides important support for decisions for the responsible.

Summary

Ice hockey is the fastest team sport and is especially aggressive and accident-prone sport. Nonetheless, soccer and American football are definitely more dangerous. The injury frequencies during game and training differ immensely with the body contact of the players being the main cause for injuries. Lesions of the medial collateral ligaments of the knee joints are the most frequent injuries. Offense players are hurt much more often than defense players or goalkeepers, and young players more often than older ones (Reid and Losek 1999). Injury frequencies of men and women do not differ significantly (Schick and Meeuwisse 2003).

The strict playing by the rules has to be indicated. Hits and pushes against the head and the so-called "checking from behind", which could lead to injuries of the cervical spine or even to paraplegia, are forbidden.

A precondition for successful ice hockey is an optimal season preparation, especially in the field of endurance and strength, as well as the training of coordinative abilities. Individually compiled training plans that have been developed especially for the individual player have proved of advantage. A close sport-medical treatment of the players in the orthopedic-traumatology and performance-diagnostic should be aimed for. The performance-diagnostic examinations should be carried out before each game season as well as during the season at intervals of about 3 months. This can provide important data especially for the structuring and perhaps modification of training. In addition to tests of performance diagnosis, also tests of the coordinative capabilities are very important in order to discover deficits and to act injury-preventively (Reid and Losek 1999).

References

Banerjee R, Palumbo MA, Fadale PD (2004). Catastrophic cervical spine injuries in the collision sport athlete, part 1. Am J Sports Med 32: 1177–1187.

Biasca N, Simmen HP, Bartolozzi AR, Trentz (1995). Review of typical ice hockey injuries: survey of the North American Hockey League and Hockey Canada versus European leagues. Unfallchirurgie 98 (5): 283–288.

Blanda M, Gallo UG (2003). Emergency airway management. Emerg Med Clin North Am 21: 1–26.

Bulter KH, Clyne B (2003). Management of the difficult airway: alternative airway: techniques and adjuncts. Emerg Med Clin North Am 21: 259–289.

Daly PJ, Sim FH, Simonet WT (1990). Ice hockey injuries – a review. Sports Med 10 (2): 122–131.

Emery CA, Meeuwisse WH, Powll JW (1999). Groin and abdominal muscle injuries in the National Hockey League. Clin J Sport Med 9 (3): 151–156.

Ferrara MS, Schurr KT (1991). Intercollegiate ice hockey injuries: a causal analysis. Clin J Sport Med 9: 30–33.

Flik K, Lyman St, Marx RG (2005). American collegiate men's ice hockey. An analysis of injuries. Am J Sports Med 33 (2): 183–187.

Groger A (2001). Ten years of ice hockey-related injuries in the German Ice Hockey Federation – A Ten Years prospective study/523 international Games. Sportverletz Sportschaden 15 (4): 82–86.

Johnston K, McCrory P, Mohtadi N, et al. (2001). Evidence-based review of sport-related concussion: clinical science. Clin J Sport Med 11: 150–160.

Karlsson J, Sward L, Andresson GO (1993). The effect of taping on ankle stability.Practical implications. Sports Med 16 (3): 210–215.

McAlindon RJ (2002). On field evaluation and management of head and neck injured athletes. Clin Sports Med 21: 1–14.

Mc Crory P, Johnston K, Meeuwisse W, Aubry M, Cantu R, Dvorak J, Graf-Baumann T, Kelly J, Lovell M, Schamasch P (2004). Summary and agreement statement of th 2nd International Conference on Concussion in Sport, Prague 2004. Br J Sports Med 39: 196–204.

Moelsae J, Kujale U, Myllyven P, Torstila I, Airaksinen O (2003). Injuries to the upper extremity in ice hockey. Analysis of a series of 760 injuries. Am J Sports Med 31: 751–757.

Pelletier RL, Montepalare WJ, Stark RM (1993). Intercollegiate ice hockey injuries. A case of uniform definitions and reports. Am J Sports Med 21 (1): 78–81.

Reid SR, Losek JD (1999). Factors associated with significant injuries in youth ice hockey players. Pediatr Emerg Care 15 (5): 310–313.

Roberts WO, Brust JD, Leonard B, Herbert BJ (1996). Fairplay rules and injury reduction in ice hockey. Arch Pediatr Adolesc Med 150 (2): 140–145.

Schick DM, Meeuwisse WH (2003). Injury rates and profiles in female ice hockey players. Am J Sports Med 31 (1): 47–52.

Stuart MJ, Smith A (1995). Injuries in junior A ice hockey: a three-year prospective study. Am J Sports Med 23: 458–461.

Tator CH, Carson JD, Edmonds VE (1998). Spinal injuries in ice hockey. Clin Sports Med 17 (1): 183–194.

Tegner Y, Lorentzon R (1991). Evolution of knee braces in Swedish ice hockey players. Br J Sports Med 25 (3): 159–161.

Tyler TF, Nicholas SJ, Campbell RJ, McHugh MP (2001). The association of hip strength and flexibility with the incidence of adductor muscle strains in professional ice hockey players. Am J Sports Med 29 (2): 124–128.

Tyler TF, Nicholas SJ, Campbell RJ, Donellan S, McHugh MP (2002). The effectiveness of preseason exercise program to prevent adductor muscle strains in professional ice hockey players. Am J Sports Med 30 (5): 680–683.

Warren WL, Bailes JE, Cantu RC (2000). Guidelines for safe return to play after athletic head and neck injuries. In: Cantu RC (ed.). Neurologic Athletic Head and Spine Injuries. WB Saunders, Philadelphia, PA.

Watson RC, Nystrom MA, Buckolz E (1997). Safety in Canadian junior ice hockey: the association between ice surface size and injuries and aggressive penalties in the Ontario Hockey League. Clin J Sport Med 7 (3): 192–195.

58 Soccer

Thomas Hess and Heinrich Hess

Soccer is the most popular sport. Considering the **injury factors**, soccer ranges in the lower third of injury statistics behind basketball, volleyball, and handball or dancing (Steinbrück 1999). About two thirds of all soccer playersmedical conditions are the result of **acute injuries**, the other third derives from **overstrain impairments** (Lees and Nolan 1998). Female soccer players show other injury frequencies and injury patterns than male soccer players (Fried and Lloyd 1992, Arendt and Dick 1995, Ireland and Ott 2004). The position on the field has no influence in this concern. (Dvorak and Junge 2000).

58.1 Pelvis and lumbosacral transgression

58.1.1 Lumbalgias, iliosacral joint syndrome

Pain at the lumbosacral junction and disorders of the iliosacral joint (IS joint), in part with pseudoradicular radiation, are frequent and persistent problems in soccer players. Mostly they are promoted by a **muscular dysbalance** with a discrepancy between well-trained leg muscles (especially extensors) and insufficient training of the autochtonous dorsal muscles. A true **radicular syndrome** must be excluded first by clinical examination and then by imaging.

An **iliosacral joint syndrome** often comes along with a **blockade**. These symptoms often occur in combination with **symphysis conditions** and **adductor problems** (Hess 2001). The physiotherapeutic stretching treatment of the mostly contracted ischiocrural muscles as well as a **correction** of the hyperlordosis are recommended, in addition to manual-therapeutic treatment.

58.1.2 Symphysis syndrome

The symphysis is subject to increased strain in soccer, especially in frequent performances of the **straddle step** under simultaneous fixation of the hip rotation in the standing leg. Occasionally, also radiological changes, such as focal osteolyses or even dehiscence of the symphysis can be detected. An involvement of the iliosacral joints should be checked and treated if necessary in addition to the temporary stress reduction and strengthening of the pelvic muscles.

58.1.3 Insertion tendinopathy of the abdominal muscles

Chronic insertion tendinopathies can develop in the insertion area of the muscles of the abdominal wall at the anterior branch of the pubic bone, especially with a **small manifestation of the rectus abdominis muscle**. In case of doubt, this diagnosis can be secured by scintigraphy (Zeitoun et al. 1995). The symptoms can almost always be controlled under **local treatments** such as transverse frictions and local infiltrations.

58.1.4 Inguinal syndrome/groin complaints

Groin conditions are typical in soccer and have a wide spectrum of causes (➤ Tab. 58.1). if the **inguinal canal** itself is the cause, a **relative insufficiency of the lateral abdominal muscles**

Tab. 58.1 Causes for groin pain in soccer players.

Causes for groin pain in soccer players soft groin
■ real inguinal hernia
■ irritation/blockade of the iliosacral joint
■ leg-length discrepancy, static changes
■ iliopsoas syndrome
■ irritation of the adductor insertion
■ changes in the hip joint
■ irritations of the lumbar roots
■ epiphysiolysis capitis femoris (in juveniles)

will mostly exist. A manifest, classic inguinal hernia does certainly not have to exist here (LeBlanc and LeBlanc 2003). The classic pain can be triggered by palpation of the inguinal canal and these symptoms allow reliable differentiation from the insertion tendinopathy of the adductors.

Conservative measures as therapy of an open groin are less effective, decision of **surgery** needs to be taken early (Hess 1980).

58.1.5 Iliopsoas syndrome

The iliopsoas syndrome is either caused by an **injury of the muscle** itself, **its tendon** or by an **irritation of the bursa iliopectinea**. The pain symptoms can be provoked by a hip flexion against resistance in the typical course of the iliopsoas tendon (and thus farther laterally than the soft groin).

The local infiltration with local anesthetics and crystal corticoid is the **therapy** of choice.

58.1.6 Abductor syndrome

The classic insertion tendinopathy of the adductors is found at the **internal side of the femur** as well as at the **lower pelvic ring**. The radiation is directed more distally and can mostly be well differentiated from the "soft groin".

The therapy of choice is first the **physiotherapeutic treatment** with local transverse friction of the tendon insertions and muscular relaxation therapy. A discission and periostomy of the tendon origins is possible at permanent inefficacy of conservative therapy.

58.1.7 Tearing of the rectus insertion

The rectus femoris muscle might avulse **osseously** at the upper socket edge of the hip joint as a consequence of **overstress** (ball kicked by two players at exactly the same time into different directions) especially in juveniles. The injury can be diagnosed clearly by **imaging**; the avulsed insertion mostly dislocated only marginally.

Usually, the **symptomatic treatment** is a sufficient therapy for the overcoming of acute pain. A refixation of the fragment is only necessary with persisting conditions (Tucker 1997).

58.1.8 Other causes of complaints in the groin and hip region

Urologic causes of groin or hip pain must be excluded. True **affections of the hip joint**, which are often overlooked (coxa vara/valga, hip dysplasia, impingement syndrome), as well as **radicular syndromes** of the layers L2/3 and L3/4 need consideration. In juveniles, an **epiphysiolysis capitis femoris lenta** always has to be considered and must be precluded at the slightest suspicion (often also knee pain) by a radiograph on two layers.

58.2 Knee joint

58.2.1 Meniscus

Especially the menisci are often hurt or degenerated in the high-pivoting sport of soccer. In addition to the classic meniscus signs, the **Thessaly test** (Karachalios et al. 2005), which has an extraordinarily high sensitivity, has proved of value in sport praxis.

Although fresh meniscus injuries are easy to diagnose by their obvious clinic and the mostly present **hematomarthros**, a **MRT** is required to detect concomitant injuries in the internal knee space. Whenever possible, repair in the sense of a **refixation** should always be intended for a traumatic injury.

Ruptures or degenerative changes that do not reach the surface (**degree II** according to Stoller) do not require therapy in the asymptomatic stadium. **Partial meniscus resection** should be indicated rapidly at **medical conditions** the same as at complete irreparable ruptures (**degree-III lesions**). Hereby the stress and sport capacity can be quickly recovered and maintained in the long term especially at lesions in the **area of the internal meniscus**. The resection should be done as sparingly as possible, because the **risk of arthritis** after partial meniscus resections increases in proportion to the resected volume (Kohn 2000).

58.2.2 Cruciate ligaments

The rupture of the **anterior cruciate ligament** is a classic soccer injury (➢ Fig. 58.1, ➢ Fig. 58.2). The indication for a **surgical substitution** is clear at the appearing of instabilities after a rupture of the anterior cruciate ligament.

> A reconstruction of the anterior cruciate ligament is generally recommended for soccer players, if they wish to continue the sport at the same level.

Ruptures of the **posterior cruciate ligament** can be treated **conservatively**, if they are isolated. If the developed instability demands a surgical stabilizing in the medium term, a **concomitant injury of dorsal capsule structures**, especially of the dorsomedial complex, will mostly be present and will have to be treated as well (Harner and Hoher 1998).

58.2.3 Collateral ligaments

Distal or proximal ruptures of the **medial collateral ligament** usually heal by conservative therapy. The internal meniscus base is often affected, as well, at intraligamentous ruptures, so that an indication for surgery will arise from this already. The proximalization of the femoral insertion is recommended at **chronic instabilities** of the internal ligament.

Lateral instabilities are expediently treated conservatively as well, in order to be able to approach remaining instabilities differently.

58.2.4 Cartilage damages

These often appear as **concomitant injuries** and are occasionally paid insufficient attention

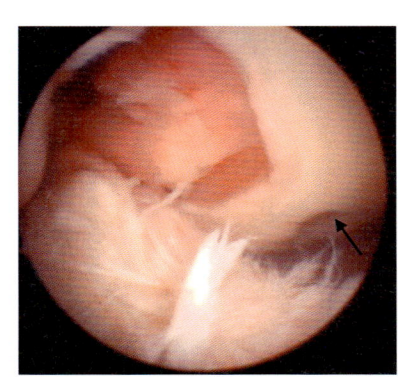

Fig. 58.1 The anterior cruciate ligament rupture are often accompanied by a cartilage impairment (arrow).

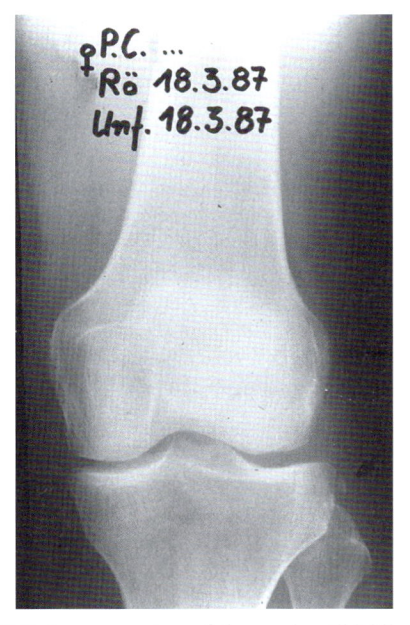

Fig. 58.2 An osseous tear of the meniscotibial ligament at the lateral tibia head (so-called Segond fracture) is nearly pathognomonic for a rupture of the anterior cruciate ligament.

to in the additional treatment of ligaments and menisci. Near full-thickness cartilage lesions usually do not show complete healing tendency (Chen et al. 1999), so that they can be monitored and at progressiveness should be transferred to **surgical therapy**, such as microfracturing, osteochondral transplantation or chondrocyte transplantation, in time. The persistent **development of effusions** is a typical clinical correlate of progressive cartilage impairment.

58.3 Ankle joint

The frequency of ankle joint conditions in soccer players lies at about 20%. The **upper ankle joint** and the **Achilles tendon** are affected in most cases. Injuries of the **lower ankle joint** are pointed out especially here, which are often differentiated insufficiently from the upper ankle joint and thus is often overlooked.

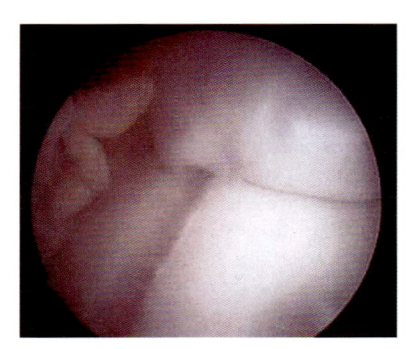

Fig. 58.3 Ventral osteophyte at the anterior tibial edge, which has already produced a cutting trace in the cartilage of the upper ankle joint.

58.3.1 Upper ankle

The rupture of the **lateral capsule-ligament apparatus** is mostly treated conservatively. The surgical treatment with reconstruction of the ligament structures is more beneficial at a complete **laceration of all three ligament structures and the capsule** in soccer players. **Mechanical and functional instabilities** at chronic conditions with persistent instability have to be distinguished carefully. Only the first should be put into surgery. The functional instability has sufficiently stable ligament structures and requires a specific proprioceptive physical therapy.

Ruptures of the **syndesmosis** and the **medial collateral ligament** (deltoid ligament) are of a long-termed process and require a strict immobilization. A securing by **arthrography** or **nuclear spin tomography** has to be carried out as fast as possible.

> An escape of contrast material at the anterior syndesmosis rupture can only be detected in the first 24 hours.

Typical affections at the upper ankle joint of soccer players are **pain in the anterior recess**.

Causes for this can be:
- a hypertrophic synovitis
- osteophytic additions at the anterior tibial edge (➤ Fig. 58.3) or talus neck, respectively, or
- formation of meniscoid-like structures at the internal side of the lateral capsule after partial ruptures.

The arthroscopic resection is a very successful method with **ventral osteophytes**.

58.3.2 Achilles tendon

In addition to the complete rupture, lesions of the Achilles tendon include especially the **achyllodynia**. Here it has to be differentiated between a **tendinosis of the tendon** itself, a **peritendinitis** and an **affection of the bursa subachillea** by sonography or MRT (Biedert 1991).

Causing factors, such as a Haglund's exostosis, contractions of the triceps muscles or impaired flexing actions, have to be clarified before the determination of the establishment regime. The **conservative therapy** consists of physiotherapeutic measures (transverse frictions, iontophoresis, stretching of the triceps surae muscle), infiltrations into the bursa subachillea and correction of the flexing actions. A resection of the bursa subachillea, a resection of the hypertrophic paratenon or the excision of necrotic tendon areas has to be considered after **persistence**.

58.3.3 Other conditions

Shin splints are insertion-tendinopathic conditions at the anterior and posterior side of the **tibia**, classically **at night** after athletic stress. The diagnosis can be confirmed by bone scintigraphy (Batt 1995). In almost all cases, a pathological flexing action of the foot is the cause and can be eliminated by according modification of the shoes.

58.4 Muscle injuries

Muscular conditions appear with structural lesions of the tissue (torn muscle fiber, muscle rupture) and without such (muscle strain, muscle contusion). In both groups, the treatment begins with the widest **reduction of the concomitant tissue swelling** by compression and ice-cooling (iced water bandages).

Further aims of therapy are the **elimination of the hematoma** (puncture, local physiotherapeutic treatment) and the **normalization of the increased muscle tonus** (electro-therapy, physiotherapeutic measures, infiltration therapy). Muscle tonus and pain level determine the further course of rehabilitation with transmission to stretching techniques and eventually sport-specific training.

Special attention deserves the **compartment syndrome**, which can develop by apparently harmless symptoms in a blunt trauma against the lower leg and which will require a fascia splitting at the appearance of a manifest compression syndrome (peroneal paresis!). But it can also appear **chronic-intermittently** as overload syndrome mainly in the dorsal and peroneal compartment.

> Immediate detumescing measures (e.g. ice-cooling) at the appearance of compression syndromes cannot be emphasized often enough!

References

Arendt E, Dick R (1995). Knee injury patterns among men and women in collegiate baskeball and soccer. NCAA data and review of literature. Am J Sports Med 23: 694–701.

Batt ME (1995). Shin splints a review of terminology. Clin J Sports Med 5: 53-57.

Bieder R (1991). Beschwerden im Achillessehnenbereich. Ätiologien und therapeutische Überlegungen. Unfallchirurg 94: 531–537.

Chen FS, Frenkel SR, Di Cesare PE (1999). Repair of articular cartilage defects: part 1. Basic science of cartilage healing. Am J Orthop 28: 31–33.

Dvorak J, Junge A (2000). Football injuries and physical symptoms. A review of the literature. Am J Sports Med 28: 3–9.

Fried T, Lloyd GJ (1992). An overview of common soccer injuries. Management and prevention. Sports Med 14: 269–275.

Harner CD, Hoher J (1998). Evaluation and treatment of posterior cruciate ligament injuries. Am J Sports Med 26: 471–482.

Hess H (1980). Leistenschmerz – Ätiologie, Differenzialdiagnose und therapeutische Möglichkeiten. Orthopädie 9: 186–189.

Hess H (2001). Fußball. In: Klmper (ed.). Sporttraumatologie Handbuch der Sportarten und ihrer typischen Verletzungen. Ecomed, Landsberg. II-21, 1–21.

Ireland ML, Ott SM (2004). Special concerns of the female athlete. Clin Sports Med 23: 281–298.

Karachalios T, Hantes M, Zibis AH, Zachos V, Karantanas AH, Malizos KN (2005). Diagnostic accuracy of a new clinical test (the Thessaly test) for early detection of meniscal tears. J Bone Joint Surg 87: 955–962.

Kohn D (2000). Das Knie. Thieme, Stuttgart.

LeBlanc KE, LeBlanc KA (2003). Groin pain in athletes. Hernia 7: 68–71.

Lees A, Nolan L (1998). The biomechanics of soccer: a review. J Sports Sci 16: 211–234.

Steinbrück K (1999). Epidemiologie von Sportverletzungen – 25-Jahres-Analyse einer sportorthopädisch-traumatologischen Ambulanz. Sportverl Sportschad 13: 38–52.

Tucker AM (1997). Common soccer injuries. Diagnosis, treatment and rehabilitation. Sports Med 23: 21–32.

Zeitoun F, Frot B, Sterin P, Tubiana JM (1995). Pubalgie du sportif. Ann Radiol Paris 38: 244–254.

59 Handball

Berthold Hallmaier

Worldwide, handball is played in 156 countries. The fascination of this sport has many attractive facets: strength, endurance, speed, coordination, technique, acrobatics, tactics, many scores, tension, dynamics, team spirit, fight, concentration and many more – this makes handball so popular all over the world.

59.1 Characteristics of the sport

Handball is a game of two competing teams with the aim of advancing the ball by hand into the opponent's goal (3 m wide and 2 m high) and to defend the own goal of the opponent's attack (➤ Fig. 59.1).

The team with most scores after the end of playing time wins. Handball is played on a field of 40 × 20 m, and the 6-m circle around each goal must not be gotten into. A hollow ball with a leather and synthetic coat of a circumference of 58–60 cm and a weight of 425–475 g is used. There are smaller versions of less weight for women and juveniles. The playing time lasts 2 × 30 min, and is accordingly shorter for juveniles.

Originally, it was developed as a game on fields of the size of soccer fields – field handball –, but has been more and more superseded by indoor handball. Nowadays, handball is played by men and women in a form different from field handball on smaller fields and almost exclusively indoors.

Every team in indoor handball consists of 14 field players and two goalkeepers, of which at a maximum only seven (6 field players, one goalkeeper) are allowed to be on the field at the same time. The game is conducted by two equal referees who are supported by a timekeeper (there is an effective playing time in indoor handball) and a scorekeeper..

General Rules

The game starts with a throw-off from the centerline.

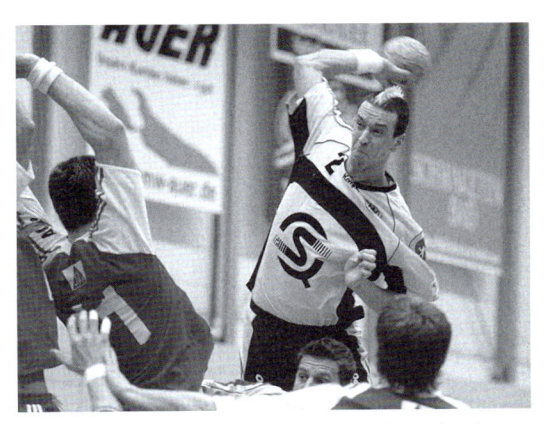

Fig. 59.1 Attack by Pascal Hens and defense by the opposing team (Germany – Poland 2005).

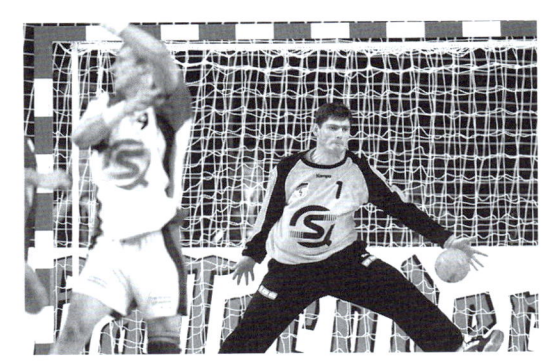

Fig. 59.2 Defense of an attack in the 6-m circle by national goalkeeper Henning Fritz under use of arms and legs (World Cup 2003).

The ball may be played by all parts of the body with the exceptions of lower leg and foot. This limitation does not apply to the goalkeeper within his goal area (6-m circle; ➤ Fig. 59.2). Outside of it, he is also considered a field player. The opponent may be blocked with the body, even if he has no ball possession. Arms and hands must only be used to acquire possession of the ball. It is forbidden to block the opponent with arms, hands and legs, or to push, hit or hold him.

Three steps at maximum may be made holding the ball in the hand (**three-step rule**). Also the ball must not be held in the hand or on the ground longer than three seconds (**3-sec rule**). Passive playing (keeping the ball in the own team without trying to score) will be punished by a free throw for the opponent. After the game break, the game will be resumed corresponding to the previous game situation; breaches of the rules and unfair behavior will be punished according to the severity by:

- a free throw
- a penalty throw, the so-called 7-meter throw (unhindered throw from the 7-m line from a standing position toward the goal of the opponent, and only the goalkeeper is allowed to defend)
- suspension from the field for 2 min (the suspended player must not be substituted)
- ejection for the rest of the playing time (the ejected player must not be substituted).

The rules of indoor handball also apply to small-field handball, which is carried out on outdoor fields (Deutscher Handballbund 2005).

59.2 Competitions and organizations

The only Olympic field-handball tournament had been carried out in 1936. Indoor handball has been accepted as an Olympic sport since the Olympic Games in Munich in 1972 and is one of the most popular disciplines.

European championships for club teams on an international level take place for national champions (for men since 1957, for women since 1961, champions' league since 1994) and cup winners (men since 1976, women since 1977), and also the EHF cup (IHF cup since 1994), similar to the UEFA cup in soccer, and the Challenge Cup (1994–2000 City Cup).

In the FRG, German handball championships have been carried out indoors since 1950. Before 1966, the championships had been carried out in play-offs of the different regional-league champions. 1966 to 1975 the first-place finishers of both federal leagues had determined the German champion in two finals. The single federal league has been in existence since 1976. German handball is organized in the German handball federation (DHB, founded in 1949 with its home in Dortmund).

The world umbrella organization is the International Handball Federation (IHF, founded in 1946, at home in Basel). The European umbrella organization is the European Handball Federation (EHF, founded in 1991, at home in Vienna).

Handball is a very young sport despite some similar forerunners (e.g. torball in Germany). The country of origin is Germany, where the first rules for field handball have been drafted in 1917. These have been adopted internationally in 1927. In 1928, the International Amateur Handball Federation had been founded, which has been changed into IHF by the omission of the word "amateur". Germany is not only considered the country of origin of handball, but the German Handball Federation with its 850,000 members is also the largest national handball umbrella organization worldwide.

The German national team of men – with the exception of the Russian one – is the only one that has earned an Olympic victory as well as a world championship title and a European championship title.

59.3 Strain profile of handball sports

The systems providing and transmitting energy on the one hand and the processes of reception and processing of information on the other hand are strained in playing handball. The strain noticeable from the outside must be distinguished from the inner strain of the player, which is determined by his individual capacity (Brack 2002, Brack et al. 2006).

59.3.1 Energetic strain

The **aerobic part of the energy supply** dominates in the most phases of the game in handball. First the ATP and CT storages will be emptied at the short velocity and springiness training. The ATP storages will be replenished oxidatively, i.e. without lactid acid development, in the game breaks or phases of low intensity.

The **anaerobic degeneration of the carbohydrates** and the concomitant increased lactid acid development will only occur in rare intensive strains of longer duration, e.g. in three directly successive speed counterblasts in the form of a fast attack (➤ Fig. 59.3). The intensive strain has definitely increased by the tactic version of the fast throw-off, which often leads to speed counterblasts. The lactate will already be degenerated in the course of the immediate recovery in low-intensive playing phases. Therefore, the immediate recovery can take effect because the relation of stress and intermissions in position offense (preparation of a shot on goal) come to 1:2 at the average.

The found lactate values in handball amount to 4–5 mmol/l of blood at the average (Brack, 2002, Brack et al. 2006).

59.3.2 Mental strain

The mental strain in indoor handball includes the demands, which are put on the player by the reception and processing of information. These demands can be of technically-tactic, or even of psychic nature (high pressure to perform).

Psychologically, these can be considered **problem situations**, because of the complex game situation, which the players are subject to in competition (Dörner 1989, Brack 2002, Brack et al. 2006):

- Multiple tasks have to be accomplished, e.g. catching the ball in sprint and sensing the team mates and opponents, as well as anticipation of the coming situation (➤ Fig. 59.4).

- Actions have to be performed under pressure of time, in order to posses the according information for solving the task in the corresponding situation. (This strain situation has occurred increasingly over the last three years because of the high variability of the defensive options.)

- Pressure to make decisions is given by the open alternatives and the high internal and external stress.

- Attention has to be paid to several things at the same time. Concentration plays an important role in three respects in the solution of this problem situation.

- Concentration in terms of mobilization goes into the direction of will powers. The catch-phrase here is "fighting".

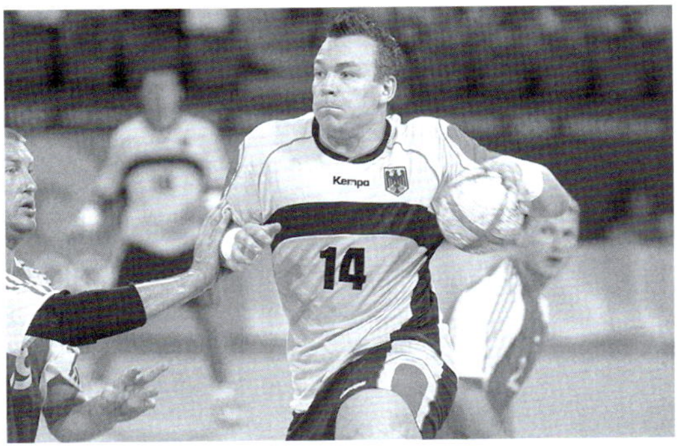

Fig. 59.3 Speed counterblast, carried out by national player Christian Zeitz (quarter-final Germany–Russia, Olympic Games 2004).

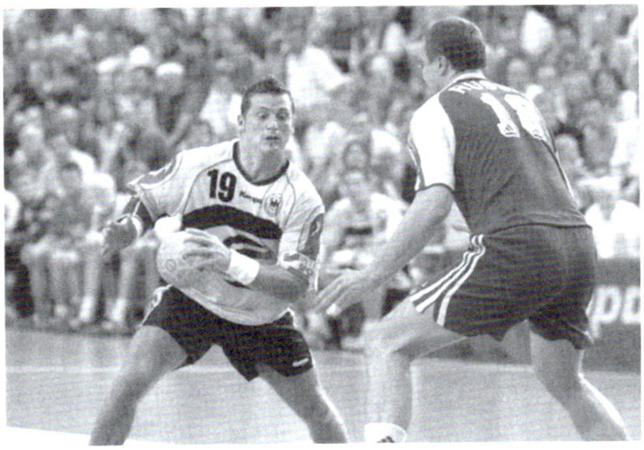

Fig. 59.4 National player Florian Kehrmann in the moment of receiving the ball and anticipation of the playing situation pressure of decision-making (quarter-final Germany–Russia, Olympic Games 2004).

- Concentration in terms of selection aims at reactive as well as active actions in complex and tactically demanding multiple tasks. The catchphrase here is "anticipation".
- Concentration in terms of shielding aims at keeping the own attention with regard to the actions that have to be carried out in order to fulfill the tasks. Catchphrases: noise, audience, mistaken whistles by the referees. (The demands have grown massively due to the increase of indoor capacities. Since the federal league plays in large gyms – numbers of spectators of up to 18,000 –, this aspect becomes more and more important.)

A game analysis by means of an action model can help to accomplish the psychic demands to the players.

Three major phases of game activity become apparent (Brack 2002, Brack et al. 2006):

- anticipation of action
- realization of action
- interpretation of action.

The quality of game activity can only be as good as the worst quality of the individual phase.

In general, the handball player reacts according to the **action model**: In the first phase of the anticipation of action, there will be the trial to perceive and to analyze the playing situation as well as to solve it mentally. The second phase of the realization of action describes the motor solving of the task by the player. In the third phase of interpretation of action, the result and the process of actions are evaluated subjectively with foreign or own information, and the received results will be stored in a part of the brain. In future, the stored information will serve the faster finding of solutions of higher quality in similar playing situations.

The third phase today is supported by decided **video analyses** of the opposing team or the individual opponent player. The video analysis will be prepared in a way that the opponent will be interpreted in their solving behavior regarding certain defensive formations at playing with superior or inferior numbers, especially with regard to solutions that are aimed at in playing situations or even stress situations. The video analysis of the individual player is an important part of the training of goalkeepers. All throwing variants of the opponent will be analyzed: in the regular case, in position attack, in an attack in small groups, his individual throwing capacity and especially which throwing variants in game-deciding situations with or without body contact are preferred by him.

The mental strain plays an important role and is more extensive than in other sports, as comparing studies have shown, because a far lower average noradrenaline/adrenaline ratio has been detected in handball players than in athletes of other sports. This ratio is considered the measurement for psychic and physical strain: the stronger the psychic strain, the lower will be this ratio, because the adrenaline level will enhance as a consequence of psychic strain in relation to the noradrenaline level (Brack 1996, Brack 2002).

59.4 Competition Equipment

Currently, the **mouthpiece** has increasingly gained acceptance – similar to boxing sport. Repeatedly, dental injuries due to body contact will occur because of the increase of dynamics in handball.

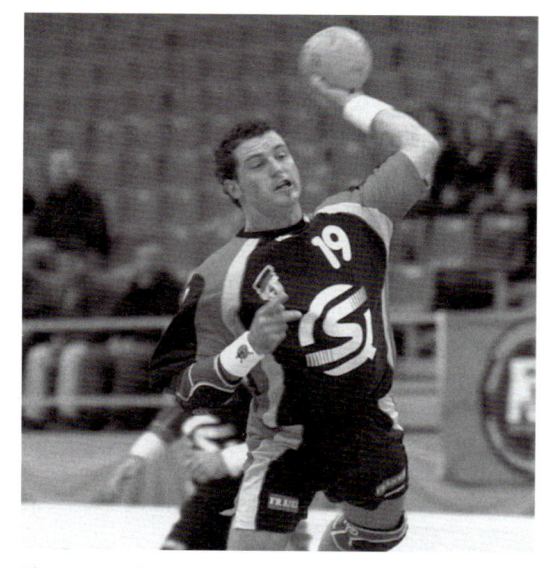

Fig. 59.5 Elbow, knee and mouth protection of a field player (preliminary Germany – Greece, Olympic Games 2004).

The **jock strap** – so far only mandatory in goal keepers – is also applied more and more in running backs and offense specialists.

Because of their special way of playing – jumping into the circle, jumping from an extreme outside position into the circle –, the players in the outfield positions and the pivot need a **fall protection** for the elbow joints and a fall protection for both knee joints, in order to avoid chronic injuries of the bursae at the elbow and knee joints (➤ Fig. 59.5). Soft-foam protectors have gained acceptance also in goalkeepers.

59.5 Injuries

At present, there are about 15 million handball players organized in federations and clubs worldwide. The German Handball Association ranks in the sixth position in number of members in the top associations of the German Sports Association. 70–80% of the sport accidents happen in the classic ball sports of soccer, handball, volleyball or basketball. In handball, the frequency of injuries amounts to 15–18% compared to other sports.

Numbers in the following statistic records the anatomical localization of handball injuries in the federal men's league in 2004/2005. It shows that the sport-specific injuries mainly affect the fingers and the ankle joints. (➤ Fig. 59.6; Lang-Jensen 1982, Leidinger et al. 1990, Langevoort 1993)

59.5.1 Diagnostics and Therapy

Injuries occurring in handball can be diagnosed broadly by the common diagnostic measures of orthopedics and trauma surgery. Special injuries, e.g. eye injuries or dental injuries, will be transferred to the according specialist.

Of course, all performance-physiological examinations as well as a complete internal health check, including an echocardiogram, are standard in the federal league. Every player of the federal league uses also biomechanical methods, e.g. for treadmill analyses and the recording of data of force measurements.

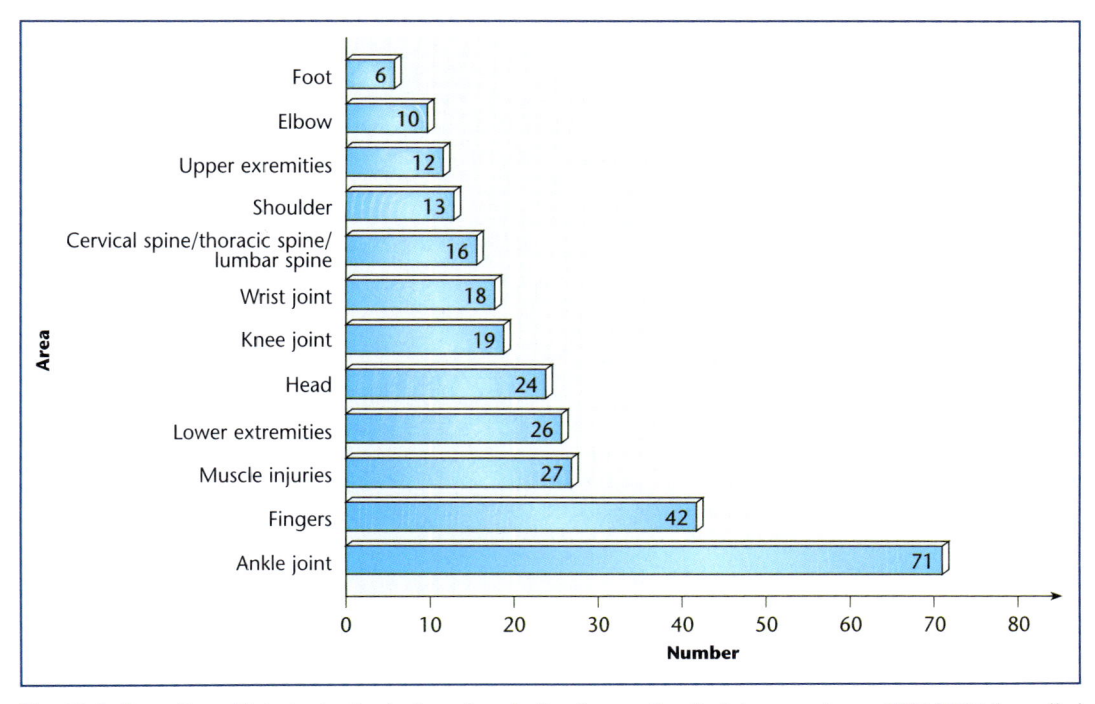

Fig. 59.6 Spreading of injuries to the body regions in the German Handball League of men 2004/2005 (compiled from the injured-cases list of the physician of the 1st German Handball League men, season 2004/2005).

Area	Number
Foot	6
Elbow	10
Upper extremities	12
Shoulder	13
Cervical spine/thoracic spine/lumbar spine	16
Wrist joint	18
Knee joint	19
Head	24
Lower extremities	26
Muscle injuries	27
Fingers	42
Ankle joint	71

Special forms of therapy or surgical procedures for handball injuries do not exist, compared to the injuries in other sports or occupational or household accidents (Jörgensen 1984, Maehlum and Daljourd 1984, Franke 1986, Nielsen and Yde 1988, Lindblad et al. 1992, Jörgensen 1993, Langevoort 1993, Münker et al. 1993).

59.5.2 Prophylaxis

Specific **whole-body strengthening and coordination programs** are carried out already in juveniles (Siewers 1996). The performance committee of the German Handball Federation determines the conception.

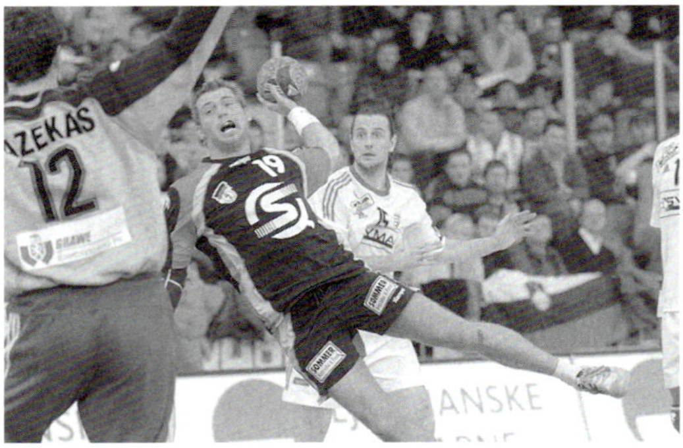

Technical training, e.g. the adhering to the correct throwing technique, is absolutely decisive for the avoidance of early chronic impairments. Juveniles tend to use an expanding, joint-stressing throwing movement (at the long lever) with the aim of a stronger throw. Injuries or impairments by improper strains of the elbow and the shoulder joint can be avoided by permanent correction. Similarly, permanent practicing of the exact technique of ball catching prevents injuries of the finger joints (Siewers 1996).

Falling exercises, at first on soft-foam mats, are important for correct falling or rolling off (➢ Fig. 59.7; Siewers 1996).

Jump exercises and exercises at the tilting board, exercises on soft-foam mats or trampolines are carried out to accustom the joints to the sport-specific strain and to automate the body's own correction procedures at collision pressure to the joints (repeated stimulation of the arthroreceptors; Siewers 1996).

The lacking **observance of regeneration periods** or relaxation phases does also have an injury-increasing effect. The recent major events, such as the European championship in Norway or the Olympic Games in Peking, have shown that the strain of the players sometimes goes to the human limit: ten games had to be absolved within 12 days, with one day, which had been planned as relaxation day, being a traveling day in Norway (8-hour bus ride) involving all inconveniences of transport, moving into a new accommodation, etc. Especially national players do not have any regeneration phases anymore because of their actions in the club, international cups, e.g. champions' league, and because of entering competitions with the national team. The German national team that has been successful since 2002 has had only 8 weeks of personal vacation altogether within these 6 years.

Regularly repeated **nutrition counseling** has been established in the federal leagues of the German handball federation. All teams receive sufficient sport-medical treatment. in special cases, there is an active **cooperation with sport psychologists**.

Fig. 59.7 Falling sideways throw with high risk of injury without automated falling technique (Germany – Hungary 2004).

References

ARAG Sportversicherung (2004). Sportunfälle.

Brack R (2002). Sportspielspezifische Trainingslehre. Wissenschafts- und objekttheoretische Grundlagen am Beispiel Handball. Feldhaus-Verlag, Edition Czwalina.

Brack R et al. (1996). Leistungstraining für Jugendliche und Erwachsene.

Brack R et al. (2006). Leistungstraining Handball, Grundlagenreferat A-Lizenz Trainerausbildung DHB.

Deutscher Handballbund (2005). Internationale Handballregeln. DHB, Dortmund.

Deutscher Handballbund (2004). Jahrbuch. DHB, Dortmund.

Dörner D (1989). Die Logik des Misslingens. Strategisches Denken in komplexen Situationen. Rowohlt Verlag, Reinbek.

References

Franke K (1986). Traumatologie des Sports. Thieme-Verlag, Stuttgart-New York.

Jörgensen U (1984). Epidemiology of injuries in typical Scandinavian team sports. Br J Sports Med 18 (2): 59–63.

Jörgensen U (1993). The epidemiology of injuries in handball. 1st IHF-Congress on Sportsmedicine and Handball. Oslo.

Langevoort Gijs (1993). Gleno-humerale Instabilität. 1st IHF-Congress on Sportsmedicine and Handball. Oslo.

Lang-Jensen J (1982). Acute sports injuries I. A one-year material from casualty department. Ugeskr laeg 144: 3603–3607.

Leidinger A, Gast W, Pförringer W (1990). Traumatologie im Hallenhandballsport. Sportverletz Sportschaden 4: 65–68.

Lindblad BE, Hoy K, Terkelsen CJ, Helleland HE (1992). Handball injuries. An epidemiologic and socioeconomic study. Am J Sports Med 20 (4): 441–444.

Maehlum S, Daljourd OA (1984). Acute sports injuries in Oslo: a one-year study. Br J Sports Med 18: 181–185.

Münker H, Gerlach I, Schreiber U (1993). Injuries in handball – an epidemiologic and traumatologic study. 1st IHF-Congress on Sportsmedicine and Handball. Oslo.

Nielsen AB, Yde J (1988). An epidemiologic and traumatologic study of injuries in handball. Int J Sports Med 9 (5): 341–344.

Sievers M (1996). Verletzungsprofil von Kaderathleten. Sport in Schleswig-Holstein.

Photographic material: Michael Heuberger.

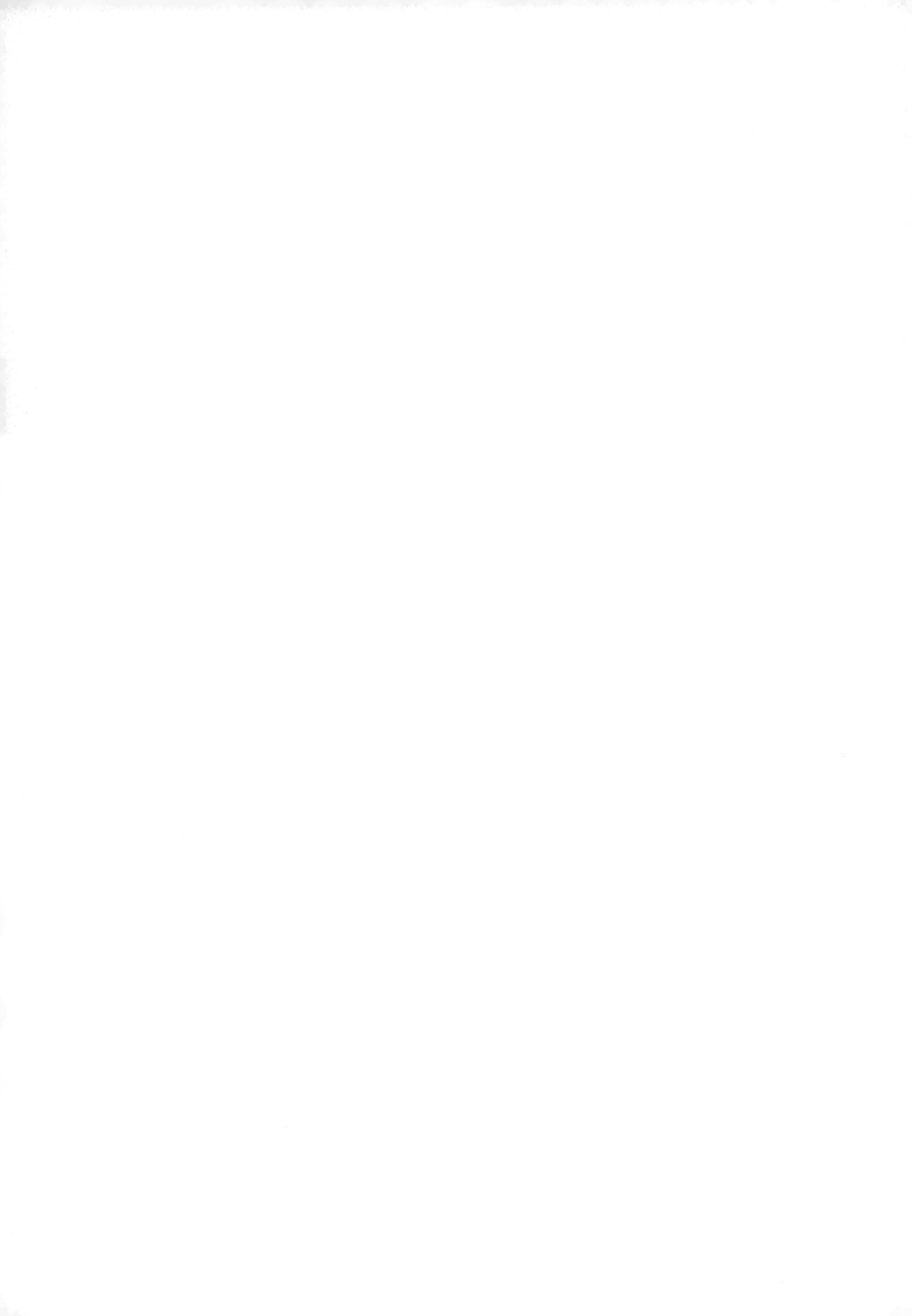

60 Field hockey

Winfried Koller

Hockey is – internationally seen – the team sport that is most successful in Germany. The successes of the national teams at the Olympic Games in Athens in 2004 (men: bronze medal; women: gold medal) and in Peking in 2008 (men: gold medal; women: 4th place) are only the most recent examples. At present, about 60,000 players in Germany play hockey actively. Still it is known far less than other team sports, such as soccer, ice hockey, basketball or handball.

60.1 Epidemiology

The **injury frequency** in hockey is given as 1.4 or 2.46%. Thus, hockey lies clearly behind soccer, basketball or even handball, but still above the average injury frequency in sport, which lies between 1.1 and 1.4%.

Half of the **injuries** (➤ Tab 60.1) are **caused** by opponent's influence, the other half by local events (fall because of the condition of the lawn) or personal negligence (lacking warm-up or insufficient physical fitness).

Lesions are caused in 23% by the stick, in 14% by the ball and in 11% by body contact with the opponent. **Goalkeepers** assume a special position. The ball affects them more than twice as often (54%). Stick injuries hardly play any role for them and the body contact with the opponent endangers them in 8%. In comparison, the fullbacks suffer lesions by the collision with the opponent in up to 19% and the forwards do so in 5%.

60.2 Typical injuries

Types of injury (➤ Tab. 60.2) do not differ too much from other sports. Minor injuries, such as distortions, contusions and especially abrasions with 80% clearly dominate, while the moderate injuries amount to 12% and only 8% are serious traumas. Fractures are found quite often at fingers and the hand region.

Hockey-specific injuries are found in the area of the upper extremity (➤ Tab. 60.3). Altogether, the relation of injuries of the upper extremity to the ones of the lower extremity is about 1:4, if the area of the head is not consid-

Tab. 60.1 Causes of injuries (according to Harlass-Neuking 1998, Eggers-Ströder 1994).

Opponent	48%	body	11%
		racket	23%
		ball	14%
Other causes (location, personal negligence)	52%		

Tab. 60.2 Injury types (according to Harlass-Neuking 1998, Eggers-Ströder 1994).

distortions	27%
contusions	14%
fractures	14%
ligament/tendon injuries	7.5%
muscle injuries	6.5%
meniscus injuries	5%
lacerations	2.1%
others	22.9%

Tab. 60.3 Injuries of the upper extremity (according to Harlass-Neuking 1998, Eggers-Ströder 1994).

fractures	61%	fingers	32%
metacarpus	16%		
forearm	3%		
clavicula	10%		
contusions	28%		
distortions	9%		
dislocations	2%		

ered. Contusions, lacerations and fractures in the **region of the fingers and the metacarpus** mostly are consequences of direct impacts by ball or stick. Fractures at the hands occur often because the hand grabs the stick firmly and therefore cannot evade when hit by stick or ball. **Mouth and tooth injuries** are mainly found in beginners. Compared to previous times, dental injuries could be clearly reduced by the mandatory wearing of a mouthpiece.

In comparison, the **injuries of the lower extremity** are not characteristic (➤ Tab. 60.4). Traumas and conditions occur in the same way as in other team sports. Distortions of the upper ankle joint are of the highest numbers, the same as in all team sports. Injuries of the knee ligaments, especially the anterior cruciate ligament, and meniscus ruptures are also found in hockey. In comparison to soccer, they only play an inferior role. Only the goalkeeper is at a risk above average, regarding the combined internal knee traumas – but also injuries in general –, by the consequences of a collision with the opponent.

Traumatically conditioned injuries of the spine are extremely rare. **Rib fractures** and **thoracic contusions** occur occasionally.

Tab. 60.4 Injuries of the lower extremity (according to Harlass-Neuking 1998, Eggers-Ströder 1994).

fractures	6%
contusions	11.5%
distortions	44%
meniscus injuries	8.5%
ligaments/tendons	12.5%
musculature	10.8%
others	3.6%

60.3 Sport-specific medical problems

Abnormalities are often detected in the yearly orthopedic preventive check-ups of the national squads: a retropatellar friction is often found. Conditions in the area of the lumbar spine are often combined with contractions of the iliopsoas muscle. Many active athletes complain of instability in the upper ankle joints. Chronic swellings of the Achilles tendons and the periost in the medial tibial edges can also be detected.

There are only few hockey-specific overstrain signs. The athletes show a number of chronic conditions (➤ Tab. 60.5) with the **lower extremity** being affected the most. Next are conditions in the region of the spine and finally the overstrain syndromes of the upper extremity.

Chondropathic conditions of the **knee** are found again and again. In addition, mainly insertion tendopathies at the tuberositas tibiae, but also at the upper and lower patellar edge appear and can be ascribed to the frequent flexed position of the knee joint in the different movement processes. Chronic meniscopathies are found occasionally, but primarily in goalkeepers. Knee ligament instabilities are

Tab. 60.5 Overstrain signs of the locomotor apparatus (multiple mentions possible; according to Harlass-Neuking 1998, Eggers-Ströder 1994).

Upper extremity	25%	shoulder	11%
		elbow	13%
		hand/fingers	15%
Spine	43.2%	CS	13.6%
		TS	2.4%
		LS	38.5%
Lower extremity	72.2%	hip	7.7%
		groin	7.1%
		knee	53.8%
		Achilles tendon	8.9%
		ankle joints	36%
		musculature	16.6%
Others	4.7%		

rather an exception. Loose **ankle joints** can be detected as often as in other sports.

Since international and also national games are played almost always on watered artificial lawns, **achillodynias and periostitides of the tibial edge** have become more frequent. Although malformations of the foot with flattening of the longitudinal and transverse arch have become common, only few athletes complain of the according conditions.

Problems of the lumbar area with **tensions of the dorsal extensors and limited mobility of the lower lumbar spine** dominate in dorsal pain. A **contraction of the iliopsoas muscle** is often found in combination with a ventral pelvic tilt. An additional cause can be the domination of the dorsal extensors over the abdominal muscles, because hockey often forces the athletes into kyphotic posture of the trunk in the defensive situations. Acute lumbagos and ischialgias are rare and therefore occur rather during the winter season. Hockey has always been described as a sport damaging the dorsum. Considering the percentages, it does not come to more frequent problems than in other sports, though.

The overstrain syndromes of the upper extremity altogether are rather rare. Impairments are caused by the **injuries in the area of the hand** that have been described before. **Pain in the shoulders** is primarily found in goalkeepers. **Epicondylitides in the elbow region** are found rather in beginners. The rule of only playing the ball by the flat side entails a permanently changing pronation and supination of the forearm at simultaneous extension of the elbow joint.

60.4 Prophylaxis

The best protection of injuries is provided by a consequent interpretation of the rules and fair play of each athlete. The field hockey rules have been clearly tightened. This had been necessary because of the frequency of head injuries. Historical records point to 39% of such traumas (Glass, 1927), today's statistics only show about 5%. Altogether, hockey is not a very risky sport, especially since most are only minor injuries. Nevertheless, prevention should also be of consideration in future.

A sensibly structured **training** is important for beginners. In addition to the running and technical qualities, emphasis has to be put on the stabilization of the trunk and the strengthening of the femoral muscles especially in juveniles. Intensive warm-up and gymnastics are sensible preventive measures. Since championships on the field as well as indoors are played in Germany, the necessary regeneration of the athletes will have to be taken into account in planning the training. This is especially problematic for the athletes of the national teams. International events have become numerous in current years (European and world championships including qualification tournaments, the Olympic Games, Champions Trophy etc.).

Altogether, the exercised condition of the athletes in hockey is excellent. In yearly examinations of the squat athletes, it is shown that hockey players belong to the best-exercised team athletes in Germany.

The **equipment** must be adjusted to new situations. The fields of artificial lawn have made hockey more rapid and faster. Therefore, it has been necessary to enhance the protection gear of the goalkeepers, and the weight could even be reduced by the use of synthetics instead of leather.

Shin splints covering the internal and external ankles are mandatory for field players. Ball and stick are often the cause of very painful bruises here. The same applies to the dental protection that can help to prevent serious injuries.

Cushioned gloves or bandages should reduce the high number of finger injuries.

Distortions in the region of the ankle joint should not be trivialized. Ligament lesions in the region are often overlooked or negated. Especially the enormously high number of chronic instabilities of the upper ankle joint requires an **exact diagnosis and adequate therapy with according rehabilitation** of each individual injury. With existing stability problems, a muscular compensation by especially exercising the peroneal muscles and a sensorimotor training should be the primary measure. Functional bandages and braces provide an additional effect.

Summary

Hockey is a sport with only very few injuries compared to other team sports. A number of the conditions will be only minor. Adhering to the rules and prophylactic measures can reduce serious injuries further.

References

Arnold A (1931). Über Hockeyverletzungen. DMW: 2175–2177.

Bolhuis JHA (1987). Dental and facial injuries in international field hockey. Br J Sports Med 21: 174–177.

Dettmer R, Nordhausen H (1981). Verletzungen und Überlastungserscheinungen am Bewegungsapparat bei Hockeyspielern. Dissertation. Heinrich-Heine-Universität, Düsseldorf.

Eggers-Ströder G, Hermann B (1994). Verletzungen beim Feldhockey. Sportverletz Sportschad 7: 93–97.

Glass E (1927). Hockeyverletzungsstatistik. DMW: 1907.

Harlass-Neuking A (1988). Verletzungen und Schäden im Hockeysport. Dissertation. Technische Universität, Munich.

Hermann B (1991). Hallenhockey: Verletzungen und Prävention. Sportverletz Sportschad 2: 85–89.

Murtaugh K (2001). Injury patterns among female field hockey players. Medicine & Science. Sports & Exercise 33 (2): 201–207.

Sherker S, Cassel E (1998). A Review of Field Hockey Injuries and Countermeasures for Prevention. Monash University Accident Research Centre – Report #143.

Thelen E (1981). Hockey. In: Pförringer W, Rosemeyer B (eds.). Sporttraumatologie. Perimed Verlag, Erlangen, pp 231–238.

Chapter 61 Rugby

Holger Schmitt

Rugby originated in the English school town of Rugby and was developed there by William Webb Ellis. In Germany, rugby has been played in clubs since 1872. In 2007, 9,738 members were registered with the German Rugby Federation.

61.1 Sport-specific characteristics

Rugby is played with an oval ball on a playing field of 100 m maximum length and 69 m maximum width. At each end there is a try area. Goal posts are positioned on the try lines: the posts are 5.60 m apart and the crossbar is 3 m above the ground. An adult rugby game lasts 2 × 40 min with a 5-minute break in between, during which the players are not allowed to leave the pitch. A team consists of 15 players: eight forwards who are positioned in three rows, a half-back, five three-quarters and the fullback. Because of their different tasks, the players in the individual positions also exhibit different physiques. Players in the front-row are very powerfully built, often weighing more than 100 kg and are at the front of so-called rucks. Players in the second row are generally very tall and aim to gain possession of the ball in the line out (➤ Fig. 61.1). Half-backs are generally small, but fast and flexible.

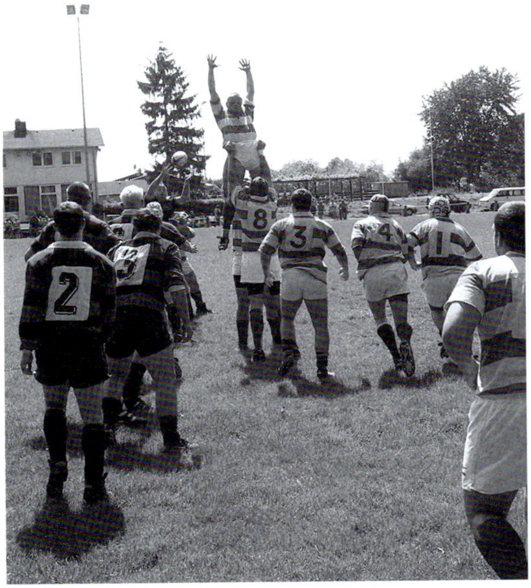

Fig. 61.1 Lifting of the player at the lateral throw-in, lineout.

61.2 Injuries and overstrain damages

The different playing positions lead to position-dependent injury patterns, which vary according to the specific physical demands of the position. Forwards playing at all standards have a higher injury rate (56.3%) than other players (43.7%), because they are subject to extra physical stress caused by the high number of collisions and tackles. The players at the back run freely over long distances.

> Forwards in rugby have a higher injury risk than all other players.

When the number of direct physical challenges between opposing professional players was looked at, it was seen that forwards are involved in 36 to 55 and the backs 19 to 29 physi-

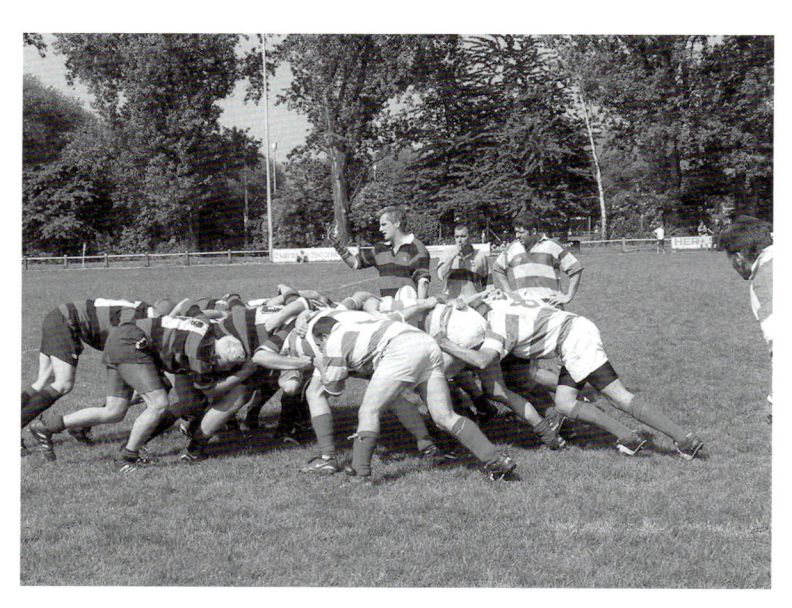

Fig. 61.2 Playing situation in the scrum.

cal challenges per game (Gissane et al. 2001). Injuries to the locomotor apparatus are frequent because of the body contact. More than 60% of injuries are caused by tackling (➤ Fig. 61.2).

A clearly increased injury risk in competition could be seen in prospective studies in comparison to training (Fuller et al. 2008). Semiprofessional athletes are at a higher risk of injuries than professionals and amateurs. When all injuries occurring during competitive games are considered, an injury rate of 214–346 injuries per 1,000 hours of competing has been calculated in professional games (Brooks et al. 2005), and amounts to 824.7 per 1,000 hours of competition in semiprofessionals. Injury rates in training amount to 26–45 injuries per 1,000 hours of training (➤ Tab 61.1; Gabbett 2003, 2004). Compared to amateur soccer players, the injury risk in rugby is more than twice as high in competition (Junge et al. 2004).

> In rugby, injuries occur in competition far more often than in training (by a factor of about 10–20).

Tab. 61.1 Localization of injuries in semi-professional rugby players (according to Gabbett 2004).

	Injuries during competition			Injuries during training		
Localization	Number	Incidence	95% CI	Number	Incidence	95% CI
thigh and calf	180	174.2	148.7–199.6	142	38.6	32.1–45.0
face	135	130.6	108.7–152.6	13	3.5	1.6–5.5
arm and hand	122	118.0	97.0–139.1	21	5.7	3.3–8.2
knee	131	126.8	105.0–148.5	47	12.8	9.1–16.5
shoulder	90	87.1	69.1–105.1	13	3.5	1.6–5.5
head and nape	89	86.1	68.3–103.9	10	2.7	1.0–4.4
thorax and abdomen	100	96.8	77.8–115.7	49	13.3	9.6–17.1
foot and ankle	91	88.1	70.1–106.1	93	25.3	20.2–30.4
others	10	9.7	3.6–15.8	1	0.3	0.0–0.8

Injuries during competition (per 1,000 hours of playing), injuries during training (per 1,000 hours of playing), 95% CI = 95% confidence interval

The lower number of injuries during training is attributed to the way in which tackles are practiced i.e. without direct opponent contact but using tackle pads (special cushions with impact protection) or padded protection vests. Cushioned scrum machines are used for practicing specific playing positions in the scrum.

In adults, injuries to the head and neck are in the most frequent in both professionals (33.3%) and amateurs (25.3%). Serious injuries with spinal cord involvement are rare, but have been observed in eight to nine players year in South Africa or New Zealand in recent years (Haylen 2004). The incidence of head injuries is 6.6 injuries per 1,000 hours of playing (Kemp et al. 2008).

> The most frequent injuries (about one third) affect head and neck. In rare cases, there are also injuries with involvement of the spinal cord.

Femur and hip are affected in about 18%, the knee joints in 10–11% and abdomen and thorax in 9–13%. Injuries to the femur and hip were frequent in semiprofessional players. Here as well as in adolescent rugby players, injuries of head and neck were only found in about 10% of cases. Different playing styles are thought to be the reason for this (Gabbett 2004).

The range of **injuries to different parts of the locomotor apparatus** is wide (➤ Tab. 61.2).

Contusions, lacerations and cerebral concussion are the primary injuries to the **cranium** and in rare cases there are also fractures. Distortions in the area of the cervical spine and rarely also discoligamentous avulsions are caused by holding and rotation stress.

In the **upper extremities**, fractures of the clavicula and rarely also of the sternum occur, along with dislocations of the shoulder joint, the sternoclavicular and the acromioclavicular joints (➤ Fig. 61.3). Distortions appear in the area of the long fingers particularly in the region of the thumb, and also some ligament ruptures caused by grabbing and traction stress in the scrum are seen.

Lateral ligament and anterior or posterior ligament ruptures are the main injuries to the **knee joint**, in some cases in combination with meniscus and cartilage lesions. Distortions or even malleolar fractures also occur at the ankle joint.

Hematomas and strains constitute about a third of all injuries in semiprofessional and professional players. In addition, there are **contusions**, **abrasions** and the joint injuries mentioned above. The latter often result in players being unfit to play or train for prolonged periods.

Tab. 61.2 Overview of injuries and overstrain impairments of the locomotor apparatus in rugby.

Localization	Type of injury
headhead	contusion or commotio cerebri skin injuries in the facial area (abrasions and lacerations) othematomas
spine	distortions up to discoligamentary tears at the CS with neurological deficits contusions and blockings of TS and LS
torso	thorax and rib contusions or rib fractures, respectively clavicular fractures and injuries of the sternoclavicular joints
upper extremitie	scontusions shoulder dislocations injuries of the rotator cuff distortions of elbow, hand and finger joints radius fractures
lower extremities	distortions in the area of the adductors (also as overstrain reaction) contusions at thigh and lower leg with hematomas muscle-tendon injuries of the thigh and the calf distortions of the knee joints with meniscus and capsule ligament injuries distortion of the ankle joints with injuries of the external ligament apparatus

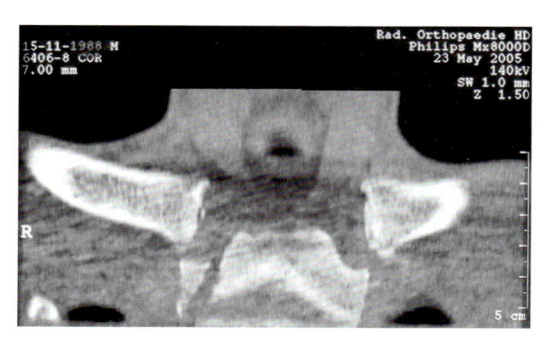

Fig. 61.3 Computer tomography: osseous chipping at the sternoclavicular joint after collision in rugby.

Injuries to the femur and hip are frequent in training. Muscle injuries (torn muscle fibers) are the most common. Forwards have an increased injury risk during training.

> Muscle and tendon injuries most often occur in training. Contusions, strains and torn muscle fibers of the femoral muscles are especially frequent because of direct collisions between opponents or because of sprint stress.

61.3 Prevention

Incidence and degree of severity of tackling injuries can be reduced by correct tackling techniques, correct falling techniques and use of protection gear (Garraway et al. 2000, Kaplan et al. 2008). The minor influence of protection gear on the injury rate was demonstrated in a cohort study in New Zealand: although mouth pieces and head protection reduced the injury risk to the ears and facial cranium, there was no influence on the occurrence of minor craniocerebral traumas (Marshall et al. 2005). Physical fitness is a risk factor in injuries. Players with less endurance suffered more injuries than those with better fitness levels (Gabbett and Domrow 2005). The injuries that appear cumulatively in amateurs in the second half of matches are in many cases caused by fatigue and can be influenced by specific training measures (e.g. endurance training) (Brooks et al. 2008).

> Correct tackling and falling techniques as well as use of protection gear can reduce the incidence and the degree of severity of injuries in rugby.

A mouthpiece with rounded security cleats are mandatory and are checked by the referee. The use of soft bandages is permitted (without any metal parts), head gear for the protection of the ears, shin guards (especially used by the "hooker" of the front-row forwards) and tape bandages; the wearing of jewelry, neck bands and guards with hard materials is forbidden.

Positioning of untrained adult players in the front-row, or of juveniles in the front and second rows, is prohibited in order to reduce the injury risk to the cervical spine.

61.4 Medical treatment

A yearly sport-medical examination is recommended and is mandatory for professional players. In order to reduce the injury risk, dangerous objects such as buckles or rings, are forbidden. The referee will decide on the suitability of clothing or equipment. Shoulder pads may only be worn after previous injuries and with the approval of the referee.

Medical assistants are only allowed onto the pitch to provide with the referee's permission. Medical treatment that takes longer than 1 min should be continued off the pitch.

Players with a diagnosed commotio cerebri should not participate in training and competition for at least three week after the injury; they have to undergo neurological examination before returning to the sport.

For all injuries to the extremities a full return to the sport with participation in training and competition is only allowed after complete healing of the injury. The attending physician must confirm full recovery of function and can then lift the restriction.

References

Brooks JH, Fuller CW, Kemp SP, Reddin DB (2005). A prospective study of injuries and training amongst the England 2003 Rugby World Cup squad. Br J Sports Med 39: 288–293.

Brooks JH, Fuller CW, Kemp SP, Reddin DB (2008). An assessment of training volume in professional rugby union and its impact on the incidence,

References

severity and nature of match and training injuries. J Sports Sci 26: 863–873.

Fuller CW, Laborde F, Leather RJ, Molloy MG (2008). International Rugby Board Rugby World Cup 2007 injury surveillance study. Br J Sports Med 42: 452–459.

Gabbett TJ (2003). Incidence of injury in semi-professional rugby league players. Br J Sports Med 37: 35–44.

Gabbett TJ (2004). Incidence of injury in junior and senior rugby league players. Sports Med 34: 849–859.

Gabbett TJ, Domrow N (2005). Risk factors for injury in sub-elite rugby league players. Am J Sports Med 33: 428–434.

Garraway WM, Lee AJ, Hutton SJ, Russell EBAW, Macleod DAD (2000). Impact of professionalism on injuries in rugby union. Br J Sports Med 34: 348–351.

Gissane C, White J, Kerr K, et al. (2001). Physical collisions in professional super league rugby, the demands on different player positions. Cleve Med J 4: 137–146.

Haylen PT (2004). Spinal injuries in rugby union, 1970–2003: lesions and responsibilities. MJA 181: 48–50.

Junge A, Cheung K, Edwards T, Dvorak J (2004). Injuries in youth amateur soccer and rugby players – comparison of incidence and characteristics. Br J Sports Med 38: 168–217.

Kaplan KM, Goodwille A, Strauss EJ, Rosen JE (2008). Rugby injuries: a review of concepts and current literature. Bull NYU Hosp Jt Dis 66: 86–93.

Kemp SP; Hudson Z, Brooks JH, Fuller CW (2008).The epidemiology of head injuries in English professional rugby union. Clin J Sport Med 18: 227–234.

Marshal SW, Loomis DP, Waller AE, Chalmers DJ, Bird YN, Quarrie KL, Feehan M (2005). Evaluation of protective equipment for prevention of injuries in rugby union. Int J Epidemiol 34: 113–118.

Badminton

Silvia Albrecht and Roland Biedert

Badminton is played with a shuttlecock; it is simple and easy to play and to learn. Therefore it has quickly become the favored hobby of many recreational athletes. Badminton is one of the most popular sports in the world and yet there is only little medical interest and surveys regarding injuries and overload syndromes are rare.

Today's form of badminton is named after an English town and has its origins in Asia. English colonial rulers brought the sport from their Indian colony back to Europe. Still, there are also indications that the Incas had already known the game with the shuttle. Since 1992 badminton has been an **Olympic sport** and is especially popular in the Asian countries. In Europe, badminton has mostly spread in Denmark and is the number-one national sport there in addition to soccer. In Switzerland, there are about 12,000 active, registered members; in Germany, there are approx. 100,000.

World and European championships, international and also national tournaments in the five disciplines of women and men singles, women and men doubles and mixed doubles – individually or as a team – are carried out regularly.

62.1 Sport-specific requirements

The physical **requirements** are very high for reaching international level. In addition to a strong will, a lot of exercising, very good flexibility, coordination and high velocity as well as a strong base of strength and endurance, but most of all a high springiness and a quick capacity of reaction are **important**. Furthermore, good hand-eye coordination, an ability to read the game and tactical awareness are of significance.

The importance of good interval endurance can be detected by the **maximum heart frequency** during the rally occasionally reaching the theoretical maximum heart rate. The average value of heart rate of a badminton match of about 28 minutes lies at approx. 15 beats under maximum heart rate. The heart rate drops during the short rest periods after maximum strain hardly ever lower than 160 beats per minute. At these high intensities, the strain during is mostly be **aerobic but alactatic** (Cabello and Gonzales Badillo 2003).

62.2 Sports equipments

In badminton, everything is about the **shuttle**, which consist of 16 goose feathers and weighs 6 g (➤ Fig. 62.1). The cutting and origin of the

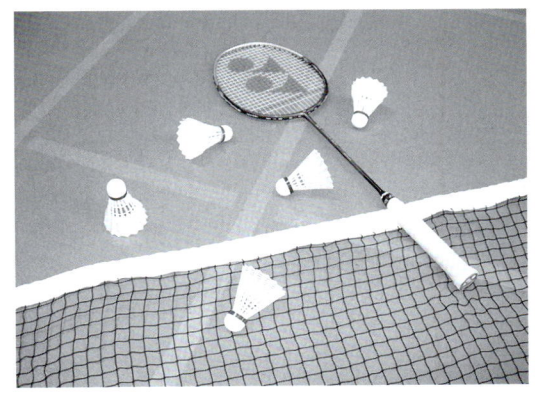

Fig. 62.1 Feather and nylon shuttles as well as further badminton equipment such as racket and net.

feathers determine the various qualities and speeds of the shuttles. Those speeds are additionally influenced by humidity and temperature in the playing arena.

The shuttle reaches speeds of more than 300 km/h from the "smash" stroke as the shuttle leaves the racket. This speed strongly decreases in the initial centimeters after leaving the racket, due to air resistance. This typical manner of flight of the shuttle is a decisive factor in the character of the game. In the recreational field, a shuttle made of synthetic material is often used which has an altogether different flying manner.

The **racket** is made of a mixture of carbon, graphite and titanium, is strung with a synthetic or natural gut (9–14 kg resistance) and weighs approx. 100 g. Balance and shaft flexibility (rigidity) are the distinctive features. There are no special rackets for women; principally, women and men, according to their own preference regarding balance and shaft flexibility, can use every racket.

Competitions are carried out on synthetic flooring with a **high friction coefficient**. Quick changes of direction can be performed due to the strongly adhesive synthetic soles of the sport shoes. Accordingly, **high de- and acceleration forces** occur in the stop-and-go movements of the game. Strong eccentric and concentric **strains in the area of knee, ankle joints and feet** develop in badminton due to the specific footwork.

62.3 Typical injuries and injury mechanisms

In 1987, Jörgensen found 26% of **acute injuries** compared to 74% of injuries by **improper strain or overstrain** in his study (Jörgensen and Winge 1987); Kluger has found 33% of acute injuries and 67% of chronic injuries (Kluger et al. 1999). **57.6%** of all acute and chronic in-

Tab. 62.1 Spreading of injuries by localization.

Localization	Kluger (1999)	Jörgensen (1987)	Hensley (1979)
lower extremity	71.0%	57.6%	69.0%
upper extremity	17.9%	30.5%	21.0%
dorsum	1.1%	10.4%	1.0%

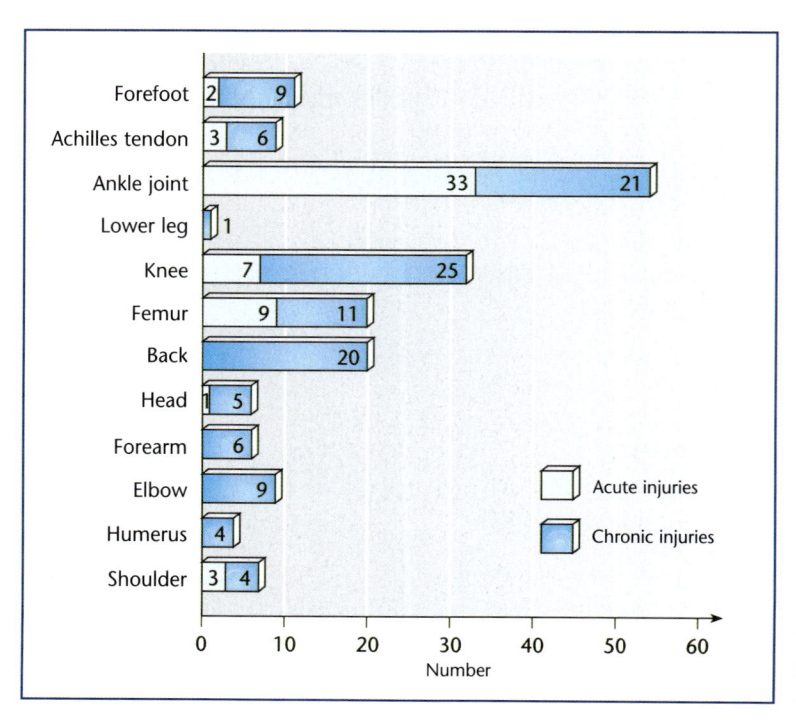

Fig. 62.2 Spreading pattern of acute and chronic injuries in badminton (Kluger et al. 1999).

Location	Acute	Chronic
Forefoot	2	9
Achilles tendon	3	6
Ankle joint	33	21
Lower leg	1	
Knee	7	25
Femur	9	11
Back		20
Head	1	5
Forearm	6	
Elbow	9	
Humerus	4	
Shoulder	3	4

juries affected the **lower extremity**, 30.5% the upper extremity, 10.4% the dorsum and 1.5% the eyes. These numbers are comparable to the studies of Kluger at al. (1999) and Hensley and Paup (1979; ➢ Tab. 62.1 and ➢ Fig. 62.2).

62.3.1 Acute injuries

Typical acute injuries are **contusions** caused by the cork of the shuttle or by the racket. In most cases, a hematoma develops which will heal out without treatment in a few days without any problems and is therefore considered a minor injury. In rare cases, lacerated contused wounds are the result and will have to be sutured. **Contusions of the eye bulbus** are considered **especially dangerous** (Barr et al. 2000), because the shuttle has a smaller diameter than the orbita.

Individual cases of losses of eyesight after contusions of the eye bulbi have been known in international badminton sport, but fortunately they are very rare.

Muscle injuries, on the other hand, are quite frequent (➢ Tab. 62.2). Slipping of the anterior foot in a lunge can strain the ischiocrural muscle (➢ Fig. 62.3). **Inversion traumas of the upper ankle joint** with a lateral ligament rupture often occur in the same accident mechanism, mostly by incorrect placing of the foot (➢ Fig. 62.4). This is the **most frequent ligament** injury in badminton (Kroner et al. 1990).

Anterior cruciate ligament ruptures are also serious injuries in badminton, which involve a long time of convalescence and rehabilitation after surgical as well as after conservative treatment. They will affect the side of the striking hand as well as the opposite side, but are more frequent at the non-striking side, probably because of the special badminton running technique. Still, they are rare and less frequent than lateral ligament ruptures at the ankle joints.

The frequency of **Achilles tendon ruptures** is similar to anterior cruciate ligament ruptures.

62.3.2 Chronic injuries

Chronic injuries are **overstrain impairments** with only few exceptions.

The most important are:

- subacromial impingement with partial ruptures of the supraspinal tendons
- tennis elbow
- achillodynia and
- jumper's knee.

As in all overhead sports, the **subacromial impingement** is conditioned by the repeated internal rotation movement of the arm in maxi-

Tab. 62.2 Spreading patterns of the injuries by kind of tissue (Kroner et al 1990).

Injured structure	Percentage
capsule/ligament	58.5
muscle	19.8
tendons	8.8
skin	5.1
bones	5.1
eyes	2.3
other	0.5

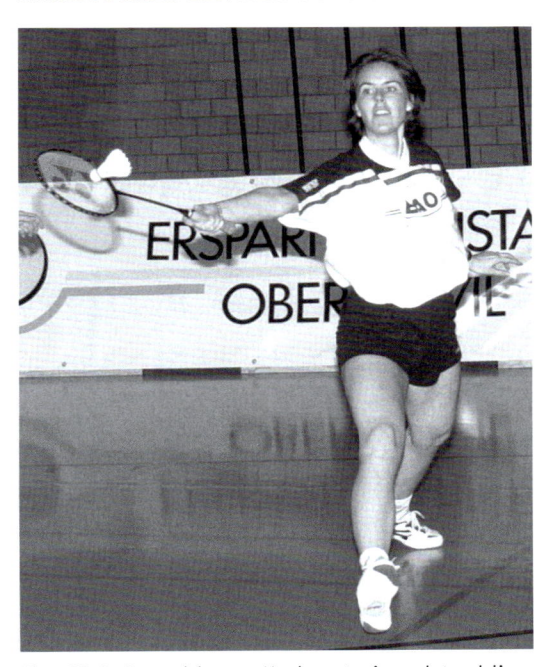

Fig. 62.3 Lateral lunge: Heel contusions, lateral ligament lesions in the upper ankle joint, and muscle lesion of the ischiocrural musculature are some of the possible injuries.

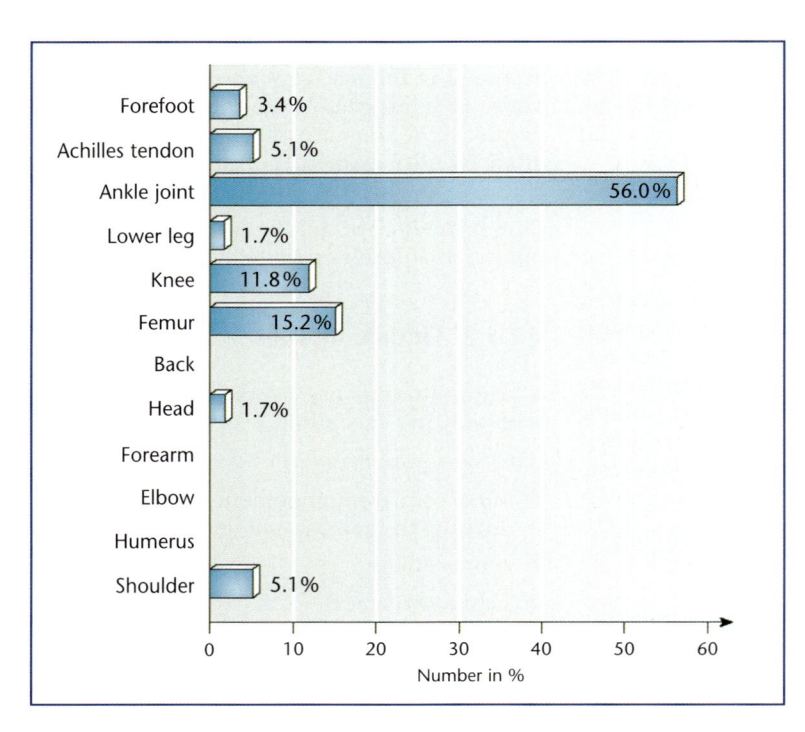

Fig. 62.4 Localization spreading of acute injuries at badminton (Kluger et al. 1999).

Location	%
Forefoot	3.4%
Achilles tendon	5.1%
Ankle joint	56.0%
Lower leg	1.7%
Knee	11.8%
Femur	15.2%
Back	
Head	1.7%
Forearm	
Elbow	
Humerus	
Shoulder	5.1%

mum flexion-abduction position of the shoulder (➤ Fig. 62.5).

The **tennis elbow** is just as frequent in badminton as it is in tennis (Kühne et al. 2004). The weight of the racket is less decisive here than the numerous repetitive, rapid movements.

Achillodynias appear in badminton quite frequently with 10–44% (Fahlström et al. 2002) and will develop especially by the increased strain at the forefoot. The **special footwork** in badminton is responsible, including sprints, forward and sideways lunges, often combined with forceful use of the heels and abrupt changes of direction, jumps to the side and fast step sequences – partly carried out on the toes – backwards with stops and changes of direction at the basic line. The **good adhesion of the shoes** to the flooring increases the strain peaks in the insertion area of the Achilles tendon. According to studies, the risk will increase with higher age and stronger exercising strain in the sense of "too much, too fast and all the time". Specific **eccentric muscle exercises for the triceps surae muscle** seem to have a

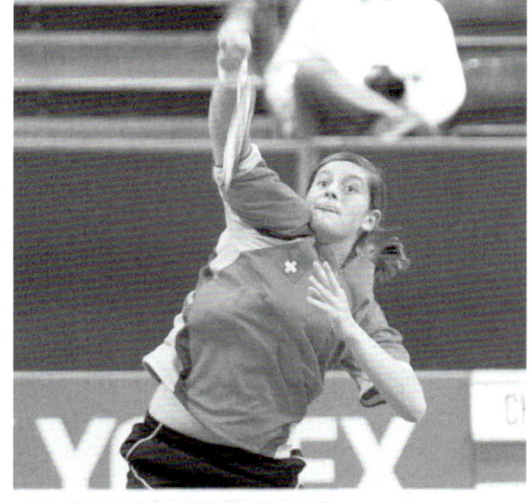

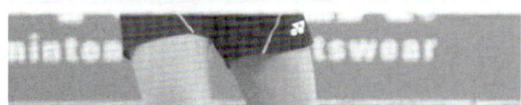

Fig. 62.5 Overhead stroke, as it is carried out hundredfold during a game and which can lead to a subacromial impingement that way.

healing and also preventive effect on achillodynias (Kluger et al. 1999, Fahlström et al. 2002).

The **jumper's knee** and patellofemoral pain in general are the most frequent chronic injuries of the lower extremity in addition to the achillodynias. These knee conditions are caused by the numerous jumps with landings on one leg and are classic overstrain conditions.

62.4 Risks by other parties

Risks by other parties occur in the **doubles disciplines** (➤ Fig. 62.6), caused by the partner or at the net because of the opponent striking over the net contrary to the rules. Altogether, these injuries are rare, mainly due to some "behavioural codes and unwritten laws" known by every player.

62.5 Injury risk

In general, the injury risk is **low** compared to other sports (Kluger et al 1999). There are reports of 4.1–5% of all sport injuries that are conditioned by badminton (Kroner et al. 1990). Most injuries are negligible and it is assumed that only a fifth of the actual badminton injuries are recorded in statistics. Jörgensen and Winge (1987) have reported an injury incidence of 2.9 injuries/player/1,000 hours of badminton.

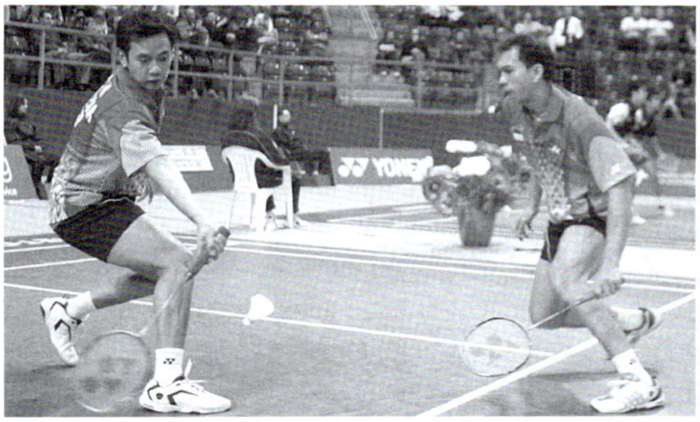

Serious injuries are relatively rare. According to Kroner et al. (1990), hospitalization had only been necessary in 6.8% of the injuries. There is a **frequency peak** of badminton injuries in January and September, corresponding to the season opening and the return after the Christmas break.

62.6 Prevention

Many of the acute injuries can be avoided by extensive **running-in** and playing-in with light stretching. **Sports goggles** are recommended for the prevention of eye injuries.

The eventuality of such consequences as **overstrain impairments** should be considered in the early years of a sport career and repetitive pain is to be taken seriously; the pain will have to be analyzed precisely and the causes will have to be eliminated, if possible. Technical mistakes, such as striking with a target point beside, instead of above the head or insufficient rotation of the body will have to be corrected in early stages. In addition, the purchase of **shoes** suitable to the feet and to the many stop-and-go movements with a sufficiently adhesive sole is recommended. **Insoles with a cushioning effect** are also advisable.

Fig. 62.6 Men's doubles: The player runs against the direction of play in the enthusiasm of the game. The danger of contusions by the racket of the opponent or by the shuttle is very high.

References

Barr A, Baines PS, Desai P, MacEwen CJ (2000). Ocular sports injuries: the current picture. Br J Sports Med 34: 456–458.

Cabello M, Gonzalez-Badillo J (2003). Analysis of the characteristics of competitive badminton. Br J Sports Med 37: 62–66.

Fahlström M, Lorentzon R, Alfredson H (2002). Painful conditions in the Achilles tendon region: a common problem in middle-aged competitive badminton players. Knee Surg Sports Traumatol Arthrosc 10: 57–60.

Fahlström M, Lorentzon R, Alfredson H (2002). Painful conditions in the Achilles tendon region in elite Badminton players. Am J Sports Med 30: 51–54.

Hensley LD, Paup DC (1979). A survey of badminton injuries. Br J Sports Med 13: 156–160.

Jörgensen U, Winge S (1987). Epidemiology of badminton injuries. Int J Sports Med 8: 379–382.

Kluger R, Stiegler H, Engel A (1999). Das Trainingsalter – ein neuer Risikofaktor akuter Badmintonverletzungen. Sportverl Sportschad 13: 96–101.

Kroner K, Schmidt SA, Nielsen AB, Yde J, Jakobsen BW, Möller-Madsen B, Jensen J (1990). Badminton injuries. Br J Sports Med 24: 169–172.

Kühne CA, Zettl RP, Nast-Kolb D (2004). Verletzungs- und Beschwerdehäufigkeit im Tennisleistungs- und Breitensport. Sportverl Sportschad 18: 85–89.

Chapter 63 Beach volleyball

Antonius Kass and Kerstin Warnke

63.1 History of beach volleyball

Beach volleyball was played for the first time in 1920 in Santa Monica, California. Initially, it spread at American beaches and became known in Europe and Asia in the 1950s and 1960s. At first, a team consisted of six players, although the type of "two against two" has become prevalent. As only few other sports, beach volleyball represents the "Californian lifestyle" of beach and sun.

In the 1970s, the tournaments became more professional and the first beach volleyball world championship was carried out in 1987. Since 1996 in Atlanta, it has been an Olympic sport and it was one of the greatest attractions at the successive Games in Sydney (at the Bondi Beach), Athens and Beijing. 2,000 professional beach-volleyball players were registered worldwide in 2004. The number of players who perform beach volleyball without having their roots in indoor sports constantly increases.

Professional beach volleyball tournaments have been carried out in Germany since 1988. These contribute to the increasing popularity in addition to Olympic reporting.

63.2 Sport-specific characteristics

Beach volleyball is played barefoot on sand by two teams of two players each, on a 8 × 8 m playing fields which are separated by a net. Since the rules changed in 2001, the beach volleyball playing field is smaller than the indoor volleyball playing field (9 × 9 m), although the height of the net is identical (2.24 m net height for women; 2.43 m for men). Two sets out of three must be won, with the first two being won with 21 points and the tiebreaker wins with 15 points and a two-point advantage. The counting is carried out in the rally-point system, i.e. every point counts. The sides will be changed in set 1 and 2 after seven and in set 3 after 5 played points. The average duration of effective playing amounts to 45 min; several games a day are common in international tournaments. It is mandatory for women to wear a bikini; the maximum side length of pants is 6 cm (FIVB 2005).

Beach volleyball has the following **characteristics** compared to indoor volleyball:

- Many outside influences, such as sun, wind and uneven sand, affect this outdoor sport.
- Timing, target point and position to the ball are often not ideal in beach volleyball, so that the player will have to attack from extreme positions and will have to counterbalance this by movements of the lumbar spine and the shoulder.
- The playing field's decreased size as a consequence of a change in the rules in 2001 has led to an extension of the average bal exchange from 6.8 sec to 7.4 sec. Jumps will be necessary every 24–36 sec in high-level men's matches.
- In the top teams, there are usually specialized block and defense players, so that the jump strain of the block players is about 75% higher than the one of the defense players (Warnke and Phieler 2006).
- The jumping behavior is different from the one in the gym due to the softness of the sand: the foot must be set down as flat as possible, in order to prevent a subsiding of

the toes at jumping. Thus, the flexion angle in the knee while jumping will is larger than than in indoor volleyball and will lead to a increased strain of the knee extension apparatus.

Studies are available regarding the **epidemiology and frequency of body injuries** with different results. In a retrospective study of the season 2001 published by the world federation FIVB, 95% of the surveyed elite volleyball players (n = 178) provided information about injuries and overstrain impairments (Bahr 2003, Reeser 2006). 54 acute injuries and 79 overstrain impairments have been documented that have resulted in absences from training and competition. Knee joint injuries amounted to 30% of these injuries, ankle joint and finger injuries to 17% each. Overstrain impairments are especially found in the area of the lumbar spine (19%), knee joint (12%) and shoulder (10%). 3.2 injuries per 1,000 hours of competition and 0.8 injuries per 1,000 hours of training have been recorded as incidence rates. This is below the frequency of soccer (4.1/1,000 hours of playing) and handball injuries (8.3/1,000 hours of playing) and at a similar frequency as volleyball injuries (1.5–4.2/1,000 hours of playing, depending on the study).

Different results have been found in a Danish study of 1997, for example, with 4.9 injuries/1,000 hours of playing of beach volleyball and 4.2 injuries/1,000 hours of playing indoor volleyball (Aagard et al. 1997) and in a published survey in Munich of 2006, in which the injury frequency has been stated with 0.08/season of beach volleyball and 0.22/year of indoor volleyball (Kugler et al. 2004).

In the comparison of **development and pattern of injuries in beach volleyball** and indoor volleyball, the following picture emerges:

- Injuries occur mainly in defense and offense. The direct net actions indoors present the higher injury risk.
- Ankle joint injuries are less frequents in beach volleyball as in indoor volleyball, where they amount to 55% of the injuries.
- Injuries in the shoulder region are more frequent in beach volleyball than in indoor volleyball, especially dislocations.
- Injuries of the fingers occur less often in beach volleyball than indoors.
- Types of injury that are unknown in indoor volleyball are present in beach volleyball: sunburn, heatstroke, incised and torn wounds by impurity of the sand and the so-called sand toe (plantar flexion trauma of the metatarsophalangeal joint of the hallux).
- Overstrain syndromes are found primarily at the shoulder and the lumbar spine, triggered by the variable movement process and because of present muscle dysbalances of the trunk and shoulder muscles.
- Overstrain syndromes of the quadriceps patellar tendon are typical for the knee extensor apparatus, correlating with the higher flexion angle in jumping off (Warnke and Phieler 2006).
- Irritations and injuries of the Achilles tendons are very rare because of the changed jumping behavior in beach volleyball.

63.3 Acute injuries

Below, the particularities of beach volleyball have been described and, in addition, the explanations of the chapter volleyball are referred to.

63.3.1 Ankle

A supination trauma of the upper ankle joint with corresponding capsule-ligament injuries will occur less often than in indoor volleyball, but still with amounts to 17% of all injuries, fractures are seldom. The trauma develops spontaneously due to landing in a supination position after offense or block (➤ Fig. 63.1) rather than due to the contact with the opponent (Warnke et al. 2006).

A major difficulty in the post treatment is that ortheses can be a hindrance on the court since the athletes play barefooted. A regular taping of the ankle joints for training and competition is recommended. Nevertheless, skin lesions can occur after a long-term treatment.

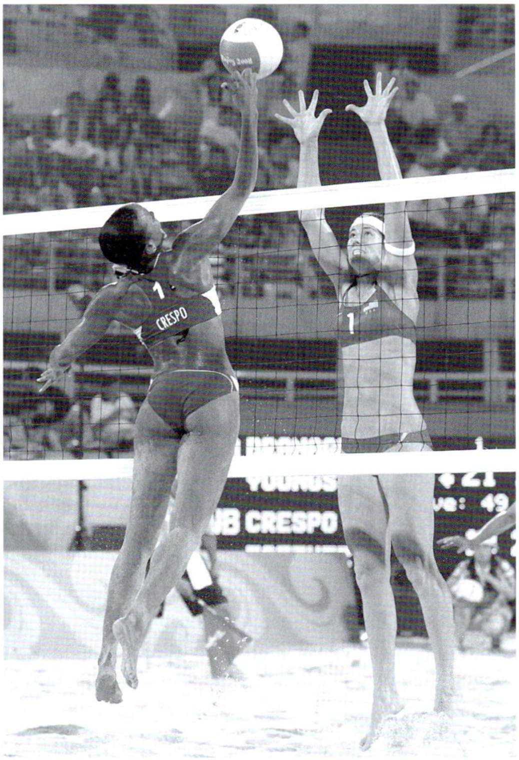

Fig. 63.1 The offensive action against the block is carried out as a "poke" here. This lob must be played with the finger knuckles (by courtesy of FIVB).

63.3.2 Knee joint

20–30% of all injuries in beach volleyball affect the knee joint and therefore are statistically more frequent than in indoor volleyball. The most frequent injury mechanism is a **locked rotation trauma** or an anteromedial buckling in the knee joint without influences from the outside, promoted by a fixation of the foot in the uneven sand. These injuries have been described as minor and will not result in a longer absence from playing (Bahr and Raeser 2003).

In addition to **sprains** and **meniscus injuries**, anterior **cruciate ligament injuries** are also a rare consequence, possibly also with involvement of the internal ligament.

Women are more frequently affected by cruciate ligament ruptures than men (factor 4–6; Petersen et al. 2005). This is due to a reduced muscular stability of the knee joint under strain, a decreased active and passive rotation stability (Wojtys et al. 2003) and an increased valgus strain during jumping (Hewett et al. 2005) in women.

A cruciate ligament rupture usually forces the volleyball player to an absence of 6–12 months; a meniscus injury that has been treated surgically requires 6–8 weeks.

63.3.3 Fingers

The incidence of finger injuries in beach volleyball has been reported to be 15–17% and is thus lower than the incidence indoors. The major amount of the injuries occurs in block actions, but the athletes can also get hurt in defense actions. Influences from the outside, such as gusts of wind and inaccurate timing in blocking, can increase the risk additionally.

Taping of the fingers is wide spread in volleyball for therapy and prevention. The affected finger will often be taped together with the neighboring finger. The resulting limitation of movement is not considered disturbing by the volleyball players.

63.3.4 Shoulder

Shoulder dislocations occure more often during volleyball than indoor volleyball. The accident mechanism is the arm getting stuck in the sand following a diving forearm pass, while the rest of the body still accelerates forwards, or a late defense of a diving forearm pass, in which the hand of the player lands on the volleyball while the body presses the shoulders down into the sand (➢ Fig. 63.2).

63.3.5 Skin

The influence of wind, sun and sand is straining to the skin in many ways. The prevention of **sunburns** and **heatstroke** is a continuous challenge of beach volleyball players. A **consequent sun protection** is absolutely necessary, as well as a **yearly dermatological examination**. Outside high temperatures strain the players extensively which can exacerbated by the lack

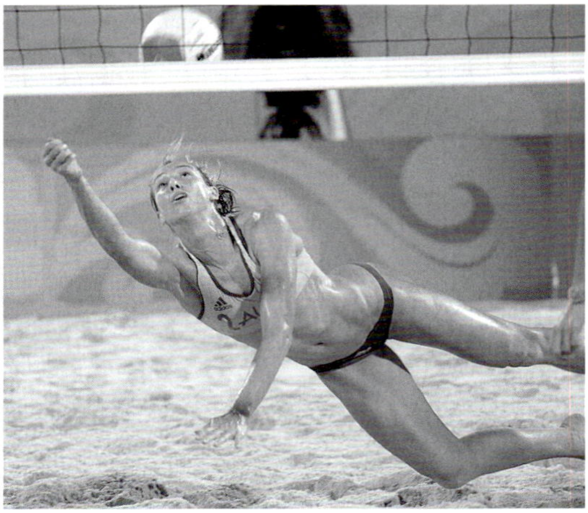

Fig. 63.2 Spectacular defensive action in deep sand (by courtesy of FIVB).

of convection in the tribunes. The temperatures of the sand had been as high as 70 °C in the Olympic Games in Athens in 2004. Cooling measures during the short breaks in the games and a sufficient amount of fluid intake are essential.

Sunglasses are recommended for the protection of the eyes.

High-class tournaments are also arranged in cities. There and also at the beaches, the **sand** will often contain **impurities**, e.g. pieces of broken glass and metal pieces. Thus, scrapes and cuts will occasionally occur.

In this context, it should be mentioned that individual cases of **parasite infestations** in players by the eggs of worms in the sand have been found.

63.4 Overstrain syndromes

63.4.1 Sand toe

An injury of the capsule-ligament structures develops by an increased plantar flexion especially in the metatarsophalangeal joint of the hallux of the bare foot in the sand. This can lead to definite function impairments for a long time afterwards in sprinting, jumping and the change of direction. A movement limitation of the dorsal flexion in the metatarsophalangeal joint of the hallux had been found in all cases in a survey of American beach volleyball professionals (n = 12); permanent conditions have been found in 42% of the cases and an unstable hallux in 17%. The average convalescence took 6 months (Frey et al. 1997).

63.4.2 Knee

The most frequent overstrain syndromes of beach volleyball players in the area of the knee joint affect the quadriceps **tendinopathy**. While the lower patellar apex syndrome clearly dominates in indoor volleyball (➢ Chapter 67), quadriceps tendinopathies are found more often in beach volleyball players. In an Austrian survey, sonographic changes have been found, such as swellings, adapted structures and calcifications of the patellar and of the quadriceps tendons, in 21–34% of the examined knee joints (n = 122; Pfirrmann et al. 2008).

The jump-off in beach volleyball occurs from the knee and not – as is mainly the case in indoor volleyball – from the ankle joint. The jump that is deeper this way with an increased flexion angle in the knee joint will lead to a rather proximally positioned force insert at the patella (Derrick 2004) and can cause a tendinopathy of the quadriceps tendon.

Therefore, the hypertrophy of the calf muscles and the hypertrophy of the quadriceps/hamstring is characteristic for beach volleyball players.

The diagnosis can be made classically and can be verified by **ultrasound and MRI**.

Therapeutically, **anti-inflammatory measures** of rest, local applications of ice, NSAR applications, if necessary, and local applications should be applied at first. A **balance of the flexor and extensor muscles** and a correct guidance of the patella through the vastus medialis muscle will have to be ensured. A **sensorimotor training program** with the stabilization of the leg axis is sensible. A surgical treatment with necrectomy and tendon reconstruction, if necessary, should be considered at the failure of a conservative physiotherapeutic therapy and will involve an absence from training and competition for several months.

63.4.3 Spine

Environmental influences, such as wind and uneven sand, will lead to incorrect passes and non-optimal target points in offensive strikes in beach volleyball. The consequences are imbalanced movements in the shoulder and a hyperlordosing and rotation in the lumbar spine. If there is a muscular dysbalance of the trunk and an insufficient segmental control of the spine muscles, an **increased strain of the small vertebral joints** will result. The resulting movement limitations can lead to **structural impairments**.

In addition to the clinical and neurological examinations, imaging procedures such as radiographs and MRI may be necessary for accurate diagnosis.

The therapy and prevention of spinal diseases present high challenges to athlete, coach, physiotherapist and sport physician. Training should start with static forms of exercise, then be increased to more complex exercises and eventually to sport-specific processes that will be implemented into the **exercise program** (Warnke and Phieler 2006).

63.4.4 Shoulder

For the reasons mentioned, the shoulder joint is not very susceptible for overstrain syndromes in beach volleyball. An incidence is indicated for shoulder injuries in 8–13% or even up to 35% (Gläser and Henke 2004).

Frequent causes are muscular dysbalances, especially in the region of the rotator cuffs (Wang et al. 2000), that will even be increased by the frequent kyphosis of the thoracic spine. There will often be a **subacromial shortage** because of a positioning of the humeral head to ventral-cranial.

The interaction of trunk and shoulder muscles is especially important in the offense and is therefore very susceptible for impairments. The most frequent consequences are **rotator cuff tendopathies** and **impingement syndromes**, **subacromial bursitides** and **irritations of the AC joint**, in few cases also limbic injuries.

In addition to the clinical examinations, radiography, ultrasound examination and – in case of doubt – MRI are necessary for diagnosis. If a limbic injury (e.g. SLAP lesion) is suspected, an arthro-MRI with intraarticular application of contrast material will be necessary.

The **healing of the inflammatory component** of shoulder pain is in the foreground in therapy. Local ice applications, balneophysical measures, NSAIDs and steroid injections, if necessary, should therefore be applied. A surgical therapy – usually arthroscopy – will be necessary following prolonged conditions or larger structural impairments.

A particularity of volleyball and beach volleyball is the **infraspinatus syndrome** or the lesion of the suprascapular nerve (➢ Chapter 67).

63.5 Prevention

- The prevention of injuries and overstrain is the most important task in a sport with intensive exercising periods and high strain in competition, such as beach volleyball.
- Knee and ankle joint injuries and spinal and shoulder impairments in the form of overstrain impairments stand out in the symptoms mentioned above as frequent conditions. A **sensorimotor exercise program for shoulder and leg axes** as well as a **segmental stabilization** will be necessary (Reeser JC et al. 2006, Warnke and Phieler 2006).

Weak points occurring frequently in beach volleyball players are:

- hyperkyphosis of the thoracic spine
- hyperlordosis of the lumbar spine with pelvic tilting
- lacking control of the segmental-stabilizing trunk muscles
- weakness of the external rotators and stabilizing muscles of the shoulder girdle
- ventral-cranial positioning of the humerus head
- weakness of the vastus medialis muscle as stabilizer of the knee joint
- weakness of the hamstrings versus the quadriceps muscles.

References

Aagard H, Scavenius M, Jorgenson U (1997). Epidemiological analysis of the injury pattern in indoor and beach volleyball. Int J Sports Med 18: 217–221.

Bahr R, Raeser JC (2003). Injuries among world-class professional beach volleyball players. The Fédération international de Volleyball beach volleyball injury study. Am J Sports Med 31: 119–125.

Derrick TR (2004). The effects of knee contact angle on impact forces and accelerations. Med Sci in Sports and Exercise 16: 832–837.

Frey C, Andersen GD, Feder KS (1996). Plantarflexion injury to the metatarsophalageal joint ("sand toe"). Foot Ankle Int 17: 576–581.

Gläser H, Henke T (2004). Sportunfälle – Häufigkeit, Kosten, Prävention. ARAG, Düsseldorf.

Hewett TE, Myer GD, Ford KR et al. (2005). Biomechanical measures of neuromuscular control and valgus landing of the knee predict anterior cruciate ligament injury risk in female athletes. A prospective study. Am J Sports Med 33: 492–501.

Kugler A, Krüger-Franke M, Schurk B (2004). Trendsportarten Beach Volleyball. Sport Orthop Traumatol 29: 235–237.

FIVB (ed.) (2005). Offizielle Beach-Volleyball-Spielregeln. 4th edition. Karl Hoffmann Verlag, Schondorf.

Petersen W, Rosenbaum D, Raschke M (2005). Rupturen des vorderen Kreuzbandes bei weiblichen Athleten. Teil 1: Epidemiologie, Verletzungsmechanismus und Ursachen. Dtsch Z Sportmed 56 (6): 150–156.

Pfirrmann CW, Jost B, Pirkl C, Aitzenmüller G, Lajtal G (2008). Quadriceps tendinosis and patellar tendinosis in professional beach volleyball players: sonographic findings in correlation with clinical symptoms. European Radiol 18 (8): 1703–1709.

Reeser JC, Verhagen E, Briner WW, Askeland TL, Bahr R (2006). Strategies for the prevention of volleyball related injuries. Br. J Sports Med 40: 597–600.

Wang HK, Cochrane T (2001). Mobility impairment, muscle imbalance, muscle weakness, scapular asymmetry, shoulder injury in elite volleyball athletes. J Sports Med Physical Fitness 41: 403–410.

Wang HK, MacFarlane A, Cochrane T (2000). Isokinetic performance and shoulder mobility in elite volleyball athletes from the United Kingdom. Br J Sports Med 34: 39–41.

Warnke K, Phieler M (2006). Trendsportarten. Deutscher Ärzteverlag Cologne, ISBN 3-7691-1207-S.

Woitys EM, Huston LJ, Schock HJ, Boylan JP, Ashton-Miller JA (2003). Gender differences in muscular protection of the knee in torsion in size-matched athletes. J Bone Joint Surg Am 85-A (5): 782–789.

Chapter 64 Squash

Ottmar Gorschewsky and Moritz Dau

64.1 History

In the late 14th century, rackets had originally been played against a front wall. Open court racket has established in Harrow school in 1822; the first indoor court had been built there presumably about 1840. That time is the actual birth of squash.

Two factors had been decisive for the initial **worldwide spread** of squash: squash had already been performed as school and university sport in England early; the graduates of Commonwealth universities took the idea of this game back to their countries. Army and naval officers stationed in India, Pakistan, Egypt or South Africa had performed squash as a **garrison sport**. Hence, squash has become popular in their home country and these countries continue to present world-class players up to today.

The **Squash Rackets Association** (SRA), founded on December 4, 1928, has set the measurements and the material of the rackets and brought out ball standards that considered the black ball only for competition. Donald Butcher had won the first official English championships over Charles Read in 1930.

In 1973, the German Squash Rackets Association (DSRV) has been founded in Hamburg. Two years later, the first German championships were carried out and more than 6,000 courts had been built in Germany within few years, where more than 2 million active people have played squash. The first four-walled glass court had been created in Cologne in October 1981 for the German Masters. In 1998, the world championship was carried out in Stuttgart.

According to the data of the World Squash Federation, squash had been played worldwide by about 15 million players in 153 countries on more than 50,000 courts around the turn of the millennium (www.worldsquash.org).

The most successful player so far is the Pakistani Jahangir Khan with six world championship titles and nine winnings in the British Open.

64.2 Particularities of Squash

Squash has some particularities that distinguish it from other rebound sports. It is a very fast game with frequent changes of direction on hard ground, and therefore it requires a lot of endurance, speed, coordination and ability to concentrate (➤ Tab. 64.1).

Very high strain peaks affect the whole locomotor apparatus. A bone-and-muscle-strengthening effect to the forearm (Ducher et al. 2005), a strengthening influence on the femoral neck (Nikander et al. 2005) and a preventive influence on post-menopausal osteoporosis (Kontulainen et al. 2001) has been shown in studies. Although an additional number of muscle groups is strained, this fastest of all racket games **does not qualify for rehabilitation sport** because of these high strain peaks and the high

Tab. 64.1 Comparison of calorie consumption during 15 minutes of sports.

Sport	Calories/15 minutes
squash	136 kcal (569 kHz)
tennis	89 kcal (321 kHz)
badminton	78 kcal (324 kHz)
table tennis	65 kcal (270 kHz)

amount of springiness (Pfoerringer and Engelhardt 1991, Goertzen et al. 1992).

Another particularity is the fact that the opponents are positioned on the same court. The closeness to the opponent, the opponent's racket and the ball hit by him cannot only affect painful injuries, but also injuries with serious consequences. The small rubber ball is of the size of an eye and can reach speeds of more than 200 km/h the hard border of the playing field also causes sport-specific injuries.

64.3 Sports injuries

About 3.2 in 100 players each year suffer an injury that has to be treated medically. Thus, the injury risk is 8 to 9 times lower than in handball or soccer and only slightly higher than in tennis (➤ Tab. 64.2). Many sport injuries developing in squash are also common in other sports, as for example:

- ankle sprains
- fibular fractures or
- knee sprains with lesions of meniscus, cruciate ligament and lateral ligament.

Furthermore, **muscle fiber lesions** often occur, especially at the lower extremity, and also Achilles tendon ruptures.

The fast game between hard concrete walls or glass walls will lead to head injuries and cerebral concussions clearly more often than other rebound sports. Dorsal contusions and cranial lacerations are caused by the **opponent's racket**. Circular, first white, then red and eventually blue, very painful spots are left by the rubber ball mostly on exposed parts of the backside of the body. Muscle soreness will develop most distinctly in the gluteal area and should not be underestimated by unexercised players.

Special attention must be paid to the squash-specific eye injuries. 7–49% of all sport-conditioned eye injuries worldwide develop by squash, dependent on source and region (Barrell et al. 1981, MacEwen 1987, Jones 1987, Loran 1992, Fong 1995 and Vinger 2000). The incidence ranges from 3.7–33.3 in 100,000 hours of playing (Clement and Fairhurst 1980, Easterbrook 1988 and Genovese et al. 1990) or 64 eye injuries in 100,000 players (Fong 1994). Although most eye injuries are not serious, they will lead to a permanent impairment or even loss of sight (Whyte 1987). The **traumatic separation of the retina** is feared most here. In a survey of 26 of such retinal separations, which partly showed serious concomitant injuries, 22 (85%) could be reaffixed, but a permanent sight impairment or loss of sight remained in 11 (42%) (Knorr and Jonas 1996).

Compartment syndromes with consecutive fascia splitting and a lesion of the axillaris nerve with complete palsy of the deltoid muscle after squash have been reported in individual cases, while the impaired nerve had to be substituted neurosurgically by the suralis nerve in order to recover the muscle function (Weber and Churchill 1996, Oberle et al. 1999).

64.4 Sport impairments

The development of an **arthritis** by squash is more frequent than in other rebound sports because of the high strain peaks. Knees, hip and ankle joints are affected mainly. The instability of the upper ankle joint as a consequence of recurrent supination traumas often can only be treated surgically. Another sign of overstrain can be a stress fracture in the area of the metatarsals.

1,047 players in New Zealand have been surveyed for specific **dorsal problems**. About 16% reported dorsal pain caused by squash, and existing dorsal pain have become worse for 10% (Macfarlane and Shanks 1998). Overstrain impairments mainly developed in the area of the lumbar spine.

Tab. 64.2 Percentage of injuries caused by hits and of traumas not caused by hits (Gorschewsky 1996).

	Caused by hits (59.1%)	Other traumas (40.9%)
head	82%	5%
torso	<1%	4%
upper extremity	13%	32%
lower extremity	4%	59%

A coracoacromial **impingement** or – at a predisposition – an anteriosuperior impingement of the shoulder will often develop in backhand players. **Tendinoses** or insertion and origin tendinitides show a wide spreading over the complete hitting arm. The epicondylitis radialis humeri develops a little less often than in tennis.

Diverse chronic overstrain impairments can appear in the region of the wrist joint. Radial-sided pain above the extensor tendon canal of the thumb is the sign of Quervain's disease. The same on the ulnar side means the subluxation of the extensor carpi ulnaris tendon. Pain at the hypotenar base points to cartilage impairments of the piso-triquetral joint (Helal 1979).

64.5 Prevention

A **thorough warm-up** is recommended because of the high strain of the locomotor apparatus in squash. The strain intensity of the organism with heart-rate peaks of more than 200 per min, the extreme fluid loss of 2 l/hour and the increase of the core body temperature to 39 °C necessitate a regular sport-medical examination and a cardiologic check-up at an age older than 40 years or at certain risk factors (Locke et al. 1997).

The use of **adequate material** can prevent sport injuries as well as impairments. Reduced racket vibration and a large sprung handle will reduce tendon insertion tendinoses. Stabilizing shoes with good cushioning should also be worn; according **protection goggles** can prevent eye injuries completely (International Federation of Sports Medicine 1989, Squash Australia 1998, Vinger 2000). Still, those goggles are unpopular amongst players, so that only 8–10% wear adequate protection goggles (Genovese et al. 1990, Loran 1992, Pardhan et al. 1995, Finch and Vear 1998, Eime et al. 2005). According to a study, only 4% of the operators in Switzerland offer adequate goggles, and only 7% point out the problem on posters (Leuba et al. 2000). In North America, it is prohibited to play without protection goggles.

The first priority in this sport is fairness. The interaction is supported by the **LET rules**. Their introduction has reduced the number of collisions with the opponents, their rackets and the hit ball.

Nowadays, Squash has already climaxed and the numbers of courts and players are **declining**. The tendency goes to the modern so-called trend sports; the squash courts nowadays become equipped with artificial rock faces and handles for the use of indoor free climbing.

References

Barrell GV, Cooper PJ, Elkington AR (1981). Squash ball to eye ball: the likelihood of squash players incurring an eye injury. Br J Sports Med 283: 393–395.

Clemett RS, Fairhurst SM (1980). Head injuries from squash: a prospective study. N Z Med J 92: 1–3.

Ducher G, Jaffre C, Arlettaz A, Benhamou CL, Courteix D (2005). Effects of long-term tennis playing on the muscle-bone relationship in the dominant and nondominant forearms. Can J Appl Physiol 30: 3–17.

Easterbrook M (1988). Eye protection in racquet sports. Clin Sports Med 2: 253–266.

Fong LP (1994). Sports-related eye injuries. Med J Aust 160: 743–750.

Fong LP (1995). Eye injuries in Victoria, Australia. Med J Aust 162: 65–68.

Genovese MT, Lenzo NP, Lim RK, et al. (1990). Eye injuries among pennant squash players and their attitudes towards protective eyewear. Med J Aust 153: 655–658.

Goertzen M, Staskiewicz B, Schulitz K-P (1992). Verletzungsprofil von Seniorensportlern in den Racketsportarten Squash und Tennis. Dtsch Z Sportmed 43: 96–102.

Gorschewsky O (1996). Sportmedizinischer Ratgeber. Fachverlag AG.

Jones NP (1987). Eye injuries in sport: an increasing problem. Br J Sports Med 21: 168.

Knorr HL, Jonas JB (1996). Retinal detachments by squash ball accidents. Am J Ophthalmol 122: 260–261.

Kontulainen S, Kannus P, Haapasalo H, Sievanen H, Pasanen M, Heinonen A, Oja P, Vuori I (2001). Good maintenance of exercise-induced bone gain with decreased training of female tennis and squash players: a prospective 5-year follow-up study of young and old starters and controls. J Bone Miner Res 16: 195–201.

Locke S, Colquhoun D, Briner M, Ellis L, O'Brien M, Wollstein J, Allen G (1997). Squash racquets. A review of physiology and medicine. Sports Med 23: 130–138.

Loran D (1992). Eye injuries in Squash. Optician Mar: 18–26.

MacEwen CJ (1987). Sport-associated eye injury: a casualty department survey. Br J Ophthalmol 71: 701–705.

Nikander R, Sievanen H, Heinonen A, Kannus P (2005). Femoral neck structure in adult female athletes subjected to different loading modalities. J Bone Miner Res 20: 520–528.

Pfoerringer W, Engelhardt M (1991). Squash-Verletzungen, vor allem an Kopf und Sprunggelenk. TW Sport u. Med.

Vinger P (2000). A practical guide for sports eye protection. Physician and Sports Medicine 28: 1–13.

Whyte JD (1987). Eye injuries. Athletic Training 22: 207–210.

World Squash Federation. www.worldsquash.org.

65 Tennis

Rüdiger Schmidt-Wiethoff, Jens Dargel and Joern W.-P. Michael

Tennis is still one of the most popular sports worldwide. About 1.8 million tennis players are organized in the German Tennis Federation. Approximately 25% of them are active tournament players and 75% play tennis on a recreational basis. Regarding the injury statistics, tennis is one of the sports with least injuries – less than one injury in 1,000 hours of playing (Thomas and Busse 2001). In the field of professional tennis, the number of injuries has remained constant in latest years according to most recent injury records of the international players' association ATP (Association of Tennis Professionals). Despite increased physical intensity and playing ability especially in competitive tennis, improvement of exercising methods as well as diagnostics and therapy have contributed to the low incidence of injuries. Furthermore, injury statistics show a positive development regarding injury prevention and sport science despite intensified striking techniques, extreme movement excursions of the strike arm and highest physical demands.

65.1 Characteristics

Tennis is a classic rebound sport, played in "singles" and "doubles". The complex movement patterns that are necessary for the playing process can be defined according to the playing situation as serve and return, baseline game and net game. In 1877, tennis had been played with today's rules for the first time in Wimbledon. It can be played on indoor and outdoor courts with different ground coatings, such as sand, grass, carpet or hard ground. Game and players are organized in single and double competitions, as well as in team competitions. Those are organized in leagues and carried out on a local, regional, national or international level. In Germany, the organization of games and tournaments are under guidance of the German Tennis Federation and its state federations which form the personal, structural and substantial preconditions of the training of coaches and coaching of the athletes. Rules, professional tournaments, and players' concerns are coordinated on an international level primarily by the player associations ITF (International Tennis Federation), ATP (Association of Tennis Professionals) and WTA (Women's Tennis Association).

65.2 Injuries

Chronic impairments and overuse syndromes mostly are acquainted in the region of the spine, the shoulder and the elbow, while acute injuries in tennis primarily affect the knee and ankle joint (➢ Fig. 65.1, ➢ Tab. 65.1). The distinction and development of sport-specific impairments to a certain extent underlies the specific strain profiles. These are mirrored in a unilateral and repetitive strain of the musculoskeletal structures.

65.2.1 Shoulder

The frequency of treatment-requiring problems in the area of the shoulder in tennis is denoted with up to 24% (Lehmann 1998). The main causes of pain are often functional deficiencies and a muscular imbalance due to unilateral strain demands.

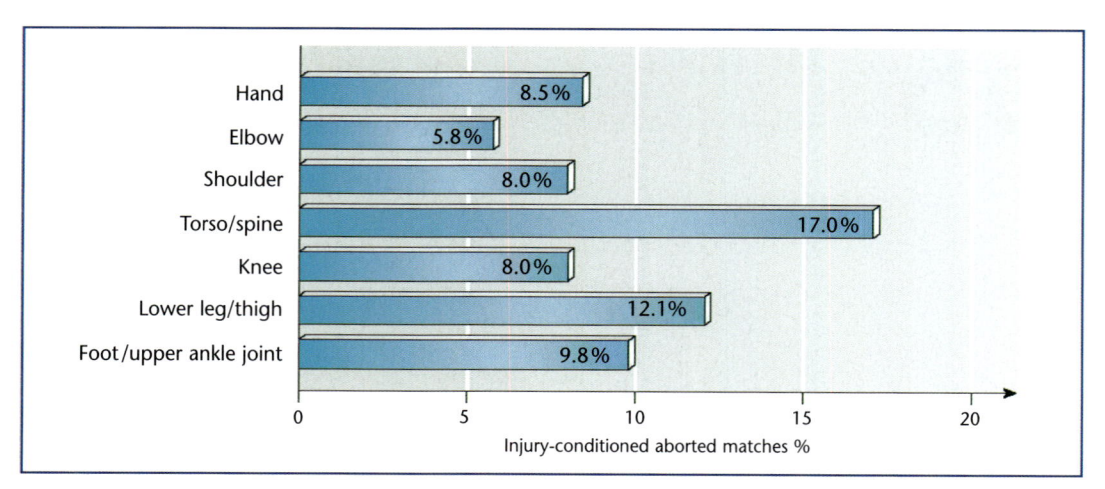

Fig. 65.1 Injury-caused game interruptions in professional tennis (ATP Tournament Physicians Conference 2002, n = 159). Internal-cardiologic causes have not been indicated in the image.

Tab. 65.1 Overview of relevant injuries in tennis.

Shoulder	postero-superior impingement micro-traumatic shoulder instability functional impingement
Elbow	lateral epicondylopathy medial epicondylopathy valgus-hyperextension overload syndrome ulnaris compression syndrome
Hand	tendosynovialitides stress fractures
Spine	muscular imbalances degenerative damages of intervertebral disks facet syndrome static impairments
Lower extremity	degenerative meniscus lesions patellar tendinosis musculo-tendineous overload syndromes sprain of the upper ankle joint

The **postero-superior impingement** has been known as a typical pathomorphological entity of tennis players by publications of Jobe and Walch (Walch et al. 1992, Davidson et al. 1993; Schmidt-Wiethoff et al. 2000). Joint-sided partial ruptures of the supraspinatus and infraspinatus tendons are found, which are caused by the compression and shearing forces of the tendon insertion at the posterosuperior glenoid rim during extreme external rotation and abduction. Degenerative lacerations are observed in the area of the posterior labrum.

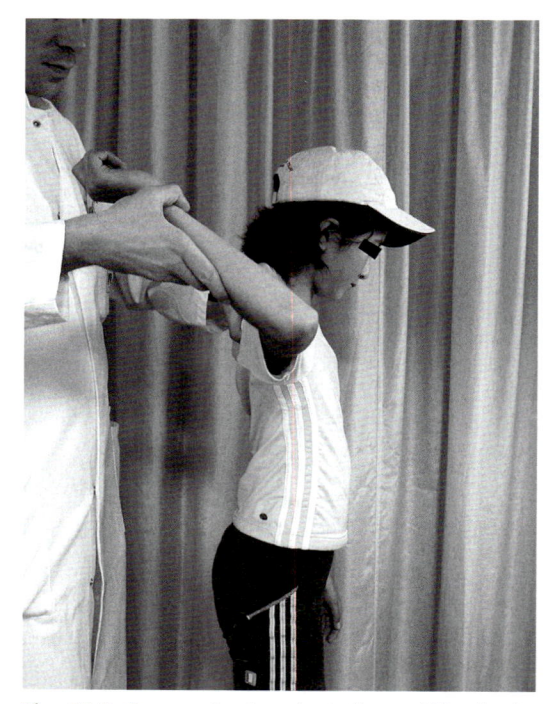

Fig. 65.2 Increased external rotation mobility in the shoulder joint of the hitting arm of a 12-year-old squad tennis player.

Racket sports present highest mechanical demands to the stability of the shoulder joint. A classical characteristic in tennis players is an increased external rotation in side-to-side comparison (➢ Fig. 65.2). On the one hand, the **in-**

Fig. 65.3 Infraspinatus atrophy with associated external rotation weakness in the area of the hitting arm in two high-performance tennis players.

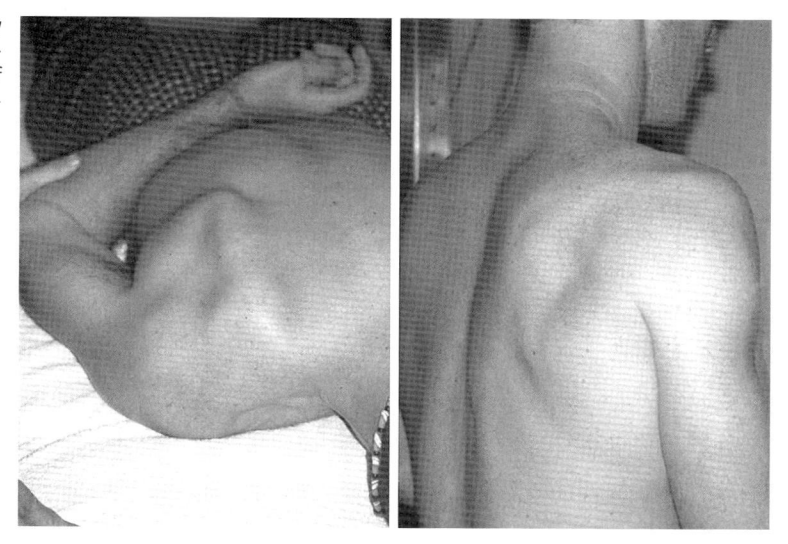

creased external rotation mobility is a precondition for maximum performance and must not be considered as pathologic, but on the other hand, it predisposes to impairment by chronic overstretching of the anterior joint capsule and thus can affect overall joint stability (Röhrrich and Kollmannsberger 1995, Steinbrück and Lehmann 1995, Radas et al. 1997). From the mechanical point of view, **chronic overstrains with plastic deformation of the capsuloligamentous stabilizers** as well as an increased A-P translation of the humeral head will result. The clinical picture shows signs of subjective instability and pathological subacromial changes.

A narrowing of the subacromial space will be caused by an insufficient depression of the humeral head because of dysfunction of parts of the rotator cuff with external rotation (➤ Fig. 65.3), deficient mechanical stability due to a capsular-ligamentous laxity and insufficient scapular rotation and stabilization. These changes may result in a so-called **functional impingement** (➤ Fig. 65.4; Habermeyer 1989, Scovazzo et al. 1991, Kibler 1994, Radas et al. 1997, Schmidt-Wiethoff et al. 2004). The consequence will be an increased anterior-superior translation of the humeral head that will cause a subacromial impingement mechanism. Finally it can lead to structural changes at the rotator cuff (Schmidt-Wiethoff et al. 1999). This problem should already be taken into account in juvenile tennis players because it will often result in painful impairments of the kinematics of the shoulder joint.

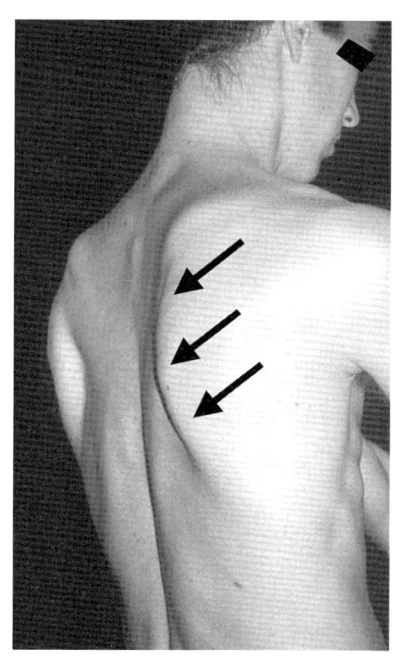

Fig. 65.4 22-year-old tennis professional: clinical picture of increased scapula protraction and lateralization ("scapula winging").

65.2.2 Elbow

The lateral and medial epicondylopathy are considered the major entity and predisposition of overstrain problems at the elbow.

The pathology of the **lateral epicondylopathy** – the tennis elbow –, generated from a chronic overstrain cascade, is often, but not exclusively, found in tennis players and represents a degenerative process of the tendon insertion of the extensor carpi radialis brevis muscle or the extensor digitorum communis muscle, respectively. The highly frequent vibration that is transmitted by the racket and the hand to the forearm is pathogenetically decisive. In the initial phase, this will lead to a painful and still reversible irritation of the wrist joint extensors at the lateral epicondyle. In the further process, pathomorphological changes of different severity will occur, depending on chronicity, degree of imbalance and exogenous factors. Although in the initial phase pathological changes respond positively to conservative therapeutic treatment, the permanent strain with inadequate treatment implicates a progression into the state of irreversible degenerative changes of the tendon insertion site. The radial extracorporeal shockwave therapy (rESWT) has been established therapeutically because of good treatment results in addition to physical and physiotherapeutical treatment approaches as well as the local application of water-soluble corticoids (Rompe et al. 2004). The tennis elbow will sometimes need surgery in case of irreversible symptomatic changes.

The **medial epicondylopathy** is clinically similar to the picture of the tennis elbow, but symptoms are localized above the epicondylus medialis humeri. The substantial pathomorphological changes are found at the insertion of the pronator teres muscle, the palmaris longus muscle and the flexor carpi radialis muscle. The treatment conforms to the one of the tennis elbow.

Another concept in the discussion of pathological elbow conditions in tennis is the **valgus-hyperextension overload syndrome** as a consequence of the extreme movement excursions and valgus forces in serve games (➤ Fig. 65.5). The pathomorphological correlate is the progressive micro-traumatic elongation of the medial collateral ligament. It will result in a medi-

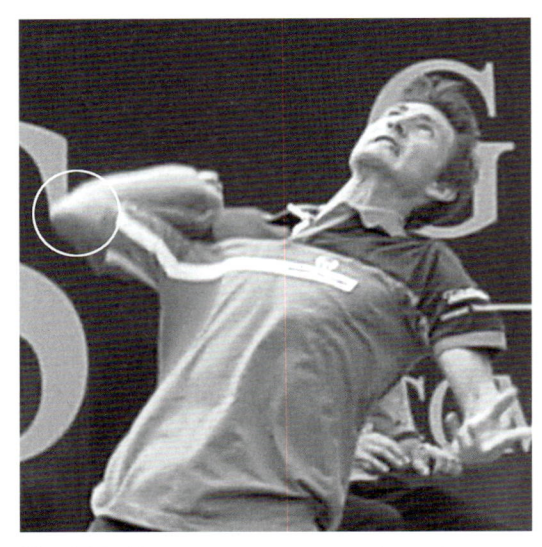

Fig. 65.5 Extreme movement excursions at serve as etiologic factor of valgus-hyperextension overload syndrome of the elbow.

al elbow instability, which can be treated conservatively by physiotherapy and stabilizing bandages, at first. The surgical tightening or reconstruction of the medial collateral ligament is carried out as a last option in therapy-resistant patients.

Another pathological substratum is the **ulnar compression syndrome** as individual entity as well as in association with a valgus instability of the elbow. The basic causes are chronic strain of the ulnar nerve with consecutive friction, irritation and compression in the sulcus ulnaris. In exceptional cases, an in-situ decompression of the nerve will be indicated.

65.2.3 Hand

Overstrain-conditioned **tenosynovialitides of the tendon of the flexor carpi ulnaris muscle** are primarily found in the region of the wrist mainly on the ulnar side, which can be treated conservatively in the initial stage (Bylak and Hutchinson 1998, Marx et al. 2001). Additionally, the optimized adjustment of the racket handle and the strings as well as a variation of the striking technique has major priority. With persisting conditions, a bandage for the wrist is recommended that will limit mobility in the end range of motion. Wrist pain localized on the radial side, which will increase with ulnar abduction, can often be due to an overstrain-conditioned inflammation of the tendons of the abductor pollicis longus muscle and the extensor pollicis brevis muscle in the region of the styloid process (Marx et al. 2001). This pathology, known as **Quervain's disease**, is treated analogously to a ulnar-sided tendovaginitis.

Osseous injuries in the area of hand and carpus, e.g. stress fractures of the os scaphiodeum or the os hamatum, are rarely found.

65.2.4 Spine

The fundamental problems of tennis-associated conditions and diseases of the spine are the **torsion, hyperextension and flexion movements** of the thoracolumbar segments (Frymoyer et al. 1983, Krahl 1994, Marx et al. 2001). The asymmetric eccentric force moments of the trunk muscles, especially developing during serve and the primarily concentric strains and high accelerations of the abdominal muscles can be made responsible for **muscular injuries at the trunk** (Marks 1988, Bylak and Hutchinson 1998, Kibler and Safran 2000). Functional adaptation processes will secondarily lead to imbalances in the area of the trunk muscles. These will manifest especially in form of an **ipsilateral paravertebral muscle hypertrophy** (side of the hitting arm). Progressive degenerative changes of the intervertebral disks and the facet joints as well as changes of the body static will be the consequences. Therapeutically, an individual and symptom-oriented segmental functional diagnosis is fundamental and will form the basis for a treatment-specific concept.

65.2.5 Lower extremities

The tennis-specific strain profile of the lower extremities is determined by a high amount of sudden stops as well as rotating and braking movements which result in high eccentric force exertions. In contrast to the upper extremity, the specific, tennis-associated problems of the lower extremities **mainly present acute injury mechanisms**. Dependent on exogenous factors such as temperature and ground coating, a high incidence of **muscle sprains** and **torn muscle fibers** is found primarily in the physically demanding competition phase. These will mostly be located in the area of the proximal hamstring muscles and in the proximal musculotendinous junction of the medial gastrocnemius muscle as a result of explosive jump and sprint movements (**"tennis leg"**; Bylak and Hutchinson 1998, Kibler and Safran 2000).

In addition to degenerative **meniscus lesions** and associated cartilage impairments, **tendinosis of the patellar tendon** are injuries and overstrain impairments of the knee joint resulting from the specific strain profile, while isolated and complex knee ligament injuries are found rarely (Lehman 1994, Schabus 1994). The therapy complies with the individual symptoms and chronicity and does not preclude surgical procedures in addition to physical and physiotherapeutic measures for treatment-resistant cases.

The dominating injury in tennis players in the area of the foot is the **sprain injury of the upper ankle joint**, with its incidence depending on the ground coating as well as on the shoe technology, as shown in ➤ Figure 65.6. Accordingly, an optimal supply of shoes and insoles contributes to the prophylaxis of ankle and knee joint injuries and can positively influence the complex of painful callosity in the area of toes and forefoot (**"tennis toe"**) as well as fungal

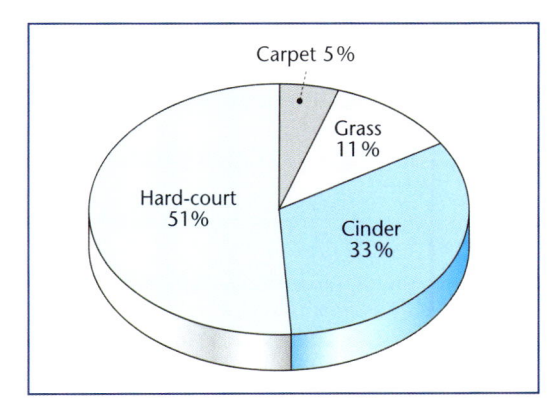

Fig. 65.6 Injuries of the lower extremity of professional tennis players depending on the ground surface (ATP Tournament Physicians Conference 2002, n = 135).

skin affections (**"athlete's foot"**), that are not to be underestimated, (Bylak and Hutchinson 1998, Kibler and Safran 2000).

65.3 Injury prevention

Injury prevention is not only an important topic in the field of top sports. Especially considering the development of performance of junior tennis players, the understanding of the specific strain profiles and the resulting overstrain impairments are significant.

Injury problems of talented junior players can be clearly reduced by comprehensive medical treatment and a professional exercise coaching. The optimal adjustment of racket handle and stringing play an important role, as well.

Regarding the individual performance development, the sports-medical squad examination will also be important. The task is to develop specified concepts for the optimization of training and coaching of performance-oriented tennis players. Efficient examination provides a precise analysis of the physical capacity, also under stimulation by different external strain factors, such as heat, humidity and height, by ergometry, cardiac ultrasound and electro-cardiography, in addition to regular lab tests, infection screenings and vaccination treatment.

Additionally, orthopedic-biomechanical examinations of body statics, achievement and performance tests and the assessment of complex movement processes provides a basis to improve the technique and injury prevention.

References

ATP Tournament physicians conference (2002). Ponte Vedra Beach, Florida, U.S.A.

Bylak J, Hutchinson MR (1998). Common sports injuries in young tennis players. Sports Med 26: 119–132.

Davidson PA, Elattrache NS, Jobe CM, Jobe FW (1995). Rotator cuff and posterior-superior glenoid labrum injury associated with increased glenohumeral motion: a new side of impingement. J Shoulder Elbow Surg 4: 384–390.

Frymoyer JW, Pope M, Clements HJ (1983). Risk factors in low back pain. J Bone Joint Surg 65-A: 213–218.

Habermeyer P (1989). Sehnenrupturen im Schulterbereich. Orthopäde 18: 257–267.

Kibler WB (1994). Current concepts of shoulder biomechanics for tennis. Tennis: Sports Medicine and Science. Walter Rau Verlag, Düsseldorf, pp. 59–71.

Kibler WB, Safran MR (2000). Musculoskeletal injuries in the young tennis player. Clin Sports Med 19: 781–792.

Krahl H (1994). Lumbar spine problems of professional tennis players. Tennis: Sports Medicine and Science. Walter Rau Verlag, Düsseldorf, pp. 120–124.

Lehmann RC (1994). Patellofemoral dysfunction in tennis players – a dynamic problem. Tennis: Sports Medicine and Science. Walter Rau Verlag, Düsseldorf, pp. 125–131.

Lehmann RC (1998). Shoulder pain in the competitive tennis player. Clin Sports Med 7: 309–327.

Marks MR, Haas SS, Wiesel SW (1988). Low back pain in the competitive tennis player. Clin Sports Med 7: 277–287.

Marx RG, Sperling JW, Cordasco FA (2001). Overuse injuries of the upper extremities in tennis players. Clin Sports Med 20: 439–451.

Radas C, Pieper HG, Quack G, Krahl H (1997). Schulterengpaßsyndrom des Überkopfsportlers – primäres oder sekundäres Subakromialsyndrom. Dtsch Z Sportmed 48: 379–384.

Röhrich F, Kollmannsberger A (1995). Atypisches Engpaßsyndrom de N. suprascapularis distal der Incisura scapulae. Nervenarzt 66: 638–642.

Rompe JD, Decking J, Schoellner C, Theis C (2004). Repetitive low-energy shock-wave treatment for chronic lateral epicondylitis in tennis players. Am J Sports Med 32: 734–743.

Schabus R (1994). Reconstructed anterior cruciate ligaments in tennis players. Tennis: Sports Medicine and Science. Walter Rau Verlag, Düsseldorf, pp. 132–137.

Schmidt-Wiethoff R, Rapp W, Mauch F, Steinbrück K (1999). Muscular imbalance and impingement syndrome of the shoulder in competitive tennis players. In J Sports Med 20-s1: 97.

Schmidt-Wiethoff R, Rapp W, Schneider T, Hass H, Steinbrück K, Gollhofer A (2000). Funkrionelle Schulterprobleme und Muskelimbalancen beim Leistungssportler mit Überkopfbelastung. Dtsch Z Sportmed 10/2000: 327–335.

Schmidt-Wiethoff R, Rapp W, Mauch F, Schneider T, Appell HJ (2004). Shoulder rotation characteristics in professional tennis players. Int J Sports Med 25: 154–158.

Scovazzo ML, Browne A, Pink M, Jobe FW, Kerrigan J (1991). The painful shoulder during freestyle swimming. Am J Sports Med 19: 77–82.

Steinbrück K, Lehmann M (1995). Sportmedizinische Aspekte von Schulterverletzungen. In: Habermeyer P, Schweiberer L (eds.). Schulterchirurgie. Urban & Schwarzenberg, Munich-Vienna-Baltimore, pp. 353–355.

Thomas M, Busse M (2001). Verletzungen und Fehlbelastungsfolgen beim Tennis. Klinische Sportmedizin 2: 73–78.

Walch G, Boileau P, Noel E, Donell ST (1992). Impingement on the deep surface of the supraspinatus tendon on the postero-superior rim: an arthroscopic study. J Shoulder Elbow Surg 1: 238–245.

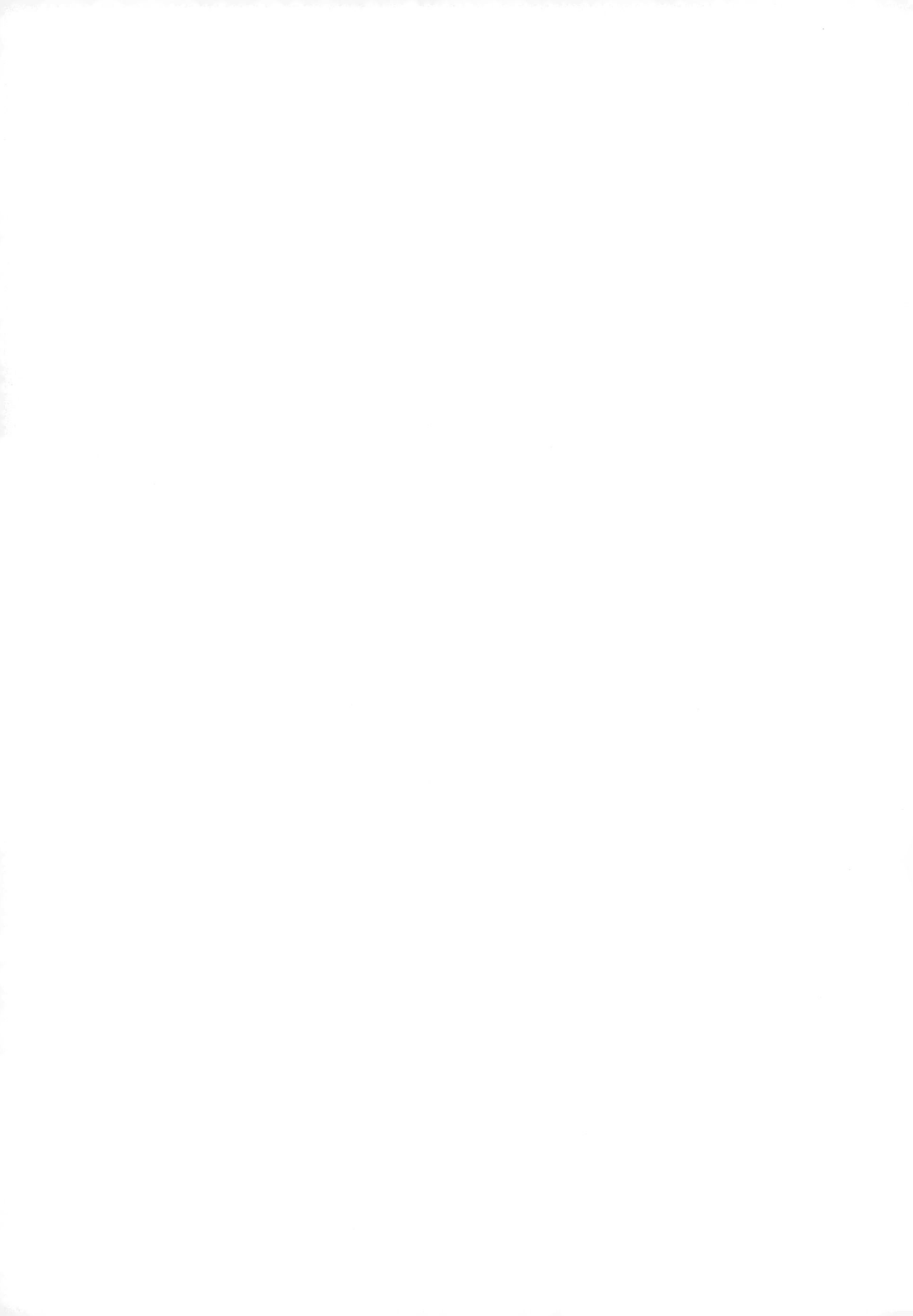

Chapter 66 Table tennis

Georg Mavridis

Table tennis is referred in the 19th century as a **East Asian sport**. The development of the **celluloid ball** by the Englishman Gibb in 1890 had been decisive for the development of this sport. First national championships were carried out in 1907 and first world championships in 1926. Since 1988, table tennis has been an **Olympic sport**. Singles and doubles for women and men are carried out. Since 2001, a game will end after four won sets; one set ends after one player has eleven points. The right of service switches after two won points.

In Germany, there are more than 700,000 players of table tennis, who are organized in clubs but a very high number of recreational players play outside of clubs.

Table tennis is one of the **fastest rebound sports**. Maximum demands are set on the ability to concentrate, on anticipation, capacity of differentiation, capacity of reaction, flexibility, springiness and endurance in the field of high performance (Stucke 1992).

The game is very fast and athletic. The **variants of hitting** are manifold. The **ball exchanges** are arrhythmic and often do not last longer than 5 sec. Different impact hardness, different kinds of racket coating, playing technique, ball speeds, ball rotation and variants of placing the balls to the table make table tennis extremely **complex** (➤ Fig. 66.2). There are already 2,000 variants of serving, alone (Zschau 1997).

The **quantity of exercising** adds up to eight to ten exercise units/week with 25–30 hours altogether on the level of national teams. High **tactical and fitness capabilities** as well as **mental strength** are necessary in order to establish in competitive sport.

66.1 Sport-specific problems

The following injuries had been recorded in the sport-medical treatment of squad athletes (A, B and C squad) in 40 athletes altogether of the German national team of table tennis over a period of 6 years (➤ Tab. 66.1, ➤ Tab. 66.2, ➤ Tab. 66.3 and ➤ Tab. 66.4):

Tab. 66.1 Typical injuries in table tennis: upper extremity and trunk (national squad, 40 athletes, observed period of 6 years).

Types of injury	Number of injuries
contusion and abrasions of hand/fingers	12
sprain supraspinatus muscle	5
sprain trapezius muscle	2
sprain quadratus lumborum muscle	1
sprain rectus abdominis muscle	1
sprain latissimus dorsi muscle	1

Tab. 66.2 Typical injuries in table tennis: lower extremity (national squad, 40 athletes, observed period of 6 years).

Types of injury	Number of injuries
sprain of the upper ankle joint	13
external ligament rupture of the upper ankle joint	1
sprain of ischiocrural muscles	2
sprain of the knee	3
strain of fibular musculature	3

Tab. 66.3 Typical overstrain problems in table tennis: upper extremity and trunk (national squad, 40 athletes, observed period of 6 years).

Clinical picture	Number of injuries
tendopathy supraspinatus muscle	12
tendopathy deltoid muscle	3
tendopathy biceps muscle	3
tendopathy latissimus muscle	2
tendopathy pectoralis major muscle	2
impingement syndrome of the shoulder	3
epicondylitis humeri radialis	8
tendopathy triceps muscle	2
tendopathy of the forearm extensor	5
tendopathy of the forearm flexor	4
dorsal pain	18
lumbago	16
humpback	12
intervertebral disk protrusion	4
slipped disks	3

Tab. 66.4 Overstrain problems in table tennis: lower extremity (national squad, 40 athletes, observed period of 6 years).

Clinical picture	Number of affected patients
fat-spray foot	16
achillodynia	4
hallux rigidus	2
periostitis of the medial edge of the tibia	5
tendinitis of the patellar tendon	3
tendinitis of the quadriceps tendon	3
tibialis anterior syndrome	2
cartilage damages of the ankle joint	1

- Hand injuries occur relatively often if hitting the play hand against the table surface.
- Shoulder and trunk injuries are triggered by high acceleration forces in forced top-spin and forehand smashes. The repeated, fast anteversion, internal rotation and adduction movement of the play hand causes frequent **tendopathies of the shoulder** with concomitant bursitis and **tendopathy of the elbow** (➤ Fig. 66.1 and ➤ Fig. 66.2).
- Dorsal muscular dysbalances are favored by high exercise strains and non-physiological basic positions (Zschau 1999). These can be avoided with consequent compensatory training (➤ Fig. 66.3).
- Ankle joint injuries often result from fast sidesteps, lunges, cross steps and two-steps or jumps. A good footwork with high capacity of springiness is a critical precondition for the reaching the ball position and ideal posture for hitting the ball (➤ Fig. 66.4).
- Irritations of the Achilles tendon or the patellar tendons are a consequence of the extensive footwork.
- Malpositions of the foot and periostitis of the medial tibial edge are especially frequent due to the extreme exercise strains and a repositioning of the body weight.

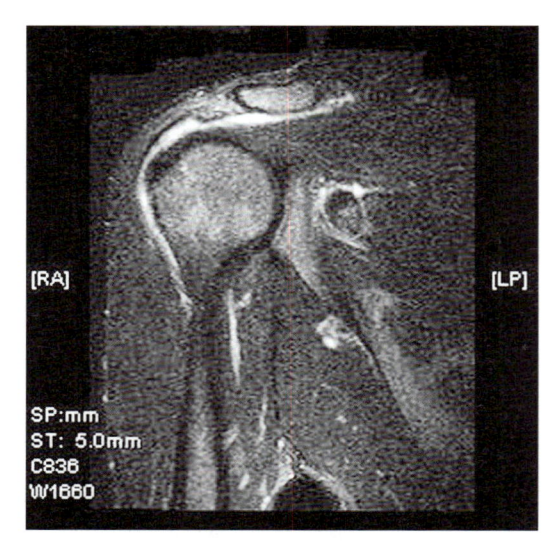

Fig. 66.1 Buristis subacromialis, right shoulder, shown in the MRI.

Absences from training and competition of more than 1 month had occurred in only three cases of the injuries and overstrain problems mentioned above. **Surgical treatments** had only been necessary in two cases (➤ Tab. 66.5).

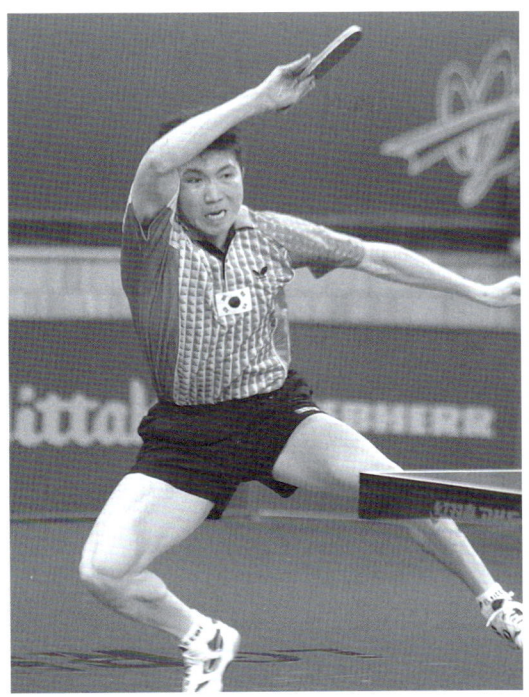

Fig. 66.2 Shoulder strain by fast anteversion movements, internal rotation movements and adduction movements (photograph: M. Schillings).

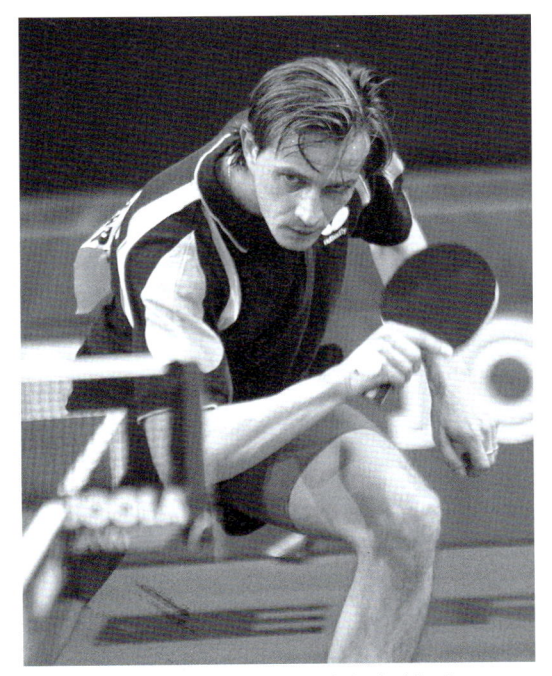

Fig. 66.3 Dorsal strain by unphysiological basic posture (photograph: M. Schillings).

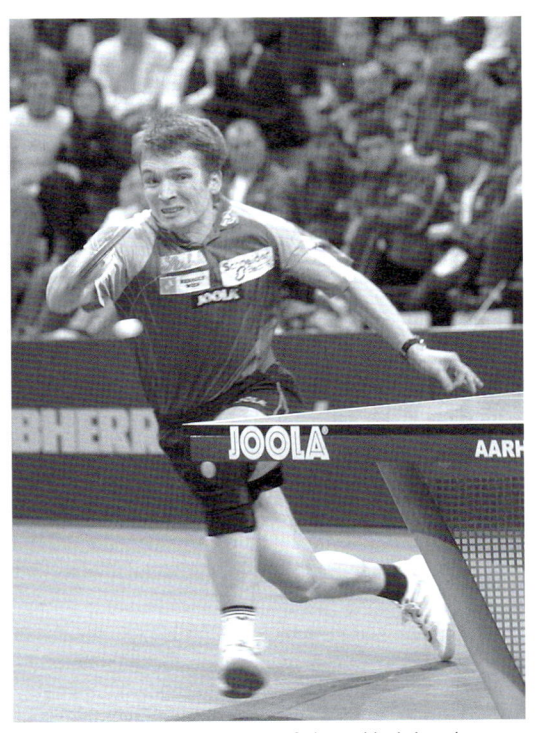

Fig. 66.4 Danger of injuries of the ankle joints because of the quick two-steps and the excessive footwork (photograph: M. Schillings).

Tab. 66.5 Surgical treatments in table tennis (national squad, 40 athletes, observed period of 6 years).

Operation	Number of patients
resection of the meniscus of the knee	1
subacromial decompression and partial synovectomy of the shoulder	1

66.2 Preventive measures

Regular sport-medical examinations, adequate exercise control, compensation training, phases of strength formation, sport-specific coordinative training, good supply of insoles, and shoes reduce the injury risk and overstrain problems.

Insoles should be provided at least once a year and **treadmill analysis** should be used (➢ Chapter 11). Adequate **physiotherapeutic measures** and sufficient **regeneration phases** should be taken care of, especially at the highest level of performance.

The strength analysis and the measuring of coordinative capabilities by force-measuring devices have proved of value in the recognition and treatment of the muscular dysbalances. Thereby, an efficient medical exercise therapy can be induced and the results of rehabilitation can be objectified.

Mental and autogenic training should be offered and promoted regularly. But a permanent exchange of information between the athletes, coaches, physiotherapists and physicians is also very important.

References

Stucke H (1992). Tischtennis. In: Ballreich R, Kuhlow-Ballreich A (eds.). Biomechanik der Sportarten. Enke-Verlag, Stuttgart.

Zschau H (1997). Tischtennis. In: Engelhardt M, Hintermann B, Segesser B (eds.). GOTS-Manual Sporttraumatologie. Huber-Verlag, Bern, Göttingen, Toronto Seattle.

Zschau H (1999). Tischtennis. In: Klümper A. Sporttraumatologie. Handbuch der Sportarten und ihrer typischen Verletzungen. Ecomed-Verlag, Landsberg, 3. Erg.-Lfg. 8/1999.

Chapter 67 Volleyball

Antonius Kass

67.1 History of volleyball

The basic idea in volleyball that the ball must not hit the ground existed already in **ancient Rome** under the name "game of trigon" (Weiler 1981). Volleyball of modern times was introduced by the PE teacher William G. Morgan at the YMCA College in Holyoke, Massachusetts, in 1885. At that time, he had been looking for a sport that could be played with less body contact than basketball. Morgan used the inner rubber bubble of the basketball in order to let his students play competitively over a 1.98 m net. This game originally called "mintonette" was re-named "volleyball" shortly thereafter and subsequently spread all over the world.

In the second half of 20th century, volleyball has become more and more popular. Since 1949, world championships have been carried out regularly and the sport became an **Olympic** discipline in 1964 in Tokyo. The Olympic Games 1972 in Munich also triggered a downright boom in Germany.

The **International Volleyball Federation** (FIVB) with 150 million members and 218 member countries is the largest umbrella sport organization in the world.

67.2 Sport-specific characteristics

Volleyball is a **rebound sport** in which two teams, each with six players face each other on two fields 9 × 9 m, separated by a 2.43 m net for men or a 2.24 m net for women. The goal of the game is to place the ball in the opponent's field. Every team is allowed to have three ball contacts (excluding the block contact). Since 2000, the "rally point system" has been effective, i.e. every point counts. The player positions of a team will rotate after every won serve. In the first four sets 25 points are needed until gaining, 15 points in the decisive fifth set. One must lead by two points to win a match. The players are specialized and a **start formation** usually consists of one setter, two middle blockers, two outside hitters and an opposite hitter. In 2001, the position of a libero has been introduced. The libero is a defense specialist who can easily be recognized by a T-shirt of contrasting colors, who acts in the back field and must not play the ball above net height into the opponent's field. This rule increases defensive actions and thus extends the the ball exchanges.

Volleyball is athletic and full of springiness. As an anaerobic, alactacid sport volleyball has a moderate endurance and low static strain and has become increasingly athletic in recent years.

The specialty of this game is the fact that most ball actions are carried out at 2.40 and 3.70 m height. This requires **extensive jumps**. In addition, the landing zone underneath the net is extremely limited. **Contact with opponents** is frequent and is the most important cause of the characteristic volleyball injury, the supination trauma of the upper ankle.

Serve, set, upper pass, attack and block, are four technical elements, which are performed overhead (Papageorgiou and Spitzley 1984). This applies heavy strain on the shoulders and the acromioclavicular joint often resulting in **overstrain of the shoulder** are found in volleyball players.

A high technical and tactic complexity is characteristic for volleyball. This results in **high ex-**

ercise intensity, not only in high level volleyball. Top teams will train 2–3 times daily. 25 hours of training a week and more are the rule; a top athlete absolves far more than 300 maximum jumps per day of training and more than 40,000 per year (Kugler et al. 1994). Thus, the players are especially prone to injuries due to fatigue and overstrain.

The incidence for injuries is average with 2.6 in 1,000 hours (Verhagen et al. 2004) as compared to other sports. About **9% of all sport injuries** are volleyball-related (Solgard et al. 1996).

67.3 Acute injuries

67.3.1 Ankle joint

41–55% of all volleyball injuries are **supination trauma** of the upper ankle joint (Hell and Schönle 1985, Verhagen et al. 2004). Jumps in the area of the center line under the net are the major cause of injury. When three players perform a block, for example, four players will jump and land within a small space at the same time (➢ Fig. 67.1). There is a high risk of landing on the foot of another player.

79% of the injuries of the ankle joints are re-injuries. The likelihood of a **fresh trauma** is 3.8 times as high with a previous injury. If the former trauma dates back less than 6 months, the risk of a new ankle joint injury increases by the 9.8-fold (Bahr 1997).

The clear increase in the rate of re-injury in the ankle joint suggests that wearing an **ankle joint orthesis** for a period of 6–12 months after the injury would be beneficial. The maximum jumping power is not reduced by wearing an orthesis.

67.3.2 Achilles tendon

Chronic irritant conditions accidents or former Cortisone shots can lead to a rupture of the Achilles tendon. More specific studies about the epidemiology of Achilles tendon ruptures in volleyball are not available. The author has observed a prevalence of **less than 5%** upon own observations. In many cases the players with a rupture of the Achilles tendon never had any trouble or irritations before.

After the surgical or conservative treatment, a return to volleyball should not be expected after 6 months at the earliest.

67.3.2 Anterior cruciate ligament

6–8% of all injuries in volleyball affect the knee joint. The most frequent accident mechanism is a **locked rotation trauma** or an anteromedial snapping in the knee joint. In addition to meniscus injuries, injuries of the anterior cruciate ligament – also with involvement of the internal ligament – will be the consequence are possible.

Women are affected by **cruciate ligament ruptures** significantly more often than men (factor 4–6, Petersen et al. 2005). The reasons are less muscular stability of the knee joint, a reduced active and passive rotation stability (Wojtys et al. 2003) and an increased valgus strain in jumping (Hewett et al. 2005). Women only achieve smaller angles in hip and knee joint flexion than men and the ground reaction forces will be higher (Lephart et al. 2003).

A cruciate ligament rupture usually forces a volleyball player to stop training for **6–9 months**, a surgically treated meniscus injury means an interruption for 6–8 weeks.

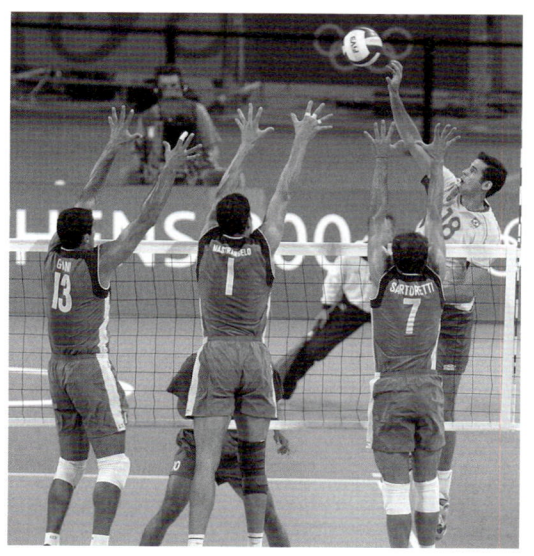

Fig. 67.1 Jump actions in volleyball in the field of the centerline.

67.3.4 Fingers

The incidence of finger injuries is inconsistent in literature with rates varying between 7% (Bahr 1997) and 22.4% (Hell and Schönle 1985). In school sports, finger injuries have been reported to be 53% (Knobloch et al. 2004). The frequency of finger injuries decreases in higher level leagues.

Finger injuries occur **especially during blocking**. Inappropriate technique and incorrect timing in blocking are typical. If the player blocks too early and is in the downward movement in the moment of the opponent's attack, he will lose the muscular tension in the fingers and will be exposed to the ball, which can accelerate up to 120 km/h.

The **taping of the fingers** is prevalent in volleyball players for therapy and prevention. The affected finger is often taped together with the neighboring finger. The resulting movement limitation is usually not perceived as disturbing by volleyball players. A setter, however, often loses the feel for the ball and the necessary precision in the upper set. Finger taping is often used for protection against bursting of the fingertips and also for an adjusted and changed feel for the ball.

67.3.5 Vascular occlusions

Arterial or venous occlusions in volleyball players have been described extensively. Acute embolisms and thromboses are induced by the impact of the ball to the arms. Schmeing (1998) has documented ten occlusions of digital arteries in the dominant hand of top volleyball players. Also thromboses of the subclavian vein (Treat et al. 2004) and the cephalic vein have been observed.

67.4 Overstrain syndromes

67.4.1 Stress fractures

Repetitive high jump strains present a permanent stimulus for the axial skeleton. Stress fractures are found in 1.9% of all injuries (Iwamoto and Takeda 2003). They are also frequently found in volleyball.

The most frequent localizations are the tibia and – less often – the metatarsals.

The diagnosis of a stress fracture is difficult and not always distinct on scout film, especially in the early phase but clearly distinguishable in MRI or in a scintigraphy.

67.4.2 Achillodynia

The high jump strain, deformations of the foot, inadequate shoes and a contraction of the calf muscles, especially of the soleus muscle, strain the Achilles tendon. Problems with the Achilles tendon are widely spread in volleyball players.

The conservative therapy includes rest, ice applications, antiphlogistics and physiotherapy with the basic aim of relaxing the fibular muscles. A surgical therapy will be indicated with persisting conditions and degenerate tissue.

67.4.3 Patellar apex syndrome

The "jumper's knee" is the **most frequent consequence of overstrain** in volleyball. An inflammation at the junction of the tendon to the bone and, in the long run, a degeneration of the tendon matrix is triggered by repetitive jumping, landing, and permanent traction force of the quadriceps in rest. Body weight, jump height and duration of the performed strength training are significant parameters for the likelihood of a patellar apex syndrome in volleyball players (Lian et al. 2003).

An **important factor for the development** of a "jumper's knee" seems to be the balance between extensors and flexors or medial and lateral amounts, respectively, of the quadriceps muscles. Thus, a significant weakness of the flexors is often found in volleyball players with patellar apex syndrome.

The clinical examination and sonography are the diagnostic tools of choice; MRI can display the extent of the structural defect.

At first, therapy is conservative and includes ultrasound therapy and injections, which should be free of steroids, in addition to the physiotherapy. A surgical therapy is sensible if conditions persist over several months and if the tendon matrix shows extensive structural impairments.

According to a survey in volleyball players, the **long-term results** of surgery are very good in 70%, good in 13%, satisfactory in 3% and poor in 10% of the cases (n = 38, Ferretti et al. 2002).

67.4.4 Spine

The spine is subject to **asymmetric mechanical strain** during the attack and the upper frontal task in volleyball. In analogy to the serve in tennis, the body is positioned in a strong hyperlordosis of the lumbar spine as well as lateral flexion and rotation to the side of the hitting arm at the end of the wind-up movement. The hitting arm will go to ventral in the swing to the ball, followed by an increased thoracic kyphosis.

These movement patterns obviously lead to characteristic adaptations in the volleyball player: The **kyphosis angle of the thoracic spine** is significantly **increased** and a **growth of the scoliosis angle** is often detected as well as **scapular malpositions** towards the dominant side (Dalichau and Scheele 2002). The segmental activation of the stabilizing trunk muscles is disturbed, medical conditions of the dorsum are the consequence (Warnke and Phieler 2006).

The spine is compressed additionally during landing. In 44% of the competitive volleyball players **nuclear spin tomography MRI** detectableshows degenerative adaptations of the intervertebral disks, such as osteochondroses and facet arthroses, as compared to 20% of a same-age control group (Bartolozzi et al. 1991). Degenerative changes have been found with 65.1% in volleyball players with high strain for several years, which is significantly more often than in players with continuously structured training and regular exercises stabilizing the spine.

A consequence is the necessity of thorough planning and a long-term structured training. Static at first, then dynamic and afterwards sport-specific exercises should be performed. Proprioceptive exercises and balance exercises will improve the segmental activation of the spinal muscles (Reeser et al. 2006).

67.4.5 Shoulder

The shoulder joint is most susceptible for overstrain syndromes in volleyball. 49% of all volleyball players complain about chronic shoulder pain (Wang et al. 2001). **Supraspinatus syndrome with impingement symptoms**, **bursitis subacromialis** and **arthrosis of the AC joint** are the most frequent diagnoses. Dislocations with injuries of the labrum are found less often.

A frequent cause for shoulder injuries in volleyball players are muscular dysbalances, especially in the region of the rotator cuffs (Wang and Cochrane 2001). These dysbalances increase with the stronger kyphosis of the thoracic spine.

X-ray and sonography will be necessary in addition to the clinical examination. MRI is sensible for certain problems, and MRI is indicated for labrum lesions or SLAP lesions.

67.4.6 Infraspinatus atrophy

Etiology and epidemiology

A volleyball-specific disease is the isolated atrophy of the infraspinatus muscle. It develops as a **compression neuropathy of the suprascapular nerve** in the sulcus suprascapularis; the dominant side is affected almost exclusively. Epidemiologic studies show an incidence of 28% in players of the first league (Eggert and Holzgraefe 1993). Setters are affected by the infraspinatus atrophy just as often as the attackers. The infraspinatus atrophy is a rarity in other overhead sports, such as handball, basketball and javelin throw. An incidence of 4.4% is found only in baseball, especially in pitchers (Pogliacomi et al. 2000, Cummins et al. 2004).

The following are discussed etiologically:

- anatomic variants with abnormal muscle fibers of the subscapularis muscle that constrain the subscapular nerve (Bayramoglu et al. 2003)
- narrowing in the sulcus suprascapilaris by increased ligamentous fiber lineaments
- existence of a spinoglenoid cyst (Weiss and Imhoff 2000)
- hypermobility of the shoulder, especially in external rotation, anteversion and protraction (shoulder girdle mobility; Witvrouw et al. 2000).

A volleyball-specific movement process is the **float serve**, in which the ball is hit without rotation. This can only be accomplished if the arm is stopped suddenly in the moment of ball contact during the serve. This can lead to a cranialization of the scapula, e.g. with an unstable shoulder girdle, and to an overstretching of the suprascapular nerve.

Clinics and diagnostics

A clearly visible dent in the area of the infraspinatus muscle is found clinically with the accompanying functional deficiencies, especially in the external rotation of the shoulder joint. A neurologic examination will be necessary to ensure diagnosis if latencies appear and decimated interference patterns is found in EMG.

Therapy

Therapy is almost exclusively **surgical** and consists of a incisura suprascapularis nerve decompression in the incisura suprascapularis. Conservative measures of therapy are not successful. **Early surgery** is **important** for a reinervation of the infraspinatus. This should be carried out 6 weeks to 12 weeks after the first symptoms. Otherwise, no improvement can be expected. The author tried CT-monitored steroid injections into the Incisura suprascapularis successfully in several cases.

If surgery is not carried out or carried out too late, the infraspinatus atrophies completely. Since the infraspinatus nerve is not needed for a technically clean performance, the only to a minor extent in then atrophy has only a limited impact on performance. Long-term effects are an **impingement syndrome** because the shoulder balance is impaired.

67.5 Prevention

Four clinical pictures are **often** found in the treatment of volleyball players (➤ Tab 67.1). **Preventive measures** are recommendable.

- The focus should be on therapy and prevention of the **ankle joint injuries**. An active stabilization program is necessary, especially for the improvement of the proprioception. The indication for orthesis treatment is given in the anamnesis with repeated ankle joint injuries.

Tab. 67.1 Prevention in volleyball.

Region	Attention should be paid to	
ankle joint	proprioception	orthesis
knee joint	flexors	vastus medialis/hamstrings
spine	trunk musculature	extension of the TS
shoulder	external rotators	balance of the muscles of the shoulder girdle

- A good balance between flexors and extensors is necessary for **conditions of the knee**. Usually, the flexors are weaker than the extensors. Specific exercise of the hamstrings as a flexor group as well as a strengthening of the vastus medialis will influence the patellar apex conditions positively.

- Regular exercise of the trunk muscles is important for the prevention of **spinal conditions**. It means to continuously train and to incorporate accompanying measures, such as static, dynamic and sport-specific exercises into the exercise program.

- A specific stabilizing of the shoulder muscles is necessary in order to avoid **shoulder conditions**. Especially the external rotators are important for the balance of the shoulder. This muscle group typically poorly exercised in volleyball players. Stabilizing exercises for the straightening up out of the thoracic kyphosis combined with a stabilizing of the external rotators, e.g. by treadmill, should be a component of every exercise session.

References

Babu R, Bahr IA (1997). Incidence of acute volleyball injuries: a prospective cohort study of injury mechanisms and risk factors. Scand J Med Sci Sports 7: 166–171.

Bartolozzi C, Caramella D, Zampa V, Dal Pozzo G, Tinacci E, Calducci F (1991). The incidence of disk changes in volleyball players. The magnetic resonance findings. Radiol Med (Torino) 82: 757–760.

Bayramoglu A, Demiryurek D, Tuccar E, Erbil M, Aldur MM, Tetik O, Doral MN (2003). Variations in anatomy at the suprascapular notch possibly causing suprascapular nerve entrapment: an anatomical study. Knee Surgery, Sports Traumatology, Arthroscopy. Official Journal of the ESSKA 11: 393–398.

Cummins CA, Messer TM, Schafer MF (2004). Infraspinatus muscle atrophy in professional baseball players. Am J Sports Med 32: 116–120.

Dalichau S, Scheele K (2002). Die thorakolumbale Wirbelsäulenform männlicher Leistungsvolleyballspieler. Dtsch Z Sportmed 53: 12–16.

Eggert S, Holzgraefe M (1993). Die Kompressionsneuropathie des Nervus suprascapularis bei Hochleistungsvolleyballern. Sportverl Sportschad 7: 136–142.

Ferretti A, Cerullo G, Russo G (1987). Suprascapular neuropathy in volleyball players. J Bone Joint Surg Am 69: 260–263.

Ferretti A, Conteduca F, Camerucci E, Morelli F (2002). Patellar tendinosis: a follow-up study of surgical treatment. Am J Bone Joint Surg 84-A: 2179–2185.

Gwinn DE, Wilckens JH, McDevitt ER, Ross G, Kao TC (2000). The relative incidence of anterior cruciate ligament injury in men. Am J Sports Med 28: 98–102.

Hell H, Schönle C (1985). Ursachen und Prophylaxe typischer Volleyballverletzungen. Z Orthop 123: 72–75.

Hewett TE, Myer GD, Ford KR et al. (2005). Biomechanical measures of neuromuscular control and valgus landing of the knee predict anterior cruciate ligament injury risk in female athletes. A prospective study. Am J Sports Med 33: 492–501.

Iwamoto J, Takeda T (2003). Stress fractures in athletes: review of 196 cases. Journal of Orthopaedic Science: official Journal of the Japanese Orthopaedic Association 8: 273–278.

Knobloch K, Rossner D, Gössling T, Richter M, Krettek C (2004). Volleyballverletzungen im Schulsport. Sportverl Sportschad 18: 185–189.

Kugler A, Krüger-Franke A, Reininger S, Rosemeyer B (1994). Der chronische Schulterschmerz des Volleyballangriffspielers. Sportverl Sportschad 8: 160–165.

Lephart SM, Ferris CM, Riemann BL, Myers JB, Fu FH (2002). Gender differences in strength and lower extremity kinematics during landing. Clin Orthop Relat Res 401: 162–169.

Lian O, Refsnes P, Engebretsen L, Bahr R (2003). Performance characteristics of volleyball players with patellar tendinopathy. Am J Sports Med 31: 408–413.

Papageorgiou A, Spitzley W (1984). Volleyball. Vom Mini-Volleyballspieler zum Universalisten. Praxis Sport vol. 8/9. Bartels und Wernitz, Berlin.

Petersen W, Rosenbaum D, Raschke M (2005). Rupturen des vorderen Kreuzbandes bei weiblichen Athleten. Teil 1: Epidemiologie, Verletzungsmechanismus und Ursachen. Dtsch Z Sportmed 56(6): 150–156.

Pogliacomi F, Perelli-Ercilini E, Vaienti E, Magnani E (2000). Atrofia isolata del muscolo sottospinoso nel giocatore di baseball. Isolated atrophy of the infraspinatus muscle in baseball players. Acta biomedica de L'Alteneo parmense organo della Società di medicina e scienza naturali di Parma 71: 127–134.

Reeser JC, Verhagen E, Briner WW, Askeland TI, Bahr R (2006). Strategies for the prevention of volleyball related injuries. Br J Sports Med 40: 597–600.

Solgård L, Nielsen AB, Møller-Madsen B, Jacobesen BW, Yde J, Jensen J (1996). Volleyball injuries presenting in casualty: A prospective study. Br J Sports Med 29: 200–204.

Schmeing P (1998). Arterielle Gefäßverschlüsse bei Volleyballspielern. University of Cologne.

Treat ST, Smith PA, Wen DY, Kinderknecht JJ (2004). Deep vein thrombosis of the subclavian vein in a college volleyball player. Am J Sports Med 32: 529–532.

Verhagen EA, Van der Beek AJ, Bouter LM, Bahr RM, Van Mechelen WE (2004). A one-season prospective cohort study of volleyball injuries. Br J Sports Med 38: 477–481.

Wang HK, Cochrane T (2001). A descriptive epidemiological study of shoulder injury in top level English male volleyball players. Int J Sports Med 22: 159–163.

Wang HK, Cochrane T (2001). Mobility impairment, muscle imbalance, muscle weakness, scapular asymmetry, shoulder injury in athlete volleyball athletes. J Sports Med Physical Fitness 41: 403–410.

Wang HK, MacFarlane A, Cochrane T (2000). Isokinetic performance and shoulder mobility in elite volleyball athletes from the United Kingdom. Br J Sports Med 34: 39–43.

Warnke K, Phieler M (2006). Trendsportarten. Deutscher Ärzteverlag, Cologne.

Weiler I (1981). Der Sport bei den Völkern der alten Welt. Wissenschaftliche Buchgesellschaft, Darmstadt.

Weiss C, Imhoff AB (2000). Sonographic imaging of a spinoglenoid cyst. Ultraschall in der Medizin 21: 287–289.

Witvrouw E, Cools A, Lysens R, Cambler D, Vanderstraeten G, Victor J, Sneyers C, Walravens M (2000). Suprascapular neuropathy in volleyball players. Br J Sports Med 34: 174–180.

Wojtys EM, Huston LJ, Schock HJ, Boylan JP, Ashton-Miller JA (2003). Gender differences in muscular protection of the knee. J Bone Joint Surg 85-A: 782–789.

68 Ballet

Gino M.M.J. Kerkhoffs and C. Niek van Dijk

Ballet pushes the locomotor apparatus – especially the lower extremity – to its extreme performance. In the 21st century, the American choreographer **William Forsythes** challenged dancers like Alina Cojocaru or Thomas Lund with technical virtuosity, choreographic requirements, and an ever increasing number of performances, tournaments and presentations. Therefore, overstrain impairments are common (in literally all athletes).

Medical conditions are primarily been found at knee (80.5%) and ankle joints (74%). The reasons are mostly landing after jumps or lifts (Arendt et al. 2003). Minor lesions can cause problems if rest periods are too short. The foot hurts, there is pain in the back, and another old strain has not healed out yet – every-day life for dancers.

Average dancers are fanatic artists and athletes, put a critical view on every movement and are continuously concerned with their body. Every difference is pointed out, maintained and placed into focus.

The central concern of the attending physician is to allow the dancer to work as physiologically and body-friendly as possible and thus to structure their career with less injuries and eventually prolon it. If a surgical treatment is indicated maintaining the largest joint function is central.

68.1 Physical aptitude

There is a range of purely anatomical preconditions that need to be fulfilled for a ballet career. The **external rotation** of the hips, which reaches 60–70° in extended standing, is fundamental. This forced external rotation is caused by an increased flexibility and not by a decreased torsion of the femoral neck. If the external rotation is less than 60–70°, an exaggerated external rotation in knee and foot compensate the reduced hip rotation to allow basic positions (Teitz 1983). Ligament instability therefore develops in the knee that predisposes meniscus impairments and arthroses (Miller et al. 1974). The medial arch is affected as well; peritendinitis of the tibialis posterior muscle and the flexor hallucis longus muscle occur.

68.2 Sport-specific diseases and possible therapies

68.2.1 Hallux joint

A dorsal extension of 90° in the metatarsophalangeal joint of the hallux is necessary for the position of relevé-à-demi-point. While this is impossible with a full hallux rigidus (Howse 1993), even a painful, slightly limited dorsal extension in case of a dorsal impingement syndrome means a high-degree impairment for a dancer (Van Dijk et al. [2] 1998). Repetitive micro-traumas on the dorsal side of the MTP-1 joint with secondary osteophyte development are the most likely cause.

We have developed an **arthroscopic method** for the removal of osteophytes (Van Dijk et al. [2] 1998). A mini-arthroscope can be brought into the metatarsophalangeal joint of the hallux from dorsomedial. The osteophytes are removed by a mini-shaver. An **osteochondritis dissecans** or a **painful sesamoid bone** can be treated similarly. The reduced scarring of the joint is of great advantage. After arthroscopic treatment, a very good result has been achieved in eight of 12 patients with a dorsal impingement syndrome, a good result in three out of four patients with osteochondritis dissecans after 2 years. Regarding the hallux rigidus or the removal of the sesamoid bones, the results have been far less positive. As in all arthroscopic treatments, the early functional therapy after arthroscopy and the early return to sport are of great advantage (Van Dijk et al. [2] 1998).

68.2.2 Ankle joint

Tendinitides of the Achilles tendon

Tendinitides of the Achilles tendon are often caused by dancing on hard ground and by wrong jump techniques. Every jump starts and ends in demi-plié. In the jump, the weight is first shifted to the heel and then to the ball of the foot. The gastrocnemius muscle is extended maximally at the jump, hence, its contraction force will be the strongest (Micheli 1983). If the dancer does not have any heel contact during the jump and thus jumps off with the ball of the foot, the contraction force of the gastrocnemius muscle will be smaller (and the jump will therefore be less powerful and not as high). This damages the fascia plantaris and the Achilles tendon. An Achilles tendon tendinitis can be triggered by too tight laces of the ballet shoes. This tendinitis affects jumping and plié.

Treatment focuses on relieving the joint; otherwise a chronic tendinitis can develop. Its full healing takes a long time and can fail completely, which is likely the result of a neovascularization of the inner tendon part. Alfredson et al. (2005) suggest a sclerosing of new blood vessels as an alternative treatment of long-term conditions. First results are promising (Kristoffersen wt al. 2005).

Bursitis retrocalcanei

A chronic bursitis retrocalcanei causes pain and a swelling of the posterior soft tissue at the front of the Achilles tendon. The prominent bursa can be palpated medially and from lateral of the insertion of the Achilles tendon. Arthroscopic removal of the bursa and resection of the prominent posterior edge of the calcaneus can be helpful (Van Dijk et al. [1] 1997). The dancer's return to the stage after this surgery is possible after 3 months on average. A retrocalcaneal bursitis is complicated by an insertion tendinosis. A partial rupture in the middle of the tendon often occurs.

Peritendinitis of the tibialis posterior muscle

This overuse syndrome is mostly based on wrong techniques: "sickling" and "rolling". In **sickling** – the turning-in of the foot in toe dance – the peronei muscles overuses in varus position, while sickling in a valgus position overuses the tibialis porsterior muscle. **Rolling** compensates for insufficient pronation of the hip (Gelabert 1980). Since the body weight stands above the medial edge of the foot in this valgus stand, the arch of the foot drops and touches the floor (= rolling).

The tibialis porterior tendinitis is treated with a combination of deep transverse frictions, ice applications and stretching exercises. If this does not help, a relapse is almost certain. If the conditions persist despite improved technique and conservative treatment, endoscopic synovectomy and a release are necessary. Under the vision of a mini-arthroscope inserted into the tendon sheath, the swollen tendon sheath can be split from the inside. The advantage is obvious: shorter periods of admission, less pain, functional after-treatment and a faster return to the stage (Van Dijk et al. [2] 1997). Additionally, tendoscopy allows diagnosis of a partial rupture. Surgery of the peroneal tendinitis is an alternative (Van Dijk et al. [1] 1998). The chance to diagnose a partial rupture is another advantage of tendoscopy.

Tenosynovitis of the flexor hallucis longus muscle

This is a common problem and pain localizes behind the medial malleolus (Kolettis et al. 1996). Pain can be induced by extending the hallux maximally dorsal. Crepitating is felt during this maneuver. The point of maximum pain and crepitating is located behind the medial malleolus, where the flexor hallucis longus runs in the tendon sheath. The cause of this irritation is an increased dental flexion of the upper ankle joint and the metatarsophalangeal joint of the hallux. This syndrome develops by repetitive exercising grand-plié and relevé-à-demi-point. The tendon needs to glide through the tendon sheath and – also conditioned by the hypertrophy – the muscle belly of the flexor hallucis longus pulls into the tendon sheath proximally of the orifice. This causes the tenosynovitis and a local fibrosis. If the patient is able to perform the grand-plié free of pain after infiltration of the tendon sheath with 1 ml lidocaine, the diagnosis is clear.

The acute tenosynovitis is treated with rest, ice massages and antiphlogistics, followed by a training without relevé, plié and jumps. Surgical treatment is indicated for a chronic tenosynovitis (Kolettis et al. 1996). The swelling at the orifice of the tendon sheath is cut out by arthroscopy, the fibrosed tendon sheath is partly removed (Van Dijk et al. [3] 1997).

Anterior impingement syndrome

A characteristic of the anterior impingement syndrome (Sammarco et al. 2000) is a constrained and painful dorsal flexion as a consequence of an inflammation of the anterior joint capsule or an osteophytic development at the talar neck or at the anterior side of the distal tibia (Van Dijk et al. [4] 1997). The surgical treatment involves the arthroscopic resection of the osteophyte.

Syndromes of the lower ankle joint

Afflictions can develop at the posterior side of the talus by compression of the posterior part of the lower ankle joint due to the increasing plantar flexion. This will especially be the case if an **os trigonum** or a **hypertrophic posterior tali process** is present. A pain will develop in the hindfoot at relevé. A pain-free relevé after infiltration of 1 ml lidocaine (under control of an image converter) is proving. Two or three infiltrations of corticosteroids could be sufficient for the elimination of the medical conditions. An excision of the os trigonum or the posterior tali process may be carried out at persistence. An open surgical treatment will show good results in dancers in 90% (Stibbe et al. 1994). For some years, this dancers' problem has been treated arthroscopically in our clinic, as well. A posterior arthroscopy will be carried out by a two-portal technique, in which the posterior part of the upper and lower ankle joint will be reached and an os trigonum can be removed (Van Dijk et al. 2000). The advantages of the arthroscopic technique for dancers will be obvious here, as well.

The posterior part of the lower ankle joint is accessible for palpation behind the medial malleolus. If the pain is localized here, a diagnostic infiltration of the lower ankle joint will be recommendable. A relevé should be performable without pain in the case of a **"dancer's heel"** (= **chondropathy of the posterior facet of the lower ankle joint**). The treatment and the result depend on the conditions and therefore also depend on potentially upcoming joint adaptations. The majority of the patients will be pain-free after one or several infiltrations of local anesthetic with/without corticosteroids. If the conditions persist, an arthroscopic nettoyage of the area by a posterior lower ankle joint arthroscopy will be indicated (Van Dijk et al. 2000).

68.2.3 Knee joint

Literature makes it clear that dancers often suffer from an **idiopathic patellofemoral syndrome**. According to a study by Winslow et al. (1995), a contraction of the tractus iliotibialis possibly underlies this pain. Therefore, it is recommendable to aspire a lengthening of the tractus at patellofemoral pain.

A **meniscus rupture** is especially diagnosed in dancers at rude landings after jumps. The most effective therapy consists of an early partial removal of the ruptured meniscus by arthroscopy. With an intensive after-treatment, a new performance can be danced after 4–6 weeks.

The **"jumper's knee"** is also a frequent lesion in dancers. Pain will occur at a jump or plié, which is caused by micro-ruptures in the patellar tendon, mostly at the insertion at the apex patellae. A fatigue fracture or an osteochondrosis can also appear in this localization. A circumscribed painful point at the patellar apex exists in the examination. The patient will be pain-free after infiltration of 1 ml of lidocaine 0.5% and the diagnosis will be confirmed. The diagnosis depends on the stage of the injury. If pain is experienced after lifting and jumping, the exercise load should be reduced first; ice massages and deep transverse frictions will have to be applied in addition to a strain reduction with run-in pain that vanishes after warm-up; a local infiltration (possibly a small amount of corticosteroid for one time) might be considered with persistent pain first. If the pain persists despite the mentioned measures, a surgical treatment will be indicated. With the experience of years of successful open surgical treatment, a 5-month-period of convalescence can be expected for the dancers. We have carried out this treatment arthroscopically with continuously good results since 1995. Here the apex patellae will be removed from intraarticular by the shaver without seriously impairing the patellar tendon.

68.2.4 Hip joint

The joint capsule of the hip is a strong structure, which surrounds the proximal femur and the acetabulum. The capsule is very important for the stability of the hip and it is sensitive with overstretching, which will find expression in pain of the hip muscles. Atraumatic instability of the hip joint is associated with generalized ligament laxity; the affected patients describe pain in running with a feeling of insecurity in the movement process. In the long term, chronic instability is conductive to an early development of an arthrosis.

Bellabarba et al. (1998) have drawn the conclusion from their results that physiotherapy alone will not be sufficient for the solution of this problem, and they recommended a posterior "plication" as temporary option. Phillippon (2001) has described an arthroscopically conducted thermal modification of the collagen of the joint capsule as another option. Good results in athletes could be achieved hereby in the short term. Still, no conclusively satisfactory treatment method has been available for this clinical picture yet.

A **low-energetic dislocation of the hip joint** is relatively rare, as Stein et al. (2002) have described.

References

Anderson H (2005). Conservative management of Achilles tendinopathy: new ideas. Foot Ankle Clin 10: 321–329.

Arendt YD et al. (2003). Injury and overuse pattern in professional ballet dancers. Z Orthop Ihre Grenzgeb 141: 349–356.

Bellabarba C et al. (1998). Idiopathic hip instability. An unrecognized cause of coxa saltans in the adult. Clin Orthop Relat Res 355: 261–271.

Gelabert R (1980). Preventing dancers injuries. The Physician and Sportsmedicine 8: 69–77.

Howse J (1993). Disorders of the great toe in dancers. Clin Sports Med 2: 499–505.

Kolettis GJ et al. (1996). Release of the flexor hallucis longus tendon in ballet dancers. J Bone Joint Surg [Am] 78: 1386–1390.

Kristoffersen M et al. (2005). Neovascularization in the chronic tendon injuries detected with colour Doppler ultrasound in horse and men: implications for research and treatment. Knee Surg Sports Traumatol Arthrosc 13: 505–508.

Micheli LJ (1983). Back injuries in dancers. Clin Sports Med 2: 473–484.

Miller EH et al. (1974). A new consideration in athletic injuries. The classical ballet dancer. Clin Orthop 111: 181–191.

Phillippon MJ (2001). The role of arthroscopic thermal capsulorrhaphy in the hip. Clin Sports Med 20: 817–829.

Sammarco GJ et al. (2000). Disorders of the foot and ankle. Foot and ankle in dance. WB Saunders, Philadelphia, p. 2483.

Stein DA et al (2002). Low energy anterior hip dislocation in a dancer. Am J Orthop 31: 591–594.

Stibbe AB et al. (1994). The os trigonum syndrome. Acta Orthop Scand 261 (Suppl): 65–66.

Teitz CC (1983). Sports medicine concerns in dance and gymnastics. Clin Sports Med 2: 571–593.

Van Dijk CN et al. [1] (1997). Tendoscopy for overuse tendon injuries. Op Techn Sports Med 1997: 170–178.

Van Dijk CN et al. [2] (1997). Tendoscopy of the posterios tibial tendon. Arthroscopy 13: 692–698.

Van Dijk CN et al. [3] (1997). Arthroscopy of the ankle joint. Arthroscopy 13: 90–96.

Van Dijk CN et al. [4] (1997). A prospective study on prognostic factors concerning the outcome of arthroscopy for anterior ankle impingement. Am J Sports Med 25: 737–745.

Van Dijk CN et al. [1] (1998). Tendoscopy of the peroneal tendons. Arthroscopy 14: 471–478.

Van Dijk CN et al. [2] (1998). Arthroscopic surgery of the metatarsophalangeal first joint. Arthroscopy 14: 851–855.

Van Dijk CN et al. (2000). A 2-portal endoscopic approach for diagnosis and treatment of posterior ankle pathology. Arthroscopy 16: 871–876.

Winslow J et al. (1995). Patellofemoral pain in female ballet dancers: correlation with iliotibial band tightness and tibial external rotation. J Orthop Sports Phys Ther 22: 18–21.

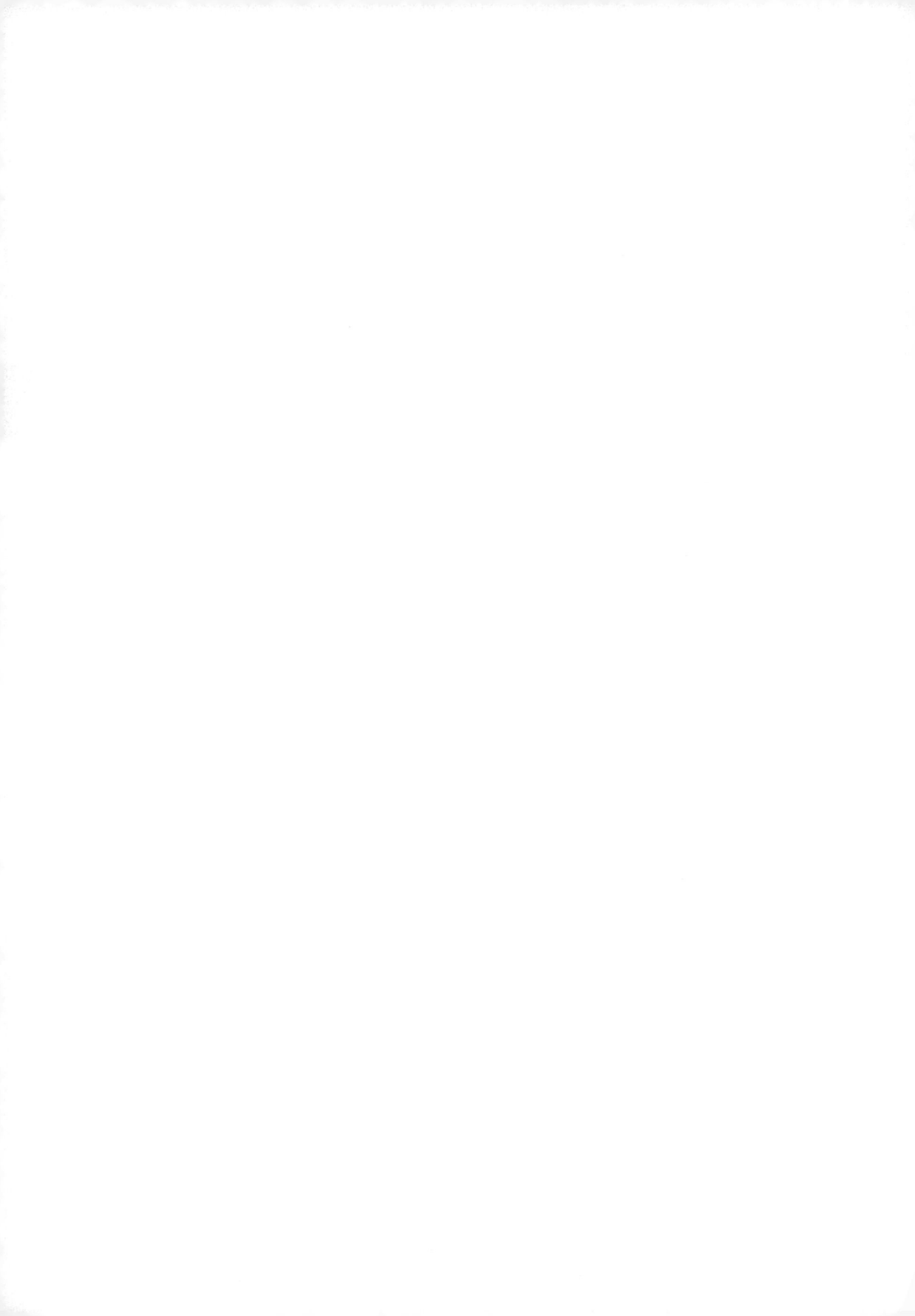

69 Figure skating

Andreas Gösele

Figure skating is a sport that combines art and esthetics with strength and athletics in a unique way. While figure skating had been considered a winter sport, it can now be practiced all year long given the growing number of skating rinks. Figure skating consists of **four disciplines**: singles (men and women), pair skating and ice dancing.

Within the last 20 years, we have registered a definite increase of the technical and athletic demands, not least because of compulsory figures have been cancelled and the **"free figures"** have moved into the foreground of training and competition. More and more complex, coordinative jumps, creative pirouettes and variations require a **more extensive training**.

Pair skating combines the classic elements, such as jumps, jump combinations, pirouettes and turns with lifts and throws, while the dance aspect with the interpretation of the music is in the foreground in **ice dancing** in addition to the purely athletic demands.

Synchronized skating (SYS) is still a very young sport, which involves a team of 16–20 skaters. Synchronization and precision of the steps, jumps, pirouettes, figures and movements in changing formations, artistic expression as an interpretation of the chosen music and the harmony of the team are the crucial criteria of this discipline.

Figure skating combines the **sport-motor characteristics** of strength, springiness, strength endurance, flexibility, esthetics, feeling for music, rhythm and "motor ensemble". The increasing technical demands can only be fulfilled by a training beginning in childhood age. The elite figure skaters will exercise up to 8 hours a day at the average, 6 times a week, between 10 and 11 months a year.

A **weekly training of 10–14 hours** already in childhood age is not rare, since the different motor capabilities have to be learned and be improved in training. Despite extensive exercising and competition, the full number of injuries regarding the hours of exercising can be considered minor. Thus, the average **incidence of injuries** amounts to 1.4 accidents in 1,000 hours of exercising.

In general, **acute injuries** have to be distinguished from **chronic and overstrain injuries**. The individual disciplines differ significantly in this respect. While overstrain injuries such as chronic tendinoses and stress fractures are in the foreground in singles' skating, acute injuries caused by falls and collisions prevail in pair skating and ice dancing (➤ Tab. 69.1).

The overstrain injuries increase in young talents. Mainly stress fractures and **tendinoses**, **pathologies near the insertions and origins**, such as jumper's knee, fasciitis plantaris and Osgood-Schlatter disease as traction apophysitis of the extensor apparatus are in the foreground (➤ Tab. 69.2).

Lower extremities are affected most often with chronic injuries and overstrain injuries, acute injuries can affect practically all regions of the body (➤ Tab. 69.3). The **spectrum of injuries** ranges from abrasions to ankle sprains to fractures and cranial injuries.

In addition to the acute and chronic injuries with overstrain phenomena of the locomotor apparatus, **psychophysical diseases**, such as the "female athlete triad" (eating disorders, amenorrhea and osteoporosis), purely psychological problems in the interrelation between athletes, coach and parents play an important role (Lipetz and Kruse 2000, Sabatini 2001, Ziegler

Tab. 69.1 Acute and overstrain-conditioned injuries of elite junior figure skaters (Dubravcic-Simunjak et al. 2003).

	Women n = 236			Men n = 233		
	Individual n = 107	Pairs n = 61	Ice dancing n = 68	Individual n = 104	Pairs n = 61	Ice dancing n = 86
acute	14.6%	60.0%	77.8%	18.6%	60.4%	58.8%
chronic	72.7%	31.7%	22.2%	68.5%	26.4%	41.2%
dorsal pain	12.7%	8.3%	–	12.9%	13.2%	–

Tab. 69.2 Overstrain-conditioned injuries of elite junior figure skaters (Dubravcic-Simunjak et al. 2003).

	Women n = 236			Men n = 233		
	Individual n = 107	Pairs n = 61	Ice dancing n = 68	Individual n = 104	Pairs n = 61	Ice dancing n = 86
jumper's knee	14.9%	3.9%	–	16.1%	1.9%	–
stress fracture	19.8%	5.9%	–	13.2%	3.8%	–
shin splints	13.9%	3.9%	–	7.5%	3.8%	1.9%
inguinal pain	7.9%	2%	1%	9.4%	2.7%	3.8%
impingement of the foot joint	2.9%	–	–	4.7%	–	–
tendinitis of the Achilles tendon	3.9%	–	1%	4.7%	–	–
Osgood-Schlatter disease	8.9%	2.9%	–	14.2%	3.8%	–
fascitis plantaris	2%	–	–	3.8%	–	–
hamstring syndrome	4.9%	–	–	2.8%	1.9%	–

Tab. 69.3 Acute injuries of elite junior figure skaters (Dubravcic-Simunjak et al. 2003).

	Women n = 236			Men n = 233		
	Individual n = 107	Pairs n = 61	Ice dancing n = 68	Individual n = 104	Pairs n = 61	Ice dancing n = 86
ankle sprains	16.8%	13.5%	3.4%	15.4%	10.8%	3.1%
ligament injuries of the knee	5.1%	1.8%	–	4.6%	3.1%	1.5%
shoulder dislocations	–	3.4%	–	–	4.6%	–
soft tissue injuries	–	13.5%	6.8%	–	7.7%	6.2%
head injuries	–	13.5%	–	–	7.7%	1.5%
humeral fractures	3.4%	6.8%	–	6.2%	3.1%	–
femoral fractures	5.1%	3.4%	–	6.2%	3.1%	–
knee injuries	–	3.4%	–	4.6%	1.5%	–
wrist fractures	–	–	–	–	4.6%	3.1%
finger fractures	–	–	–	–	1.5%	–

et al. 1998 [a], 1998 [b], 2002, Jonnalagadda et al. 2004).

A cooperation of the individual groups is a decisive measure for success in the medical follow-up and the athletics, especially with complex disorders being of variable and multiform causes.

69.1 Acute injuries

Sprains are the most frequent acute injuries (16.8%) in figure skating. Injury of the **supination and pronation chain** with capsule-ligament injuries or even fractures appear (Smith and Ludington 1989). **Skin and head injuries** and acute **knee injuries** (3.4%) appear often, but not as often as ankle joint injuries (Dubravcic-Simunjak et al. 2003).

69.2 Chronic injuries and overstrain damages

Stress fractures are the majority of the chronic injuries with up to 20% of all injuries. About 53% of the stress fractures affect the **foot** (Pecina et al. 1990). **Low-risk (LRF), high-risk fractures (HRF)** and their combination and multiple localizations are common. The LRF (e.g. metatarsal heads) are characterized by uncomplicated progress of disease with a short healing time of 6–8 weeks and can primarily be treated conservatively. The HRF (e.g. os naviculare pedis; ➤ Fig. 69.1) show a prolonged healing process of 8–16 weeks, tend to develop pseudarthrosis and often have to be treated surgically (➤ Fig. 69.2). Muscular fatigue combined with a **reduction of the "stress protection"** is stated in current literature as the cause of stress fractures of the lower extremities.

In addition to the stress fractures of the foot (53%), the **tibia** is affected primarily by stress fractures with 35% of the cases. The remaining stress fractures spread over the fibula and the femur; the spine is affected only rarely.

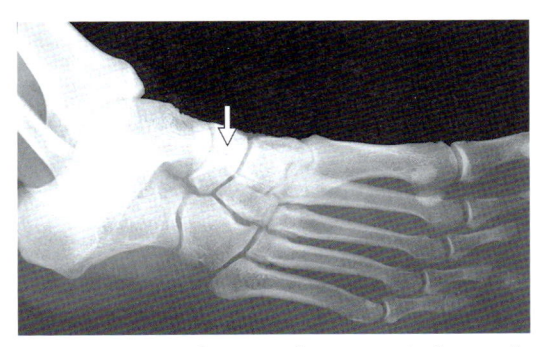

Fig. 69.1 Stress fracture of an os naviculare pedis (high-risk fracture) preoperatively.

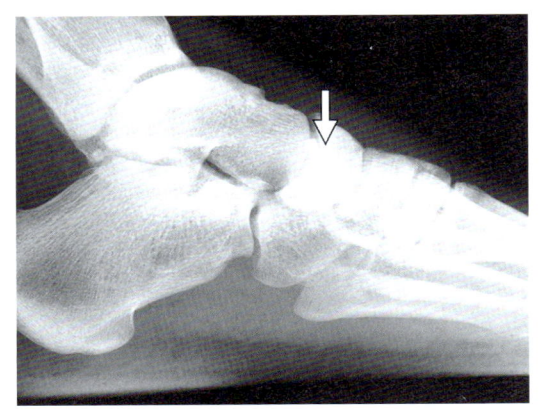

Fig. 69.2 Screw osteosynthesis at a stress fracture of an os naviculare pedis (high-risk fracture).

69.2.1 Tendon injuries

Another frequent chronic injury is the "anterior knee pain" and jumper's knee (14%) as an expression of a chronic painful **disease of the knee joint extensor apparatus**. A chronic overload by jumps and by landing with massive eccentric strain peaks (Lockwood and Gervais 1997) is the cause and the combination of strain with muscular imbalances and disturbances of the flexor-extensor relation.

Intrinsic factors (Q-angle, patellar shape and patellar index) and **extrinsic** factors (exercise intensity, amount and exercise ground) are included in etiologic discussions. **Variants** of pure inflammation with full continuity up to partial or total ruptures have been observed (➤ Fig. 69.3). **Degenerative** processes seem to play a much more important role here than in-

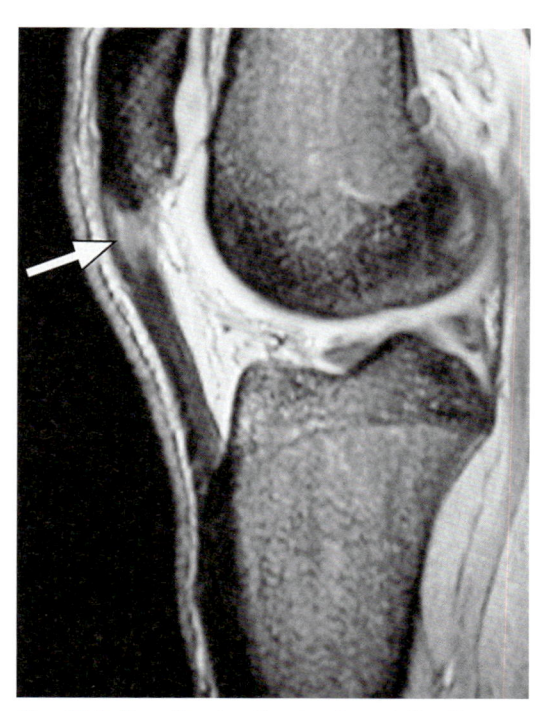

Fig. 69.3 Insertion tendinosis of a patellar ligament (jumper's knee) with tendon edema and partial lesion.

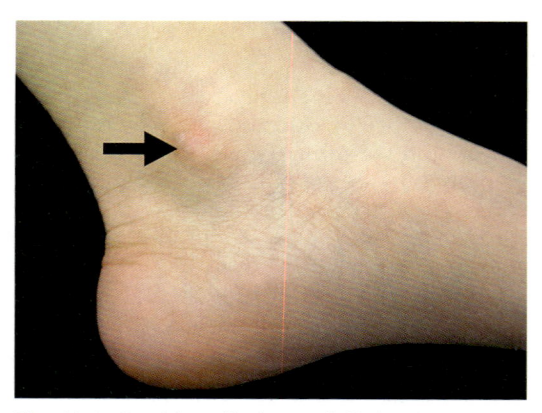

Fig. 69.4 Bursitis malleolus medialis by chronic pressure of the ice skate.

flammatory processes, at least from a histological point of view (Smith et al. 1991).

Injuries and diseases of the Achilles tendon as well as the plantar aponeurosis (maximally 4%) play a minor role, because the shoes practically do not allow any turning moment in the upper and lower ankle joint. In contrast, **tendon diseases near the insertion**, such as apophysis injuries are more frequent, because figure skating is carried out to a large amount and with high intensity already in childhood age. The **Osgood-Schlatter disease** of the tuberositas tibiae partly appears in up to 14% of the cases with boys and young men being affected especially (Smith 2000).

69.2.2 Bursitides

A rare, but extremely unique disease is the **bursitis of the malleolus medialis**. **Chronic pressure** of the shoe in combination with an **expansive malleolus medialis** can lead to the development of a clearly prominent, partly asymptomatic and also partly inflammatory bursa (➤ Fig. 69.4). The bursa serves as protection and as layer of shifting and primarily does not present pathology. A **conservative treatment** with antiphlogistics, cushioning and partly also adjustment of custom shoes is carried out only in the case of an inflammation. A surgical treatment is rarely necessary.

69.3 Prevention

Acute injuries in figure skating can only contingently be influenced. Helmets and protectors reduce injuries. But since they are not used in competition because of esthetic reasons, their acceptance has to be doubted in the first place. In training, on the other hand, certain **protectors** adapted to the sport are applied and reduce injuries. In individual cases, this method has already been practiced but data collection of this primary prevention has not been available yet.

Avoiding **muscular imbalances and mal distributions** between agonist and antagonist seem to play a significant part for **chronic injuries** and overstrain impairments. Variants for the set-up of training, alternative training stimuli combined with active measures of rest should become established especially in sports with such intensive training. Not least, stress fractures can be reduced by a specific **advanced muscular training**, by active measures of regeneration and by an improvement of the muscular "stress protection".

The **cooperation** of coach, athlete, sport-physician and also psychologists is indispensible especially in such a weight- and figure-accentuating sport as figure skating for the **prevention of eating and nutrition disorders**. It mirrors the complexity of individual injuries and diseases and complex attempts at their solution.

> Figure skating promotes different motor characteristics in children and juveniles, despite intensive physical strain and a high time expenditure. Figure skating still presents only a relatively low injury risk compared to other sports.

References

Dubravcic-Simunjak S; Pecina M, Kuipers H, Moran J, Haspl M (2003). The incidence of injuries in elite junior figure skaters. Am J Sports Med 31(4): 511–517.

Jonnalagadda SS, Ziegler PJ, Nelson JA (2004). Food preferences dieting behaviors, and body image perceptions of elite figure skaters. Int J Sport Nutr Exerc Metab 14(5): 594–606.

Lipetz J, Kruse RJ (2000). Injuries and special concerns of female figure skaters. Clin Sports Med 19(2): 369–380.

Lockwood K, Gervais P (1997). Impact forces upon landing single, double, and triple revolution jumps in figure skaters. Clin Biomech (Bristol, Avon) 12(3): 11.

Pecina M, Bojanic I, Dubravcic S (1990). Stress fractures in figure skaters. Am J Sports Med 18(3): 277–279.

Sabatini S (2001). The female athlete triad. Am J Med Sci 322(4): 193–195.

Smith AD (2000). The young skater. Clin Sports Med 19(4): 741–755.

Smith AD, Ludlington R (1989). Injuries in elite pair skaters and ice dancers. Am J Sports Med 17(4): 482–488.

Smith AD, Stroud L, McQueen C (1991). Flexibility and anterior knee pain in adolescent elite figure skaters. J Pediatr Orthop 11(1): 77–82.

Ziegler PJ [a], Khoo CS, Kris-Etherton PM, Jonnalagadda SS, Sherr B, Nelson JA (1998). Nutritional status of nationally ranked junior US figure skaters. J Am Diet Assoc 98(7): 809–811.

Ziegler PJ [b], Khoo CS, SS, Sherr B, Nelson JA (1998). Nutritional status of nationally ranked junior US figure skaters. Int J Eat Disord 24(4): 421–427.

Ziegler PJ, Jonnalagadda SS, Nelson JA, Lawrence C, Baciak B (2992). Contribution of meals and snacks to nutrient intake of male and female elite figure skaters during peak competition peak competitive season. J Am Coll Nutr 21(2): 114–110.

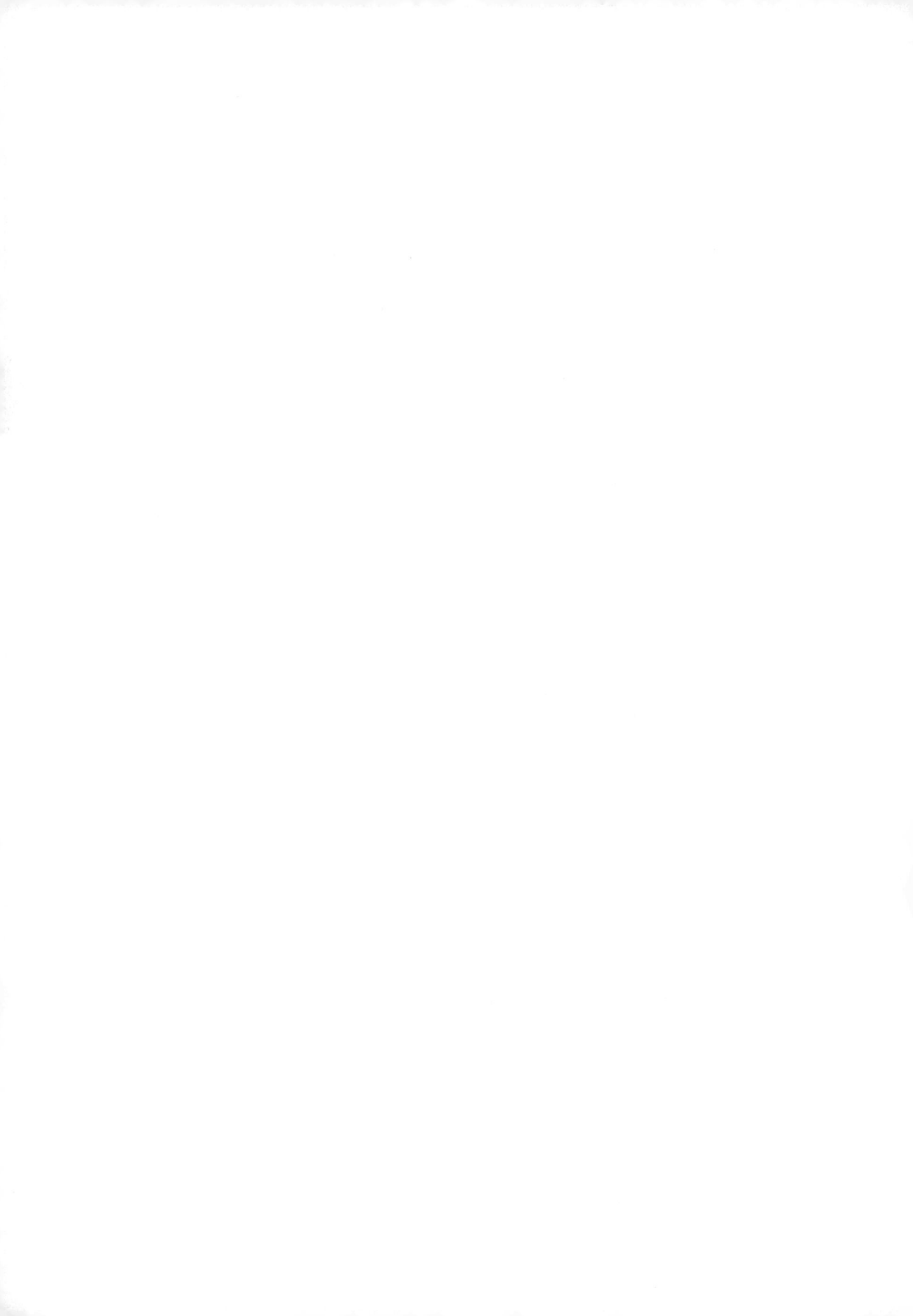

Chapter 70 Artistic gymnastics

Hans-Peter Boschert

70.1 History of artistic gymnastics

Artistic gymnastics dates back in Germany to the 16th and 17th century. Johann Christoph Guts Muths (1759–1839), Friedrich Ludwig Jahn (1778–1852), Karl-Friedrich Friesen (1784–1814) and Adolf Spieß (1810–1859) had been the most important forerunners. Artistic gymnastics developed in Germany by political restraints and prohibitions to what gymnastics had represented until the end of 19th century. Gymnastics had become more and more influenced by the state and was supposed to serve the **national physical education** after the failed 1848 revolution. Progressively, "gymnast artists" developed separately, which resulted in a controversy of **"artificial gymnastics"** and **"natural gymnastics"** in late 19th century. The consequences of the fight between gymnastics and sport reach back to the time of National Socialism. Even today, there are still discussions between supporters and opponents about the competitive nature of the sport. However, both belong together inseparably and profit from each other.

Today's gymnastics does not share with the original idea of its ancestors. **Acrobatics**, risk, spectacular gymnastics and pushing the body to its limits are in the foreground of today's top sports. New benchmarks are set by the **"apparatus specialists"**. The traditional multi-discipline athlete therefore moves more and more into the background.

70.2 Description of the sport and its demands

Artistic gymnastics in its current form is characterized by a high degree of **specification**. It has developed into a dynamic sport, which puts high demands to the athlete as a technical-compositional sport regarding **basic motor skills** (strength, strength endurance, flexibility), **psychomotor basic skills** (motor learning aptitude, motion remembrance, precision of movement, movement adaptation, psychodynamic abilities, cognition), **coordination** and **concentration** (Martin 1985).

Artistic gymnastics has been part of the **Olympic program** since 1896 for men and 1928 for women with the disciplines of vault, balance beam, uneven bars and floor for women, and floor, pommel horse, still rings, vault (jump will be carried out over a vaulting table – previously "transversely or longitudinally placed horse"), parallel bars and high bar for men. Competitions of the individual apparatuses and multi-discipline competitions are carried out, which are evaluated according to the "code de pointage", the international regulations of assessment. The International Gymnastics Federation (FIG) has been requested by the IOC to change the **assessment regulations** after the controversial assessments at the Olympic Games in Athens in 2004. Therefore, the old assessment system with the highest score of 10.0 points and the marks A and B has been retired. The A-mark relates to the degree of difficulty of the exercise and sums up 10 elements that have constant values according to their degree of difficulty. Therefore, the A-mark is open to the top and will reach values of up to 7.7 in the top field. The B-mark for the technical execution is calculated by the average of the deductions by the 6 B-judges, starting from the highest value of 10.0. Thus, the sums in the absolute top field even amount to 16.8.

The German men belong to the absolute top of the world; the leading nations are China, Japan and the U.S.A.

70.3 Strain profile and biomechanical specialties

Regarding the performance development, artistic gymnastics has experienced another immense boost in current years. There has been an **increase of the degrees of difficulty** of individual exercises and parts of exercises. Constantly new and more difficult exercise elements have been invented and new techniques have been developed or old ones have been improved. Sports science contributes essentially to this, because new elements and techniques have been improved or developed with the help of computer simulation, modern video and computer technology, with no end in sight yet.

Flying elements at the high bar have increasingly developed into most difficult artistic-acrobatic elements with simultaneous multiple turns of the longitudinal and lateral axes. In 1987, a triple somersault on the floor was shown for the first time and a quadruple somersault at the high bar seems possible (Knoll 1992).

Another progress exists in the neo-construction and **improvement of the apparatuses**:

- Gymnastic exercises on the floor are performed on strain-reducing, elastic constructions.
- Sponge pits allow the training of difficult flying parts, vaults and take-offs.
- Double-elastic springboards and landing mats with strong damping characteristics reduce the strain and injury risk.
- Grips with worked-in dowel rods protect the skin and improve the grip on the rings, the high bar and the uneven bars ("hook effect").
- Miscellaneous support equipment allows a methodic training of exercises.

From the **anthropometric** point of view, there are special characteristics in artistic gymnastics. The athletes are of a **small size and a low body weight**. Since 1972, there have not been any drastic changes in the anthropometry of men.

Special **biomechanical aspects** of artistic gymnastics (Brüggemann 1995):

- mechanical loads:
  - high passive impact forces on the supporting and locomotor apparatus, which can not be compensated muscularly, as well as active forces in vaults and landing
  - acceleration and centrifugal forces to the upper extremities of up to 12 G at the rings (Nissinen 1992)
  - ground reaction forces of up to 12–15 G in landing from the high bar (Amadio and Baumann 1990)
  - compression, torsion and shearing forces to the elbow and wrist joints of the double or triple amount of the body weight (Brüggemann and Rühl 1995)
- fast and high force increases
- short strain periods of 100–300 ms
- high-rate vibrations at the frame of the rings and the parallel bars
- high strain repetitions
- high amounts of exercising (2–3 exercise units daily and 30–35 hours of exercising a week in top sport)
- strained supporting and locomotor apparatus surpassing the physiological movement limit.

70.4 Sport-specific injuries and consequences of improper strain

Artistic gymnastics belong to the rather risky and potentially injury-prone sports. The individual risk-taking, technical and the fitness levels of the athlete play an important role. **Muscle injuries** hardly play any role because of the good extensibility and the balanced musculature.

There are numerous **external and internal influences**, which have an effect on the risk of an injury and/or impairment:

- methods of exercising, movement technique, equipment, gym
- training group, physical preconditions, age (sensitive puberal phase)
- training preparation, fatigue, general state of health (e.g. infections)
- psychological make-up, coach.

Artistic gymnastics are characterized by a low to middle **absolute and relative injury frequen-**

cies (Steinbrück 1997). Ball sports and martial arts have a higher injury risk. The injury and impairment pattern in artistic gymnastics shows several particularities, which are not present in other sports.

70.4.1 Acute injuries

Lower Extremities

Ankle joint injuries (➤ Fig. 70.1) amount to 34.5% of all **injuries** at the locomotor apparatus. Felländer-Tsai and Wredmark (1995) have stated the injury frequency of the lower extremities with 59%. Primarily, these are **capsule-ligament injuries**, occurring mostly on the floor and in landing from the apparatuses due to twisting of the ankle at the edges of the mats or in take-offs. Currently, a significant amount also occurs when playing soccer!

The remaining injuries spread in equal amounts to all other regions of the body. Serious injuries such as **cruciate ligament ruptures** with and without meniscus injuries are rather rare and mostly develop after vaults or landing after incomplete turns of the longitudinal axis. Hyperextension trauma develop, if the athlete lands first on the heel due to rotations of lateral axis in forward jumps with extended knee joints.

Upper extremities

Discus lesions primarily occur at the **wrists** in performing the pommel horse, if an overturn to ulnar or a slipping off the pommels at a spindle in handstand occurs. High torsion forces affect the joint simultaneously.

Forearm fractures close to the joint, so-called grip lock injuries and capsule-ligament injuries of the carpal joints are typical injuries in performing **high bars**, caused by getting caught in the leather grip Samuelson et al. (1996) give an incidence of 0.2% per year for this type of injury. These types of fractures had neither been known to them nor to us before the introduction of grips with dowel rods. An injury mostly occurs if the leather thins out and is overexpanded and thus cannot withstand the strain anymore. The built-in dowel rods wrap around the bar, and release is literally impossible.

Fractures and dislocations of the **elbow** develop almost exclusively by falls at the apparatus or off the apparatus in the attempt to break the fall by outstretched arms. At the parallel bars, avulsion fractures are typical at falls to the upper arms with flexed elbows.

Finger joint injuries develop mostly because of improper gripping in the handstand at the pommel horse or the parallel bars; they occur quite often.

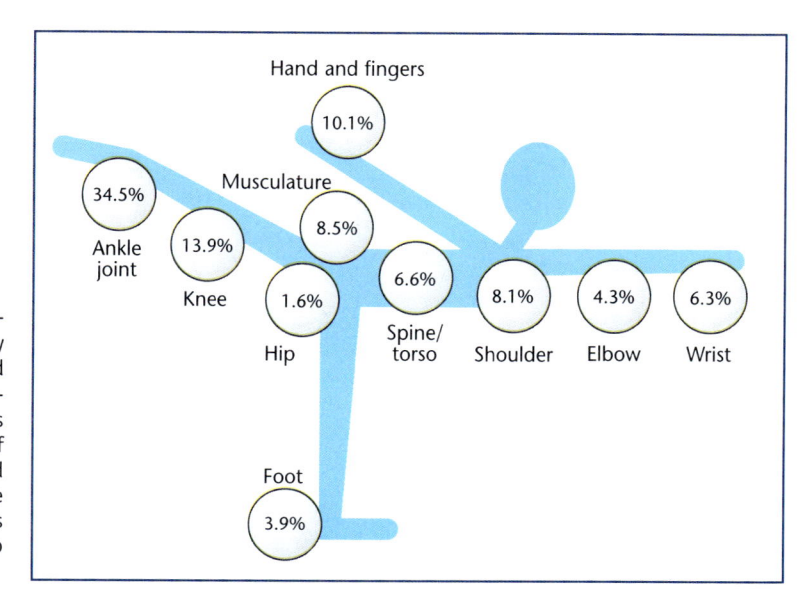

Fig. 70.1 Frequency of injuries of the individual body regions of the supporting and locomotor apparatus (own retrospective analysis of "sports traumatology in Mooswald" of 185 gymnasts of the A, B, and C squads as well as diverse national squads of the years 1988–1996; according to Boschert et al. 1998).

Hand and fingers 10.1%
Ankle joint 34.5%
Musculature 8.5%
Knee 13.9%
Hip 1.6%
Spine/torso 6.6%
Shoulder 8.1%
Elbow 4.3%
Wrist 6.3%
Foot 3.9%

The **shoulder joints** are subject to particularly high strain at the still rings and the high bar. Therefore it is astonishing that the number of injuries is very low in contrast to the forces. Injuries of the shoulders mostly develop, if the fall ends on the side, i.e. if the circling-in did not fully succeed, at the high bar.

Spine

Serious injuries of the spine are **rare**. Still, hyperflexion or hyperextension traumas of the spine can cause serious injuries of the lower segments of the cervical spine with mostly permanent impairments due to a fall to the head or neck. **Mild traumas of the cervical spine** can relatively often lead to **early degenerative adaptations** of the vertebral joints, intervertebral disks or neuroforamina. The causes mainly are falls off the apparatus and one-and-a-half forward somersaults on the floor, which lead to insufficient rotation and are not be intercepted by the hands, but the lower segments of the cervical spine (Elsässer 1997). A high injury risk is present at the vaulting table at double somersaults backwards, if they end on the neck due to insufficient rotation.

70.4.2 Overstrain impairments

The largest amount of problems of the supporting and locomotor apparatus by far in artistic gymnastics involves the overstrain impairments or the consequences of improper strain (➢ Fig. 70.2). In the mentioned period of time, we have carried out 600 treatments of diverse overstrain conditions. These developed as a consequence of chronic and improper overstrain and resulted in **relapsing microtraumas**.

Lower extremities

The **hyperextension-pronation trauma** at an insufficient circling of the lateral axis with subsequent landing in a forward posture (counterposing of the feet) is one of the most frequent impairment mechanisms in artistic gymnastics. An anterior end position with **tibiotalar impingement** is caused by a missing muscular compensation, e.g. fatigue or exceeding the compensation limit. This can impact on cartilage. Contusions, bone bruises, and cartilage flakes to **osteochondrosis dissecans** (OCD) are characteristic conditions. In addition, these traumas affect the **Achilles tendon** or the deep flexor tendons in the dorsomedial part of the upper ankle joint. Lately, meniscua injuries at the knee joint have become more frequent, mostly caused by forward vaults with $2\,^1/_2$ circles of the longitudinal axis.

Upper extremities

In almost two thirds of the cases (61%) altogether, the upper extremities are affected due to excessive strain. Almost one third of all impairments affect the shoulder or wrist joints. All others spread equally over the remaining body regions.

Hypermobilities/instabilities towards anterior and/or inferior at the **shoulder joint** with **tendinitides**, especially of the supraspinal tendon and the long biceps tendon are frequent. Remarkably **Partial capsule separations of the AC joint** corresponding to Rockwood type II or Tossy I–II appear. Studies have shown similar results for the shoulder (Boschert 1992, Wülker et al. 1995). Functional-anatomical and biomechanical inappropriate joint position result in extreme tensions of the ligament of the AC joint and the glenohumeral ligaments in exercising at the still rings.

Overstrain at the **elbow joints** often occur as **epicondylitis radialis et ulnaris** or rarely also as cartilage impairments or osteochondrosis dissecans of the capitulum humeri (Panner's disease). The highest strain develops in the **iron cross** and other static-dynamical strength elements with mostly hyperextended elbow joints at the still rings.

In addition to the shoulder joints, the **wrist joints** represent another frequent problem of artistic gymnastics, which is often interrelated with restricted exercising and impairments. **High strain in stands** at the pommel horse (especially in flat stand) in combination with rotation and shearing forces often lead to cartilage strain of various degrees. A very typical strain consequence is the **tendovaginitis flexor carpi ulnaris** after frequently performed exercises at the pommel horse, which are carried out as a circular motion over one arm in hand stand.

Fig. 70.2 Overuse damages of the individual body regions of the supporting and locomotor apparatus (own retrospective analysis of "sports traumatology in Mooswald" of 185 gymnasts of the A, B, and C squads as well as diverse national squads of the years 1988 to 1996; according to Boschert et al. 1998).

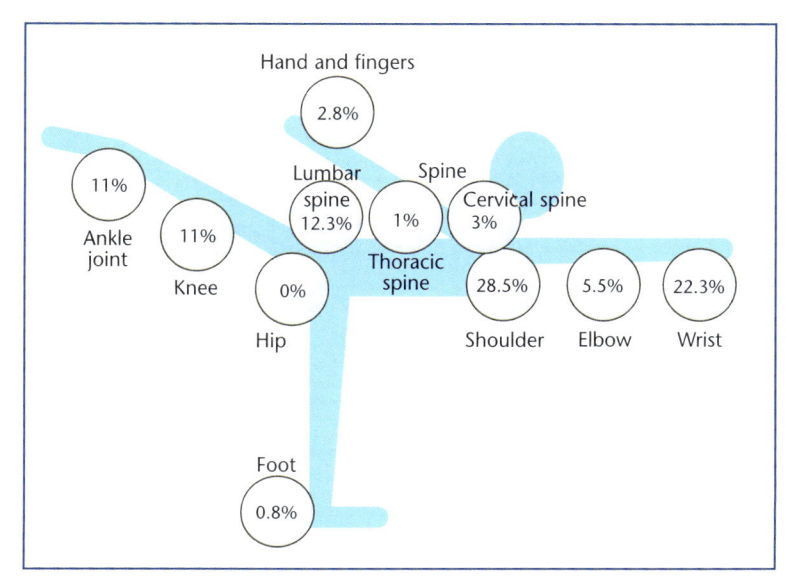

- Hand and fingers 2.8%
- Lumbar spine 12.3%
- Spine 1%
- Cervical spine 3%
- Ankle joint 11%
- Knee 11%
- Thoracic spine 0%
- Hip 28.5%
- Shoulder 5.5%
- Elbow 22.3%
- Wrist
- Foot 0.8%

Spine

In previous years, **spondylolyses and spondylolistheses** in artistic gymnastics have been reported. Schietholz and Liebig (1979) reported a 12% average (2.7–32%), Konermann and Sell (1992) more than 42% as compared to the incidence in general population of 2–7%. Islebe (1993) describe a frequency of 3.7% in female artistic gymnasts of the B and D squads and of 7.1% in the male gymnasts. Gradinger et al. (1991) mention a frequency of 16% in gymnasts. Our analysis resulted in 14% spondylolyses and 7.6% spondylolistheses as a lower average value, compared to literature, although it should be considered that those had been selected patients and not a longitudinal study.

Hypermobilities and segment loosening of the lower **lumbar spine** lead to medical conditions. These are not apparatus or exercise-specific, but rather result from diverse functional limitations or improper strain. Thus, a **missing harmonious mobility** of the full spine as well as the shoulder and hip joints are a possible cause. A compensatory hyperlordosis and more or less selective peak loads occur lumbosacrally in reclination movements, e.g. at a limited extension in the thoracic region with the consequences mentioned above. In my view, **too weak deep dorsal muscles** and **unbalanced muscles of the trunk** play a key role.

We have found early degenerative adaptations of the cervical spine or the lumbar spine in 16%, which had nearly all been triggered after a compression trauma or frequent falls to the neck.

Cartilage ossification disorders

Cartilage ossification disorders in **juvenile gymnasts** (➤ Fig. 70.3) are responsible for compulsory exercise limitations or training breaks. 217 cartilage ossification disorders have been treated during the mentioned period with the focus on the **joints of the upper extremity**. Almost a third have affected the **epiphyses of the wrist**, a fifth have affected the **thoracic and lumbar spine** as well as a slightly smaller amount the **epiphysis of the humeral head**. Mafullin et al. (1992) have reported similar changes at the growing skeleton. We deliberately do **not** speak of osteochondonecroses since no such changes in the majority of the cases have been detected.

Furthermore, the **diagnostic classification** is very different. The following examples have been known:

- enchondral dysostoses
- epimetaphyseal enchondral dysostoses

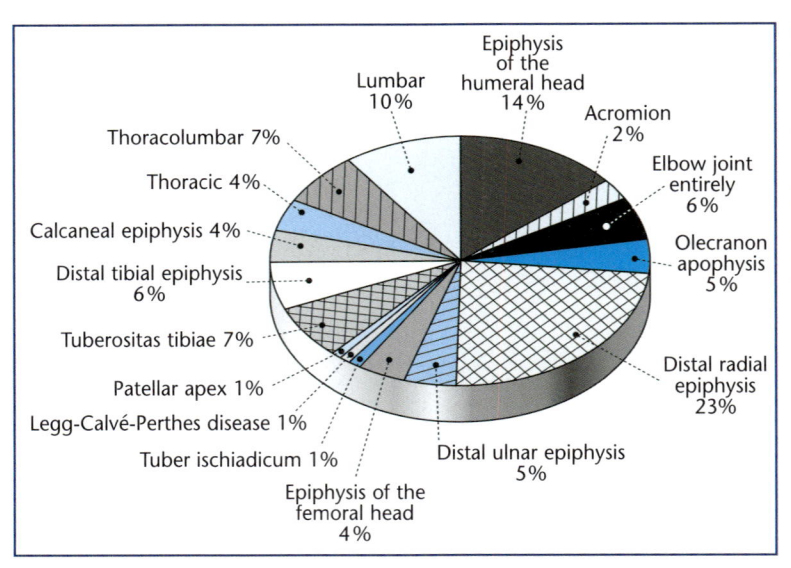

Fig. 70.3 Cartilage ossification disorders of the individual body regions of the supporting and locomotor apparatus (own retrospective analysis of "sports traumatology in Mooswald" of 185 gymnasts of the A, B, and C squads as well as diverse national squads of the years 1988–1996; according to Boschert et al. 1998).

Pie chart values:
- Thoracolumbar 7%
- Thoracic 4%
- Calcaneal epiphysis 4%
- Distal tibial epiphysis 6%
- Tuberositas tibiae 7%
- Patellar apex 1%
- Legg-Calvé-Perthes disease 1%
- Tuber ischiadicum 1%
- Epiphysis of the femoral head 4%
- Distal ulnar epiphysis 5%
- Distal radial epiphysis 23%
- Olecranon apophysis 5%
- Elbow joint entirely 6%
- Acromion 2%
- Epiphysis of the humeral head 14%
- Lumbar 10%

- Scheuermann's disease
- juvenile osteochondrosis or
- disorders in the apophyseal structure.

Primary changes of the spine affect the cores of the ventral marginal ridge of the lower thoracic and upper lumbar segments, which can affect one or vertebral bodies. Simmelbauer (1992) found such changes in the thoracic and lumbar spine in 68% of the gymnasts, who had been A, B and C squad members of the DTB from 1977 to 1987. In our studies, we recorded only the clinically symptomatic gymnasts. He sees the **cause** in the **mechanically** induced cartilage ossification by the repetitive "strike-on-the-back" phenomenon. High pressure and shear forces with missing optimal flexibility of the spine, unbalanced muscles, and insufficient compensatory forces can possibly contribute to these changes.

In advanced cases, we often find:

- widening of the vertebral bodies in the sagittal
- insufficient ventral development of the vertebral bodies or
- downright edge defects with formation of wedge-shaped vertebrae.

Lohrer et al. (1996) hold these responsible for the development of the **"gymnast's hump"**.

However, most gymnasts show a more or less distinct round back and wedge-shaped vertebrae are not present in all cases. The majority of so-called "gymnast's humps" could also be caused by a limitation of the thoracic extension, simultaneous contraction of the pectoralis major muscle, and an attenuated the scapular fixations.

According to Lohrer et al. 1996, the initial phase can be diagnosed clinically by the so-called "flexibility test" above the spinous processes of the according motion segments, even before radiological signs are visible. Positive tested gymnasts can be recognized early; training breaks and specific therapeutic exercises can be initiated.

> The flexibility test should be carried out routinely in all juvenile gymnasts.

A definite reduction of overstrain in almost all regions of the body, and particularly in the shoulder joints, could be achieved by a **consequent application of preventive measures** in exercise routine (especially specific strength programs for the shoulder girdle and trunk, muscle stretching and mobilization of joints and spine actively and passively). Nevertheless, this only applies to senior athletes. During the last 2 years, we have observed a large discrepancy between gymnasts of the A/B squad and C or D squad, respectively. Massive functional deficits partly exist in almost all regions of the body, especially in junior athletes. A possible cause can be the inconsequent prevention programs due to lack of time.

70.5 Clinical findings

Since all elements in artistic gymnastics require an extraordinarily high measure of movement technique, optimal physical preconditions are necessary for the correct performance and eventually prevention or reduction of overstrain impairments. **Stretching and strengthening programs** need to be part of the routine training program. Since adaptation of the training program, we find far fewer problems of the supporting and locomotor apparatus in the German federal athletes. However, medical check-ups are still needed.

➢ Table 70.1 shows the most important clinical findings, of which some are specific for artistic gymnastics and present unfavorable factors regarding the development of injuries. The most frequent abnormalities occur in juvenile athletes of the C and D squads, which did not consequently follow the preventive training program.

Contractions of the scapulohumeral musculature and of the pectoralis major muscles are found regularly in many gymnasts. This is accompanied with simultaneous **weakening of the scapular fixations** and limited extension of the thoracic spine. This decreases the mobility of the shoulder joints; a compensatory hypermobility of other spine segments, in particular lumbosacral segments, develops. The imbalance between muscle length (possible motion amplitude) and muscle tonus, i.e. the aspects of the muscle function (strength – endurance – recreation – coordination) are suboptimal and can affect the elementary movements of a joint.

Muscle contractions of the **ischiocrural** and the **iliopsoas muscle** in combination with muscular **dysbalances of the abdominal and deep dorsal muscles** lead to static and dynamic malpositions of the lumbar spine/pelvis with sacroiliac or iliosacral dysdunctions. They cause ascending and descending compensations at the supporting and locomotor apparatus.

Further frequent abnormalities are the splayfoot and the **valgoplanus splayfoot**, which develop as a consequence of the **weak muscles of the foot** or the musculature transcending the ankle joint in combination with high stress and strain of the feet by thousands of vaults and landings.

Limited dorsal mobility of the wrists and hypomobilities of the carpus are common. This often leads to wrist problems particularly in flat stand on the pommel horse.

Betz et al. (1993) have found a similarly high number of muscle contractions of the iliopsoas muscle and the ischiocrural musculature in an examination of muscle functions of the musculature of the trunk and the extremities in 1,866 14-year-old children.

Tab. 70.1 Typical clinical findings (source: own examinations of 75 squad athletes – A, B, C, and D squads – of the years 2004 and 2005).

Clinical findings	Frequency
shortening of the scapulohumeral musculature	95.0%
limitation of TS extension	62.6%
hypermobility of lower LS (L5 > L4)	55.9%
■ contraction of the iliopsoas muscle and/or ischiocrural musculature (juvenile artistic gymnasts, above all)	48.6%
■ splayfoot or valgoplanus splayfoot	48.6%
weak posture (hollow-back)	43.9%
hypomobility of the wrists/carpus	42.6%
weakening of the deep spinal musculature	37.3%
weakening of the scapular fixators	33.3%
hypermobility/instability of the shoulder joints	27.9%
hypermobility/instability of the ankle joints	24.0%

70.6 Profile of athletes and coaches from a medical perspective

An **initial examination** (e.g. X-ray) and yearly check-up of the **supporting and locomotor ap-**

paratus should be carried out with beginning competitive sport. We recommend medical checks from 8 years on. This allows detection of existing or developing problems and medical appropriate recommendation – if needed stop of competitive sport.

Trained coaches – in cooperation with physiotherapists and physicians – are required to guarantee an **optimal motion development** with focus on:

- strength, strength endurance and fitness
- ability to spread and good movement technique
- achieving of movement control in time and space
- development of balance and control of muscle tension.

The all-round **strengthening of the complete trunk muscles** is needed in the daily exercise program. To allow full capacity and physical movement of all spinal segments, **strengthening of all muscles transcending the joints, including the gluteal muscles** is needed.

> Consistent stability and mobility, including optimally stretched muscles, are of significant meaning.

This is particularly important if relatively "pointy" forces, e.g. in the region of the lumbar spine occur in sudden hyperlordosings. These can only be counterbalanced with a **perfect movement technique** and an optimally developed and functioning musculature. A harmonious mobility of the full spine, shoulder and hip joints is necessary.

The **puberal phases** require special attention, because maturation, growth and differentiation of biological systems affect the entire organism. The **maturing bones** are vulnerable in this critical phase; **muscle and ligament insertions** are equally sensitive.

Training must be increased carefully after injuries or training breaks, in order to provide sufficient periods of time for adaptation of the passive supporting apparatus (bones, cartilage, tendons, capsules, ligaments). **Taking training breaks** in time at fatigue and/or overstrain for the prevention of injuries and impairments requires a high attention by the gymnasts. Athletes need to respect natural warning signals of the body; coaches should know the individual physical limits of their athletes.

Maintained **exercise and competition equipment**, especially grips of still rings or parallel bars are the own responsibility of the athlete. They are also responsible for **relaxation baths**, sauna or massages; the coach needs to supervise younger gymnasts to minimize the risk of an injury or impairment.

Apparent minor injuries need immediate attention and need medical supervision. This helps to avoid subsequent impairments (see spinal injuries).

> **Important for the prevention of sport-specific injuries or overstrain impairments:**
> - medical examinations at the start of competitive sports and yearly check-ups
> - physical, technical, coordinative and specific movement formation
> - cooperation of staff qualified in the sport
> - full-body gymnastics, application of the prevention program
> - strain reduction in sensitive puberal phases
> - slow strain setup after injuries or breaks in exercising
> - sufficient warm-up phases in the beginning of exercising and cool-down at the end of exercising
> - taking breaks from exercising in time at fatigue and/or overstrain
> - precaution (well maintained exercise and competition equipment) and relaxation (massages, sauna, hot baths)
> - immediate and specific treatment of minor injuries
> - sufficient compensation and regeneration phases

References

Amadio AC, Baumann W (1990). Kinetics and electromyographical analysis of the triple jump. In: Brüggemann G-P, Rühl IK (eds.). Technics in Athletics. Conference Proceedings Vol. 2. Cologne.

Betz M, Schiffer E, Klimt F (1993). Muskelfunktionsstörungen im Kindesalter. Praktische Sporttraumatologie und Sportmedizin.

Borrmann G (1974). Geräteturnen. Sportverlag, Berlin.

Boschert HP (1992). Ursachen von Veränderungen im Akromioklavikulargelenk bei Kunstturnern. In: Klümper A (ed.). Osteologie und Sporttraumatologie 2. Verlag Johannes Krause, Freiburg.

Boschert, Elsässer, Lohrer (1998). Kunstturnen. In: Klümper A (ed.).Sporttraumatologie. ecomed-Verlag, Landsberg.

Brüggemann GP, Rühl IK (1995). Belastungen und Risiken im Kunstturnen. Zwischenbericht BISp.

Elsässer HP (1997). Besteht ein Zusammenhang zwischen degenerativen Veränderungen der HWS und der Periarthritis humero-scapularis? In: Klümper A (ed.). Osteologie und Sporttraumatologie 6. Verlag Johannes Krause, Freiburg.

Felländer-Tsai L, Wredmark T (1995). Injury incidence and cause in elite gymnasts. Arch Orthop Trauma Surg 114: 344–346.

Fröhner G (1995). Retrospektive Studie ehemaliger Turnerinnen. In: Information/Dokumentation Sport: Begegnung zwischen Theorie und Praxis. Aktuelle Forschungsergebnisse Kunstturnen und Rhythmische Sportgymnastik. IAT, Leipzig.

Gradinger R, Flock K, Träger J, Scheyrer M, Hipp E (1991). Sportfähigkeit bei Spondylolyse und Spondylolisthese. Praktische Sporttraumatologie und Sportmedizin.

Islebe V (1993). Wirbelsäulenveränderungen und -schäden bei Turnern, Turnerinnen und Gymnastinnen des Bundes- und Landeskaders Baden-Württemberg. Magisterarbeit in Sportwissenschaft. Eberhard-Karls-Universität, Tübingen.

Knoll K (1992). Zum biomechanischen Wirkungsmechanismus und Flugelementen aus vorbereitenden Bewegungen und Ableitungen für die Technik von Rondat und Flickflack am Boden. In: Brüggemann GP, Rühl JH (eds.). Biomechanics in Gymnastics. Cologne.

Konermann W, Sell S (1992). Die Wirbelsäule – eine Problemzone im Kunstturnhochleistungssport. Sportverletz Sportschad.

Krug J (1995). Entwicklungsaspekte der Trainingssysteme im Kunstturnen und in der Rhythmischen Sportgymnastik. In: Information/Dokumentation Sport: Begegnung zwischen Theorie und Praxis. Aktuelle Forschungsergebnisse Kunstturnen und Rhythmische Sportgymnastik. IAT, Leipzig.

Lohrer H, Alt W (1997). Kunstturnen. In: Engelhardt M, Hintermann B, Segesser B (eds.). GOTS-Manual Sporttraumatologie. Verlag Hans Huber, Bern.

Maffullin N, Chan D, Aldrige J (1992). Overuse injuries of the olecranon in young gymnasts. J Bone Joint Surg 74-B (2).

Martin D (1985). Die psychomotorische Leistungsfähigkeit von Kindern – Voraussetzung für das Geräteturnen. In: Schwerdter HP (ed.). Sport und Sportmedizin Kunstturnen. Perimed-Verlag, Erlangen.

Müller-Gerbl M, Putz R, Hodapp N, Schulte E, Wimmer B (1989). Computed tomography-osteoabsorptiometry for assessing the density-distribution of suchondral bone as a measure of long-term mechanical adaptation in individual joints. Skel Radiol 18: 507–512.

Müller-Gerbl M, Putz R, Hodapp N, Schulte E, Wimmer B (1990). Die Darstellung der subchondralen Dichtemuster mittels der CT-Osteoabsorptiometrie (CT-OAM) zur Beurteilung der individuellen Gelenkbeanspruchung am Lebenden. Z Orthop 128: 128–133.

Nissinnen M (1992). Kinematische und dynamische Analyse der Riesenfelge an den Ringen. In: Brüggemann GP, Rühl IK (eds.). Biomechanics in Gymnastics. Conference Proceedings. Cologne.

Samuelson M, Reider B, Weiss D (1996). Grip lock injuries to the forearm in male gymnasts. Am J Sports Med 24: 1.

Schierholz U, Liebig K (1980). Spondylolyse bei Kunstturnerinnen. In: Cotta H (ed.), Stein W. Die Belastungstoleranz des Bewegungsapparates. Grundlagenforschung in der Sportmedizin. 3. Heidelberger Orthopädie-Symposium 1979. Thieme Verlag, Stuttgart-New York.

Schweizer L (1992). Unpublished study by the Institute for Sport and Sport Sciences of the University of Freiburg about the anthropologic development of world-class gymnasts.

Simmelbauer B (1992). Knorpelverknöcherungsstörungen der Brust- und Lendenwirbelkörper bei Hochleistungsturnern. In: Klümper A (ed.). Osteologie und Sporttraumatologie 1. Verlag Johannes Krause, Freiburg.

Steinbrück K (1997). Epidemiologie. In: Engelhardt M, Hintermann B, Segesser B (eds.). GOTS-Manual Sporttraumatologie. Verlag Hans Huber, Bern.

Wülker N, Rössig S, Morell M, Thren H (1995). Die dynamische Stabilität des Glenohumeralgelenkes. Eine biomechanische Untersuchung. Sportverletz Sportschad.

Chapter 71 Rhythmic gymnastics

Jens Enneper

Rhythmic gymnastics is a relatively young sport, which has developed in the late 1940s in the former Soviet Union (Lissizkaja et al. 1985). Rhythmic gymnastics have become more and more popular and the first world championship was in Budapest in 1963. It has been part of the **Olympic program** since the Summer Olympic Games in Los Angeles in **1984** (Lissizkaja et al. 1985, Schwabowski et al. 1992).

71.1 Characteristics

Rhythmic gymnastics, which had formerly been called "esthetic gymnastics", is carried out in the gym on a gymnastics surface of 12 × 12 m to music (Lissizkaja et al. 1985, Schwabowski et al. 1992, Lohrer et al. 2002). Diverse exercise elements of **dance, music and acrobatics** (jumping, walking, swinging and circling) are combined with a ball, rope, ribbon, hoop and clubs. These handheld equipments are bounced, rolled, flexed, rotated, thrown and caught. There is a time limit of 60–90 sec for freestyle exercises (Lissizkaja et al. 1985, Schwabowski et al. 1992, Lohrer et al. 2002).

This sport is only carried out by **female athletes**. In addition to the **individual gymnasts**, there is the **team competition** with six athletes. The handheld apparatuses for a group exercise are mixed (e.g. three clubs and three hoops) and can be rotationally exchanged. Groups and individual gymnasts are equally evaluated. 30 points are the maximum. Maximally ten points are awarded for technical precision consideringthe different difficulties. Ten points can be achieved for the esthetic performance, music, choreography, composition of exercise and originality etc., and another ten points for the execution of the complete exercise. Points are deducted respectively for mistakes (Lissizkaja et al. 1985, Lohrer et al. 2002).

71.2 Physical prerequisites

A number of talents are needed for a successful gymnast. The mobility of spine, shoulder, hip and ankle joints, coupled with a very good co-ordination of movements are very important basic prerequisites (Lissizkaja et al. 1985, Schwabowski et al. 1992). In addition, the exercises require musicality, velocity and spatial orientation. Static malpositions (distinct spinal deformation, varus or valgus axis), a disproportionate physique, and overweight are inappropriate (Lissizkaja et al. 1985, Lohrer et al. 2002).

71.3 Preparation for training and competition

The optimal **start age** is between 5 and 7. The first fundamentals are set with 1–2 hours of exercise about twice a week (➤ Tab. 71.1). The **performance training** begins at about eight years with three to five exercise units a week of 2–3 hours each. According to the performance, athletes may switch to **high-performance training** at the age of 12, with a maximum age of 25 years. 3–7 hours of exercising are needed nearly every day, in order to perform the exercises to the point (➤ Tab. 71.2). Specific training for several days is needed to adapt to a new (competition) environment (height, light of

Tab. 71.1 Training contents of rhythmic gymnastics (single and group).

- promotion of mobility and agility
- rhythmic instruction
- posture improvement
- preventive athletics
- complex choreographies

Tab. 71.2 Age and amount of training of rhythmic gymnastics (Lissizkaja et al. 1985, Schwabowski et al. 1992, Lohrer et al. 2002).

	Optimal age (years)	Amount of training (hours)
age of entry/learning	5–7	2–4/week (2 × training)
beginning performance training	8–9	6–15/week (3–5 × training)
maximum performance training	12–25	15–42/week (5–6 × training)

the gym, etc). The exercise areas are switched according to a tight schedule. Important impressions are already conveyed for the actual competition.

71.4 Special orthopedic aspects

Chronic overstrain impairments are common in rhythmic gymnastics whereas acute injuries in training or competition are rare. **Spinal diseases** and conditions of the **lower extremities** are characteristic (Hume et al. 1993, Schneyder et al. 1993, Congeni et al. 1997, Engelhardt et al. 1997, Huchinson 1999, Tanchev et al. 2000, Hasler et al. 2002, Lohrer et al. 2002, Schmitt et al 2002).

For every kind of symptoms, the growth and development of the individual gymnast needs special consideration (Schwabowski et al. 1992).

71.4.1 Spine

Spondylolysis and spondylolisthesis

Spondylolyses of the pars interarticularis and associated slipping of a vetebra (spondylolisthesis) appear in about 5–7% of the normal population (Engelhardt et al. 1997, Renström 1997, Schmitt et al. 2002). This is often observed in rhythmic gymnastics because of the frequent hyperextension and rotation movements. Biomechanical studies conclude that hyperextension movements lead to a high shear strain to the pars interarticularis, which is increased with lateral flexion (Engelhardt et al. 1997, Renström 1997, Schmitt et al. 2002). Therefore, an increased risk of **acquired spondylolysis** exists (Engelhardt et al. 1997, Renström 1997, Schmitt et al. 2002). Mostly, the **lumbar spine** is affected, which starts with an unspecific back pain. Later, radiating conditions can supervene and affect the daily routine.

At the **clinical examination**, paravertebral myogelosis and hyperlordosis posture of the lumbar spine are often detected. If a slipping of vertebral segments has already occurred, overlapping bones in the region of the spinous processes of vertebrae are possible. This applies especially to higher degrees of spine instability (Engelhardt et al. 1997).

Overstrain of the facet joints, ligamentoses and beginning ostoechondroses need consideration (Schmitt et al. 2002).

X-ray of the lumbar spine in two layers is usually sufficient for initial diagnosis. If a spondylolysis is suspected, transverse X-rays or MRT are needed. The spondylolisthesis can be differentiated into four degrees according to Meyerding (Niethard et al. 1997). A complete slipping is called spondyloptosis.

The **sport capability** derives from the following criteria (Engelhardt et al. 1997, Schmitt et al. 2002):

- lysis (uni- or bilateral) of the pars interarticularis without clinical symptoms:
  - semiannual check-up (clinical and radiological)
  - no sport restriction, but increased attention in exercising (cave: hyperextension and rotation)
- spondylolisthesis (<50%) asymptomatic:
  - moderate sport restriction
  - additional conservative therapeutic measures
  - exercises for the stabilization of the trunk

- spondylolisthesis (>50%):
  - limited athletic capacity
  - conservative and also surgical therapeutic measures, if necessary
  - no competitive sport.

71.4.2 Hip

The hip joints are subject to specific demands in rhythmic gymnastics (Lissizkaja et al. 1985, Schwabowski et al. 1992). The loosened capsule-ligament apparatus allows a massive over-flexibility of the hip joints. A standing or vaulting oversplit on the floor is only possible only because of this over-flexibility. **Soft-tissue injuries** (musculotendinous overstrain, soft groin, hernias etc.) are often found at the hip joint. The **hip joint dysplasia** presents a sports contraindication (Lohrer et al. 2002), because relapsing conditions are frequent and the demands of training and competition cannot be fulfilled anymore. Another clinical picture typical for gymnasts is the **lesion of the acetabular labrum** (Lohrer et al. 2002). Impaction symptoms can be caused by a hypermobility of the labrum. The gymnast describes a sudden limitation of movement, which can be associated by a piercing inguinal pain. In exceptional cases, the acetabular labrum can be injured massively. Stress reactions of the femoral neck and the epiphysiolyses can also be observed in rare cases.

71.4.3 Shank and ankle

The exercises of modern rhythmic gymnastics strain the lower extremity, in particular the lower leg and ankle joints. **Periosteal irritations of the tibia**, functional **compartment syndromes**, **tendovaginitides** of the Achilles tendon and the hallucis longus tendon are found during intensive exercise phases (Lohrer et al. 2002).

Ankle joint conditions in gymnasts can be acute and chronic. The hypermobility of the joint can lead to **arthritides** and **cartilaginous abrasions** or **supination traumas**.

71.4.4 Feet

The feet are massively strained in rhythmic gymnastics, because most exercises are performed on the forefoot. Osseous stress reactions or even **stress fractures** might appear in the region of the midfoot bone V and the os naviculare. Typical late consequences can be cartilage impairments at the metatarsophalangeal joint of the hallux, which can develop to the full clinical picture of the hallux rigidus (Lohrer et al. 2002).

71.4.5 Bones

Many gymnasts are still in the phase of growth. This can be associated to typical conditions in the area of the **epiphyseal plate** (Niethard et al. 1997). Those are mostly minor conditions, which can be reduced by adjusting training strain. **Aseptic bone necroses** occur less often. Florid bone necroses present an absolute contraindication for the performance of rhythmic gymnastics (➤ Tab. 71.3). In addition to an insertion tendinopathy, apophysitis calcanei should be taken into account in differential diagnosis of the heel.

Tab. 71.3 Absolute contraindications for rhythmic gymnastics.

Absolute contra indication	Relative contra indications
florid aseptic necroses	ship joint dysplasia
acute general diseases	light cartilage damages
acute trauma	static abnormalities

References

Congeni J et al. (1997). Lumbar spondylolysis. A study of natural progression in athletes. Am J Sports Med 25: 248–253.

Engelhardt M et al. (1997). Spondylolyse und Spondylolisthese im Sport. Orthopäde 26: 755–759.

Hasler C et al. (2002). Spondylolysis and spondylolisthesis during growth. Orthopäde 31: 78–87.

Huchinson MR (1999). Low back pain in elite rhythmic gymnasts. Med Sci Sports Exerc 31(11): 1686–1688.

Hume PA et al. (1993). Predictors of attainment in rhythmic sportive gymnastics. J Sports Med Phys Fitness 33(4): 367–377.

Lissizkaja TS et al. (1985). Rhythmische Sportgymnastik. Sportverlag, Berlin.

Lohrer H et al. (2002). Rhythmische Sportgymnastik; Sportärztliche Untersuchung und Beratung. 3rd edition. Spitta-Verlag, Balingen, pp. 250–251.

Niethard FR et al. (1997). Kinderorthopädie. Thieme-Verlag, Stuttgart.

Renström PAFH (1997). Sportverletzungen und Sportschaden. Deutscher Ärzteverlag, Cologne.

Schmitt H et al. (2002). Sportliche Belastungsfähigkeit bei orthopädischen Deformitäten der Wirbelsäule im Kindesalter. Dt Z Sportmed 53(1): 6–10.

Schneyder J et al. (1993). Correlation between intensive sports activity in athletes. Ped Ex Science 5: 467.

Schwabowski R et al. (1992). Rhythmische Sportgymnastik. Meyer & Meyer Verlag, Aachen.

Tanchev PI et al. (2000). Scoliosis in rhythmic gymnastics. Spine 25(11): 1367–1372.

Chapter 72 Dance

Christoph Raschka

Dancing is a technical-compositional sport. In contrast to ballet or aerobics, only few scientific studies focus on dance. The German dance sport federation (Deutscher Tanzsportverband e.V.) coaches the disciplines of Standard and Latin dancing as individual couples and formation (8 couples) dance. Wheelchair dance represents a specialty, in which a person in a wheelchair and a "walker" dance together.

The **standard dances** are slow waltz (three-quarter time, length of 90–120 sec, 30 measures/min), the tango (two-quarter time, length of 90–120 sec, 33 measures/min), Viennese waltz (three-quarter time, length of 60–90 sec, 60 measures/min), slow foxtrot (four-quarter time, length of 90–120 sec, 30 measures/min) and quickstep (four-quarter time, length of 90–120 sec, 52 measures/min). They all have the close dance positions in common. The partners hold each other in their arms, which implies excessive strain to shoulders and arms. In contrast to this, Latin dances are performed in an open posture with the men leading the women mostly with just one hand, or the dance is performed without body contact.

The **Latin dances** are samba (two-quarter or four-quarter time, length of 90–120 sec, 53 measures/min), cha-cha-cha (four-quarter time, length of 90–120 sec, 32 measures/min), rumba (four-quarter time, length of 90–120 sec, 28 measures/min), paso doble (two-quarter time, length of 90–120 sec, 62 measures/min) and the jive (four-quarter time, length of 60–90 sec, 44 measures/min).

The first world championship in dancing had been carried out in 1909 in Paris; the first German championship had occurred in 1919, and the first European championship in 1927. Since 1964, there have been German formation championships, and world championships in formation dance since 1973.

Other dance types are jazz and modern dance, which are usually danced barefooted, tap-dance, boogie-woogie and rock 'n' roll as well as guard dance.

According to Burger and Hesemann-Burger (2002), a reduced joint mobility (e.g. ankyloses, contractures), overweight, missing basic endurance, but also unharmonious body proportions are performance limiting. Dancers have bodies of a distinctly harmonious shape (Raschka 2006). Partners should have equal physiques, harmony, and musicality. Optimal age of entry is the age of 9 to 11 years (Burger and Hesemann-Burger 2002). Performance training, 2–3 hours 3–5 times/week, should not be started before the age of 13. The period between 19 and 25 years is the age of highest performance for the standard dances; 18 and 24 for Latin dances.

72.1 Energy consumption and cardiovascular strain

According to Léger (1982), the average use of energy during a 90-minute night of disco dancing (twist, disco fox and others) amounts to approximately 4,350 kJ in men and 2,850 kJ in women and thus is twice as high as foxtrot or waltz. The gender difference is conditioned by the higher body weight of men. Regarding the intensity, it can be compared to running or cross-country skiing with speeds of 8 or 9 km/h, to swimming with 2.5–3 km/h or cycling with 20–25 km/h.

> Regarding the intensity of exercise, a night of dancing can be compared to common endurance sports.

Dancing to different musical rhythms does not induce change performance. Paradoxically, Léger (1982) has even found higher heart rates in slower music. The pulse reaches 135 beats/min on average (72% of the maximum heart rate).

Blanksby and Reidy (1988) have determined a medium energy consumption of athletes performing Latin dance of an amount of 36.1 kJ/min (women) and 54.0 kJ/min (men). In comparison, a male dancer of modern dance requires 54.1 kJ/min; a female dancer of modern dance will need 34.7 kJ/min. According to Blanksby and Reidy (1988), male and female Latin dancers will reach maximum heart rates of 168 and 177 beats/min; in modern dance, on the other hand, they will reach 170 and 173 beats/min. According to Böhmer and Ambrus (1981), the heart rates in competition ballroom dance amount to 160–180 beats/min with peaks of more than 190, with the pulse rate of women being higher than the one of men. The strain intensity in competitively performed Latin dances amounts to more than 80% of the maximum oxygen absorption for both genders (Blanksby and Reidy 1988).

According to Oldörp (1992), the aerobic capacity of top-class competition ballroom dancers amounts to values in the range of 50 to 60 ml/kg/min.

In addition, Rohleder et al. (2007) have documented increases of the cortisol levels during stressful competitions of ballroom dance, which had been independent of the physical strain.

72.2 Injuries

According to Horn (1977), dancing is at the 26th place in the spectrum of sport-accident frequencies with an incidence rate of 0.11 accidents in 100 athletes each year.

> The accident rate in dancing is low and amounts to 0.11 accidents in 100 athletes per year.

78 dancers of the (top) C to S classes in the dancing types of Latin, standard, formation and ten dance had injuries at knee joints (16%), femur (14%), feet (13%), ankle joints (11%) and lower legs (10%) (Strauß and von Salis-Soglio 1997). According to Steinbrück and Cotta (1983), the ankle joint had even been affected in 27% of the cases.

> The lower extremity is affected in 66% of cases.

Contusions prevail with 34%, followed by pulled muscles (16%) and sprains of the ankle joints (11%). Serious injuries such as internal meniscus lesions (5%), patellar dislocations (3%), shoulder dislocations, ruptures of the anterior cruciate ligaments, coccygeal fractures, finger or rib fractures are much less frequent (Strauß and von Salis-Soglio 1997).

Interestingly, the amount of distal radius fractures caused by dance accidents (n = 225) has been relatively high with 8.9% in a Scottish clinic in Edinburgh, but no further details are given (➤ Fig. 72.1; Lawson et al. 1995).

Considering **injury mechanism**, Wirth (2002) found that adolescent dancers often cannot sufficiently control the movement of their arms and thus collide more often with obstacles (usually the bodies of other dancers), which can lead to carpal sprains and subluxations. According to Strauß and von Salis-Soglio (1997), collision with other dancers dominate in general, followed by slipping on the dance floor, as well as overcrossing of the feet; Latin dancers are affected more often than standard dancers.

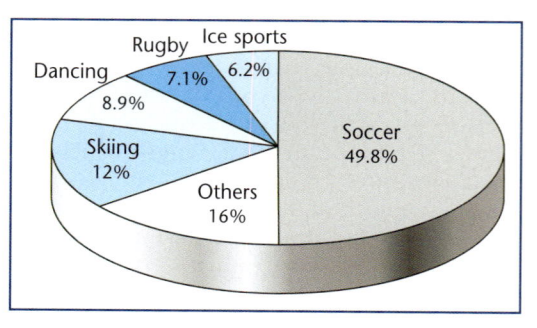

Fig. 72.1 Relative spreading of the distal radius fractures (n = 225) to the affected sports in a Scottish clinic (Lawson et al. 1995).

> The most frequent injury mechanism is the collision with another dancer.

According to Burger and Hesemann-Burger (2002), the knowledge of functional bandages for ankle and knee joints is essential for the attending sport physician.

72.3 Overstrain impairments

According to Wirth (2002), consequences of overstrain and improper strain, such as blockades of the small vertebral, costotransversal and iliosacral joints, but also myogeloses and myoscleroses of the shoulder musculature as well as tendinoses and peritendinoses of the shoulder region dominate in comparison to acute traumas.

Overstrain and improper strain are much more common than acute injuries.

Burger and Hesemann-Burger (2002) have highlighted the inconvenient long breaks during tournaments, in which the athletes are often wearing their sweaty and scarcely air-permeable clothes. They recommend a change of clothes during the breaks as a measure of prevention.

Muscle cramps often occur in longer competitions because of mineral loss by sweating (Böhmer and Ambrus 1981).

Wirth (2002) and Burger and Hesemann-Burger (2002) have described capsule and tendon irritations (rarely coxitis) in the region of the hip, patellar chondropathies, patellar apex and patellar tendon syndromes, capsule dilations and meniscus impairments at the knee joint and the tibial edge syndrome at the lower leg. Sprains of the ankle joints in competitive dancers had not appeared more often than in other sports despite the high heels of the women's shoes. Medical conditions occurred more frequently because of splayfeet, hallux valgus, tyloses at the feet as well as irritations of the plantar aponeurosis. Burger and Hesemann-Burger (2002) emphasize here the effect of frequent torsion movements in the foot, knee and hip joints.

Kukowski (1993) presents a case history of a 25-year-old semi-professional Latin dancer who had suffered a distal impairment of the suprascapular nerve due to the repetitive arm movements with rotation and abduction.

> Overstrain impairments in dancing affect primarily the feet (shoes!) as well as the lower and upper segments of the spine (torsion movements).

High and partially pointed heels of the women change body posture, with the pelvis tilting forwards and artificial lumbolordosis (Burger and Hesemann-Burger 2002). According to Wirth (2002), extreme hyperlordoses of the lumbar spine are typical in Latin dancers.

Tsung and Mulford (1998) have traced back the radiculopathy in the segments C7 of a female standard dancer to the frequent hyperextensions and lateral rotations of the cervical spine in the movements of the neck in dancing.

Strauß and von Salis-Soglio (1997) name splayfeet (13%), increased plantar tyloses in the region of the forefoot (11%), hyperlordoses of the lumbar spine (7%) as well as hardenings of the dorsal extensor muscles and patellar symptoms (7% each) as the most frequent findings. Böhmer and Ambrus (1981) have pointed out the specific strain of the complete ankle joint as well as Chopart's joint line, if additional foot malformations are present. Burger and Hesemann-Burger (2002) recommend wearing of special dancing shoes with adhesive, roughened soles for exercising and competition, and Böhmer and Ambrus (1981) advise a frequent changing of the shoes with high and low heels during the course of a day.

References

Böhmer D, Ambrus AP (1981). Tanzsport. In: Pförringer W, Rosemeyer B, Bär HW (eds.). Sporttraumatologie – Sportartentypische Schäden und Verletzungen. Diagnostik – Therapie – Prävention. Vol. 15. Perimed Fachbuch Verlag, Erlangen, pp. 356–358.

Blanksby BA, Reidy PW (1988). Heart rate and estimated energy expenditure during ballroom dancing. Brit J Sports Med 22: 57–60.

Burger HJ, Hesemann-Burger U (2002). Tanzsport. In: Clasing D, Siegfried I (eds.). Sportärztliche

Untersuchung und Beratung. Spitta Verlag, Balingen, pp. 252–254.

Horn W (1977). Unfallhäufigkeit und Ursachen im Vereinssport. In: Clauss A (ed.). Unfallursachen und Unfallverhütung im Sport: Infektionen und sportliche Belastung. Beiträge zur Sportmedizin, vol. 7. Perimed Fachverlag, Erlangen, pp. 50–51.

Kukowski B (1993). Suprascapular nerve lesion as an occupational neuropathy in a semiprofessional dancer. Arch Phys Med Rehabil 74: 768–769.

Lawson GM, Hajducka C, McQueen MM (1995). Sport fractures of the distal radius – epidemiology and outcome. Injury 26: 33–36.

Léger LA (1982). Energy cost of disco dancing. Res Q Exerc Sport 53: 46–49.

Oldörp Th (1992). Tanzen – gesunder Breitensport mit Hochleistungsspitzen. TW Sport und Medizin 4: 425–429.

Raschka C (2006). Sportanthropologie. Sportverlag Strauß, Cologne.

Rohleder N, Beulen SE, Chen E, Wolf JM, Kirschbaum C (2007). Stress on the dance floor: the cortisol stress response to social-evaluative threat in competitive ballroom dancers. Pers Soc Psychol Bull 33(1): 69–84.

Steinbrück K, Cotta H (1983). Epidemiologie von Sportverletzungen. Dt Z Sportmed 6: 174–186.

Strauß B, von Salis-Soglio G (1997). Sportverletzungen und Sportschäden im Tanzsport. Sportorthopädie Sporttraumatologie 13(3): 173–176.

Tsung PA, Mulford GJ (1998). Ballroom dancing and cervical radiculopathy: a case report. Arch Phys Med Rehabil 79(10): 1306–1308.

Wirth T (2002). Tanzsport. In: Klümper (ed.). Sporttraumatologie. II-59: 1–7. Ecomed, Landsberg.

Chapter 73 High diving

Sabine Krüger

The history of high diving can be traced back to **antiquity**. The art of swimming and high diving has been perfected later by the Salters of Halle/Saale, Germany, who inevitably had been connected to the water. Generally, these jumps had been performed in order to show courage (Priewe 1962). The first **German championship** of diving was carried out in **1886**.

73.1 The sport

High diving belongs to the technical-compositional sports and is divided into springboard diving and platform diving. In **springboard diving**, the jumps are carried out from a **flexible springboard**, which is affixed by its back-end and rests on an adjustable roller. In competition the athletes jump from heights of 1 m and 3 m. In contrast, the **platform diving** jumps are performed from a **stable platform**, which will be at least 6 m long and 1–2 m wide; a width of 3–3.20 m is required for synchronized diving. In the group of grown-ups, the athletes usually jump from the 10-m platform.

There are **dry-land diving facilities** (boards, platforms), which end in foam pits, and trampoline facilities with lunge systems, acrobatic tracks or strength equipment for the optimal preparation of the dives. Girls/women and boys/men always dive separately. Since 1995, there have also been competitions for **paired synchronized diving**, which are also divided into fancy diving and platform diving.

73.2 Sport-specific risks

Specific **consequences of improper strain or injuries** can appear because of the structure of the sport and the fact that sport-specific exercising usually start at early age and the growing organism have to compensate high physical demands in phases of relatively low capacity. The causes are found directly in the process of exercising and/or the shape of the biological systems and functions of the active athlete (Strauzenberg et al. 1990). Etiologically, there is the distinction of subjective and objective causes of injuries.

Objective causes of injuries are:

- unavoidable accumulation of vertically operating forces
- sport-specific movements in clear space with the available amount of time being predefined by take-off
- sudden increase of the resistance by 850 times at the change of the surrounding medium (air or water, respectively) due to the plunge
- deficiencies of the sites of exercise
- deficiencies in the organization of loads in exercise and competition (qualification often taking hours and long breaks).

Subjective causes of injuries are:
- condition of central-neural fatigue
- indiscipline
- disturbed movement pattern of a learnt element (e.g. by fear)
- unfocused approach of simple movements
- insufficient warm-up

- inappropriate preconditions of the supporting and locomotor systems for the movement structures
- high rate of micro-traumas, because every failed attempt will lead to shear forces appearing at the spine at the plunge
- high psycho-neuronal demands.

The mental dealing with the demands of exercise or competition requires mental performance-enhancing or confining characteristics. This should not be underestimated as a risk factor for injuries and improper strain. In addition, indirect **consequences of injuries and improper strain** can further develop depending on previously impaired tissue or endogenously conditioned causes (Strauzenberg et al. 1990).

The latter ones are, for example:

- wrong posture or positional errors of extremities or trunk
- phases of accelerated growth
- retardation of fitness development
- distinctly strong hypermobility
- exercising at the condition of fatigue.

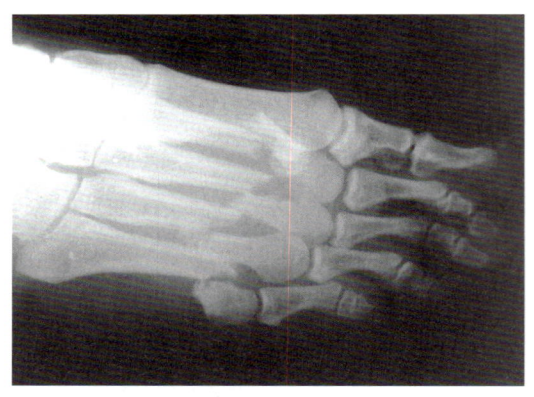

Fig. 73.1 Fractures of the metatarsalia II-V with dislocation after incorrect board reception of a 19-year-old diver.

73.3 Most frequent injuries and consequences of improper loads

Traumas of head or body after collisions with the board or the platform are common (Arndt 1992). Lacerations and less often craniocerebral traumas of a higher degree have been reported. Contusions, bruises or fractures in the region of **midfoot and hand** result from impact on board or the platform (➤ Fig. 73.1).

Bruises/contusions of the **trunk and the extremities** result from unsuccessful attempts by striking the water with the body. This is independent of diving height. In addition, **shoulder dislocations** (dives starting with a handstand or unsuccessful plunges) occur occasionally in platform diving. Sprains and **ligament ruptures** in the region of **knee and ankle joints** are rather found in **springboard divers** or as a consequence of traumas in dry-land exercises (e.g. acrobatic exercises). Typical injuries are shown in ➤ Fig. 73.2.

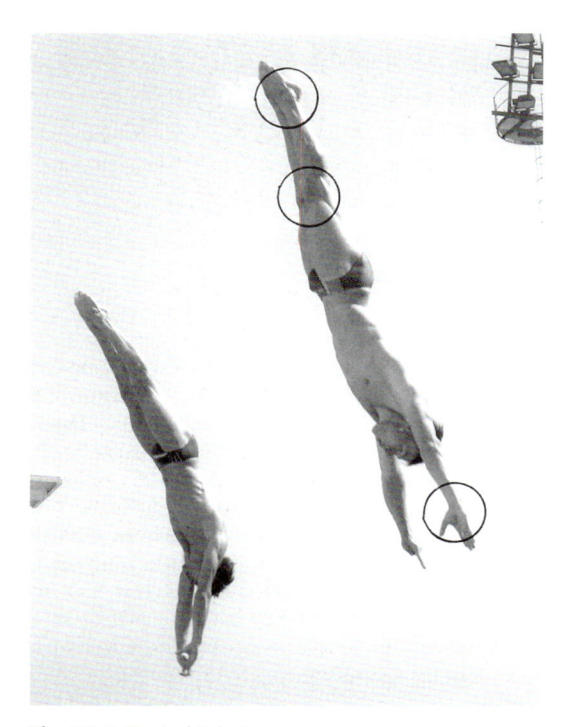

Fig. 73.2 Typical injuries.

> Lesions of hands and feet, including knee and ankle joints belong to the most frequent injuries in diving. Spinal injuries are rare and rather appear in the recreational diving.

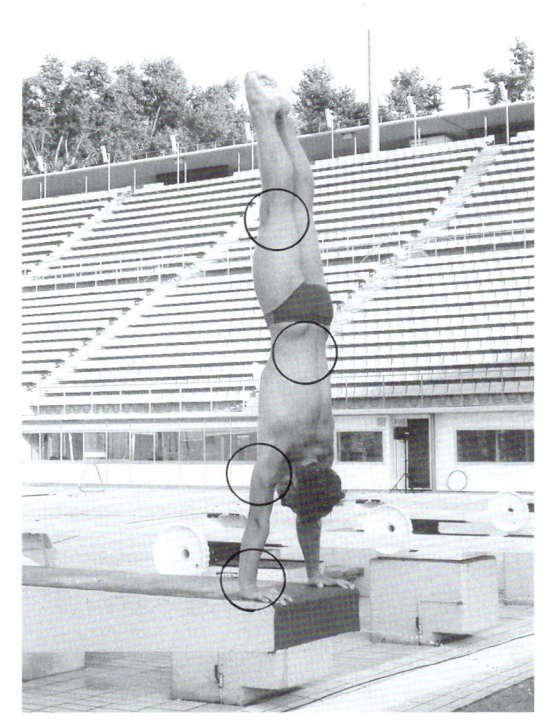

Fig. 73.3 Typical consequences of improper strain.

Improper strain (➤ Fig. 73.3) also develops in high diving by an imbalance of strain and capacity. The problem of the sport is the complex psychophysical strain, which has to be processed in the different functional circles of the organism. **Inadequate exercise conditions** as well as too much exercising (**overtraining**) in addition to athletic failures will often lead to **overstrain impairments** of the locomotor apparatus and to **functional disorders** in the area of psychosomatic and psycho-vegetative processes (Geiger 1991).

Improper strain leads to:

- impairments of the retro patellar cartilage
- chronic irritations of the tendon sheaths of the extensor pollicis longus muscle
- teno-osseous insertion pain of the extensor carpi radialis longus and brevis muscles and
- instabilities in the area of the saddle joint of the thumb even up to arthrosis.

Because of the strain structure of the sport, we also often find:

- subacromial impingement syndromes as well as
- **insertion tendinoses** of the supraspinatus and infraspinatus muscles and the pectoralis major muscle.

Relapsing functional disorders in the region of the **cervicothoracic junction**, the first rib and the thoracic spine are often involved causatively. Impairments by improper strain can also develop in the area of the lumbar spine, which is subjected to high axial pressure and **hyperlordosings** during plunging. Based on this, instabilities and – depending on duration and intensity of the disorders – also early **degenerative adaptations** (e.g. also in the area of the intervertebral disks) can be caused by frequent functional disorders. Appearing or deteriorating **aseptic necroses** (e.g. Scheuermann's disease) need to be considered at an existing predisposition in high diving (Schmidt 1988).

> Typical consequences of improper strain appear in the regions of the shoulder, hand and knee joints as well as in the area of the lumbar spine.

73.4 Diagnostics and therapy

The diagnosis of **acute injuries** usually does not present any problems as witnesses are mostly found at the site of the accident (physician or coach). Further diagnosis and therapy will of course is carried out according to the general standards. The knowledge of the sport-specifics is essential for the diagnosis of **impairments by improper strain**. Primarily, the technical demands of the sport need to be considered for therapeutic considerations. A comprehensive knowledge of the biological subsystems and their reactions to strain is as necessary as the knowledge of individual biological properties (Strauzenberg et al. 1990), in order to be able to induce specific measures.

The diving behavior of the athlete plays a significant role in the assessment of **improper strain in the region of the wrists**. Different hand positions and thus postures in the wrist are practiced depending on the body structure to achieve a plunge creating as little splash as possible. They range from hyperextension with or without gripping of the thumb and opened fingers to maximum volar flexion and fist clenching (Krüger 2000). Most problems develop by hyperextension with gripping of the thumb. Especially the knowledge of the diving technique of the respective athlete is of decisive importance in the assessment of consequences of improper strain in the area of the wrist.

In general, therapy is often **conservative** and adaptation of the sport-specific technique and an optimization of the prophylactic measures is required. Individually customized ortheses for the reduction of strain effects in exercising and competition have been of value. Surgical measures result from the kind of injury or overstrain impairment.

References

Arndt K-H (1992). Sportmedizinische Betreuung bei Sportveranstaltungen. Johann Ambrosius Barth, Leipzig.

Geiger L (1991). Überlastungsschäden im Sport. Vieweg, Bad Feilnbach-Braunschweig.

Krüger S (2000). Wasserspringen. In: Klümper A (ed.). Sporttraumatologie. Ecomed-Verlagsgesellschaft, Landsberg/Lech.

Priewe K-H (1962). Zur Vor- und Entwicklungsgeschichte des internationalen Kunst- und Turmspringens. Staatsexamensarbeit der Philosophischen Fakultät der Universität Rostock

Schmidt H (1988). Orthopödische Grundlagen für sportliches Übern und Trainieren. Johann Ambrosius Barth, Leipzig.

Strauzenberg SE, Gürtler H, Hannemann D, Tittel K (1990). Sportmedizin. Johann Ambrosius Barth, Leipzig.

Chapter 74 Inline skating

Jörg Jerosch and Cornelius Heck

Conventional roller skates have been known for more than 200 years but only the **market introduction of inline skates in 1980** has revolutionized skating on rolls. Inline skating receives has reached such a **popularity** based on the combination of physical exercise and a fast way of transport with affordably priced equipment. In contrast to most other trend sports such as skateboarding or wakeboarding, inline skating attracts people of all ages. Although teenagers still share the highest percentage (77%), every fourth inline skater is adult (Hoffmann and Tambotino 1996. Speed skating, skater hockey or aggressive skating arose recently and come with a higher risk of accidents (Anderson and Kirkpatrick 2002, ➢ Fig. 74.1).

74.1 Equipment

Inline skating accidents are preventable **technically flawless equipment**. The quality of the skates need to match own skating abilities and should meet international **technical inspection agency** standards.

German consumer safety groups (Stiftung Warentest) surveyed inline skates for pricing, performance, handling and stability. Acceptable inline skates are already available for as little as 50 Euros, with professional skates reaching 8 to 10 times as much.

Boot stability is equally important. Tight but comfortable fit reduce sprains in the upper ankle joint. In addition, functional **stoppers** at the heel of the skates, which allow breaking, are critical for safety (➢ Fig. 74.2).

Also the ball bearings will have to be adapted to the individual capabilities. Beginners can mostly be satisfied with **ABEC** (**A**nnular **B**earing **E**ngineers **C**ommittee)-3 ball bearings, while at least ABEC-5 ball bearings should be used by advanced skaters with higher demands to their sport equipment. Today's professional inline skates have ABEC-9 ball bearings with optimal rolling characteristics that will allow extremely high speeds (➢ Fig. 74.3).

The appropriate choice of **protective clothes** is probably the most important piece of equipment for the prophylaxis of inline-skating accidents. Basically, the wearing of long pants and shirts is recommended in order to reduce abrasion caused by falls due to covering the endan-

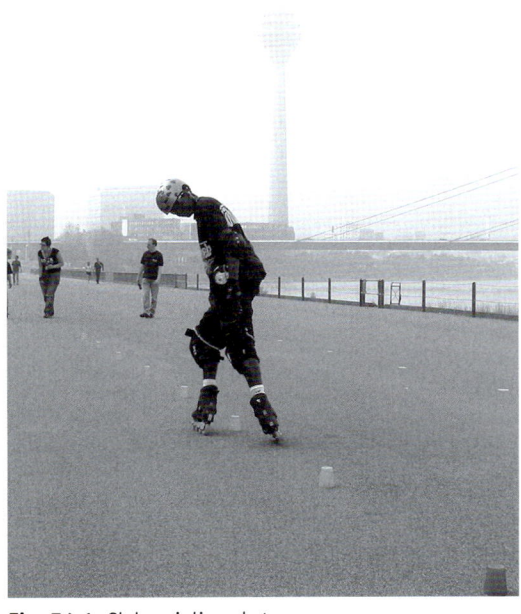

Fig. 74.1 Slalom inline skater.

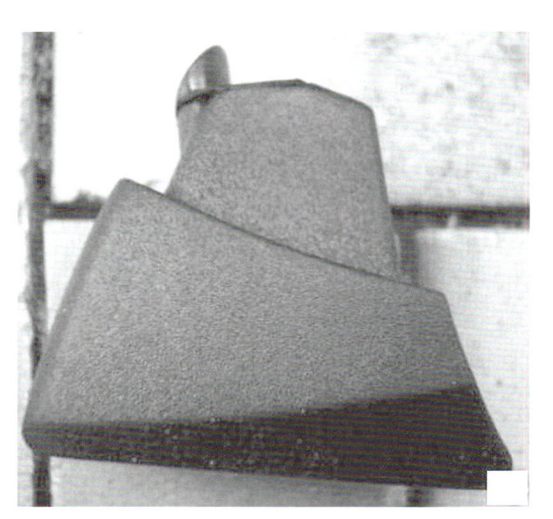

Fig. 74.2 Stopper of inline skates.

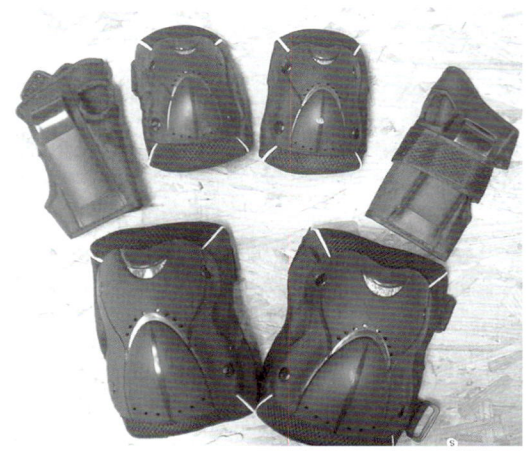

Fig. 74.4 Protective equipment for inline skating.

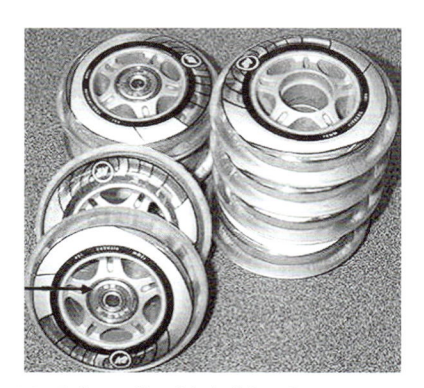

Fig. 74.3 Inline rolls with ball bearings.

gered skin parts. But the **protective equipment** especially developed for inline skaters is still more important, because of the specific protection of the endangered joints. **Protectors** for the wrists, elbows, knees and the head are available, which can also cover additional parts, depending on the manufacturer, e.g. knee protectors with integrated shin guards for players of roller hockey (➢ Fig. 74.4). Prices vary from 30 Euros for beginner kits (wrist, elbow, knee) to 250 Euros for complete protective equipment for skater hockey.

The wearing of all available protectors is recommended for safe inline skating, including a **protective helmet**. The wearing of helmets has been mandatory in some countries already; recreational skaters in Germany are only seen rarely wearing this piece of protective equipment (Jerosch et al. 1998). The wearing of head protection has been mandatory only for inline-specific sports yet (➢ Fig. 74.5).

Wrist protectors are especially important for the prevention of injuries with sudden extreme hyperextension in the wrist joint. They will additionally dampen the impact and will reduce local burns of the skin in fall-conditioned sliding by the integrated volar plates, which are mostly made of plastic or metal. Helmets, elbow protectors and knee protectors are recommended for **shock resorption** in the case of falls.

74.2 Injuries

The common opinion of inline skating not only having bio-positive effects on the cardiovascular system, but also leading to an increased joint strain could be refuted in a study. The strain in **knee and hip joint** at different ground conditions had been observed and compared to other sports in this survey. It has shown that only a minor acceleration and strain to the joint have been recorded for inline skating in contrast to sports as skiing or gymnastics (Jerosch et al. 1998).

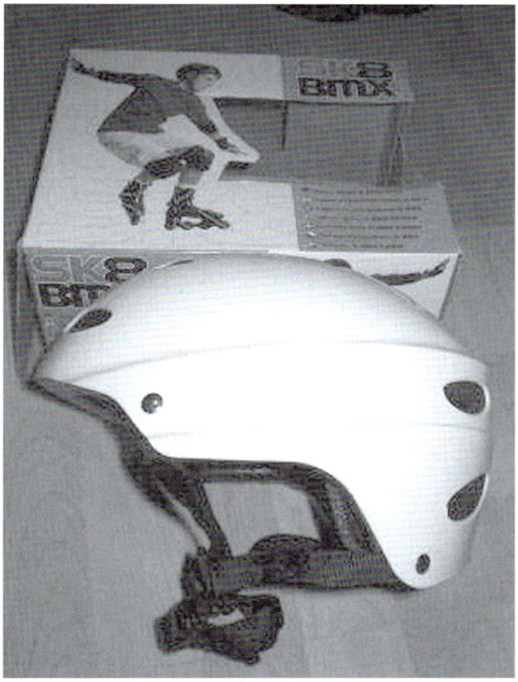

74.2 Injuries

Fig. 74.5 Protective helmet for inline skaters.

Tab. 74.1 Types of injury in inline skating (CHIRPP 1998).

Type of injury	Frequency in %
fractures	47.6
superficial abrasions	19.6
sprains	15.8
open wounds	7.7
smaller head injuries	3.3
joint dislocations	1.4
tooth injuries	1.1
nerve and muscle injuries	1.0
cerebral concussion	0.6
intracranial injuries	0.3
internal injuries	0.2
contusions	0.1
other injuries	0.5
no injuries detected	0.7

Tab. 74.2 Most frequent fractures in inline skating (CHIRPP 1998).

Localization	Numbers in %
distal radius	45
carpus	23
finger	9
metacarpus	4
lower leg	4
elbow	4
ankle joint	3
humerus	2
clavicula	2
face/head	1
foot/toes	1
hip/groin/knee	1
spine	0

A distal radius fracture is by far the most frequent fracture in inline-skating accidents.

Another survey has shown that the **values of foot pressure** measured during skating are comparable to the ones in regular walking and lie clearly below the ones of running. That implies that no severe overstrain impairments are to be expected from the view of plantar strain of anatomical structures in the region of the foot in inline skating (Eils and Jerosch 2000).

Regarding the injuries caused by falls, inline skating is considered one of the most dangerous sports. The spread of injuries in inline skating has been investigated in several studies. The upper extremity, especially in the region of the distal forearm and the wrist, is the part of the body endangered most. The frequency of fractures lies between 25 and 57% (Young et al. 1996, Jerusch et al. 1998, Hilgert et al. 2004, Kassel-Inline-Club).

Based on further surveys in Canada, it has been found that nearly every second person had suffered a distal radius fracture, followed by carpal fractures (23%), finger fractures (9%) and metacarpal fractures (4%); ➢ Tab. 74.1 and ➢ Tab. 74.2; CHIRPP).

Tab. 74.3 Studies about the use of protective equipment at inline skating.

Study	Design	Duration	Number	Used equipment (%)				
				Helmet	Knee	Elbow	Wrist	None
Calle and Eaton (1993)	■ injured persons ■ retrospective	6 months	501	–	–	–	20	80
Ellis et al. (1995)	■ injured persons ■ pediatric ■ prospective	2.33 years	194	2.1	–	–	–	88.0
CHIRPP	■ injured persons ■ time of injury ■ prospective	15 months	121	18.6	38.1	28.0	44.9	45.8
CHIRPP	■ injured persons ■ normally used equipment ■ prospective	15 months	121	28.0	48.3	33.9	54.2	30.5
Jacques and Grzesiak (1994)	pure observation	1 day	89	9.0	41.6	27.0	65.2	–
Schieber and Branch-Dorsey (1995)	■ case control ■ injured persons ■ retrospective	19 months	161	20.0	45.0	28.0	33.0	46.0
Young and Mark (1995)	■ unsuspicious ■ observation	3 months	1.5	2.6	30.0	15.1	64.5	31.7
Young et al. (1996)	■ survey ■ retrospective		134	8.0	34.0	21.0	52.0	–

Type and extent of injuries in inline skating depend on different factors. Some can be influenced by the skater him- or herself (insufficient skating skills, inappropriate equipment), others are conditioned by outside circumstances (wet track, dense traffic). The main reason for the high number of inline skating injuries seems to be the neglected wearing of protective equipment, especially of the wrist protectors (➤ Tab. 74.3). It has become obvious that the abandonment of wrist protectors increases the injury risk by the 10.4-fold, while the not-wearing of elbow protectors increases the risk of an elbow injury by the 9.5-fold (Accident Research Center 2003).

In recent years, the willingness to wear protectors has increased only gradually (Young and Mark 1995). The wearing of protectors can reduce the accident consequences, but it cannot preclude them completely. Some injury patterns – such as forearm fractures above the wrist guard – are even conditioned by the build of the protective gear (Eingartner et al. 1997).

The causes for the abandonment of protective clothes have been surveyed by Young et al., who have found out that 42% of the surveyed persons had considered the wearing uncomfortable, 34% had not regarded it necessary, another 22% have admitted that they had neglected it for optical reasons and the protective clothes had just been too expensive for 15% of the skaters (Young et al. 1996).

> The abandonment of wrist protectors increases the injury risk in inline skating by the 10-fold.

References

Accident Research Center: Facts on fall injury among skaters, Jan. 2003 (www.monash.edu.au/muarc/VISAR/falls/skatfact.pdf).

Anderson G, Kirkpatrick MA (2002). Variable effects of a behavioral treatment package on the performance of inline roller speed skaters. J Appl Behav Arial 35(2): 195–198.

Callé SC, Eaton RG (1993). Wheels-inline roller skating injuries. J Traum 35: 946–951.

CHIRPP (Canadian Hospitals Injury and Prevention Program): www.phac-aspc.gc.ca/injurybles/chirpp/injreprapbles/inline_e.html

Eils E, Jerosch J (2000). Plantare Druckverteilung beim Inline-Skating auf Geraden. Sportverl Sportschad 14: 134–138.

Eingartner C, Jockheck M, Krackhardt T, Weise K (1997). Verletzungen beim Inline-Skating. Sportverl Sportschad 11: 48–51.

Ellis JA, Kierulf JC, Klassen TP (1995). Injuries associated with inline-skating from Canadian hospital reporting and prevention program database. Can J Public Health 86(2): 13–136.

Hilgert RE, Besch L, Behnke B, Egbers HJ (2004). Injury pattern caused by aggressive inline skating. Sportverl Sportschad 18(4): 196–203.

Hoffmann J, Tambotino I (1996). Verletzungsrisiko beim Inline-Skating. Sporttraumatologie 12: 287–290.

Jacques LB, Grzesiak E (1994). Personal protective equipment use by inline roller skaters. J Fam Pract 34: 486–488.

Jerosch J, Heck C (2005). Verletzungsmuster und Prophylaxe beim Inline-Skaten. Orthopädie 34: 441–447.

Jerosch J, Heidjahn J, Linnebecker S, Throwesten L (1996). Defizite in der Verletzungsprophylaxe beim Inline-Skating. Dt Z Sportmed 47: 570–573.

Jerosch J, Heidjahn J, Throwesten L (1998). Gelenkbelastung beim Inline-Skating – eine biomechanische Untersuchung. Sportverl Sportschad 12: 1247–1253.

Jerosch J, Heidjahn J, Throwesten L (1998). Injury pattern and acceptance of passive and active injury prophylaxis for inline skating. Knee Surg Sports Traumatol Arthrosc: 644–649.

Kassel-Inline-Club online: www.kassel-inline.de/aboutinline/tipps.php

Schieber RA, Brache-Dorsey CM (1995). Inline-skating injuries. Epidemiology and recommendations for prevention. Sports Med 19: 427–432.

www.stiftung-warentest.de/online/freizeit_reise/test/1027837/1027837/1030336/907837.html

Young CC, Mark TH (1995). Inline-skating. An observational study of protective equipment used by the skaters. Arch Fam Med 4: 19–23.

Young CC, Mark TH, Reichert RM et al. (1996). Inline-skaters: a survey of protective equipment. Med Sci Sports Exerc 28 (suppl 5): 178.

Chapter 75 Kitesurfing

Karl-Heinz Kristen

Kitesurfing is a new water sport that allows surfing with the power of a power kite. After a short learning phase of 3–7 days, surfing at a high speed level, as well as several meters high jumps are already possible. Kitesurfing combines the use of a stunt kite and sail boarding. The expression of kitesurfing for riding the waves and surfing the wind has become prevalent (➢ Fig. 75.1).

The radical maneuvers and spectacular jumps of 5–10 m height explain the keen interest in this sport. The flying phases often last several seconds. But there have been concerns of possible risks to other water athletes and potential **dangers** have already led to prohibitions and restrictions.

In 2007, about 10,000 Austrians have carried out this water sport. About 2,000 active kitesurfers have been performing this sport regularly. Athletes are 12 to 75 years with a median range of 20 to 40 years. Each year, more people start kitesurfing with an average increase of about 30%, which is similar in Europe and the US. A far less extensive development can be expected of kitesurfing on land – carried out by skis or snowboard.

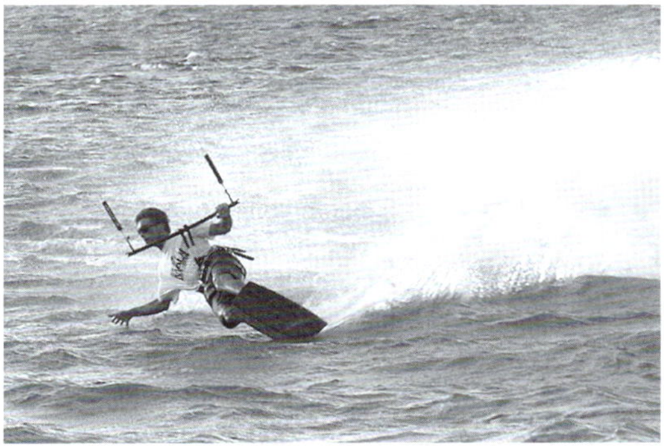

Fig. 75.1 Kite surfing. Spectacular banks similar to water skiing are possible in addition to high jumps. Rider: Reinhard Elischka, Maui/Hawaii (photograph: Haimo Sunder Plassmann).

75.1 History

Although the sport of kitesurfing is a new sport, it is not a new invention. People have used this concept for a long time. People have used the concept of using a kite to use the power of the wind for a long time. According to reports, fishermen in Polynesia and Indonesia have used kites for locomotion of their boats already in the 12th century. The kite, which has been fixed and controlled by strings, has been successfully used and presented by the British inventor G. Pocock in 1926 (GB 5420). Kitesurfing in its current sense has begun its development in 1987; the first **kitesurfing world cup** has been carried out in 1991. The windsurfers Manu Bertin, Laird Hamilton and Roby Naish (from Hawaii) put this sport on the market, which initiated today's worldwide spread and popularity.

75.2 Equipment

Just as in other sailing sports, a high technical expense and development standard are necessary for kitesurfing. The kitesurfing material consists of several parts.

75.2.1 Power kite

Power kites are kites with a wing profile. They do not have a lot in common with the usual toy kites. They are made of special, ultra lightweight, water-repellent and airtight **sailcloth**. With softer winds, 12–18 m² kites are used; smaller kites of 5–10 m² are reserved for

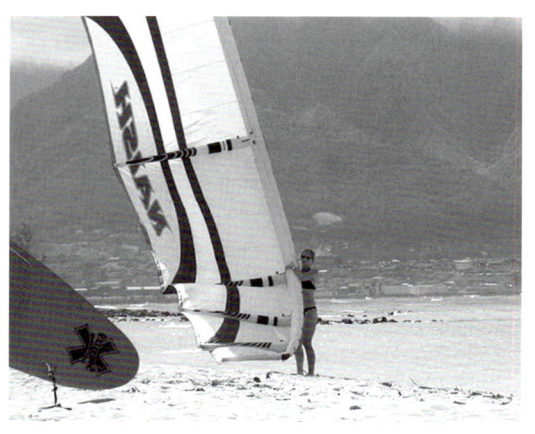

Fig. 75.2 Tube kite (total surface of 16 m²) at the start. The assistant holds the kite in the correct position for the start in the land zone (see ➢ Fig. 75.4). The kite is held at the leading edge.

allow a firm stand (➢ Fig. 75.3). The classical surfboard with grips and fins and a length of 1.5–2.0 m is mostly used without the deck grips (unstrapped) for kiting in the wave.

75.2.3 Further equipment

The kite is controlled with tear-proof, smooth surface texture lines (2 mm **Spectra flying lines**, ultimate load 2,000 N). The lengths of the lines and thus the action radius of the stronger winds (more than six knots). The most frequently used **tube kites** are navigated with four lines, while two lines serve the control of the flight direction and two lines are used to change the angle of the kite. A recent development is the use of a fifth line, which has proved successful as protection system and allows immediate "de-powering" (taking pressure off the kite; ➢ Fig. 75.2).

75.2.2 The board

The kite boards are 100–140 cm long. They have the shape of wakeboards. Two deck grips

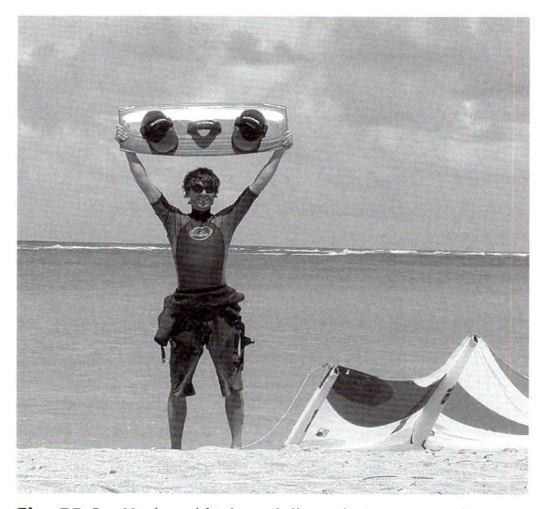

Fig. 75.3 Modern kiteboard (length 95–185 cm).

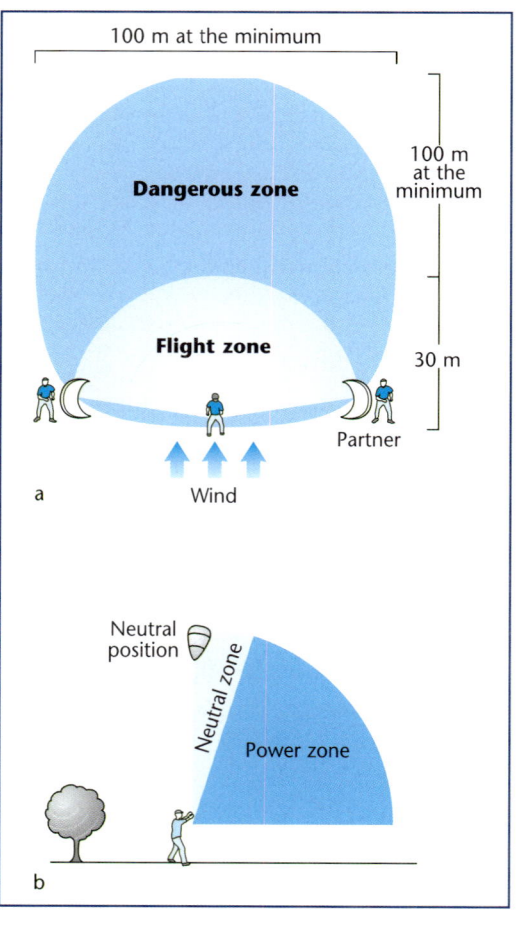

Fig. 75.4 a: Zones of danger in kitesurfing. The partner/support should always stay laterally of the kiter at the recommended safe distance. The safety zone to lee (downwind side) towards other persons should be kept by every responsible kite surfer.
b: The positioning of the kite in the air determines the direction and strength of traction. The traction forces will be lowest in the neutral position (photographs: instruction material of the VDWS).

kite is 20–35 m. This is also the safety distance the kiter needs to lee (downwind side), to both sides and above (➤ Fig. 75.4 a). A **bar** of a width of 40–70 cm, to which lines are attached, is used as a control device. The arms control the flight direction of the kite. The surfer wears a **trapeze harness** similar to windsurfing. This relieves the arms and frees them for other tasks, e.g. to set the board for start. The harness controls the depower function – the changing of the angulation of the kite towards the wind.

This combination of different functions turns the control and mastering of the kite into a complex task: wind direction and wind strength influence the positioning of the kite in the air, which determines the position of the kite determines the direction of traction and the amount of force the kite can develop (➤ Fig. 75.4 b).

75.3 Overstrain syndromes and injuries

75.3.1 Localization

International Collective, Competition world cup 2000–2011

The author was the sport-medics of a kitesurfing world cup event in 2000 to 2011. Injury data was collected and analyzed for the period 2002 to 2005 (Kristen 2005). The multi-national collective of the top kitesurfers had been surveyed by a standardized questionnaire. Current or recent injuries had been medically examined and treated. 154 data sets had been recorded during the period of 2002 to 2005. About a third of the athletes had been attainable for follow-up, conditioned by the natural fluctuation of the starter fields during the time period of 4 years. The rest had not been actively represented in the world cup anymore, conditioned by their performance, injuries or for of other reasons, and had therefore been substituted by young and talented athletes.

The examination of the kitesurfing professionals has led to the following results: 58 injuries were documented over four years including 50 minor injuries and overstrain, and eight serious injuries and fractures. The most frequently affected body parts were **ankle joints, knees, shoulders and thoraxes/ribs**. Five fractures (4× ribs, 1× ankle joint), 19 capsule/ligament lesions (6× knee, 5× ankle joint, 8× shoulder), 21 overstrain impairments of the spine (11× cervical syndrome with radicular irritation, 9× lumbago), two constriction injuries and 4 contusions had been recorded (➤ Tab. 75.1). The distinctive change of the injury pictures during the course of the observed period can be explained by the adjustment of the sport technique and by the changed environmental and wind conditions.

Tab. 75.1 Sports medical evaluation of the injuries and overstrain syndromes in the course of the Kitesurfing World Cups 2002–2005.

Year	2002	2003	2004	2005	Sum
number of athletes	22	37	42	53	154
injury localization					
head	0	0	0	0	0
cervical spine	0	1	6	4	11
shoulder	0	1	6	1	8
ribs	4	0	0	0	4
ankle	1	3	0	3	7
knee	2	2	1	1	6
lumbago	2	0	5	2	9
constriction injuries	0	1	0	1	2
others	3	3	1	5	12
severe injuries	7	1	0	0	8
minor injuries	5	9	19	17	50

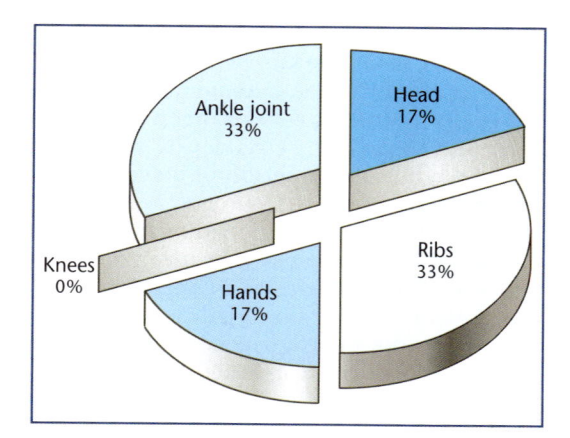

Fig. 75.5 Spreading of the injury localization with beginners and advanced kitesurfers (according to Kristen and Kröner, 2001).

Austrian Collective 2000–2001

The authors have surveyed a national (Austrian) collective of 50 kitesurfers of differently skilled levels ranging from beginners to advanced athletes (Kristen and Kröner 2001, Kristen and Kröner 2002a, 2002b). The data have been recorded retrospectively by a standardized questionnaire over a time period of 2 years (2000–2001). The injured persons have been medically examined in the course of the survey.

The following data have been recorded: four fractures (both at the lower costal arch, 8th-10th rib), two contused lacerations (head), two finger injuries (constriction injury), three sprains (ankle joint) and an ankle joint fracture. Injury localizations had been **head** (17%), **thorax and ribs** (33%), **hand** (17%) and **ankle joint** (33%; ➢ Fig. 75.5).

German collective 2000–2001

Prospective studies (Petersen et al. 2002, Nickel et al. 2004, Petersen et al. 2005) could provide evidence of a general **injury risk** of four to seven injuries in 1,000 hours of sport performance in a mixed collective. The survey has considered data of the German-speaking world from 2000 to 2001. The kite that could not be separated from the trapeze harness in critical situations was responsible for 56% of all injuries.

75.3.2 Risk factors

The **insufficiently developed safety-release system** has been demonstrated as a dominant risk factor. The kitesurfers had been dragged behind the kite, which had run out of control, without any chance to reduce the traction of the kite. A decisive step in the direction of a better release system is the **use of the fifth line**, which will allow a distinct de-powering. The handling of the safety mechanisms must be exercised accurately because otherwise they will not be used correctly in case of emergency. The dominant personal risk factor is the overestimating of one's own skills and the disregard of critical wind and weather situations.

75.3.3 Injury mechanisms

Abrasions, bruises and constrictions: the typical beginners' injuries, which develop by **falls** on the beach, near the beach or against firm obstacles near the water. Unpracticed handling and entangling fingers in the thin and extremely tensile lines causes constriction injuries.

Bounces after jumps of several seconds, which are possible due to the upwards traction of the kite, lead to ankle joint or knee injuries (➢ Fig. 75.6). These joints are also affected by **hard landings** (ligament lesions, fractures). The optimal landing should be a soft touching and

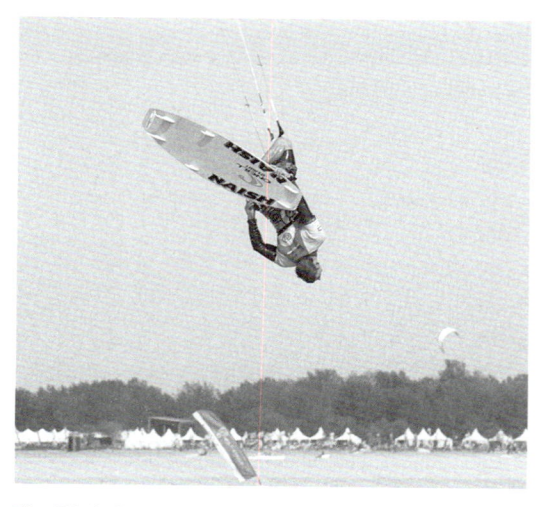

Fig. 75.6 Bounce with kite (Podersdorf/Neusiedlersee).

floating to the ground – this requires a lot of skill and feeling in the control of the kite during the flight phase.

A sport-specific overstrain impairment is the stress fracture of the ribs, primarily of the 7th and 9th rib. Cause of those rib fractures is the **pressure of the trapeze harness to the waist**, combined with **high traction and rotation forces**.

75.4 Sport-specific strains and demands

General preconditions

Not the strength but the sport technique is the decisive criterion of this sport. A high measure of balance is necessary for the control of the board. The largest effort is the control of the kite in the wind. Good knowledge of the weather and a feeling for the force of the wind are key issues. Indispensable basic physical conditions are the abilities to perform pull-ups and adequate swimming skills.

Spine

The lumbar spine is subject to **extreme rotation and flexion strain**, because the traction of the kite is transmitted via arms and trapeze to the legs. Kitesurfing is therefore a good exercise for the trunk muscles. The axial strain of the lumbar spine is reduced obliquely upwards. The cervical spine is highly strained, especially beginners control the position of the kite in the air with the eyes in a "back-tilted head position". **Whiplash injuries of the cervical spine** cannot be avoided at spinning falls with high speeds. The over the bar fixed shoulder girdle has an intensifying effect.

Shoulder joints

Subluxations and **dislocations** can appear even in shoulder joints with well stabilized muscles because of the high and often sudden traction strain to the arms – a critical situation in the water without outside help. The recent development in competitive kitesurfing with "handle pass" maneuvers (the bar will be handed from one hand to the other during a jump – a trick from show waterskiing) has led to a clearly increased incidence of shoulder injuries of top athletes. A strong shoulder girdle and **good shoulder-stabilizing muscles** are the precondition of kitesurfing.

Danger to others

The power kite as well as the **tensed lines** can become not only a risk for the athlete himself, but also a risk for other water athletes and bathers, if they are used by an unpracticed or irresponsible athlete. The German Federation of Windsurfing and Watersport Schools has set up **rules** for this new sport. The **adherence to safety distances** must be urged especially for the prevention of a danger to uninvolved persons. A crash is possible in areas with dense traffic, because the safety radius in kitesurfing with a line length of 20–30 m amounts to 100 m to lee (downwind side) and 50 m to the side

> **Summary**
>
> Kitesurfing is a sport that includes a **third dimension** in watersports. It conveys the feeling of floating over the water, only driven by the force of the wind, due to the upward traction of the kite. The **large requirement of space** of kitesurfers reduces the territories, especially in Central Europe, to only few spots. The long lines and the kite itself present a **risk for bathers and other water athletes**, if the flight of the kite is not mastered or if the athlete does not act responsibly. New safety functions (e.g. safe and fast depowering systems) have been developed. 80–90% of all rescue efforts in water athletes (referring to all watersports) are necessary, because the own abilities and fitness had been overestimated (Exadaktylos et al. 2000). The following **precautions** are recommendable for kitesurfers:
>
> - attendance of a kitesurfing class with according safety exercises
> - mastering the kite; estimating the risk zone as well as maintaining the safety distance to the side and to lee
> - knowledge of the territory: this includes the maintaining of safety distances to surrounding areas in addition to the knowledge of wind and streams.
>
> An important step has been taken by the further development of the safety release system of kite and kiteboard. But further work and custom-oriented test are needed.

References

Exadaktylos AK, Sclabas GM, Swemmer K et al. (2005). The kick with the kite: An analysis of kite surfing-related off-shore rescue missions in Cape Town, South Africa. Br J Sports Med 39(5): e26.

Kristen K-H (2005). Kitesurfen In: Grifka J, Engelhardt M et al. (eds.). Sportverletzungen – Sportschäden. Praxiswissen Halte- und Bewegungsapparat. Thieme-Verlag, Stuttgart, pp 180–185.

Kristen K-H, Kröner A (2001). Kitesurfing. Sportorthop Sporttraumatol 17(4): 253–259.

Kristen K-H, Kröner A (2002a). Orthopädische Checkliste: Kitesurfing/Kiteboarding – Surfen mit Lenkdrachen. Sportorthop Sporttraumatol 18: 204–205.

Kristen K-H, Kröner A (2002b). Riskieren Kitesurfer Kopf und Kragen? Medical Tribune 37, volume 31: 10.

Nickel C, Zernial O, Musahl V, Hansen U, Zantop T, Petersen W (2004). A prospective study of kitesurfing injuries. Am J Sports Med 32(4): 912–917.

Petersen W, Nickel C, Zantop T, Zernial O (2005). Kitesurfing injuies. A young sport. Orthopäde 34(5): 419–425.

Petersen W, Hansen U, Zernial O, Nickel C, Prymka M (2002). Mechanism and prevention of kitesurfing injuries. Sportverletz Sportschad 16(3): 115–121.

76 Mountain biking

Markus Arnold

A group of young Americans around Gary Fisher and Joe Breeze pioneered the new sport Mountain biking in the early 1970s. Starting in 1973 they raced their bikes in Marin County, North of San Francisco, using heavy, scarcely modified Schwinn cruisers. They began to adjust their bikes to off-road usage since they felt limited by the existing bicycles design.

In 1980s the commercial breakthrough succeeded and mountain bikes became the stars on bicycle fairs. But it still took some time until the boom in the early 1990s fully developed. The **technical evolution** of the bikes has brought forth awesome materials and designs. The improvement of the riding comfort by better **suspension systems**, the development of efficient and affordable **disk brakes** and the diversification of very different bike types are the most impressive. Purpose and budget decide the choice of the individually ideal bike.

In the year 2000, 13.4 million Americans owned a mountain bike and more than half of them had ridden their bikes off road (Gluskin and Edmondson 2000). Apart from the general stagnation on the market, incremental rates had been noticed especially in the middle and upper market segments in Switzerland in 2003 and 2004 (Stettler 2005).

76.1 Disciplines

Competitive bike sport is described in different disciplines defined by the "Union Cycliste Internationale" (UCI). The most popular are:

- **Cross-country (XC):** has been an Olympic discipline since the Games in Atlanta in 1996. These races with mass starts last about 2 hours, lead along a round course that has to be ridden several times over a distinctly undulated profile through the country on dirt and forest roads, partly also over meadows. All passages must be possible to ride at all weather conditions; the total altitude difference amounts to 1,500 m (➤ Fig. 76.1).

- **Long-distance races (marathon):** In contrast to XC, the ride is done from A to B or in a large loop. The racing time will last 4 hours at the least, the minimum distance is 80 km. Such races lead across several Alpine passes, for example, and total altitude differences of 5,000 m are common; the bike will have to be carried for some parts of the distance.

- **Downhill (DH):** This single-start procedure aims for a downhill ride of 1,500–3,500 m within 3–5 min as fast as possible, demanding technical skills. The ride leads across roots, sticks and rocks with a high speed; top speeds of 100 km/h are common (➤ Fig. 76.2).

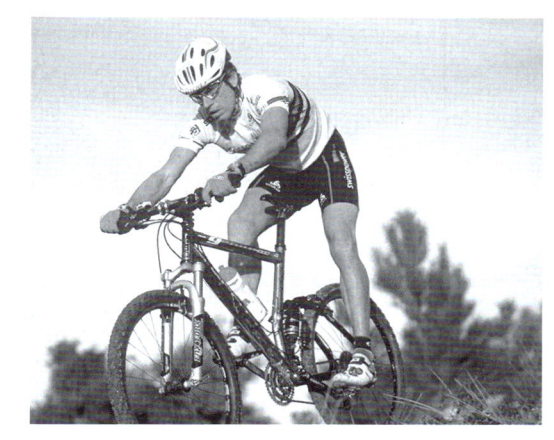

Fig. 76.1 Typical downhill posture of cross-country world champion Th. Frischknecht. Protection clothes: helmet, glasses, gloves (photograph: Stephan Bögli).

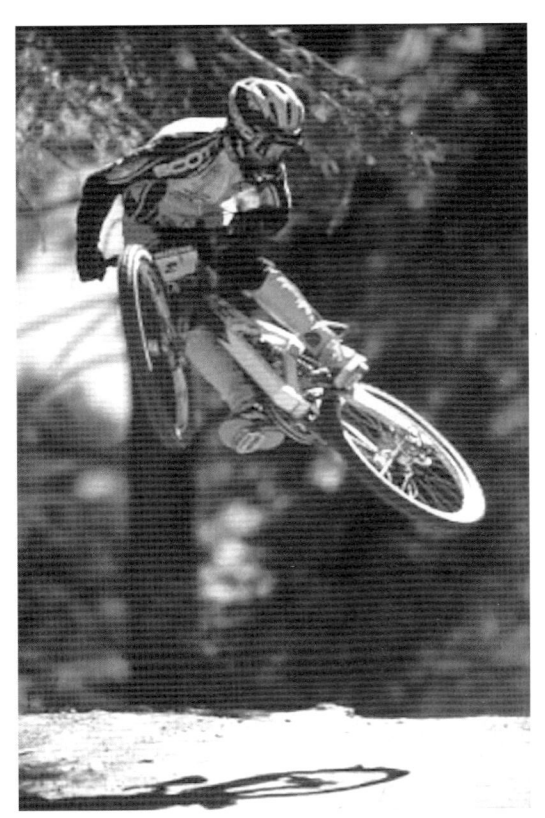

Fig. 76.2 Scene of a descent: DH rider with integral helmet, motocross glasses, chest and back protectors, full-fingered gloves, protectors for the elbows, knees and lower legs (photograph: Stephan Bögli).

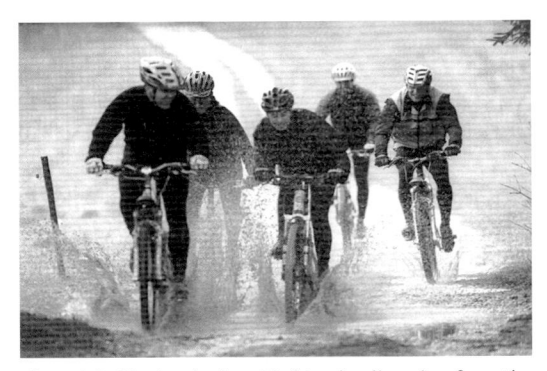

Fig. 76.3 Weekend trip with friends: diversion from the "sterile" daily routine (photograph: Thomas Ulrich).

- **Recreational biking** is usually similar to a short marathon, where a loop on forest and dirt roads with uphill and downhill parts are ridden. The aim is to find peace of mind under one's own power and away from everyday stress (➤ Fig. 76.3).

76.2 Most frequent injuries

In **mountain biking**, there is a **risk** of 6.8 injuries for men and 12.0 injuries for women in 1,000 hours of performing the sport, and this is comparable to the risk of Alpine skiing (Requa et al. 1993, Pfeiffer 1994). Mountain bikers tend to be individualists and are not organized in a larger federation, which complicates a systematic data collection. Therefore, a "selection bias" is practically unavoidable. Most studies of recent years have focused on racing athletes (Kronisch and Rubin 1994, Pfeiffer 1994, Kronisch et al. 1996, Arnold et al. 1999). Only few have recorded data of non-racers (Gaulrapp et al. 2001).

According to a large-scale survey of the subscribers of the largest European journal "bike" based on questionnaires, only 10% of the bikers had never suffered an injury, but all others have averagely reported **2.3 injuries in each biker**. 85% of those had been minor injuries that could be treated on an outpatient basis, they only caused exercise breaks of 3 weeks at a maximum (Gaulrapp et al. 2001). Abrasions and bruises are frequent; the recorded 2.8% or 187 cyclists with a cerebral concussion in their history are an important subgroup.

76.2.1 Top bikers

Experiences in the treatment of the Swiss National Mountain Biking team and the Scott World Cup Teams of 1993 to 2001 form the basis for the following data (Arnold and Biedert 2000). The National Team consisted of 45 athletes on an average, the professional team of 12 athletes. **XC riders** of this class always perform the sport wearing **helmets and gloves**, **DH riders** additionally wear **protectors** for elbows, knees and lower legs and often also a light back protector.

Injuries had to be reported to the team-doctor if either surgery had been necessary or the exercising had to be reduced significantly for at least

76.2 Most frequent injuries

Fig. 76.4 Injury patterns of a group of international top bikers, 1993–2001.

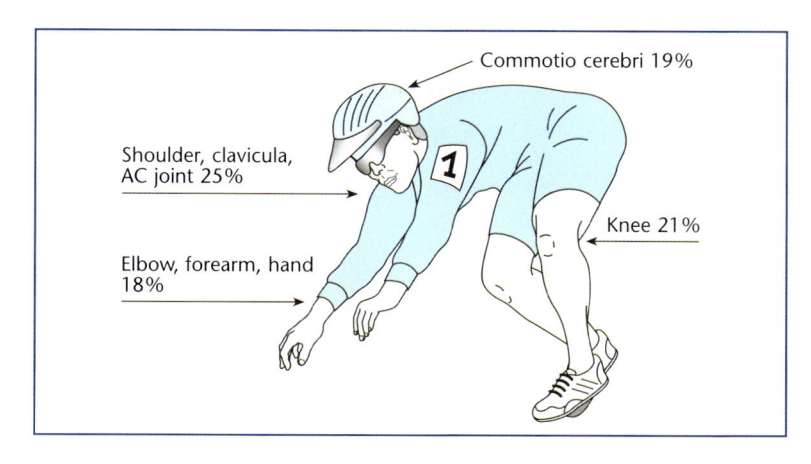

- Commotio cerebri 19%
- Shoulder, clavicula, AC joint 25%
- Knee 21%
- Elbow, forearm, hand 18%

Fig. 76.5 Injury patterns of the SUVA insured bikers of Switzerland, 1995 to 1998 (figures: Stefan Gut).

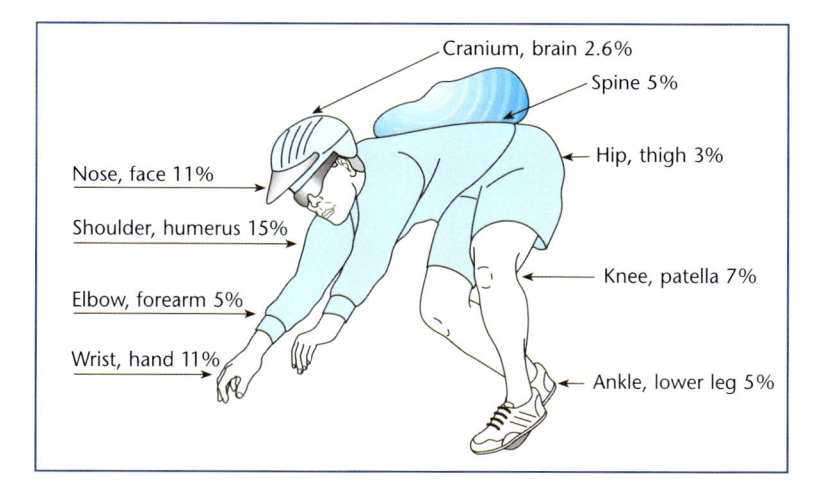

- Cranium, brain 2.6%
- Spine 5%
- Hip, thigh 3%
- Nose, face 11%
- Shoulder, humerus 15%
- Knee, patella 7%
- Elbow, forearm 5%
- Wrist, hand 11%
- Ankle, lower leg 5%

1 week. Therefore, the list of injuries primarily consisted of **fractures, dislocations and ligament ruptures**. Altogether, 116 relevant injuries had been recorded (➤ Fig. 76.4). Additionally, **sprains of the cervical spine** with long-term consequences had been registered in three athletes, serious **abdominal traumas** in two athletes and a **pertrochanteric femur fracture** in one athlete. The most **frequent accident causes** had been falls at downhill rides. 19% of the top bikers had suffered a **concussion** despite the consequent wearing of helmets.

76.2.2 Recreational bikers

The wearing of helmets had not been common for recreational bikers for a long time, although a **correctly worn helmet** demonstrably provides protection of head injuries (Williams 1991). According to records of the Swiss information center for accident prevention, the average percentage of bikers wearing helmets has increased from 4% in 1990 to 17% in 1999 and has reached 53% in 2003 (Unfallverhütung BfU 2004).

As most Swiss employees are insured in an obligatory accident insurance an overview of the spread of the most relevant injuries in recreational bikers can be easily estimated (➤ Fig. 76.5). On average 2,155 accidents a year had been recorded during the period of 1995 to 2002 (minimum of 1,585 in 1995, maximum of 2,821 in 2001). 2.6% **craniocerebral traumas** per year (56 cases a year) had had been serious enough to be recorded in the database. These numbers confirm the results of the study by Gaulrapp et al. (2001).

The recorded injuries consisted of:

- 9.1% fractures
- 3% dislocations
- 21.3% sprains and ligament and tendon injuries (SUVA Unfallstatistik).

76.3 Prevention

76.3.1 Passive protection from concussion

The risk of further brain concussions increases after a first cerebral concussion (Guskiewicz et al. 2003); the symptoms tend to be stronger after a re-injury and it will take longer until the freedom of symptoms (Collins et al. 2002, Guskiewicz et al. 2003).

This topic has been surveyed and described multidisciplinary already for contact sports, such as ice hockey (Williams 1991, Barnes et al. 1998, Aubry et al. 2002, Biasca et al. 2002, Andersen et al. 2004). A current clear principle is that an athlete after a concussion should not be permitted to perform the sport until all symptoms have completely disappeared, so that even performing the sport flat out no more symptoms have occurred. Young athletes (<18 years) must be given special consideration because regeneration can take longer in this group. The still maturing brain is more susceptible for the so-called second impact syndrome with a second concussion within few hours up to weeks after the first one, which can lead to catastrophic consequences (Guskiewicz 2003).

> The risk of troublesome long-term consequences after cerebral concussion must not be underestimated. Young athletes are extremely vulnerable for this devastating injury.

76.3.2 Active prevention

Mountain biking has technically only little in common with the cycling on hard-surfaced ground. Sliding, jumping, landing, the controlled cornering technique on steep downhill rides are skills specific for mountain biking and can be acquired in mountain bike classes (Hayman 2005).

> **Summary**
>
> Mountain biking is about as risky as alpine skiing. Most mountain bikers have accidents during downhill rides. The wearing of helmet, glasses and gloves needs to be popularized further. The cerebral concussion is a serious injury and needs to be treated accordingly, especially in the young athletes.

References

Andersen TE, Amason A, Engebretsen L Bahr R (2004). Mechanisms of head injuries in elite football. Br J Sports Med 38: 690–696.

Arnold MP, Biedert R (2000). Mountainbiken – Trendsportart in der Gefahrenzone. Med Praxis: 2–5.

Arnold MP, Biedert R, Friedrich NF (1999). Das Verletzungsmuster von Spitzenbikern. Sportverl Sportsch 15: 3–6.

Aubry M, Cantu R, Dvorak J, Graf-Baumann T, Johnston K, Kelly J, Lovell M, McCrory P, Meeuwisse W, Schamasch P (2002). Summary and agreement statement of the First International Conference on Concussion in Sport, Vienna 2001. Recommendations for the improvement of safety and health of athletes who may suffer concussion injuries. Br J Sports Med 36: 6–10.

Barnes BC, Cooper L, Kirkendall DT, McDerott TP, Jordan BD, Garrett WE, Jr. (1998). Concussion history in elite male and female soccer players. Am J Sports Med 26: 433–438.

Biasca N, Wirth S, Tegner Y (2002). The avoidability of head and neck injuries in ice hockey: an historical review. Br J Sports Med 36: 410–427.

Collins MW, Lovell MR, Iverson GL, Cantu RC, Maroon JC, Field M (2002). Cumulative effects of concussion in high school athletes. Neurosurgery 51: 1175–1181.

Gaulrapp H, Weber A, Rosemeyer B (2001). Injuries in mountain biking. Knee Surg Sport Traumatol Arthrosc 9: 48–53.

Gluskin E, Edmondson B (2000). The cycling consumer of the new millennium. Costa Mesa (CA). National Bicycle Dealers Association.

Guskiewicz KM (2003). Assessment of postural stability following sport-related concussion. Curr Sports Med Rep 2: 24–30.

Guskiewicz KM, McCrea M, Marshall SW, Cantu RC, Randolph C, Barr W, Onate JA, Kelly JP (2003). Cumulative effects associated with recurrent concussion in collegiate football players: the NCAA Concussion Study. Jama 290: 2549–2555.

Hayman F (2005). Fliegen lernen. bike: 68–72.

Kronisch RL, Chow TK, Simon LM, Wong PF (1996). Acute injuries in off-road bicycle racing. Am J Sports Med 24: 88–93.

Kronisch RL, Rubin AL (1994). Traumatic injuries in off-road bicycling. Clin J Sport Med 4: 240–244.

Pfeiffer RP (1994). Off-road bicycle racing injuries – the NORBA pro/elite category. Clin Sports Med 13. 207–218:

Requa RK, DeAbilla LN, Garrick JG (1993).Injuries in recreational adult fitness activities. Am J Sports Med 21: 461–467.

Stettler A (2005). Persönliche Mitteilung. Inhaber XX.S Sports.

SUVA unfallstatistik UVG 1998–2002. www.unfallstatistik.ch.

Unfallverhütung BfU (2004). Bulletin: Tragquote der Schutzausrüstung beim sportlichen Radfahren, 2003.

Williams M (1991).The protective performance of bicyclists' helmets in accidents. Accid Anal Prev 23: 119–131.

Chapter 77 Paragliding

Michael Bohnsack

Paragliding is a young sport and developed from parasailing with ram air parachutes in the 1970s. In 1979, the German hang-gliding federation (DHV) has been founded and has become today's umbrella organization of hanggliders and paragliders in Germany. About 32,000 pilots (86% men, 14% women) exercise this sport actively in Germany at the present time (DHV 2004).

The paraglide pilot needs a state flight certificate and indemnity insurance. The **minimum age** is 14 years (with parents' consent). A medical certificate is not needed. Special permits in addition to the flight certificates such as winch launch and passenger flight exist. The cost for such training is approximately 1,000 Euros.

The German Paragliding Federation has created a department of security in 2000 in order to evaluate the registered flight accidents and to introduce necessary material and training guidelines. Introduction of **security and performance training** further reduced the risk of accidents (➤ Fig. 77.1).

77.1 Equipment and security

Today's paragliders have elliptic 20–30 m^2 wings with ram air filled chambers, which stiffen the paraglider. The pilot is connected to the paraglider by **painters** running down from the bottom side of the wing and the **harness** (➤ Fig. 77.2 a and b). The **emergency parachute** is attached to the harness; wearing a **helmet** is mandatory. The equipment altogether weighs approximately 15 kg and can be carried in a backpack at mountain hikes without any problems. More and more **instruments** are used at thermal or long-distance flights, such as the variometer (control of climb and descent rates, flying altitude) and the GPS (satellite navigation).

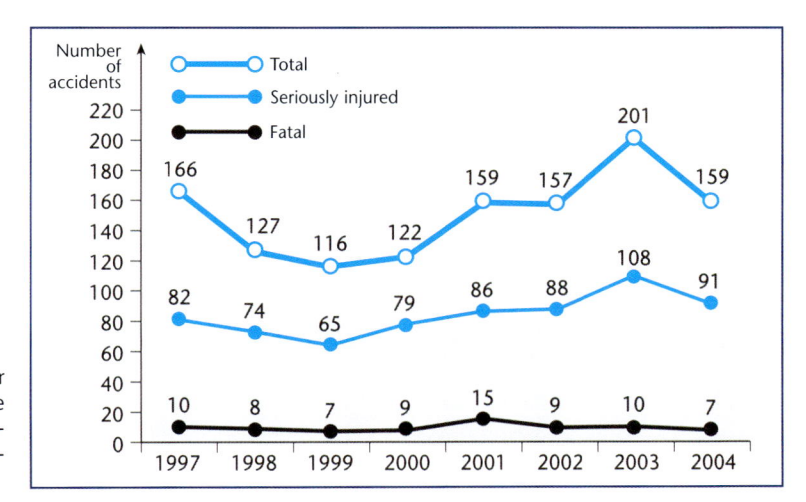

Fig. 77.1 The relative number of accidents has halved since 1997, measured by the increasing number of German paragliding pilots.

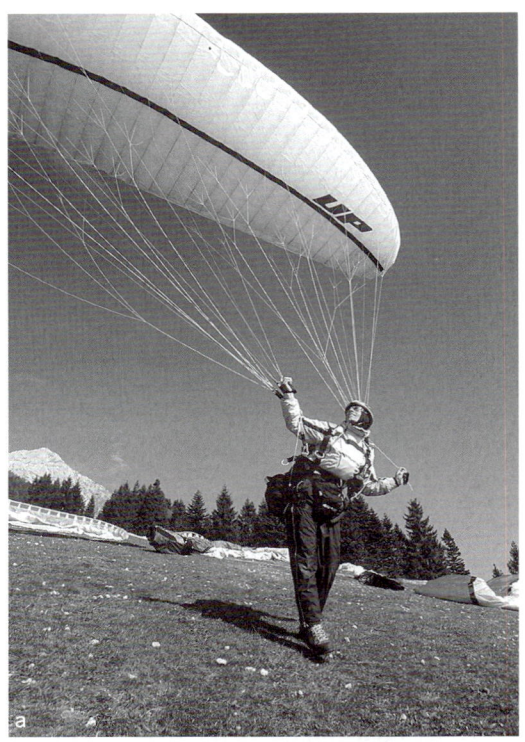

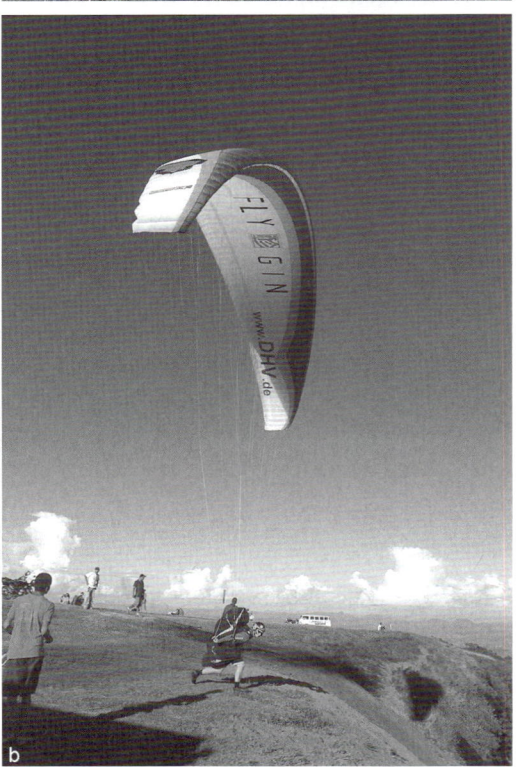

A right and a left suspension line is used as a brake on the posterior edge of the paraglider control the paraglider. A simultaneous traction on both suspension lines will reduce the flying speed. The **gliding performance** of modern paragliders lies at about 1:8 (kites: 1:13, gliders: 1:60), the **trim speed** amounts to about 37 km/h at a **maximum speed** of up to 55 km/h. Thermal flights lasting for hours and long-distance flights of more than 100 km are possible with modern paragliders without any problems. The **distance world record** is 423 km, flown by the Canadian William Gadd in Zapata, Texas, in 2002.

The **adherence to the security standards** and flying rules and self-discipline of all pilots are the basis of flight security especially in highly frequented flying areas and at "thermal weekends" (➤ Fig. 77.3). Additionally, every paraglider is equipped with a **seal of approval** as a guarantee for material stability, processing and flying characteristics. This seal of approval is renewed every two years, similar to a technical inspection certificate.

> Security standards, flight rules and self-discipline of all pilots are the basis of safe paragliding.

77.2 Physical strains in paragliding

In paragliding, an **increase of the catecholamine release** and – depending on the situation, also in very experienced pilots – **heart rates** of more than 180 beats per minute might occur (Gomez-Huerga et al. 1988, Tusk 1995). The top and permanent strains regarding stress and circulation must not be underestimated in paragliding, because there is no underlying muscle activity.

Sudden deaths occur in this sport with a frequency of 1/100,000 (Raschka and Parzeller 2002). Pilots with a known **disease of the cardiovascular system** should therefore perform

Fig. 77.2 a and b: The paraglider is pulled forwards or backwards with crossed lines against the wind at a slope. Before starting, the pilot checks the equal filling of the chute and the correct array of the control lines.

Fig. 77.3 The declared flying areas will be strongly frequented on "thermal days", especially on weekends. A focused defensive flying behavior under strict observance of the rules for the right of flight is necessary in order to avoid dangerous collisions.

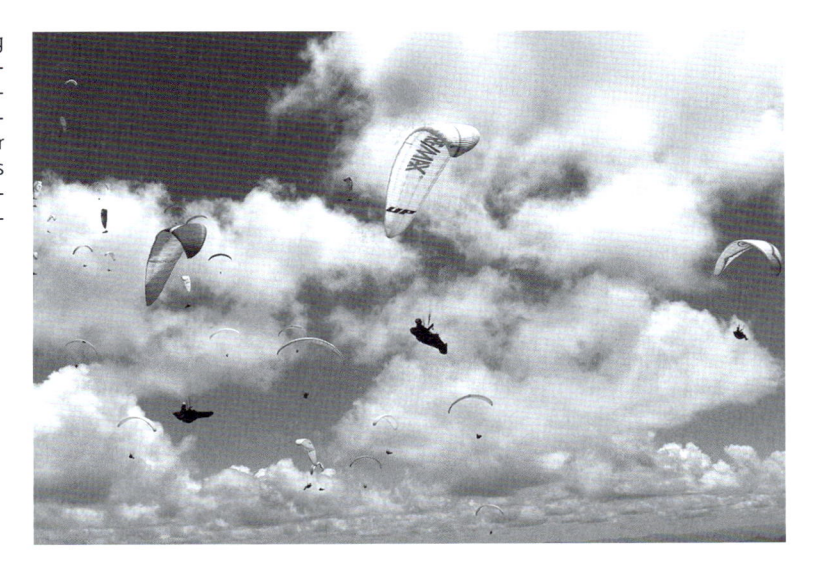

paragliding only after detailed examination and consultation (exercise echocardiography).

A central blood loss due to the strong increase of the centrifugal forces of up to 3 G at the "steep spiral" (descent support with a maximum descend speed of > 15 m/s) can lead to **impaired vision** and **temporary unconsciousness**. Short and sudden accelerations occur occasionally during the thermal flight and in turbulences, which can lead to **nausea and back aches**.

The frequent change of the flight altitude with the quickly **changing atmospheric pressure**, the increased **UV radiation** and the **cold** in high air levels present a special challenge for the thermal and long-distance flyer. With increasing flight altitude, the temperature falls 6.5°C by 1,000 m in standard atmosphere. Achievable flight altitudes with environmental temperatures below the freezing mark can be expected at strong thermal in summer.

Oxygen deficiency restricts the physical and mental capacity – often unnoticed by the affected person – and leads to the following symptoms:

- hyperventilation
- tingling paresthesias
- vertigo
- changed color perception and field of vision
- euphoria and drowsiness.

A regular **intake of fluids** is stringently required for all longer flights with altitudes of more than 3,500 m in order to avoid dehydration due to the altitude-conditioned sinking of humidity. The high intensity of the UVA and UVB radiation to the skin can lead to **radiation injuries**, if no sufficient light protection is used.

> High cardiovascular strain triggered stress and a centrifugal force is possible in paragliding.

77.3 Causes of accidents

About 30% of the accidents occur in "standard situations" such as start, landing approach and landing. The most frequent serious **start accidents** (14 accidents in 2002; Slezak 2003) are triggered by insufficient breaking the paraglider. In steep starting areas, the pilot takes off with a frontally infolded wing. A fast rotation movement of the wing with occurs due to a unilateral in-folding.

A mistake in the **landing** (paraglider must be landed against the wind) can lead to a fast turn near the ground and the risk of a unilateral compressor stall or an overflying of the landing field with outside landing (trees, houses, water). At **tree landings**, serious injuries only occur in 20% of the cases due to direct colli-

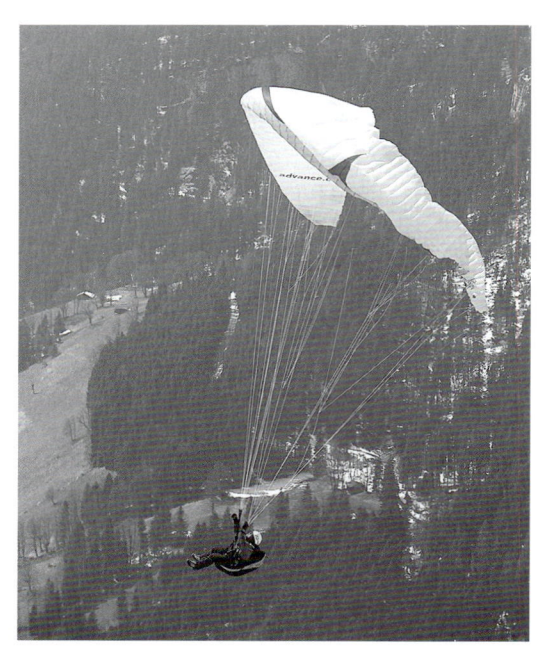

Fig. 77.4 Mistakes or strong thermic can collapse the wing. This requires a controlled reaction of the pilot. A collapsed during flight because of flying maneuver or strong thermal, will require a controlled reaction of the pilot. A stable flight situation is can be achieved by a shifting the body weight and measured use of the brakes, so that the paraglider fills again.

sions of the pilots with the tree trunk or a fast rotation around the trunk.

Strong (32% of the accidents) and **thermal wind** (35% of the accidents) can cause turbulent flight conditions within seconds; this requires a high level of flying technique. **Lateral in-folders** are considered the most frequent accident cause in paragliding (➤ Fig. 77.4). The pilot is unable to control the sudden rotation movement of the wing or provokes a unilateral stall by excessive counter-steering.

Flying should not be performed at foehn wind conditions, thunderstorms, a gathering cold front or strong gusty wind and precipitation because of the increased accident risk. 64% of the pilots having an accident have shown a deficiency in training; 84% of the accidents have occurred at a distance from the ground of less than 50 m.

> Most flying accidents occur with strong wind and thermal conditions.

77.4 Injury patterns

Spinal injuries are the most frequent injuries in paragliding (Ballmer and Jakob 1989, Cereghetti and Martinoli 1990, Krueger-Franke et al. 1991, Lautenschlager et al. 1992, Krauss and Mischkowsky 1993, Exadaktylos et al. 2003).

Zeller et al. (1992) have found 125 (26%) **thoracolumbar fractures** (n = 30, 25% L1; n = 22, 19% Th12) in an analysis of 489 paragliding accidents with injury. Schulze et al. (2002) have found 62% of **spinal fractures** as the most frequent reason for in-patient treatment of paragliding athletes (n = 64). The reason is the flyer's sitting position in the harness. At a "hard" landing, the pilot tries to support his body weight with his legs. If this is unsuccessful or the pilot falls on his back, the spine is compressed and shearing forces occur. Depending on to the fall position, load peaks at the thoracolumbar junction occur. The amount of spinal injuries has decreased in Germany from 39 to 31% since **back protectors** have become **mandatory** in Germany and Austria in 2000 (Slezak 2004).

The most frequent injuries in paragliding affect the **lower extremities** (➤ Fig. 77.5). These have been 45% of all injuries (n = 376) (Zeller et al. 1992), with **fractures or ligament injuries at the ankle joint** in 120 cases (32%), **fractures of the lower leg** in 39 cases (10%) and **meniscus and ligament injuries at the knee joint** in 34 cases (9%). Schulze et al. (2002) have found injury rate of the lower extremities of 36 com-

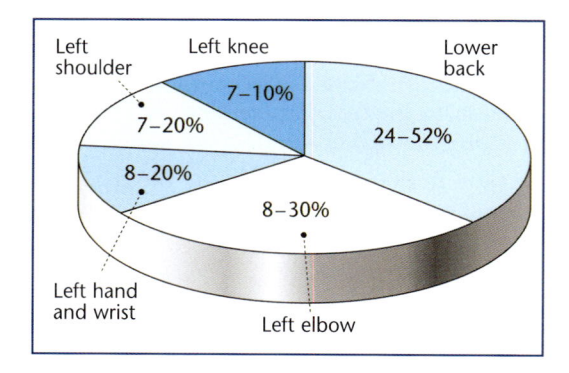

Fig. 77.5 Reported injuries in paragliding in Germany (Slezak 2003). Fractures (65%) and sprains (20%) were most frequent.

pared to the accident statistics of the DHV security department with 39% for 2003 (Slezak 2004).

Usually, falls at takeoff in steep territories, landings in uneven territories and landings on the feet with high speeds caused by the influence of tail wind or a "stalling" of the wing are responsible for this kind of injury. The wearing of ankle-high, cushioned boots with treaded soles and the training of falling techniques in landing are recommended as preventive measures.

Injuries of the upper extremities, caused by the straight sitting position and the lifted arms with permanent contact to the toggles, occur far less often with 13–23% of all injuries in paragliding (Krüger-Franke et al. 1991, Zeller 1992, Schulze et al. 2002, Little 2004, Slezak 2004).

Typical injury patterns are:

- anterior shoulder dislocations at launching
- ruptures of the rotator cuffs at falls to the lifted and abducted arm
- wrist and forearm fractures by breaking reactions of land falls as well as
- injuries of the elbow joint.

Head injuries with only 4% are the exception in paragliding in Germany because of the **helmet requirement**, which has been mandatory since the beginning (Little 2004, Slezak 2004).

Pelvic fractures (about 3%), thoracic injuries (2–7%) and injuries of the internal organs (about 4%) are **rare injuries**. These injuries demand high impact energy or a contusion by obstacles on emergency or tree landings.

In addition to spinal injuries, injuries of the lower extremities occur in paragliding.

References

Ballmer FT, Jakob RP (1989). Gleitschirmunfälle, Verletzungsmuster und Unfallanalyse. Schweizerische Zeitschrift für Sportmedizin 37: 247–249.

Cereghetti C, Martinoli S (1990). Gleitschirmunfall: Epidemiologie und Klinik. Zeitschrift für Unfallchirurgie und Versicherungsmedizin 83: 159–167.

Exadaktylos AK, Sclabas G, Eggli S, Schoenfeld H, Gygax E, Zimmermann H (2003). Paragliding accidents – the spine is at risk. European Journal of Emergency Medicine 10: 27–29.

Gomez-Huerga O, Blanc D, Decombaz J, Guignard T, Moesch H (1988). Hormonal and electrocardiographic studies in acrobatic and passenger hang-gliding flights. Schweizerische Zeitschrift für Sportmedizin 36: 21–28.

Krauss U, Mischkowsky T (1993). Der schwerwiegende Gleitschirmunfall. Analyse von 122 Fällen. Unfallchirurg 96: 299–304.

Krueger-Franke M, Siebert CH, Pfoerringer W (1991). Paragliding injuries. Br J Sports Med 25: 98–101.

Lautenschlager S, Karli U, Matter P (1992). Multizentrische Gleitschirm-Unfallstudie 1990. Zeitschrift für Unfallchirurgie und Versicherungsmedizin 85: 90–95.

Little J (2004). 2003 U.S. Paragliding accident summary. http://www.ushga.org/safety/PG2003 AccidentSummary.pdf (epub).

Raschka C, Parzeller M (2002). Akuter Myokardinfarkt beim Sport. Sportorthop Sporttraumatol 18: 275–276.

Schulze W, Richter J, Schulze B, Esenwein SA, Büttner-Janz K (2002). Injury prophylaxis in paragliding. Br J Sports Med 36: 365–369.

Slezak K (2003). Unfallstatistik Gleitschirm 2002. DHV-Info http://www.dhv.de/typo/fileadmin/user _upload/monatsordner/2004-06/Ausbildung/Unfallstatistik_2002_Gleitschirm.pdf (epub).

Slezak K (2004). Gleitschirmunfallstatistik 2003. DHV-Info 128: 49–56.

Tusk I (1995). Sportmedizinische Aspekte des Gleitschirmfliegens. Med. Dissertation, Johann-Wolfgang-Goethe-Universität, Frankfurt am Main.

Zeller T, Billing A, Lob G (1992). Injuries in paragliding. International Orthopedics 16: 255–259.

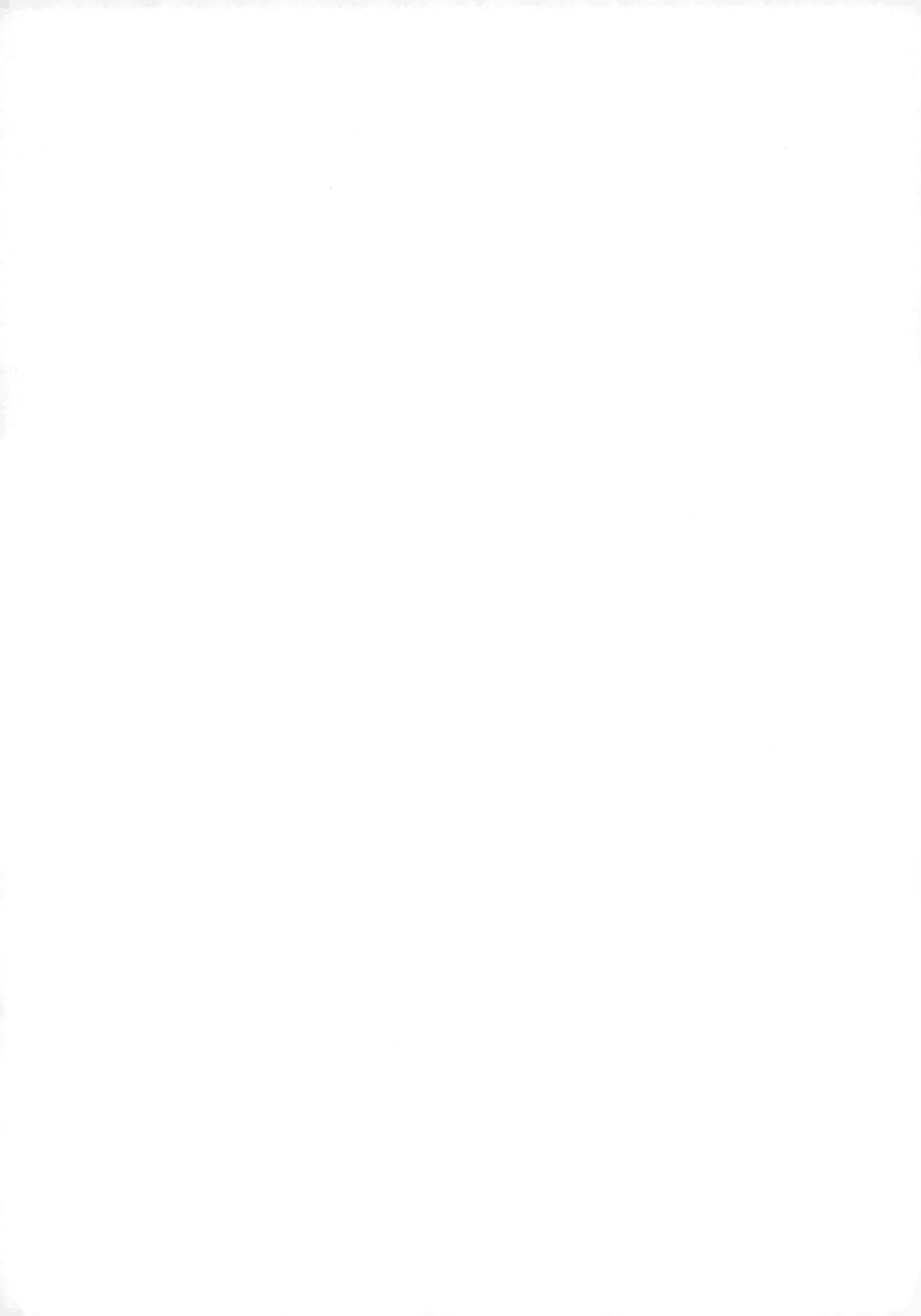

78 Snowboarding

Klaus Dann

78.1 History

Sherman Poppen invented in 1963 the "snurfer", a snow surfer, which was a water ski with a curved up shovel and a line for steering. At that time, nobody had ever expected to ride high alpine territories with tilts of more than 50°. Meanwhile, even Mount Everest has been snowboarded. The Americans Jake Burton, Tom Sims and Dimtrij Milovich were snowboard pioneers in the US. The brothers Strunk with the swing bow and the freestyle skier Fuzzy Garhammer constructed the European "snow surfer".

Since the mid-1980s, this sport has experienced an enormous booming in America and in Europe. The boards have become controllable with the invention of steel edges, coatings and high-back binding systems. Snowboarding has developed into a trend sport for young winter athletes. Snowboarding has become an **Olympic** discipline in 1998 in Nagano with the two disciplines of half pipe and GS carving. At the Olympic Games in Turin in 2006, the snowboard cross (SBX) was introduced. Meanwhile, there are 10 million snowboarders worldwide. Snowboarding moves away from competitive stress towards free riding, just as in any other fun sports. The best snowboarding experience is the riding through deep powder snow and the jumping over hilltops into the soft snow (➤ Fig. 78.1).

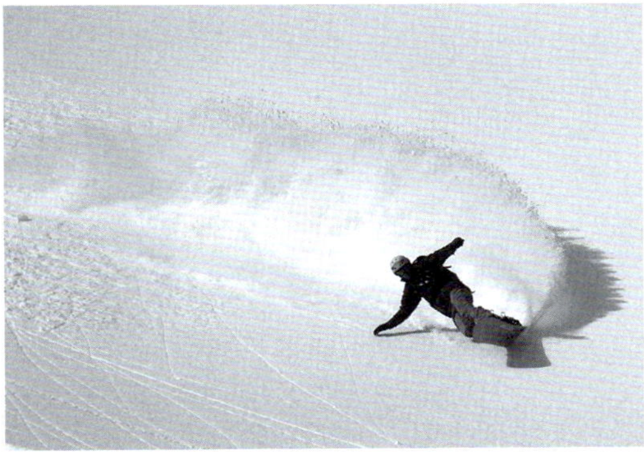

The majority of snowboarders now favor riding in free territories and in deep powder snow as well as in fun parks (trend: "Off piste – out to the country side or fun park!").

78.2 Sport-specific strain/demand profile

Snowboarding requires a permanent change from front-side to backside, which puts a strain on the extensor and flexor of the lower extremity. This is different to skiing, where the balance can be spread on both legs and, thus, riding is energy saving (Knöringer et al. 1998). Each snowboard discipline uses different foot positions with different angles to the longitudinal axis of the board. This allows a better spread of the body weight, especially in freestyle and free-riding, which have different positions as alpine race disciplines.

> The permanent change from front-side to backside requires fitness, coordination and a good sense of balance.

78.3 Epidemiology of injuries

The risk behavior of juvenile snowboarders matches the age. The major **risk group** is found

Fig. 78.1 Perfect freeride (freerider: Gerry Ring/location: Val Grisenche).

in juvenile male snowboarders at the age of 13–19 years (Kemeny 1989, Dann et al. 1996 and 1997, Made and Elmqvist 2004, Xiang et al. 2005). Thus, the injury risk for 16-year-olds is 9 times higher than for 25-year-old athletes (Dann et al. 1996 and 1997). They mainly ride in soft boots on freestyle boards and prefer the **half pipe** as favorite territory. The light snowboard helmets now commercially available is urgently recommended for beginners (Hagel et al. 1999, Tilburg 2000, Made and Elmqvist 2004).

In contrast, the injury risk of girls increases significantly after the age of 25. But beginners with rented equipment and ski boots – that are completely inappropriate for snowboarding – are at a risk of injury (Boldrino and Furian 1999).

78.3.1 Accident mechanisms

The **fall** is in 90% of the cases **self-induced**. Collisions only occur rarely (9.8%) and the majority are collisions with fixed objects. Collisions with skiers and with snowboarders are rare (Dann et al. 1997).

Most falls occur forwards (40.5%), followed by falls to the side (27.2%) and backwards (18.2%). Forward falls over the board shovel lead to injuries:

- of the upper extremities (39%)
- of the lower extremities (30%)
- of the spine as well as the head (11%) and
- of the thorax (9%).

78.3.2 Snowboard injuries in course of time

Lower extremities

At the beginning of snowboarding, many injuries were triggered by insufficient training and defective materials. Since improved materials, in particular binding and shoes, injury risk has decreased. Previous studies reported up to 55% of the injuries of the lower extremities, especially in the **region of ankle joints, lower legs and knee joints** (Pino and Colville 1989, Berghold and Seidl 1992, Campbell et al. 1992/1003, Janes and Fincken 1993, Shealy 1993, Zollinger et al. 1994, Oberthaler et al. 1995, Wambacher et al. 1995, Dann et al. 1997). The development of appropriate **snowboard boots** and tear-proof binding inserts has led to a reduction of injuries of the lower extremities.

This reduced the injury risk of lower extremities from 41.6% in 1988 (Wambacher et al. 1995) to 19.3% in 2004 (Wambacher et al. 2001,

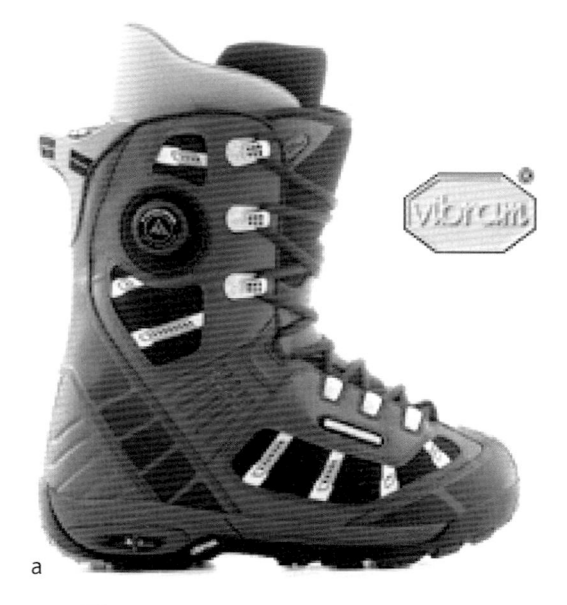

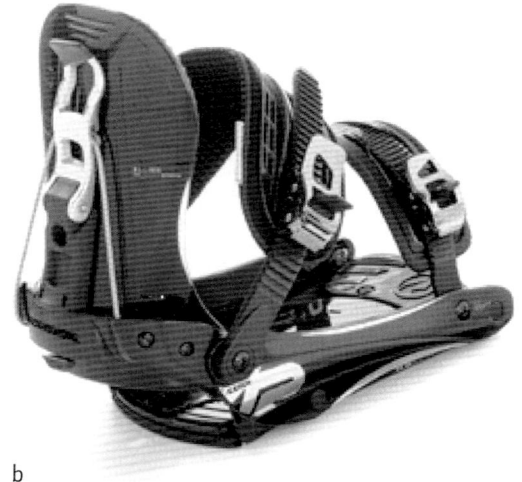

a

b

Fig. 78.2 Soft slip-in system (company: K2, type cinch).

Made and Elmqvist 2004, Xiang et al. 2005). Nevertheless, knee injuries (9.2%) have been related to **hard boots** (Wambacher et al. 2001). These boots are worn nearly exclusively in alpine racing sport. About 95% of the snowboarders wear soft boots either combined with ratchet bindings or step or slip-in bindings, respectively (➢ Fig. 78.2 a and b).

Upper extremities

Injuries of **arms and shoulders** have clearly increased. The most frequent injuries are **injuries near the wrist** (36%), they constitute up to 53% of all serious injuries especially in beginners (Ferrara et al. 1999, Idzikowski et al. 2000, Machold et al. 1999 and 2002, O'Neill and McGlone 1999, Sacco and Sartorelli 1998, Shorter et al. 1999, Xiang et al. 2005).

A prospective randomized trial with 5,029 snowboarders in Norway demonstrated that **wrist protectors** in snowboard gloves reduce the injury risk at the wrist significantly (Ronning et al. 2001). Their usefulness was proven in an independent study (Staebler et al. 1999); the use of these extensor-and flexor-sided protectors had similar beneficial effects (Machold et al. 2002, O'Neill 2003, Made and Elmqvist 2004, Matsumoto et al. 2004). Industry has reacted and started production of adapted **gloves** (➢ Fig. 72.3; Dann et al. 2002).

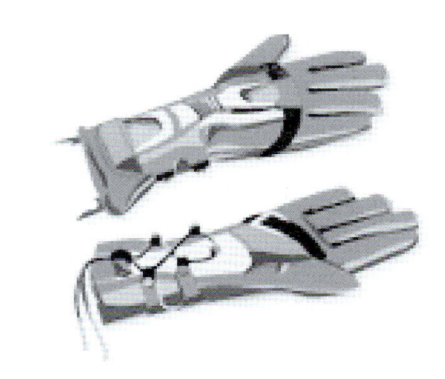

Fig. 78.3 Wristguards (company: Ziener GmbH).

Torso and spine injuries

Japanese studies show that beginners of snowboarding show significantly more spinal injuries with and without impairment of the spinal cord or even **paraplegia** (Seino et al. 2001, Yamakawa et al. 2001). This is different to beginners of skiing. There have been reports of **serious craniocerebral injuries** even with **fatal** cases (Naguchi et al. 1999).

Interestingly, Genital injuries in Japanese female snowboarding beginners had developed by **falls on the buttocks and collisions** with the high-backs of the posterior soft binding (Kanai 2001).

In summary, these studies show that serious injuries mainly affect beginners, which is explained by lack of **training and experience**. Serious spinal injuries and cases of death occur typically in high-alpine territories, where falls over rocks, steep areas and avalanche accidents have led to polytraumas with lethal consequences (Gabl et al. 1991, Tarazi et al. 1999).

> Two thirds to three quarters of all injuries are close to the wrist and can be prevented with extensor and flexor wrist protectors. Back protectors and snowboard helmets are urgently recommended for beginners, but also for advanced snowboarders.

78.3.3 Chronic injuries

35% of the examined snowboarders complained about permanent conditions in snowboarding. The **knee joint** had been affected with 34.2%, followed by the shoulder joint with 14.5% and the upper ankle joint with 9.4%. The lumbar spine as well as fingers and wrist had been next (Dann et al. 1997). Furthermore, many snowboarders reported **shoe pressure problems** (Kristen and Dann 1996).

78.4 Snowboard competition disciplines and their injury patterns

The following snowboard competition disciplines are distinguished:

- alpine competition disciplines with
  - parallel slalom (PS)
  - giant slalom also as a parallel competition (PGS)
- freestyle competitions with super, half and quarter pipe (snowboarding in artificially constructed obstacles, similar to skateboarding)
- straight jump or big airs (BA): jump disciplines, in which width (up to 40 m) and altitude of the jump (15 m) and performance are rated
- Snowboard cross (SBX) as latest competitive discipline – a fused competition of alpine and freestyle elements. After the joint start, several boarders ride through an artificially constructed course
- Free riding as most original snowboard discipline (riding in unprepared territories, surfing in deep powder snow); this is also performed as tour snowboarding or backcountry snowboarding with climbing supports such as snow shoes, short skis and split boards.
- Extreme free riding: a fully autonomous scene and competitive risk discipline of snowboarding sport is the snowboarding of extremely steep slopes with tilts of more than 50°.

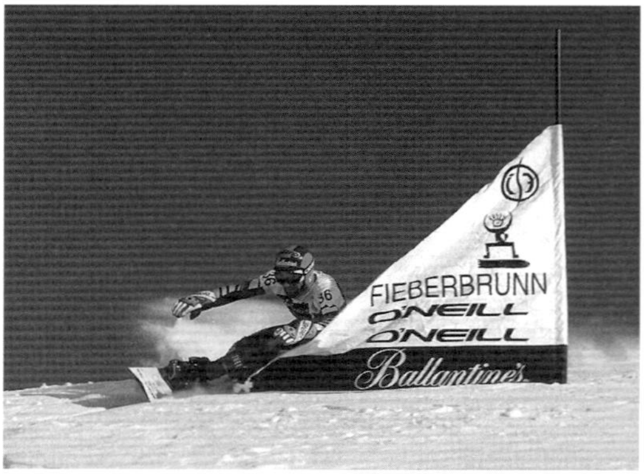

Fig. 78.4 Alpine racing: perfect carving technique (Gerry Ring/photograph: private).

78.4.1 Alpine disciplines

The alpine disciplines (racing, parallel slalom and parallel giant slalom) lost their appeal within the last 5 years, although GS carving has been chosen as an Olympic discipline in Nagano. Triangular gates adapted for snowboarding are passed similar to ski giant slalom. Symmetrical, stiff racing boards and hardboards are used for this (➤ Fig. 78.4). There are only few injury surveys of professional top snowboarders.

In a study of former ISF professionals (International Snowboard Federation; Kristen and Dann 1996, Dann et al. 2002), the **most common serious injuries** are:

- lower extremities in up to 39%
- upper extremities in 26%
- spine in 23% and
- cranium in 10%.

The most frequent localizations of serious injuries have been the **shoulder** with 12%, the **knee** with 11% and the **cervical spine** with 11%. The injuries of **hands and fingers** caused by contacts to the gates poles account for 37%, shoulder and knee joints for 36% or 33%, respectively, and ankle joints for 28% of injuries in professional snowboarders (Schrank et al 1999). Four in 1,000 injuries have been recorded in competitive runs (Torjussen and Bahr 2005); dorsal, knee as well as forearm and wrist injuries were mostly affected.

78.4.2 Freestyle

The freestyle disciplines in the **classic half pipes** refer to a trend, which is very popular amongst young people. Freestyle is a game with the own body, in which **individuality, creativity and style** are expressed. It has become an Olympic discipline; individual runs are evaluated by difficulty level, performance and overall impression in competition by an independent jury.

Snow parks with half pipes are meanwhile widespread in many skiing areas. **Insufficient techniques** and **self-overestimation** often lead to serious falls and injuries.

Half-pipe snowboarding has 8.6% higher injury risk than piste snowboarding (Dann et al. 1996).

Previously, loss rates of 18% per season in men and 11% in women had been typical even in professional snowboarders (Dann et al. 1996).

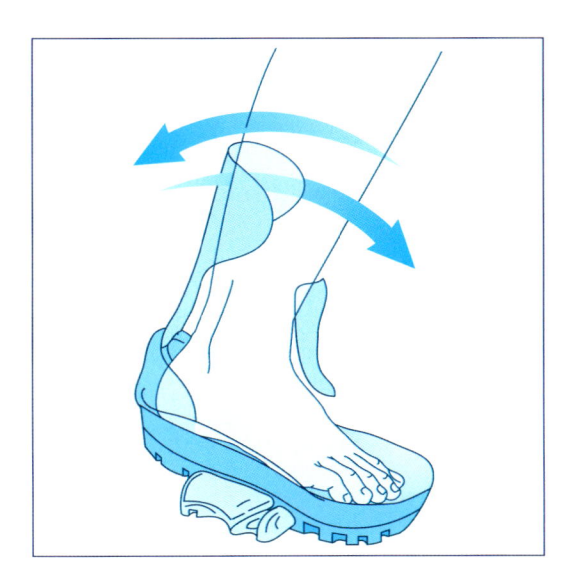

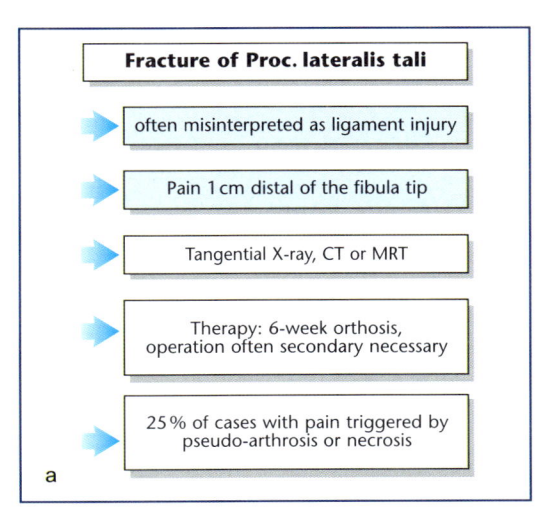

78.4 Snowboard competition disciplines and their injury patterns

Fig. 78.5 Soft step-in system, injury mechanism of snowboarder's ankle.

Serious injuries of the **lower extremities** and **knee joint** occurred in 19.4% (primarily internal ligament and internal meniscus lesions). In recent years, **cruciate ligament injuries** increased. 10 m jumps are possible over the half-pipe edge. Landing in the flat part of the pipe presses the lower leg being into an "anterior drawer" (quadriceps tension in dorsal position and stiff high backs of the soft bindings), which ruptures **the anterior cruciate ligament**. **Tibial plateau fractures** with complex ligament injuries have also been observed.

The most frequent injury at the ankle joint of the freestylers is the **fibular ligament rupture** (50%), followed by 14% of external ankle fractures with and without involvement of the internal ankles and 7% each of midfoot and talus fractures.

Especially the fracture of the processus lateralis tali, described for the first time in 1996 as **"snowboarder's ankle"** is often ignored and affects 15% of all ankle joint injuries (Bladin and McCrory 1996, Kirkpatrick et al. 1998, Boldrino and Furian 1999, Estes et al. 1999, Platz and Sommer 2000). This injury mainly occurs at the anterior ankle in dorsal extension and hyperpronation if **landing** with soft boots (➤ Fig. 78.5; Kirkpatrick et al. 1998, Boldrino and Furian 1999, Estes et al. 1999, Platz and Sommer 2000). This injury is often misinterpreted and treated as fibular ligament lesion. It can be visualized by **tangential radiographs X-ray**, tomography or CT (➤ Fig. 78.6 a and b).

Fracture of Proc. lateralis tali
- often misinterpreted as ligament injury
- Pain 1 cm distal of the fibula tip
- Tangential X-ray, CT or MRT
- Therapy: 6-week orthosis, operation often secondary necessary
- 25% of cases with pain triggered by pseudo-arthrosis or necrosis

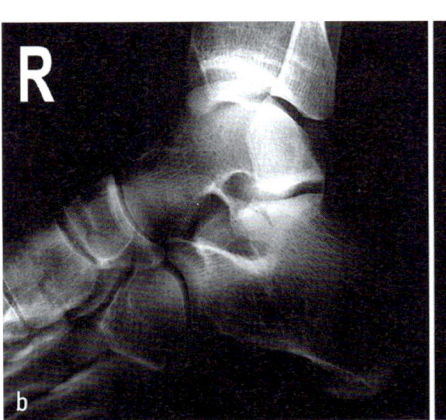

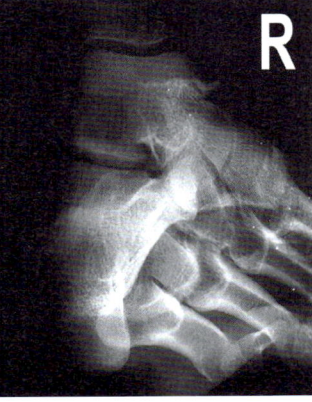

Fig. 78.6 Snowboarder's ankle (photograph: Dann).

78.4.3 Snowboard cross

Snowboard cross is a very popular and spectacular type of competition. It has been introduced to the tour program of the ISF and has also been accepted as competition by the FIS.

The snowboard cross presents a fusion of race disciplines and freestyle. Obstacles, such as rollers (ground waves), kickers (jump ramps), banks (heightened curves) and the boarders conquer corner jumps in a certain period of time. Typically, four participants mostly attempt to run the course together. The two fastest of the four are promoted to the next run. **Collisions** and **falls** often occur due to the **high velocities**, **far jumps** and difficult obstacles (➢ Fig. 78.7).

Serious **incisions** have been reported at first competitions. The loss rate amounted to 25% in men in the first season of the ISF pro tour.

The ISF has introduced **full-body protectors** (protection of back and extremities) and **helmets** in 1998/1999. This reduced the loss rate to 7% for men and to 5% for women in the following season.

Since 1999/2000, only snow **boards** with **rounded** tails and noses are allowed. **Distinct border-cross boards** have been produced and bindings and boots have been adapted to the demands of this discipline. Snowboard cross requires **good stability in boot and binding** for pick-hard courses and **flexibility of boots** to secure landing without jamming. 95% of all snowboard crossers ride on such strengthened soft boots with **step or slip-in bindings** with high-backs (spoilers) and firm toe abutments (➢ Fig. 78.2 a and b).

Medical consulting 2003 snowboard world cup in Murau

15 physicians had been present at the snowboarding world cup in Murau/Styria in 2003. 17 serious or moderate injuries resulted from a very inhomogeneous starter field with 350 athletes from 39 nations.

The world cup disciplines were alpine, parallel and parallel giant slalom, freestyle half pipe and big air and snowboard cross. The degree of injuries at this event had been significantly higher than at events of the former (International Snowboard Federation; Dann et al. 1996, Schrank et al. 1999).

Numerous ligament injuries at the knee and shoulder joints, complex fractures at the arms, numerous lacerations and incisions, cerebral concussions, and internal injuries had been treated and diagnosed.

Most injuries had appeared in the freestyle disciplines of half pipe, snowboard cross and big air, while the classic alpine competitions of parallel slalom and parallel giant slalom had only few injuries. For that reason, the Society of Orthopedic Traumatologic Sports Medicine (GOTS) suggested an improved safety for the athletes in cooperation with the snowboarding coordinator of the FIS.

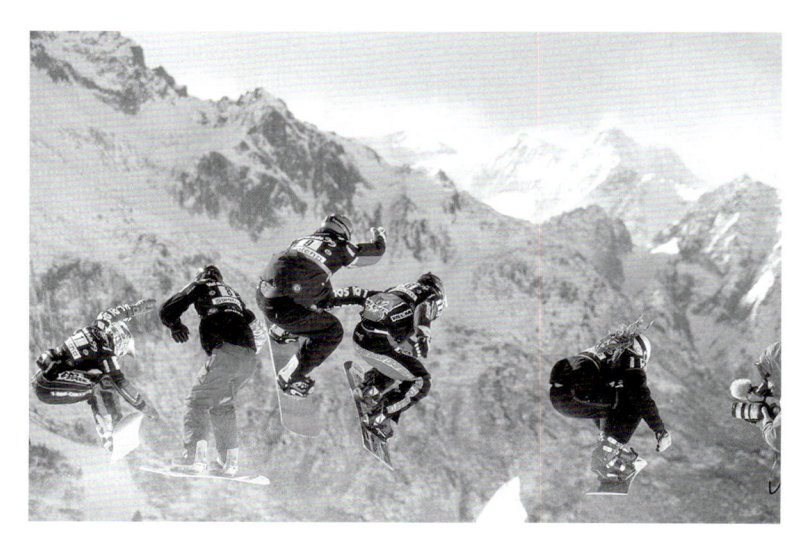

Fig. 78.7 Snowboard cross (photograph: ISF).

78.5 New materials

Injury prophylaxis in snowboard competitions:
- helmets and back protectors (mandatory for alpine and freestyle competitions)
- additional full-body protectors for SBX
- rounding of the boards with protective caps at top and rear for SBX
- harmonization of athletes' levels
- separated difficulty degrees of men and women
- technical improvements of the half pipes and jumps with diverse fall and security precautions
- The attending physician may withdraw an injured athlete from competition against the will of the responsible trainer.

78.4.4 Extreme snowboarding

Media and industry encourage young and recreational athletes to imitate spectacular rides.

Extreme snowboarding rides over steep cliffs and requires an optimally exercised fitness level of highly experienced professional alpine athletes, combined with an exact knowledge of the territory. Weeklong documentation and observation of downhill runs and planned jumps allow exercising this sport. **Full-body protectors** consisting of protection vests and pants with synthetic plates are passive protections. **Protectors of the extremities** are also used. Basic **avalanche equipment** is mandatory and the backpack also serves as an additional back protection (Knöringer 2000).

78.5 New materials

Soft boots with step or slip-in bindings improved the strength transmission to the board and displaced hard boots almost entirely. The lock mechanism resembles clipless bicycle pedals.

The advantage of these systems is the convenient opening/closing of the binding and better strength transmission. They are suitable as **all-terrain solution**, especially for snowboarding in free, difficult territories with deep or compact

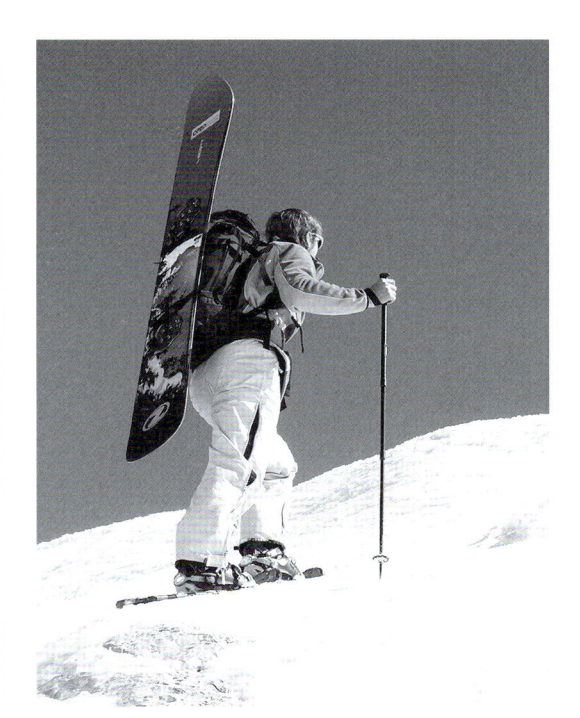

Fig. 78.8 Basic equipment for freeriding (freerider: Gerry Ring).

snow and hard pistes. The classical **ratchet bindings** is still used and very popular with the hardcore boarders and freestylers.

The **boards** tend to become longer. Experienced snowboarders in free territories and in deep powder snow ride 2 m and longer boards. The **"swallow tails"** are used for powder boards.

Riding in free territories requires **basic freeride equipment**, endurance and skills. The basic equipment consists of the board and binding system mentioned above and also of avalanche beacon, probe, shovel and emergency equipment with first-aid kit and bivouac sack (➤ Fig. 78.8).

Summary

Since the Olympic Games in Nagano in 1998 snowboarding has turned from a trend sport to a winter sport of young people. More than 50% of all serious injuries are fractures near the wrist. Wrist splints integrated into the snowboarder's glove can reduce this injury to a quarter. The torso and extremity protector systems are of value for the alpine, freestyle, and snowboard-cross competitions. Young people now accept the helmets and they make sense in competition – especially in freeriding – and for children and teenagers. Beginners on rented equipment with inappropriate skiing boots are at highest risk of injuries. Injury risk is nearly similar to skiing. The injury risk of beginners is clearly higher.

References

Berghold F, Seidl AM (1992). Snowboardunfälle in den Alpen, Risikodarstellung, Unfallanalyse und Verletzungsprofil. Prakt Sport Traumatol Sportmed 1: 2.

Bladin C, McCrory P (1996). Fractures of the lateral processus of the talus: a clinical review, "snowboarder's ankle". Clin Sports Med 6(5): 124–128.

Boldrino C, Furian G (1999). Risikofaktoren beim Snowboarden. Eine empirische Studie. Institut „Sicher Leben des österreichischen Kuratoriums für Schutz und Sicherheit".

Campbell L, Soklic P, Ziegler W, Matter P (1992/93). Snowboardunfälle. Multizentrische schweizerische Snowboardstudie unter Mitwirkung der bfu. In: Matter P, Holzach P, Heim D. 20 Jahre Wintersport und Sicherheit-Davos.

Dann K, Kristen KH, Boldrino C (1996). Verletzungen von Snowboardprofis. Sportorthop Sporttraumatol 12(4): 257–260.

Dann K, Boldrino C, Kristen KH (1997). Verletzungsrisiko und Risikofaktoren beim Snowboarden. TW Sport and Medizin 9: 128–132.

Dann K, Boldrino C, Ring G (2002). Handgelenksverletzungen beim Snowboarden. Sportorthop Sporttraumatol 18: 171–174.

Estes M, Wang E, Hull ML (1999). Analysis of ankle deflection during a forward Fall in snowboarding. J Biomech Engineering 121: 243–247.

Ferrera PC, McKenna DP, Gilman EA (1999). Injury patterns with snowboarding. Am J Emerg Med 17: 575–577.

Gabl M, Lang T, Pechlaner S, Sailer R (1991). Snowboardverletzungen. Sportverletz Sportschad 5(4): 172.

Hagel BH et al. (1999). Skiing and snowboarding injuries in the children and adolescents of southern Alberta. Clin J Sports Med 9: 9–17.

Idzikowski JR, Janes PC, Abbot PJ (2000). Upper extremity snowboarding injuries. Am J Sports Med 28: 825–832.

Janes PC, Fincken GT (1993). "Snowboarding Injuries". Skiing Trauma and Safety: American Society for Testing and Materials.

Kanai M, Osada R, Maruyama K, Masuzawa H, Shih HC, Koinishi I (2001). Warning from Nagano: increase of vulvar hematoma and/or lacerated injury caused by snowboarding. J Trauma 50(2): 328–331.

Kemeny P (1989). Methoden und kritische Betrachtung der Unfallanzeige als Datenerhebungsinstrument für die Sportunfallforschung. In: Rümmele E, Kayser D (eds.). Sicherheit im Sport – Eine Herausforderung für die Sportwissenschaft. Sport und Buch Strauß, Cologne.

Kirkpatrik DP et al. (1998). The snowboarder's foot and ankle. Am J Sports Med 26: 271–277.

Knöringer M, Schaff PS, Rosemeyer B (1998). Muscular dysbalance during snowboarding. EMG and video analysis. Sport Orthop Traumatol 4: 206–210.

Knöringer M (2000). Extreme freeride snowboarding. Sport Orthop Traumatol 16: 3–6.

Kristen KH, Dann K (1996). The Occurrence of Retrocalcaneal Bursitis at Alpine Snowboarding. Paperpresentation, 2nd World Congress on Sport Trauma/ Aossm 22nd Annual Meeting/Florida.

Machold W, Kwasny O, Eisenhardt P, Kolonja A, Bauer E, Lehr S, Mayr W, Fuchs M (2002). Reduction of severe wrist injuries in snowboarding by an optimized protection device: a prospective randomized trial. J Trauma 52(3): 517–520.

Made C, Elmqvist LG (2004). A 10-year study of snowboard injuries in Lapland Sweden. Scand J Med Sci Sports 14(2): 128–133.

Matsumoto K, Sumi H, Sumi Y, Shimizu K (2004). Wrist fractures from snowboarding: a prospective Study for 3 seasons from 1998 to 2001. Clin J Sport Med 14(2): 64–71.

Nakaguchi H, Fujimaki T, Ueki K, Takahashi M, Yoshida H, Kirino T (1999). Snowboard head injury: A prospective study in China, Nagano, for two seasons from 1995 to 1997. J Trauma 46(6): 1066–1069.

Oberthaler G, Primavesi Ch, Niederwieser B (1995). Snowboardunfälle 1991–94 – eine Analyse. Sportverl Sportschad 4(9): 118.

O'Neill DF, McGlone MR (1999). Injury risk in first-time snowboarders versus first-time skiers. Am J Sports Med 27(1): 94–97.

O'Neill DF (2003). Wrist injuries in guarded versus unguarded first time snowboarders. Clin Orthop Relat Res (409): 91–95.

Pino EC, Colville MR (1989). Snowboard injuries. Am J Sports Med 17(6): 778.

References

Platz A, Sommer C (2000). Eine typische Snowboarderverletzung – die Fraktur des Processus lateralis tali. Therap Umschau 57: 756–759.

Ronning R, Ronning I, Gerner T, Engebretsen L (2001). The efficacy of wrist protectors in preventing snowboarding injuries. Am J Sports Med 29(5): 581–585.

Sacco DE, Sartorelli DH (1998). Evaluation of alpine skiing and snowboarding injury in a northeastern state. J Trauma 44: 654–659.

Schrank C, Gaulrapp H, Rosemeyer B (1999). Verletzungsmuster und -risiken von Profisportlern im Snowboardsport. Sportverl Sportschad 13: 8–13.

Seino H, Kawaguchi S, Sekine M, Murakami T, Yamashita T (2001). Traumatic paraplegia in snowboarders. Spine 26(11): 1294–1297.

Shealy EJ (1993). Snowboard vs Downhill Skiing Injuries. Skiing Trauma and Safety: Ninth International Symposium, ASTM STP 1182. In: Johnson RJ, Mote Jr. CD, Zelcer C (eds.). American Society for Testing and Evaluation, Philadelphia.

Shorter NA, Mooney DP, Harmon BJ (1999). Snowboarding injuries in children and adolescents. Am J Emerg Med 17: 261–253.

Staebler MP, Moore DC, Akelman E, Weiss AP, Fadale PD, Crisco JJ 3rd (1999). The effect of wrist guards on bone strain in the distal forearm. Am J Sports Med 4: 500–506.

Tarazi F et al. (1999). Spinal injuries in skiers and snowboarders. Am J Sports Med 27: 177–180.

Tilburg C (2000). In-area and backcountry snowboarding: medical and safety aspects. Wilderness Environ Med 11: 102–108.

Torjussen J, Bahr R (2005). Injuries among competitive snowboarders at the national elite level. Am J Sports Med 33(3): 370–377.

Wambacher M, Benedetto K-P, Gabl M, Wischatta R (1995). Verletzungsmuster beim Snowboarden. Sportorthop Sporttraumatol 11(4): 230.

Wambacher M, Hausberger K, Wischatta R, Gabl M (2001). Einfluss der Ausrüstung auf das Verletzungsmuster von Knie- und Sprunggelenk beim Snowboarden. Sportorthop Sporttraumatol 17(2): 115, Abstract 39, 16. Jahreskongress der GOTS.

Xiang H, Kelleher K, Shields BJ, Brown KJ, Smith GA (2005). Skiing- and snowboarding-related injuries treated in U.S. emergency departments. J Trauma (1): 112–118.

Yamakawa H, Murase S, Sakai H, Iwana T, Katada M, Niikawa S, Sumi Y (2001). Spinal injuries in snowboarders: risk of jumping as an integral part of snowboarding. J Trauma 50(6): 1101–1105.

Zollinger H, Gorschewsky O, Cathrein P (1994). Verletzungen beim Snowboardsport – eine prospektive Studie. Sportverl Sportschaden 31.

Chapter 79 Golf

Dietolf Hämel

The **origin** of golf has not been clarified yet. A possible forerunner of this sport had occurred in the third pre-Christian century in China. Golf has been mentioned as a Scottish national game in a document of 1457, but a game called "chole" was already mentioned in the Netherlands in 1353. Here, the word "hole" is found as well as "pat" or "kolt". The **birth** of modern golf sports is the "Honourable Company of Edinburgh Golfes" in 1744 and the building of the court of Saint Andrew in 1754, on which the 1st open had been carried out in 1860. The **German Golf Federation** has been in existence since 1907. Nevertheless, golf had already been played for the first time in 1889 in the spa park of Hamburg.

In modern times, golf has become the **most frequently exercised sport worldwide** before volleyball and basketball. The reasons of the popularity are probably multi-faceted: There is an increased health consciousness in addition to an increased recreational need in our prosperous society. In addition to physical and mental fitness, there is also the endeavor to free from everyday stress by exercising a sport in a nice environment and fresh air.

Golf is a sport, which can be exercised **at any age** and is well adapted to individual preconditions. Persons who are suffering diseases of the locomotor apparatus or the cardiovascular system can exercise golf.

79.1 Basics

Facts about the physical and mental strain are only limited.

The following **physical strain** have been described:

- A **standard golf course** has 18 holes with distances varying between 200 and 435 m. This results in a **full length** of hole distances of about 6,000 m. The actual **distance** covered by the athlete may range between 6.5 and 10 km.
- The athlete bruns approximately **1,500 kcal** in every round. He can lose as much as 1 kg of body weight.
- One round in tournaments lasts approximately **5 hours**; the measured **pulse rates** during this time range between 100 and 150 beats per minute.
- The considerably increased **muscle activity** during the time of competition is reflected in the 100% increase of the **creatine-kinase**. Such an increase is only found in sports with high muscle strain, e.g. rowing. An increase of only 5% of the creatin-kinase values has been detected in the caddies of the athletes, who actually cover the same distances.
- Golf players have shown a 20% higher **pulmonary function tests** capacity as compared to unexercised persons.
- The **blood-fat values** of golf players are 15% lower.

Altogether, golf provides a **permanent load** without risky strain peaks, but with high **coordinative and mental demands**.

> Golf is an appropriate sport for persons with cardiovascular problems. There is a low injury risk, but high permanent demands of the supporting and locomotor apparatus might cause specific orthopedic problems.

79.2 Injuries

Serious injuries are extremely **rare**. They mainly affect **torso and cranium** by the impact of the golf ball. In rare cases, serious injuries are caused by the **impact of the golf club**. Rib fractures, however, are often caused by faulty technique (especially by beginners) with chopping strokes into the ground.

The majority of injuries are **minor** contusions and sprains at extremities, the shoulder girdle, back and trunk muscles.

79.3 Consequences of improper loads

Chronic conditions primarily affect the **opposite upper extremity** (e.g. the left arm and left shoulder girdle for right-handers) and the **lower part of the dorsum** (lumbar spine and lumbosacral junction/IS joint). In contrast, the lower extremities are rarely affected. The **non-dominant side** of the player is usually affected as well (mostly the knee joint; ➢ Fig. 79.1).

79.3.1 Golfer's shoulder

Affected structures: long biceps tendon, rotator cuff, bursa subacromialis, acromioclavicular joint.

Cause: overstrain syndrome by motion stereotypy of golf sport, additional degenerative adaptations of the affected structures.

Diagnosis: clinical shoulder examination, especially manual examination techniques; **sonography and nuclear spin tomography** are the examination procedures of choice. X-rays and CT only serve as clarification of osseous causes, which are rare.

Therapy: physiotherapy with manual therapy, friction massages, electrotherapy including phonophoreses, classical acupuncture treatment, therapeutic local anesthesia (TLA), temporary rest.

Prophylaxis: optimization of the swinging technique.

79.3.2 Golfer's elbow

Clinical picture: epicondylitis humeri radialis (left-sided), epicondylitis humeri ulnaris.

Cause: overstrain as a consequence of cramped, faulty holding of the club.

Diagnosis: primarily anamnestically-clinically (local tenderness on palpation at a typical point, indication of pain in movements against resistance).

Therapy: therapeutic local anesthesia, physical measures (phonophoreses, iontophoresis, ice or mild warmth, depending on tolerance), physiotherapy including friction massages, temporary immobilization, acupuncture.

Prophylaxis: optimization of the gripping technique ("over-lap" – interlocking baseball grip), improvement of the swinging technique.

79.3.3 Wrist

Clinical picture: mainly tendinitides and synovitides, especially of the extensor carpi ulnaris and radialis muscles and the extensor digiti

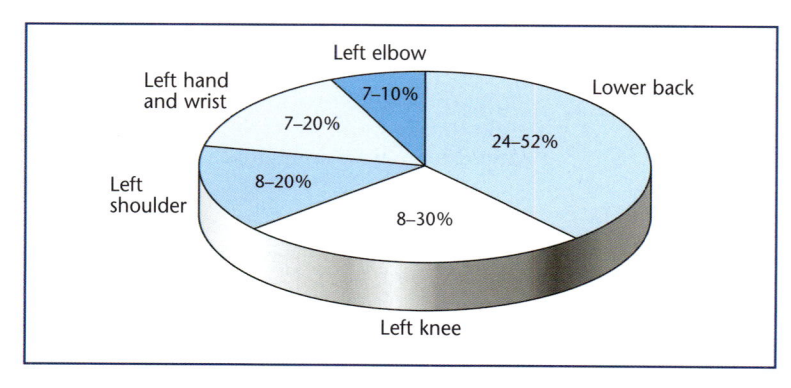

Fig. 79.1 Spreading of consequences of improper strain in golf sports (for right-handers).

79.3 Consequences of improper loads

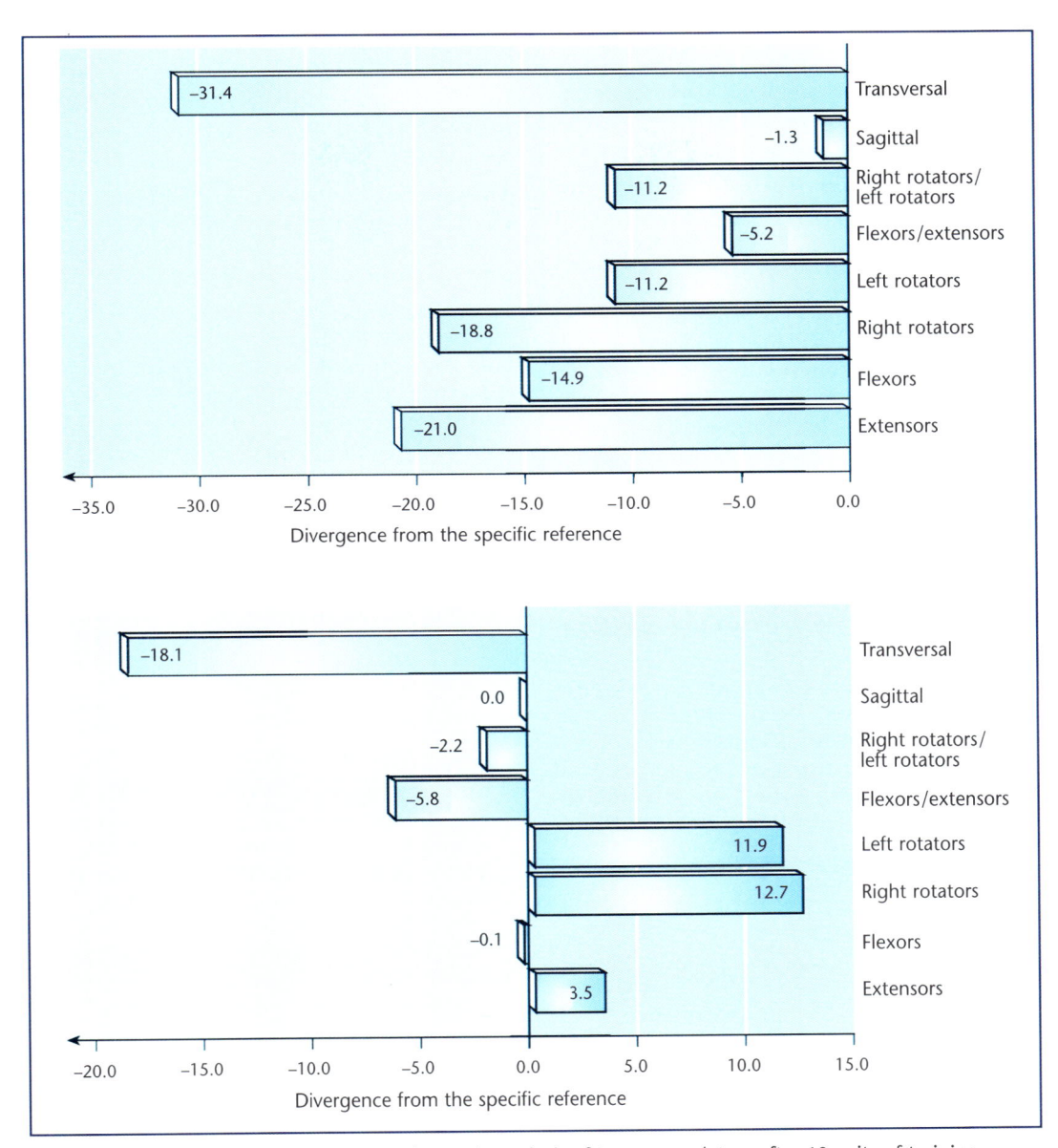

Fig. 79.2 a: Initial analysis of torso musculature, b: analysis of torso musculature after 12 units of training.

minimi muscle. What has been said above applies to **causes, diagnosis, therapy and prophylaxis**. The rupture of the discus articularis and ligament connections of the radioulnar joint and **osteoporosis-conditioned** fractures of the os hamatum, which occur rather seldom, are **traumatically** conditioned causes for medical conditions of the wrist.

79.3.4 Spine

The spine is the most strained body part in golf sport. Primarily the **lumbar spine**, followed by the spinal segments of the cervicothoracic junction is affected.

Causes: improper postures of the spine in line with the golf-specific movement procedures (especially the ones related to the spinal rotation), combined with pre-existing improper postures (e.g. hyperkyphosis, hyperlordosis), pre-existing **degenerative** changes especially in older athletes.

Diagnosis: scout film and – if necessary – nuclear spin tomography in addition to the anamnesis and clinical examination (especially techniques of manual therapy). An extensive assessment of findings should be considered especially for **athletes of a higher age** in terms of prophylaxis. This will also apply to an **analysis of the muscle functions** of the **dorsal and abdominal muscles**. An improvement of the handicap by muscle strengthening can be detected in all golfers (➤ Fig. 79.2 a and b).

Therapy: physiotherapeutic measures and methods of physical therapy, medical exercising therapy, therapeutic local anesthesia, acupuncture, implementation of non-steroid antirheumatics or other analgesics depending on the strength of present pain in the acute phase.

Prophylaxis: muscle-strengthening exercises considering especially the strengthening of antagonistic/contralateral muscle groups, improvement of the stroke technique, removal of existing functional (e.g. muscle dysbalances) or anatomic disorders (leg-length differences).

79.3.5 Lower extremities

Clinical pictures:

- hip joint: tendopathies at the trochanter major, bursitis trochanterica
- knee: internal meniscus irritation or ruptures, irritations of the internal ligament
- upper ankle joint: stretching of the fibular collateral ligament
- Achilles tendon: tendinoses.

Causes: Movement processes typical for the golf swing, here the triggering of chronic impairments by faulty swing with consecutive malposition (e.g. valgus position with external rotation of the knee joint) as cause of meniscus irritations and irritations of the internal ligament; meniscus tears as a consequence of abrupt movements and rotations are rather rare.

Diagnosis: anamnesis/clinical findings, further imaging procedures as required (sonography, X-ray, MRI).

Therapy: rest/immobilization according to the conditions, physical methods, NSAIDs in the acute phase, TLA or acupuncture for chronically therapy-resistant conditions.

Prophylaxis: muscle-strengthening exercises especially for the muscles guiding the hip and knee joints in addition to the optimization of the stroke and swing techniques, general coordination exercises.

79.4 Golf after surgeries of the locomotor apparatus

Golf sport is possible after surgeries at the locomotor apparatus, especially artificial joint substitution at hip and knee joint, and after surgeries of the intervertebral disks or conservatively treated herniated intervertebral disks.

The following should be considered:

- Sport-specific exercises and strain should be integrated carefully in the therapy – according to the constitution of the patient – in line with the (in-patient?) rehabilitation already 3–4 weeks after the surgical treatment. Special attention should be paid to a modification – adapted to each disease – of the postures and movement processes the athlete had been used to previously.

- Increase loads can be accomplished after reaching full capacity and good muscular stability also regarding the sport-specific movement processes (up-swinging to "finish", avoiding a lordosis).

The **precondition** for this is the physician's and the physiotherapist's sufficient knowledge of the sport and its strain as well as sufficient sport-medical knowledge by coach and professionals. The **technical training** should be adjusted to the according clinical picture after consultation with the physician. A **resumption** of playing golf can be thought of with a generally uncomplicated healing process and a quickly starting golf-specific exercise program already 4–6 months after surgery or a herniated disk.

79.5   Further aspects

The success in playing golf is based to 90% on **mental factors** in addition to physique and technique, which have been treated before. It is therefore also the task of the sport physician to support the athlete by means of **mental training**.

Golf as one of the modern trend sports is of increasing **relevance** for the sports physician – also in **mass sports**. There are still substantial deficits of knowledge regarding the physical as well as the mental demands.

Further efforts should be made to improve the sport-specific and sport-medical treatment.

References

Boomer P (1998). On learning golf. Random House, New York.

Chamberlain P (1999). Golf-Rezepte – 72 schwierige Situationen meistern Hürden. BLV-Verlagsgesellschaft, Munich.

Cochran A, Stoobs J (1968). The search for the perfect swing. Triumph Books, London.

Hamster R (2003). Golf. BLV-Verlagsgesellschaft, Munich.

Hebron M (1993). Golf Mind, Golf Body, Golf Swing. Smithtown Landing Country Club, New York.

Kölbing A (2001). Richtig gutes Golf. BLV-Verlagsgesellschaft, Munich.

Rotella B (1999). Golf ist Selbstvertrauen. BLV-Verlagsgesellschaft, Munich.

Tomasi T J (2001). The 30-Second Golf Swing. Harper Resource, New York.

Motorsports

Bernd Rosemeyer

The first car race of the world was carried out in 1887 in Paris – with only one participant – and Georges Bouton established the **first speed record** during this event. He reached an average speed of **26 km/h** on the Paris-Versailles distance on a steam tricycle of the "De Dion Bouton Trepardoux" type. This date is considered the beginning of speed records and car races. A race from Paris to Rouen took place in 1894 over a distance of 126 km with some more participants. Since that time, the events have become more regular, more extensive and more difficult. They have always been used as a test of the state-of-the-art automobiles. Until today, innovations developed for motor sports are adapted to serial production.

Every type of motor sport is intriguing for the active athletes and spectators who in everyday-life use cars as well. The motor racer shows currently achievable limit of a vehicle. Some figures: a **formula one car** can accelerate from 0 to 200 km/h (124 mph) in less than 5 sec, which requires a distance of 149 m. The deceleration from 200 km/h to 0 will take 1.9 sec at a distance of 55 m (!) with triple engine power. Gravitational deceleration forces reach up to 5 G! The deceleration is much more powerful for the pilots of formula cars and drivers and co-drivers in rally sports than the possible acceleration.

Mastering these powerful forces is fascination but always carries the potential danger of an **accident with serious injuries**. Unfortunately this is **also true for the audience**. On June 11, 1955, the Mercedes of Pierre Levegh flew into the crowd at the 24-hour-race of Le Mans. 82 spectators and Levegh died. This tragedy has slowed down substantially the technophilia of car races and has changed the security awareness of people visiting racing events. Fortunately, not every spectacular accident is dangerous for the driver. Rollovers and turns will annihilate a lot of energy! Senna and Ratzenberger had been victims to the last deathly accidents in 1994.

Crash tests for the frontal and lateral parts, **black box** and many more are mandatory nowadays.

80.1 Definition

Motor sport involves many fields and other formulas in addition to Formula 1 (including the US).
Races on high-speed ovals are of a different fascination and present different problems than races on our rather curvy rounds. This also applies for pure **acceleration competitions** (dragster races), which are carried out in different vehicle classes according to special rules. The **German Touring Car Masters** (DTM) is carried out with cars, which look similar to our everyday cars even though they are pure racing cars. **Rally sport** has provided spectacular driving scenes in the past and present. **Motocross races** and events with "all terrain vehicles" have their own fans but remain small. **Motorcycle racing** is a sport for "tough guys" with a special attraction and its own problems.

> The driving speed itself is not problematic, but the interval of speed changes and potential possible curve speeds.

The **sport-medical problem** and **solution** remain always identical:

- improve the active security with optimal physical fitness
- passive protection of the driver
- avoid long decelerations in accidents by setting passive brake elements along the racing courses
- optimize medical and technical support after accidents.

80.2 Equipment

In the 1930s, cars were equipped insufficiently according to today's safety standards. Nonetheless, cars had been driven fast on dangerous speedways. In 1937, the top speed of grand prix vehicles on the round track (AVUS in Berlin) amounted to 380 km/h (236 mph). At a world record attempt in 1938, my father had an accident in an open car at 440 km/h (273 mph) on a 9 m (30 ft) wide expressway made of concrete slabs.

At that time, drivers had no seat belts; only dust caps and racing goggles. The racetracks run through cities along houses and thick tree trunks, which had only been protected by bales of straw – with the consequence of serious or even fatal injuries.

The speed is the basic problem – today even more than in old times. 330 km/h (200 mph) on a straight road is no problem for experienced pilots. It becomes difficult if the **speed changes drastically within a short period of time**. Racetracks without runout zones or guard rails along houses and trees have been and still are extremely dangerous.

This is still valid in a modified way for the **high-speed ovals** in America that are limited by walls. The passive protection systems are effective, although the accidents look spectacular. If the vehicle impacts an obstacle in a steep angle without braking, the forces occurring in deceleration are so strong that they cannot be compensated even by the best passive protection systems. The limit of our body that mainly consists of water is easily reached; serious injuries are the consequence.

One case of death per year has been recorded **until 2001**, although the equipment had clearly improved with the introduction of Formula 1. **Every sixth** of the active formula-one racers died at that time in an accident.

Today's security standards are very high. They include (but are not limited to):

- optimal fitness of the driver
- passive safety within the vehicle and speedway:
  - survival cell, enlarged and cushioned cockpit opening, six-point safety belts, protective clothes
  - energy-absorbing steering post, safety tanks (coming from aircraft construction), dual fire fighting system
  - HANS system (head and neck support system)
  - seat that is rescued together with the driver
  - Kendrick Extrication Device (KED)

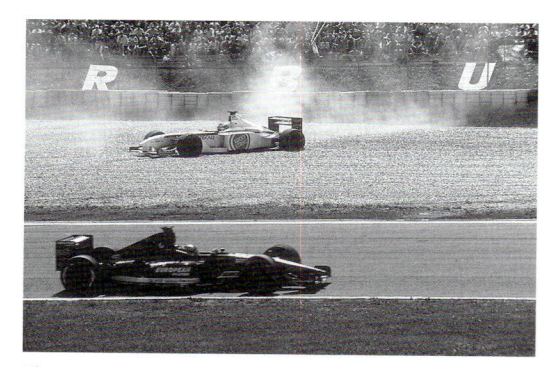

Fig. 80.1 Run-off area with gravel trap and multi-row tire barriers drastically reduce collision speed.

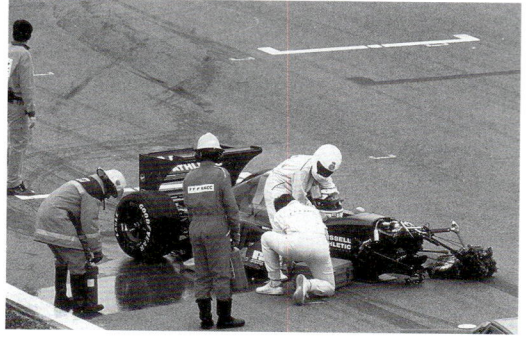

Fig. 80.2 Security squad at work. Fast intervention of an inter-disciplinary team.

- computer simulation of the speedway (how much fall space and gravel bed is necessary, in order to reduce the impact?)
- piles of tires (➤ Fig. 80.1), safety squad (➤ Fig. 80.2), rescue helicopters
- medical centers for first aid of injured persons.

Stefan Bellof has lost his life in the famous full-speed passage "Eau Rouge" 20 years ago. Schneider, however, was protected by a safe car, larger fall spaces, four rows of piled-up tires and the HANS system despite flying off with a speed of 232 km/h (144 mph). He got out of his fully destroyed car without any injuries.

80.3 Most frequent injuries and overstrain impairments

The range of injuries is large and depends on the size and the effect of the occurring forces.

Main injuries are:
- cervical spine (➤ Fig. 80.3)
- cranial base
- wrists and
- feet (➤ Fig. 80.4).

The cervical spine carrying head and helmet is not able to cope with the forces occurring in racing sport – even with a maximum exercise of the neck and cervical muscles. The **weight of the head with the helmet** can increase up to the 80-fold. No matter how well exercised the muscle corset is, such forces cannot be compensated.

This led to the development of the **head and neck support system**. It has been tested and accepted by the FIA (Fédération Internationale de l'Automobile) in 2002. Its use is implemented worldwide since 2003 for Formula 1, DTM, Formula 3, cart races, NASCAR and other races. This measure drastically reduced the incidence of serious injuries of the cervical spine and fractures of the cranial base, which had been the most frequent cause of death in racing sport.

Accidental injuries of the **spinal segments** became worse during rescue of the driver. This led to the development of **seats that are rescued together with the driver**.

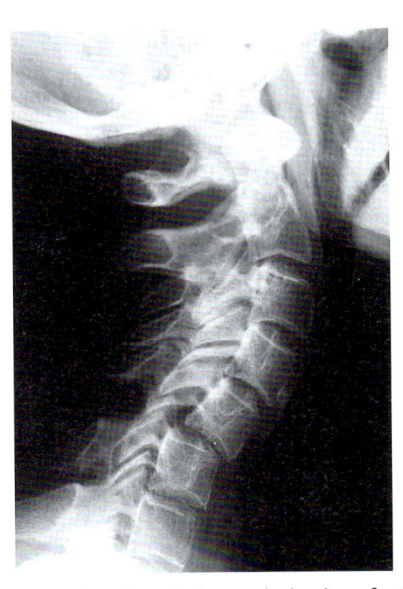

Fig. 80.3 Subluxation of the cervical spine of a formula-1 driver in movement segment C5/6 after a collision with an obstacle at 220 km/h (136 mph).

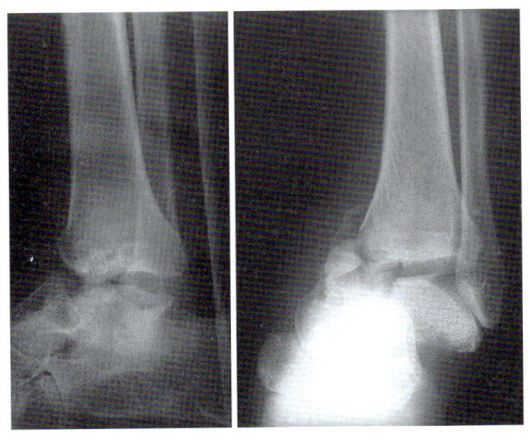

Fig. 80.4 Internal malleolus dislocation fracture and "luxatio sub talo" of a rally driver after an accident in the forest at 190 km/h (118 mph).

In order to limit the tech race of the teams, a very **complex set of rules** with standardized tires, standardized electronics, limited race time etc. has been **introduced in 2008**.

The combination of unconsciousness and unstable spine after an accident is extremely dangerous for the neural spinal cord structures.

At frontal collision, the **wrists** are particularly exposed to the forces transmitted over the steering wheel. **"Hands off the steering wheel and wait!"** is the golden rule for all uncontrolled accidents in Formula 1.

The **lumbar spine** is the primary target of overuse impairments. Different curving increases the internal pressure of the intervertebral disks (Anderson et al. 1974). The constricted space of the cockpit does not allow for drivers with a large physical size. But even small drivers are forced to compromises regarding body posture. The driver are rather in a lying than sitting position with legs higher than the buttocks, although the seat is adjusted individually with a lot of effort (➢ Fig. 80.5).

Hence, the **spine** is less compressed by compression forces (which would be physiological) than by **shear forces**. Formula 1 has only the advantage over long-distance races and rallies: the time of the uncomfortable sitting position is only very limited and easier tolerated.

Linke described an increased incidence of **relapsing dorsal conditions** of 89.5% in touring-car drivers and 66.7% in formula-three-race drivers compared to 35.5% of matched control group race drivers (Linke 2001).

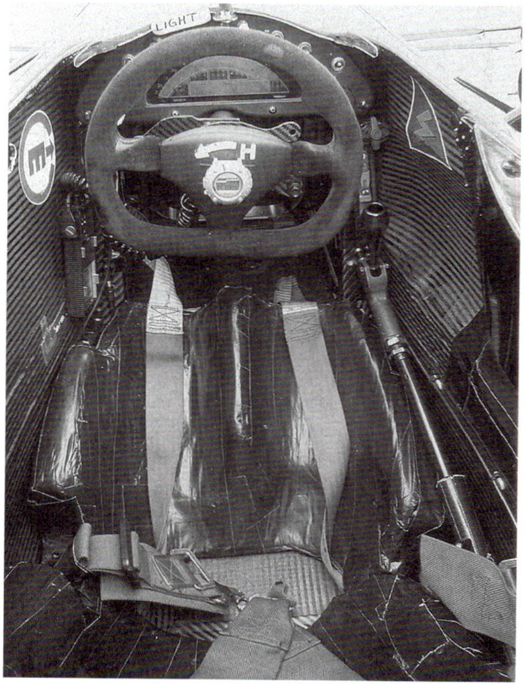

Everybody following up with race drivers knows these problems. The **non-physiological sitting position** enforced by the spatial constrictions causes problems (Rosemeyer 1975). The athletes are generally young, have only few degenerative changes in the lumbosacral motion segment, are well exercised, and perform their sport with so much commitment that they tolerate these problems.

The **psychophysical strain** of the race drivers plays an important role as well (Scheidt 1993). Motor sports are high-performance sports, they cannot be carried out successfully without comprehensive and specific training. The physical strain to the driver is very high at start and precarious situations. Interestingly, the co-driver in rally sports is much more affected than the driver. Increased tension reduces performance.

> The number of racing accidents increases with too few regeneration.

Systematic endurance exercises and **psychological training** can reduce body tension.

The situation in **motorcycle racing** is different. Only **few passive elements for accident protection** can be built into the motorcycle. For a long time, the speedways of motorcycles had only a limited fall space. The motorcycle itself also presents a danger for the driver. While uncontrolled slipping despite large dynamics usually passes without serious injuries (if the driver does not collide with an obstacle), a slipping 'controlled' by some act of the driver often lead to overreactions. The motorcycle straightens up and throws the driver off (**"highsider"**). The driver falls from 2 m directly in front of the motorcycle. Serious injuries are usually the consequence.

Uncontrolled driving situations are also the highest risk for the driver in dragster races, pure acceleration competitions. However, serious injuries occur mostly by the unsuccessful try to gain control of the situation. Experienced pilots know that and activate the deceleration parachute.

Motor sport, which had formerly been marked by a high injury risks, has not lost its fascina-

Fig. 80.5 Orthopedic unfavorable, half-lying sitting position in Formula 3 racing cars (photograph: Linke).

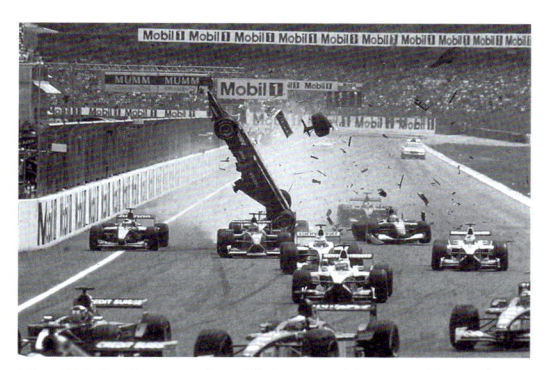

Fig. 80.6 Rear-end collision accident at Formula 1. None of the involved drivers was injured.

tion. It is not life threatening anymore and the risk of serious injuries has decreased significantly (➤ Fig. 80.6). Ideas developed on the raceway still enter serial production, despite today's simulation techniques. Finally, also the national pride to build the best car and to be able to drive faster than the competitors continue to play an important role.

References

Anderson B J G, Örtengren R, Nachemson A, Elfström G (1974). Scand J Rehab Med 6: 128–133.

Linke RD (Dissertation 2001). Wirbelsäulenbeschwerden im Automobilrennsport.

Rosemeyer B (1975). Schädigung des Bewegungsapparates durch falsche Haltung im Autositz. Z Orthop 113: 653–655.

Scheidt S (1993). Die psycho-physischen Belastungen des Autofahrers im Straßenverkehr und im Rennsport und die sich hieraus ergebenden präventiven und trainingswissenschaftlichen Konsequenzen. Diplomarbeit Deutsche Sporthochschule Köln.

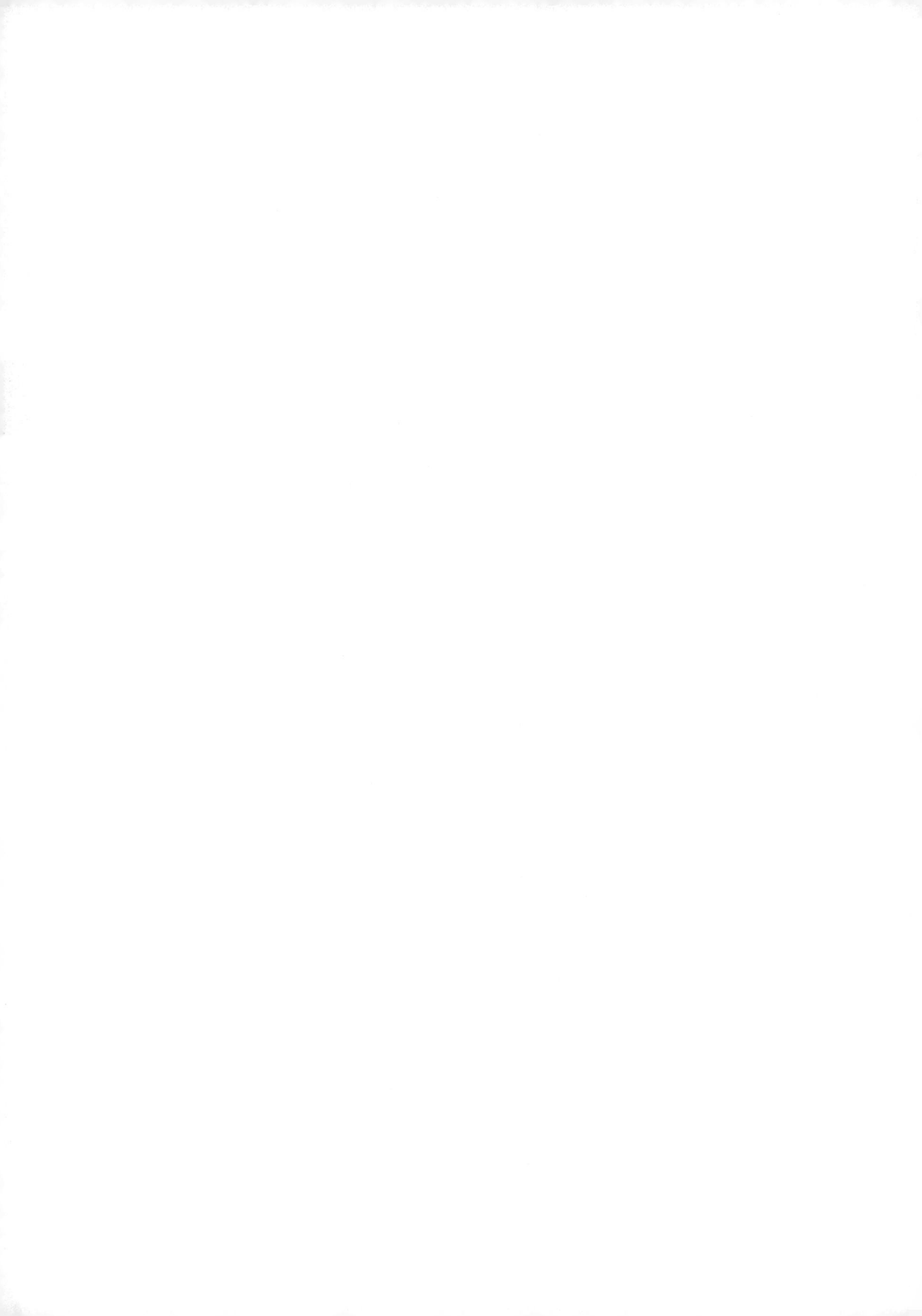

Chapter 81 Equestrianism

Thomas Rodt, Lisette Rodt and Gerhard Sybrecht

Equestrianism can be divided in the Olympic disciplines of dressage, show jumping and eventing and horse racing, endurance riding, western riding, and polo (➤ Tab. 81.1). **Elderly** can perform equestrian sport if horses are well-trained and show a controlled, safe behavior. This animal-man partnership is a particularity and special opportunity of equestrian sport, but the risk of accident can never be excluded completely. Prevention in equestrianism is possible with training **general fitness, coordination, flexibility, and concentration**. A **cardiopulmonary protection** is not mandatory (Sybrecht 1991). Equestrianism offers a movement dialogue between rider and horse and the possibility of life-long activity on the horseback (Sybrecht 1991).

Equestrianism has an immense economic meaning given its yearly sales of more than 5 billion Euros in Germany alone (IPSOS 2001).

Tab. 81.1 List of some equestrian disciplines and their estimated risk of injuries.

Discipline	Typical injuries	Injury risk
dressage	■ chronic dorsal complaints ■ myositis ossificans	+
show jumping	■ adductor strain ■ rib contusions/fractures ■ craniocerebral traumas ■ osseous injuries of the extremities	++
eventing	■ rib contusions/fractures ■ craniocerebral traumas ■ osseous injuries of the extremities ■ injuries of the pelvic ring ■ spine injuries	+++
horse racing	■ rib contusions/fractures ■ craniocerebral traumas ■ osseous injuries of the extremities ■ injuries of the pelvic ring ■ spine injuries	+++
vaulting	■ ligament injuries and fractures, of the ankles and the knee joints above all	+
recreational horseback riding	■ osseous injuries of the extremities ■ craniocerebral traumas	++
endurance riding	■ chronic dorsal conditions ■ myositis ossificans	+

81.1 Injury patterns, mechanisms and frequencies

Acute injuries and to a minor extent also **chronic overstrain impairments** can be found in equestrianism (Heipertz 1997). Injury patterns, mechanisms and frequencies have been studied. However, general conclusions regarding the etiology of the injuries and overstrain impairments should be interpreted with caution given the relatively small number of cases and methodological differences (Biener 1992, Braun 1993, Ceroni et al. 2007, Schmidt et al. 1994, Heipertz 1997, Petridou et al. 2004). A substantial amount of the accidents (up to 35%) happens when preparing the horses and not during riding itself (Thomas et al. 2006); beginners are at a higher risk of injuries (Mayberry et al. 2007). The number of potentially avoidable injuries – false behavior or wrong equipment – is considerably high. A relevant amount of injuries is related to the use of alcohol or drugs (Carillo et al. 2007).

Head injuries are the most frequent injuries in equestrianism caused by

- falls off the horse
- the horse's head surging up during riding, and
- the horse's kicking in daily routine.

There is a wide field of possible injuries – ranging from a **simple commotio cerebri** even to a **serious craniocerebral trauma** that is occasionally overlooked at first sight. Special attention is therefore needed when clarifying apparently trivial head injuries.

Injuries of the shoulder girdle and the upper extremities (➢ Fig. 81.1 a and b), especially clavicular fractures and fractures of the forearm, and dislocations belong to the frequent injuries (Turner et al. 2008). **Finger amputations** at holding and leading the horses are rare and can be avoided with correct technique, e.g. avoiding a slinging of the rope.

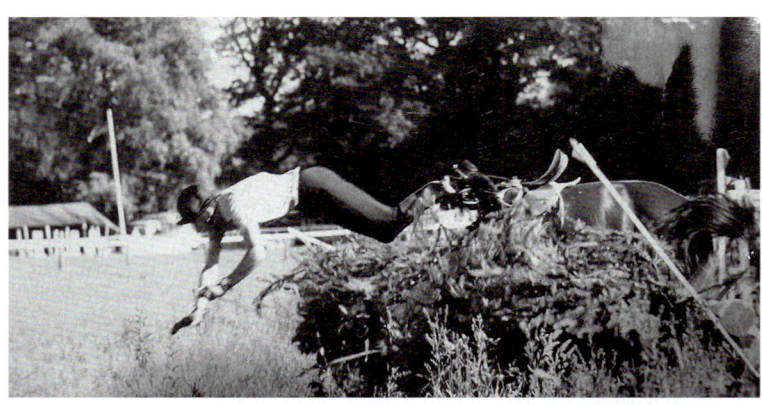

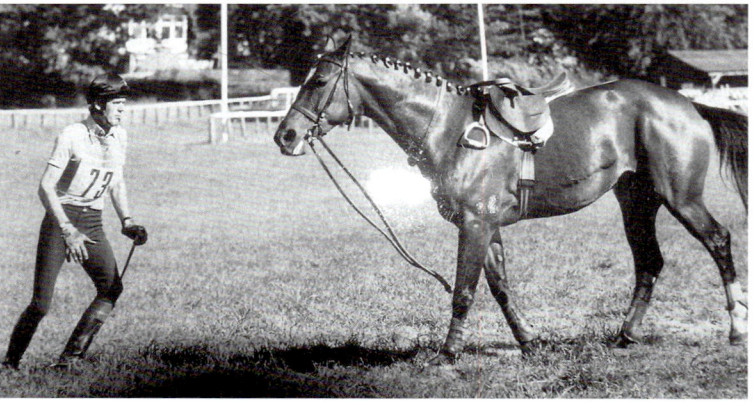

Fig. 81.1 Fall mechanism, which can lead to injuries of the shoulder girdle and the upper extremity. Fall at the eventing race track, because the horse refuses to jump. The rider falls off and away from the horse because of the high initial speed, and therefore is safe. Even spine fractures may be a result at an unfavorable landing because of the high acceleration. In the presented case, horse and rider were on their legs again at once and were able to continue the ride without injuries.

Serious injuries of torso, pelvis and spine can occur if **being run over** given the horses' weight of approximately 600 kg (➤ Fig. 81.2 a and b). This can also lead to **fatal falls**. The frequency and seriousness of thoracic traumas is often underestimated (Ball et al. 2007).

The **foot caught** in the stirrup at a fall leads to traction to the leg (➤ Fig. 81.3 a to c) and is a dangerous fall mechanism of the lower extremity. The cuboid fracture after abduction of the forefoot is another typical injury pattern (Ceroni et al. 2007). The kicking of closely standing horses can cause **fractures of the lower leg**. **Soft-tissue injuries and fractures in the region of the forefoot** also appear frequently during the care and leading of the horses. Steel-toed safety boots provide protection.

81.2 Overstrain impairments

Correct riding is a good prevention of the widespread back pain, the resonating spine on the horseback has prophylactic effects. **Chronic back pain** often develops especially in profes-

Fig. 81.2 Fall of rider and horse at a jump in the water with slow speed. The rider does not fall off and away from the horse because of the low speed. The horse that is also falling will overroll the rider. Severe blunt injuries of thorax and abdomen may be caused by this fall mechanism and, because of the severity of the trauma, also fractures of spine and pelvis. This highly dangerous fall mechanism is slightly lessened here by the damping effect of the water.

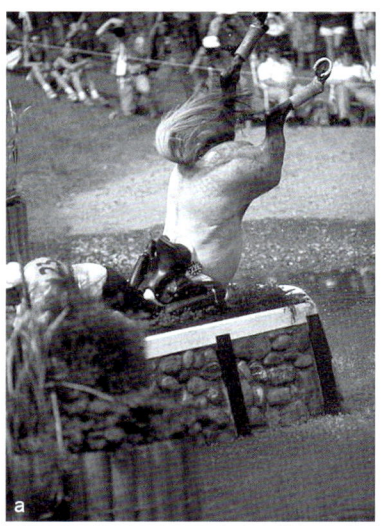

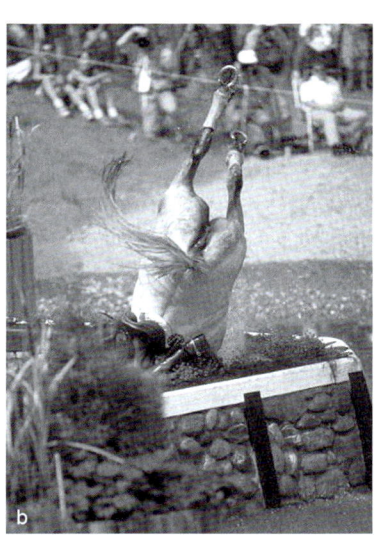

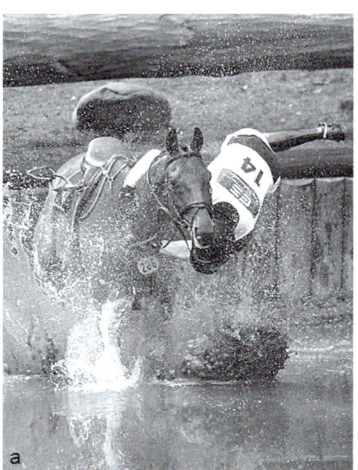

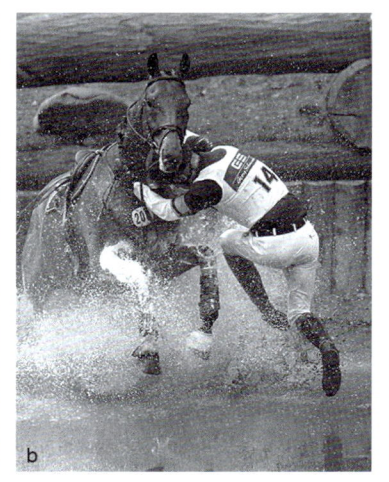

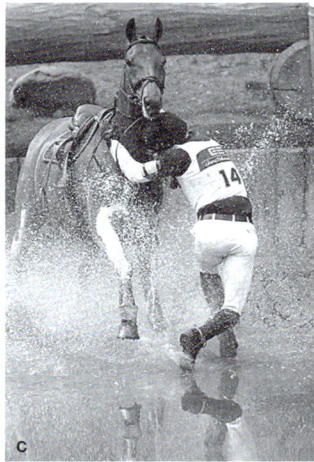

Fig. 81.3 Fall of the rider because of the sudden deceleration of the horse at the water-entering jump. The foot of the rider does not get stuck in the stirrup; but due to the landing on both legs, rotation and sprain traumas with injuries of the ligament structures or fractures of the lower extremity may result from this fall mechanism, though.

sional horse riders. This is mostly due to **repeated microtraumas** and **improper posture of the spine**. **Degenerative changes** of the spine or other causes of lumbalgia or lumboischialgia can occur, which have no direct relation to riding but are emphasized by the present strain. A detailed anamnesis, clinical examination and – if necessary – imaging diagnostics are recommended.

Painful **myositis ossificans** can be caused by **repeated microtraumas** in the region of the femoral **adductors**. Imaging is recommended.

Sonographic examinations of horse riders have hardly shown any significant differences (more frequent varicoceles/hydrocele) compared with other patients (Turgut et al. 2005).

81.3 Safety equipment

Safety helmets, which are mandatory for eventing and races, provide protection of serious head injuries (➤ Fig. 81.4 a). They have to fulfill international standards; this equally applies to **back and shoulder protectors**. Protectors have recently been available that are only triggered during fall and are inflated by a rip line – similar to airbags in cars. A **medical card** attached to the arm provides important medical background information about the potentially unconscious horse rider (Whitlock 1999). Knee protectors and helmets with face guard are used in **polo sport** (Renström 1997).

Safety stirrups have been developed to avoid the rider getting caught in the stirrup and being dragged along after a fall. These stirrups allow the foot to slip out of the stirrup. Another type of safety stirrup, which separates the stirrup at rotation similar to ski binding, has not gained general acceptance. The stirrups are usually fixed to the saddle by a safety spring and allow slipping out at traction (➤ Fig. 81.4 b).

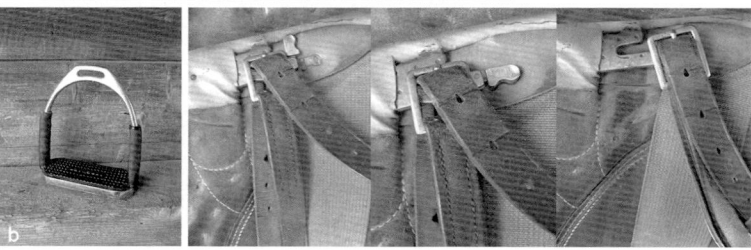

Fig. 81.4 a: Safety equipment in eventing, consisting of crash-helmet, back protector with shoulder protection and Medical Card. b: Security stirrups and spring mechanism at the saddle, which are supposed to prevent the getting stuck in the stirrup and the rider being dragged along.

The wearing of **shoes with heels** is absolutely necessary to prevent the foot from slipping through the stirrup to the front. Sturdy shoes are recommended for the handling of the horses to prevent feet injury. The equipment requires good quality to prevent falls caused by damaged material such as defective cinches, reins and brackets. Falls in **traffic** are especially dangerous. **Reflectors worn by rider and horse** are important in **twilight** for the prevention of accidents.

Concentration on the behavior of the horses in the everyday care is essential for the assessment of dangers and risks triggered by the behavior of the horse.

81.4 First aid at the site of the accident

A **medical stand-by team** is now standard in equestrian tournaments. Nevertheless, many accidents do not occur in sport events, but in the everyday handling of the horses.

The **potential danger of further injuries** of rider and assistants caused by the horse need to be considered, because the horses can show unpredictable behavior due to the event of the fall (Renström 1997). Otherwise, the emergency treatment in equestrian sports is no different from the treatment of other emergencies. Nonetheless, **minor craniocerebral traumas** have to be emphasized given their frequency and underestimation by the riders – often they wish to continue the competition.

The **spine** should always be considered for fall injuries in equestrian sport. A respective **positioning** is need at the suspicion of such injuries (Gerner 1991).

Mobile safety equipment is needed for eventings and experienced physicians should be attending to treat potentially serious injuries (Renström 1997).

References

Ball CG, Ball JE, Kirkpatrick AW, Mulloy RH (2007). Equestrian injuries: incidence, injury patterns, and risk factors for 10 years of major traumatic injuries. Am J Surg 193: 636–640.

Biener K (1992). Sportunfälle: Epidemiologie und Prävention; Lehre, Forschung, Verhütung. Verlag Hans Huber, Bern, Göttingen, Toronto.

Braun K (1993). Unfälle im Pferdesport, Unfallhergang, Verletzungen und Prävention. Dissertationsschrift, Universität des Saarlandes.

Camillo EH, Varnagy D, Bragg SM, Levy J, Riordan K (2007). Traumatic injuries associated with horseback riding. Scand J Surg 96: 79–82.

Ceroni D, De Rosa V, De Coulon G, Kaelin A (2007). Cuboid nutcracker fracture due to horseback riding in children: case series and review of the literature. J Pediatr Orthop 27: 557–561.

Gerner HJ (1991). Reitsport – prädestiniert für gravierende Wirbelsäulenverletzungen? TW Sport und Medizin 3: 270–274.

Heipertz W (1997). Reiten. In: Engelhardt M (ed.). GOTS Manual Sporttraumatologie. Verlag Hans Huber, Bern.

IPSOS (2001). Marktanalyse des FN zum Pferdesport. Deutsche Reiterliche Vereinigung e.V.

Mayberry JC, Pearson TE, Wiger KJ, Diggs BS, Mullins RJ (2007). Equestrian injury prevention efforts need more attention to notice riders. J Trauma 62: 735–739.

Petridou E, Kedikoglou S, Belechri M, Ntouvelis E, Dessypris N, Trichopoulos D (2004). The mosaic of equestrian-related injuries in Greece. J Trauma 56: 643–647.

Renström PAFH (ed.) (1997). Sportverletzungen und Überlastungsschäden: Prävention, Therapie, Rehabilitation; Eine Veröffentlichung der Medizinischen Kommission des IOC in Zusammenarbeit mit der FIMS. Dt. Übersetzung und Bearbeitung. Dt. Ärzteverlag, Cologne.

Schmidt B, Mayr J, Fasching G, Nöres H (1994). Reitsportunfälle bei Kindern und Jugendlichen. Unfallchirurg 97: 661–662.

Sybrecht GW (1991). Faszinosum Reitsport – stimmt das Image? TW Sport und Medizin 3: 266–268.

Thomas KE, Annest JL, Gilchrist J, Bixby-Hammett DM (2006). Non-fatal horse-related injuries treated in emergency departments in the United States, 2001–2003. Br J Sports Med 40: 619–626.

Turgut AT, Kosar U, Kosar P, Karabulut A (2005). Scrotal sonographic findings in equestrians. J Ultrasound Med 24: 911–917.

Turner M, Balendra G, McCrory P (2008). Payments to injured professional jockeys ind British horse racing (1996–2006). Br J Sports Med. Apr 1. (Epub ahead of print)

Witlock MR (1999). Injuries to riders in the cross country phase of eventing: The importance of protective equipment. Br J Sports Med 33: 212–216.

Chapter 82 Shooting sports

Stefan Nolte und Martin Bauer

Shooting has been an **Olympic sport** since the games of modern times and is now represented with 15 disciplines. Team competitions are carried out in national leagues (air gun and pistol, bow).

The **German Gunners Association** as umbrella organization unites 1.5 million members and also includes the 3,000 summer biathletes now. 900 persons have been registered in the section "gunners" in the **German Federation of Disability Sports**.

82.1 Sport-specific demands

Mental and sensomotor contorl is key in top shooting sports. The **performance-determining factors** are:

- sharp sight with minor fatiguing
- precise fine motor skills (e.g. trigger of the rifle of top athletes by 20 g)
- ability to concentrate permanently, e.g. for 120 shots in three position air gun (lying, standing, kneeling), possibly with participation in the finals and play offs
- sensitive perception (e.g. target acquisition, strike position, wind and light conditions), perception of the own body, so-called "internal aiming position" and
- mental stability.

These skills are objectified in practice-oriented **tests** as qualification for certain disciplines. **Motor skills** and **mental components** (relaxation techniques, concentration programs) can be exercised. The cooperation with sport psychologists plays an increasingly important role in recent years.

Shooting is performed competitively by **severely disabled** (e.g. wheelchair drivers) as well as by **visually impaired persons** (even blind persons!) at the Paralympics.

82.2 Sport equipment

Standardized sport **guns** (rifles, pistols, muskets, bows, crossbows) with different projectiles and "missiles" (pellets, rounds, lead shots, arrows, bolts) are common, which have a different **propulsion** (gas pressure, powder, tension of cross bow/bow) and hit different **targets** (stationary or mobile targets, discuses as so-called clay pigeons; ➤ Fig. 82.1).

The shooting **clothes** (jacket, pants, shoes) minimize the body's oscillation and are subject to strict controls. Stabilizing bandages are not

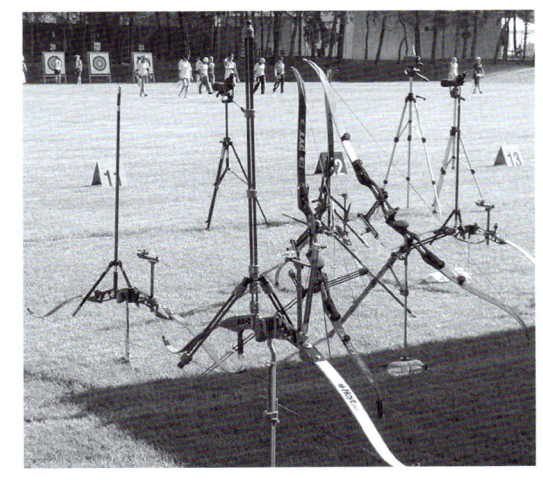

Fig. 82.1 Piece of sport equipment: recurve bow, during a shooting break.

allowed. **Shooting goggles** are adjusted to the **aiming procedure**, since notch, bead sight and disk must not be represented sharply at the same time.

Summer biathlon is run without a gun, and the shooting is performed lying or standing.

82.3 Overstrain occurrences, dangers, injuries

Sport shooting shows no susceptibility regarding sport-specific injuries – with the exception of **hearing impairments**.

However, the unilateral strain of the locomotor apparatus are problematic. This **improper strain** is the result of the primarily static aspects of many disciplines (➤ Fig. 82.2, ➤ Fig. 82.3 and ➤ Fig. 82.4):

- high intensity of exercises
- duration of the competition (up to 2 hours in qualification)

- weight of the gun (maximum weight of the guns, e.g. air rifle 5.5 kg, small calibercaliber rifle men 8 kg, rapid fire pistol 1,400 g; tension force of the bow up to 18 kg).

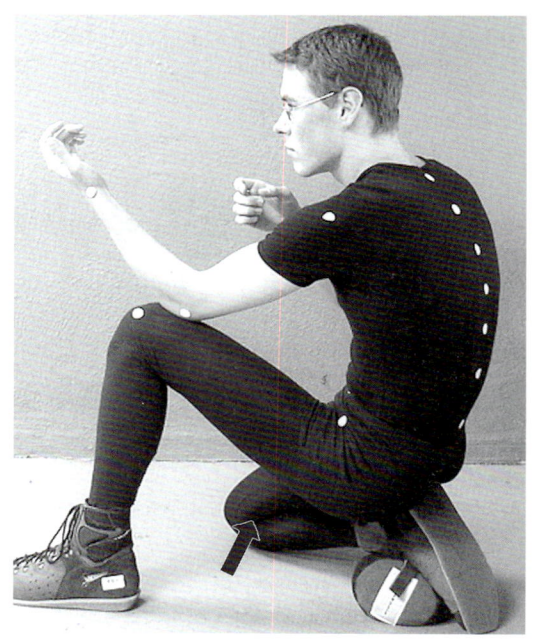

Fig. 82.3 Posture with the so-called kneeling-position rifle. Please note the strain to knee and ankle joint!

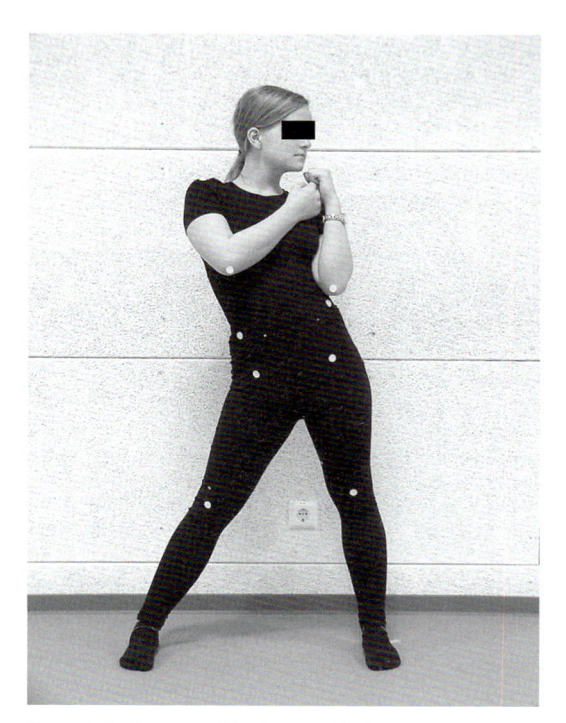

Fig. 82.2 Posture with the so-called standing-position rifle.

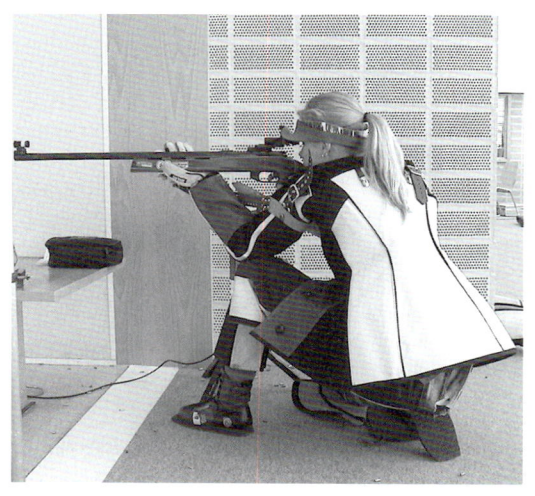

Fig. 82.4 Kneeling aiming position with shooting clothes.

82.3.1 Typical overstrains

Pistol: tendinoses of arm and shoulder (epicondylitides, overstrain of the rotator cuff and of wrist and carpal joints).

Rifle:
- Standing: overstrain syndromes of the spine (which is "locked" for to minimize the body's oscillation solely by rotation, sideways tilting, and hyperlordosing in the lumbar region). Ligamentoses and faceted strain are common here in addition to myogeloses.
- Lying: bursitis olecrani due to the rested elbow (pressure up to 12 kp on the elbow in the discipline of small caliber rifle), compression to the humerus by the shooting strap (neuropathy of the radial nerve).
- Kneeling: maximum knee flexion triggers paresthesias due to compressed vessels and nerves of the popliteal fossa, pain at disposed knee joints (retropatellar, tuberositas tibiae, posterior meniscal horns).

Bow: pain in the shoulder-nape area and at the rest of the spine due to muscular dysbalances. Tendinoses and subacromial irritation are often an indication of a too ambitious pretension of the bowstring or too much exercising.

Shotgun: contusions in the area of the AC joint and the rotator cuff as well as the anterior surface of the shoulder, humerus and cheek caused by repulsion of the gun (wrong technique). Very painful segmental blockades often appear at the junction of cervical and thoracic spine.

Summer biathlon: Prophylaxis and therapy are similar to classic running disciplines. The high competition density of winter biathletes often leads to crucially shortened regeneration times due to their participation in summer biathlon competitions. Tendinoses, muscle injuries and also fatigue fractures can develop at midfoot and tibia.

Hearing loss: The bang of shots close to the unprotected ear permanently impairs **hearing** (high-frequency lowering) – especially, if the vulnerable internal ear is affected. An acute, non-repairable hearing loss can develop after extreme deafness by shock waves ("white noise").

The intensity of top pressure, duration, the number of acoustic trauma and the duration of breaks in-between (relaxation) determine the extent of **deafness by shock waves**.

> The danger of a permanent impairment of the internal ear (and therefore hearing loss) is always a risk in shooting sports!

High-frequency lowering remains **unrecognized** at first, because the hearing loss is not that intense in the beginning.

Hearing impairments can also occur in shooting small caliber rifles (three position air gun) without any hearing protection at several exercise units per week in addition to the noise exposure of occupational and leisure-time noise.

Extent of noise exposure:
- air rifle: 112 dB
- small caliber rifle: 130 dB
- large caliber rifle: 160 dB
- in comparison: jet propulsion: 140 dB.

82.3.2 Preventive measures

Athletes, coaches, audience and competition attendants need **sufficient hearing protection**!

Electronically supported ear protectors are forbidden for athletes. Empty bullet casings stuffed into the auditory canals should actually be an obsolete measure, but they are still better than no protection!

A damping of as much as 30 dB can be achieved by **ear plugs** of wax, rubber, cotton or plastics, and **capsule ear protectors** even achieve more than 40 dB. The **otoplastics** – an individually produced "silicone drain" of the ear with special acoustic filters – can provide a damping of 25 dB over the complete frequency range. This has the advantage that the "closing effect" of common ear protections is minimized and speech can be understood in an undistorted way. A hearing test is demanded at beginning and if the athlete was exposed to noise.

Recreational sports balance the unilateral demands to the locomotor apparatus. Endurance sport as well as appropriately dosed strength training can help to prevent muscular dysbalances.

82.3.3 Endangering others

Shooting injuries are **extremely rare** as a consequence of the practiced care, storage, use and transport of the sport equipment "gun". Nevertheless, they occur.

> Sufficient hearing protection and recreational sport are the most important preconditions for the prevention of consecutive impairments in shooting sports.

82.4 Doping

Beta blockers are forbidden in shooting sports in addition to the common prohibited substances (WADA list, see also ➢ Chapter 4). Additionally, **alcohol** is prohibited **in bow sport** (more than 0.1 g/l in competition).

Beta blockers and **stimulants** (especially ephedrine) are typical "positive" controls. However, the doping rate is altogether very low and is mostly pure thoughtless use of **cold medicine**. **Older athletes** are also often found in high-performance shooting sport in contrast to other sports. Therefore, a high blood pressure treatment by beta blockers or diuretics may be needed. Adjusted medication rules of WADA remain desirable for this group of athletes.

References

Lösel H (1999). Leistungssteigerung im Schießsport, Bd. 1 u 2. Deutscher Schützenbund, Wiesbaden.

Reinkemeier H (1994). Vom Training des Schützen (Gesamtausgabe). Westfälischer Schützenbund 1861 e.V.

Important internet links

Deutscher Schützenbund: www.dsb.de

International Shooting-Sport Federation (ISSF): www.issf-sports.org

Fédération Internationale de Tir à l'Arc (FITA): www.archery.org

Nationale Anti-Doping-Agentur (NADA): www.nada-bonn.de

World Anti-Doping Agency (WADA): www.wada-ama.org

83 Sailing

René Schwall

Sailing is a competitive sport on all waters, over distances of any length ranging from a few miles to global circumnavigations. The success in sailing depends on material and the technical and tactical skills of the crew. The **optimally coordinated actions of the crew** are key. Experience, openness to risks, practice and a high physical and mental capacity are some necessary preconditions to optimally use a yacht or dinghy. The smaller the boat, the higher the physical strain to the sailors.

83.1 Boat classes and regattas

The classification into boat classes allows comparison of the athletic achievements. The **standard class** sails and equipment. Variations within certain limitations are possible within a **construction class**. Today, **Olympic classes** described by the ISAF (International Sailing Federation) and so-called **international classes** are distinguished. A **sailing regatta** consists of several races. In a race, the participants of one boat class follow a defined course and receive points according at arrival at the goal. The average time period of regattas is 4 days. Two races are sailed each day.

83.2 Sport-specific demands

The individual boat classes – from keel boat to dinghy to windsurfer – expose each athlete with different physical strain.

The increasing professionalism of this sport leads **junior work** starting earlier and earlier (average beginning of competitive sailing is 7 years) and triggered a discussion of the **prevention** of acute injuries and chronic impairments.

The duration of an individual sailing competition ranges between 45 min and 2 hours, with the exception of long-distance regattas. Besides such long-term performance, individual situations require **short-term maximum strength**. Intensive muscle contractions with **high heart rates** and **blood pressure** and relatively **low breathing frequencies** are typical for sailing (Shephard 1997).

To increase speed, every sailor aims to sail his boat as straight as possible. The sailor counters the wind with a **torsion moment** that increases at high wind speeds. This torsion moment results from the body's center of gravity and midship line interplay. If wind gust comes up, the sailor moves the body's gravity center farther away from the midship line, so that the torsion moment increases (Rieckert and Sievers 1999).

Thus, **knee and spine**, **femoropatellar joint and the lumbar spine** are particulary affected (Bettermann 1988).

83.3 Most common injuries and overstrain impairments

83.3.1 Acute injuries

They occur most often **in tacking or jibing** during **capsizing** (➤ Fig. 83.1), less often by collisions of the boats.

Typical acute injuries are:

- incised wounds and lacerations
- hematomas
- bruises.

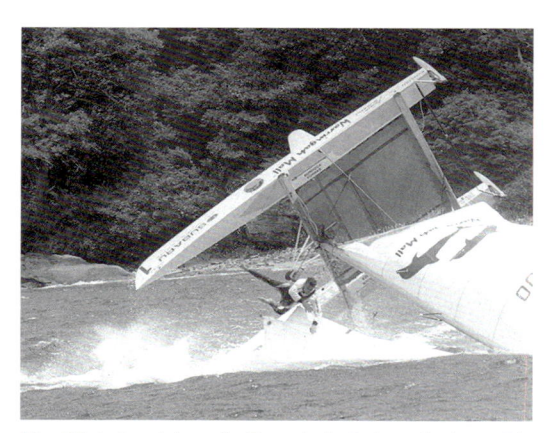

Fig. 83.1 Capsizing of a Tornado in Sydney Harbour, followed by injuries.

Therapy and prevention

The treatment is usually **conservative**; about 20% require. Permanent conditions are rare.

The exact **technique** of standard maneuvers is the best preventive measure in addition to the **cushioning sharp edges** of the boat fittings.

83.3.2 Muscle injuries

They develop most often in **tacking/jibing**, less often in capsizing and in the so-called **pumping with the sails** (pumping = repeated fast and strong pulling at the sheet to increase propulsion).

Typical muscle injuries are:

- strains of autochtonous dorsal muscles
- overstrain of the flexor muscles of the fingers at the forearm, especially in wind surfing (ischimia)
- tensions/strains of the neck and nape muscles.

The quadriceps muscle and the peronei muscles are injured rarely.

Therapy and prevention

Usually, these injuries are treated conservatively. Surgical measures are rare.

A specific **strength and muscle coordination** training can reduce the risk of muscle injuries.

83.3.3 Tendon injuries

The so-called hiking, i.e. moving the crew's body weight away from the midship line cause tendon injuries. Different maneuvers, capsizing and other events lead to acute tendon injuries (➤ Tab. 83.1).

Typical chronic tendon injuries are:

- patellar apex syndrome and insertion tendinitis of the patellar ligament, especially in singlehanded dinghies that accomplish the hiking of the boat without trapeze wire, e.g. in the classes of finn, Europe and laser (➤ Fig. 83.2)

Tab. 83.1 Most frequent localizations of sailing-specific tendon injuries (n = 65).

Localization of the tendon injuries	Number
Patellar ligament	26 (41%)
extensor carpi radialis muscle	11 (17%)
distal tendon of biceps brachii muscle	6 (10%)
peroneus longus and peroneus brevis tendons	5 (7%)
rotator cuff of the shoulder	5 (7%)
adductor longus tendon	1 (3%)
flexor digitorum longus tendon	1 (3%)
Achilles tendon	1 (3%)

The results of tables 83.1 and 83.2 are based on a sportmedical study in which 65 athletes of the Olympic sailing competitions in Sydney in the year 2000 participated.

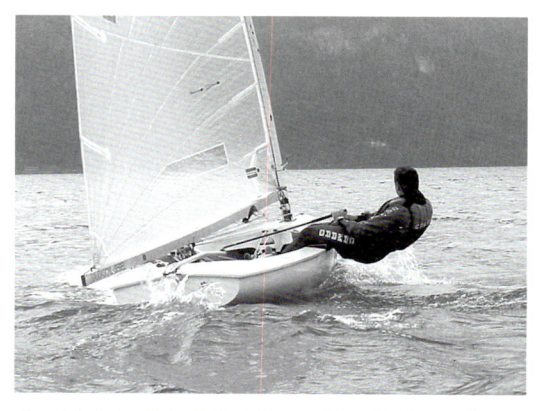

Fig. 83.2 A pilot of the Olympic finn dinghy at the so-called hiking.

- epicondylitis humeri radialis as a consequence of overstrain after intensive "sheet traction".

> The patellar apex syndrome and the epicondylitis humeri radialis are typical chronic tendon injuries in sailing.

Therapy and prevention

The therapy of tendon injuries consists of physiotherapy and massage combined with stretching exercises. Physical therapy (e.g. stimulation current) and infiltrations are indicated in individual cases. 65% of the high-performance sailors describe **permanent conditions** after tendon injuries.

A **long-term strength training combined with stretching exercises** is necessary for the preparation of the **patellar tendon** and the **quadriceps tendon** for a high and static long-term exposure. The epicondylitis humeri radialis can be prevented by **improving sailing technique** and by changing sheet leading angle, if permitted.

83.3.4 Joint impairments

Joint impairments develop **acutely during maneuvers**, e.g. at tacking/jibing, capsizing and at collisions. Injuries often occur during competition, and less often in exercising. **Chronic joint impairments** can also be caused by overstrain in hiking (➤ Tab. 83.2).

Typical acute joint injuries are:

- acute meniscus lesions, LCL and MCL lesions of the knee
- sprains and subluxations/dislocations of the shoulder
- sprains of the radiocarpal joint
- sprains of the finger joints.

Typical chronic joint injuries are:

- lumbalgias: They are the result of high **permanent strain of the autochtonous dorsal muscles** in nearly all boat classes (Aagaard et al. 1998, Allen 1999). These muscles have to perform isometric static effort for several hours during competition. A **muscular imbalance** appears in the forced hiking posture. The ventral trunk, hip flexor and leg musculature much more affected than the antagonizing long dorsal extensors, the gluteal muscles, the ischiocrural muscles and the gastrocnemius muscles. Sailors can counter this imbalance by specific strength training.
- Anterior knee pain at chondromalacia patellae.

Therapy and prevention

Interruptions of training and competition often support therapy. Physiotherapy, manual therapy, massages, fango treatments and NSAIDs are primarily used. Intraarticular injections and surgeries are rare.

Specific **strength training** is key for prevention. Antagonist training, i.e. by a training of the autochtonous dorsal musculature, the gluteal musculature and the ischiocrural muscles can avoid relapsing lumbalgias. A combination of **concentric and eccentric exercising** and regular **muscle-coordination training** are the best supporting success factors.

The **patellar guidance** and the Q angle have to be checked with retropatellar conditions. A specific training of the vastus medialis muscle is recommended at a tendency of lateralization. Specific strength training for the antagonists should be carried out in addition to **stretching exercises** for the **quadriceps muscles**.

The wearing of warm sailing clothes, a different movement and changes in the design on board are **additional measures** for the prevention of a reoccurrence of these conditions. A

Tab. 83.2 Most frequent localizations of sailing-specific joint injuries (n = 65).

Localization of the joint injuries	Number
spine	26 (40%)
knee joints	19 (29%)
shoulder joints	10 (15%)
wrists	4 (6%)
finger joints	1 (2%)
elbow joints	1 (2%)

change of functions in the crew – e.g. from presheeter to steerer – can reduce physical strain.

> Typical chronic consequences of sailing are relapsing lumbalgias caused by muscular imbalance and anterior knee pain due if hiking the boat.

References

Aagaard P, Beyer N, Simonsen EB, Larsson B, Magnusson SP, Kjaer M (1998). Isokinetic muscle strength and hiking performance in elite sailors. Scand J Med Sci Sports 8 (3): 138–144.

Allen JB (1999). Sports medicine and sailing. Phys Med Rehabil Clin N Am 10 (1): 49–65.

Bettermann AA (1998). Zwei typische Leiden des Segelsportes. Praktische Sport-Traumatol und Sportmed 3: 19–24.

Riekert H, Sievers M (1999). Sportmedizinische Aspekte beim Segeln. Deutsches Ärzteblatt 96, Issue 9: 542–546.

Shephard RJ (1997). Biology and medicine of sailing, an update. Sports Med 23 (6): 350–356.

Chapter 84 Sport diving

Wilfried Gfrörer

Sport diving has lived an enormous boom in the past 15 years. In Germany, approximately 300,000 sport divers had been active in 1993, their number has been exponentially grown to 1.5 million in 2003 (Klingmann and Weidauer 2004). Both scuba diving (SCUBA = self containing underwater breathing apparatus) and apnea diving (apnea = Greek for "without breathing") became more and more popular. The age limits shifted downwards and upwards. Travel to the Red Sea (➤ Fig. 84.1) or to the Pacific Ocean is popular for fans of diving. The accident risk with 0.015% per dive is relatively low compared to other sports and diving can thus be considered as safe (Almeling et al. 1999, Ehm et al. 2003). Diving under certain preconditions has even been offered to handicapped.

84.1 Underwater-diving sports

Free diving

Diving by holding one's breath has been a method of performing activities under water for ages. Free diving is practiced in different disciplines in swimming pools with saltwater or fresh water.

In general, the competitive disciplines such as **underwater rugby**, **static apnea diving** and different **distance competitions** in diving with or without fins or scuba are carried out **in swimming pools**.

Two competing teams play underwater rugby with six players each, who will try to place a ball filled with salt water into the opponent's basket on the ground of the swimming pool. Only swimsuits, fins, diving masks, snorkels and head covers with ear protectors are allowed. The

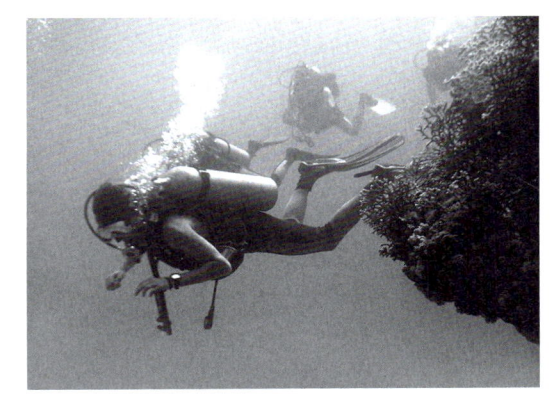

Fig. 84.1 Scuba diver in the Red Sea.

static apnea divers lie motionlessly with their faces in the water and hold their breath.

The disciplines carried out **in free water** focus on **deep diving**, for which there are no competitions but only record lists. The best-known discipline is probably no-limit apnea diving, where technical equipment is permitted such as a sled, on which the athlete glide into the depth, and air cushions carry him back to the surface. The current world record is at the unbelievable depth of 214 m (700 ft), held by the Austrian Herbert Nitsch.

Scuba diving

Scuba diving usually means diving in free waters, using compressed air as breathing gas. But also **special breathing gas mixtures** with an increased amount of oxygen (nitrox) or with partial or full substitution of the nitrogen in the air by **helium** (trimix or heliox) – depending on the planned diving depth – are available. Pure oxygen is often breathed for decompression. This is also called **technical diving**.

Rebreather diving is another kind of diving. The dive is carried out with pure oxygen and a CO_2 cutter in a closed-circuit breathing apparatus.

84.2 Physical specialties

Hydrostatic pressure

Everybody can feel the pressure to the ears if submerging the water. This is the result of a higher density and an increased pressure by about 1 bar (= 100 kPa) per 10 m (30 ft). This compresses the gases carried in the body. The volume of a gas in constant temperature decreases proportionally with increasing depth according to the **Boyle and Mariotte law**. Gas expands correspondingly at the ascent from the depth (decompression; ➤ Fig. 84.2). Within a closed body, 1 l of air breathed at 3 meters depth expands to 4 l at the surface. This triggers so-called **barotraumas** (see below).

Tissue satiety

Henry's law describes the physical dissolution of a gas in liquids under pressure. The saturation and desaturation speed of a gas in a liquid is proportional to the surface of a volume and the difference of the partial pressure between gas and solution. Gas bubbles develop in the liquid at quick pressure reduction, as in case if ascending too rapidly. An example is the fizzing upon opening a bottle of sparkling water.

> Development of gas bubbles can lead to diseases or long-term impairments or even to traumatic lesions.

84.3 Diving-specific injuries

84.3.1 Due to physical specificities

Barotrauma

So-called barotraumas develop because of the pressure changes in submerging and emerging; this affects all gas-filled cavities of the body. Even inadequate dental fillings can cause barotraumas. But primarily the cavities of the ENT region are affected in diving routine.

If pressure compensation does not work immediately **at submerging**, a farther submerging is

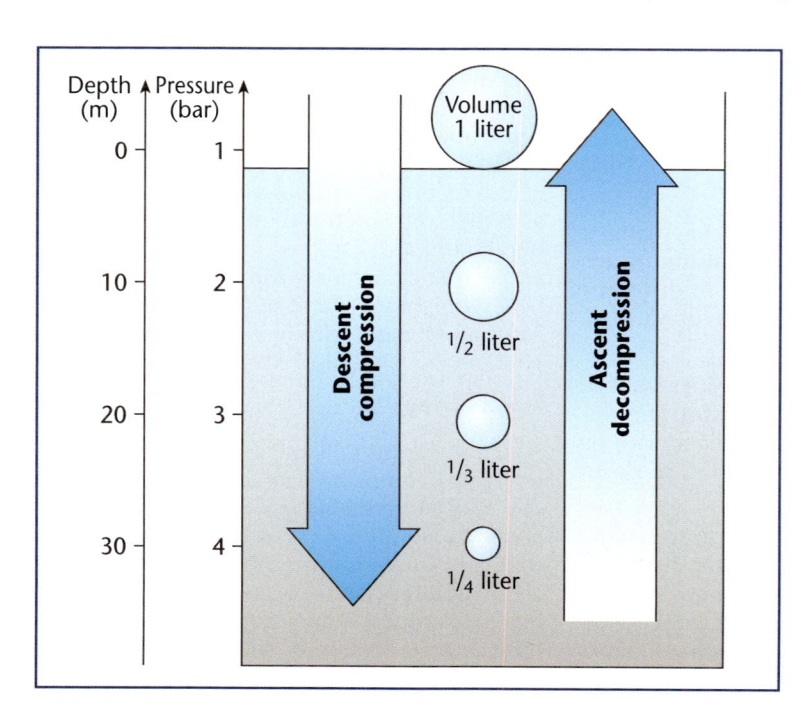

Fig. 84.2 Simplified representation of compression or expansion of gases under pressure according to the law of Boyle and Mariotte. 1 l of secluded air on the surface condenses to $1/4$ l at a descent into a depth of 30 m. A volume of 30 l of air inhaled in a depth of 30 m will expand to a volume of up to 4 l in the ascent to the surface.

excluded. A further pressure compensation with relatively reduced pressure is not possible anymore. The so-called **internal or external morbus caerulescens** (exudation of body liquids conditioned by negative pressure) develop. An **eardrum rupture** with an inflow of cold water into the ear can occur in extreme cases and result in caloric rotator vertigo.

Overstretching and ruptures of tissue might also develop at the seclusion of gas-filled cavities **in emerging** due to the expansion of the secluded gas, e.g. pulmonary alveoli at pulmonary emphysemas with consecutive **pneumothorax** or **arterial gas embolism**.

Decompression sickness

> The human body consists of different tissues and compartments, e.g. muscles, nerve cells, skin, bones, fat etc., which are differently supplied with blood. At submerging, these tissues take up breathing gas – especially nitrogen.

If the environmental pressure is reduced too quickly so that the gases dissolving, gas bubbles develop in the venous system of the lung. The lung has an additional parenchymatous vessel system, thus, blood perfusion continues without tissue damage. **Arterial gas bubble embolisms** (e.g. AGE) develop, if gas bubbles form in the arterial branch. This activates the coagulation cascade at the border surface of the gas bubbles/blood. A thrombus forms and blocks circulation, which leads to tissue necroses. Emphysemas develop at a **gas-bubble formation in the interstitium**, which heals without sequelae in most cases.

Different saturation and desaturation kinetics are available for the individual body tissues (Bühlmann et al. 2002). These are used to calculate decompression time in computer models. If a gas-bubble formation still form, there is a risk of **decompression sickness** (DCS).

Previously, the following classification system was used:

- DCS type I with itching skin (so-called diver's fleas) or joint pain (so-called bends) and
- DCS type II with involvement of the CNS, the internal ear or the cardiovascular organs or other organ systems.

This traditional classification of decompression sickness has recently been replaced by a **descriptive classification system**. Besides symptoms, the following is now considered as well:

- temporal dynamics
- moment of the beginning of the symptoms in relation to the end of the dive
- involved organ systems
- present barotraumas.

Furthermore, the diving profile is considered to assess the strain of the body with inert gas (Klingmann and Tetzlaff 2007). Nevertheless, our own current examinations with bone makers and echocardiography indicate that persons with identical diving profiles may or may not develop micro-bubbles (Gfrörer et al. 2006, Gfrörer et al. 2008 [1]). This requires further investigation.

Dysbaric osteonecroses

Aseptic osteonecroses – the so-called dysbaric osteonecroses – can develop at an accumulation of micro-bubbles. These occur especially at the **long bones of the large joints**. Aristotle has already described skeletal changes for Greek sponge divers in 332 B.C. These changes have been accepted as **a disease** in professional divers. Necrosis **proceeds without any symptoms** and is not directly related to decompression sickness. The embolisms in the bone caused leads to an interrupted blood supply and successive necrosis. **Symptoms** are **joint pain, movement limitations and joint swellings** – similar to arthritis.

Nitrogen narcosis

Sport divers often want to dive deeply. Usually dry atmospheric air is used as breathing gas. It consists to 79% of N_2, traces of argon and neon and 20.9% O_2. An **excessive pressure of N_2** impairs the brain function. An N_2 pressure of 3.9–4.7 bar, which conforms to a diving depth of 40–50 m, can already cause a **euphoria** – the "depth rapture". The diver becomes **loses orientation** and keeps descending instead of ascending. There is a high risk of drowning.

Pure oxygen has the same effect in diving. If the O_2 pressure is higher than 1.6 bar, which conforms with a diving depth of 6 m at a 100%-breathing of O_2, a **sudden unconsciousness with tonic-clonic seizure** are caused by the **oxygen toxicity**. The diver loses the mouth piece of his breathing device and drowns if not rescued in time.

Shallow water blackout

The so-called shallow water blackout appears in apnea diving. An acute hypoxia and eventual unconsciousness caused by the reduced CO_2-conditioned breath stimulus occurs after hyperventilation before diving.

Calf cramps

The locomotor apparatus is much less influenced by the physical conditions under water than the air-filled body cavities. Movements with the fins against water resistance induce an unfamiliar strain for muscles, tendons and joints, which require increased force. Therefore, calf cramps appear primarily **in unexercised athletes** and **with dehydration**.

84.3.2 External influences

Injuries in sports carried out in swimming pools usually occur only in underwater rugby. Those are mostly injuries of the eardrums caused by another player's fin impacting the ear. They usually heal without complications after an according splinting.

Injuries caused by the stings of sea urchins can be caused at sea diving. These stings are often hard to remove, since they mostly consist of chalk and therefore break easily and cause inflammations. The use of citric acid poultices over night is a domestic remedy, which mostly dissolves the sting.

Injuries caused by **animal attacks under water** are extremely rare. Keeping the so-called flight initiation distance to the animals usually avoids them.

The **danger of falls when leaving the water after diving** – especially apparatus diving – exists. The muscle tone is strongly reduced in diving. The diver has to carry the full weight of the equipment after exiting the water, which often weighs more than 50 kg including the weight belt. All kinds of fall injuries are possible here.

Further accident causes that can partly be fatal are indicated in ➤ Chapter 86.2.4.

84.4 Prevention

A **diving-fitness assessment** by a trained physician should be carried out before starting diving and then regularly in order to minimize the risks of diving. This examination should national rules every 3 years in 30-year-olds, every 2 years in the 30–40-year-olds and every year for athletes older than 40 years. A spirometry, an ECG and an ear mirroring with valsalva maneuver for the assessment of the ear tube function should be carried out in the fitness assessment in addition to a comprehensive anamnesis and investigation. An additional exercise ECG is recommended beginning with the 40th year of age. A divers' physician should be consulted for individual questions of diving capability after diseases or injuries.

A fundamental theoretical and practical **diving training of the athlete** is obligatory. This can be absolved with different sport federations or professional suppliers.

The loss of body fluids in the course of a dive amounts to 2 l because of the so-called immersion dieresis and sweating (Gfrörer et al. 2008 [2]). Thus, **sufficient amounts of liquids have to be drunk** before and after every dive.

It is also recommended to perform **safety decompression stop** of 3 min at 3 m at the decompression times suggested by the diving computers (also for zerohour dives) in order to reduce the development of micro-bubbles.

Obviously, an endurance training program 2 hours before diving – as has been publicized by Blatteau and colleagues (2007) – cannot protect of bubble development. Regular, general **fitness exercising** with is highly recommended.

References

Almeling M, Böhm F, Welsla W (1999). Handbuch der Tauch- und Hyperbarmedizin. ECOmed-Verlag, Landsberg.

Blatteau J-E, Bossuges A, Gempp E, Pontier J-M, Castagna O, Robinet C, Galland F-M, Bourbon L (2007). Haemodynamic changes induced by submaximal exercise before a dive and its consequences on bubbole formation. Br J Sports Med 41: 375–379.

Bühlmann AA, Völlm EB, Nussberger P (2002). Tauchmedizin. Springer-Verlag, Berlin.

Ehm OF, Hahn M, Hoffmann U (2003). Tauchen noch sicherer. Müller Rüschlikon, Stuttgart.

Gfrörer W, Fusch G, Müller C, Fusch C, Ekkenkamp A (2006). Verursacht moderates Sporttauchen Osteoporose? Abstract, Sport-Orthopädie Sport-Traumatologie 22; 2: 101.

Gfrörer W, Hansel J, Horstmann T, Nieß A, Tetzlaff K, (2008) (1). Intravasale Blasenbildung bei einem 50 m Druckkammer Simulationstauchgang. 11. Wissenschaftliche Tagung der GTÜM. Heidelberg 18.–20. 04. 2008.

Gfrörer W, Fusch G, Ekkenkamp A, Horstmann T, Nieß A, Tetzlaff K, Hansel J (2008) (2). Tauchen verursacht eine erhebliche Dehydration. 11. Wissenschaftliche Tagung der GTÜM. Heidelberg 18.–20. 04. 2008.

Klingmann Ch, Tetzlaff K (2007). Moderne Tauchmedizin. Gentner Verlag, Stuttgart.

Klingmann Ch, Weidauer H (2004). Tauchmedizin aktuell. Gentner Verlag, Stuttgart.

V Rehabilitation

85 Rehabilitation after athletic injuries 687
85.1 Occupational groups involved in rehabilitation 687
85.2 In-patient and ambulant rehabilitation 687
85.3 Biomechanical performance diagnostics 688
85.4 Aims and limitations of rehabilitation 688
85.5 Latest approaches in rehabilitation 689
85.6 Physiotherapy 691

Chapter 85 Rehabilitation after athletic injuries

Jürgen Freiwald

This chapter gives a short overview over **physiotherapy** after sports injuries. Only an overview related to practice can be provided; references indicate further subject-related reading.

> The rehabilitation after sport injuries provides the optimal recovery of the functional and athletic capabilities by indication-specific treatment of injuries and the compensation of injury-conditioned functional deficits.

The recent rehabilitation model of the World Health Organization (WHO), **"International Classification of Functioning, Disability and Health"** (ICF) takes into account that the injured athletes have suffered structural impairments and is restricted in many areas of life. Other factors, which exceed the purely structural findings, have to be considered for a successful rehabilitation.

85.1 Occupational groups involved in rehabilitation

In recent years, rehabilitation after sport injuries has developed analogously to recent conservative and surgical treatments.

The principles that the rehabilitation is based upon have changed. Now **structural deficits** of injuries and diseases and **psychological and social components** are recognized factors that influence rehabilitation.

The professional groups of (sports) physicians, sports scientists and physiotherapists have to work hand in hand in rehabilitation; (sports) psychologists can additionally be called in, if required. This can be especially necessary, if the sport is the personal focus of life and if the income depends on the athletic performance in the professional field.

All persons involved in rehabilitation must have competent knowledge of the functional and performance-related diagnostics and the treatment of diseases. In addition, the range and the giving of indications of physical therapy (physiotherapy, exercise therapy) for curative, rehabilitative and preventive purposes must be known for physical therapy.

Especially in competitive sports, all involved in the rehabilitation of the athlete must be sufficiently experienced in the interaction with injured athletes and must have a positive attitude towards (competitive) sports.

85.2 In-patient and ambulant rehabilitation

It depends on the **seriousness of the injury**, the **social environment** and the **insurance-legal terms**, whether an in-patient or ambulant rehabilitation process is chosen.

> The following legal policy is valid: ambulant treatment above in-patient treatment.

Ambulant rehabilitation prevails for cases of sports injuries of mostly young persons.

The **technical qualification** of therapists and coaches and the **equipment of the rehabilitation facility** are both important for rehabilitation. Exercise equipment, water basins, the gym and preferably outdoor facilities (terrain exercises) are necessary for sport-specific re-integration, depending on the injury and the rehabilitation protocol.

85.3 Biomechanical performance diagnostics

Furthermore, a biomechanical performance diagnosis by trained staff – especially in the field of competitive sports – is preferred (➤ Fig. 85.1).

Many clinics and ambulant facilities have accordingly equipped departments.

Following analyses should be viable:

- cardiopulmonary capability (performance ergometry)
- strength diagnosis of the large muscle groups (isokinetics, isometry, concentricity, eccentricity)
- measurements of ground reaction force (gait analysis, jump analysis)
- videographic measurements (motion analysis)
- electromyographic measurements (activation patterns of the superficial musculature).

Nonetheless, a biomechanical performance diagnosis should only be carried out if its results are implemented in the following therapy and exercise planning.

85.4 Aims and limitations of rehabilitation

Impairments remain after serious sport injuries despite intensive rehabilitation; a restitutio ad integrum as condition of healing with complete recovery will be the exception.

> A "restitutio ad integrum" is the full recovery of original structure and function or of the original-capabilities and the social role, respectively, while the "restitutio ad optimum" is defined as the largest possible recovery of original structure and function or capabilities and the social role, respectively (BAR 2000).

The athlete nevertheless can mostly perform the sport also after serious injuries and impairments due to a successful rehabilitation, often on a lower, the same or – at long-term training processes – even on a higher level (Engelhardt et al. 1997, Renström 1997, Engelhardt et al. 2005).

Since a restitutio ad integrum will not always be possible with serious sport injuries, the recovery of capability based on **changed neuromuscular and structural conditions** will be attained.

> Changed structural and neuromuscular conditions, e.g. after substitution of the anterior cruciate ligament:
>
> Minor torsion moments of knee extensor muscles and a reduced possible activation of the vastus medialis muscle remain also in the long term after the substitution of the anterior cruciate ligament by the patellar tendon.
>
> Only minor torsion moments of the knee flexor muscles remain often and for the long term after the substitution of the anterior cruciate ligament by a gracilis or semitendinosus transplant.

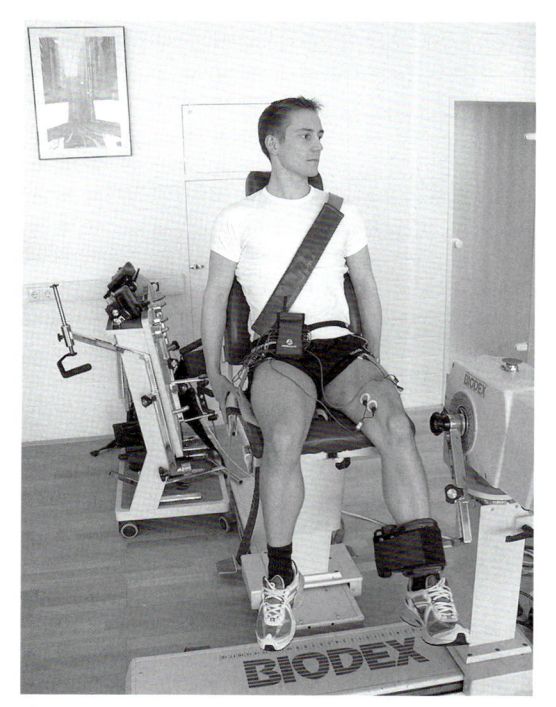

Fig. 85.1 Isokinetic measurements of torsion moments combined with telemetric EMG measurement.

Still the affected athletes will mostly be able to perform the sport again, in many cases even on a high (competitive) level.

Therefore, not only the question arises in rehabilitation of how injured structures can be set back into their original condition by medical-therapeutic influences, but also whether the methods of rehabilitation are sufficient for the recovery of the original functionality without accepting secondary and tertiary impairments.

85.5 Latest approaches in rehabilitation

The ICF of the World Health Organization (WHO) combines the views of a rather traditionally aligned medicine, which is primarily focused on **structural impairments**, with the ones of an individual-related, psychosocial point of view. The newer view thus is more strongly oriented on the **subjective condition** of the patients and their **social integration**.

A renunciation of a purely structural assessment of exclusively clinical parameters, such as extent of motion, strength and pain, is carried out due to the definition of functional health (Schüle and Huber 2004, Stein and Greitemann 2005).

85.5.1 Classification of Functioning, Disability and Health (ICF)

According to International Classification of Functioning, Disability and Health (ICF), persons will be functionally healthy, if they:
- conform in their bodies' functions and structures the ones of healthy persons,
- do or can do everything expected of persons without any health problems,
- can unfold their being in all areas of life that are important to them in a way and extent that would be expected of people without health problems in their body functions or structures or the activities (concept of participation).

The parts of functional health are defined as follows (DIMDI 2004):

- **Body functions** are the physiological functions of body systems (including psychological functions).
- **Body structures** are anatomical parts of the body, such as organs, extremities and their components.
- **Lesions** are the impairments of body functions or structures, such as a substantial difference or a loss.
- An **activity** describes the performance of a task or an action by a person.
- **Participation** is being involved in a life situation.
- **Impairments of activity** are difficulties a person can have in the performance of an activity.
- **Impairments of participation** are problems a person experiences at the involvement in a life situation.
- **Environmental factors** project the material, social and attitudinal environment, in which humans live and unfold their being.

➤ Figure 85.2 clearly shows the problems by a fictional example of a ski racer with a serious knee lesion (patellar fracture). It also becomes obvious that the therapeutic attention to exclusively physical structures and functions only presents a partial aspect of a successful rehabilitation. The recent rehabilitation model is also to be explained and the consequences are to be shown.

Example 1: ICF – skiing accident and rehabilitation

A skier of the A squad has a serious skiing accident. He suffers a transverse fracture of the patella. The joint surface of the patella cannot completely be reconstructed; a retropatellar cartilage lesion will remain.

Structural lesion/functional disorder:
- This lesion is serious. No restituto ad integrum is possible. A restituto ad optimum is aspired.
- The impairment concerns two categories: the impairment of the body structures (patella, cartilage) and impairments of the body functions, while the latter ones can again include physiological (athlete cannot participate in training and competition) and mental (athlete is depressed and lacking in drive) functions.

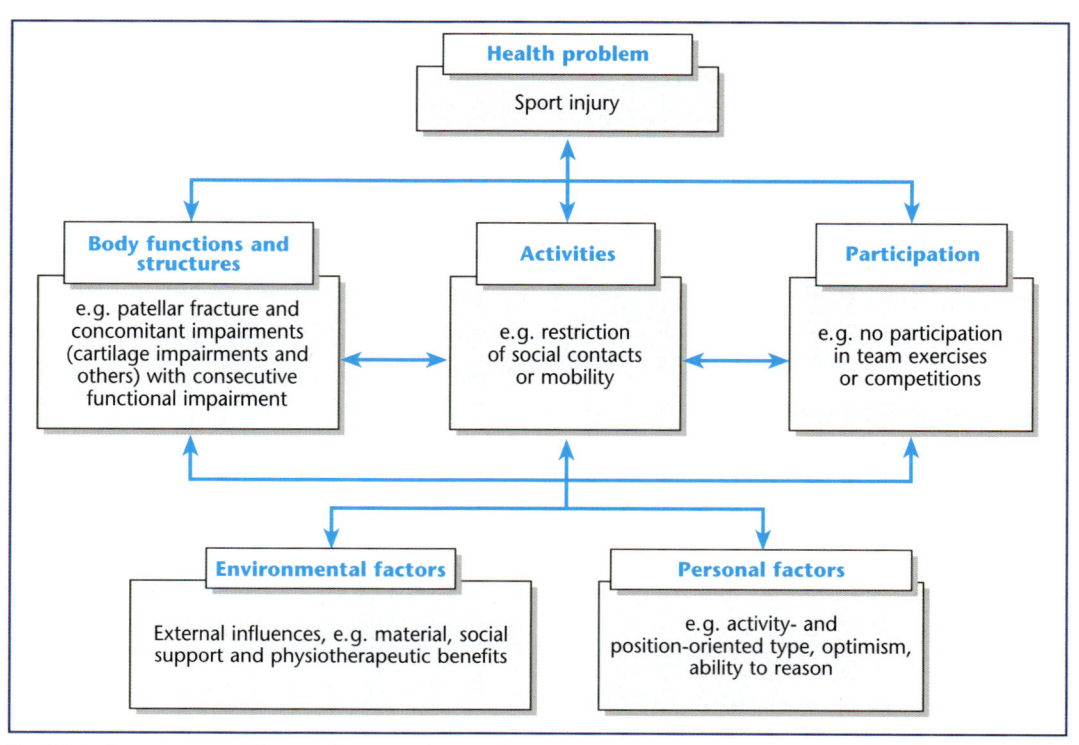

Fig. 85.2 Components and interactions according to the criteria of ICF at the example of a skier after fracture of the tibial plateau (changed according to DIMDI 2004).

- The impairment is to be cured or to be minimized by acute-medical treatment and surgically. In the present example, the patella is repositioned and the fracture lines are fixed preferably in optimal positioning.

Activity/impairment of activity:

- The activity impairment is deduced from the accident and the surgical treatment. The skier can only move forward by help of walking aids because of the partial immobilization. No athletic exercises should be considered during this phase. The capacity and action of the injured athlete therefore are impaired in all areas of life.
- During rehabilitation, it has to be tried to regenerate the structural impairment with the support of the healing processes as fast as possible and to minimize or even cure the resulting functional impairments.
- Physician and orthopedic technician have to cooperate and they have to define the most adequate ortheses treatment and further details (partial weight-bearing, movement extent, and others) and all further treatment measures and principles.
- The physiotherapist postoperatively begins with the first treatment measures. This applies to the gait training by use of walking aids, training in the use of the orthesis as well as first physical methods, which are to prevent secondary impairments and concomitant diseases.

Participation/impairment of participation:

- The injured (professional) athlete is impaired in his professional, social and private involvement. He cannot practice his occupation, contacts to coaches and sport comrades lessen, and there is the danger of social retreat. Psychological disorders are also possible, e.g. the development of depressions.
- Disturbances of participation must be counteracted by a rehabilitation plan adapted to the individual situation of the athlete.
- A strategy consists of the reintegration of the athlete into competitive sport as fast as possible and preferably in an optimal condition.

> In addition to the treatment of the structural impairments, contacts to coaches, officials and comrades are made and the circle of friends and the family will be involved in order to optimize the phase of rehabilitation.
> - If the prospects of a full recovery are only minor and a future participation in (competitive) sports is unlikely, the athlete will have to be prepared by appropriate measures – psychological treatment, and others – for a life, in which the own athletic capacity is not in the central focus anymore.

85.5.2 Orientation values (norm values)

The usual difference between normal and abnormal findings is not conclusive in rehabilitation after sport injuries. The original capability is often recovered by surgical treatment also after serious injuries.

It would be helpful for physicians and therapists to orientate themselves by norm values. Norm values are presented as measurement parameters in the border areas (e.g. laboratory values, mobility values or force values). They are deduced from the measurement of healthy, preferably representative population groups, which for example correspond to the age and gender of the population to be compared.

The norm values, which describe healthy persons as well as rather unexercised population groups, are only restrictedly applicable for the orientation in rehabilitation of athletes who have an injury and belong to a specially exercised population as well.

The **sport-specific conditions** have to be considered especially in the assessment of athletes by normative values. Every sport leads to the development of very different special values (Dalichau 2001).

> **Example 2: Orientation values – soccer players and ballet dancers**
>
> Soccer players and ballet dancers are clearly different in their strength and mobility values. The unequal strength and mobility values result from:
> - different baseline values already at childhood age (genetic dispositions)
> - different athletic interests already in childhood and juvenile age (social selection)
> - different athletic demand profiles and exercise procedures (exercise-conditioned, specific adaptations).
>
> Considering the mentioned aspects, the soccer player cannot participate in training during rehabilitation, different from ballet dancers. The soccer player always have to differentiate from the ballet dancer in their physical capabilities and characteristics for the successful performance of a sport.
>
> No abstract norm values but norm values adapted to the individual, the sport and the injury will have to be used for orientation in rehabilitation.

In the rehabilitation of top athletes – regarding the use of orientation values –, the additional problem occurs that no orientation values for the rehabilitation after sport injuries are available because of the low number of top athletes in the particular sport, but only individual findings exist. Therefore, it will be left to the experience and the therapeutic skill of physicians and therapists in the specific situation of action to orientate by the action field because of their long-term experiences and to treat the athletes successfully.

85.6 Physiotherapy

Physiotherapy is a branch of physical medicine and contains procedures of medical gymnastics, movement therapy and the physical therapy. In practice, it is almost impossible for the sports physician to keep the overview of the multitude of the diverse procedures of physiotherapy. Therefore, only the most important procedures, which are of sports-medical relevance are introduced shortly and their mechanisms of action discussed.

Physiotherapeutic methods can be classified as follows:

- medical gymnastics
- massage
- electrotherapy
- hydro- and thermotherapy
- light therapy.

Physiotherapeutic methods are natural healing methods. **Passive** – e.g. led by the therapist –

and **active** – independently performed – movements of the person are used for the recovery of his health and capability.

The use of physiotherapeutic methods serves the **prevention** of sports injuries as well as the **support of self-regulating forces** after sports injuries. The physiotherapy can be applied **alternatively or complementary** with the medicamentous or surgical therapy.

> A lot of the physiotherapeutic methods have not been tested for their effectiveness yet. Still, that does not mean that these therapies are ineffective.

85.6.1 Active principles of physiotherapy

The application of physiotherapeutic methods requires the knowledge of the active principles on each organ system and the functions.

The **effects** of physical methods base on:

- irritation-reaction patterns (adaptations)
- regulation patterns.

The natural healing procedures are stimulated by physiotherapeutic methods influencing **metabolism**. Adaptations on the organ level are achieved by appropriate physical stimuli.

The **functional** capacities (e.g. improvement of coordination) will be increased and – with according stimulation – so will also the **morphologic** capacities (e.g. muscle growth) due to physiotherapy, and thus the capability will be increased.

Not all processes in the organism run synchronously. The adaptation mechanisms and their timely processing will have to be known in order to plan physiotherapeutic measures sensibly and to be able to assess their effects appropriately. The time requirements of the relaxation, healing and adaptation processes are presented in ➢ Table 85.1.

85.6.2 Sports physiotherapy

The sports physiotherapy is a branch of physiotherapy. The use of the title "sport physiotherapist" is coupled with extensive **advanced training**.

The German Sport Federation issues the license of "DSB sport physiotherapy" after the

Tab. 85.1 Systematic and timely course of adaptation processes (modified according to Hildebrandt 1998).

Adaptation modus	Functional and morphologic level	Timely course
cortical-autonomous adaptation	learning, behavioral changes	spontaneously up to years
plastic adaptation	adjustment of specific performing and protecting tissue (e.g. muscle, connective and bone tissue)	weeks up to years
trophic adaptation	<ul><li>increase of energy storages</li><li>adjustment of the of the supply and secretion capacity (e.g. secretion performance)</li></ul>	seconds up to months
functional adaptation	economization, normalization, increase of general quality and time coordination (e.g. environmental synchronization, spread of the range of adjustment)	hours up to years
habituation	shift in target value and adaptation of excursion (e.g. damping of the formatio reticularis, physical and mental regulatory circulation mechanisms)	hours up to years
nerve adaptation	changes of afferent stimulation patterns (e.g. restraint of noxious afferences on a local, spinal or central-nervous level)	seconds up to months (years)
cellular adaptations	optimization of protective mechanisms (e.g. lowering of the critical oxygen step, increase of the cellular myoglobin content, enzymatic adaptations within the cell, e.g. of the aerobic metabolism)	milli-second up to weeks (months)

passed final exam. It is the aim of the training to teach masseurs and physiotherapists special praxis-relevant techniques and abilities, which are adjusted to the requirements of athlete treatment in modern competitive sport.

On the orders of the German sport federation (segment of competitive sports), only therapists with the license of the German Sport Federation will be employed for central events of the top federations.

The subject of sports physiotherapy is the **prevention and treatment** of sports injuries, the **treatment** of athletes during training and competition as well as **rehabilitation** after sports injuries in cooperation with sports physicians.

Not only is the treatment of injuries in the foreground in sports physiotherapy, but also the **assessment of the physical and mental condition** of the athlete. The sports physiotherapist therefore must understand sports-medical examinations and be able to plan and attend exercise procedures.

Furthermore, the sports physiotherapist must be able to contribute to the **prevention** of sports injuries. This aim can be achieved by **exercise advice** (optimization of the warm-up and cool-down phases, methods going along with exercising, e.g. compensation training, regeneration methods, nutrition methods and others) and by advice for sport-specific **equipment** (protective gear, such as helmet, shin guards).

85.6.3 Medical gymnastics

Medical gymnastics is a part of physical therapy (➤ Fig. 85.3). It bases on a specific, measured, methodically planned application of movement processes (Stein and Greitemann 2005).

Medical gymnastics is indispensable in orthopedic-traumatologic rehabilitation after sports injuries. Its effects base on an individually adapted, active or passive physical exercising. The therapy plans of medical gymnastics are characterized by a planned, systematic and stepped **treatment structure**. It is structured for the support of the healing process, depending on the injury or the disease, and to regain preferably the full capacity of the athlete as soon as possible. There is a multitude of **different conceptions** in medical gymnastics. They can be used together but also alternatively or in combination with other physical treatment methods or psychological influences.

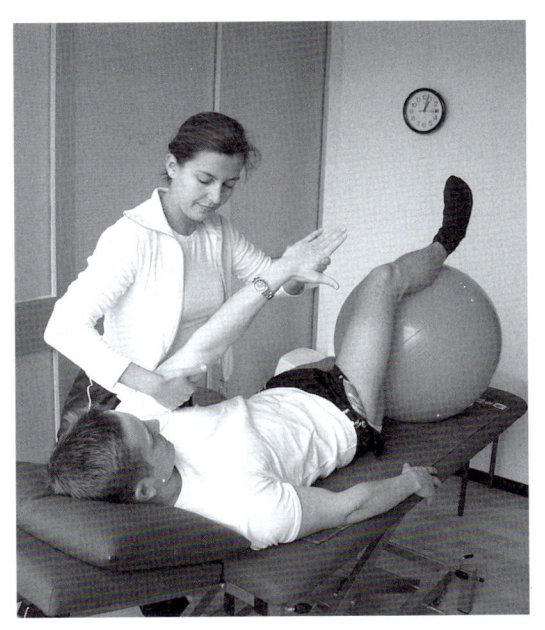

Fig. 85.3 Physiotherapeutic therapy.

The therapies of medical gymnastics that are important for traumatologic sport medicine – without any claims of being complete – are listed in ➤ Table 85.2. The regarding **contraindications**, which have not been listed here, are also to be thought of with regard to the different application fields and indications.

The **assessment of the effectiveness** of the medical-gymnastic methods is problematic. Scientific evidence is mostly missing; in some fields, it is more esoteric than subject-related. Here, the experienced and scientifically trained physician will be required to sort the wheat from the chaff. The proof of a positive effect under scientific criteria could be brought forth only for few techniques of medical gymnastics compared to other procedures/exercises (Gutenbrunner and Weidmann 2004).

> Most medical-gymnastic methods have not been tested scientifically yet for their effectiveness.

Tab. 85.2 Physiotherapeutic therapy concepts being significant in orthopedic-traumatologic rehabilitation.

Physio-therapeutic therapy concepts	Description	Areas of application in sports medicine (selection)	Remarks
organ-specific exercise and therapy concepts	breathing therapy	■ support of the athletes' ability to breathe ■ exercising of the breathing muscles ■ regulation of breathing	none
exercising therapy concepts	isokinetic muscle exercising	■ specific muscle growth exercises with isometric, concentric and eccentric forms of muscle contraction (all large joints) in open and closed kinetic chains ■ bio-feedback training: strength employment ■ bio-feedback training: capability of angle reproduction	Isokinetic muscle training is also part of the medical exercising therapy, which is planned by PE teachers, and others.
physiotherapy with apparatus	specific exercising of the basic motor abilities under specific use of adequate training and exercise equipment	Training by help of apparatuses is also part of the medical exercising therapy, which is planned by PE teachers, and others.	
medical exercising therapy	specific exercising of the basic motor abilities under specific use of adequate training and exercise equipment	■ the term of "medical exercising therapy" has become established, but is still controversial ■ the medical exercising therapy is planned and carried out by a team of PE teachers, physiotherapists and physicians	
manual therapy	manual medicine (chirotherapy)	■ reversible articular dysfunctions ("blockades") ■ reversible segmental dysfunctions	■ the substrate of a blockade is just as little ensured clearly as the treatment successes under consideration of scientific criteria despite often reported positive effects in practice ■ the treatment of blockades should only be carried out by trained and experienced therapists, because serious incidents – especially in treatments of the cervical spine – have been reported
manual therapy (according to Maitland)	■ functional disorders of the support and locomotor apparatus ■ limited joint mobility ■ acute and chronic irritations of joints and spine ■ irritation of neuro-meningeal structures	First scientific surveys support the effectiveness of the Maitland therapy.	

Aims and effects of physiotherapeutic treatment

Medical gymnastics is supposed to contribute to the economization of movement processes in rehabilitation. It is to help analyzing movement procedures at partial functional losses, make suggestions regarding the optimization as well as to develop movement strategies, which can help to compensate the partial deficiencies.

Especially during the phase of rehabilitation, the patients will be responsive to a special degree regarding **behavioral changes**. But they will also be especially sensitive and depressed in this phase. Thus, it will also be the task of the physiotherapist to provide **mental** support and to put the athlete into a confidential and positive mood.

Further **purposes** of medical-gymnastic therapists are:

- communication of realistic purposes (length of rehabilitation, duration of the absence from sport etc.)
- behavioral change in everyday life (eating behavior, regime of life etc.)
- change of behavior in sport (information regarding warm-up and cool-down, introduction and practice of compensational gymnastic methods, information of adapted regeneration, information of sport-specific nutrition etc.)
- communication of trust into the own abilities of the patient and initiation of a positive basic mood.

It will be sensible in many cases to work with **different** medical-gymnastic methods and to combine these with other methods of physical therapy (massages, electrotherapy), depending on each functional disorder and the capacity of the patient.

The athletes should carry medical gymnastics out daily during rehabilitation in order to achieve sufficient therapeutic effects. The adjustment of exercises or training will require several exercise units per week for competitive athletes (Gutenbrunner and Weimann 2004).

Nevertheless, caution should be exercised. Some surveys show that capacity of the organism is clearly reduced after surgeries. The multitude of new and unfamiliar exercises as well as the concomitant physical therapy (warmth, cold, electricity and others) can lead to massive **overstrains reactions**; they will be easily visible in the **hemogram**.

Typical changes are found (Viru and Viru 2001, Clasing and Siegfried 2002):

- change of the testosterone/cortisol ratio (overtraining)
- increase of muscle and serum enzymes (CK, CPK and others; tissue demise)
- changed leucocytes (including an increase at overstrained muscles)
- changes of the electrolytes (tendentiously higher values in athletes)
- changed ureal values (overtraining)
- changed level of uric acid (gout, conditions at the tendon insertions and slide bearings, insufficient supply of liquids and others)
- changed lipid metabolism (risk assessment, metabolic lapses).

It is suitable to carry out an internal monitoring parallel to the orthopedic-traumatologic intervention especially in the rehabilitation of competitive athletes and to implement the results into the prescriptions. Latent factors (internal diseases, mistakes in exercise planning, nutrition problems including liquid intake, and others) interfering with the recovery can be recognized, which is another advantage.

> Normal laboratory values can fluctuate inter-subjectively in healthy athletes. The normal laboratory values change in many cases also in healthy competitive athletes.

In order to assess the values of competitive athletes appropriately, adequate literature should be used for help.

Active physiotherapeutic methods

Active medical-gymnastic exercises require the **cooperation of the patient**.

The direct therapeutic aims are the improvement of coordination and strengthening of the actively exercised muscles as well as the regain and optimization of coordination. The further classification into medical gymnastics on a neurophysiologic base does not seem appropriate. Neurophysiologic processes are to be established in motion (also in every passive method). If such a distinction is to be made, it will have to be done on the level of naming these methods.

Passive physiotherapeutic methods

Passive methods, in which the patient will develop **no own motor activity** (deliberate muscle activity), are:
- positioning (e.g. stepwise positioning)
- mobilization (e.g. continuous passive motion)
- extension and traction (e.g. manual therapy, sling table).

Indication and prescription

The **fields of indication** for medical-gymnastic treatments in sports medicine are manifold:
- structural and functional disorders of the locomotor system (joint dysfunctions, muscular atrophies, neuromuscular dysbalances, and others)
- structural and functional disorders of the nervous system (peripheral nerve injuries, disorders and diseases of the central nervous system, coordination disorders, and others)
- structural and functional disorders of the cardiopulmonary system
- functional disorders of the intestinal and genitourinary system
- mental indications.

The **prescription** of medical gymnastics is a physician's performance. Medical gymnastics must be **dosed correctly**, just as a medication. Therefore, every prescription should contain the following data:
- exactly specified diagnosis and performance symptoms
- exact purpose (description of the function to be improved)
- description of the methods of medical gymnastics that are to be used
- number of treatments

- specification, whether an individual or a group treatment is necessary
- specification of the interval between treatments (frequency of stimulations, e.g. daily or 3 times a week)
- specification of combinations with other physiotherapeutic methods or measures
- description of existing or concomitant medication (for information).

Contraindications

Medical gymnastics will only not be indicated in exceptional cases.

Relative contraindications towards (active) medical gymnastics are (changed according to Gutenbrunner and Weimann 2004, Stein and Greitemann 2005):
- acute inflammatory processes (e.g. feverish infect, myocarditis, rheumatic episode, florid infections)
- most serious decompensated heart diseases (NYHA III and IV)
- respiratory insufficiency
- unstable angina pectoris – malign hypertension
- decompensated respiratory insufficiency
- strain-conditioned cardiac dysrhytmia of high degree
- oncologic diseases at their final stages
- myositis ossificans (regional contraindication)
- regional inflammatory diseases
- unstable fractures
- disturbances of consciousness
- certain psychoses.

85.6.4 Massage

Massage is a very old, if not even the **oldest treatment method** for human persons in general (Kladny 2005). Massage is defined as the mechanical, systematic, layered work-through of the external tissue layers for healing purposes and relaxation as a procedure of physical therapy. Massage has physiologic effects, which have often been underestimated (➤ Tab. 85.3).

Tab. 85.3 Overview of the most significant massage techniques (modified according to Kladny 2005, Kohlrauch 2005, Roche Lexikon Medizin 2003, Weimann 1993).

Classic massages

Massage technique[1]	Execution	Indications[2]	Effects and remarks
stroking (effleurage)	Stroking (effleurage) describes expansive movements from peripheral to central in main areas over certain muscle groups by only little skin shifts.	■ muscular hypertonus as tissue tone or as contractive tone (myogeloses) ■ acute and chronic pain syndromes of the spine ■ arthroses ■ inflammatory rheumatic diseases ■ soft-tissue rheumatic pain conditions ■ after subsiding of the acute phase – posttraumatic and post-operative conditions ■ psycho-vegetative dysfunctions ■ pre- and after-treatment of athletic performances	■ exciting the cardiovascular system (increased venous back circuit to the heart, increased arterial circulation, increase of the heart rate and/or the stroke volume depending on the massage technique) ■ humoral reactions (release of histamine and acetylcholine, other vasoactive substances) ■ liquid shifts in the tissue with effect to the local metabolic milieu (pH value, and others) ■ improvement of the blood circulation and trophism of the massaged tissue (acceleration of the transport of nutrients) ■ increase of the lymph flow (backflow promotion) ■ increase of the venous return ■ acceleration of the healing process (with correct indication; detaching of adherences in the connective tissue) ■ pain relief (by increase of the blood circulation, normalization of the cell milieu with an increase of the pH value, release of pain-reducing substances, etc.) ■ initiation of neuro-reflectory long-distance effect to vessel systems and internal organs (relations between dermatomes and myotomes, head or Mackenzie zones, segmental effects, reflexology) ■ increase of metabolism, e.g. by axon reflexes ■ triggering of reflexes and adjustments of the actual values of the musculature by the influence of longitudinal receptors (muscle spindles, and others) and stretch receptors (Golgi organs and others) ■ adjustment of the normal value and loosening of hardened muscles (physical and mental influences) ■ relaxation by support of physiological relaxing processes of metabolism ■ vegetative regulation (activation of the sympathicus or parasympathicus, depending on the massage technique) ■ emotional relaxation
vibrations (hand vibrations, finger-pad vibrations)	Vibrations are delicate swinging movements of the flat hand with a frequency of 10–15/sec. They will be perceived as very pleasant by the patient and will lead to a relaxation of the musculature.		
tapping	Tapping is a variation of knocking.		
knocking	Depending on the force of knocking, a tone increase (hard knocking grips) or a tone decrease (soft rhythmic knocking) will be achieved.		
chopping	Chopping is a variation of knocking.		
slapping	Slapping is a variation of knocking.		
kneading (one-hand, two-hand, two-finger kneading)	Kneading and flexing (petrissage) are stretching, twists or pressing of muscle tissue reaching deeply and inserting obliquely to the run of the fibers		
skin irritation grips (frictions and shifting grips)	Frictions present intensive, small, circular, elliptic gripping techniques by the thumb or finger tips. These grips mean a strong impulse to the muscles and the connective tissue.		

Tab. 85.3 Continued.

Classic massages			
Special forms of massage			
Massage technique[1]	Execution	Indications[2]	Effects and remarks
sport massage	activating or sedative techniques, depending on the purpose	■ for pre- and after-care of athletic performances (exercising and competition)	■ sport Massage can be combined with a preparing and postprocessing "muscle check", and – if necessary – first therapeutic measures can be applied (e.g. loosening of hardenings). ■ For other effects, please see last column of ➢ Tab. 85.3 of current massage effects. **Please note:** Sport massage has proved to be an indispensable component of the athletic performance development in competitive sports.
connective tissue massage	massage in three segments of connective tissue: ■ skin technique (area between epidermis and subcutis – upper shifting layer) ■ subcutis technique (area between subcutis and fascias – deep shifting layer) ■ fascia technique: effects on the peripheral arterial blood circulation are possible	■ increased tension of tissue segments (connective tissue zones) ■ diseases of the respiratory organs ■ functional disorders of the gastro-intestinal and genitourinary tract ■ increased blood circulation ■ vessel diseases (arteriosclerosis, PAOD) ■ complex regional pain syndrome (Sudeck's atrophy)	■ reflex-therapeutic procedures ■ influencing the internal organs by use of segmental reflex arcs ■ existing tissue adhesions are to be loosened by the gripping techniques ■ normalization of the tissue elasticity ■ pain relief by relaxation ■ influencing the autonomic nervous system (cave: extreme fatigue appearing 1–2 hours after treatment has been known for connective tissue massages.) **Remark:** At the connective tissue massage, there have only been theories so far about the exact processes of the body during and after the therapy, which have not withstood any scientific examination yet.
reflexology	massage of reflex zones for the specific influence on the organs belonging to these zones	■ influence on the internal organs by use of reflexive connections (reflex zones) ■ treatment of pain syndromes	Reflexology consists of: ■ connective tissue massage ■ foot reflexology ■ segmental massage ■ periosteal treatment ■ muscle reflexology ■ colon massage

	Reflexology of the foot is based on the thought that an analogy of shape exists between the foot and a sitting person. This form of therapy belongs to the alteration and order therapies.		**Remark:** At reflexology, there have only been theories about the exact processes of the body during and after the therapy, so far, which have not withstood any scientific examination yet.
periost massage (periosteal treatment)	circumscribed, punctiform pressure massage at certain adequate periosteal localizations	■ acute and chronic pain conditions	■ local hyperemic treatment ■ stimulation of the cell regeneration (periosteal tissue) ■ the effect mechanism is focused on the nerval influence on organic functional procedures **Remark:** As in the complete field of reflexology, periosteal massages so far have only been considered regarding the exact processes of the body during and after the therapy, which have not withstood any scientific examination yet.
manual lymph drainage (decongestion therapy)	The lymphatic vessels will be stroked out manually, which will activate the lymphatic vasomotion, stimulate the lymphatic lymphatic flow and wick away the tissue fluid. The removal of tissue fluid is promoted by: ■ sufficient and pumping grips ■ spiral and circular grips (by help of thumb and fingers, so-called scoop grips, turn grips). The skin will be shifted gently against the subcutaneous tissue. The treatments start centrally, near the orifices of the lymphatic vessels in the angulus venosus (venous angle), and then will extend to more distant regions of the body. The necessary capacity for the fluid removal will thus be created in the according segment of the lymphatic vessels from peripheral.	■ primary lymphatic edema ■ secondary lymphatic edema (posttraumatic, postoperative) ■ secondary lymphatic edema (after surgical tumor resection, at swellings caused by a venous edema or a lipedema) ■ regional pain syndrome (lymphatic drainage proximally of the lesion) ■ headaches and migraine will respond to this therapeutic procedure	**Remark:** ■ The effect of the MLD is not only to be understood mechanically. It will lead to a transposition of the organism up to relaxation and regeneration by way of the autonomic nervous system. ■ The lymphatic drainage will only make sense, if a compression therapy by application of an elasto-compressive bandage or compression stocking follows directly. ■ It will usually be applied in combination with other methods (bandages, skin care, movement exercises, decongesting posture etc.; see also decongestion, massage therapy). ■ Manual lymph drainage has proved effective in the phase of recovery after sport injuries.

Tab. 85.3 Continued.

Classic massages			
Special forms of massage			
Massage technique[1]	Execution[2]	Indications	Effects and remarks
brush massage	By hand brushes as dry brushings or by wet brushes (can also be carried out by massage gloves made of hemp or terrycloth). The brush massages will be carried out with different body positions (erect, lying; cf. Heisel 2005).	■ peripheral blood circulation disorders ■ vegetative dysfunctions ■ peripheral rheumatism (soft tissue rheumatism) ■ venous and lymphatic congestions ■ inurement (at susceptibility for infections)	Brushing will work as a reflex to the blood circulation of the skin as well as stimulating to cardiovascular functions as well as their regulative abilities: ■ improvement of the venous backflow ■ improvement of the lymphatic drainage ■ improvement of the skin functions (skin elasticity) ■ Central relief will be caused by an essential hypertension at centrifugal stroke of the brush (Heisel 2005).
acupressure (acupressure massage, rod massage)	The finger pressure massage will be carried out as a variant of acupressure, i.e. as a puncture massage under the consideration of the meridians, segmental, supraspinal and central mechanisms (for more specific descriptions, see mentioned specialist literature).	■ chronic pain (headaches, migraine, cervical syndrome) ■ degenerative spinal conditions, ischialgias ■ degenerative joint adaptations ■ diseases of rheumatic forms ■ insertion tendopathies ■ scar treatment ■ soft-tissue rheumatic conditions (fibromyalgia, myofascial pain syndrome and others) ■ functional disorders at the locomotor apparatus with secondary vegetative dysfunctions ■ weak immune system	■ The rod massage (acupuncture massage) is based on the assumptions of the traditional Chinese medicine and meridians running through the body. ■ The findings and the treatment of disorders will also be possible at the auricle, which – according to classic Chinese medicine – presents a mirror image of the human body.
under-water pressure jet-massage	circulatory application of a water jet controllable in its intensity	In principle, the indications of under-water pressure jet-massage are similar to the ones of classical massage: ■ muscular hardenings ■ postacute radicular lumbar syndromes, ankylosing spondylitis (Bekhterev syndrome), chronic relapsing lumbar syndromes ■ coxarthrosis	■ The under-water pressure jet-massage combines the massage effect with the advantages of the warm bath (water temperature of 34–40°C, upwelling, hydrostatic pressure, mental aspects, relaxation). ■ The under-water pressure jet-massage is especially well applicable with hirsute patients. The disadvantage of the under-water pressure jet-massage compared to the classical massage are the worse possibilities of localization and dosage.

85.6 Physiotherapy

	A special form of under-water pressure jet-massage is the **whirlpool** (**hot Jacuzzi**) – it is appropriate for concomitant after-treatment of orthopedic-traumatologic impairments. A distinctly relaxing effect (mental regeneration) can also be observed with he application of the whirlpool.	■ muscular inactivity atrophy (concomitant measure) ■ complex regional pain syndrome (stage II and III) ■ neurological clinical pictures (s/p poliomyelitis, flaccid paralysis, Parkinson's disease, and others)
segmental massage	The segmental massage will primarily be applied to the region of the back (for the exact techniques of segmental massage compare Heisel 2005). At first, the caudal, and afterwards the cranial segments will be treated. First, the superficial, afterwards the deeper located layers will be treated.	■ spinal syndromes ■ reactive muscular disorders depending on the impairment (muscular dysbalances) ■ headaches, migraine ■ ischialgias ■ functional disorders, climacteric conditions ■ sympathetic reflex dystrophies ■ arterial and venous disorders of the blood circulation ■ after-treatment of pneumonias, bronchial asthma, pulmonary emphysema ■ (early recognition of disorders of the internal organs) ■ (differential diagnosis of arthrogenic and visceral conditions) ■ (normalization of the activity and the functional condition of the internal organs by the removal of [perhaps painful] superficial tissue changes; c.f. Heisel 2005)
	■ The segmental massage is based on the thought that all regions of the body as well as all tissue layers between skin and periost interact via neural and humoral controlling circuits. ■ Disorder focuses in an area will affect other body segments (reflex principles). ■ The treatment will be carried out segmentally with modified grips of the classical massage. ■ Treatment is also diagnosis. ■ Segmental changes appear first clinically as muscular changes, and only afterwards reactions of the connective tissue will follow. ■ Reflex changes (disorders) will occur at an earlier time than analgetic irritations. **Please note:** Segmental massage in sports shows (by experience) good results in many forms of neuromuscular dysbalances, in the prevention and treatment of (neuro-)muscular problems (muscle strains, insertion tendinoses, etc.) as well as in connective tissue dysfunctions (irritations). **Remark:** As with the full area of reflexology, only theories about the exact processes in the body during and after the therapy have existed until today, which have not withstood any scientific examination yet.	

---

[1] References are given for the modalities of application (techniques); only a general overview is to be provided here.
[2] The indications will always have to be made individually.

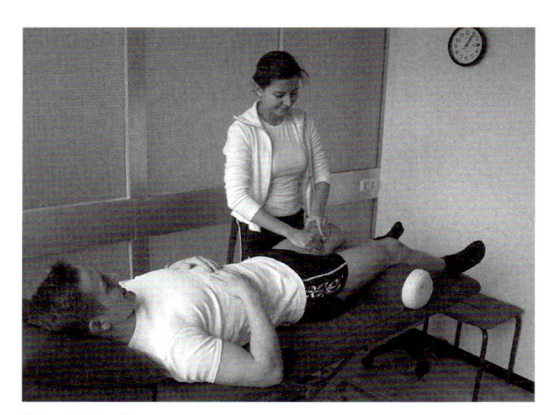

Fig. 85.4 Sport massage.

Massage is not only very useful in older persons who often cannot carry out active forms of therapy, but also in athletes – whether in the course of exercise and preparation/post-processing of competition or in the field of therapeutic treatment, e.g. after sports injuries, at conservative as well as after surgical treatment (➤ Fig. 85.4).

Massages can be carried out as a **partial or as full body massages**. Liquid or ointment-like massage lotions such as petrolatum or special oils facilitate them.

It is sensible to combine passive techniques – to which massage is counted – with active forms of therapy (e.g. medical gymnastics, medical exercise therapy) especially in phases of rehabilitation after sport injuries.

Massage techniques

Massage techniques will lead to the mechanical influencing of the skin and the soft tissue near the skin (musculature, fatty tissue, connective tissue, periost) by pressure, traction, vibration, friction to different physiologic reactions.

They are differentiated into:

- classical massage techniques: Primary purpose is the transversely striate musculature.
- special forms: These will influence different target locations.

The common massage techniques and their special forms are listed in ➤ Table 85.3. Indications, application and effects are listed in short terms. An optimal treatment success can be achieved by the indication-specific combination of grip techniques.

Indication and prescription

As for medical gymnastics, the physician prescribes the massage, which needs correct **dosing** like medication.

Therefore, every prescription should contain the following **data**:

- exactly specified diagnosis and performance symptoms
- exact purpose (description of the function to be improved)
- description of the methods of massage that are to be used
- number of treatments
- specification of the interval between treatments (frequency of stimulations, e.g. daily or 3 times a week)
- specification of combinations with other physiotherapeutic methods or measures
- description of existing or concomitant medication (for information).

The prescribing physician must consider that the different massage techniques require different time expenditures. While partial massages are carried out for ca. 20–30 min, lymphatic drainages will be carried out in about 60 min, possibly several times a day (Weimann 1993).

Contraindications

Contraindications of massage are (changed according to Weimann 1993, Gutenbrunner and Weimann 2004, Stein and Greitemann 2005):

- **absolute contraindications:**
  - feverish diseases
  - local and generalized inflammations (abscesses, lymphangitis, thrombosis, phlebitis, osteomyelitis, myositis)
  - fresh fractures, ligament injuries and dislocations in the area of the injury
  - condition after fresh myocardial infarction
  - arterial circulation impairments in stages III and IV

- **relative contraindications:**
  - impaired blood coagulation
  - tumor diseases, consuming processes
  - distinct or decompensated heart insufficiency
  - thromboses (danger of an emboly)
  - distinct arteriosclerosis and seriously impaired blood coagulation
  - direct condition after surgical treatments
  - direct condition after muscle injuries
  - distinct hematomas (in the hematoma area)
  - complex regional pain syndrome (CRPS, Sudeck's atrophy: The clinical picture can deteriorate by mechanical irritation!)
  - gravidity (especially under-water pressure jet-massage)
  - older persons (careful with minor stressable tissue, osteoporosis of a high degree)
  - neurologic diseases (e.g. neuralgias, distinct impairments of skin sensitivity).

85.6.5 Electrotherapy

In the electrotherapy, an electrical current will be used for therapeutic purposes. Electrical currents can be used very well for therapy, because **chemo-electrical procedures** are very significant in the body.

Electrotherapy is to be classified generally by the frequency spectra (Jenrich 2000):

- galvanization 0 Hz
- low-frequency therapy 1–1,000 Hz
- medium-frequency therapy 1,000–100,000 Hz
- high-frequency therapy >100,000 Hz
- ultrasound therapy ≥ 800,000 Hz.

Indication and prescription

The prescription of electrotherapy is to be done by the physician, because it will have to be **dosed correctly**.

Every prescription should contain the following data:

- exactly specified diagnosis and performance symptoms
- exact purpose (description of the function to be improved, problems, e.g. pain)
- description of the methods of electrotherapy that are to be used (dosage, intensity)
- number of treatments, length and interval between treatments of electrotherapy
- specification of combinations with other physiotherapeutic methods or measures
- description of existing or concomitant medication (for information).

Indications for electrotherapy are:

- pain conditions of the nervous system (analgesia)
- pain conditions of the locomotor organs (analgesia)
- myalgias
- non-activated arthroses (high frequency, ultrasound)
- arthroses with secondary myotendinoses (ultrasound)
- posttraumatic and postoperative conditions of the locomotor apparatus (bruises, strains, joint effusions and others)
- tendopathies, tendinoses
- arterial impairments of blood circulation (promotion of blood circulation)
- prevention of inactivity atrophies (e.g. during immobilizations)
- increasing the chance of activation and the blood circulation of myasthenias and tensions (by pathologic joint afferences at segmental impairments)
- chronic-inflammatory diseases
- treatment of edemas
- muscular atrophies (inactivity and immobilization atrophies)
- muscular atrophies (peripheral nerve injuries).

Contraindications

The contraindications for electrotherapy are to be understood as general contraindications.

They will **not be the same for all forms of electrical current and all locations**; for closer information please see mentioned reference literature (Weimann 1993, Jenrich 2000).

Contraindications can be:
- metal in the body (area of treatment)
- cardiac pacemaker
- impaired skin sensitivity
- skin diseases
- wounds
- pregnancy (relative contraindication)
- hemorrhages and risk of hemorrhages (impaired blood coagulation)
- thromboses and danger of embolies
- fever
- Sudeck's atrophy
- edemas (relative contraindication, especially at high frequency).

Medical electrolysis

Jenrich explains that medical electrolysis is the therapeutic application of en electrical current with constant power and direction, i.e. frequency = 0 Hz (Jenrich 2000, p. 21).

Medical electrolysis causes a **polarization of the tissues** and it affects especially the **skin**, the **fascias** and the **tendons**. Furthermore, the diffusion and osmosis processes in the tissues increase, which will improve the metabolic rate and thus the ability to regenerate.

Effects:
- analgesic (major effect), especially under the anode
- promotion of the percutaneous substance transport of ionized substances and adequate medication (iontophoresis)
- regional increased blood perfusion and – depending on the polarity – increase or decrease of the motor susceptibility and sensitivity
- palliation or covering of neuralgic and myalgic conditions.

Low-frequency therapy

Nerves and muscles can be stimulated **selectively** by low-frequency currents. The physiotherapist must prove his skills in the indication-specific choice of the **adequate current parameters** (power, abruptness of increase, lengths of impulse and break).

Low-frequency currents are:
- diadynamic currents
- ultra-stimulation current according to Träbert
- two-phase currents as well as
- transcutaneous electric nerve stimulation (TENS).

Effects:
- especially pain relief
- prevention of e.g. muscular atrophy in immobilization due to stimulation of nerve-muscle systems by help of two-phase impulse sequences and by surge-current application.

Medium-frequency therapy

Nerve-muscle systems can be stimulated by medium-frequency therapy and **muscular atrophies** can be **prevented**.

Effects:
- Promotion of the local muscle endurance in particular by the application of medium-frequency currents. In general, the patient will tolerate the medium-frequency currents for muscle contraction better than the low-frequency currents.
- An improved nutritional state of the contracted muscle tissue will occur concomitantly to the electrically stimulated muscle contraction.

High-frequency therapy

The therapy with high-frequency currents is carried out with higher current intensities. Therapeutically effective warmth will develop in the skin and in the deeper tissue layers because of the absorption of the provided electric energy in the tissue. **Different depth effects** can be achieved by the specific selection of current frequencies. High-frequency therapy is often considered a **thermotherapy** because of its warmth effects.

Effects:
- hyperemia and increase of the local metabolism; no motor stimulation effect
- positive influence, especially on muscle tensions
- positive influence on nervous processes, such as increase of excitability, shortening of the

chronaxy and increase of the conduction speed (Jenrich 2000).

Ultrasound therapy

Ultrasound therapy has proved valuable (Jenrich 2000) especially for:
- tendopathies and tendinoses as well as
- arthroses with secondary myotendinoses.

Effects:
- increased blood perfusion
- accelerated metabolism and
- higher pain threshold in the treated tissues.

85.6.6 Hydro- and thermal therapies

Hydrotherapy

Hydrotherapy is the treatment of patients by application of **water** in multiple variants (➤ Tab. 85.4). The physical characteristics of water are used for therapy: hydrostatic pressure, buoyancy resistance effect.

The following **applications** are distinguished:
- by cloth (washings, compresses, wet packs)
- by running water (showers, douching)
- by hydrostatic pressure (partial and full immersion baths)
- bath treatment without hydrostatic pressure (sauna, steam baths).

Baths are classified with regard to their medium (Weimann 1993):
- by their hydrostatic effect (full, three-quarter and partial immersion baths)
- by the used medium (water baths, perhaps with additives, baths of pultaceous consistence, gas and steam baths)

The hydrotherapeutic effects can be increased by **combination with electric currents** (e.g. four cell baths), by the use of special **curative waters** (e.g. mineral or mud baths) or by the application of **additives** (e.g. carbonic acid).

Thermal therapy

The treatment with **warmth** or **cold** is called thermal therapy.

It can be differentiated into:
- measures procuring warmth and
- measures withdrawing warmth.

The thermal therapy is mostly used in **combination with hydrotherapy**. Interchanging applications of warmth and cold are often used by means of a stimulation therapy.

Effects of hydrotherapy and thermal therapy

The hydrotherapy and thermal therapy often work as **stimulation therapy** by mechanical, thermal and chemical influences. The **hydro-**

Tab. 85.4 Hydrotherapeutic applications classified by strength of stimulus (changed according to Stein 2005, Weimann 1993).

Mild hydrotherapeutic stimuli	Medium-strong hydrotherapeutic stimuli	Strong hydrotherapeutic stimuli
- washings, attritions and brushings - partial baths, alternating baths - rising foot and forearm baths - cold knee affusions, facial, nape and arm affusions - femoral affusion - water treading - packings - wet onlays - boiling vapor bath	- rising partial bath and half bath - dry brushes - water treading, dew walking, snow walking - alternating-temperature hip baths - alternating-temperature affusions of arms, knees and crus - half baths - temperature-increasing partial baths - arm affusion with breast affusion - torso packings - sauna	- hyperthermia bath - three-quarter baths and full baths with cold dowsing - contrast hip baths - hot lumbal affusion - full affusion (cold), power showers - three-quarter or full poultice - large packing, hay sack

static pressure – combined with thermal stimuli – can be used for compression, especially with swellings.

Cryotherapy is still indispensible with acute sports injuries in the course of **first care**. "Hot ice" (iced water) in combination with compressions still is the standard treatment for **acute traumas**. The local and global application forms of cold and warmth are listed in ➤ Table 85.5.

The warmth will be transmitted over the skin, e.g. by conduction, convection or radiation. Warmth and cold receptors will be activated by the physical stimuli and neural-reflexive effects will be triggered.

The receptor density at the extremities is $3–6/cm^2$. The temperature, which stimulates the cold receptors to a maximum, ranges between 15 and 34 °C, or 38 and 48 °C for the warmth receptors. Lately, there have been

Tab. 85.5 Local and global forms of warmth and coldness applications (changed and amended according to Weimann 1993).

Measures	Application	Remarks
packings, formentations	circularly directed, tight-fitting wraps	warmth or coldness, corresponding to the indication
poultice	wraps of the whole body or of individual parts (duration approx. 20–30 min)	warmth or coldness, corresponding to the indication e.g. peloids (mud, turf, mineral mud, fango)
warm or cold onlays, compresses	covering of body regions	■ warmth or coldness, corresponding to the indication ■ Suitable compresses are also offered ready-for-use by industry.
hot role	will be rolled over and impressed on the region to be treated (thermal effect and mechanical stimulus)	primarily refectory effects
ice cube therapy	with ice cubes or ice cones	■ The ice therapy will be well integrated into other physiotherapeutic exercises. ■ The skin should be protected of cold injuries by applying wet cloth that has been plunged into salt water beforehand.
partial ice bath	short-time partial ice baths of the extremities (10–60 sec)	mixture of ice and water in the relation of 2:1
cooler spray	on-spraying of cooling chemical substances	■ suitable for the first cooling with sports injuries ■ also to be applied as spray-and-stretch technique as well as in the treatment of trigger points ■ The unqualified application of cooler spray may lead to severe tissue damages.
cold air	cold air generated by special devices, which will be specifically applied to the regions to be treated	There will be the risk of tissue damages also with cold-air applications.
heated air	■ sauna and vapor bath as global application ■ alternatively, apparative-local application	Sauna and vapor bath will have a specifically positive effect on the immune system; if applied appropriately, they will support the athlete's regeneration.
cold chamber	cold-air chamber with up to –110 °C (–160 °C)	Cold-chamber applications will only be possible at few locations because of the limited availability and the high costs.

stronger scientific findings of the cold in edema treatment being rather ineffective. The edemas can even be increased. The cold perhaps influences the system of the lymphatic vessels negatively (van den Berg 2003).

The impulse rate of cold receptors, which occur more often in the tissues than the warmth receptors, clearly ranges above the impulse rate of warmth receptors.

The use of the **buoyancy effect of water** supports the weight relief, e.g. with knee injuries. Early loads will therefore be possible In the water (e.g. aqua jogging), which would strain the injured structures too much on land.

Due to the **resistance effect** of the water, the setting of impulses will already be possible at an early point of time at the therapeutic use in swimming pools, and it will train the muscle strength and the muscle strength endurance.

The thermal therapy – depending on the warmth or cold application – has the following effects:

- **warmth effects:**
  - increase of temperature and metabolism
  - increased blood perfusion (vasodilatation)
  - increase of the body (core) temperature (global application)
  - spasmolysis
  - pain relief
  - antiphlogistic effect at chronic and proliferative inflammations
  - mental well-being
  - triggering of vessel reactions (arterial and venous vessel enlargements with hyperemia and skin erythema)
  - warmth-conditioned change of plasma viscosity
  - influence on the contractile and viscoelastic muscular tone
  - support of the muscle stretching
  - cardiovascular reactions (increased pulse rate, increase of the cardiac output, reduction of the peripheral vessel resistance, blood pressure descent)
  - influence on the immune system.

- **cold effects – short-term cold stimuli (≤ 5 min):**
  - rather superficial effect
  - local algesia by desensitization
  - locally restricted vasoconstriction
  - inhibited blood perfusion by timely restricted local vasoconstriction (counter-regulation hyperemia)
  - influence on the contractile and viscoelastic muscular tone.

- **cold effects – longer-termed cold stimuli (>15–20 min):**
  - depth effect
  - intramuscular temperature reduction
  - intraarticular temperature reduction
  - reduced metabolism (cell metabolism)
  - reduced enzyme activity
  - antiphlogistic effect in the cooled area
  - influence on the contractile and viscoelastic muscular tone.

- **cold effects – cold chamber:**
  - neuronal stimulation with consecutive pain relief
  - antiphlogistic effect (rheumatism, ankylosing spondylitis)
  - preparation of athletic top performances, especially under heat conditions.

Indications

Hydrotherapy and thermal therapy provides a wide application field in the treatment of athletes. **Indications** are (Stein 2005, Weimann 1993):

- impairments and diseases of the supporting and locomotor apparatus (myotendinoses, insertion tendopathies, periostoses)
- diseases of the rheumatic spectrum disorder
- chronic conditions of the postural and locomotor apparatus (especially warmth)
- injury-caused conditions
- postoperative conditions
- degenerative and non-inflammatory joint impairments and diseases
- soft-tissue rheumatism (especially warmth)
- during postoperative rehabilitation
- after endoprothetic treatment

- subacute and chronic pain of the joints (joints of spine and extremities)
- postoperative rehabilitation after orthopedic or emergency-surgical spine surgeries including surgeries of the vertebral disks
- vertebrogenic structure defect, instability and degeneration
- spastic conditions
- myosclerosis (warmth)
- physical-mental weak performance (prophylaxis of overtraining, and others)
- vegetative-neural regulation disorders (in overtraining, amongst others).

Contraindications

The contraindications of cold and warmth treatments are mostly relative contraindications. The assessment of the **individual case** is decisive.

Warmth effects an **increased blood perfusion**, for example, and thus promotes the development of **edemas**.

This will lead to contraindications at:
- acute injuries
- acute inflammatory processes as well as
- hemorrhages.

Further relative contraindications for hydrotherapy and thermal therapy are:
- heart decompensation
- angina pectoris syndrome with rest symptoms
- coronary heart disease
- cardiomyopathy
- hyperthyreosis
- badly adjusted diabetes mellitus
- cerebral seizures
- pulmonary tuberculosis
- infectious-bacterial intestinal diseases
- mucosal ulceration with hemorrhaging tendency
- arterial occlusive disease
- acute inflammations
- varicosis
- lymphatic congestions and swellings after trauma or surgery.

85.6.7 Light therapy

Light therapy is the application of **natural or artificial light sources** for therapeutic purposes. In sports medicine, light therapy can also be used for the support of regeneration and training processes.

The mood-lifting, **anti-depressive effect** of UV radiation has been known, as well as the clearly improved **efficiency of strength training** under UV radiation.

The **protection of the eyes** (retina) by adequate glasses is important. The **dose** of light therapy is to be increased slowly depending on sensitivity and purpose.

Classification of light therapy (changed according to Weimann 1993):
- infrared waves (range of frequency 780 to 5,000 nm)
- visible light (range of frequency 400–780 nm)
- ultraviolet radiation (range of frequency UVA 315–400 nm, UVB 280–315 nm).

The infrared waves are applied as the thermal therapy (warmth).

Effects

Infrared waves: Infrared radiation is sensible especially for **superficial inflammatory processes**, such as boils, abscesses or paranasal sinusitis (Weimann 1993) by:
- generating a superficial warmth effect
- increasing the skin perfusion
- pain reduction as well as
- implementation of reflexive-regulative processes.

UV light:
- reduction of the serum bilirubin by the blue amount (425–475 nm)
- pigmentation
- stimulation of the vitamin-D synthesis
- stimulation of immunologic processes
- influence on the autonomic nervous system in the sense of a normotrophic regulation
- antiseptic, disinfecting effect

85.6 Physiotherapy

- effect to the cell nuclei and enzyme systems
- supporting measures in competitive sports for training and regeneration processes, e.g. for the protection of susceptibility for infections.

> Burns of the skin, overdosing especially in the UVA and UVB radiation can cause preterm skin aging and dermal cancer. Therefore, the doses should only be increased slowly; treatments should be in blocks.

Indications

- psoriasis (UVB)
- neurodermatitis
- acne (UVA)
- myocosis fungoides
- atopic dermatitis (UVA)
- vitiligo (UVA)
- superficial ulcers
- vitamin-D deficiency
- osteoporosis
- seasonal forms of depression (winter depression)
- vegetative adaptation
- for the preparation of training and competition in climate zones with high UV exposition (pre-pigmentation, UV hardening).

Contraindications

- increased light sensitivity ("being pale-skinned" and due to light sensitivity increased by medication)
- existing sunburn
- sensitivity disorders of radiated areas
- acute inflammatory processes (infrared)
- impairments of the porphyrin metabolism.

References

Bundesarbeitsgemeinschaft für Rehabilitation (BAR) (2000). Rahmenempfehlungen zur ambulanten Rehabilitation bei muskuloskeletalen Erkrankungen.

Clasing D, Siegfried I (2002). Sportärztliche Untersuchung und Beratung (3rd ed.). Balingen: Spitta-Verlag.

Dalichau S (2001). Der Einfluss sportmechanische Belastungsprofile auf die thorakolumbale Wirbelsäulenform. Butzbach: Afra-Verlag.

Engelhardt M, Hintermann B, Segesser B (eds.) (1997). GOTS-Manual Sporttraumatologie. Bern: Hans-Huber-Verlag.

Engelhardt M, Krüger-Franke M, Pieper H-G, Siebert C-H (eds.) (2005). Sportverletzungen – Sportschäden. Stuttgart: Thieme-Verlag.

Gutenbrunner C, Weimann G (eds.) (2004). Krankengymnastische Methoden und Konzepte. (1st ed.). Berlin: Springer-Verlag.

Heisel J (2005). Physikalische Medizin. Stuttgart: Thieme.

Hildebrandt G (1998). Therapeutische Physiologie. In: Gutenbrunner C, Hildebrandt G (eds.). Handbuch der Balneologie und medizinischen Klimatologie. Berlin: Springer-Verlag.

Jenrich W (2000). Grundlagen der Elektrotherapie. Munich: Urban & Fischer Verlag.

Kladny B (2005). Massage und Thermotherapie. In: Stein V, Greitemann B (eds.). Rehabilitation in Orthopädie und Unfallchirurgie. Methoden, Therapiestrategien, Behandlungsempfehlungen. Heidelberg: Springer-Verlag.

Kohlrausch A (2005). Passive Techniken. In: Gutenbrunner C, Weimann G (eds.). Krankengymnastische Methoden und Konzepte. Berlin: Springer-Verlag.

Renström PAFH (ed.) (1997). Sportverletzungen und Überlastungsschäden. Köln: Deutscher Ärzte-Verband.

Roche Lexikon Medizin (ed.) (2003). 5th edition. Munich: Urban & Fischer Verlag.

Schüle K, Huber G (eds.) (2004). Grundlagen der Sporttherapie. Prävention, ambulante und stationäre Rehabilitation. (2nd ed.). Munich: Urban & Fischer Verlag.

Stein V, Greitemann B (eds.) (2005). Rehabilitation in Orthopädie und Unfallchirurgie. Methoden, Therapiestrategien, Behandlungsempfehlungen. Heidelberg: Springer-Verlag.

van den Berg F (ed.) (2003). Schmerzen verstehen und beeinflussen. (vol. 4). Stuttgart: Thieme-Verlag.

Viru A, Viru M (2001). Biochemical Monitoring of Sport Training. Champaign: Human Kinetics.

Weimann G (1993). Physikalische Therapie. Stuttgart: Hippokrates-Verlag.

VI Deaths in sports

86 Deaths in sports 713
86.1 Deaths by natural causes in sports 713
86.2 Unnatural deaths in sports 715
86.3 Preventive aspects 720

Chapter 86 Deaths in sports

Markus Parzeller, Peter Schmidt and Christoph Raschka

The chances to depart one's life in performing physical exercises are nearly unlimited. Cyclists race against trees, skiers crush against rocks, mountain hikers break their necks (source: Der Spiegel 11/1996).

The **manners of death** in sports can primarily be classified into **natural**, **unnatural** and **unexplained** deaths (➢ Tab. 86.1; Bux et al. 2008, Schmidt et al. 2008, Turk et al. 2008). The relation of natural and unnatural deaths is estimated as approximately 10 : 1–2 (Jung and Schäfer-Nolte 1982, Berghold 1986, Raschka et al. 1996, Parzeller et al. 1998).

The **yearly incidence** of traumatic deaths amounts to 0.3/100,000 and of cardiovascular deaths to 1/100,000 in male club athletes in Germany (Parzeller et al. 1998). 2,969 deaths of German club athletes have been analyzed over a time period of 20 years in SAUDIS ("sudden and unexpected deaths in sports", ➢ Tab. 86.2; Parzeller and Raschka 2003).

86.1 Deaths by natural causes in sports

Individual regions and certain age groups show different causes of natural deaths in sports. **Myocardial infarctions** or a **coronary heart disease** are diagnosed as the most common cause of death in athletes older than 35 years (➢ Tab. 86.3; Maron et al. 1996, Raschka et al. 1999, Tafur et al. 1999, Bux et al. 2004, Bux et al. 2008, Turk et al. 2008).

However, there have been different data of the most frequent causes of death in younger athletes. **Hypertrophic cardiomyopathy** has been described as most common cause of death in young athletes in the U.S. (Goble 1999, Weiner 1999, Maron et al. 2002), while the myocardial infarction and the coronary heart disease have been dominant also in younger athletes in Europe (Basso et al. 1999, Raschka et al. 1999, Bux et al. 2004, Parzeller et al. 2006, Bux et al. 2008, Turk et al. 2008). The diagnosis of cardiac genetic defects of potentially lethal ion channel diseases has recently become more and more important also for natural deaths in sports (Kauferstein et al. 2008). Especially in water sports, the so-called bathing fatalities and the sudden death in water by natural causes will have to be distinguished from **drowning accidents**. **Bathing fatality** is a sudden immersion and death caused by **vagal reflexes** triggered

Tab. 86.1 Definition of death.

Manner of death	Definition
natural death	Death occurs only due to diseases, dysplasias or biologically conditioned decrepitude caused by pathological internal reasons. There is no evidence for third party fault, such as medical errors in treatment, active medicide, etc.
non-natural death	Death occurs because of an accident, suicide, an unlawful action or other external influences. Third party fault is not essential.
unexplained manner of death (not predefined for all states in Germany)	This specification only shows that the manner of death cannot sufficiently be ascertained at the moment of post mortem and with the information and measures available for the necropsy. Further investigations and an autopsy, if required, as well as additional examinations are necessary.

Tab. 86.2 Sport- and age-based analysis of deaths.

Sport	Number of deaths	Average age	Sport	Number of deaths	Average age
soccer	919	37.1	parachuting	6	34.3
tennis	209	51.7	squash	6	37.2
cycling	187	47.7	surfing	5	34.2
gymnastics	132	52.6	boxing	5	30.8
handball	123	34.1	billiard	4	39.3
table tennis	121	46.8	motorboat	4	47.5
ninepins	108	56.6	kayak	4	34.8
track and field	100	47.3	prellball	4	57.8
equestrianism	85	34.1	hockey	4	30.5
disabled sports	76	58.6	golf	4	49.9
gliding	67	40.3	bowling	3	29
aviation sports	64	49.3	hang gliding	3	45
canoeing	62	41.3	weightlifting	3	22
swimming	59	48.5	rugby	3	42
functionary	54	49.2	ballooning	2	40
volleyball	45	41.3	bobsleighing	2	32
trimming	40	52.7	triathlon	2	35.5
alpine skiing	38	38.6	ultralight aviation	2	42.5
shooting sports	36	39.9	motorcycle racing	2	41.5
jogging	34	52.9	YMCA	2	50.5
sports fishing	30	48.7	water polo	2	14.5
hiking	29	57	aikido	2	46
rowing	28	38.3	fencing	2	62.5
gymnastics	24	56	curling	2	30
underwater diving	23	37.5	stock sport	1	65
sailing	22	47.6	taekwondo	1	34
fistball	22	52	baseball/softball	1	17
badminton	21	39.7	vasity team	1	56
company-facilitated sports activities	21	45.1	American football	1	21
basketball	15	37.3	water ski	1	32
judo	14	28.3	ice hockey	1	15
German Catholic Sports Federation (DJK)	10	53.3	bocce	1	50
motor sports	10	33.1	sleighing	1	22
dance sports	9	52.9	German Ju-Jutsu	1	52
chess	9	57.9	kickboxing	1	15
mountaineering	9	31.2	inline sports	1	12
karate	8	27	miniature golf	1	34
cross-country skiing	8	49.9	ice sports	1	33
wrestling	6	21.3			

Tab. 86.3 Age and natural causes of death after athletic activity (autopsy material of Forensic Medicine Frankfurt/Main from Jan 1972–Aug 2008: n = 124 (0.37%) of approx. 33,700 autopsies; mod. according to Bux et al. 2008).

Cause of death	Number
coronary heart disease	39
myocardial infarction (initial manifestation)	31
reinfarction	26
myocarditis or suspicion, respectively	6
right heart failure	3
cardiac dysrhythmia	2
heart anomalies	2
unclear cause of death	2
ruptured aortic aneurysm	2
non-obstructive hypertrophic cardiomyopathy	1
dilatative cardiomyopathy	1
aneurysm of the heart wall	1
chronic abacterial endocarditis	1
other cardial causes	4
bronchial carcinoma	1
nephrorrhagia	1
acute influenza	1

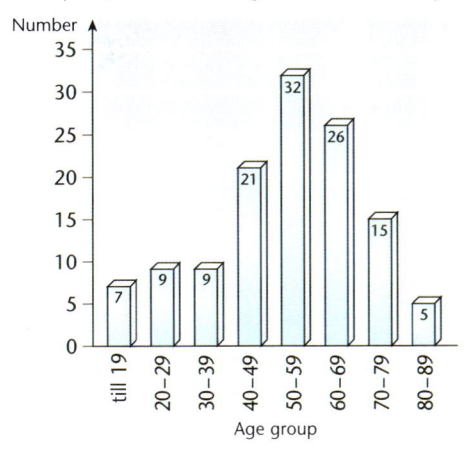

under water. The Ebbecke or dive reflex, which is triggered by the contact of the facial skin with the cold water, comes into question as well as reflexes due to the irritation of the vagal part in the superior laryngeal nerve. Valsalva mechanisms, cold, urticaria and laryngospasms have also been described as causes.

The term of **"sudden death in the water by natural cause"** describes a sudden death by a **disease**, which only accidentally occurs at the same time as the stay in the water. Especially diseases of the cardiovascular system or epileptic seizures with agonal drowning are causes of death (Keil 2003, Brinkmann 2004).

86.2 Unnatural deaths in sports

Deaths in sports can appear in all different disciplines with most traumatic deaths in flying and water sports – according to a Frankfurt autopsy study – and in cycling and riding – according to a Frankfurt insurance study (Parzeller and Raschka 2003, Schmidt et al. 2008). Swimming, cycling and riding dominate as affected sports disciplines in regional comparison in a Hamburg autopsy study (Turk et al. 2008). Unnatural deaths can be influenced by the **weather** or **local conditions** in all sports carried out in the open air. Thus, deaths by lightning have been described in golf very often (Cherington 2001). Parachuters can suffer deathly current surges by contacts to the power lines. Trauma-conditioned causes have often occurred in the months of spring and summer (Koch et al. 2002).

86.2.1 Team sports

In principle, traumatic deaths can occur in every team sport with possible unfortunate **body contacts** between the players, e.g. basketball (Friedmann et al. 2001). Soccer as a team sport and also as a most commonly practiced sport has the top position of injury frequencies in most sport-traumatologic surveys in Europe. Fatal soccer accidents only play a minor role, though (Biener 1985).

The **mortality rate in soccer** amounts to 0.6–1.2 in 100,000 players according to a survey of the time period from 1938 to 1959 (Fields 1989) with more than one third of the deaths being caused by craniocerebral traumas.

> **Lethal injury mechanisms in ball sports:** collision with another player (Varga and Takács 1990, Raschka et al. 1995, Raschka 2008), collision with posts or boards, direct ball impacts to the head or torso (contusio cordis; Parzeller and Raschka 2003), headers.

Four traumatic deaths have been reported in high school and college soccer players in the U.S.A. in the period from 1982 to 1988 (Mueller and Cantu 1990). A death can also be caused in soccer by the injury mechanism of a **commotio or contusio cordis** (Maron et al. 2002, Parzeller and Raschka 2003) with a possible underlying circulatory disorder with coronary spasm and resulting ventricular fibrillation (Raas and Hörtnagel 1983). The smaller the impact surface and the faster the trauma, the more disastrous are the consequences.

The cases reported in literature involve soccer balls, golf balls, baseballs or hand balls (Dickman et al. 1978, Abrunzo 1991) and softballs (Froede et al. 1979, Green et al. 1980) shot from close by as a **trigger**. Especially children and adolescents are at a risk, because their thoracic walls are still very elastic (Maron et al. 2002). The puck in ice hockey can also induce a lethal commotio cordis (Deady and Innes 1999).

Deaths have also been reported after sport-conditioned leg injuries with a phlebothrombosis followed by a **pulmonary embolism**.

American football, which has developed in 1869 from the English rugby, involves more dangerous situations. Injuries in this sport are already conditioned by the performance of the game itself. 18 athletes died in 1905, which has led to consecutive rule changes for the protection of the athletes. However, these changed rules could not prevent an increase of the violence of the game. The requirement of helmets has only been introduced in 1939. 497 fatal accidents with involvement of the CNS have been documented for American football in the period from 1945 to 1999 (Cantu and Mueller 2003).

The **causes of death** have been brain injuries in 69% of the cases and traumas of the cervical spine in 16% of the cases. 61% of the deaths occurred during competition with 75% of them in high schools. The number of high school football players amounts to more than 1 million, though, of college players to approximately 75,000 and of the professionals to approximately 2,000. In addition, 18 high school or college players have died since 1995 after a **heat stroke** during the game.

86.2.2 Individual sports

The term "individual sports" summarizes different disciplines of track and field athletics as well as ball sports that are not performed in the team compound, e.g. tennis, table tennis or squash. Larger retrospective studies (Hawley et al. 1990, La Harpe et al. 1995) consistently document that those are primarily **sudden natural deaths** and only exceptionally injury-conditioned traumatic deaths.

Sudden deaths in **running** have mainly been described for **track and field athletics**. These apply primarily to **male athletes older than 40 years**. The direct cause of death is usually a fresh **myocardial infarction** (with or without coronary thrombosis). Findings such as distinct cardiac hypertrophies, infarction scars or a pronounced calcifying and stenosing coronary sclerosis often indicate acute complications of an existent chronic ischemic heart disease.

Traumatic deaths have only been documented as **individual observations** in larger series without a precise description of the injury patterns (Hawley et al. 1990). Only three cases had been of traumatic genesis in an analysis of 197 deaths in tennis, table tennis, squash and badminton (Parzeller and Raschka 1995).

Another survey of 60 sudden deaths in **squash** presented a nearly identical image. 59 of 60 cases had been men with an average age of 46 years. A **coronary heart disease** had been the cause of death in more than 80% of the cases. It also has to be mentioned that 75% of the deceased had previously shown **prodromal clinical symptoms**, especially thoracic pain.

Traumatic deaths were not observed in this examination series (Northcote et al. 1986). Conclusions drawn from these few observations suggest that these deaths do not seem to be characterized by the specific conditions of each athletic performance. An example is a jogger colliding with a car. The description and reconstructive interpretation of the injury pattern would have to comply with the regularities of car-pedestrian-collision in such a case (Wehner 2003).

86.2.3 Martial arts

A progression of rougher martial arts has begun with the development of full-contact karate and kick boxing as well as the establishment of the Muay Thai in the western world. Fighters of all disciplines of martial arts encounter each other in a cage almost without any rules in the so-called ultimate or **cage fights**.

The Brazilian **vale tudo** is also extremely injury-prone. So-called free fights are carried out in the Netherlands, which present certain rules despite being very violent. The 31-year-old U.S. American Douglas Dedge was the first martial arts athlete who lost his life in ultimate fighting in a Ukrainian tournament in early 1998.

Koiwai (1987) mentions 13 fatal incidences caused by **choke holds** by police officers in the U.S.A., while it has been emphasized repeatedly that correctly performed **judo** has not caused any serious complications by the use of these techniques since 1882 (also see Parzeller et al. 2008). Pressure values of 250 or 300 mmHg – according to a cable haulage of 5 kg – are only necessary for the occlusion of the carotids of a grown-up man. **Concomitant injuries** of the cervical structures by enormous force effects (laryngeal and intervertebral disk injuries) have been documented for all cases. A significant alcohol and drug influence to the choked had also been present in many cases.

One death has been documented for **"vo et vat"** – an extremely rough variant of judo – that had occurred in the teaching of the choking technique of gyaku-juji-me: A 34-year-old trainer of this martial art lost his life due to a choke hold lasting several minutes that had been applied without his defense by one of his own trainees (Koiwai 1987).

The average number of deaths in boxing in the time period from 1918 to 1983 has amounted to 9.9 per year and to 4.0 in the period from 1970 to 1985 (Ryan 1987). 20 deaths have occurred in professional boxing in Great Britain, while there had been none in amateur boxing (Carter and Green 2000). According to their data, the **subdural hemorrhage** (➢ Chapter 12) in the middle cranial fossa presents the major cause of death. Nowadays, the major cause is being attributed to repetitive prolonged punches, while a single impact to the jaw had previously been considered the trigger due to its force transmission to the cranial content via the temporomandibular joint. The practice of **"making weight"** before competition also contributes to this, because a consecutively "shrunken" brain exposes itself to an increased traumatic risk of its emissary veins.

86.2.4 Water sports

The most common cause of death in diving is **unconsciousness** under water followed by drowning. The used diving method or diving equipment substantially determines causes of death and fatal accidents.

The breath is being held under water for a longer period of time in so-called **free diving** with or without the use of mask, fins or snorkel. Duration and depth of the dive as well as perhaps a preceded hyperventilation determine the extent of a possible hypoxia.

The most common cause of death is the **aspiration of water** by the snorkel in unpracticed divers. The partial O_2 pressure can fall below the level of consciousness at the end of a long dive, before the level of the breath stimulus has been exceeded again by the increase of carbon dioxide in the blood, if there had been hyperventilation before the dive and thus CO_2 had been breathed (so-called **shallow water blackout**).

The so-called **shallow water unconsciousness** is caused by O_2 insufficiency after deep diving under apnea with a rapid reduction of the partial O_2 pressure as a consequence of the pressure relief in ascending. **Ear drum ruptures** due to neglected pressure compensation can eventually lead to an impairment of the sense of balance and to a loss of orientation in the water (➢ Chapter 14). **Environmental influences**, such as hypothermia in cold waters, heat stroke under a wet suit, bites by water animals or toxic influences are also possible causes of death.

Only **intoxications** (O_2, CO_2, CO or other gases) as well as **decompression sickness** are to be mentioned here as the accidents in **scuba diving**. Decompression sickness means the appearance of nitrogenous gas bubbles after too quick pressure relief at the end of the dive. Cardiac, pulmonary or cerebral **gas embolisms** are usually the cause of death.

Individual factors of each diver's personality predisposing for fatal accidents include pre-existing diseases of the cardiovascular system, the lung and the respiratory passages as well as psychiatric symptoms that do not call the diving capability into question primarily. Insufficient diving experience, fatigue, panics, false behavior of the victim or of the diving partners as well as influences by alcohol, drugs or medication should also be mentioned here (Fischer et al. 1978, Fechner and Püschel 1986, Keil 2003, Müller 2004).

Fatal accidents at the jump into the water can occur in platform or cliff diving or with too low water depth. **Craniocerebral injuries** or **injuries of the cervical spine** are usually the cause of death. The autopsy findings and information provided by eyewitnesses usually allow a conclusive reconstruction and assessment. Unusual **absorption of alcohol** can impair the attention and critical faculty of the athletes and thus contribute to the fatal processes (Carter and Green 2000).

597 accidents by drowning or sinking have been registered in 1999 in Germany alone, and 97 of these accidents affected children younger than 10 years of age. This example documents the impact of death by drowning (see also Schmidt et al. 2008, Turk et al. 2008). The fatal conditions are listed in ➢ Table 86.4.

Tab. 86.4 Causes for drowning.

Environmental factors	Drowning victims
■ depth of water ■ temperature ■ current ■ surf ■ tides	■ insufficient swimming skills ■ overheating ■ alcoholization/use of centrally effective substances ■ pre-existing diseases ■ prostration and collapse tendency ■ panic

The process of drowning is said to take approximately 4–5 min. **Reanimation** is usually successful if a drowning victim is rescued from the water **within less than 3 min**. The drowning accident usually ends with death, if the time of immersion is longer than 5 min (Pearn and Nixon 1977). The **drowning foam**, i.e. the issuing of hemorrhaging foam of fine bubbles from the breath openings, is a characteristic symptom that can be found in the external examination of drowned persons. The drowning foam consists of a mixture of air, water, edema fluids and bronchial mucus hypersecreted during the process of drowning.

The possibility of a postmortem development must be considered in differential diagnosis for **injuries** found in a body rescued from the water. Drift injuries (especially at the back of hand and foot and at the prominent parts of the face) and injuries by screw propellers, rocks or by the feeding of animals come into question.

The screw of the outboard engine can cause injuries or strangulations by the tow rope in **water skiing**. There is the possibility in all high-speed water sports that an athlete might be flung to the beach, lose consciousness and is drawn back into the water by the tide and then drowns (Carter and Green 2000).

86.2.5 Air sports

The **statistics for aerial accidents** excluding accidents of aviation sports have brought forth 70 dead persons and 160 injured persons in aviation accidents in the nationwide yearly average during the time period from 1955 to 1999 (since 1990 including the newly formed German states; source: hazard analysis for the state of Hesse by the Hessian Ministry of the Interior and for Sport 2000). 95% of these had been accidents of small aircrafts and helicopters. The maximum number of dead persons has come to n = 118 (1992), of injured persons to n = 321 (1993). The German Federal Bureau of Aircraft Accidents Investigation has provided a differentiated list.

No fatal accidents of aircrafts of more than 5.7 t and of aircrafts between 2.0 and 5.7 t, and 15 fatal accidents of aircrafts up to 2.0 t (2003: n = 17), in which 30 persons (2003: n = 32) have lost their lives, had been documented in 2004 in Germany. Only one fatal **helicopter accident**, in which three occupants had been killed, was registered in 2004. One fatal accident of a **motor glider** was registered in 2004. The bonnet had opened during the start and the motor glider thus came into ground contact and the pilot suffered fatal injuries. Nine accidents happened in 2004 with **sailplanes** (2003: n = 17), in which nine persons (2003: n = 19) died. Fatal sports accidents in aviation sports happened in 28 cases (motor plane: n = 22, sailplane: n = 5, paraglide: n = 1) according to a Frankfurt autopsy study (Schmidt et al. 2008).

No fatal accidents had been found with **free balloons** and **aeronautics** in the time period from 2000 to 2004. Two deaths resulted from 98 free balloon accidents in Great Britain from 1976 to 2004 (Hasham et al. 2004).

The registration of accidents in **hang-gliding and paragliding** is far more difficult. Reported aviation sport accidents or data of mountain rescues or hospitals form the basis for the statistic evaluation. Lautenschlager et al. (1992) have documented one fatal paragliding accident by 86 accidents in 1990 in a multi-center survey of 12 hospitals in Switzerland, for example.

A rate of 6 deaths in 100,000 jumps (0.005%) has been stated for **amateur parachuting** in Denmark (Ellitsgaard 1987). Averagely 29 parachuting athletes are killed in accidents every year in the U.S.A. **Causes of these accidents** are pulling the rip cord late, collisions, landing problems, faulty responses to disturbances. Faster parachutes ("high-performance parachutes") and more aggressive flying practices have led to an increase of fatal parachute jumps in the United States (Hart and Griffith 2003). 25 deaths and 19 serious brain injuries have been registered in a study of 106 accidents in **hang-gliding** (Mang and Karpt 1977).

The **risk** of suffering a fatal accident in aviation sports is **20 to 40 times higher** than the overall average of all sports. This has been shown by the data of the insurance survey SAUDIS ("Sudden and unexpected death in sports", Parzeller et al. 1998) regarding deaths in aviation sports in relation to the number of members. The risk of soccer, for example, is 100 times lower than the risk of aviation sports. **Contrary weather conditions** and **faulty human behavior** are often significant general influences to lethal aviation accidents. The aviation athletes (n = 14: motor plane pilots = 5, sailplane pilots = 8, parachuting athletes = 1) are dominant in the primary traumatic deaths (n = 33) in an international autopsy survey (Germany, Austria, Switzerland) about the causes of sudden death in sports. No organ-pathologically comprehensible cardiovascular failure had preceded the actual accident in any of these cases (Raschka et al. 1999, Schmidt et al. 2008).

86.2.6 Winter sports

The range of mortality is dominated by deaths in skiing. The mortality risk has been estimated to one death in 3.3 million days of skiing sport in a retrospective 5-year study in the U.S.A. and has thus been categorized as markedly **low** (Weston et al. 1977). The amount of natural deaths ranges between 25 and 50%, depending on the survey series (Sherry et al. 1988, Ambach et al. 1992). The **ischemic heart disease** and its complications are in the foreground in the range of the causes of death also for this sport, according to the uniform picture of sudden death during physical exercise. **Craniocerebral injuries** or **injuries of the spinal cord** are dominant causes of death in fatal accidents (Sherry et al. 1988, Ambach et al. 1992).

The **accident processes** include especially **headlong falls** onto the iced, hard surface of the snow cover (Weston et al. 1977) or the **collision** with a firm obstacle – usually a tree. High speeds, freezing-over of the snowy surface or avalanches have been identified as favoring environmental factors (Weston et al. 1977). A possible alcoholization must not be underestimated by the athletes as a causative factor, which leads to the dangerous contrast between subjective overestimation of the own capabilities and insufficient cautiousness in assessing dangerous situations on the one hand and the actual limitation of the psychophysical performance or athletic skill on the other hand.

Deaths by hypothermia also belong to this array in winter sports (Sherry et al. 1988). Findings in the external examination of the dead persons include local freezing and also light red coloring of the postmortem lividity as well as blue-red, edematous, diffusely confined swellings circumscribed nodularly or by pads at the extensor sides of the knee joints, fingers and toes (so-called perniones). Dead persons having taken off their clothes partially or completely before being found might have been subject to a subjective feeling of warmth despite sinking body temperature before time of death (so-called paradoxical undressing). Ensuring the diagnosis involves the ruling out of other causes of death and the toxicological examinations for alcohol, medications and drugs in order to clarify the death circumstances (Lignitz 2003).

86.2.7 Bicycle and motor sports

Retrospective studies regarding fatal bicycle accidents in general (Schmidt et al. 1991) prove a clear dominance of the **male gender** with **children and older persons** primarily being endangered due to their own riding errors and cyclists of the ages of 19 to 46 years due to accident opponents (Rowe et al. 1995). Approximately one third of the cases are single-vehicle accidents without involvement of others, i.e. **falls**. Two thirds are **collisions**.

> The procedure of turning and the crossing of roads are especially accident-prone.

The amount of fall injuries is clearly higher in clinical examinations of survived bicycle accidents. About 10% of the cyclists killed in an accident had been under substantial **influence of alcohol**. A **craniocerebral trauma** can be ensured as sole cause of death in half of the cases, a polytrauma with involvement of a craniocerebral injury in another 25% of the cases (Schmidt et al. 1991). Lethal injuries of mountain bikers have been conditioned by craniocerebral traumas in most cases, as well (Shang 1994).

86.2.8 Equestrianism

About **one fourth** of all fatal sport accidents in Germany occur in equestrianism (Hebecker and Piek 2003). One horse-riding accident in 1 million inhabitants has been stated as yearly rate (Pounder 1984). A retrospective study of 53 fatal horse-riding accidents (Ingemarson et al. 1989) with the aim of identifying special risk factors has shown that especially **girls** or young women are endangered in the group of children and adolescents (younger than 25 years; also see Turk et al. 2008); **men** are endangered primarily at a higher age. Fatal accidents happen clearly less often, if older horses are ridden.

Craniocerebral injuries dominate the causes of death. The analysis of a database of fatal accidents of children in Australia (NPTD, New South Wales Pediatric Trauma Death Registry) with reference to horse accidents of children, especially, has stated six deaths for the time from January 1988 to December 1999, with a craniocerebral trauma being the cause of death in five of the cases. 65% of the 232 children with horse-riding injuries in a clinical examination series have been girls. Injuries of the cranium or the arms caused by falls have led to the stay in hospital in about 75% of the cases. Only 40% of the accident victims had worn a helmet and only 23% had been under parental supervision at the time of the accident. An **important preventive conclusion** has been drawn from the findings of this study: the **wearing of helmets** can reduce the severity of craniocerebral injuries (Holland et al. 2001, Schmidt et al. 2008, Turk et al. 2008).

86.3 Preventive aspects

Preventive approaches often apply to the **equipment** of the athletes. A specific **protection helmet** belongs to the sport-specific gear of **cyclists**, for example. The wearing of protection helmets has unfortunately not become prevalent yet. Thus, 1,300 cyclists died in the U.S.A. only in 1985. A definitely protective effect has been proved for the wearing of protection helmets by cyclists according to a case control study in the U.S.A. (Thompson et al. 1989). A 6.6 times **higher risk** of head injuries and an 8.3 times higher risk of brain injuries have been registered for **persons not wearing helmets**. At the same time, the conclusion has been drawn that a quantitative and qualitative minimization of 85% of all head injuries and 88% of all brain injuries would have been possible by wearing hard-shelled bicycle helmets. A survey of 111 cyclists has shown that 4 cyclists without the protection of a helmet died of the consequences of craniocerebral traumas, while all cyclists protected by helmets have survived the accident (Kelsch et al. 1998). Analogue conclusions apply to **inline skating** as well as **equestrianism accidents** (Parzeller et al. 1998, Schmidt et al. 2008, Turk et al. 2008).

The wearing of **helmets** (Aronson and Tough 1993) and **training of sufficient extent by experienced horse-riding trainers** as well as the restriction of **rides into open country limited** to experienced riders only are suggested preventive measures **in equestrianism** (Holland et al. 2001). An optimization of the equipment has been demanded after the analyses of (fatal) accidents in harness racing (Boglioli et al. 1987).

A significant decrease of intracranial hemorrhages has been registered after the improvement of the **special helmets in American Football** with face masks, but so has also a crucial **increase of injuries of the cervical spine** with tetraplegias (Torg et al. 1979). The cause had been the use of the helmet as a battering ram in tackling and blocking. Cantu and Mueller (2003) have analyzed fatal brain injuries in American football from 1945 to 1999 and have found the highest incidence in a 5-year period from 1965 to 1969 and the lowest within the two decades from 1975 to 1994. They ascribe this significant reduction to the establishing of an optimized helmet standard, on the one hand, and to the **changes of the rules** in 1976, on the other hand, forbidding the initial contact of head and face in blocking and tackling. The amount of severe football accidents could be reduced by 74% and the incidence of serious head injuries could be reduced from 4.25/100,000 to 0.68/100,000 due to the improvement of the helmet standard, according to Levy et al. (2004).

Janda et al. (1995) suggest the use of **padded goal posts** in **soccer**, which can significantly reduce the impact forces by 63%, since fatal soccer accidents often result from the contact with the goal posts. The use of so-called **safety balls** in **baseball** could minimize the risk of a commotio cordis, compared to the use of regular balls (Link et al. 1998).

The availability of a **defibrillator on the sidelines**, as has been demanded by Deady and Innes (1999) for ice hockey, and the use of a special **chest protector** (Maron et al. 2002) are further measures for the prevention of a lethal commotio cordis. This measure could also be applied analogously to handball, hockey, baseball or soccer.

The preventive and responsible function of the **physician on site** contributes significantly to the prevention of fatal accidents in **martial arts**, considered from a sport-medical point of view.

References

Abrunzo TJ (1991). Commotio cordis: The single, most common cause of traumatic death in youth baseball. Am J Dis Childr 145: 1279–1282.

Ambach E, Tributsch W, Henn R (1992). Epidemiologie von Todesfällen beim alpinen Schisport. Beitr Gerichtl Med 50: 333–336.

Aronson H, Tough SC (1993). Horse-related fatalities in the province of Alberta. Am J Forensic Med Pathol 14: 28–30.

Basso C, Corrado D, Thiene G (1999). Cardiovascular causes of sudden death in young individuals including athletes. Cardiol Rev 7: 127–135.

Berghold F (1986). Der plötzliche Tod im Sport. Sportpraxis 27: 35–38.

Biener K (1985). Fußball. Sportmedizin, Sporternährung, Sportunfälle. Habegger-Verlag, Derendingen-Solothurn, Schweiz.

Boglioli LR, Taff ML, Lukash LI (1987). Harness racing injuries and deaths. Report of a fatal accident and review of 178 cases. Am J Forensic Med Pathol 8: 185–207.

Brinkmann B (2004). Tod im Wasser. In: Brinkmann B, Madea B (eds.). Handbuch Gerichtliche Medizin. Springer-Verlag, Heidelberg-Berlin, pp. 797–823.

Bux R, Zedler B, Schmidt P (2008). Plötzlicher natürlicher Tod beim Sport. Rechtsmedizin 18: 155–160.

Bux R, Parzeller M, Raschka C, Bratzke H (2004). Vorzeichen und Ursachen des plötzlichen Todes im Zusammenhang mit sportlicher Betätigung. DMW 129: 997–1001.

Cantu RC, Mueller FO (2003). Brain injury-related fatalities in American Football, 1945–1999. Neurosurgery 52: 846–852.

Carter N, Green MA (2000). Injury and death in sports and recreational activities. In: Mason JK, Purdue BN (eds.). The Pathology of Trauma. Arnold Publishers, London, pp. 283–299.

Cherington M (2001). Lightning injuries in sports: situations to avoid. Sports Med 31: 301–308.

Deady B, Innes G (1999). Sudden death of a young hockey player: case report of commotio cordis. J Emerg Med 17: 459–462.

Dickman GL, Hassan A, Luckstead EF (1978). Ventricular fibrillation following baseball injury. Phys Sportsmed 6/7: 85–86.

Dingerkus ML, Martinek V, Kölzow I, Imhoff A (1998). Verletzungen und Überlastungsschäden beim Mountainbiken. Dtsch Z Sportmed Special Issue 1 49: 273–275.

Ellitsgaard N (1987). Parachuting injuries: a study of 110,000 sports jumps. Br J Sports Med 21: 13–17.

Fechner G, Püchel K (1986). Pathologisch-anatomische Untersuchungsbefunde von Todesfällen beim Sport. Dtsch Z Sportmed 37: 35–40.

Fields KB (1989). Head injuries in soccer. Phys Sports Med 17: 69–73.

Fischer H, Masel H, Sigl W (1978). Tödliche Unfälle mit Preßlufttauchgeräten. Z Rechtsmed 81: 157–162.

Friedman JA, Meyer FB, Nichols DA, Coffey RJ, Hopkins LN, Maher CO, Meissner ID, Pollock BE (2001). Fatal progression of posttraumatic dural arteriovenous fistulas refractory to multimodal therapy. Case report. J Neurosurg 94: 831–835.

Froede RC, Lindsey D, Steinbronn K (1979). Sudden unexpected death from cardiac concussion (commotio cordis) with unusual legal complications. J Forensic Sci 24: 752–756.

Goble MM (1999). Sudden cardiac death in young athlete. Indian J Pediatr 66: 1–5.

Green ED, Simson LR, Kellerman HH, Horowitz RN, Sturner WQ (1980). Cardiac concussion following softball blow to the chest. Ann Emerg Med 9: 155–157.

Hart CL, Griffith JD (2003). Rise in landing-related skydiving fatalities. Percept Mot Skills 97: 390–392.

Hasham S, Majumder S, Southern SJ, Phipps AR, Judkins KC (2004). Hot-air ballooning injuries in the United Kingdom (January 1976–January 2004). Burns 30: 856–860.

Hawley DA, Slentz K, Clark MA, Pless JE, Waller BF (1990). Athletic fatalities. Am J Forensic Med Pathol 11(2): 124–129.

Hebecker R, Piek J (2003). Schädel-Hirn-Verletzungen durch Reitunfälle. Notfallmedizin 29: 304–309.

Holland AJ, Roy GT, Goh V, Ross FI, Keneally JP, Cass DT (2001). Horse-related injuries in children. Med J Aust 175: 609–612.

Ingemarson H, Grevsten S, Lhoren L (1989). Lethal horse-riding injuries. J Trauma 29: 25–30.

Janda DH, Bir C, Wild B, Olson S, Hensinger RN (1995). Goal post injuries in soccer. A laboratory and field testing analysis of a preventive intervention. Am J Sports Med 23: 340–344.

Jung K, Schäfer-Nolte W (1982). Todesfälle im Zusammenhang mit Sport. Dtsch Z Sportmed 33: 1–11.

Kauferstein S, Kiehne N, Neumann T, Pitschner HF, Bratzke H (2009). Pötzlicher Herztod bei jungen Menschen durch kardiale Gendefekte. Dtsch Ärztebl Int 106: 41–47.

Keil W (2003). Tod im Wasser. In: Madea B (ed.). Praxis der Rechtsmedizin. Springer-Verlag, Berlin-Heidelberg, pp. 166–170.

Kelsch G, Helber MU, Schmid K, Ulrich C (1998). Sind schwere Kopfverletzungen durch einen Fahrradhelm vermeidbar. Dtsch Z Sportmed Special Issue 1 49: 279–284.

Koch H, Raschka C, Parzeller M (2002). Saisonale Schwankungen plötzlicher Todesfälle im Vereinssport. Versicherungsmedizin 54: 176–178.

Koiwai EK (1987). Deaths allegedly caused by the use of "choke-holds" (Shime-waza). J Forensic Sci 32: 419–432.

La Harpe R, Margairaz C (1995). Rechtsmedizinische Aspekte des plötzlichen Todes beim Sport. Arch Kriminol 195:159–165.

Lautenschlager S, Karli U, Matter P (1992). Multizentrische Gleitschirm-Unfallstudie 1990. Z Unfallchir Versicherungsmed 85: 90–95.

Levy ML, Ozgur BM, Berry C, Aryan HE, Apuzzo ML (2004). Birth and evolution of the football helmet. Neurosurgery 55: 656–661.

Lignitz E (2003). Kälte. In: Madea B (ed.). Praxis der Rechtsmedizin. Springer-Verlag, Heidelberg-Berlin, pp. 181–186.

Link MS, Wang PJ, Pandian NGI, Bharati S, Udelson JE, Lee MY, Vecchiotti MA, Van der Brink BA, Mirra G, Maron BJ, Estes NA (1998). An experimental model of sudden death due to low-energy chest-wall impact (commotio cordis). N Engl J Med 338: 1805–1811.

Mang WR, Karpt PM (1977). Verletzungen beim Drachenfliegen. Fortschr Med 95: 1575–1579.

Maron BJ, Gohman TE, Kyle SB (2002). Clinical profile and spectrum of commotio cordis. JAMA 287: 1142–1146.

Maron BJ, Thompson PD, Puffer JC (1996). Cardiovascular preparticipation screening of competitive athletes: a statement for health professionals from the sudden death committee (clinical cardiology) and congenital cardiac defects committee (cardiovascular disease in the young). Circulation 94: 850–856.

Maron BJ, Poliac LC, Kaplan JA, Mueller FO (1995). Blunt impact on the chest leading to sudden cardiac death from cardiac arrest during sports activities. N Engl J Med 333(6): 337–342.

Mueller FO, Cantu RC (1990). Catastrophic injuries and fatalities in high school and college sports, fall 1982–spring 1988. Med Sci Sports Exerc 22: 737–741.

Müller P (2004). Tod im Wasser – Tauchen. In: Brinkmann B, Madea B (eds.). Handbuch gerichtliche Medizin. Springer-Verlag, Heidelberg-Berlin, 819–824.

Northcote RJ, Flannigan C, Ballantyne D (1986). Sudden death and vigorous exercise – a study of 60 deaths associated with squash. Br Heart J 55: 198–203.

Parzeller M, Ramsthaler F, Zedler B, Raschka C, Bratzke H (2008). Griff zum Hals und Würgen des Opfers – Juristische, rechts- und sportmedizinische Bewertung. Rechtsmedizin 18: 195–201.

Parzeller M, Schmidt P, Bratzke H (2006). Die Funktion der Rechtsmedizin bei der Aufklärung von Kapitalverbrechen, insbesondere Tötungsdelikten (medizinische und rechtliche Grundlagen). In: Anders D, Bratzke H, Gotthardt H, Parzeller M (eds.). Praxishandbuch Kapitalverbrechen. Boorberg-Verlag, Stuttgart.

Parzeller M, Raschka C (2003). Auswertung von 2969 Todesfällen im Vereinssport anhand einer 20-jährigen Erhebung. Dtsch Z Sportmed 53: 415.

Parzeller M, Raschka C (2003). Locked-in-Syndrom bei einem Fußballspieler nach Contusio cordis mit tödlichem Verlauf. Sportorthopädie Sporttraumatologie 19: 111–113.

Parzeller M, Raschka C (1999). Der plötzliche und unerwartete Tod im Vereinssport der Bundesländer Berlin und Brandenburg (Januar 1992–April 1997). Versicherungsmedizin 51: 157–160.

Parzeller M, Raschka C et al. (1998). Der traumatische Tod bei der Sportausübung: Ursachen, Inzidenzen und präventive Ansätze. Dtsch Z Sportmed Special Issue 1 49: 285–289.

Parzeller M, Raschka C (1995). Death in sports: comparison between tennis, table-tennis, badminton and squash. In: Krahl H, Pieper HG, Kibler WB, Renström PA (eds.). Tennis: Sports medicine and science. Rau-Verlag, Düsseldorf.

Pearn J, Nixon J (1977). Bathtub immersion accidents involving children. Med J Austral 1: 211–213.

Pounder DJ (1984). "The grave yawns for the horseman". Equestrian deaths in South Australia 1973–1983. Med J Austral 141: 632–635.

Raas E, Hörtnagel H (1983). Gefahren für Herz und Kreislauf durch unsachgemäße Sportausübung. Wien Klin Wschr 95: 13–137.

Raschka C (2008). Unfälle bei großen Mannschaftssportarten – Schwerwiegende bis tödliche Verletzungen und deren Mechanismen. Rechtsmedizin 18: 167–172.

Raschka C, Parzeller M, Kind M (1999). Organpathologische Ursachen des akuten Sporttodes. Eine internationale Autopsiestudie (Deutschland, Österreich, Schweiz). Med Klin 94: 473–477.

Raschka C, Parzeller M, Gläser H (1996). Todesfälle im Vereinssport in der Bundesrepublik Deutschland. Dtsch Z Sportmed 47: 17–22.

Raschka C, Roth J, Sitte T, Gödecke A, Haas JP, Hammar CH (1995). Ein tödlicher Fußballunfall als unglückliche Kollisionsfolge. Sportverl Sportschad 9: 24–26.

Rowe BH, Rowe AM, Bota GW (1995). Bicyclist and environmental factors associated with fatal bicycle-related trauma in Ontario. Can Med Assoc J 152: 45–53.

Ryan AJ (1987). Intracranial injuries resulting from boxing: a review (1918–1985). Clin Sports Med 6: 31–40.

Schmidt P, Zedler B, Bux R, Raschka C, Parzeller M (2008). Tödliche Sportunfälle. Rechtsmedizin 18: 161–166.

Schmidt P, Haarhoff K, Bonte W (1991). Fatal bicycle accidents in Düsseldorf 1980–89. Analysis of autopsy cases. J Traffic Med 19: 113–118.

Shang E (1994). Studie Mountainbike-Verletzungen. Mountainbike 5–6: 158–163.

Sherry E, Clout L (1988). Deaths associated with skiing in Australia: a 32-year study of cases from the Snowy Mountains. Med J Austral 149: 615–618.

Tabib A, Miras A, Taniere P, Loire R (1999). Undetected cardiac lesions cause unexpected sudden cardiac death during occasional sport activity. A report of 80 cases. Eur Heart J 20: 900–903.

Thompson RS, Rivara FP, Thompson DC (1989). A case-control study of the effectiveness of bicycle safety helmets. N Engl J Med 320: 1361–1367.

Torg JS, Truex R Jr, Quedenfeld TC, Burstein A, Spealman A, Nichols C 3rd (1979). The national football head and neck injury registry. Report and conclusions 1978. JAMA 241: 1477–1479.

Turk E, Riedel A, Püschel K (2008). Natural and traumatic sports-related fatalities: a 10 year retrospective study. Br J Sports Med 42: 604–608.

Varga M, Takács P (1990). A fatal accident on the football field. In J Leg Med 104: 47–48.

Wehner H-D (2003). Der Verkehrsunfall. In: Madea B (ed.). Praxis Rechtsmedizin. Springer-Verlag, Heidelberg-Berlin, pp. 466–478.

Weiner HR (1999). Preventing sudden death in student athletes. Compr Ther 25: 151–154.

Weston JT, Moore SM, Rich TH (1977). A five-year study of mortality in a busy ski population. J Forensic Sci 22: 222–230.

VII Accompanying measures

87	**Nutrition**	727
87.1	Energy requirement in competitive sports	727
87.2	Carbohydrates	728
87.3	Hydration	732
87.4	Protein absorption	733
87.5	Vitamins	734
87.6	Minerals	741
88	**Sportswear**	751
88.1	Introduction	751
88.2	Thermoregulation	751
88.3	Post exercise chill	753
88.4	Properties of Sportswear	753
88.5	Special applications – Compression clothing	754
88.6	Care	755
89	**Athletic Footwear**	759
89.1	Introduction	759
89.2	From "Turnschuh" to technical athletic footwear	759
89.3	Components of sport shoes	760
89.4	Concluding remarks	766
90	**Ortheses**	769
90.1	Ankle joint ortheses	769
90.2	Knee joint ortheses	771
90.3	Spine ortheses	776
90.4	Elbow ortheses	778
90.5	Thumb and wrist ortheses	778
90.6	Hip joint ortheses	779

ated for more than 2 hours.
Chapter 87 Nutrition

Georg Neumann

87.1 Energy requirement in competitive sports

Maintaining muscular capacity requires filled energy reservoirs and a regular energy metabolism. This is dependent on the duration and intensity of the athletic performance.

The natural **glycogen depots** in muscles and in the liver provide an athlete with energy reserves for 90–120 min. No food is required during this period. In contrast, liquid needs to be provided already after 15 min at heat. Food is only necessary after exercises of more than 2 hours.

Exposure of several hours is possible because of the increased **free fatty acids (FFA) metabolism** and the additional gluconeogenesis of amino acids, glycerol and lactate. A lactate concentration of less than 3 mmol/l triggers FFA metabolism. The energy is gained from aerobic and anaerobic glycogenic degradation. FFA oxidation is suppressed almost completely at more than 7 mmol/l lactate.

At present, long-distance runners free their body fat, i.e. the athletes starve off the weight and become almost anorexic. To prevent impaired performance and metabolic lapses, **body fat** should not be less than 7% for both genders. Body fat is best measured with a skin fold caliper at ten measure points. The assumption that every additional kilogram of body mass impairs the running performance is a misconception of body weight.

Runners are classified as underweight if the body fat falls below 6%. **Body mass index** (BMI) should be **more than 18** for competitive athletes.

Eating disorders are relatively frequent in female juvenile runners. Anorexia nervosa and bulimia are predominant (➤ Tab. 87.1). The

Tab. 87.1 Consequences of eating disorders of female and male athletes and the options of influence (modified according to Clasing 1996).

Consequences of eating disorders
Eating disorders can lead to severe health impairments, power stagnation and reduced performance. The disturbed eating behavior massively influences physical functions and leads to the following problems in performance training: ■ The energy storages (glycogen) decrease and hypoglycemic conditions increase in training. ■ The permanent protein deficiency leads to reduction of muscle mass. The sport-specific propelling force (strength endurance) decreases. ■ The energy deficiency weakens the immune system; the susceptibility for virus infections increases. ■ The undersupply of electrolytes increases the frequency of muscle cramps and cardiac dysrhythmias. ■ The estrogen deficiency of women leads to reduced metabolism and decreased energy conversion. Amenorrhea is almost obligatory. ■ The decrease of osseous minerals promotes the development of an osteoporosis. Stress fracture will increase at highly strained bones.
Measures
■ BMI (kg/cm^2) and growth speed ought to be defined with a suspected eating disorder. The normal BMI of female endurance athletes must exceed 18.0 kg/cm^2. The growth speed at the age of childhood and adolescence amounts to more than 4 cm/year. ■ Attentive psychic guidance of the athletes and reduction of stress or temporary training breaks are necessary. ■ Doctor's advice: substitution of micro-nutrients, amino acids and possibly hormones will must be induced. The treatment of these complex psychophysical disorders is complicated; the intervention of several specialists will be required.

performance stagnates and disorders accumulate with every kind of malnutrition. The appearance of stress fractures is often an indication of insufficient diet.

87.2 Carbohydrates

Aim of the following chapters is to review individual nutrition components; detailed reviews of sports nutrition are available in the literature (Brouns 1993, Konopka 2001, Neumann 2003, Jeukendrup and Gleeson 2004, Berg and König 2008 etc.).

87.2.1 Absorption of carbohydrates and carbohydrate abstinence before running

Principally, endurance strain can start with an empty stomach since the glycogen depots provide sufficient initial energy. One study showed that FFA concentration is higher if **running with an empty stomach** (Hottenrott and Sommer 2001). Carbohydrate absorption has a minor effect on fat metabolism in less exercised runners and exercising with empty stomach only trains the fat metabolism. A long low carbohydrate diet with 5.7% carbohydrates, 56.3% fat and 37% proteins is needed (Johnson et al. 2003) to maintain the triglyceride depots in muscles. **Increased triglyceride depots** are a **primary condition** for **long endurance for several hours**.

Glycogen depots are not refilled if no food is absorbed 6 to 12 hours prior to start. 200–350 g carbohydrates 6 hours before the start sufficiently refill glycogen depots. This is the rational of pasta parties before endurance events, which sufficiently refill **glycogen depots** the night before competition.

Every kind of food intake before long endurance exposure is of advantage; nutrients with a fast turnover in the stomach are preferred (➤ Tab. 87.2).

The **absorption of carbohydrates before running** can show two effects: suppression of fat metabolism in trained athletes and reduction of the blood glucose. Hypoglycemia can be avoided if glucose (1 g/kg of body weight) is absorbed about 30 min before start (Tokmakidis and Volakis 2000). Blood glucose values of 3.6 mm/l (65 mg/dl) on average are typical prior to strain if glucose is absorbed 60 to 90 min before start (➤ Fig. 87.1). ➤ Table 87.3 summarizes effect of carbohydrate intake. Increased insulin secretion as a consequence of glucose absorption before or during exposure is physiologically limited and low in exercised persons.

Tab. 87.2 Recommended ingestion before running*.

Retention time in the stomach	Food and beverages
1	■ water (without carbonic acid, still water) ■ tea, coffee, nonalcoholic beer, cola beverages ■ carbohydrate solutions, protein hydrolysate, amino acids ■ energy bars with carbohydrates
2	■ milk, cocoa, yoghurt, meat broth ■ light bread, bread rolls ■ granola, bananas ■ fine vegetables, rice ■ trout ■ energy bars with proteins
3	■ rye-wheat bread, cookies, buttered bread rolls ■ potatoes ■ eggs, beef and lamb, chicken ■ vegetables, apples
Conditionally recommended	
4	■ sausage, ham ■ roast veal, beefsteak, turkey, pork ■ nuts
Not recommended	
5	■ legumes (peas, beans) ■ roasts (poultry, game) ■ cucumber salad ■ French fries
6	■ bacon ■ herring salad, tuna fish ■ mushrooms
7	■ sardines in oil, eel ■ roast goose, knuckle of pork

* The more intensive a load or the shorter the contest distances are, the less food should be ingested. Liquid food or gels should be preferred with a stomach sensitivity, indisposition or stress before starting.

Fig. 87.1 Optimal point of time for glucose absorption before the start.

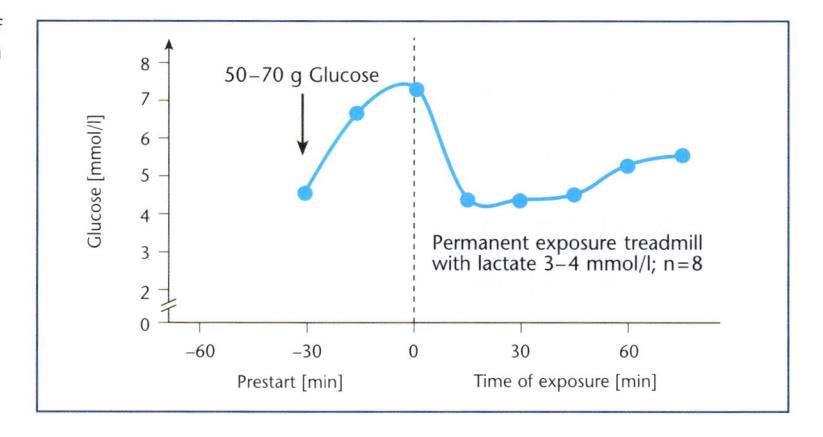

Tab. 87.3 Effect of carbohydrates (CH) on the endurance strain.

Carbohydrate absorption before endurance strain:
If 140–330 g CH are absorbed no later than 3–4 hours before exposure, this is sufficient for the filling of muscle and liver glycogen (Coyle et al. 1985, Chryssanthopoulos and Williams 1997). Performance can be increased with filled glycogen depots (Wright et al 1991).
Carbohydrate absorption directly before the start:
The point of time of the last CH absorption before the start influences the blood-glucose level before the start of strain. Glucose absorption provokes an insulin secretion; thus, the blood glucose will be reduced. CH absorption (1 g/kg of body mass) is most convenient about 30 minutes before the start (Tokmakidis and Volakis 2000). Glucose absorptions 90–60 minutes before the start reduces blood glucose before the start.
Carbohydrate absorption during strain of a duration of up to 60 minutes:
CH absorptions within the first 60 minutes cause a glycogen saving effect; the absorbed glucose is oxidated preferentially. The transmission of long-chain fatty acids into mitochondria decreases (Horowitz et al. 1997). The glucose absorption in the first hour of strain will not influence the performance capability (Marmy-Conus et al. 1996, Hargreaves 1999).
Carbohydrate absorption during strain of a duration of more than 60 minutes:
The increasing exhaustion of the glycogenic storages of the body (muscle and liver) reduces the oxidation rate of CH (Hargreaves 1999). The Speed cannot be kept at clearly reduced CH oxidation; fatigue and decreased performance after 90–120 minutes are the consequence. CH absorption becomes objectively necessary after 90 minutes in order to maintain the speed. 30–50 g CH every hour or 10–15 mg CH every 3 km in running should be absorbed after the 70th minute of load. Regular CH absorptions increase the performance of endurance or allow strain with duration of several hours. If the glucose absorption is combined with a fructose absorption in the relation of 2:1, a higher oxidation rate of CH and an improvement in performance will be achievable at the same time (Currell and Jeukendrup 2008).

Insulin peaks 45 min after glucose absorption under resting conditions. It peaks, however, after 20 min of strain, if glucose is absorbed 30 min prior to start. The adrenaline increase at the beginning exposure causes an increase of blood glucose.

Time and amount of glucose intake prior to start determine the insulin peak.

Obviously, above observations do not apply to type 2 diabetics.

87.2.2 Nutrition during competition

Absorption of carbohydrates during strain maintains exercise capacity and extends endurance. Glucose intake is particularly performance enhancing in the last third of endurance (Coggan and Swanson 1992). Dosed glucose absorption does not deplete muscle glycogen. Glucose intake during trainings increases the rate of glucose oxidation and thus the moment of fatigue.

30 g of carbohydrates per hour of strain are recommended (Brouns 1993). The lower limit of glucose absorption during running performance is approx. 20 g/h. This prevents further drastic decrease of blood glucose. The carbohydrate absorption effect can be neglected at performances up to 70 min or runs up to 20 km.

Glucose, fructose and maltose cause a similar increase of blood glucose. The rate of carbohydrate oxidation can be increased during performance by combined glucose and fructose (2:1 ratio) absorption (Jentjens et al. 2004).

Unlike other sugars, fructose absorption has **no influence on the insulin release** from the pancreas. Thus, fructose absorption during performance is recommended. However, concentrations of more than 3.5% cause diarrhea.

Not all carbohydrate solutions are stomach-compatible. Therefore, the tolerance or the carbohydrate mixtures – no matter which shape/company – should be checked prior to important starts.

Maltose is very stomach-compatible. The small particle size of **maltose** allows a quick resorption even at higher concentration (up to 15%). The slow absorption of oligo- and polysaccharides makes them ideal supplements for long-term endurance.

87.2.3 Carbohydrate absorption during long strain

8–12 g every 15 min or 32–48 g per hour of carbohydrates absorption (energy bars, gels, glucose-enriched drinks, dextrose, natural products, and others) allow continued performance during long endurance (Coyle et al. 1983, Ivy et al. 1983, Hargreaves et al. 1984 and 1987, Hargreaves 1999, Neumann and Pöhlandt 1994, and others). Even larger amounts of carbohydrates suppress fat metabolism. The **limit of reabsorption** of glucose or carbohydrates during exposure amounts is ~70 g/h.

The first intake of carbohydrates should be at 1 hour of strain, this starts the carbohydrate and fat metabolism. Until that time point carbohydrates and fatty acids are regulated via the glycogen depots.

The gradual increase of FFA blood concentration is a sign of increased fatty acids turnover. Fat metabolism is not influenced, if 35 g carbohydrates/h are administered (Neumann and Pöhlandt 1994). The intake of 35–45 g of carbohydrates per hour increases the blood glucose level by 0.5–1 mmol/l (9–18 mg/dl). Carbohydrate absorption increases performance time by about 20% (➢ Fig. 87.2).

Singular intakes of 70–80 g of carbohydrates increase the carbohydrate turnover and lengthen the endurance exposure.

The hormones **insulin** and **glucagon** act reversely in longer exposures. The insulin activity in the blood decreases and glucagon increases after 30–60 min of endurance strain. Glucagon increases FFA metabolism. The homeostasis of

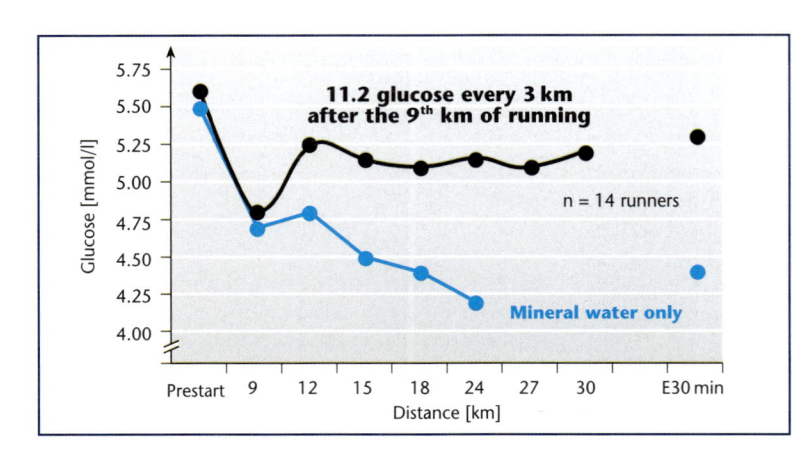

Fig. 87.2 Runners received either water after 9 km of running or 11.2 g (≈45 g/h) glucose solution every 3 km. Blood glucose decreased for runners with water absorption, and they finished the default speed 6 km earlier at the individual threshold (own data).

the blood glucose is ensured by the additional gluconeogenesis. The respiratory quotient (RQ) remains unaltered at 40 g carbohydrates/h.

> Muscular fatigue does not correlate with blood glucose level and only depends on exercise.

Nevertheless, **hypoglycemia** – neglected glucose absorption or low glucose availability in exposures of more than 2 hours – reduce **performance**. Glucose insufficiency reduces the motor impulse of cerebrum and cerebellum. The brain metabolism depends on glucose and requires a constant glucose supply for full functionality.

87.2.4 Carbohydrate absorption after strain

A refill of emptied glycogen depots in muscles and liver is the aim of the carbohydrate absorption after long strain. The preconditions for the composition of glycogen and the infiltration of amino acids into the muscle cells are most favorable 1–2 hours after the end of strain. The enzyme of the glycogen formation – the glycogen synthethase – is even active in increased condition, and this can be used by immediate glucose absorption. Additional absorption of amino acids accelerates the glycogen repletion.

A nutrition rich of carbohydrates 1–2 hours after strain has advantages over the mixed diet. The intake of high-fiber food, which is carrier of vitamins and minerals in vegetables and fruit at the same time, should be delayed.

The **infusion of glucose solutions** in early regeneration or short relaxation after the end of exposure is physiologically justified for performances in stages (cycling, running), which lead to a strong energy and regeneration deficit at chronic glycogen insufficiency for the prevention of a too strong protein catabolism and a disorder of the immune system. This way, a long-distance trip by bicycle (RAAM) over 4,701 km straight through the U.S. has led to a daily energy intake of 9,612 ± 1,500 kcal, but also to an actual consumption of 17,965 ± 21, 650 kcal. Thus the energy deficit has amounted to 8,259 kcal over 9 days (Knechtle et al. 2005).

Depleted emptied glycogen depots cannot be filled completely after 24 hours even with specific carbohydrate absorption of approximately 6 g/kg of body weight. The refilling of the glycogen depots after intensive endurance strain takes longer than generally expected; it can take as long as 4 days after marathon runs (Sherman et al. 1983, Blom et al. 1986).

The muscle has capacity even without full glycogen filling, as analyses of extreme runs have shown. The muscles cannot regenerate completely anymore at stage runs in which daily distances of 40–100 km have to be run to a final load of 4,000 km. The decomposition products of mechanically destroyed contraction proteins appear in the blood with deceleration. This applies to the myosin heavy-chain fragments and the troponin 1 (Koller et al. 1998). The **decomposition products of muscle fiber** reflect the persistent fatigue and the reduced muscle strength. They can be detected distinctly longer than the CK (Prou et al. 1996).

The aerobic energy potential in the mitochondria is partly destroyed at **extreme running strain** (marathon, long-triathlon, 100-km-run, iron man, etc.). Changes of the form of the mitochondria, density changes in the internal space of the mitochondria and mitochondria demises caused by the persistent need of energy occur here (Sherman et al. 1983). The period of regeneration after these long-term exposures clearly exceeds the one necessary for the refilling of the muscular glycogen depots.

The **glucose** is more suitable for the refilling of the muscle glycogen than the fructose is. The **fructose** can be used better for the reconstruction of the liver glycogen. The amount of carbohydrates to be absorbed depends on the energy consumption (➤ Tab. 87.4).

An **energy** amount of 1,170–1,365 kcal/h is **necessary** for a competitive runner with a body mass of 65 kg maintaining a speed of 5–5.5 m/sec for 1 hour.

The oxygen absorption has a decisive influence on the energy turnover. It is understandable that a recreational athlete turns over clearly less energy per time than a top runner, because the oxygen absorption depends on the intensity of strain (speed). Additional energy is won in intensive permanent loads of 90 min by the anaerobic energy turnover.

Tab. 87.4 Energy consumption during walking and running in persons of 70 kg.

Energy consumption increases by 1 kcal/min with a mass increase of 5 kg.

Strain duration (hours)	Walking (6 km/h or 10 min/km)	Running (12 km/h or 5 min/km)
1	600 kcal	870 kcal
2	1,200 kcal	1,740 kcal
3	1,800 kcal	2,610 kcal
4	2,400 kcal	3,480 kcal
5	3,000 kcal	4,350 kcal
6	3,600 kcal	5,220 kcal
8	4,800 kcal	6,960 kcal

87.2.5 Diabetics and endurance strain

Diabetics (type 2) can also perform endurance exercises of **as much as 1 hour** without dangerous consequences. There is a higher risk of hypoglycemia in longer strain, e.g. marathon. Diabetics can run a marathon, if they measure the blood glucose regularly during the run or combine the food intake by measuring the glucose values.

Diabetics **reduce their insulin requirement** and decrease the insulin resistance of the muscle cells. The intake of large amounts of glucose at once is to be avoided by diabetics, especially after strain. A long-lasting glucose level of more than 10 mmol/l is to be expected with the application of 100 g of carbohydrates to a diabetic of type 2.

87.3 Hydration

There is no drink which is appropriate for all situations in sports. The liquid absorption is influenced by:

- the mineral content (e.g. sodium chloride, bicarbonates, magnesium)
- the carbohydrate concentration
- the temperature
- the amount of drinking.

Industrially produced sports drinks with defined amounts of carbohydrates and mineral content have proved to be performance-enhancing. The combination of carbohydrate drinks with minerals (electrolytes and trace elements) has no influence on tolerance and reabsorption.

Electrolyte solutions with a low amount of carbohydrates (hypotonic solutions) are to be preferred with **strain in heat conditions**.

Low amounts of carbohydrates in the sports drinks encourage the water absorption in the intestines (Brouns 1993). This effect is valid for glucose drinks to 8%. Carbohydrate concentrations of more than 10% slow down the gastric emptying and stimulate the emission of liquids from the blood into the intestines. The osmotic gradient determines the direction of the stream of liquids.

Hypertonic liquids must be diluted before their reabsorption in the intestines. This involves a temporary water deprivation of the

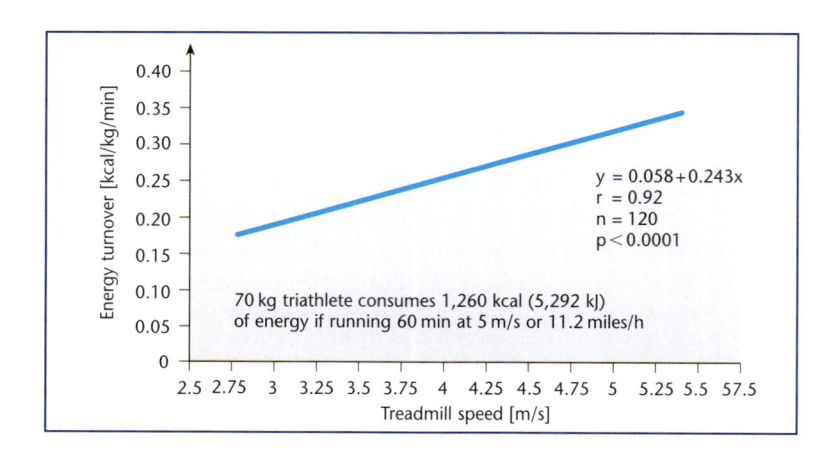

Fig. 87.3 The triathletes used altogether 1,260 kcal (5,292 kJ) of energy in a run of 60 minutes at a speed of 5 m/sec (18 km/h). At the maximum, an aerobic-anaerobic energy conversion of 28.6 kcal/min or 1,716 kcal/h, respectively, or 0.41 kcal/kg/min will be possible.

$y = 0.058 + 0.243x$
$r = 0.92$
$n = 120$
$p < 0.0001$

70 kg triathlete consumes 1,260 kcal (5,292 kJ) of energy if running 60 min at 5 m/s or 11.2 miles/h

body for the diluting of these solutions. The dilution of the carbohydrates in the intestines does not influence the capacity at normal outside temperatures (up to 20 °C). The intake of concentrated drinks at heat with the condition of dehydration can lead to an additional liquid loss. This also applies to low-salt liquids (tap water). A condition of **water intoxication** can appear with longer strain, if the athlete has absorbed a lot of hypotonic tap water (Noakes 1992).

Sodium has to be drawn off the blood before the water can be reabsorbed from the intestines. **Salt deficits** repeatedly appear in extreme runs or in long-triathlon in Hawaii. Blood sodium of less than 125 mmol/l causes dangerous coordination disorders in running or cerebral edemas with a loss of orientation. Salt should be added into own drink solutions at the relation of 1–1.5 g per 1 l of liquid as a precaution. The liquid might taste a little salty then.

The nourishment of the cerebral nerve cells with glucose is not adequately ensured anymore, if the blood glucose drops to an amount lower than 3.5 mmol/l (63 mg/dl) during strain. Loss of motivation and motor disorders are consequences of the glucose insufficiency in the brain (➤ Tab. 87.5).

Less stress develops if carbohydrates are absorbed in dosages and regularly during long-term strain. Disorders of the immune system are reduced with an even energy balance. The intake of carbohydrates reduces the increased protein catabolism in the muscles.

Tab. 87.5 Movement disorders (ataxia) with hypoglycemic runners or triathletes.

- disorder of running coordination
- irregular stride (dysmetria)
- unsteady running (imbalance)
- runner begins to walk
- athlete cannot change the movement failure (slow walking, basing oneself on an attendant, crawling)
- slow reactions and actions on acclamation

87.4 Protein absorption

Long-term endurance performances do not cause glycogen depletion, but an increased gluconeogenesis. Amino acids are released preferably in long-term exposures. The free amino acid depot has only an amount of 110 g. The antibodies which act immunologically can be utilized energetically in emergency situations. Highly strained athletes often show a **concentration of immunoglobulin** (Ig) at the bottom limit; this involves IgG especially.

The main amino acids that are brought up for the gluconeogenesis are the branched-chain amino acids as well as glutamine and alanine. About 0.6 g of glucose develops in metabolism from 1 g of amino acids. As much as 10% of the needed energy can be supplied by the oxidation of amino acids during long-term strain. The higher the protein catabolism, the longer takes the recovery. As is generally known, the athlete recovers faster after a run of 10 km than after a marathon. The absorption of branch-chain amino acids or essential amino acids during long-term strain or in altitude training leads to an improved performance (Parry-Billings et al. 1992, Bigard et al. 1993, Lucà-Moretti et al. 2003). The protein synthesis is depressed for as long as 48 hours after long-term strain, and thus a pointed absorption of proteins or amino acids makes sense in this period (Rennie and Triptom 2000).

Summary

It is not contradicted anymore that nutrition can influence the performance. There is a difference between the nutrition before performance, during exposure and in the early period of recovery. A final intake of carbohydrates should happen about 30 min before the start. This form of energy absorption has no hypoglycemic effect before the start. The intake of carbohydrates during strain does not influence the capacity within the first hour of strain. The carbohydrate absorption should be started only after 70 min of strain. It reduces an increased protein catabolism in exposures of several hours. The continuous carbohydrate absorption of 30–50 g/h is better tolerated in general than the singular consumption of a larger amount (60–80 g). The tolerance for the products is to be checked at an own supply before important starts. Liquid must be supplied from the beginning at conditions of heat; salt has to be added to the drinks here (~ 1.0–1.5 g/l). Approximately 100 g of carbohydrates combined with amino acids or protein hydrolysates conduce to the acceleration of the glycogen development in the first two hours of recovery after strain, whereas the triglyceride depots can only be refilled by a fat-containing mixed diet.

87.5 Vitamins

Vitamins are micronutrients of organic origin and are essential for the organism. Growth and the processes of important life functions would not be possible without vitamins. The human organism cannot generate them itself. Vitamins are neither construction material nor are they energy suppliers, and they enfold their effect as co-enzymes or hormone-like substances.

Information on the **need of vitamins** bases on experience and the knowledge of the necessary amount of vitamins for the prevention of health impairments. The amounts recommended by the German Society of Nutrition (DGE) are average data for the whole population. People engaged in sport activities have an energy turnover twice or three times as high as the one of unexercised people and thus also a higher need of vitamins, depending on the exercise loads.

The additional intake of vitamins is common in competitive training; the objective limitation of the amounts is open, though. Even highly dosed vitamin absorptions do not increase the athletic capacity. The adjustment to exercise strain and the process of regeneration are only possible without many disorders, if there is an optimal supply of vitamins.

The individual requirement of vitamins cannot be predicted. Signs and diseases of insufficiency or undersupply of vitamins known so far are no reliable benchmark of orientation for the person engaging in sport activities.

The quantity of vitamins needed is influenced by:

- the amount of exercise (hours/week)
- stress situations
- gastrointestinal function

Tab. 87.6 Vitamin demand of untrained persons and competitive athletes.

Vitamins	Daily demand		Minimal toxic dose
	unexercised persons*	competitive athletes**	
A (retinol)***	5,000 IU	13,000 IU	25,000–50,000 IU
beta-carotene (precursor of vit. A)	3 mg	4.5 mg	30 mg
D (calciferol)	400 IU (10 µg)	800 IU (20 µg)	5,000 IU (1.2 mg)
E (tocopherol)	10 mg	50 mg	1.2 g
K (phylloquinone)	80 µg	150 µg	2 g
B_1 (thiamin)	1.5 mg	6–8 mg	300 mg
B_2 (riboflavin)	1.8 mg	8 mg	300 mg
B_3 (niacin)	20 mg	30–40 mg	1 g
B_4 (folic acid)	300 µg	400 µg	400 mg
B_5 (pantothenic acid)	≈10 mg	20 mg	10 g
B_6 (pyridoxine)	2.1 mg	6–10 mg	2 g
B_{12} (cobalamin)	3 µg	6 µg	20 mg
C (ascorbic acid)	75 mg	300–500 mg	> 5 g
H (biotin)	0.1 mg	0.3 mg	50 mg
Q_{10} (ubiquinone)	10 mg	30 mg	uncertain

* recommendations of the German Nutrition Society (Deutsche Gesellschaft für Ernährung – DGE) of 2000
** higher amounts for power and power endurance training as well as for altitude training
*** one IU of vit. A equals 0.3 µg all-trans-retinol (vit. A_1)

- diseases (e.g. infections)
- condition of regeneration
- phase of growth
- pregnancy and others.

The recommendations for the vitamin absorption supply a safety margin as to avoid undersupplies (➤ Tab. 87.6). There is no difference in the effect of industrially produced and of natural vitamins. Nevertheless, the **natural vitamins are more advantageous**, since they still contain important secondary plant compounds.

The traditional classification of vitamins is slightly abstruse due to the discovery of new essential substances the organism depends upon. Such substances are, for example, antioxidants, bioflavonoid, omega-3 and omega-6 fatty acids as well as beta-carotene.

The vitamins are classified by their dissolving behavior into water-soluble and liposoluble vitamins.

Vitamin A, vitamin D, vitamin E and vitamin K belong to the **liposoluble vitamins**.

Vitamin B_1, vitamin B_2, vitamin B_6, vitamin B_{12}, folic acid and pantothenic acid are the **water-soluble** vitamins.

Water-soluble vitamins cannot be stored; they are excreted at an excess.

87.5.1 Vitamin A (retinol)

Vitamin A is only found in animal source foods. The precursor beta-carotene exists in plants. 7 times as much beta-carotene has to be absorbed to achieve the effect of vitamin A. Liver, butter and egg yolk have the highest vitamin A content. Cheese, margarine (additive) and sea fish are also important sources.

Vitamin A has significant **effects** on growth and differentiation of skin and mucous membranes as well as on the process of vision (➤ Tab. 87.7). The body has only a small depot

Tab. 87.7 Physiological effects and demands of liposoluble vitamins in competitive sports.

Vitamin	Effects	Recommended absorption/day
vitamin A (retinol)	- development and preservation: skin, mucosa - vision process (scotopic vision) - stabilization of immune defense - growth regulation (promotion of protein synthesis) Resources will last for 3–6 months.	- 1.5–4.5 mg retinol equivalents (5,000–15,000 IU vit. A) - maximum dose: 25,000 IU, 15,000 IU at pregnancy
beta-carotene	Effective antioxidant. Only reaches 15% of the effect of vitamin A	2–4 mg retinol equivalent Overdosage recognizable by the yellow color of the skin (harmless)
vitamin E (alpha-tocopherol)	- strong antioxidant for unsaturated fatty acids, vitamin A, hormones and enzymes - arteriosclerosis protection Resources last for 2–6 weeks.	20–400 mg (higher dosages are not recommended anymore)
vitamin D (calciferol)	- growth and development of bones and cells - promotion of the absorption and utilization of calcium and phosphor - hormone-like effect Resources last for 2–6 weeks.	5–10 µg vit. D_2 or D_3 Overdosage possible, starting with 25 µg (1000 IU)
vitamin K (phylloquinone)	- initiation of the synthesis of blood coagulation factors - involved in the carboxylation of proteins Resources will last for 2–6 weeks.	70–140 µg vit. K_1 (phylloquinone)
vitamin Q (ubiquinone)	- antioxidant (in combination with vitamins E, C and beta-carotene) - electron conveyor in the respiratory chain - key function for cellular energy development	10–30 mg coenzyme Q_{10}

of vitamin A which is located in the liver. The depot is sufficient for about 6 months.

The daily **need** of vitamin A is estimated to be 1 mg. The need in competitive sports is 4 to 5 times higher than for unexercised persons. Impaired twilight vision is a sign of deficiency. An overdose is possible in the intake of vitamin A, but not in the intake of beta-carotene.

87.5.2 Vitamin D (calciferol)

Vitamin D consists of several substances – the calciferols. The prohormone 7-dehydrocholesterol is transformed into the effective vitamin D_3 in the human skin by UV-radiation (sun, sunlamp). The latter one is contained mainly in animal source products (butter, cheese, liver) and abounds in sea fish and codliver oil. The common mixed diet is low of vitamin D_3.

The self-generation of 7-dehydrocholesterol from cholesterol is the major source for vitamin D in humans. Adults get along with the generation of vitamin D_3 by the sun radiation. It is transformed into calcitriol in the kidneys, which regulates the calcium need of the body.

Vitamin D forms the precursor for hormone-like substances that affect the **calcium and phosphate household**. D-vitamins are determining for the mineralization of the bones. Sunlight deficiency and largely cloaking clothes in childhood and adult age lead to impaired bone augmentation.

Athletes exercising in the open and exposing themselves to the sun rays have no problems with D-vitamin supply 10 IU (0.25 µg) of vitamin D are generated from 7-dehydrocholesterol in 1 hour at a sun radiation of 1 cm^2.

Hall sport athletes, swimmers or athletes exercising in protection gear (e.g. fencers) have a **higher need** of vitamin D that amounts to ~ 10 µg per day.

87.5.3 Vitamin E (alpha-tocopherol)

Alpha-tocopherol enfolds the major effect of vitamin E. Tocopherols are generated in plants. Plant oils therefore contain large amounts of vitamin E. It is also found in meat, fish and dairy products. Cereals and cereal products, however, provide the most.

Tab. 87.8 Vitamin E (alpha-tocopherol) in sports.

Effect	■ protection of membrane lipids, lipoproteins and depot fats from dissimilation by lipidperoxidation ■ synergistic effects with vitamin C at the protection of cell membranes ■ protection of multiply unsaturated fatty acids (e.g. linoleic acid), vitamin A, hormones and enzymes from oxidative destruction
Recommended daily demand (1 mg alpha-tocopherol = 1.49 IU)	■ untrained persons 10–15 mg ■ children, adolescents 10–12 mg ■ pregnant women 12–17 mg ■ fitness athletes 20–40 mg ■ competitive athletes 100–200 mg* ■ top athletes at stress exposures 300–400 mg*
Aliments with high vitamin E content	■ margarine and vegetable oils (soy, sunflower, olive, corn) ■ cheese ■ wheat germ ■ brown rice ■ oatmeal ■ fruit, vegetables (asparagus, spinach, Brussels sprouts, broccoli) ■ potatoes ■ eggs ■ milk
Pharmaceuticals	50–500 mg in the form of alpha-tocopherol

* High dosages are evaluated controversially at present.

The strong **antioxidant effect** is the common mechanism of action of the tocopherols. Vitamin E also influences the protein synthesis, the immune function and the neuromuscular system.

The aerobic gain of energy only proceeds effectively in the presence of vitamin E. It protects the strained muscle's cell membranes from the destruction by oxygen radicals and stabilizes their structure. Several grams of vitamin E can be stored in the fatty tissue of the liver.

The exact **vitamin-E demand** is not known. A daily absorption of 15–20 mg (15–20 IU) of alpha-tocopherol is recommended for adults (➤ Tab. 87.8). The vitamin-E demand of competitive athletes is usually 10–20 times higher than normal. The additional absorption of vitamin E increases the muscular capacity and alleviates sore muscles.

87.5.4 Vitamin B_1 (thiamine)

Vitamin B_1 (thiamine) exists in food of animal source as well as of vegetal origin. Cereal products (wheat, rye, oatmeal), corn and rice include a large amount of vitamin B_1. Beef only contains one third of the vitamin-B_1 compared to pork. The major thiamine providers in vegetables are peas (0.3 mg/100 g) as well as potatoes and carrots (0.1 mg/100 g each).

Thiamine is a component of enzymes in the aerobic and anaerobic carbohydrate metabolism. It is not heat-stable and is destroyed in cooking since it is a water-soluble vitamin. The **vitamin-B_1 need** increases with the higher energy turnover. The demand of unexercised persons amounts to 0.5 mg thiamine per 1,000 kcal of food consumption or 1.2–1.4 mg/day. Thiamine is also necessary for the function of the nervous system and in gluconeogenesis.

87.5.5 Vitamin B_2 (riboflavin)

Vitamin B_2 (riboflavin) is widely spread in the animal and vegetal field. A sufficient supply is provided by milk and dairy products. Meat is rich of riboflavin (0.2 mg/100 g), especially liver of beef (3 mg/10 g). Peas, beans and cabbage contain 0.1–0.2 mg/100 g of vitamin B_2.

The riboflavin content of the grains of wheat, corn and rice amounts to 0.1 mg/100 g.

Excessive riboflavin is excreted, which can be recognized by yellow coloring of the urine. The riboflavin reserves are enough for 2–6 weeks. It is the co-enzyme of a large number of reducing substances that are called flavoproteins or **flavoenzymes** because of their yellow color. It is a component of the enzymes of the respiratory chain in the mitochondria and is therefore permanently necessary for the aerobic energy metabolism.

The **demand** is 1.8–2.5 mg/day in unexercised persons and increases in performance exercise (➤ Tab. 87.9). 0.6 mg/day of riboflavin should be supplied to the body with each energy absorption of 1,000 kcal. 6–12 mg of vitamin B_2 should be absorbed daily with high exercise strain (more than 20 hours/week). This demand can be satisfied with high-caloric and balanced mixed diet. Riboflavin cannot be overdosed.

87.5.6 Vitamin B_6 (pyridoxine)

Vitamin B_6 (pyridoxine) is widely spread. Fish and meat have amounts of 0.4–0.8 mg/100 g; cereal, corn and rice have amounts of 0.2–0.6 mg/100 g. Smaller amounts of pyridoxine are found in fruit and vegetables (0.1–0.3 mg/100 g). The loss in cooking amounts to 20–40%. There will be no deficits in vegetarian nutrition, if there is a sufficient intake of cereal products.

Pyridoxine is the coenzyme of many enzymes in protein metabolism. The **protein synthesis** in the organ growth, muscle growth and muscle regeneration would not be possible without pyridoxine. In addition, it works as an antioxidant. Pyridoxine is necessary for the remethylation of methionine and prevents an increase of the homocysteine in combination with vitamin B_{12} and folic acid.

The **demand** of vitamin B_6 depends on the protein turnover and increases with the absorption of large amounts of protein and of fatty acids. Highly strained athletes should absorb > 6 mg/day of vitamin B_6 because of the significance of this vitamin for the protein metabolism. Undersupplies are possible with abun-

Tab. 87.9 Effects and recommended dosage of water-soluble vitamins in performance training.

Vitamins	Effects	Absorption/day
B_1 (thiamin)	■ aerobic energy metabolism ■ heart and nerve function	6–10 mg
B_2 (riboflavin)	■ anaerobic and aerobic energy metabolism ■ metabolism for skin, hair and nails	6–12 mg
B_3 (niacin)	■ energy metabolism ■ biosyntheses	30–40 mg
B_5 (pantothenic acid)	■ aerobic energy metabolism ■ antioxidant ■ hair growth; skin resurfacing	4–7 mg
B_6 (pyridoxin)	■ protein metabolism ■ antioxidant ■ averts homocystein increase	6–15 mg
B_{12} (cobalamin)	■ cell formation; DNA synthesis ■ L-carnitine synthesis ■ immune system ■ averts homocystein increase in combination with B_6 and folic acid	2–6 µg
C (ascorbic acid)	■ antioxidant (protects vitamins A, B_2, E and pantothenic acid of oxidative destruction as radical scavenger) ■ cell protection; resistance to infections ■ development of skin elasticity	300–500 mg
biotin (H)	■ synthesis of fatty acids ■ gluconeogenesis ■ T- and B-cell-mediated immune defense	50–100 µg
folic acid (M)	■ cell formation; DNA synthesis ■ immune system ■ blood coagulation ■ impedes homocystein increase	400–800 µg

dant alcohol absorption and with the use of contraceptives. Dry skin, inflammations of the labial angles and the tongue are signs of undersupply.

87.5.7 Vitamin B_{12} (cobalamin)

Vitamin B_{12} (cobalamin) appears in animal source food. Beef and pork liver contain 70 or 30 µg. Flesh includes definitely less cobalamin (2–3 µg/100 g). The fish with the highest content of cobalamin is the herring (10 µg/100 g).

Eggs, cheese and whole milk (2–0.4 µg/100 g) are further vitamin-B_{12} sources. Vegetal food does not contain vitamin B_{12}, which leaves vegetarians undersupplied.

The absorption of vitamin B_{12} is bound to the **intrinsic factor** in the intestines. A lack of cobalamin occurs, if vitamin B_{12} is missing, and this leads to the symptoms of the "pernicious anemia".

Vitamin B_{12} is effective in the reducing systems of the mitochondria, in the formation of the fatty acids and the amino acids in metabolism. It supports the degeneration of the branch-chain amino acids and is necessary for the cell formation as well as the synthesis of deoxyribonucleic acid (DNA). It is also decisive for the formation of blood in the bone marrow. Vitamin B_{12} is required for remethylation of methionine and prevents an increase of the homocysteine, in combination with vitamin B_6 and folic acid. A vitamin B_{12} deficiency causes impairment in the formation of the erythrocytes and thus a reduced oxygen transport.

The daily **demand** of vitamin B_{12} amounts to 2 µg with an increase by the factor 3 for competitive athletes. There is no risk of deficiency with regular consumption of meat. The depot of vitamin B_{12} suffices for 3–4 years. Vitamin B_{12} has to be supplemented in vegetarian nutrition.

87.5.8 Vitamin B_7 (biotin, vitamin H)

Biotin had previously been called vitamin H. This vitamin is widely spread in nature. Main providers are liver, kidneys, milk, eggs and meat. 30–100 µg/200 g of biotin are found in liver. Soy beans, on the other hand, contain 60 µg/100 g, chicken eggs 25 µg/100 g, bananas and grain of wheat 5–6 µg/100 g and meat 2–5 µ/100 g. Vegetal biotin is water-soluble; the biotin in animal source food appears in a water-insoluble (protein-bound) form.

Biotin is a coenzyme in several metabolic processes and is necessary for the key enzymes of the **gluconeogenesis** and the **synthesis of fatty acids**. It is also important for the dissimilation of the branch-chained amino acids. Furthermore, it is involved in the cellular immune defense (B and T cells).

The daily **demand of biotin** is 50–100 µg, and it is covered easily by a normal mixed diet. A disturbed cell metabolism of skin and hair (hair loss, skin inflammations) is an indication for an undersupply. Muscle pain and sleepiness appear as a result of an insufficiency. 200–1,000 µg of biotin have to be absorbed daily with a possible undersupply. Overdoses have not been known.

87.5.9 Folic acid (vitamin M)

Folic acid comes with vegetal and animal source foods. Leafy greens, tomatoes, cereal and liver are rich of folic acid. Low amounts are found in meat, fish and fruit. Chicken liver (1,880 µg/100 g), cereal grains (1,800 µg/100 g) and brewer's yeast (1,800 µg/100 g) have the highest content of folic acid. Distinctly less is found in eggs (70 µg/100 g), leaf salads, beans, spinach, asparagus and tomatoes (20–160 µg/100 g). Milk and cheese contain 5–20 µg/100 g of folic acid. The folic acid absorbed with food is bound (folates) and is reabsorbed only to 40%.

Folic acid forms an important coenzyme in the metabolism of the amino acids and of the nucleic acids. It functions as acceptor and transmitter of activated formaldehyde and formic acid. The **neoformation of cells** depends on folic acid. Formic acid is additionally involved in the immune function and the blood coagulation. It is necessary for the remethylation of methionine and prevents an increase of the homocysteine, in combination with vitamin B_6 and B_{12}.

50% of the full amount of folic acid (5–10 mg) is deposited in the liver. Excessive folic acid is excreted.

There is a **demand** of approximately 400 µg/day and twice as much is needed by pregnant women and breast-feeding mothers. Folic acid is absorbed with the food as free and bound folic acid (total folate).

An undersupply of folic acid is possible in sport; the effects cannot be defined clearly, though. A sufficient supply of folic acid is necessary, because a deficit is often connected to an undersupply of vitamin B_{12} and it encourages anemia. The increased homocysteine level, which is considered an own risk factor for cardiovascular diseases, is caused by a lack of folic acid and the vitamins B_{12} and B_6. The undersupply of folic acid becomes effective after about 4 months.

87.5.10 Niacin (nicotine acid and nicotinamide)

Nicotinic acid and nicotinamide in combination are called niacin. Both substances have the same effect, because they can be transferred into each other in metabolism. Niacin is no proper vitamin, because it can be synthesized out of **tryptophan** by the body.

Niacin deficiency – known as pellagra – causes fatigue, mucosal inflammations and inefficiency.

Nicotinamide is found in all animal source products. Niacin is basically found in plants in form of nicotinic acid, although the amount here is definitely smaller than in liver and meat. It is almost completely reabsorbed from meat products, but only to 30% from plants. 1–2 mg of niacin are combined in one cup of coffee.

Niacin is an important coenzyme in **energy metabolism**. The NAD-dependent dehydrogenases are primarily effective in the mitochondria. They provide hydrogen to the respiratory chain for oxidation and gain of energy. The process of glycolysis and the synthesis of fatty acids require niacin.

60 mg of tryptophan are necessary for the creation of 1 mg of niacin. Highly dosed niacin absorption increases the carbohydrate oxidation and suppresses the fat metabolism.

The **demand** is denoted in nicotinic equivalents that consider the tryptophan content of food. The daily demand is assumed to be 15–20 mg. The niacin amount of various foods is different; thus, 200 g of beef, 750 g of peas or 1.25 kg of potatoes correspond to a supply of 15 mg of niacin. 8–17 mg of niacin and 0.5–1.0 g of tryptophan are absorbed daily with a mixed diet. Conditions of niacin deficiencies have not been known in athletes.

87.5.11 Pantothenic acid

Almost all foods contain pantothenic acid. Liver (7 mg/100 g), innards (2.7 mg/100 g) and meat (0.6 mg/100 g) are rich of pantothenic acid. 1–1.6 mg/100 g are found in wheat grains, eggs, broccoli and cauliflower.

The pantothenic acid is a component of important substrates in the **energy metabolism** as well as the activated acetic acid (acetyl-coenzyme A). It is involved in all composition and degradation processes in the carbohydrate, fat and amino acid metabolism. It is also needed for the synthesis of steroids (cholesterol, sexual hormones), hemoglobin or cytochromes in the mitochondria.

The demand is estimated 8 mg/day. About 10 mg of pantothenic acid are absorbed by a usual mixed diet. Increased consumption of food and stress situations in sport increase the demand. Excessive pantothenic acid is excreted.

87.5.12 Vitamin C (ascorbic acid)

Important nutritional **vitamin-C providers** are:
- citrus fruit (~ 50 mg/100 g)
- peppers (140 mg/100 g)
- cabbages (45–115 mg/100 g)
- fruit (20–100 mg/100 g)
- potatoes (14 mg/100 g).

Furthermore, fruit and vegetable juices – especially of sea buckthorn, black currants, gooseberries and citrus – are profitable vitamin-C sources. During preparation of food (cooking) and storage is destroged a large amount (30 to 100%) of the oxidation-sensitive ascorbic acid.

Vitamin C can only be stored restrictedly because of its water-solubility. The storages are enough for 2–6 weeks. Excessive vitamin C is excreted.

Vitamin C belongs to the very effective **antioxidants**, because it intercepts free radicals and thus protects the cell walls. Vitamin C protects the vitamins E, A, thiamin and riboflavin from destruction. It is involved in numerous metabolic processes.

More iron is reabsorbed in the presence of vitamin C. The stability of the intracellular iron depot ferritin is ensured by vitamin C. It is also assigned tumor-suppressing and vessel-protective effects. An increase of the athletic capacity by highly dosed vitamin-C absorption has not been proved. The disposition for infections can be reduced, though, by regular vitamin-C absorption.

Indications of the demand range from 75 mg to even several grams per day. The high dosage is especially promoted by orthomolecular medicine. A regular supply of more than 1 g/day for athletes is not necessary, regarding all advantages of vitamin-C absorption 300–500 mg of vitamin C per day are usually enough.

The stored vitamin C amounts to approximately 3 g and is exhausted in 2 weeks of exercising. A supplementation with vitamin C during the season of competition provides advantages, because it functions as antioxidant and promotes regeneration.

An overdose of vitamin C is not possible, because it is excreted in oxidized condition, i.e. it has fulfilled its antioxidant function.

Major arguments for the increased absorption of vitamin C in competitive sports are:

- muscle cell protection by the antioxidant effect
- ensured immunologic disposition of defense
- support of the capacity of the connective tissue
- encouragement of the iron absorption
- reduction of the stress disposition (production of hormones), as well as
- compensation of losses by sweat.

Latent undersupplies find expression in an increased disposition for infections, gingival hemorrhages, impaired wound healing, fatigue, increased stress disposition and other functional impairments. A deficiency of several vitamins (e.g. vitamin E, D, folic acid) is mostly present in these conditions. The willingness for exercising decreases and the need of sleep increases.

87.6 Minerals

Minerals are inorganic substances that are essential for the preservation of life. They are needed as supporting and hard substances for the growth of bones, teeth and tissues. Viability is bound to balanced minerals. Competitive sports training can disturb this balance in the body and can lead to an undersupply of individual minerals.

A decrease of minerals in food as well as in fruit and vegetables has been found in recent years attributable to modern cultivation methods in agriculture. Fast food and cola drinks also contribute to the undersupply. Natural orange juice and whole-wheat bread have a high density of nutrients, since they contain many vitamins and minerals. Permanent sweating in performance-oriented training leads to an increased loss of minerals (> Tab. 87.10).

87.6.1 Sodium

Sodium is basically stored in body fluids. The stored sodium amounts to ~100 g (4,348 mmol/l) in men and ~77 g (3,348 mmol/l) in women. 23 mg conform to 1 mmol/l of sodium. The sodium concentration in the blood amounts to 135–145 mmol/l.

The **water balance** is decisively maintained by sodium. The aldosterone-angiotensin-renin system and the atrial natriuretic protein control the sodium balance. The sodium concentrations in tissue and blood influence the blood pressure, the osmotic balance, the acid-base balance and the muscular excitability. The kidneys control the sodium excretion.

A permanent sodium loss by sweating happens in exercising. One liter of sweat contains averagely 1 g of sodium. Common salt (NaCl) con-

Tab. 87.10 Daily demands of minerals and trace elements.

Mineral	Daily demand		Minimal toxic dose
	unexercised persons	athletes	
salt (NaCl)	8 g	15 g	>100 mg
potassium	2.5 g	5 g	12 g
calcium	1 g	2 g	12 g
phosphor	1.2 g	2.5 g	12 g
magnesium	400 mg	600 mg	6 g
iron	18 mg	40 mg	>100 mg
zinc	15 mg	25 mg	500 mg
copper	2 mg	4 mg	100 mg
iodine	0.15 mg	0.25 mg	2 mg
selenium	70 µg	100 µg	1 mg
chromium	100 µg	200 µg	2 mg

sists of 40% of sodium and 60% of chloride. The daily **demand** of common salt amounts to ~6 g. Tap water is low of sodium and cannot be reabsorbed as easily as sodium-rich mineral water or salty drinks. Isotonic liquids that contain 0.5–1.2 g/l NaCl are absorbed best. Liquids taste slightly salty with these concentrations.

There is a risk to health in the decrease of the blood sodium lower than 130 mmol/l, which appears in numerous triathletes at the ironman competition in Hawaii (Hiller et al. 1985, Hiller 1989). A **hyponatremia** can develop with dehydration and also due to excessive drinking of low-sodium tap water. Recreational athletes exude about 3.5 g of common salt in 1 l of sweat, while competitive athletes exude only 1.6 g/l. Well exercised athletes sweat less than recreational athletes at comparable speeds and also lose smaller amounts of the minerals.

The need for the intake of salty food or the adding of salt to the food is a typical indication for the salt deficit after strain.

It is often assumed that muscle cramps are caused by sodium deficiency. The muscle cramp is probably caused by a circulation disorder with a deficit of several minerals, such as magnesium, calcium and sodium.

87.6.2 Potassium

The concentration of potassium in the cell is 40 times higher than outside the cell. The intracellular potassium concentration comes to an amount 155 mmol/l, the extracellular concentration, on the other hand, only comes to an amount 4 mmol/l. The regular blood potassium level is 3.8–5.5 mmol/l.

Potassium ensures the:

- stability of the cell membrane
- nerve impulse transmission
- muscle contraction
- regulation of the blood pressure.

It is involved in the carbohydrate, protein and fat metabolism.

The intracellular potassium content influences the aerobic **energy metabolism** in the mitochondria. The exchange of potassium with the external cell space happens via the potassium channels of the cells. The potassium and sodium concentration of the cell membrane represents the membrane potential. The potassium strives to leave the inner cell. Therefore, it must be redirected from the outside to the inside under expenditure of energy by the sodium-potassium pump.

The potassium depot contains 140–150 g in men and 90–120 g in women. The daily potassium demand is 2–3 g for unexercised people and 3–4 g for exercised people. Large amounts of potassium function diuretically, as is found after consumption of fruit.

Bananas, potatoes, spinach, tomatoes, dried fruit and fruit are profitable **potassium sources**.

Up to 10 g of potassium are absorbed daily in a vegetarian diet. The major amount of potassium is excreted via the kidneys. Only a small amount of potassium (0.1–0.2 g/l) is exuded by sweat. The potassium demand definitely increases after diarrhea and vomiting as well as after increased absorption of carbohydrates.

87.6.3 Magnesium

Magnesium is an essential mineral that is stored in the organism with 24–28 g (584–684 mmol/l). An amount of 60% of the magnesium is stored in the bones and 39% are found in the muscles. The magnesium stored in the bones is usually not available. Thrice as much magnesium as in the serum is found in the erythrocytes. The usual magnesium concentration in the blood serum is 0.8–1.3 mmol/l.

The **importance** of magnesium results from its effect in more than 300 magnesium-containing enzymes. The magnesium demand of unexercised men is 330–400 mg/day and of unexercised women 255–310 mg/day; the demand can be attained by a regular mixed diet.

Magnesium is necessary for the:

- energy supply
- energy transmission
- signal transmission at muscle contraction
- muscle relaxation
- blood circulation
- hormonal effect and other functions.

The permeability of cell membranes increases with an undersupply of magnesium. This leads to a decreased density of the sodium-potassium pumps. The ATP activity with a magnesium undersupply is lower and thus a general performance reduction or muscle function disorders are to be expected.

Sweat development and increased urine excretion in competitive training are the main causes for the magnesium loss. Sweat loss of 2–3 l/day means an exudation of 437–656 mg of magnesium/day.

Muscle cramps and reduced performance give reason for measuring the magnesium concentration in the blood. An undersupply is to be expected in sport at a decrease of the magnesium in the blood to under 0.75 mmol/l. The decrease of the blood magnesium in performance training appears 2 months earlier than in the muscle cell.

Indications of an **undersupply** are:
- muscle trembling
- calf cramps
- nervousness
- fatigue or decreasing capacity.

Magnesium absorption of 0.5 g/day over a longer period is necessary in this case.

Whole-wheat products and dairy products, liver, poultry and fish, potatoes, vegetables and soy beans, berries, bananas and oranges **provide magnesium**.

The food preparation causes losses. Magnesium-containing mineral waters are to be preferred (➤ Tab. 87.11). Magnesium absorption of more than 3–5 g/day causes diarrhea.

87.6.4 Calcium

Calcium is an essential mineral. 98% of the calcium depot of 1,000 g is placed in the bones. The stability of bones and teeth depends on the calcium content. The calcium in the blood serum amounts to 2.3–2.7 mmol/l (92–108 mg/dl). The calcium balance is regulated hormonally. Only half of the calcium is in an actively physiological function; the rest is bound to plasma proteins. Definitely less calcium is stored intracellularly than extracellularly.

Tab. 87.11 Aliments containing magnesium (modified according to Holtmeier, 1995).

Aliment	Magnesium content (data in mg by 100 g)
cocoa	414
wheat germs	336
soy flour	235
brewer's yeast	231
peanuts	182
almonds (sweet)	170
hazelnuts	156
oat meal	139
beans (white)	132
walnuts	129
rice (unpolished)	119
peas (peeled)	116
chocolate	104
lentils	77
crispbread	68
noodles	67
raisins (dried)	65
herring fillet	61
wholemeal wheat bread	59
wholemeal rye bread	45
banana	36
potatoes	25
mineral water	20–160 mg/l

Calcium is effective in:
- the stabilization of the cell membrane
- the intracellular signal transmission
- conduction in the nervous system
- signal transmission at the motor endplate (neurotransmitter function) as well as in the blood coagulation.

The calcium demand ensures the parathormone by the activation of the osteoclasts in the bones and the bone substance. Exercising does usually not lead to a calcium deficiency. The **estrogen deficiency** in young female athletes is an exception, because it encourages the demineralization of the bones. The ossification disorder caused by estrogen deficiency and combined with minor calcium absorption encourages the development of **stress fractures**, which is often found in young female runners and female triathletes. The early demineralization can lead to a successive osteoporosis.

Maximum calcium retention in the bone is only reached at 900 mg/day (Matkovic and Heaney 1992). The calcium demand is higher in competitive training of juveniles and amounts to 1,200–1,500 mg/day.

Important **calcium sources** are dairy products, low-fat milk, vegetables and specific mineral waters (> 100 mg/l of calcium). The calcium absorption can be impeded by several factors. The high protein content of milk, phytates, oxalates, lignins and phosphates (cola drinks) reduce reabsorption. The influence of these nutritional components on the bio-availability of calcium is only minor. Vitamin D encourages reabsorption. Calcium is exuded by sweat at amounts of 5–50 mg/l.

87.6.5 Trace elements

Trace elements are the minerals that are absorbed by amounts of 20 mg/day. Iron, copper, zinc, selenium, chromium and vanadium are those of the 14 known essential trace elements that are related to physical strain.

Iron

Iron is a trace element with a depot of 3–5 g in the body. About 60% of it are bound to hemoglobin, 25% in ferritin and hemosiderin and 15% in myoglobin and enzymes of the anaerobic metabolism (cytochromes, catalases, peroxides). The functional iron depots spread into 2.3 g of hemoglobin, 0.32 g of myoglobin and 0.18 g of iron-containing enzymes. 700 mg are bound in the iron depot of ferritin. The largest iron depot is the liver.

The serum concentration of iron amounts to 0.6–1.45 mg/l (10.7–26 µmol/l) in women and 0.8–1.68 mg/l (14.3–30 µmol/l) in men.

The normal range of ferritin in the blood has an amount of 30–400 µg/l in male athletes and 30–150 µg/l in female athletes. The determination of ferritin in the blood is a standard procedure for the assessment of the iron supply in competitive sports, because the ferritin concentration within the blood is connected closely to the iron depots in tissue.

A medium ferritin concentration in the blood of 30–150 µg/l is to be aspired in endurance athletes.

The average iron absorption in Germany amounts to 11 mg in women and 13 mg in men. Competitive athletes objectively have a higher demand. An **iron undersupply** appears in competitive athletes, if the serum ferritin drops below 30 µg/l (➤ Tab. 87.13). Iron supplementation increases the anaerobic capacity also with normal hemoglobin (Agawal 2007).

The endurance training leads to an increase of the plasma volume by 10–20% and affects a pseudo-decrease of hemoglobin by 1–2 g/dl. This pseudo-anemia should not mislead to a wrongly diagnosed iron deficiency. Hemoglobin in male competitive athletes must not fall below 13 g/dl and below 12 g/dl for female athletes at normal hematocrit (➤ Tab. 87.14).

Contributors to the development of a low ferritin balance are:

- exercise-conditioned hemodilution
- increase of the muscle myoglobin
- increase of the erythrocyte mass in the blood
- insufficient iron absorption (vegetarians)
- microhemorrhages in the gastrointestinal tract
- loss of iron by sweating
- loss of iron by urine (loss of erythrocytes by the liver)

Tab. 87.12 Trace elements in the human organism.

Essential	Non-essential	
chromium*	aluminum	mercury
iron*	antimony	rubidium
fluorine	arsenic	silver
iodine	barium	strontium
cobalt	beryllium	tellurium
copper*	lead	thallium
manganese	boron	titanium
molybdenum	bromine	
nickel	cadmium	
selenium*	cesium	
silicon	noble gases	
vanadium*	gold	
zinc*	lithium	
tin	platinum	

* These trace elements are related to physical strain.

87.6 Minerals

- large iron storage in the liver
- menstruation blood of women (15–30 mg/cycle)
- unbalanced vegetal nutrition (vegetarians).

A **main cause** for the loss of iron is the mechanical destruction of the erythrocytes in the soles of the feet by running on hard ground.

The daily iron loss in competitive training is about 2 mg. The reabsorption of iron (non-hem iron) at vegetarian nutrition amounts to only 3–8% in comparison with meat nutrition (hem iron) of 15–22%.

The iron depots are exhausted after 5–8 months of iron undersupply. The decrease of 1 µg/l of serum ferritin conforms to the loss of about 10 mg of depot iron. Absorption of 100–200 g/day of bivalent iron for 2–3 months is necessary for the increase of the ferritin depot.

An **iron undersupply** is **indicated** by:

- unfamiliar fatigue
- early exhaustion
- lacking tolerance of intensity
- no performance development

Tab. 87.13 Main causes for undersupply with minerals in performance training.

Mineral undersupply	Signs of undersupply	Recommended food
magnesium: serum concentration < 0.75 mmol/l	calf cramps; nuchal pain; paresthesias in hands and feet; vagotonic function conversion; cardiac dysrhythmias; organ and vessel cramps	soy beans; milk chocolate; oatmeal; wholewheat bread; milk; fish; mineral water; pharmaceuticals: magnesium preparations 0.3–0.5 g/day
iron: • serum ferritin: < 12 µg/l: iron storage exhausted • 12–15 µg/l: diminished iron storage • 35 µg/l: below normal value men (M) • 23 µg/l: below normal value women (W) • Hemoglobin: < 12 g/dl W, < 13 g/dl M serum iron insecure (< 60 µg/l / < 11 µmol/l W, < 80 µg/l / < 14 µmol/l M)	fatigue; increased feeling of exertion; decreasing endurance potential at higher speeds; procrastinated recovery; anemia	liver; kidneys; red meat; legumes; chocolate; wholewheat bread; liver paste; nuts; pharmaceuticals: 1–2 months of iron absorption of 100–200 mg/day (preferably bivalent iron and gastro compatible preparation)
zinc: serum concentration < 12 µmol/l	tasting and smelling disorders; absence of appetite; weight loss; fatigue; skin lesions; clear increase of infections	cheese, whole milk; meat; eggs; oysters (zinc in legumes and cereals is hardly applicable because of contained phytates); pharmaceuticals: zinc preparations of 15–20 mg/day
Potassium: serum concentration < 3.5 µmol/l	muscle insufficiencies; decreasing reflex responses; diarrheas; tiredness and training aversion; cardiac dysrhythmias	fruit, vegetables; cereal products; meat; pharmaceuticals: potassium-magnesium aspartate (50–100 mmol/l potassium)

Tab. 87.14 Normal blood values and deviations due to endurance training ("athlete's anemia").

Normal values in high-performance sport	Men	Women
hematocrit (%)	46 (39–50)	41 (35–47)
hemoglobin (g/dl)*	15.5 (13.3–17)	13.7 (11.7–16)
serumferritin (µg/l)**	30–400	30–150
"athlete's anemia"		
hematocrit (%)	< 40	< 35
hemoglobin (g/dl)	< 13	< 12
serumferritin (µg/l)	< 30	< 20

* Hemoglobin g/dl × 0.6206 = mmol/l. The indicated maximum values (17 or 16 g/dl) are the upper limits designated by the doping agency WADA, which causes an examination corresponding to EPO, if transgressed.
** 1 µg/l serumferritin is equivalent to 8–10 mg stored iron.

- intensified breathing in strain
- accumulation of infections of the upper respiratory tracts.

Zinc

Zinc also belongs to the trace elements. The body stores 1.3–2 g of zinc primarily in bones, skin and hair. The blood concentration of 4–7.5 mg/l or 61–114 mmol/l is a small depot. 90% of the zinc is kept in erythrocytes and is available for metabolic processes. A continuous absorption is necessary, because the zinc depots are small.

Zinc fulfills numerous important **functions** in the protein, carbohydrate, fat and nucleic acid metabolism. it is also a part of hormones, receptors and functions in the immune system. It is part of more than 200 enzymes. Zinc is lost by sweat and urine during strain. Competitive athletes with versatile nutrition can usually ensure the daily demand of 10–15 mg of zinc. About 30% of the zinc content in food is reabsorbed.

Generous consumption of calcium impairs the reabsorption of zinc. The regular zinc supply for athletes ensures the capacity and helps to prevent muscle cramps. Zinc has a stabilizing effect on the immune system. The sufficient supply of zinc helps to prevent infections. Zinc is necessary for the protein synthesis. **Zinc absorption** of 20–25 mg/day is sufficient for endurance athletes.

Copper

The copper depot contains 80–100 mg. The daily **demand** is 1–1.5 mg or 11 µg/kg of body weight. Copper is a part of 16 metallo-enzymes that are **antioxidants**. The copper-containing coeruloplasmin intervenes in the oxidation of iron.

Nutrients rich of copper are: cereal products, liver, fish, nuts, cocoa, coffee, tea and legumes. Copper is essential for the organism. An undersupply leads to health impairments, disorders in the tissue-structuring and limited enzyme activities. The development of connective tissue, the function of the central nervous system and blood production are not possible without copper.

Selenium

Selenium also belongs to the essential trace elements and should be absorbed in amounts of 30–70 µg/day. The **selenium demand** is estimated to be 50–100 µg/day. The medium supply is 30–50 µg/day in Europe and 30–40 µg/day in Germany. A selenium amount of 70–100 µg/day should perhaps be absorbed by competitive athletes to ensure the antioxidant capacity.

Selenium functionally plays a central role in the **antioxidant defense** in a synergy of vitamin E. A selenium deficiency is equal to symptoms of a sodium deficiency, because selenium is a part of the deiodases. The deiodases are necessary for the transformation of thyroxin (T_4) into the active thyroid hormone T_3.

The iodine deficiency developing simultaneously with a selenium undersupply is indicated by cold sensitivity, low blood pressure, gain of weight, changes of skin and hair as well as the development of a crop.

Sea fish, meat, chicken eggs, liver, cereal products, yeast, nuts, lentils and asparagus are **nutrients** providing selenium.

The soil in Germany is poor of selenium. A selenium supplementation of 180 µg/day leads to an increase of the antioxidant capacity. The bio-availability of inorganic selenium (e.g. sodium selenite) is better than the one of organic connections. Organic selenium is part of nutritional supplements, while the inorganic selenium is used for medication.

Chromium

Chromium is effective in the carbohydrate, protein and fat metabolism and exponentiates the effect of insulin in the stimulation of the absorption of glucose, amino acids and triglycerides in the cell (Anding et al. 1997). The storing of glycogen is enhanced by chromium.

The insulin increases and hypoglycemic conditions or disturbed glucose tolerance can appear caused by a **chromium undersupply** (< 20 µg/day). No improved performances or increased strength have been found with absorption of chromium picolinate (200 µg/day). The consumption of chromium as a supplement can amount to 50–200 µg/day. The absorption of chromium combined with picolinate is presently not allowed in Germany.

Iodine

The prohormone thyroxin (T_4) is transformed into the active thyroid hormone (T_3) by help of iodine. The decisive enzyme here (iodine thyronine deiodase) includes iodine and selenium.

The iodine depot in the body contains 10–20 mg with the largest amount of it being placed in the thyroid gland (8–15 mg). Iodine absorption of 200 µg/day causes the thyroid gland to absorb 15% in 24 hours. The iodine absorption in the thyroid gland is increased by self-regulation, if the iodine supply drops. Excessive iodine is excreted.

Germany is a region of iodine deficiency with a north-south divide. Iodine deficiency leads to an enlargement of the thyroid gland (crop).

The **daily iodine absorption** should be as much as 2 µg/kg of body weight at the minimum. Competitive athletes have a potentially higher iodine demand. Iodized salt is to be used regularly in training regions in southern Germany, because there is an endemic region of iodine deficiencies. The weekly fish meal (sea fish) increases the natural iodine absorption.

87.6.6 Supplementation of selected agents

More and more additional substances are consumed in addition to the absorption of vitamins and minerals in competitive and recreational sports. The additional supply of substances by nutritional supplements and their use is subject to controversial assessments.

Nutritional supplements are isolated, mostly chemically defined substances or mixtures of substances that are of a nutritional character or have physiological effects, according to the guidelines of the EU. But they have no pharmacological effect. Their effect relates to vitamins, minerals and protective substances (secondary plant products), and others.

Potential healing effects of nutritional supplements shall not be advertised in certain countries (e.g. Germany), whereas in the US claimed healing effects can be advertised but are – in the absence of randomized controlled trials – not supported by the FDA.

Medications are substances and preparations of substances that are designed to heal, alleviate, prevent or recognize diseases, ailments, impairments or pathological conditions at the or in the human body. They influence the structure, condition or function of the body or the mental conditions.

The opinions regarding the additional consumption of vitamins and minerals in sports or in stress situations differ. There is a large tendency to the treatment with vitamins, trace elements and minerals in the shape of nutritional supplements or individual preparations in the **U.S.A.** The problem is that there are no compulsory recommendations regarding the actually necessary amounts of these micronutrients for athletic activity.

Performance-orientated training leads to an increased loss of sweat, so that a supplementation with **minerals** can be justified at a weekly training of more than 12 hours. The diverse indications in literature recommend higher absorptions of minerals for athletes.

The energy density marks the energy content (kcal) per 100 g of nutrient. Nutrients that show 12–30 kcal/100 g are low of energy. Fast-food nutrition has a high energy density compared to fruit and vegetables. The energy content of "Monster Thickburgers" is 1,420 kcal, of a "Double Whopper" 980 kcal and of a "Bic Mac" 580 kcal.

References

Agarwal R (2007). Nonhematological Benefits of Iron. Am J Nephrol 27: 565–571.

Anding JD, Wolinsky I, Klimis-Tavantzis DJ (1997). Chromium. In: Wolinsky I, Riskell JA (eds). Sports Nutrition: Vitamin and Trace Elements. CRC Press, Boca Raton U.S.A.

Berg A and König D (2008). Optimale Ernährung des Sportlers. 4th edition. Hirzel Verlag, Stuttgart, Leipzig.

Bigard AX, Satabin P, Lavier P, Cannon P, Taillander D, Guezennec CY (1993). Effect of protein supplementation during prolonged exercise at moderate altitude on performance and plasma amino acid pattern. Eur J Appl Physiol 66: 5–10.

Blom P, Vollestad NK, Costill DL (1986). Factors affecting changes in muscle glycogen concentrations during and after prolonged exercise. Acta Physiol Scand 128 (Suppl. 556): 67–74.

Brouns F (1993). Die Ernährungsbedürfnisse des Sportlers. Springer Verlag, Berlin.

Chryssanthopoulos C, Williams C (1997). Pre-exercise carbohydrate meal and endurance running capacity when carbohydrates are ingested during exercise. Int J Sports Med 18: 543–548.

Clasing D (1996; ed). Die essgestörte Athletin. Spot und Buch Strauß, Köln.

Coggan AR, Swanson SC (1992). Nutritional manipulation before and during endurance exercise: effects on performance. Med Sci Sports Exerc 24: 331–335.

Coyle EF, Hagenberg JM, Hurley BH, Martin III, WH, Ehsani AA, Holloszy JO (1983). Carbohydrate feeding during prolonged strenuous exercise can delay fatigue. J Appl Physiol 15: 466–471.

Coyle EF, Coggan AR, Hemmert MK, Lowe , Walters TJ (1985). Substrate usage during prolonged exercise following a preexercise meal. J Appl Physiol 59: 429–433.

Curell K, Jeukendrup A (2008). Superior endurance performance with ingestion of multiple transportable Carbohydrates. Med Sci Sports Exerc 40: 275–281.

Hargreaves M, Costill DL, Coggan AR, Fink WJ, Nishibata I (1984). Effect of carbohydrate feedings on muscle glycogen utilization and exercise and performance. Med Sci Sports Exerc 16: 219–222.

Hargreaves M (1999). Metabolic responses to carbohydrate ingestion effects on exercise performance. In: Lamb DR, Murray R (eds). The Metabolic Basis of Performance in Exercise and Sport. Cooper Publ. Group, Carmel, U.S.A.

Hiller WDB (1989). Dehydration and hypoatremia during triathlons. Med Sci Sports Exerc 21: 219–221.

Hiller WDB, O'Toole ML, Massimino F, Hiller RE, Laird RJ (1985). Plasma electrolyte and glucose changes during the Hawaiian Ironman triathlon. Med Sci Sports Exerc 17: 219–221.

Holtmeier HJ (1995). Gesunde Ernährung von Kindern und Jugendlichen. 3rd edition, Springer, Berlin.

Horowitz JF, Mora-Rodriges R, Byerley LO, Coyle EF (1997). Lipolytic suppression following carbohydrate ingestion limits fat oxidation during exercise. Am J Physiol 273: 768–775.

Hottenrott K, Sommer HM (2001). Aktivierung des Fettstoffwechsels in Abhängigkeit von Nahrungskarenz, Kohlenhydratkost und Ausdauerleistungsfähigkeit. Dtsch Z Sportmed 52 (Sonderheft): 7–8.

Ivy JL, Miller W, Dover V, Goodyear LG, Sherman WH, Williams H (1983). Endurance improved by ingestion of a glucose polymer supplement. Med Sci Sports Exerc 15: 466–471.

Jentjens RLG, Moseley L, Waring RM, Harding LK, Jeukendrup AE (2004). Oxidation of combined ingestion of glucose and fructose during exercise. J Appl Physiol 96: 1277–1284.

Jeukendrup A, Gleeson M (2004). Sport Nutrition. Human Kinetics, Champaign, IL.

Johnson NA, Stannard SR, Mehalski K, Trenell MI, SachinwallaT, Thompson CH, Thompson MW (2003). Intramyocellular triacylglycerol in prolonged cycling with high-and-low-carbohydrate availability. J Appl Physiol 94: 1365–1372.

Knechtle B, Enggist A, Jehle T (2005). Energy turnover at the Race Across America (RAAM) – a case report. Int J Sports Med 26: 499–503.

Koller A, Mair J, Schobersgerger W, Wohlfarter TH, Haid CH, Mayr M, Villinger B, Frey W, Puschendorf B (1998). Effects of prolonged strenuous endurance exercise on plasma myosin heavy chain fragments and other muscular proteins. J Sports Med Phys Fitness 38: 10–17.

Konopka P (2001): Sporternährung. 8th edition. BLV-Verlag, Munich.

Levine L, Evans WJ, Caderette BS, Fisher EC, Bullen BA (1983). Fructose and glucose ingestion and muscle glycogen use during submaximal exercise. J Appl Physiol 55: 1767–1771.

References

Lucà-Moretti M, Grandi A, Lucà E, Mariani E, Vender G, Arigotti E, Ferrario M, Rovelli E (2003). Comparative results between two groups of track and field athletes with or without the use of Master Amino Acids Pattern as protein substitute. Adv Ther 4: 195–202.

Marmy-Conus N, Fabris S, Proietto J, Hargreaves M (1996). Pre-exercise glucose ingestion and glucose kinetics during exercise. J Appl Physiol 82: 853–857.

Matkovic V, Heaney RP (1992). Calcium balance during human growth; evidence for threshold behavior. Am J Clin Nutr 55: 992–996.

Neumann G (2003). Ernährung im Sport. Meyer & Meyer Verlag, Aachen.

Neumann G, Pöhlandt R (1994). Einfluss von Kohlenhydraten während Ergometerausdauerleistung auf die Fahrzeit. Schriftenreihe Angewandte Trainingswissenschaft. IAT Leipzig 1: 7–26.

Noakes TD (1992). The hyponatremia of exercise. Int J Sports Nutr 2: 205–228.

Parry-Billings M, Budgett R, Koutedakis Y, Blomstrand E, Brooks S, Williams C, Calder PCPilling S, Baigrie R, Newsholme EA(1992). Amino acid concentration in the overstraining syndrome: possible effects on the immune system. Med Sci Sport Exerc 24: 1353–1358.

Prou E, Margaritis I, Tessier F, Marini JF (1996). Effects of strenuous exercise on serum myosin heavy chain fragments in male triathletes. J Sports Med 17: 255–276.

Rennie MJ, Tripton KD (2000). Protein and amino acid metabolism during and after exercise and the effects of nutrition. Annual Review Nutrition 20: 457–483.

Sherman WM, Costill DL, Fink WJ, Hageman FC, Armstron LW, Muray TF (1983). Effect of 42.2 km footrace and subsequent rest or exercise on muscle glycogen and enzymes. J Appl Physiol 55: 1219–1224.

Tokmakidis SP, Volakis KA (2000). Pre-exercise glucose ingestion at different time periods and blood glucose concentration during exercise. Int J Sports Med 21: 453–457.

Wright DA, Sherman WM, Dernbach AR (1991). Carbohydrate feedings before, during, or in combination improve cycling endurance performance. J Appl Physiol 71: 1082–1088.

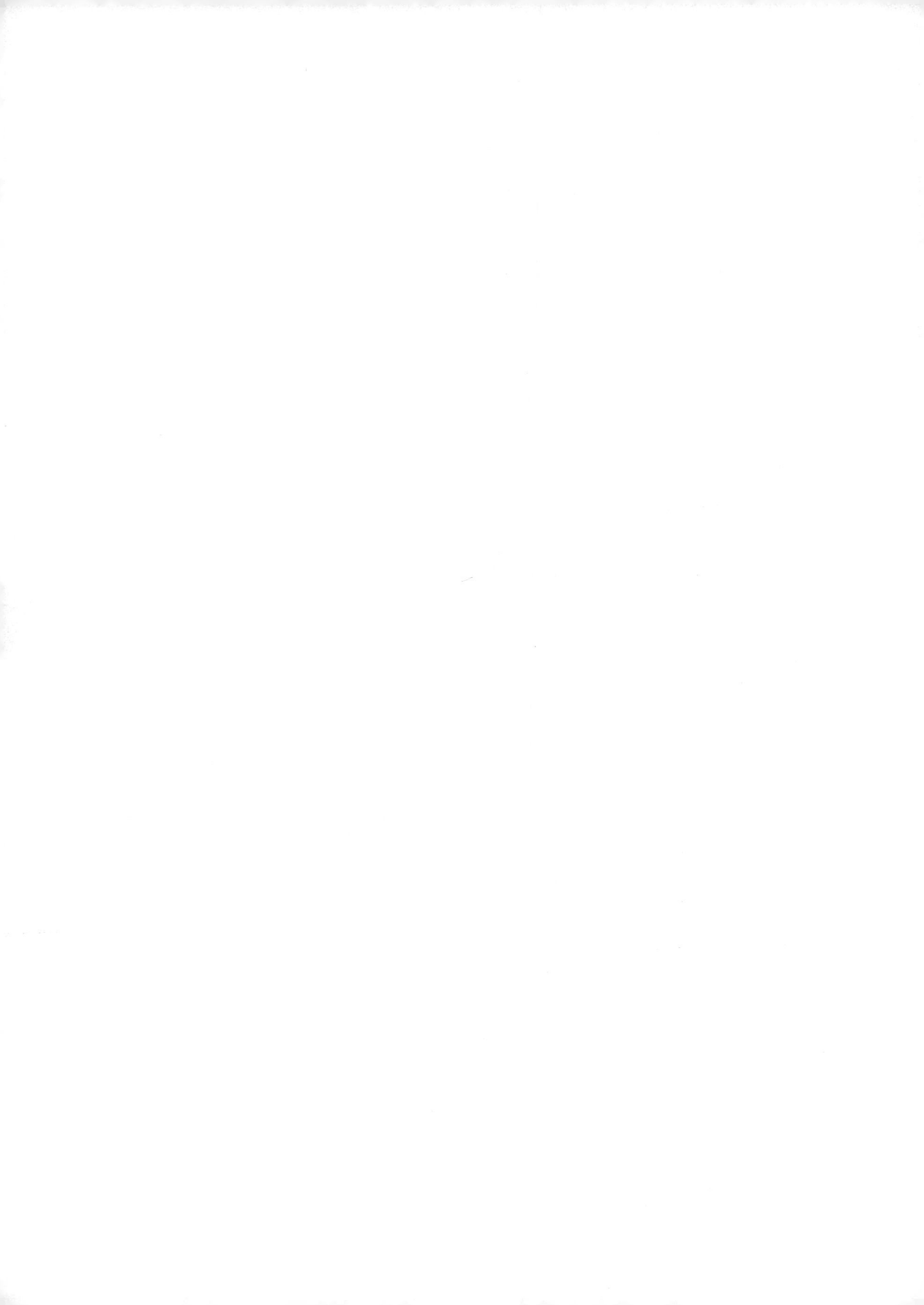

Sportswear

Gregor Deitmer and Andreas Gösele

88.1 Introduction

Modern functional textiles allow athletes to practice their sports under multiple conditions with a maximum of comfort in order to achieve the best performances as possible.

The effective support of the own body thermo regulation is hereby the most important attribute of functional clothing. That demands diverse qualities of the textiles, dependent on the kind of impact, its intensity and the dominant environmental conditions.

Under cold a fast evacuation of sweat from the skin is desirable. Under heat the sweat is only able to cool the body effectively, if it vaporizes on a surface as large as possible.

For an optimal functionality the choice of the right textiles is extremely important. Every athlete should be informed about the basic properties of the different materials and clothing concepts in order to be able to find the best adopted clothing for his/her demands.

Another important function of sport textiles beside thermoregulation is the protection against environmental influences such as cold, heat, humidity, wind and UV-radiation.

Today, via the adoption of special membranes or a specific configuration of tissue fibres protective attributes can be integrated into breathable and functional textiles without problems.

Dependent on the kind of sports, the clothing can be equipped with supplementary elements such as compression materials or supporting padding elements and can in this way even offer protection against bodily injuries. Such clothing is used e.g. in mountain biking, motocross or in different team sports.

By particular coating of fibres or the integration of specific materials into the fibres the textiles can get various properties. Antibacterial properties can be usefully applied in textiles that are difficult to clean such as professional swimsuits, shoes or functional underwear and socks. UV-absorbing or -reflecting materials allow a high UV-protection even for light summer wear.

The compression clothing represents an own class of sportswear. In professional as well as in leisure sports it enjoys increasing popularity. The spectrum of application reaches from compression socks for running (Berry et al., 1987, Chatard et al., 2004, Ali et al., 2007, Kemmler et al., 2009) up to full body combinations for cycling, triathlon and team sports (Duffield; Portus, 2007, Scanlan et al., 2008)

In the future we will see in which way „intelligent materials" will adapt to changing demands and in which way „wearable technologies" will find their way into our sportswear. Adaptive materials are able to accomplish their function fast and reversibly. They integrate mechanical, electronic, optical and chemical characteristics on a microscopical level.

With these advanced materials jackets will be developed that improve their isolating properties independently with decreasing temperatures or functional shirts that emit cooling substances according to temperature or transpiration. Even electric circuits or sensors for measuring heart rates e.g. can be integrated directly into textiles.

88.2 Thermoregulation

The metabolic activities of our body depend on a stable core temperature. The production of heat amounts to about 75% of the energy expenditure so that large amounts of heat have to be released under physical impact. Only by this way, a constant core temperature of the body of about 37–40°C [98.6–104 F] can be assured.

The heat is transported to the body surface via the blood circulation and there it is released primarily via the evaporation of sweat (Armstrong; Maresch, 1989). Further procedures of heat release such as heat conduction, heat convection or heat radiation do not play an important role under physical impact (Fortney; Vroman, 1985). For the heat release a mostly high temperature gradient between the inner body and the surface and between the corporal surface and the environment is indispensable. The environmental temperature, the air humidity, the wind speed and the temperature of the skin determine the degree of delivery of heat. The temperature of the skin depends essentially on the temperature of the environment whereas the core temperature of the body is primarily influenced by the intensity of the impact.

The clothing can influence the bodily thermoregulation decisively as it influences directly the heat exchange with the environment (Gleeson, 2009). That is why each sportswear should possess two properties regardless of whether it is destined for the comfort orientated or for the competitive athlete: a high breathing activity that supports optimally the heat and humidity exchange and good redrying abilities to avoid the cooling of the body after physical exercise. Furthermore isolating properties play a major role in cold weather.

Transfer of heat to and from the environment:

- **Conduction:** transfer of heat from one solid material to another through direct molecular contact
- **Convection:** transfer of heat by the motion of gas or liquid across the heated surface
- **Radiation:** heat transfer by infrared rays (primary method of heat release in the resting body)
- **Evaporation:** heat transfer by fluid evaporation (primary way of heat dissipation during exercise)

88.2.1 Heat

If the temperature gradient between the body surface and the environment decreases because the heat transport is hindered, the result will be an overheating. If the core body temperature increases from normally 37–39 °C [98.6–102.2 F], the result will automatically be a mental and physical loss of efficiency (Hargreaves; Febbraio, 1989).

Sweating is the most important factor of the thermal regulation under heat. The sweat vaporizes and evaporating cooling develops on the skin. By this procedure the temperature gradient between body core temperature and surface is maintained actively.

For the permanent functioning of evaporation a gradient of the water saturation of the air is essential as well. That means the water vapor must be able to escape from the body surface with the help of breathable materials.

Beside high heat, high humidity is one of the most frequent causes of a heat exhaustion in sports because the gradient of water vapor is diminished accordingly.

The loss of liquids under physical exercise caused by heat is enormous. Dependent on the intensity up to three liters of water per hour can be lost. At 20 °C [68 F] of environmental temperature there is only a loss of about 0.5 to 1 liter. Under impact the heart rate increases proportionally to the loss of liquid and the increase of the core temperature of the body. Per liter of liquid loss an increase of the heart rate of about eight beats per minute can be supposed. This fact points up the supplementary stress of the liquid loss caused by heat on the cardiovascular system and the thermoregulation.

Besides an adequate supply of liquid the exercise intensity in training has to be reduced accordingly.

88.2.2 Cold

Hypothermia will occur if the core temperature of the body decreases to under 35 °C [95 F]. It sprouts with a negative heat balance, if the loss of heat is bigger than the heat production.

The most frequent causes are insufficiently isolating or not windproof clothing. The mecha-

88.4 Properties of Sportswear

Tab. 88.1 Wind-chill equivalent temperature chart.

Wind speed (km/h)	Air temperature (°C)		
	−10	−15	−20
5	−13	−19	−24
10	−15	−21	−27
15	−17	−23	−29
20	−18	−24	−30
25	−19	−25	−32
30	−20	−26	−33

nism leading to a cooling of the body is simple. During the resting state a thin isolating layer out of warmed-up air or water is formed round about the body. If this layer is broken, there will be an accelerated delivery of heat because the temperature gradient between the skin and the environment increases. Wind can bring the body to cooling (wind-chill) as well as water that leads heat 25times better than air. That is why swimmers are particularly endangered by undercooling (Wade; Venghte, 1977).

88.3 Post exercise chill

A „post-exercise chill" is the cooling of the body after training. During the physical impact only a part of the humidity is transported to the environing air. The humidity in the close to the body layers continues to evaporate in the rest phase and cools the skin although a further cooling is no longer necessary.

As to the after-cooling effects synthetic materials represent clear advantages in comparison to cotton ones. In contrast to materials such as cotton, wool and viscose they only have a drying time of some minutes because they store much less humidity.

The classic cotton, once sweated, remains humid for at least half an hour. That is why it is no longer used in functional underwear.

88.4 Properties of Sportswear

Modern sports textiles are based on a layer principle. We differentiate between three layers with each one posessing different properties. The so-called first layer regulates the climate on the skin and is characterized by a high breathing activity. The second layer possesses particularly isolating properties and certain thermal properties of the clothing. The third layer is the most exterior one and appoints the protective properties of the clothing.

The three layers can be arranged by particular pieces of clothing and therewith adapted individually. One possibility e.g. would be the combination of functional underwear, a fleece-shirt and a windbreaker offering as such a maximum of flexibility. However, the three layers can also be integrated in one single piece of clothing such as a functional jacket. Therefore membranes are used that are breathable and at the same time wind- and waterproof. GoreTex^{TM} made these membranes popular in the early eighties. The membranes are connected to a laminate by a medium material. For a three-layer laminate the membranes are inserted between the top cloth and the lining fabric. As all three layers are connected tightly one to each other, the membrane is protected against friction. So the three-layer laminate is very tough and robust.

88.4.1 First Layer – Breathing activity

The clothing parts of the comfort layer (first layer) are cut close to the body, they have a direct contact with the skin and transport the sweat quickly in order to keep the body dry or they contribute actively to the dispersion of the sweat so that it can vaporize on a surface as large as possible.

In which extent a material supports the evaporation cooling on the skin depends on its properties related to the water affinity.

Generally we differentiate between hydrophobic, hydrophilic and hygroscopic materials. Underwear out of a hydrophilic material such as polypropylene e.g. extracts only little energy and heat out of the body. The fibers do not imbibe any humidity, but transfer it immediately to an absorbing layer afar from the skin. That is why it is suited for winter sports e.g. where a dry and warm climate on the skin is desirable to protect against cooling.

A hydrophilic material such as polyester is able to store sweat on the surface. The sweat is kept near the skin where it then evaporates. The evaporation coldness is able to extract large quantities of heat out of the body. In this case the athlete's core temperature of the body increases less quickly than with a product out of hydrophobic material. A high cooling capacity is demanded above all in summers with warm temperatures or with indoor-sports.

A good anatomic fit is typical for the first-layer clothing. A tight fitting to the skin is a pre-condition for the above mentioned functional properties and should be considered in the selection.

88.4.2 Second Layer – Isolation

The isolating layer (second layer) stores the heat of the body and transfers humidity outwards at the same time. With deep temperatures a good isolation is important. As immobile air is the best heat insulator, textiles are recommended which imbed much air. Fabrics with technical fibers and voluminous materials with a high capacity of air storage characterize these products. Alternatively insulating coatings on the fabrics such as kevlar can be used as even thinner, tight fitting clothing such as compression clothing can be insulated effectively.

With warm environmental temperatures in summer, the isolation has to be as little as possible. The material should dispose of good heat conductivity and the transfer of water vapor has to be highly efficient. The MVTR-value is a measure for breathing activity. It indicates the quantity of water evaporating in one square meter of fabric within 24 hours. Very good values are more than $10.000 \text{ g/m}^2/24\text{h}$.

88.4.3 Third Layer – Protection

The third layer is the outward protection layer that has to support the humidity transfer of the two other layers outward and to hinder the infiltration of water and wind. Membranes, laminates and microporous coatings are applied here.

Basically there exist two kinds of membranes: The microporous and the poreless ones, hydrophilic membranes. Microporous membranes such as GoreTex™ are 10 to 25 micrometres thin and are out of polytetrafluorethylene (PTFE), a material that frying pan coverings are also made of. The pores of the membranes are such small that even tiniest rain drops cannot go through. However, steam molecules can pass off them unhindered. By this they become breathable.

Hydrophilic membranes do not possess any pores. The body sweat in form of steam molecules is attracted actively by the material of the membranes and diffuses through them. In combination with hydrophobic fibers results an excellent humidity transport.

Dependent on the range of application materials with different water tightness come into use. That is why it is important for the selection to watch the degree of water tightness. The water head measures the degree of water tightness. It determines the point of compression, measured in millimeters, where the material begins to let pass water. Following the DIN standard a fabric between 400 mm and 1,300 mm is hold as hydrophobic and from 1,300 mm on as waterproof. As compressive stress by sitting or kneeling already causes decisively higher compression, most producers of functional clothing only define a material as waterproof from a water head of 10,000 mm.

88.5 Special applications – Compression clothing

The principle of gradual compression is at the base of good compression clothing. An improved performance by compression wear can be explained by an improved peripheral tissue perfusion and an increased venous backflow. The pressure on the skin causes a decrease of the vessel diameter in the superficial venous system. A pressure of 15mHG at the lower extremities leads to a reduction of about 20% already (Litter,1952). The result is a volume deferral of the blood into the deep venous system (Meyerowitz; Nelson, 1942, Stanton et al., 1949). A further result is the mechanical functional improvement of the venous valve and –

by this – a higher venous backflow (Bergan; Sparks, 2000). In persevering performances this volume shift increases the O_2 disposal in the capillary bed of the musculature (Gandhi et al., 1984, Lawrence; Kakar, 1980). The increased O_2-offer might lead to a heightening of the oxidation of lactate and thereby to a decelerated exhaustion of the musculature.

Until now it has not been possible to prove definitely the evidence of a positive impact on the lactate metabolism and of a factually improved performance.

The results of the studies concerning compression wear are partly contradictory and are discussed controversially.

Tight fitting compression wear has found its way especially to competitive and amateur athletes in persevering sports such as middle-distance and long-distance running and triathlon. Users estimate above all the wearing comfort and a subjectively accelerated regeneration of the musculature.

Athletes from diverse kinds of sports report a significant decrease of injuries when using compression wear. This applies particularly for team sports such as football, handball and rugby. That is why compression wear is employed widespread in professional sports.

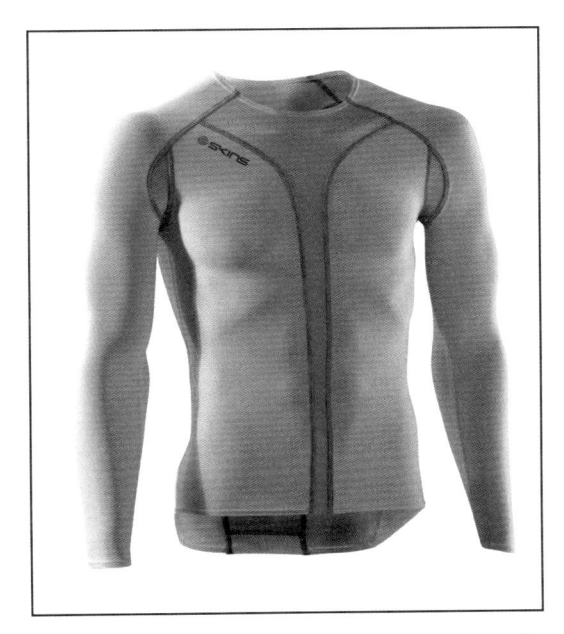

Fig. 88.1 Functional compression shirt (source: Skins™)

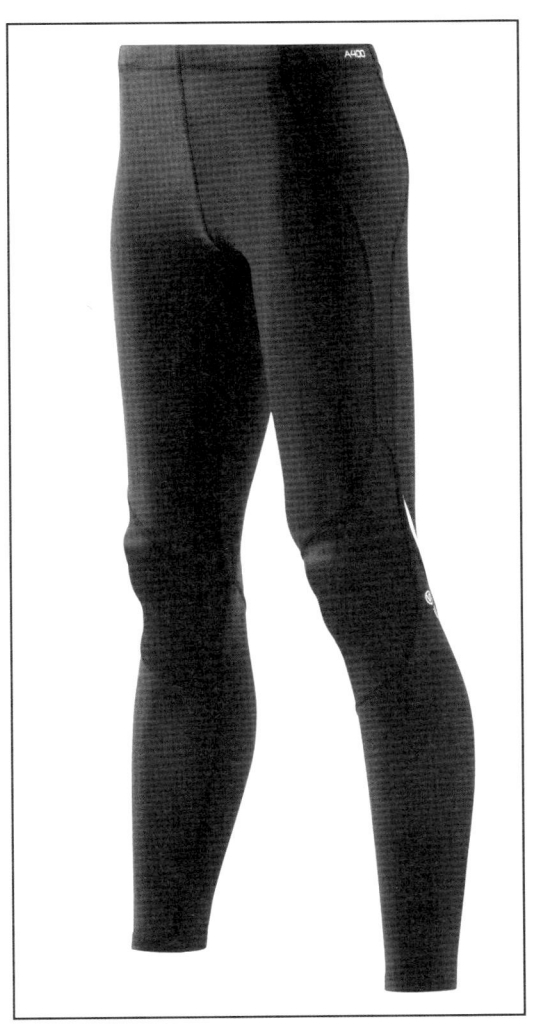

Fig. 88.2 Compression tight witch gradual compression (source: Skins™)

88.6 Care

For the cleaning of functional wear the use of special cleaning agents is recommended.

Fabric softeners and brighteners, which can be contained in conventional detergents, are stored on the fibers and limit their functional properties. It is also important that no detergent residues remain on the fabric because they have a hygroscopic effect. A supplementary rinse cycle will help. However, only cleaning is not sufficient for functional wear, especially for weather protecting clothing, to conserve its function in the long term. Chemical preparations of the fibres use them up with the time by wearing, by washing or also by the UV-radiation. The functional properties are reduced by the time. That is particularly the case for hydrophobic equipments, but also for hydrophilic materials, e.g. in functional underwear.

The better water rolls off the surface of a material the higher are its breathable properties.

If the outer cloth of a jacket absorbs water, the partial pressure gradient decreases and the breathing activity may be reduced drastically. There will be a condensation of water vapor in the inside of the jacket and wetness will develop. If the outer cloth absorbs water, more cold will penetrate from outward to inward.

The more a textile has lost its hydrophobic efficiency, the more difficult it will be to re-establish it. That is why a re-impregnation should be started in time.

Impregnations for textiles can be sprayed or a liquid additive can be used (wash-in). The disadvantage of the wash-in is that the hydrophilically treated inner layers will also be impregnated and this will have a negative effect on their function.

Certain impregnations can be reactivated by a heat treatment in the laundry dryer or by ironing with low temperatures. In this context the recommendations of the producers must be respected.

References

Ali A, Caine MP, Snow BG (2007). Graduated compression stockings: physiological and perceptual responses during and after exercise. J Sports Sci 25: 413–419.

Armstrong LE, Maresh CM (1998). Effects of training, environment, and host factors on the sweating response to exercise. Int J Sports Med. 19 Suppl 2: S103–S105.

Bergan J, Sparks SR (2000). Non-elastic compression: an alternative in management of chronic venous insufficiency. J Wound Ostomy. Cont Nurs 27: 83–89.

Berry MJ, McMurray RG (1987). Effects of graduated compression stockings on blood lactate following an exhaustive bout of exercise. Am J Phys Med 66: 121–132.

Chatard JC, Atlaoui D, Farjanel J, Louisy F, Rastel D, Guezennec CY (2004). Elastic stockings, performance and leg pain recovery in 63-year-old sportsmen. Eur J Appl Physiol 93: 347–352.

Duffield R, Portus M (2007). Comparison of three types of full-body compression garments on throwing and repeat-sprint performance in cricket players. Br J Sports Med 41: 409–414.

Fortney SM, Vroman NB (1985). Exercise, performance and temperature control: temperature regulation during exercise and implications for sports performance and training. Sports Med. 2(1): 8–20.

Gandhi DB, Palmar JR, Lewis B, Schraibman IG (1984). Clinical comparison of elastic supports for venous diseases of the lower limb. Postgrad Med J 60: 349–352.

Gleeson M (1988). Temperature regulation during exercise. Int J Sports Med 19 Suppl 2: S96–S99.

Hargreaves M, Febbraio M (1998). Limits to exercise performance in the heat. Int J Sports Med 19 Suppl 2: S115–S116.

Kemmler W, von Stengel S, Kockritz C, Mayhew J, Wassermann A, Zapf J (2009). Effect of compression stockings on running performance in men runners. J Strength Cond Res 23: 101–105.

Lawrence D, Kakkar VV (1980). Graduated, static, external compression of the lower limb: a physiological assessment. Br J Surg 67: 119–121.

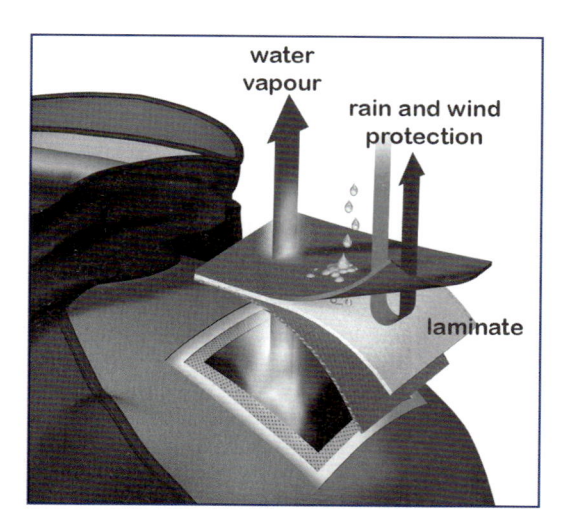

Fig. 88.3 Three-layer laminate providing breathability, water resistance and wind protection (source: Gore-Tex™, modified by the authors).

References

Litter J (1952). Thromboembolism; its prophylaxis and medical treatment; recent advances. Med Clin North Am 36: 1309–1321.

Meyerowitz BR, Nelson R (1964). Measurement of the velocity of blood in lower limb veins with and without compression. Surgery 56: 481–486.

Scanlan AT, Dascombe BJ, Reaburn PR, Osborne M (2008). The effects of wearing lower body compression garments during endurance cycling. Int J Sports Physiol Perform 3: 424–438.

Stanton JR, Freis ED, Wilkins RW (1949). The acceleration of linear flow in the deep veins of the lower extremity of man by local compression. J Clin Invest 28: 553–558.

Wade CE, Veghte JH (1977). Thermographic evaluation of the relative heat loss by area in man after swimming. Aviat Space Environ Med 48(1): 16–18.

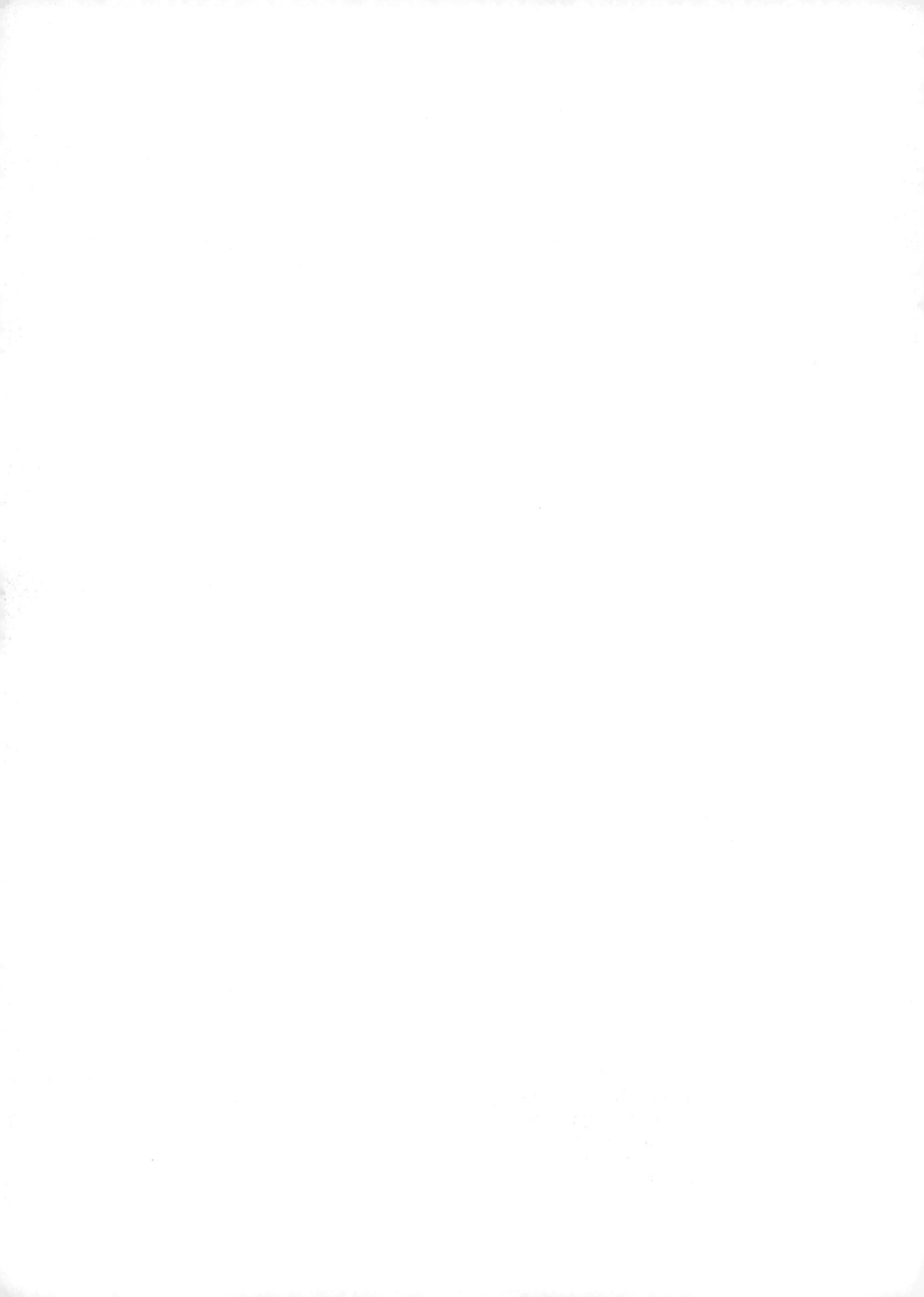

Athletic Footwear

Andreas Gösele, Hardy Hüttemann and
Gerd-Peter Brüggemann

89.1 Introduction

Athletic footwear comprises all kind of shoes or shoe-like equipment which is used in sports and physical activity by professional and non-professional athletes, by young and older subjects, by male and female athletes, by elite and novice performers, by frequently active athletes and occasional users in leisure sports. Movements executed in physical activities and sports such as running, jumping, cutting, skating, cycling or skiing and the corresponding forces acting on the athlete's body are widely different. At the same time the functional capacity of the biological structures of the users of athletic footwear vary extremely from strong tissue of the competitive athlete to low or even very low of the occasionally physical active. Therefore, sports and applications specific concepts and designs have been developed to meet the demands of functional footwear for specific activities, sports and the different customers.

Recently corresponding to the discussion on barefoot running or moving shoes have been designed to re-define the mechanical loading of the muscular skeletal system of the lower limb and to train skeletal muscles and increase proprioception. This novel idea to use the shoe as a training tool led to completely new footwear designs sometimes opposite to what manufacturers advertised for decades.

Due to the variety of footwear for the different applications this chapter will, instead of just listing the shoes or the shoe-like equipment, offer a concept structuring athletic footwear from a view of the major goals of the customer: injury prevention, performance enhancement and increasing the functional capacity of biological tissue or in other words training. The major technical features of athletic footwear in general will shortly be explained before the three categories will be elaborated using few representatives of specific sport shoes. Consequently this chapter will not present all kinds of shoes, which are used in the different sport disciplines. A selection of athletic footwear will explain the major features, concepts and technical solutions. Many special designs e.g. of long jump, shot put or rock climbing shoes can not even mentioned or listed.

89.2 From "Turnschuh" to technical athletic footwear

Due to the facts that running shoes have been widely used as training footwear in general and that the category running and training had the highest frequency of sales the focus in the technical development was mainly on technical running shoes. Athletic footwear in general evolved from the simple "shoe" into a high tech product. Since Wait Webster applied rubber to the sole of his shoe in 1832 and developed the first running shoe, the trainer or the running shoe industry has gone through various phases of development to help athletes achieve greater performance or to decrease the risk of injury. To date the major brands have invested a huge amount of money into research and marketing with the view to develop shoe that alter running mechanics, improve lower limb function and to reduce the frequency of injuries.

The development of running footwear has seen many changes, starting out as a basic plimsoll and advancing to shoes that claim to address impact forces, prevent excessive rearfoot motion, improve stability and increase performance. Remarkably the effects of cushioning in a shoe have not contributed to lower the peak ground reaction force or the resultant joint forces of the lower limb on impact; instead runners modify their running style to accommodate for the change in loads. However cushioning or midsole hardness is greatly associated with comfort and muscle function and is featured in most of running shoes. Motion control is a key characteristic for many shoes with brand specific features, all of which are designed to be supportive to the medial aspect of the shoe with duel density midsoles and altered midfoot support. The aim of this feature is to reduce excessive foot pronation and related tibial internal rotation at midstance with the goal to decrease the risk of overuse and injury. One should also note that running shoes need to be lightweight and breathable as the material content of the upper plays a key part in comfort of the shoe.

Such functional factors (comfort, performance and injury prevention) and also less-functional factors (e.g. price, fashion, and durability) have been relevant for the design of athletic footwear.

89.2.1 Athletic footwear categories

From the functional factors, the major applications and goals of athletic and the customers expectations shoes one can differentiate three principle categories of athletic footwear:

- Protection footwear (PF)
- Performance enhancement footwear (PEF)
- Training footwear (TF)

The prime goal of PF is to control and/or decrease the mechanical loading of the muscular skeletal system and the biological tissue during all kind of sport activities like running, jumping, or skiing in order to decrease the risk of injury. The most established concepts are cushioning or shock attenuation at impact, motion control or avoidance of excessive joint motion, and joint moment control or decrease of excessive joint torques.

Performance enhancement footwear (PEF) is designed to permit and/or increase sport performance. PEF offers the possibility the enhance performance. Such PEF shoes minimize loss of energy during performance (e.g. through minimum mass), store elastic energy and re-utilize this energy, and/or optimize muscle function by offering an optimum muscle length and velocity of the contractile elements. PEF shoes sometimes build the basis or the prerequisite to play the given sport e.g. like skiing or skating.

In opposite to protection or injury prevention footwear TF shoes are designed to increase the mechanical loading of biological tissue and the stimulus to the muscular-skeletal system to adapt. Such shoes increase instability by enlarging the lever arms of the ground reaction forces (e.g. by the height of the midsole; MBT) or increase the range of joint motion and the muscle work (e.g. Nike Free).

The selection of the appropriate shoe is strongly related on the demands of the user and the purpose of its use.

89.3 Components of sport shoes

Shoes build the interface between the human foot and the physical environment or abutment (e.g. the running track, the playing ground or the ski and its binding).

Casual and street footwear sport shoes contain two main pieces: The upper part (the "upper") and the lower part (the "base"), which contains the midsole and the outer sole. The upper consists usually of several layers that could be divided into inner, intermediate and outer upper. Furthermore, the upper integrates the heel cap and the toe box. The lower part the sole is divided into the insole or the sockliner, the midsole and the outer sole. The purpose of the upper is to ensure the positioning of the foot on the midsole which contains the mechanical properties of a functional shoe. Therefore the upper provides the prerequisite to couple the foot and the shoe and to allow force and torque transmission to the ground or the equipment (e.g. ski). The outer sole, the interface to the ground, ensures the force transmission to the abutment, gives the proper traction, and prevents slips.

The upper is built on the "last", the mechanical representative of the foot. The last defines the shape and the volume of the shoe. It should be noted that human feet vary considerably. Differences are reported from young to old, male and female but also within different ethical groups. To meet the large variations of the different foot shapes various manufacturers offer different models based on different lasts and also different widths. It is evident that the last is responsible for the fit of the shoe, which is a major factor for its functional capacity. Brand-specific characteristics such as "narrow" or "wide" lasts are known in the market and well recommended. Recently customized athletic footwear is not restricted to top athletes for which the individually manufactured last was used since decades. Modern 3D scanning technology (e.g. Infoot, Iware Inc.) creates a 3D model of the individual foot, compares this model with existing lasts, selects the best fitting last or mills an individual last. In the very next future such technologies and athletic footwear customization will be available not only for professional athletes but also for all users of sporting shoes. The individual last is undoubtedly the best solution for the fit of the shoe, which is the prime factor for the function of the shoe and its technical features.

The upper material: The choice of material depends on the sport, the purposed use and weather requirements. Therefore, the competition shoe of a marathon runner differs from a training shoe in design, weight, and material properties. In general, materials like nylon fabric, breathable membranes, leather, artificial leather, plastics, cords and rubber are used. The different areas of the shoe are adjusted to the sport-specific requirements. Therefore the toe box is larger in the running shoe whereas it is tiny in the climbing shoe. The locking systems also vary considerably. Classical lacing, buckles, straps, BOA-Systems or combinations of those different systems are available.

Soles: Insole or sockliner, midsole and outer soles can be identified in most of the athletic footwear. In some cases the midsole build the basis to attach cleats (in the soccer shoe) or spikes (in the sprint shoe) or include the attachments to the binding e.g. of a ski or to the runner of an ice skating boot. In some special shoes the outer layer of the upper and the midsole can hardly divided. In ski boots the upper and the sole build one solid part or in road cycling shoe only an insole and a midsole.

Insoles: Next to the last the insole is primarily responsible for the comfort. It should be removable, antibacterial, lightweight, thin, yet comfortable. Any medial support of the foot through the inner sole should only in the region under the sustentaculum tali. In special cases insoles should be replaced with custom-made, individual orthopaedic orthotics.

Midsole: The midsole forms the technical potential of a sport shoe. The midsole re-distributes the ground reaction forces and is therefore responsible for the plantar pressure under the foot. It modifies and controls the point of force application, has the capacity to modulate the force signal, contributes to shock attenuation and has the potential to dissipate energy. A midsole can store elastic energy and has the principal potential to return this energy to the foot. Depending on the application more or less elastic and damping materials are placed at different regions. Especially In the running shoe, the midsole is the core element of the shoe. Related to the application plastics (e.g. in ski boots) or polymers such as EVA (ethylene vinyl acetate) or PU (polyurethane) are used. The different materials and the geometry (e.g. heel area, flex grooves) determine the biomechanical properties (flexibility, shock attenuation, energy dissipation, energy storage and return, modulation of force signal from the ground, point of force application, lever arms of ground reaction forces to ankle and knee joint) of the shoes significantly.

Outer sole: As in all other areas, the outer sole depends on the application of the footwear. The major purpose of the outer sole is to provide sufficient friction in order to allow to transmit horizontal forces to the ground and to prevent slips. To meet this aim synthetic rubber is used in most technical solutions. In combination with different shapes the outer sole provides the required grip, allows controlled turns in pivot sports and has to withstand multiple and long tem use. Durability is an important feature for the outer sole. Rubber is heavy; therefore, todays outer sole does not fill the entire midsole. It is separated and only regions with contact to the ground are covered with outer sole material. In addition the outer sole should not decrease the functions and especially the flexibility of the midsole. Technically this goal is solved by separation and cuts.

89.3.1 Protection footwear

Protection footwear (PF) is focused on prevention of overload and injuries. Therefore in addition to protect the foot from heat or cold, from water or stones, from asphalt and broken glass PF should provide sufficient protection from excessive impact peak forces, excessive peak plantar pressure, excessive joint excursion at ankle and knee joints, excessive joint moments at knee and ankle joints in all planes of motion. Protection footwear is typically the running shoe which is used in long distance running with a high number off repetitive impact loadings and external force application of up to three times body weight which is related to internal joint loading at ankle and knee joints of five to six times body weight. The protection footwear concept has also been applied to shoes for long lasting activities in difficult physical environment like trekking or walking with moderate force application or to shoes designed for sports with high force application like basketball.

The running shoe is often used as basic or cross training shoe. It is the most frequent used shoe and the most sold footwear. Therefore the "running shoe" will be used as representative of protection footwear.

Running shoes: Significant changes can be identified in the design of running shoes since the introduction of the first special shoe for running. Many of these changes have been driven by the reports that, depending from the study, 37 to 56% of runners have been injured during the period of one year. Pre injuries, excessive training volume, training mistakes, but also excessive impact forces, excessive pronation or excessive knee joint moments (adduction-abduction moments, external rotation moments) have been proposed as major reasons for the development of overuse injuries. Footwear was assumed to influence impact forces, foot pronation and knee joint movements. This led to technical developments in which as a first modification, cushioning materials were used in the mid sole in order to reduce the impact forces. Bizarre sole sizes and shapes, high heel to forefoot ratio and wide outsoles characterized this attempt. As a consequence of these technical changes an increased instability at ankle and knee joint occurred and mechanical stress of the fore- and hind foot and subsequently of the ankle, knee and hip joints increased. In order to counteract the instability and the resulting medical concerns the concept of motion control was introduced into the development of athletic footwear design. One can observe that over the last twenty years the percentage of motion control shoes increased in the different footwear companies. However, results of more recent studies challenged the proposed association between skeletal alignment, foot pronation and running injuries. Remarkably the frequency of running related injuries did not change significantly in the last three decades during which the cushioning and motion control concepts built the guidelines in running shoe design. Even the injury distribution and location were not affected. One can conclude that the purely mechanical concept of impact cushioning and motion control by cushioning midsole devices and duo density midsole technology did not meet the expectations to decrease the risk of injuries. The skeleton changes its path of movement for a given task only minimally and non-systematic when exposed to a mechanical intervention. The locomotor system seems to choose a strategy to keep a minimal resistance movement path. An optimal or ap-

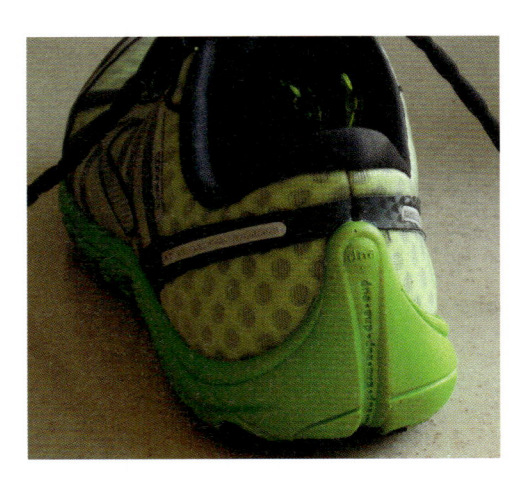

Fig. 89.1 Rounded heels to minimize lever arms.

Fig. 89.2 "Natural motion" footwear with minimum ground contact areas.

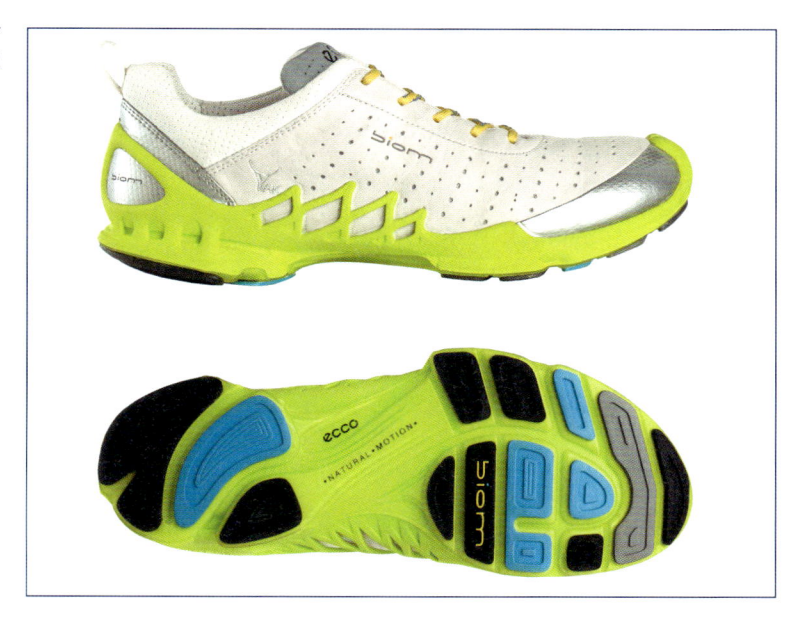

propriate shoe concept would affect muscle activity and muscle force potential rather than a mechanical support.

Novel running shoe concepts are based on the consideration to allow and support the natural and preferred joint's path of motion. The technical concept minimizes the lever arms of the external ground reaction force to the joints of the foot and the tibiotalar joint allowing relative segmental motions in all planes. Technical solutions of a minimization of lever arm of the ground reaction forces by sole geometry and material are shown in ➤ Figure 89.1.

In a controlled, randomized, intervention study with footwear designed on the preferred joint motion or natural motion concept (lower to ground, less heel lift, no stiff heel counter, higher torsional flexibility, rounded and asymmetric heel, elastic and non energy dissipating mid sole material, no medial support by duo density material, minimal ground contact area, mimicking barefoot ground contact) a re-definition of neuromuscular loading as well as a re-learning of running patterns was shown within six weeks of training using the novel footwear (➤ Fig. 89. 2). Runners decreased stride width and reduced the medio-lateral ground reaction forces in the early and midstance phase. The lever arm of the ground reaction forces to the ankle joint and the knee joint in the frontal plane was significantly reduced. Calcaneal eversion angular velocity decreased. The resupination during push off was clearly increased and showed a more barefoot like behaviour with the natural motion footwear. In the sagittal plane the lever arm of the ground reaction forces was reduced during initial plantar flexion and the ankle joint de-coupling was significantly decreased. This leads to a more stable ankle joint, an increased joint stiffness and consequently to a more efficient use of the potential of elastic energy storage and return of the muscle tendon units of plantar flexors in the stretch-shortening cycle. The stiffness of the knee joint is reduced with the natural motion concept, which is related to a decrease of axial knee joint loading. Knee adduction moments, which are strongly related to knee joint overuse and injuries are reduced in average of about 20% in the 6 weeks, experiment by wearing the natural motion footwear.

Modern running footwear has in comparison to the past a lower midsole, less cushioning material, less heel spring, less stiff heel counters and less medial support. It is characterized by rounded soft heels, separated lateral heel areas, less torsional stiffness, medio-lateral and longitudinal deep flex grooves separating the medial and the lateral rays and a wide forefoot base of support. Small lever arms to ankle and knee joints lead to a more natural joint loading and running patterns.

89.3.2 Performance enhancement footwear

Performance enhancement footwear (PEF) is designed to offer the potential to increase sport performance and/or to permit specifics sports transmitting forces and moments to apparatus or equipment with minimum loss of energy. PEF shoes compromise four major strategies that can be summarized as

- Minimum loss of energy during performance (e.g. through minimum mass of a racing flat),
- Storage and return of elastic energy (e.g. in a ski boot), and/or
- Optimization of muscle function by generating an optimum muscle length and velocity of the contractile elements (e.g. by a clap skate boot). And
- Transmission of forces and moment from the foot to the equipment and further on the ground.

The list of performance enhancement shoes is numerous and a complete list will contain summer and winter sports, team and individual sports, track and field sports. A few examples explain the variety:

Long distance running flats, sprint spike, middle distance spike, long jump shoes, high jump shoe, shot put shoes, javelin shoes, discus shoes, ski boots, snowboard boots, trekking shoes, hockey boots, ice skating boots, figure skating boots, short track boots, field hockey shoes, team handball shoes, cycling shoes.

As representatives the ski boot for alpine skiing and the cycling shoe have been chosen to explain the special demand, designs and technical features.

Cycling shoes: In cycling we differentiate three main shoes: road bike shoes, mountain bike shoes and casual or all round training shoes (➢ Fig. 89.3).

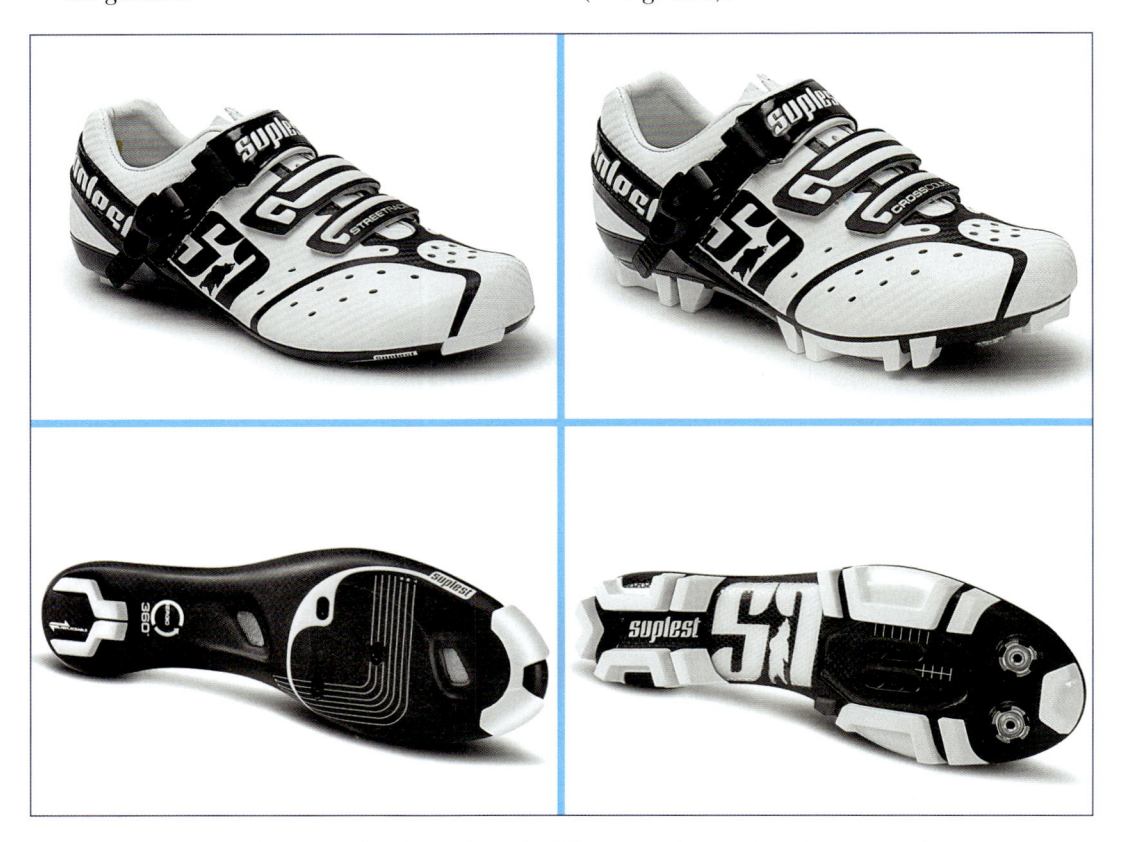

Fig. 89.3 Road Bike and Moutain Bike Shoes. The main difference is the outsole and the inserts for cleats.

Road bike shoes: The requirements of a modern road shoe are clear, simple and defined. The shoe must be light and stiff and the sole should be as thin as possible. The goal is to implement the muscle strength in pedal power without significant loss of energy. Of course, the shoe should fit well also, what is an important criterion for the choice of shoes. Especially in professional cycling with a training volume of quite 30,000–35,000 km per year fitting and comfort are important.

The heel to forefoot ratio can differ from manufacturer to manufacturer. The upper varies often and materials such as leather and nylon, as well as combinations thereof should apply. The closing systems vary from straps to buckles or combinations of both. Micro adjustable BOA-Systems are also very popular, even though they are often found in the top-of-the line models.

Mountain bike shoes: The requirements of a contemporary mountain bike shoes are similar to those of a racing shoe. In addition to the required attributes such as stiffness and weight, also a non-slip sole is demand. Especially in the alpine area with slide and carrying sections an adequate sole is important. Cleats in the toe area, similar to football boots, are also used, as well as reinforcement in the heel and ankle region.

Casual shoes: Casual shoes, or skateboarding shoes were used in downhill cycling. Here it would be too dangerous to use cleats, because off the high risk of accidents and the short re-action time. Instead big pedals and shoes with a good grip (normally used for skateboarding) were preferred.

Ski boots: For decades the most important demands to a ski boot were stiffness and transmission of forces through the binding to the skies. These demands are still important and the bases of a good ski boot, but other additional demands were added.

Nowadays a ski boot should be flexible, light and the sole should provide walking ability. Flexible areas in the midfoot region are introduced to increase the elastic module in this part of the shoe and also increasing the sensomotor interaction between the skier and the ski.

Skiing techniques changed since carving skies were introduced and also freeriding and back-

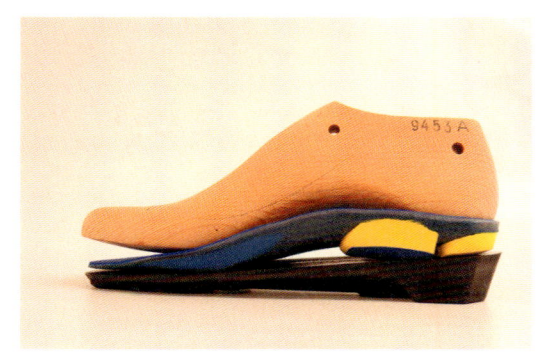

Fig. 89.4 Last, orthopedic insole and midsole for ski boots.

country skiing are very popular. The flex factor of a modern ski boot varies between 90 to 120 for freeriding and recreational skiing, however we find shoes with flex factors over 150 in professional ski racing.

A wide variety of brands and models are on the market. In addition the to different shoes, we have the possibility to adept every shoe individually if necessary by adding orthopedic insoles (➤ Fig. 89.4) and liners or even customize the whole boot. People with ankle, midfoot or toe problems no longer have sty away from skiing. A very important factor of modern skiing ist he adjustment of the boots shaft ankle, called canting adjustment. This allows the correction of varus or valgus axis of the legs leading to plain ski position on snow.

Comfort plays an important role especially in recreational skiing. Micro adjustable buckles as well as self molding liners provide a maximum of different possibilities to find a perfect mixture between fitting and force transmission.

In the future we will find even lighter, partly sensomotoric boots that will help us to enjoy skiing all day long.

89.3.3 Training footwear

In contrast to protection or injury prevention footwear, TF shoes are developed to increase the mechanical loading of biological tissue. With the controlled increase of mechanical loading the stimulus to the muscular-skeletal system increases and should lead to a morphological and/or functional adaptation. The so-called barefoot shoes are not elements of the PT category because they only cover the foot in order to protect it, they do not allow to move barefoot and they do not provide any technical feature to increase the mechanical tissue loading. PT shoes are designed on two strategies: (1) Increase of instability by decreasing the base of support and by increasing the lever arms of the ground reaction forces and (2) increase of the range of joint motion and related muscle work. Representative of the first strategy is the MBT (Masai Barefoot Technology). As most recommended representative of the second strategy the Nike Free is chosen.

MBT: Through the extreme height of the midsole the lever arm of the ground reaction forces to the ankle and knee joints and the related lateral instability increase significantly (➤ Fig. 89.5). The rounded midsole leads to a minimization of the base of support in the sagittal plane and therefore an increasing demand to the stabilizing and balancing muscles. Standing on a MBT shoe is comparable to wobbling board training. As expected the use of MBT leads to a significant increase in the balancing capacity and a higher activation of extensor and flexor muscles during walking. If the increase of mechanical loading of the muscle tendon units is sufficient to strengthen muscle or adapt volume is not yet reported.

Nike Free: The so-called minimal shoe mimics barefoot walking and running on grass and was designed to increase neuro-muscular loading of the intrinsic and extrinsic foot and shank muscle. The shoe is built on an anatomical last which contains an anatomical plantar surface representing the plantar foot surface. The midsole of the shoe is flat and consists of a series of flexible connected platforms. The shoe allows unrestricted movements (➤ Fig. 89.6) of the metatarsal phalangeal joints in flexion and extension. It was scientifically shown in a longitudinal study that using the Nike Free for five months muscle strength and even muscle volumes of the foot muscle increase significantly. A reduction in recovery time after plantar fasciitis has already been reported.

89.4 Concluding remarks

Athletic footwear is designed for different applications and goal. Different sports and related movement generate different demands to

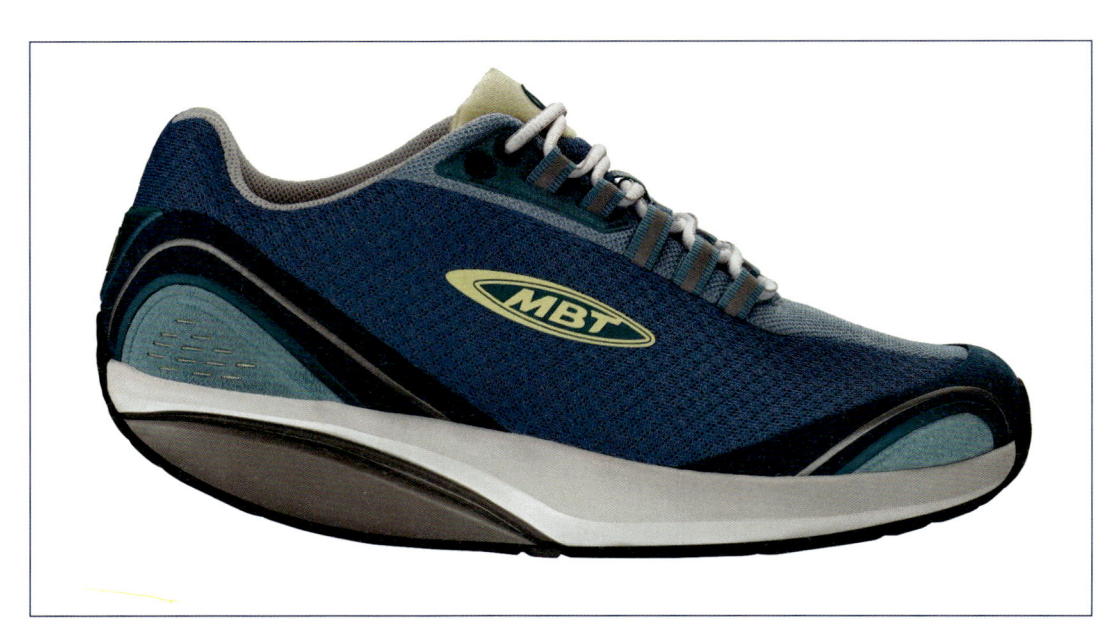

Fig. 89.5 MBT with high and rounded midsole.

Fig. 89.6 Nike Free: Shoe and sole with maximal flexibility.

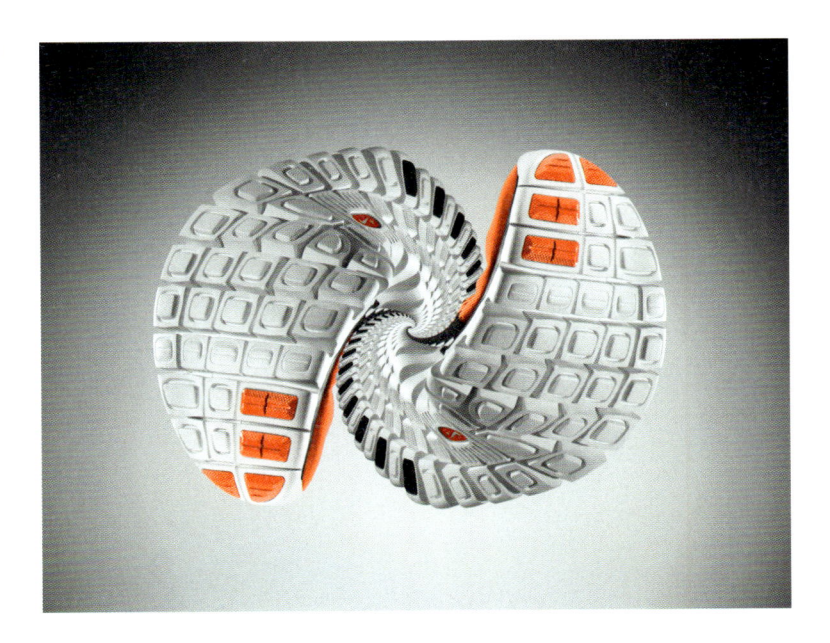

the footwear. We propose to differentiate between (1) protection footwear (PF), (2) performance enhancement footwear (PEF) and (3) training footwear (TF). There is some overlapping between these categories but mixing up the aims of shoes and create an overall solution is a contradiction per se. PF has to decrease mechanical loading while TF increase load, stress and strain of the biological structures. PEF approaches the enhancement of performance, increase the kinetic energy and the general mechanical loading. Such footwear should consider some aspects of loading control and decrease if this is not related to performance enhancement.

The customer and his or her consultant have to decide for which purpose in which sport under which circumstances he or she wants to use the footwear. After such decision one can identify the proper technical solution.

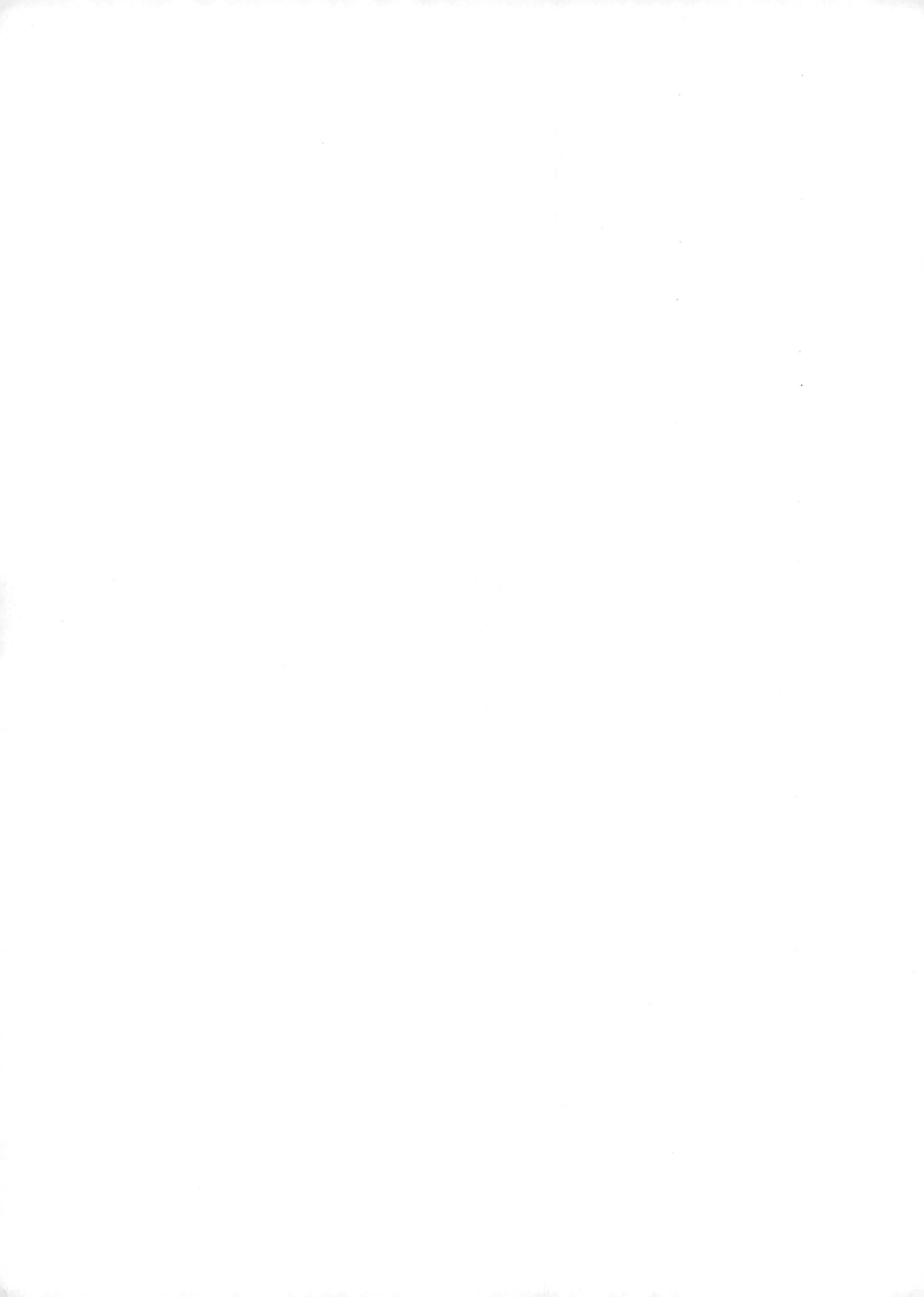

Chapter 90 Ortheses

Rolf Haaker

In sport ortheses can be used for prophylaxis and also for therapy. They have a **long tradition** as orthopedic treatment with the aspect of splinting being in the foreground first. Amédée Bonnet (1809–1858) described an orthesis as a treatment of knee instability, which had been inserted distally into a shoe and had been equipped with two stiffening girders, a central joint and three fixation straps, for the first time in his book "Traité dé thérapeutiqué des maladies articulaires" in 1853 (Bonnet 1853, Pässler 1993, quoted from Grifka).

The **negative effect of immobilization** – not only to the osseous skeleton and the musculature, but also to the tendons and ligaments – is no problem anymore nowadays. The significance of **proprioception** for the muscular protection of the joint becomes more and more obvious. Jerosch has demonstrated the improvement of proprioception by different ortheses in several studies (Jerosch et al. 1997, Jerosch and Porten 2000, Jerosch and Schoppe 2000).

Diverse ortheses can be implemented in sports. **Knee and ankle joint ortheses** are naturally in the foreground of interest because of their importance. The ones that are used in sports are to be treated here in the order of frequency of their application. There will be neither a claim to completeness of this not even remotely comprehensible multitude of ortheses, nor shall the indications of their use be understood as "mere recipe". The scientific principles – as far as known – shall be demonstrated as comprehensively as possible, so that each prescriber will be able to develop a personal strategy for their application.

90.1 Ankle joint ortheses

The most common injury in sports is the **sprain of the upper ankle joint** with facultative laceration of the external ligament apparatus, the syndesmosis or even the deltoid ligament. Ankle joint bandages have gained very high significance within the last 10–15 years, because **fibular ligament ruptures** are mostly treated conservatively nowadays. Ankle joint ortheses appropriate for the **direct posttraumatic phase** are distinguished from ankle joint bandages that are **rather used in the further process** of the treatment of ankle joint injuries.

90.1.1 Ankle-joint ortheses for the immediate post-traumatic use

An extensive **prevention of pronation and supination movements** in the ankle joint must be demaded of these ankle joint ortheses. A group of brace strap systems and a group that binds the foot joint region in a planar mode by textile material exist. The **dorsal and plantar flexion** in the ankle joint is to be influenced only marginally. A padding of the splint individually adapted to the situation has to be taken care of because of the **varying conditions of swelling**. The **aircast splint** (➢ Fig. 90.1) with its lateral air chambers for the individual filling with air via a valve gear has proved successful in current years.

The implementation of a similar product – called **airloc splint** – has recently increased (➢ Fig. 90.2). The inflexible **connection part of the sole** of the aircast splint and the flexible one of the airloc splint form the difference between these two splints that both provide the option of individual filling of the ankle chambers with air. The wearing of these splints is limited to the use in **sport shoes**.

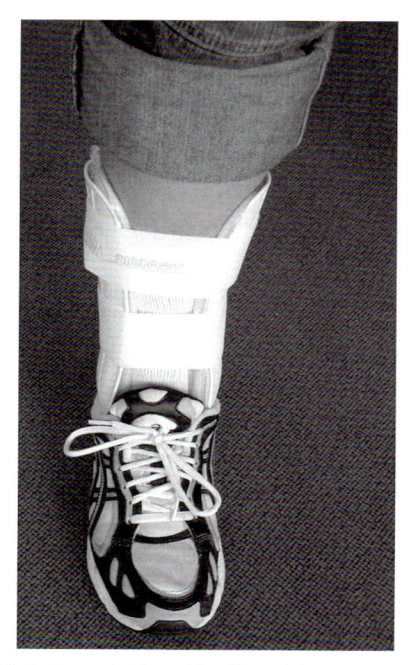

Fig. 90.1 Example for a U-splint with presentation of the spatial requirement in sports shoes. Here: aircast splint.

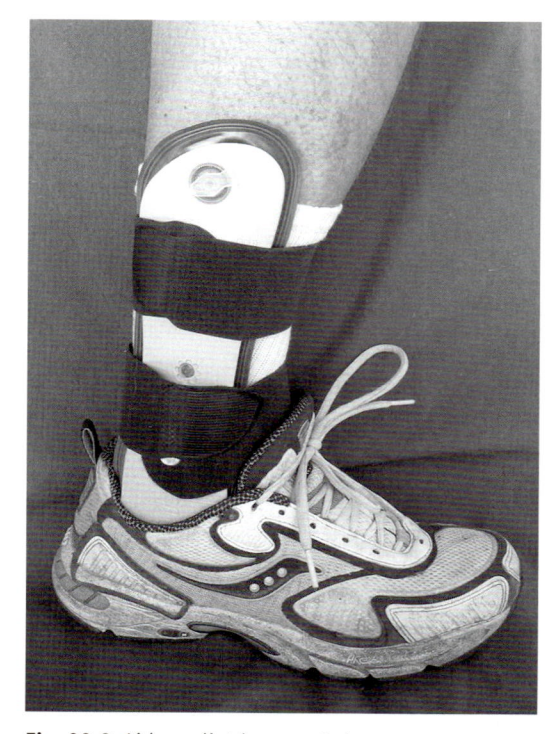

Fig. 90.2 Airloc splint in a sport shoe.

90.1.2 Ankle-joint ortheses for the sub-acute post-traumatic use

There are multiple ankle joint ortheses with different Velcro and semi-shell constructions for the stabilization of the upper ankle joint and the use in the further posttraumatic phase **after the detumescence** of the joint. The **Malleoloc orthesis** has been used for a long time (➢ Fig. 90.3). It is characterized by a very small design, so that it can be worn easily in every sport shoe and even in **ready-to-wear shoes** (Hoffmann et al. 1987, Zwipp et al. 1994).

All ortheses of this type are also applicable for the **prophylaxis** of ankle joint injuries. Critical as well as positive reports about this application have been published within the last 10 years. Thus, the prophylactic application of the Mikros bandages in the 1980s and 1990s in U.S. basketball had been widely spread. However, the frequency of ankle joint injuries while wearing these bandages for prophylaxis has been higher than in relinquishing them – according to publications of the insurance companies.

Especially Jerosch and his colleagues could prove in German literature that the proprioception in the upper ankle joint is even improved by the wearing of an ankle joint bandage.

> Prophylactic tape bandage or the wearing of an orthesis suitable for sports is recommended for chronic ankle joint instabilities.

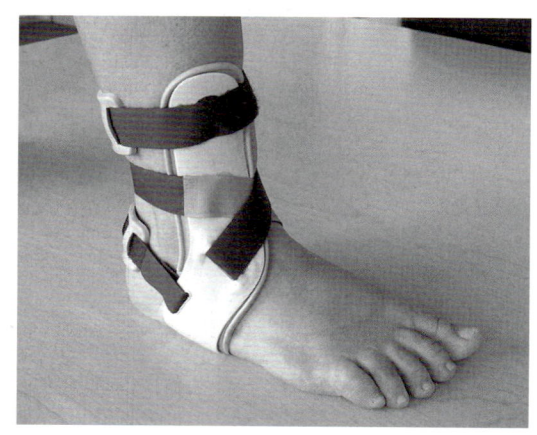

Fig. 90.3 Malleoloc splint with blocking of the talus and support of the external ridge of the foot.

90.1.3 Compression stockings with facultative padding in the area of the external ankle or the Achilles tendon friction bearing

Bandages have to be distinguished from the ankle joint ortheses. Usually, they have **no inflexible elements** for mechanical stabilization, but partly have strap constructions that are supposed to counter a supination (e.g. figure-of-eight bandage). The prevailing effect is based on the **compression** and **proprioceptive stimulation**.

The so-called **compression stockings** are usually suitable for the treatment of **chronic swelling conditions** in the upper ankle joint or for the treatment of achillodynia. A stabilizing effect of these compression stockings to the external ligament apparatus cannot be expected.

The **Malleotrain bandage** is a typical representative of these bandage types (➤ Fig. 90.4). On the one hand, it is padded in the area of the friction bearing of the Achilles tendon, and the bandage can be combined facultatively with a removable heel cushion for the elevation of the heel. A **mechanical friction massage** of the soft tissue around the Achilles tendon is expected here, which can be helpful with an existing paratendinitis. The temporary **elevation of the heel** will lead to a relief of the tendon and can be removed again after a variable period of treatment.

Similar compressive stockings have a U-shaped **gel cushion in the area of the external ankle**. Their primary application field is to be found in chronic ankle joint swellings, because the massage effect will rather support the reduction of the swelling. It is to be pointed out again that both types of bandages are not suitable for the stabilization of the ligament apparatus. The peroneal tendon dislocation could be perhaps an additional indication for the bandage with external ankle padding.

90.1.4 Heel cushion with individual padding

The wide range of insole treatment, which would require an own chapter, is not to be gone into here. But the heel cushion with asymmetric longitudinal-oval padding for the **treatment of the calcaneal spur** is to be mentioned here. The asymmetric soft padding extending in the direction of the longitudinal arch of the foot must be placed analogously to the position of the calcaneal spur on the medial side of the heel cushion and should have a longitudinal-oval extent, because not only the calcaneal spur itself but also the longitudinal ligament of the foot is to be padded softly in its area of origin in the calcaneum. Such heel cushions are suitable for the treatment of the calcaneal spur in its **acute phase**.

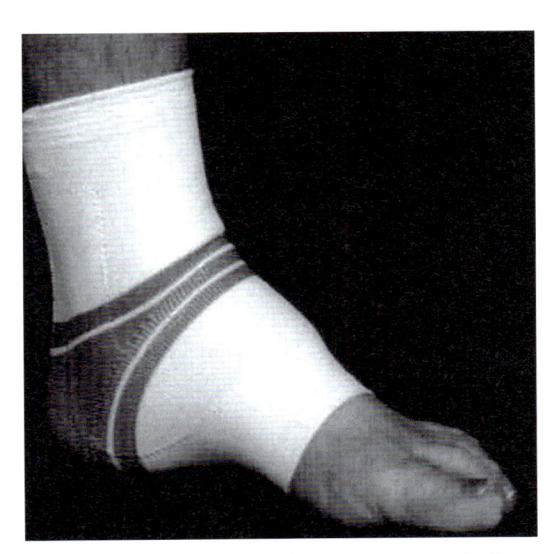

Fig. 90.4 Malleotrain bandage as an example for a stocking bandage with truss padding in the external malleolus area.

90.2 Knee joint ortheses

90.2.1 General basics

Two theses are discussed in general in orthotics of the knee joint:

- The cruciate ligament is not only to be considered a passive holding structure, but also a carrier of proprioceptors.
- The collagenic structure of all presently used transplants changes after approximately 6 months and is organized completely anew.

The current discussion regarding orthesis rehabilitation after stabilizing knee joint surgeries is not concerned with the justification of early mobilization anymore, but rather with the proper point of time and the amount and appropriate performance level being suitable for mobilization. The more aggressive the after-treatment is, the more the reconstruction has to be protected of an early overuse.

Classification of the knee ortheses

According to the American Academy of Orthopedic Surgeons (1988), ortheses are classified into constructions for.

- rehabilitative
- prophylactic and
- functional major tasks.

About the kinematics of the knee joint and the ortheses

The knee joint presents a special challenge to orthesis treatment because of its **complex motion processes**. The components had been unclear for a long time, because the basic mechanical structures are far more complex than the ones of other spheroidal and hinge joints.

The **contact faces** of the joint components are relatively small in comparison to the circumference of the joint. The **menisci** work as additional stabilizers in terms of circular brake pads. The **securing of the joint** is carried out by passive (tendons, ligaments) and active structures (muscles). The cruciate ligaments guide the joint mechanically and use the system of a projected quadrangle for orientation (the lines AD and BC correspond to the course of the cruciate ligaments; ➤ Fig. 90.5).

The gait pole curve of a natural knee joint arises from the detection of the point of intersection of the lines (cruciate ligaments) in every flexed degree of the knee joint (➤ Fig. 90.6).

The joint receives a smaller or larger **freedom of rotation** depending on the degree of flexion, and this amounts to 40° externally and 30° internally, according to Lanz and Wachsmuth. It is most distinctively recognized as end rotation in the last knee extension phase (the feet show 15° externally in standing). This is also conditioned by the differently sized condyles.

The femur can be distally compared to a **crank lever** mechanically, i.e. the radius of the condyle is larger in the 90° flexion than it is in extension. This leads to a rise of the femoral sheath in flexion and results in the lengthen-

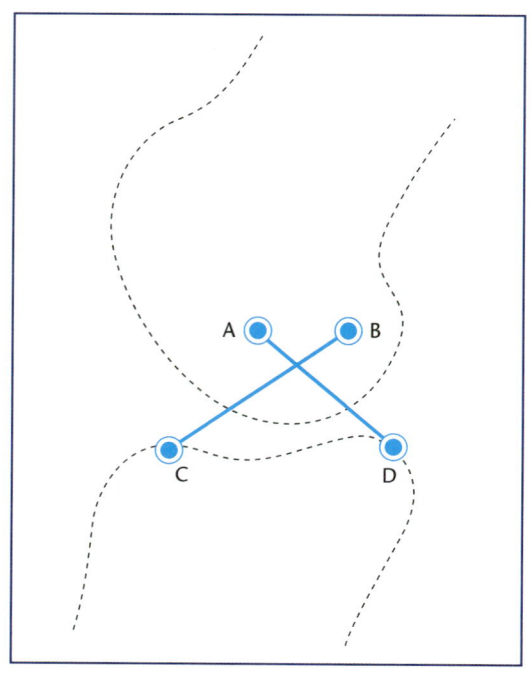

Fig. 90.5 Pattern of the cruciate ligament function in the knee joint (two-dimensional simplification; according to Kapandji 1984).

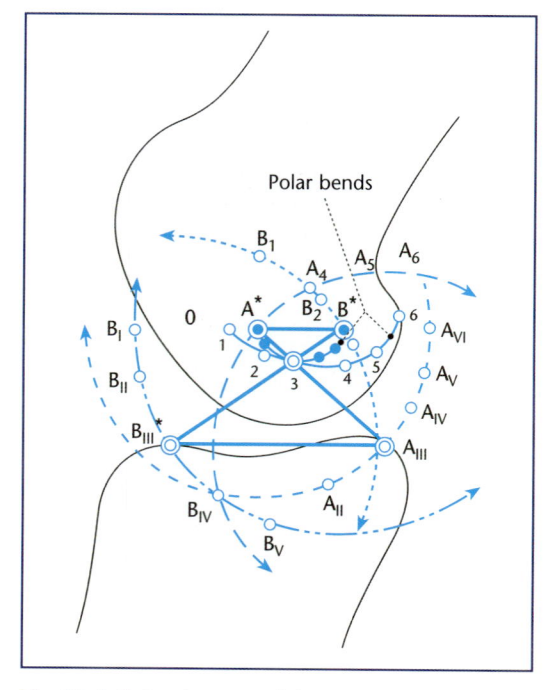

Fig. 90.6 Gait pole curve of the natural knee joint.

90.2 Knee joint ortheses

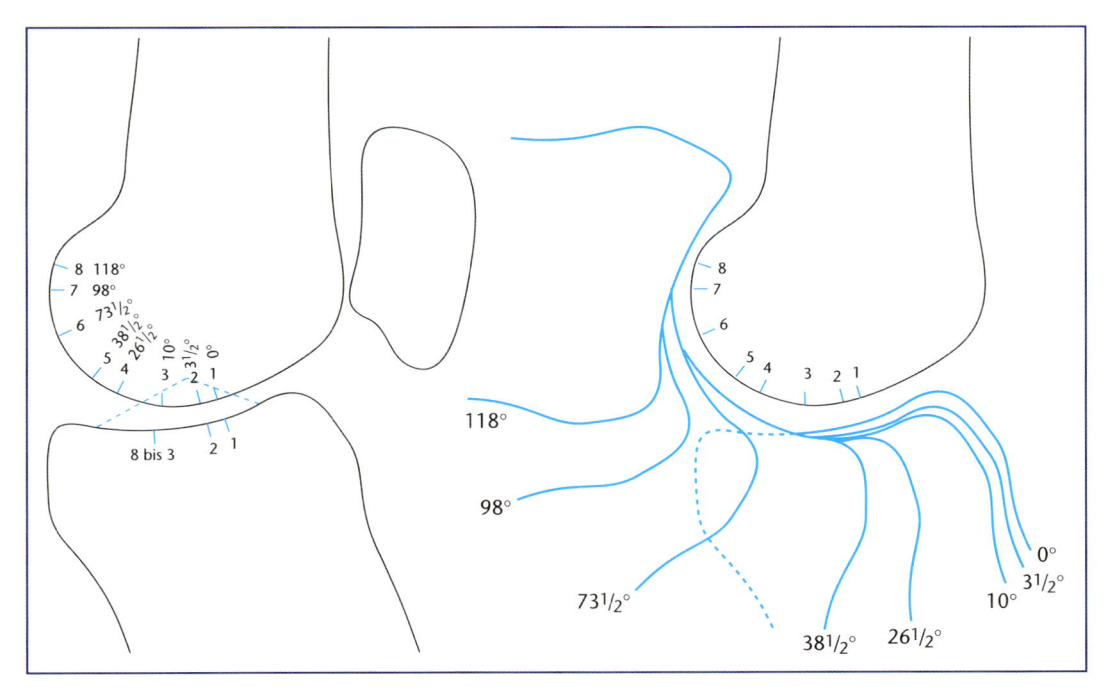

Fig. 90.7 Points of contact between femur and tibia during movement with the resulting compromise axis (according to Nietert 1975, Weiskopf et al. 1995).

ing of the leg at the same time (Bähler 1989). This leads to a so-called **parallel shift** in the joint with inappropriate orthesis treatment.

Exact records of the points of contact between femoral condyle and tibial plateau (Menschik 1975 and Müller 1982, quoted from Grifka 1995 1nd 1996, Kapandji 1984) prove a so-called roll sliding in the joint. The relation between rolling off and sliding is 1:2 in the beginning of flexion and 1:4 in the end (➤ Fig. 90.7). The transmission of this principle to the elliptically shaped femur shows the existence of a **pivot point** that hardly rises or lowers up to the flexion of 90°, but only shifts **backwards** (compromise axis, according to Niebert 1975).

Ortheses types

In general, we distinguish **four types of ortheses**:

- system splints with back-shifted axis by 16/22 mm (back-shift/shift of the axis by 16 mm is the precondition for the prescription potentiality of the orthesis)
- double-joint splints with tooth guidance
- physiological joint splints
- four-axle cruciate ligament splints (only works if the axes correspond to the four corner points of the projected quadrangle).

The more the axis of the mechanical joint has been shifted backwards, the deeper the axis has to sit so that the side of the splint remains parallel to the thigh in the flexion of 0–90° (the one-axle joints with a shift of 16/22 mm came off best in comparison).

The shift of the axis must not be too large in order to compensate the lengthening in flexion or the shortening in extension (a shift of 22 mm has led to a lengthening of 16 mm in a flexion of 90°). A lengthening of 10 mm is negligible!

Nonetheless, the **parallel shift** is of a higher meaning, because it leads to an incongruence of the motion behavior between splint and leg. Lengthening/shortening problems in turn lead to a pumping of the orthesis at the leg.

> **Demands:**
> - The thigh part of the splint or shell must shift upwards during flexion of up to 90° at the same amount as the femur is repositioned upwards due to the elliptic shape of the condyles.
> - The shift of the femoral condyles opposing the tibial plateau at a flexion of more than 90° has to be reconstructed backwards and downwards.
> - The joint construction has to lengthen during the flexion. The knee joint can be treated orthopedic-technically well by the available mechanical joints. The adjustment of the orthesis is at least as important as the kinematics of the joint.

The knee orthesis that **adamantly** clings to the thigh and lower leg has a larger influence on the construction of the joint than an orthesis that partly enfolds the leg by **adaptive elastic bands**. The firmly adjoining part of the prosthesis with elastic bands is relocatable in flexion and extension.

As a consequence, a one-axle joint shifted backwards or a double joint can thus be used without disadvantages for the joint with the use of elastic bands. Nevertheless, Johnson has proved inappropriate effects of the preliminary knee ortheses in 1992 and has won the Elisabeth Winston Lanier Award for this at the congress of the American Academy of Orthopedic Surgeons in New Orleans in 1994.

Own examinations

The products "Lennox-Hill", "Don-Joy" and "CTI Brace" have been compared in our clinic.

The following **problems** have been found:
- restricted flexion
- pressure marks
- unsteady truss pad pressure of the joint construction with soft splints (e.g. Don-Joy)
- separation from the thigh and lower leg in flexion because of insufficient compensation of the lengthening and parallel shifting effect in flexion.

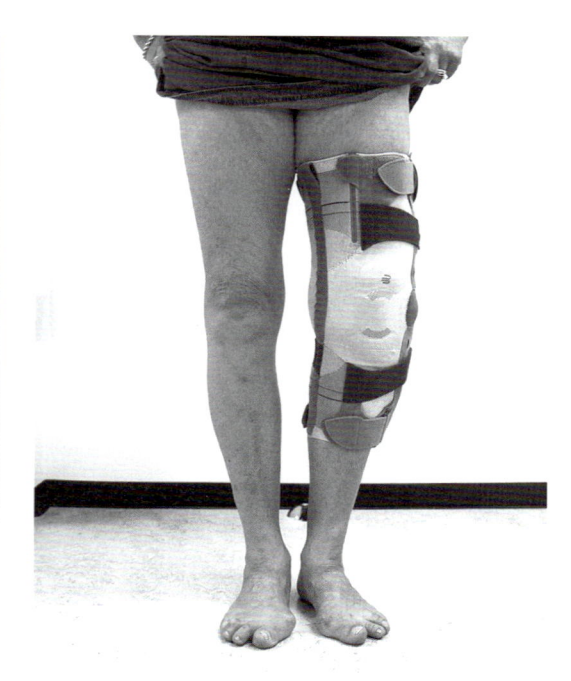

Fig. 90.8 SoftecOA splint with three-point principle for arthrosis treatment.

This survey was carried out in 1994, though, and modern splint systems do not show theses separations of the thigh and lower leg parts anymore (➤ Fig. 90.8).

Prophylactic ortheses

Teitz carried out a controlled study of college students **in 1987** with football players wearing prophylactic ortheses suffering **more injuries** than a control group without ortheses. In 1991, Tegner has described serious ligament injuries in Swedish ice hockey players despite prophylactically worn ortheses.

It can be concluded from these available studies that the **prophylactic wearing** of an orthesis should be handled very **cautiously**, in general.

Functional ortheses

Functional ortheses are used for uni-compartmental arthroses or a varus or valgus instability. An according varization and valgization are achieved by the active three-point principle as a compensation of such varus or valgus instabilities.

Pro and contra ortheses

Pro

- Siebert et al. (1993) have reported a minor **reduction of the translation** of the tibial head in the one-leg-hop test by use of EMG, use of a video analysis system for three-dimensional movement analysis and isokinetic measurements. The strain to a tendon transplant is significant in the first 30° of a flexion. The **risk of translation** is present in a flexion of 30° to 60°.
- A **bad compliance** of the patient (athlete) should lead to the indication of an orthesis, even if it is only a psychological support.
- It is a protection for the transplant in the **early postoperative phase** (first 3 months).

Contra

- **Persisting extension inhibitions** have been observed especially after too long limitation of the extension according to the old pattern of 0–30–60° and 0–20–90°.
- Anglo-American studies (Beynnon 1992 and 1993 as well as Liu et al. 1993, quoted from Grifka) have put the value of the limited motion ortheses into perspective. It was shown for the first time under in-vivo conditions that the ortheses used most worldwide (Don-Joy, Lennox-Hill, CTI Brace) help to safely prevent a tibial shift **up to a force effect of only 100 N**. All ortheses fail at a force effect of 450 N, which already occurs in simple ADL ("activities of daily living"), such as climbing stairs. Loads of up to 2,200 N are reached in sports.
- The **tear strength** of the patellar tendon transplant and also the semi-tendinosus tendon transplant amounts to 1,200 or 1,000 directly postoperatively. The **remodeling** of the tendon transplant begins in the phase between the **6th and 12th postoperative month** and not in the first 3 postoperative months.
- More than 60 cruciate ligament plastics **without orthesis after-treatment** have been observed in the frame of the advanced ambulant therapy: There had been no extension inhibition, no loosening of implants or transplants and no increase of instability.

It has to be pointed out that especially **coordination training with PNF** (proprioceptive neuromuscular facilitation) is important. **Quadriceps training** in the open movement chain, i.e. with freely movable lower leg (leg curler, isokinetic exercise equipment) significantly induces higher strain to the transplant than exercises in **closed movement chains**, i.e. with fixed foot (leg press, e.g. Hackenschmitt equipment; squats). The latter also lead to definitely lesser tibial shift. Tilting forward of the upper body during a squat leads to an activation of the ACL agonists (ischiocrural musculature; Ohkoshy et al. 1991, quoted from Grifka).

> An orthesis treatment is stringently required for a meniscus suture or a meniscus replacement as well as for an insufficient transplant fixation. An orthesis treatment should be carried out especially after the removal of patellar tendon transplants with the risk of a fracture of the donor (patella).

> **Summary**
> The attending physician should decide in individual cases whether he induces an orthesis treatment. A general assessment is not possible despite the available surveys. The approval of stress and motion amount in order to prevent an extension inhibition is the aim of each after-treatment with or without orthesis. An optimal after-treatment is not only marked by the wearing of an orthesis, but also by the concomitant measures such as physical therapy, medical exercise therapy etc.

90.2.2 Knee-joint bandages

Knee joint bandages with lateral stabilizers

Stocking-shaped bandages with various truss padding and partly removable **stabilizers in the lateral ligament area** are available for the knee joint, similar to the ankle joint bandages. It has to be stated that these bandages – the same as ankle joint bandages – are not sufficient for the stabilization of a ligament rupture of any extent.

A **massage effect** at chronic knee joint effusions is to be expected of these stocking-shaped bandages primarily with every step; the relief of the medial compartment can also be expected in the consequent performance of the three-point principle at beginning varus gonarthrosis or a cartilage damage in the medial joint compartment.

A typical representative of these knee joint bandages is the **Genutrain bandage** with annular **patellar padding**. This reduces the pressure to the sensitive lateral area of the retinaculum, on the one hand, and it has a massage effect in the area of the knee cap, on the other hand, which can support the reduction or **prophylaxis of a knee joint effusion**. Many different manufacturers offer knee joint bandages with removable lateral stabilizers.

Knee joint bandages for the treatment of varus gonarthrosis

A therapeutic effect can be expected **in individual cases** of a bandage working intransigently by the three-point principle at a beginning varus gonarthrosis. Truss padding at the point of the external joint cavity is to be combined here with two straps in the distal femoral region and the proximal region of the lower leg, which can develop a traction effect individually adjustable by a Velcro fastener.

Knee joint bandages for the treatment of patellar apex syndrome

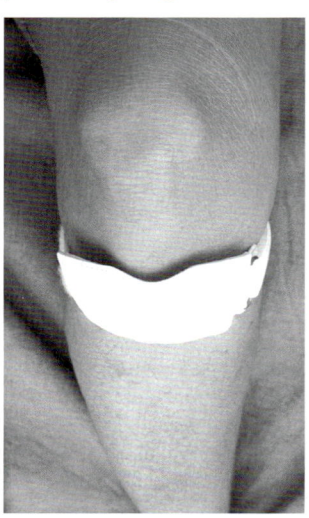

The patellar apex syndrome is an **overstrain situation of the patellar tendon** at its origin – the patellar apex. Shortening of the knee extensor muscles or a muscular imbalance between extensor and flexor muscles can be the **cause**. But also direct repetitive traumas such as a dive in volleyball are blamed. A bursa is possibly found in the area of the apex of the knee cap (bursitis) with chronic pain. The Kassel bandage of the Sporlastic Company with its effect mechanism to be looked for in the change of the angle of incidence of the tendon is appropriate for conservative therapy (➢ Fig. 90.9).

Fig. 90.9 Kassel bandage.

90.3 Spine ortheses

90.3.1 General basics

Pain reduction and **increase of capacity** of the axial organ are the primary aim of an ambulant rehabilitation of posttraumatic spinal injuries and also in the after-treatment of disk prolapses.

Specific orthotic adjustments are used, which – in agreement with the American Academy of Orthopedic Surgeons (AAOS) – are classified into

- **long ortheses** as thoraco-lumbosacral ortheses (TLSO)
- **short ortheses** as lumbosacral ortheses (LSO) and
- **sacroiliac ortheses** or pelvic belts (SIO).

The classification of Morris (1981) only distinguishes **correcting ortheses** and immobilizing or **supporting ortheses**.

It has been known since the primary studies by Norton and Brown in 1957 that long ortheses effect a good fixation of the lower thoracic spine and the thoracolumbar junction, but as compensation rather lead to an **increase of mobility** in the segment L4/L5 and in the lumbosacral hinge. Norton and Brown had carried out tests after the implantation of Kirschner wires into the spinous processes of vertebra in voluntary patients with and without ortheses, in which they checked the angles of the wires (Haaker 2001).

Also the rotation-impairing effect of a **lumbosacral orthesis** (LSO) is ascribed to the higher positioned segments, according to Lumsden and Morris, and – rather to the contrary – leads to a **rotation increase at exposure** in the lumbosacral hinge (Lumsden and Morris 1968). They had implanted Steinmann nails into the spinous process L5 and into the spina iliaca posterior superior. Transducers have measured the rotation of L5 against the pelvis with and without ortheses. More rotation in the lumbosacral hinge has been found here with an orthesis than without one in fast walking.

Waters and Morris have also disproved the permanent hypothesis of a reduction of muscle activity in 1970, who have at least found **no effect to the electrical muscle activity** in EMG. An increase of muscle activity has been found in the region of the dorsal muscles. On the other hand, the authors have found a reduction of the activity in the region of the abdominal muscles (obliquus internus and externus muscles).

Even recent surveys by Rohlmann and Bergmann (Rohlmann et al. 1999 [1], [2]) confirm these findings. They have found no strain-reducing effect of the examined ortheses (Boston overlap brace, three-point-reclination orthesis and Lumbotrain bandage of Bauerfeind) with measurements in a specifically developed internal spine fixator.

90.3.2 Lumbar relief orthesis in sports

The lumbar relief orthesis (LRO) in sports is used primarily after surgeries of prolapsed disks in terms of a **reminder bandage** (Gutenbrunner et al. 1998). The best known representative is the modular multifunction orthesis Soft Tec-Lumbo of Bauerfeind (➤ Fig. 90.11) in addition to the DiscoFlex and LumboFlex bandage of Basko (➤ Fig. 90.10). These lumbar relief orthoses are of course only **conditionally applicable in early rehabilitation** about 6 weeks postoperatively for running sports and shall prevent an excessive inclination and reclination. Höfer et al. could prove the efficiency of these kinds of ortheses for the first time in their publication in 2008.

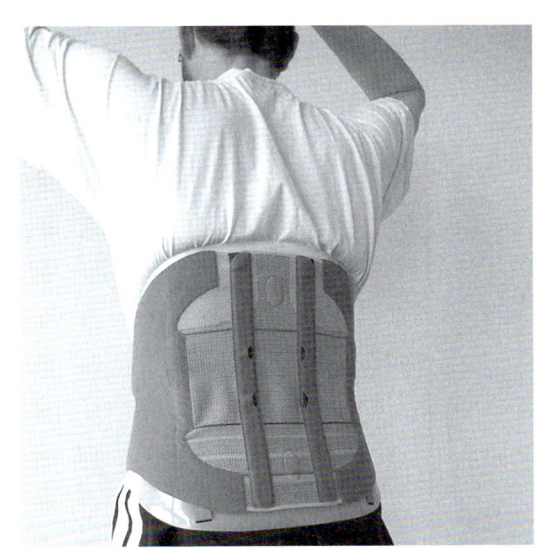

Fig. 90.11 SoftTec Lumbo bandage as a typical representative of LRO for the after-treatment of spinal surgeries.

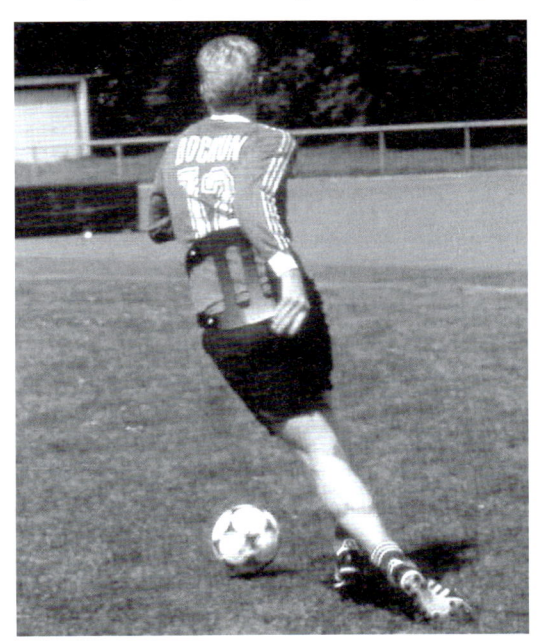

Fig. 90.10 DiscoFlex bandage (Basko) as delicate LRO, which is suitable for sports.

90.3.3 Sacroiliac ortheses in sports

Sacroiliac ortheses **in the form of bandages** are widely used in sports. They are supposed to have a **massaging effect** to the paravertebral dorsal extensors by their facultative equipment with a lumbar gel pad either with knobs or of another structure. A significant stabilization in the area of the iliosacral joints or a prophylactic wearing with a spondylolisthesis is certainly doubtful (Rohlinger et al. 1996).

The Lumbotrain bandage is a typical representative of these bandages (➤ Fig. 90.12).

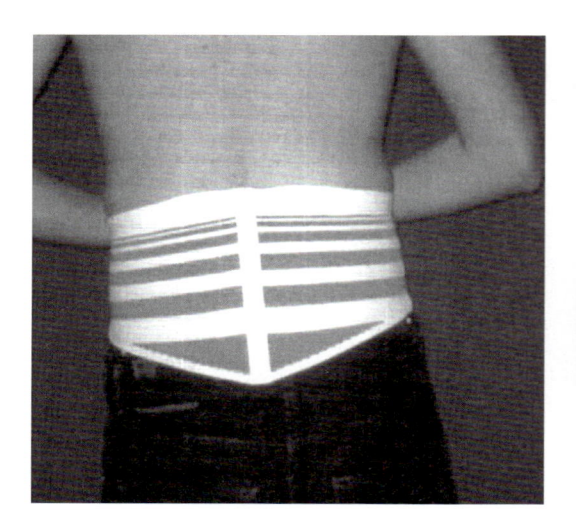

Fig. 90.12 Lumbotrain bandage as iliosacral orthesis or bandage, respectively.

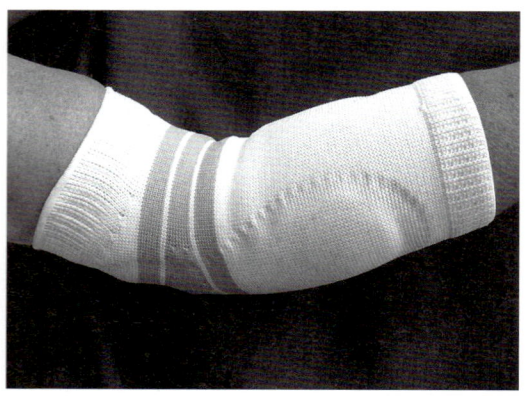

Fig. 90.13 Epitrain bandage with typical truss padding.

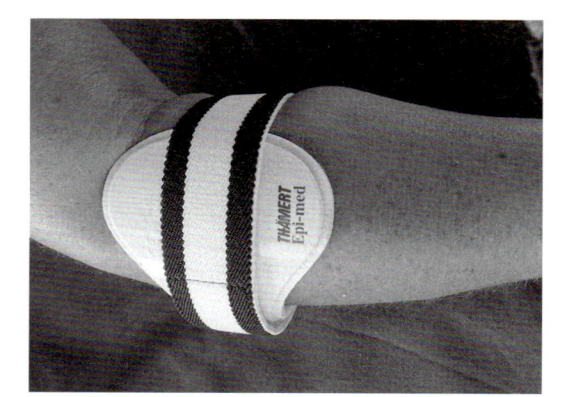

Fig. 90.14 Tennis elbow brace.

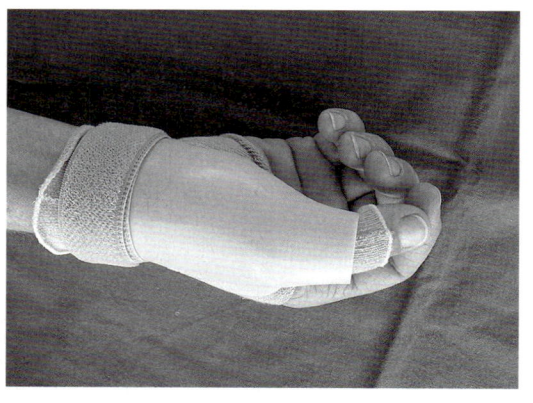

Fig. 90.15 Sporlastic thumb orthesis for the treatment of a skier's thumb.

90.4 Elbow ortheses

The therapy of elbow joint injuries – especially the tennis and the golfer's elbow – is in the key. **Stocking-shaped bandages** are available affecting the epicondyles in terms of a **massage effect** by the involvement of according gel pads, e.g. the Epitrain bandage (➤ Fig. 90.13).

Furthermore, there are the so-called **epicondylitis braces** (➤ Fig. 90.14). These are semicircular ortheses of stiff plastic or copper materials for the adaptation of the angle of incidence of the muscle insertions at the radial or ulnar epicodyle. **Different successes inefficiency** have been reported for these ortheses.

90.5 Thumb and wrist ortheses

Different indications are found in sports for the treatment of sports injuries at the metacarpal of the thumb and the hand. The after-treatment of the so-called **skier's thumb** is to be mentioned here after the generally surgical treatment of the rupture of the ulnar collateral ligament facultative with osseous avulsion in the metacarpophalangeal joint of the thumb. The **thumb shell** from Sporlastic is suitable (➤ Fig. 90.15).

90.6 Hip joint ortheses

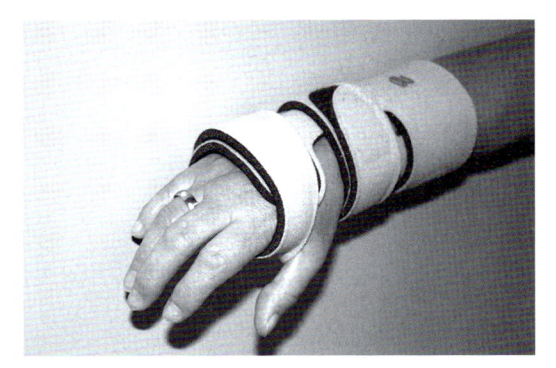

Fig. 90.16 Manuloc bandage for the treatment of complex hand injuries.

The **Manuloc bandage** of Bauerfeind can be applied for the treatment of different **instabilities in the carpal region**, such as scapholunate dissociation (➢ Fig. 90.16).

90.6 Hip joint ortheses

Although hip joint ortheses only play a minor role in athletes without endoprothetic treatment, the **bandage treatment** after surgeries because of coxa saltans (snapping hip), bursitis trochanterica or a partial avulsion of the gluteus medius off the trochanter major is carried out routinely.

The orthesis treatment of the hip joint with dislocations or for protection after extensive exchange surgeries gains in importance, because more and more **wearers of hip prostheses** wish to be athletically active. The **SofTec coxa** fills a gap here between stiff orthesis and bandage with a two-dimensionally adjustable stable aluminum joint. This makes the adduction and the abduction adjustable in the range of 0 to 6° as well as the extension and flexion (Haaker and Engelhardt 2008). This orthesis with a good fitting also under the exercising clothes has achieved a good acceptance and compliance (➢ Fig. 90.17 a and b).

Summary

- **Ankle joint ortheses:** brace strap systems for the direct acute treatment after supination injuries, shell strap systems for the immediate therapy (e.g. aircast, airloc). Subacute treatment and prophylaxis, if necessary, after detumescing with stiff brace strap system without padding.
- **Ankle joint bandages:** mostly without rigid elements for the mechanical stabilization, but with multiple variants of truss padding (external ankle, Achilles tendon) or half-elastic strap constructions (figure-of-eight dressing) for the prophylaxis of the supination movement. The effect is based on compression and proprioceptive stimulation.

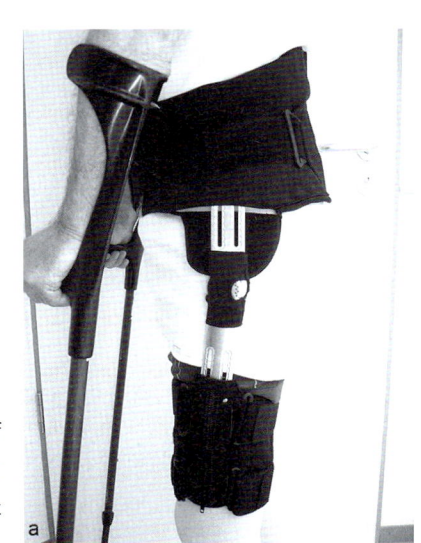

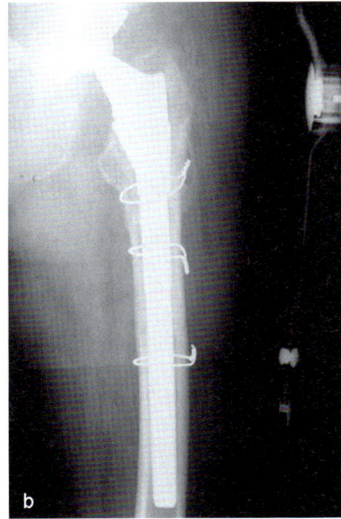

Fig. 90.17 SofTec coxa of a wearer of a hip endoprosthesis. a: lateral view. b: radiograph with the centering of the joint to the trochanter major.

- **Heel pads:** for the relief of the Achilles tendons or the soft padding of the plantar calcaneal spur.
- **Knee joint ortheses:** brace shell systems for the stabilization of ligament injuries at the knee joint and after-treatment of cruciate ligament plastics (double-joint splint with gear wheel guidance or four-axle joint splints).
- **Knee joint bandages:** tricot bandages with different (patellar) truss padding and belt applications for special application fields. The essential effect also bases on compression and proprioceptive stimulation. Bandages with strap systems according to the three-point system are also used for the treatment of the varus gonarthrosis. Simple belt systems for the treatment of patellar apex syndrome.
- **Spinal ortheses:** thoraco-lumbosacral (TLSO), lumbosacral ortheses (LSO) as well as sacroiliac ortheses (SIO). LSO and SIO are mainly used in sports in terms of a reminder bandage after disk prolapses.
- **Elbow joint ortheses:** brace-like, semicircular ortheses for the adaptation of the angle of incidence of the radial or ulnar epicondyle.
- **Elbow joint bandages:** with variable truss padding for the treatment of the same clinical picture or relapsing effusions due to compression or proprioceptive stimulation.
- **Hip ortheses:** ortheses with pelvic girdle and femur part for the prophylaxis of dislocation and flexor-adductor contraction.

References

Bähler A (1981). Das Kniegelenk und seine orthetische Versorgung. Orth Technik 32.

Bähler A (1989). Die biomechanischen Grundlagen der Orthesenversorgung des Knies. Orth Technik 2: 52–59.

Grifka J (1995). Systematik der Kniegelenkorthetik. Orth Technik 5: 390–397.

Grifka J (1996). Kniegelenksorthesen, Jahrbuch der Orthopädie. Biermann-Verlag, Zülpich.

Gutenbrunner C, Hildebrandt HD, Gercke HA (1998). Katamnestische Untersuchungen über die Wirksamkeit der Verordnung einer dynamischen Kreuzstützbandage bei Patienten mit chronischem Lumbalsyndrom. Orth Praxis 34: 383–390.

Haaker R, Engelhardt M (2008). Klinische Ersterfahrungen und Indikation für eine neuartige Hüftorthese. Med Orth Technik 128(5): 75–80.

Haaker R (2001). Differenzialindikation der lumbalen Entlastungsorthesen. Orth Praxis 37(12): 805–808.

Höfer S, Siemsen CH (2008). Biomechanischer Wirkungsnachweis einer Lendenwirbelsäulen-Entlastungsorthese zur Kreuzschmerzbehandlung. Z Orthop Unfall 146: 439-443.

Hoffmann R, Zwipp H, Kretek C, Tscherne H (1987). Zur funktionellen Behandlung der frischen fibularen Bandruptur. Unfallchirurg 90: 441–447.

Jerosch J, Porten M (2000). Einfluss von Stabilisierungshilfen am oberen Sprunggelenk auf sensomotorische und sportpraktische Fertigkeiten. Orth Praxis 37: 313–326.

Jerosch J, Schoppe R (2000). Langfristige Auswirkungen von Sprunggelenkbandagen auf sensomotorische Fähigkeiten. Orth Praxis 36: 38–46.

Jerosch J, Thorwesten L, Frebel T, Linnenbeckers S (1997). Influences of external stabilizing devices of the ankle on sport-specific capabilities. Knee Surg Sports Traumatol Arthrosc 5: 50–57.

Kapandji IA (1984). Funktionelle Anatomie der Gelenke. Enke-Verlag, Stuttgart.

Lumsden RM, Morris JM (1968). In vitro study of axial rotation and immobilisation at the lumbosacral joint. J Bone Joint Surg 50A: 1591–1596.

Morris JM (1981). Biomechanics of corsets and braises for the low back: American Academy of Orthopedic Surgeons: Symposium on the lumbar spine, Braun FW (ed.), Mosby CV Company, St. Louis, Toronto, London.

Nietert M (1975). Untersuchungen zur Kinematik des menschlichen Kniegelenks im Hinweis auf ihre Approximation in der Prothetik. Dissertation TU Berlin.

Rohlinger I, Kinsger M, Eckhardt P, Tilscher H (1996). Orthesenversorgung der Lenden- und Beckenregion, Teil II. Man Med 34: 280–287.

Rohlmann A, Bergmann G, Graichen F, Neff G (1999) (1). Braces do not reduce loads on internal spinal fixation devices. Clin Biomech 14: 97–102.

Rohlmann A, Bergmann G, Graichen F, Weber U (1999) (2). Die Belastung des Wirbel-Fixateur-interne. Orthopädie 28: 451–457.

Weiskopf M, Nusie HR, Siebert WE (1995). Erfahrung mit der dynamischen Bewegungsanalyse zur Beurteilung einer Knieeorthese. Med Orth Tech 112: 103–108.

Zwipp H, Gottschalk F, Tscherne H (1994). Die konservativ-funktionelle Behandlung des knöchernen Bänderrisses hat sich bewährt: 5-Jahres-Ergebnisse. Med Orth Tech 114: 122–126.

Index

A
Acceleration 143
Acetabular labrum lesions 256
– Classification 257
– Clinical tests 257
Acromioclavicular joint 213, 225
Adaptation 3
Adductor snydrome 270
Adjustment to training 4
Adolescents 9
Age-associated diseases 11
Age-specific aspects 9
Aikido 455
American football 495
Analgesics 34
Anamnesis 49
Ankle instability 312
– lateral 312
– medial 316
– subtalar joint 317
Ankle ortheses 769
Annular ligament injury 246
Anterior cruciate ligament rupture 279
Anterior interosseus syndrome 169
Anterior knee pain 287
Anti-Doping rules 31
Apophyseal avulsion fractures 251
Apophyseal damages 11
Arterial hypertension 31
Arthroscopy 97
– Equipment 97
– Indications 100
– Pre-operative preparations 101
– Knee 102
– Shoulder 106
– Hip 109
– Ankle 111
Arthrosis 23
Artistic gymnastics 597
Asthma bronchiale 33
Athletic footwear 759
Athletics 425
– Jumping disciplines 426
– Throwing disciplines 426
Autologous chondrocyte transplantation (ACT) 345
Axillary neuropathy 165
Axonotmesis 162

B
Badminton 549
Ballet 585
Bandages 775
Bankart surgery 217
Barotrauma 680
Baseball 499
Basketball 507
Beach soccer 515
Beach Volleyball 555
Biathlon 361
Biceps tendon rupture 228
Bobsleigh 413
Bodybuilding 417
Boxer's fracture 462
Boxer's knuckle 463
Boxing 461
Brachial plexus 162
Brain injuries 149
Bristow-Latarjet 220
Bursitis praepatellaris 289
Bursitis subachillea 357
Buttonhole deformity 246

C
Calcaneus fractures 293
Calcium 743
Calf cramps 682
Cam impingement 258
Canoeing 369
Capsular shrinking 209
Carbohydrates 728
Carpal tunnel-Syndrome 169
Cartilage-bone transplantations 344
Cartilage 341
– Composition 341
– Biomechanics 342
– Healing process 342
– Imaging 343
Cartilage cell transplantation 345
Cartilage injuries 283
– Conservative treatment 341
– Surgical treatment 342
Carving Ski 441
Cauliflower ear 474,493
Central nervous system 141
Cervical soft-tissue 204
Children 9
Chondroitin sulfate 343
Chondromalacia patellae 287
Chondropathia pateallae 12
Chopart's joint 218
Chromium 747
Classification of Functioning, Disability and Health (ICF) 689
Climbing 451
– Free climbing 451
– Soloing 451
– Bouldering 451
Clincal biomechanics 115
Compartment Syndrom 175, 331
Compression clothing 754
Concussion 151, 519
Conduction 752
Congenital hip dysplasia 11
Contusion, cerebral 150
Convection 752
Copper 746
Coracoid transfer 220
Cross-body-test 164
Cross-country biking 631
Cross-country skiing 403
CT 73
– Bones 80
– Spine 80
– Shoulder 83
– Elbow 85
– Hand 87
– Hip 89
– Knee 91
– Foot 92
Cubital tunnel Syndrome 167
Cuboideum fractures 295
Cutaneus femoral nerve 170
Cycling 387
Cycling shoes 764

D
Dance 611
Dancer's heel 587
Deaths in Sports 713
Decompression sickness 681
Decorin 330
Diabetes mellitus 32
Diagnostic procedures 47
Disability 39
Disabled sports 39
Discoid meniscus 12
Distal biceps tendon rupture 228
Downhill 631
Dynamometry 130
Dysbaric osteonecroses 681
Dystonia 175

E
Ears 199
Eden-Hybinette 219
Elbow dislocation 227
Elbow orthesis 778
Elderly persons 18
Electromyography 121.134
Electrotherapy 703
Energy requirement 727

Entrapmentsyndrom 164, 268
Epicondylitis 230
Epidural hematoma 144
Epiphysiolysis capitis femoris 11
Equestrianism 665
Evaporation 752
Examination 49
Extensor digitorum longus 308
Extensor hallucis longus 308
Eyes 181
– Children and adolescents 181
– Non-competitive sports 183
– Competitive, high-performance sports 186
– Sport-specific injuries 187

F
Facial Cranium 201
Facial fractures 144
Femoral fractures
– Distal 284
Femoral nerve 171
Femoroacetabular impingement 257
– Arthroscopic surgery 259
– Open surgery 259
Figure skating 591
finger joint injuries 243
Finger pulley injuries 452
Finkelstein's test 247
Flexor digitorum longus 308
Flexor hallucis longus
– Tenosynovitis 307
– Tendon rupture 308
Foot and Ankle
– Fractures 291
– Ligament injuries 310
Footwear 759
Forearm fracture 227
– Fractures 291
Free diving 679
Functional disorders 39
Functional orthesis 774

G
Gait ad treadmill analysis 125
Gerber, latissimus-dorsi transfer 224
Glasgow-Coma Scale 150
Glenoid reconstruction 219
Glucocorticosteroids 34
Glucosaminglycan 343
Golf 653
Golfer's elbow 654
Golfer's shoulder 654
Groin 263
– Weak groin 264
Growth factors 35
Growth hormones 35

Growth-associated diseases 11
Gymnast's hump 602
Gymnastics 597

H
Hallux 319
Hamilton's test 307
Hamulus fracture 238
Hand joint 235
Handball 531
Head injuries 142
– Acute management 151
– Return to sports activity 151
– Cumulative effects 153
Hearing loss 673
Herbert screw 238
Hernias 264
High diving 615
Hip injuries 255
– Dislocations 255
– Fractures 255
Hip ortheses 779
Hockey
– Field 539
– Ice 517
Humerus fracture 214
Hyaluronic acid 344
Hydration 732
Hydrotheraphy 705

I
Ice hockey 517
Iliopectinea bursa 268
Iliotibial friction syndrome 289
Impingement
– Posterosuperior 212
– Anterosuperior 212
Infiltrations 34
Infraspinatus transfer 224
Injections 34
Inline Skating 619
Instability impingement 210
Intersection syndrome 248
Intracerebral hematoma 145
Intramedullary hemorrhage 158
Intravenous/infusions 34
Intrinsic-plus position 239
Iodin 747
Iron 744
Isokinetics 119

J
J-Chip plastic 218
Jersey finger 245
Jones fracture 295
Judo 471
Jump tests 120

K
Karate 477
Kinematic motion analysis 116
Kitesurfing 625
Knee
– Anatomy 273
– Biomechanics 274
– Injuries 275
– Medial collateral ligament 278
– Lateral collateral ligament 278
– Anterior cruciate ligament 279
– Posterior cruciate ligament 280
– Osseous ligament avulsion 281
– Cruciate ligament injuries at open epiphyseal plate 281
Knee orthesis 771
Knee bandages 775
Knockout 464

L
Labrum-biceps-tendon complex 212
– Andrews lesion 212
– SLAP-lesion 212
Lateral femoral cutaneous neuropathy 172
Latissimus-dorsi-transfer 224
Le Fort Classification 144
Light therapy 708
Lisfranc joint 295, 319
– Dislocation fractures 295
– Ligament instability 319
Little Leaguer's elbow 232
Local anesthetics 35
Long thoracic nerve 164
LT ligament lesions 242
Luge 431

M
Magnesium 742
Malleolar fractures 292
March fracture 333
Massage techniques 696, 702
Median nerve 168
Medical gymnastics 693
Medication 31
Meniscus
– Injuries 275
– Resection 275
– Refixation 276
– Replacement 278
Metacarpal fractures 239
Metatarsalia fractures 295
Microfracturing 344
Minerals 741
Morphine 35
Mortonmetatarsalgia 174

Motion analysis
- 2D 127
- 3D 128

Motorsports 659
Mountain biking 631
MRT 73
- Tendons and muscles 76
- Neurons 78
- Bones 80
- Spine 80
- Shoulder 83
- Elbow
- Hand 87
- Hip and groin 89
- Knee 91
- Foot 92

Muscle damage, exercise-induced 175
Muscle injuries
- Classification 324
- Healing 324
- Diagnostics 327
- Acute treatment 327
- Conservative treatment 328
- Chronic 330
- Prevention 331

Muscular dysbalances 331
Musculocutaneous nerve 165
Myositis ossificans 330

N

Naviculare fracture 295
Neer, ventral capsule plastic 220
Nerve impairments 247
Neurapraxia 162
Neuromuscular imbalance 332
Neuropathy, suprascapular 164
Neurotmesis 162
Neviaser, infraspinatus transfer 224
Nike free 766
Nitrogen narcosis 681
Nutrition 727
Nutritional supplements 747

O

Oburator nerve 171
Orienteering 381
Orthesis 769
Os tibiale externum 306
Osgood-Schlatter disease 11, 288
Osteochondrosis 14
Osteochondrosis dissecans 12, 283

P

Paragliding 637
Patellar apex Syndrom 288
Patellar dislocation 13
Patellar fractures 285

Patellar neuropathy 172
Patellar tendon rupture 283
Pectoralis major transfer 225
Pedography 133
Pelvic belt 255
Pelvic fractures 253
Pelvic injuries 251
Pelvis 251
- Stress fractures 253
- Anterior ventral pelvic ring instability 254

Performance enhancement footwear 764
Peripheral nervous system 161
Peritendinitis 354
Peroneal nerve 173
Peroneal tendinitis 302
Peroneal tendon
- Dislocation 302
- Rupture 303

Perthes syndrome 11
Phalangeal fractures 239
Physiotherapy 691
- Aims and effects 695
- Active methods 691, 696

Pincer impingement 258
Plantar pressure measurement 116
Platelet-Derived Growth Factor (PDGF) 330
Plica syndrome 287
Post exercise chill 753
Posterior cruciate ligament rupture 280
Posterior cutaneous femoral nerve 170
Potassium 742
Processus lateralis tali-fracture 647
Projection radiography 71
Prophylactic orthesis 774
Protection footwear 762
Protein 733
Pseudotumor 253
Psoas syndrome 267
Pudendal nerve 170

Q

Quadriceps tendon rupture 283
Quadriplegia 159
Quervain's disease 247, 569

R

Radial nerve 166
Radiation 752
Recreational biking 632
Rectus femoris muscle
- Avulsion of the reflected part 253

Regeneration 4
Rehabilitation 687
- Aims and limitations 688
- Ambulant 687

Resch, pectoralis major transfer 225
Rhythmic gymnastics 607
Rockwood-classification 213
Rotator cuff rupture 210, 221
Rowing 391
Rugby 543
Running 375
Running shoes 762

S

Sacroiliac ortheses 777
Sailing 675
Sand toe 552
Saphenous neuropathy 172
Scaphoid fracture 237
Scapula protraction 567
Scapula winging 567
Sciatic nerve 169
Scoliosis 13
Scuba diving 679
Second impact syndrom (SIS) 152
Selenium 746
Sesamoid fractures 296
Shallow water/blackout 682
Shooting sports 671
Short track speed skating 361
Shoulder 207
- Dislocation and instability 207
- Arthroscopic stabilization 208
- Capsular shrinking 209
- Open surgery procedures 217
- Posterior instability 221

Sinding-Larsen-Johansson-Syndrome 12
Skeletal muscle 323
Skeletal muscle relaxants 35
Skeleton 437
Ski, Carving 441
Ski-boots 765
Skier's thumb 244
Ski-jumping 447
Skull fractures 143
SL ligament lesions 240
SLAP lesion
- Snyder classification 213

Snowboarder's ankle 647
Snowboarding 643
- Hard boots 645
- Soft boots 649

Soccer 525
Sodium 741
Sonography 55
- Shoulder 56

- Elbow 60
- Hand 61
- Hip joint 63
- Leg musculature 64
- Knee joint 65
- Foot 67

Spinal cord injuries 154
- Sport-specific injuries 155
- Classification 158
- Assessment 159

Spinal edema 158
Spinal contusion 158
Spinal shock 158
Spine, overuse injuries 160
Spine ortheses 776
Spondylolisthesis 14
Spondylolysis 14
Sports after endoprothetic treatment 24
Sports and arthrosis 23
Sport and Rockclimbing 451
Sport diving 679
Sportsban 16
Sportshoes 760
Sportsphysiotherapie 692
Sportswear 759
Stack splint 245
Strength diagnostics 118
Stress fractures 333
- Etiology 333
- Diagnostics 334
- Diffential diagnosis 334
- Therapy 337
- Prevention 338
- Foot 297

Stress reactions 333
Subarachnoid hemorrhage 146
Subdural hematoma 145
Sumo 487
Suprascapular neuropathy 164
Sural nerve 174
Swan-neck deformity 245
Swimming 399
Symphysis instability 255
Syndesmosis injuries 314

T

Table tennis 573
Taekwondo 491
Talus fractures 293
Tendon injuries 245, 351
- Causes 354
- Ruptures 354
- Partial lesions 355
- Tendinopathies 356
- Luxation 357
- Flexor tendon 245
- Extensor tendon 245
- Foot 301

Tendovaginitis stenosans de Quervain 247
Tennis 565
Tennis leg 569
Tennis toe 569
TFCC injuries 242
Thermal therapy 705
Thermoregulation 751
Thrower's elbow 232
Thumbortheses 778
Tibia head fractures 284

Tibial nerve 174
Tibialis anterior tendon
- Rupture 306

Tibialis posterior tendon
- Dysfunction 304
- Rupture 305
- Dislocation 306

Tissue engineering 347
Toe fractures 296
Toe joints 319
Tossy-classification 213
Training footwear 765
Triathlon 407
TUE 35
Turf toe 319

U

Ulnar nerve 167

V

Video and 2D motion analysis 127
Vitamins 734
Volleyball 577

W

Weber, subcapital derotation 220
Weightlifting 421
Whiplash injury 155
Women 17
Wrist joint 235
- Overstrain syndroms 248

Wrist ortheses 778

Z

Zinc 746
Zurich guidelines 150